Oxford Textbook of
# Suicidology and Suicide Prevention

# Oxford Textbook of
# Suicidology and Suicide Prevention

## A GLOBAL PERSPECTIVE

Edited by

**Danuta Wasserman and
Camilla Wasserman**

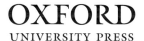

OXFORD
UNIVERSITY PRESS

# OXFORD
UNIVERSITY PRESS

Great Clarendon Street, Oxford OX2 6DP

Oxford University Press is a department of the University of Oxford.
It furthers the University's objective of excellence in research, scholarship,
and education by publishing worldwide in

Oxford  New York

Auckland Cape Town Dar es Salaam Hong Kong Karachi  Kuala Lumpur Madrid Melbourne
Mexico City Nairobi  New Delhi Shanghai Taipei Toronto

With offices in

Argentina Austria Brazil Chile Czech Republic France Greece  Guatemala Hungary Italy Japan
Poland Portugal Singapore  South Korea Switzerland Thailand Turkey Ukraine Vietnam

Oxford is a registered trade mark of Oxford University Press
in the UK and in certain other countries

Published in the United States
by Oxford University Press Inc., New York

British Library Cataloging in Publication Data

Data available

Library of Congress Cataloguing in Publication Data

ISBN 978–0–19–857005–9 (hbk)

10 9 8 7 6 5 4 3 2 1

Typeset in Minion
by Cepha Imaging Private Ltd, Bangalore, India
Printed in Italy
by L.E.G.O. S.P.A.

Whilst every effort has been made to ensure that the contents of this book
are as complete, accurate and up-to-date as possible at the date of writing,
Oxford University Press is not able to give any guarantee or assurance that
such is the case. Readers are urged to take appropriately qualified medical
advice in all cases. The information in this book is intended to be useful to
the general reader, but should not be used as a means of self-diagnosis or
for the prescription of medication.

# Foreword

Every year a million people kill themselves and at least ten times as many attempt to do so, frequently ending up disabled by the psychological, physical and social consequences of their attempts. A large proportion of this loss of human life could be prevented, but this does not happen. One of the reasons for this is that the information about the magnitude of the problem and about ways to reduce it, as well as the results of research done to explore the causes and consequences of suicidal behaviour, are not sufficiently well known.

It is easy to understand this. The prevention of suicide requires access and use of many sources of information. The media, schools, health services, social services, authorities dealing with labour and many others who should be involved in the prevention of suicide, and in the evaluation of methods used to do this, are distant from one another and belong to different worlds. There is little or no sharing of information among them. Data remain in the parts of the society in which they were produced. Highly interesting positive and negative experiences obtained in programmes of suicide prevention by one social agency or one country are often not published in widely read journals, neither in the country in which they were obtained nor in other countries.

What is true for the difficulties in obtaining information is even more disturbing when it comes to collaboration between agencies and countries in programmes of suicide prevention. Declarations of intent to work together are numerous and recommendations to do so even more frequent: yet in most countries there is no serious and lasting intersectoral collaboration on any topic—including the prevention of suicide. The same problem is a major hurdle to any programme aiming to help those who have attempted suicide but did not complete it.

The magnum opus that Danuta and Camilla Wasserman and their colleagues prepared attempts to deal with the first of these two problems. It brings together information about suicide in different cultures and at different stages of life; about the relevance and role of religion in the prevention of suicide; about political and socio-economic determinants of suicide; about the psychiatric and somatic diseases and their relationship with suicidal behaviour. The volume explores the theories of suicidal behaviour and provides a cogent review of methods that help in the recognition of suicidal risks and in the prevention of suicide. The strategies of the health care system, and the ways in which health services can make a contribution to the prevention of suicide and to the alleviation of the consequences of suicidal behaviour, are examined critically. The impact of suicide on those who are left behind, and an estimation of the economic cost of suicide to society, are discussed along with the arguments for action that can be successful, as examples from many countries clearly demonstrate.

The large number of contributors to the volume is a witness to the size and excellence of the network that Professor Wasserman and her colleagues working in the field of suicide have established: more importantly, however, it demonstrates that suicide and its consequences are a global problem that is likely to become even more important in the future for a variety of reasons, ranging from changes of the demographic structure and the growing prevalence of chronic mental and physical disorders (often occurring together, thus worsening the prognosis of both types of disorders), to the increase of alcohol consumption and of other risk factors for suicide, and the many forms of social disruption leading to the reduction of sources of support in times of stress and destructive anomie.

I wish to be the first among the many who will wish to express thanks to the editors of this work. They give us a volume that is unique in its coverage of the field—both in geographical and in epistemological terms—and remarkable because of the excellence of its many contributors who give us hope that the major public health problems created by suicidal behaviour can be reduced by concerted action. They show us that this can be done by describing successful programmes, which give us information that is often difficult to access, yet can be of great importance for the understanding of suicidal behaviour and for the development of programmes to prevent suicide and its consequences. It is to be hoped that the book will be read by many and that the information that has been so skilfully presented will be used in developing programmes against suicide: in that lies the usefulness of this effort and, in that, would be the greatest reward for the editors and the contributors to this extraordinarily valuable book.

Professor N. Sartorius, M.D., Ph.D.

# Preface

The subject of suicide is old, yet still suicide prevention remains an uncharted territory. Only in the last decades has the World Health Organization recognized suicide as a serious problem not sufficiently addressed by the clinical and public health sectors. Emerging research and knowledge about the predicaments surrounding suicide calls for action on all continents. Conventionally, much research on suicide has been geographically and culturally confined to Europe, North America, Australia and New Zealand; however, in recent times, suicidology and suicide prevention in Africa, Asia and Latin America has emerged on the international scene, and consequently this textbook reflects a large range of research across all continents.

Each year approximately one million people across the world commit suicide and ten million attempt to do so. Estimates indicate that these numbers will increase if preventive and treatment efforts will not be forcefully supported by legislative and economical measures.

Understanding risk and protective factors on the individual, family, structural and sociocultural levels is necessary in order to tailor suicide preventive actions. Suicidal behaviours vary widely across the lifespan. One example is the ratio of suicide attempts to completed suicides which is generally around 20 or even 30 to 1 in young people and 3 or less to 1 in the elderly. Risk factors for suicide are only partly dependent on psychiatric diagnosis and even if illness is an important component in suicide, it is a challenge to understand what makes a minority of people who have suicidal thoughts within any given diagnostic category, suicidal. The underlying causes of attempted and completed suicide are extremely complex and the body of research presented in this textbook shows that the recognition of the problem, appropriate intervention and prevention is not an easy task. Yet they are possible. Prevention is superior and preferable to therapy as shown in many fields; therefore a focus on prevention and early recognition of suicidal behaviours should direct its attention to much earlier stages of the suicidal process.

This textbook is written by the foremost international scholars in suicidology, presenting the latest developments in the field, while allowing for an extension into fields closely related to suicidology and suicide prevention. The book offers a comprehensive review and synthesis of data regarding suicidal behaviour and suicide prevention across the lifespan as well as in different countries, encompassing both health care and public health perspectives on all continents. Thus, all references have been carefully selected by the authors with such objectives in mind. The textbook is intended for researchers but also for clinical and public health care practitioners. The two major approaches in suicide prevention, through general health care and public health, are described against the background of the sufferings and the cost of suicide and suicide-prevention strategies. Across the world, suicide is deeply tied up with human beings' existential and social conditions. Consequently, we decided to open the reading of this textbook with chapters examining religious expressions and practices across the world, so allowing the reader to contemplate people's attitudes to and representations of suicide. The chapters discussing representations of suicide in film and other media give room for unbound associations and new initiatives on how preventive efforts can be tailored. In the final sections, examples of suicide-preventive activities on all the continents are given together with descriptions of the major actors and organizations in the field. These chapters provide the readers with resources and options for future developments of suicide preventive activities. The content of the chapters has been updated until the very last submission before publishing: consequently they contain the most up to date clinical psychiatric perspectives, including all aspects of pharmacological, psychotherapeutic and other treatment methods, as well as public health perspectives with all existing strategies described extensively.

Since the field of suicidology and suicide prevention comprises themes bordering on sociocultural and structural contexts, as well as functions of the central nervous system (CNS) to the molecular biological level, we as editors were privileged to collaborate in the preparation of this textbook with our complementary competences. Danuta Wasserman with experience from medicine, psychiatry, psychoanalysis and public health was in charge for parts of the book covering the psychiatric, psychological and somatic determinants of suicide and suicide prevention. Camilla Wasserman, on the other hand, with a background in social anthropology, political science and public health was responsible for chapters covering the sociocultural, religious, political, economical and organizational determinants of suicide and suicide prevention.

Many people deserve our deepest thanks for their help and advice in preparing this book. We would like to acknowledge the wholehearted and considerable support from all the contributors, their administrative staff and all the staff at NASP (The National Swedish Prevention of Suicide and Mental Ill-Health) at Karolinska Institutet, Stockholm, Sweden, with special gratitude to Ana Nordenskiöld (Information Officer), Tony Durkee (Research Assistant), and Gergö Hadlaczky (Research Assistant) whose hard work and dedication have proven momentous, without which the book would have not seen the light of day.

Special thanks are directed to Professor Jerzy Wasserman for his never failing support, inspiring discussions filled with valuable suggestions and for participating creatively in the book's conceptual evaluation.

Notwithstanding the fact that treatment of suicidal people and prevention of suicide is a difficult task, this book is filled with evidence showing that such efforts are in fact effective. Therefore it is important to try to continue to decrease suicide's toll. This textbook is not only an extensive forum for discussion across continents, disciplines and themes of research, but can also be seen as a platform for future research and joint action.

Before commencing your journey into this book, we will leave you with a saying open to your own interpretation:

*To save one life is as if you have saved the world.*

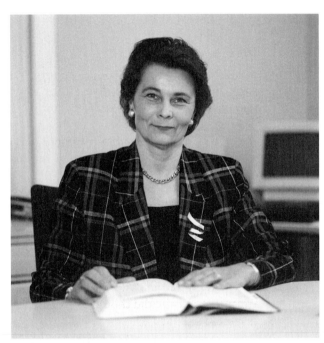

Photo by Solveig Edlund, Stockholm, Sweden

Danuta Wasserman
Karolinska Institutet and Karolinska University Hospital,
Stockholm, Sweden, 2009

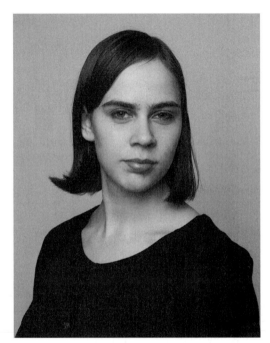

Photo by Hannah Whitaker, NYC, NY, USA

Camilla Wasserman
Columbia University, New York State Psychiatric
Institute, New York, USA, 2009

# Contents

# Contributors

**Paulo Alterwain** MD, Full Professor of Psychiatry, School of Medicine, Montevideo, Uruguay; Past Director of Mental Health, Uruguayan Ministry of Public Health; Founder of the Uruguayan Federation for Suicide Prevention (UNAPS); Past Member of the Board of Directors of the World Federation for Mental Health (WFMH); Member of the Suicide Section of the WPA, Montevideo, Uruguay

**Rubén Alvarado** MD, MPH, PhD, Assistant Professor, School of Public Health, Medical Faculty, University of Chile, Santiago, Chile

**David Althaus** MD, Psychologist, Competence Network 'Depression, Suicidality', Department of Psychiatry, University of Leipzig, Leipzig, Germany

**Martin Anderson** Associate Professor in Mental Health, School of Nursing, University of Nottingham, UK

**Karl Andriessen** MA Suicidology, Coordinator of the Suicide Prevention Program of the Community Mental Health Centres (FDGG-VVI) in Flanders-Belgium; Co-founder of the Flemish Working Group on Suicide Survivors (Verder); Belgian National Representative in IASP and Co-Chair of the IASP Postvention Taskforce

**Alan Apter** MD, Professor and Chairman of the Department of Psychiatry at Sackler School of Medicine, Tel Aviv, Israel; Director of the Feinberg Child Study Center and the Department of Child and Adolescent Psychiatry at Schneiders Childrens Medical Center of Israel; Foreign Adjunct Professor at the National Swedish Prevention of Suicide and Mental Ill-Health (NASP) at Karolinska Institutet, Stockholm, Sweden

**Kiminori Arai** Priest of, Chichibu Shinto Shrine, Chichibu, Japan

**Victoria Arango** PhD, Professor of Clinical Neurobiology, Columbia University and New York State Psychiatric Institute, New York, New York, USA

**Suichi Awata** MD, PhD, Department of Neuropsychiatry and Center for Dementia, Sendai City Hospital, Sendai, Japan

**Hélène Bach-Mizrachi** PhD, Assistant Professor of Clinical Neurobiology, New York State Psychiatric Institute, Columbia University, New York, New York, USA

**Kristen Batejan** Graduate student, Suffolk University, Department of Psychology, Boston USA

**Gaspar Baquedano** MD, Professor of Psychiatry and Masters of Social Anthropology, University of Yucatan; Coordinator of Integrated Program for The Attention of Suicide (IPAS), Hospital Psiquiatrico Yucatan, Mexico; Founder of the suicide prevention programmme 'Let's Save a Life', Chablekal, Yucatan, Mexico

**Sergio A Perez Barrero** MD, Professor of Psychiatry, Granma University, Cuba; Member of IASP, WSN, WPA Suicidology Section, AITS (International Association of Suicidology and Thanatology), Suicidology and Thanatology Section, Cuban Psychiatry Society

**Franz Baro** MD, PhD, Professor emeritus of Psychiatry, Catholic University Leuven (KUL); WHO Mental Health Expert, Chair of the WHO Collaborating Centre for Health and Psychosocial and Psychobiological Factors Brussels, Belgium

**Héctor Basile** MD, Professor of Psychiatry of Children and Adolescents, School of Medicine, Buenos Aires, Argentina; President of the Chapter of Psychiatry of the Child and Adolescent at the Argentinean Association of Psychiatrists (APSA), Buenos Aires, Argentina

**Jens Baumert** PhD in Mathematics and Statistics, Institute of Epidemiology – Helmholtz Zentrum München, German Research Center for Environmental Health, München-Neuherberg, Germany

**Annette Beautrais** PhD, Associate Professor and Principal Investigator of Canterbury Suicide Project, Christchurch School of Medicine, Canterbury, New Zealand; Editor-in-Chief of the journal *Crisis*

**Per Bech** MD, Professor of Psychiatry and Applied Psychometrics and Head of Psychiatric Research Unit, Frederiksborg General Hospital, Hillerød, University of Copenhagen, Copenhagen, Denmark

**Lanny Berman** PhD, Executive Director of AAS, Washington DC, USA

**José M Bertolote** MD, PhD, Professor, Department of Neurology, Psychology and Psychiatry; Director of the Post Graduate Programme in Public Health, Botucatu Medical School, São Paulo State University, São Paulo, Brazil

**Jan Beskow** MD, PhD, Professor Emeritus of Psychiatry, Section for Psychiatry and Neurochemistry, Gothenburgs University, Gothenburg, Sweden; Member of IASR

**Astrid Palm Beskow** MD, PhD, Honorary Vice President of the Society for Coaching Psychology; Founder and Member of the Board of the Center for Cognitive Psychotherapy and Education, Gothenburg, Sweden

**Dinesh Bhugra** Professor of Mental Health and Cultural Diversity Health Services Research Department, Institute of Psychiatry, King's College London, London UK

**Eric Blaauw** PhD, Senior Researcher and Manager Forensic Health Care, Addiction Health Care, The Netherlands

**Jed Boardman** PhD, FRCPsych, Senior Lecturer in Social Psychiatry, Health Service and Population Research Department, Institute of Psychiatry, Consultant Psychiatrist, South London and Maudsley NHS Foundation Trust, London, United Kingdom

**Neury J Botega** MD, PhD, Professor of Medical Psychology, Faculty of Medical Sciences, State University of Campinas, Campinas, Brazil

**David A Brent** MD, Professor of Psychiatry, Pediatrics and Epidemiology, University of Pittsburgh School of Medicine Pittsburgh, USA; Academic Chief of Child and Adolescent Psychiatry, Western Psychiatric Institute and Clinic; Endowed Chair in Suicide Studies, University of Pittsburgh School of Medicine; Director, Services for Teens at Risk

**Beth S Brodsky** PhD, Assistant Clinical Professor of Medical Psychology in Psychiatry at Columbia University; Research scientist in the Silvio O Conte Center of Neurobiology of Mental Disorders, New York State Psychiatric Institute, Department of Neuroscience, New York, New York, USA

**Thomas Bronisch** MD, PhD, Associate Professor of Psychiatry and Head of Open Unit at the Max-Planck-Institute of Psychiatry, Munich, Germany; Member and Treasurer of IASP, Member of IASR and AAS

**Anat Brunstein Klomek** PhD, Assistant Professor of Clinical Psychology in the Division of Child and Adolescent Psychiatry Columbia University, Department of Psychiatry, New York, USA; Schneider Children's Medical Center of Israel, Petah Tikva, Israel

**Stephanie Burrows** PhD, Centre for Research and Intervention on Suicide and Euthanasia, Université du Québec à Montréal, Montréal, Canada

**Cendrine Bursztein** PhD-student, at the National Swedish Prevention of Suicide and Mental Ill-Health (NASP) at Karolinska Institutet, Stockholm, Sweden; Researcher at Feinberg Child Study center, Schneider Children's Medical Center of Israel, Petah Tikva, Israel

**Gérard Camy** Director of Audiovisual Public and Professional High School in Cannes; President of the Association 'Cannes Cinema'; Historian of Cinema; Journalist for weekly 'Telerama' from 1994 to 2004; Author of several influential books about cinema

**Silvia Sara Canetto** PhD, Professor of Psychology, Department of Psychology Colorado State University, Fort Collins, USA

**Chris Cantor** MD, PhD, Senior Lecturer Department of Psychiatry, University of Queensland, Noosa Heads, Australia

**Vladimir Carli** MD, PhD, Research Assistant at the Department of Health Sciences, University of Molise, Campobasso, Italy; Member of IASP; Treasurer of the EPA Section of Suicidology and Suicidal Behaviours

**Ying-Yeh Chen** MD, ScD, Assistant Professor at the Institute of Public Health and Department of Public Health, National Yang-Ming University, Taipei, Taiwan; Attending Psychiatrist at Taipei City Psychiatric Centre, Taipei City Hospital, Taipei, Taiwan

**Qi Cheng** MD, PhD, Professor of Epidemiology and Neurology, and Deputy Director for School of Public Health, Shanghai Jiao Tong University, Shanghai, China

**Paula J Clayton** MD, Medical Director, American Foundation for Suicide Prevention

**John F Connolly** MD, FRCPsych, Secretary of The Irish Association of Suicidology; Former Editor-in-Chief of the journal *Crisis*

**Doina Cozman** MD, PhD, Professor of Psychiatry and Mental Health, and Head of the Department of Clinical Psychology and Mental Health at Iuliu Hatieganu University of Medicine and Pharmacy, Cluj-Napoca, Romania; Head of the 3rd Psychiatry Clinic, Cluj Clinical Emergency County Hospital; National Representative for Romania in IASP

**Dianne Currier** PhD, Staff Associate, Division of Molecular Imaging and Neuropathology, Department of Psychiatry, Columbia University, New York, New York, USA

**Diego De Leo** MD, PhD, DSc, FRANZCP, Professor of Psychiatry at Griffith University, Brisbane, Australia; Director of Australian Institute for Suicide Research and Prevention, The National Centre Of Excellence in Suicide Prevention, and WHO Collaborating Centre for Research and Training in Suicide Prevention; Editor in Chief of *Crisis*; Former President of IASP and IASR

**Sandra Dietrich** MA, Research fellow, Department of Psychiatry, University of Leipzig, Leipzig, Germany

**Carlos Felipe Almeida D'Oliveira** MD, Ministry of Health of Brazil, São Paulo, Brazil

**Brian Draper** MBBS, MD, FRANZCP, Conjoint Associate Professor, University of New South Wales, Sydney; Senior Staff Specialist, Academic Department for Old Age Psychiatry, Prince of Wales Hospital Randwick New South Wales Australia

**Edward J Dunne** PhD, Psychotherapist, Director of Survivor Initiatives for Suicide Prevention International Foundation; Senior Faculty Member of the Ackerman Institute for the Family, Former President of AAS and Former Director of its Survivor Division, New York, USA

**Karen Dunne-Maxim** RN, MS, Former President of AAS, Former Coordinator for New Jersey Suicide Prevention Project at the University of Medicine and Dentistry of New Jersey - University Behavioral Health Care at Piscataway, NJ, USA

**Tony Durkee** PhD-student, and research assistant at the National Swedish Prevention of Suicide and Mental Ill-Health (NASP) at Karolinska Institutet, Stockholm, Sweden

**Øivind Ekeberg** MD, PhD, Professor, Department of Behavioral Sciences in Medicine, University of Oslo; Senior Psychiatrist, Department of Acute Medicine, Oslo University Hospital, Norway

**Natalia Erazo**  PhD in Psychology, Department of Psychosomatic Medicine and Psychotherapy, Technische Universitaet Muenchen, Munich, Germany

**Christianne Esposito-Smythers**  PhD, Adjunct Faculty, Center for Alcohol and Addiction Studies, Brown University, Providence, RI, USA; Assistant Professor of Clinical Psychology, George Mason University, Department of Psychology, Fairfax, VA, USA

**Elmar Etzersdorfer**  MD, Univ.-Doz, Medical Director of the Furtbachkrankenhaus, Hospital for Psychiatry and Psychotherapy, Stuttgart, Germany; Chairman of the German Association for Suicide Prevention

**Jan Fawcett**  MD, Professor of Psychiatry University of New Mexico School of Medicine, New Mexico, USA

**Marcello Ferrada-Noli**  MD, PhD in Psychiatry, Karolinska Institute; Professor Emeritus of Public Health Sciences, University of Gävle, Sweden; Head, Research group International and Cross-cultural Injury Epidemiology, Section of Health and Safety Promotion, Div of Social Medicine, Dept Public Health Sciences, Karolinska Institute, Sweden; Affiliate Professor, School of Public Health, Medical Faculty, University of Chile

**Alexandra Fleischmann***  PhD, World Health Organization, Geneva, Switzerland

**Francisca Florenzano**  Sociologist, MPH; Assistant Professor, Department of Sociology, Catholic University of Chile

**Daniel Fränkel**  Professor of Sociology, University of Buenos Aires, Argentina; Past Associate Director of the Interzonal Neuropsychiatric Hospital Dr. Domingo Cabred, Buenos Aires, Argentina

**Robert Gebbia**  Executive Director, American Foundation for Suicide Prevention

**Sheree Gibb**  PhD-student, Department of Psychological Medicine, University of Otago, Christchurch, New Zealand

**Tresha Gibbs**  MD, Psychiatry Resident, Columbia University, New York, New York, USA

**Mark J Goldblatt**  MD, Assistant Clinical Professor of Psychiatry, Harvard Medical School; Faculty Member, Boston Psychoanalytic Society and Institute; Supervisor and Faculty Member, The Center for Psychoanalytic Studies at Massachusetts General Hospital; Clinical Associate, McLean Hospital

**Jacki Gordon**  Independent consultant in health improvement planning and evaluation, Scotland; Formerly (2004-2007) National Information Manager, Choose Life

**Madelyn S Gould**  PhD, MPH, Professor, Division of Child Psychiatry and Department of Epidemiology, Columbia University; Research Scientist, New York State Psychiatric Institute (NYSPI), New York, New York, USA

**Onja T Grad**  PhD, Professor of Health Psychology at Medical School, University of Ljubljana; Psychotherapist and Supervisor, Head of the Centre for Suicide Prevention at the University Psychiatric Hospital, Ljubljana, Slovenia; President of the Slovenian Associaltion for Suicide Prevention, chief-editor for the journal *Pogled/The View – Acta Suicidologica Slovenica*, the director of the Centre for psychological counseling in Ljubljana, Slovenia

**Jaime Greif**  Full Professor of Law and Past Director of the Law Process Department at the School of Law, Uruguayan Republic University; Founder of the Uruguayan Federation for Suicide Prevention (UNAPS), Montevideo, Uruguay

**Marc Vande Gucht,**  Founder and Chair of 'Go for Happiness' Non-profit Organization for Prevention of Depression and Suicide, Gooik, Belgium

**David Gunnell**  PhD, Professor of Epidemiology, Department of Social Medicine, University of Bristol, UK; Member of the National Suicide Prevention Advisory Group, England; South Asian Clinical Toxicology Research Collaboration (SACTRC)

**Ann P Haas**  PhD, Director of Prevention Projects, American Foundation for Suicide Prevention

**Gergö Hadlaczky**  PhD-student, Lecturer and Research Assistant at the National Swedish Prevention of Suicide and Mental Ill-Health (NASP) at Karolinska Institutet, Stockholm, Sweden

**Ulrich Hegerl**  MD, Professor of Psychiatry, Chair and Medical Director, Department of Psychiatry, University of Leipzig, Germany; Head of Competence Network 'Depression, Suicidality'; Principal Investigator for the European Alliance Against Depression (EAAD); Head of OSPI-Europe (Optimised Suicide Prevention Programs and Their Implementation in Europe)

**Gregor Henderson**  Director of Scotland's National Programme for Improving Mental Health and Wellbeing from 2003-2008 and Senior Fellow, the Institute of Psychiatry, Kings College, London

**Herbert Hendin**  MD, Professor of Clinical Psychiatry, New York Medical College; Chief Executive Officer and Medical Director of Suicide Prevention International

**Silvia Hernandez**  PhD, Epidemiology Specialist, Department of Public Health, Montevideo, Uruguay

**Chia Boon Hock**  MD, MBBS, DPM, FRANCZ, Consultant Psychiatrist, The Chia Clinic, Singapore, Singapore

**Christina W Hoven**  DrPH, MPH, Associate Professor, Department of Epidemiology and Division of Child Psychiatry, Director, Child Psychiatric Epidemiology Group, College of Physicians and Surgeons and Mailman School of Public Health, Columbia University; Research Scientist, New York State Psychiatric Institute, New York, New York, USA

**Maya Iohan-Barak**  PhD, Psychologist, Bar Ilan University Department of Psychology, Ramat Gan, Israel; Department of Child and Adolescent Psychiatry at Schneider Children's Medical Center of Israel, Petah Tikva, Israel

**Rachel Jenkins**  Professor of Epidemiology and International Mental Health Policy; Director of the WHO Collaborating Centre; Head of Section of Mental Health Policy, Institute of Psychiatry, Kings College London; Director of International Affairs, Royal College of Psychiatrists, UK

---

*  This author is a staff member of the World Health Organization. She alone is responsible for the views expressed in this publication and they do not necessarily represent the decisions, policy or views of the World Health Organization.

**Guo-Xin Jiang** MD, PhD, Researcher, Epidemiology and Neurology, National Swedish Prevention of Suicide and Mental Ill-Health (NASP) at Karolinska Institutet, Stockholm, Sweden

**Jennifer Jones** Instructor of Clinical Psychology, Columbia University, Department of Psychiatry, New York, New York, USA

**Brigita Jurišić** MSc student, University of Minho, Braga, Portugal

**John Kalafat** PhD, Professor in the Rutgers Graduate School of Applied and Professional Psychology; Former President of American Association of Suicidology; Fellow in the Society for Community Research & Action and Psychotherapy divisions of APA (Deceased)

**Yoshihiro Kaneko** PhD, Director of Department of Empirical Social Security Research, National Institute of Population and Social Security Research, Ministry of Health and Welfare, Tokyo, Japan

**Chiaki Kawanishi** MD, PhD, Associate Professor at the Department of Psychiatry, Yokohama City University School of Medicine, Yokohama, Japan

**Brendan Kennelly** B Comm, M Econ Sc, Lecturer, National University of Ireland, Galway, Ireland; Visiting Professor at Department of Economics at Lehigh University, Pennsylvania, USA; Member of Mental Health Economics European Network

**Ad Kerkhof** PhD, Professor of Psychology, Department of Clinical Psychology, Vrije Universiteit, Amsterdam, The Netherlands; Member of IASP; Associate Editor of the journal *Crisis*

**Murad M Khan** MRCPsych, Professor & Chairman, Dept of Psychiatry, Aga Khan University, Karachi, Pakistan; Chair, Council of National Representatives, IASP; Member, IASR; Member of Editorial Board, *Crisis*

**Robert A King** MD, Professor of Child Psychiatry and Medical Director, Tourette's/OCD Clinic, Yale Child Study Center, Yale University School of Medicine, New Haven CT, USA

**Dejan Kozel** BSc, Comunity Health Centre Ljubljana, CINDI Slovenija, researcher, Ljubljana, Slovenia

**Valery Krasnov** MD, Professor of Psychiatry and Director of Moscow Research Institute of Psychiatry, Moscow, Russia; President of the Russian Psychiatric Society

**Orit Krispin** PhD, Clinical Psychologist-supervisor, Chief Psychologist, Schneider Children's Medical Center of Israel, Petach-Tikva, Israel

**Karolina Krysinska** PhD, Australian Institute of Suicide Research and Prevention, Griffith University, The National Centre of Excellence in Suicide Prevention, and WHO Collaborating Centre for Research and Training in Suicide Prevention; Brisbane, Australia

**Karl-Heinz Ladwig** MD, PhD, Professor of Psychosomatic Medicine and Medical Psychology, Institute of Epidemiology -Helmholtz Zentrum München German Research Center for Environmental Health München-Neuherberg, and Department of Psychosomatic Medicine and Psychotherapy, Technische Universitaet Muenchen, Munich, Germany

**Antoon Leenaars** PhD, CPsych, Windsor ON, Canada; Faculty member of University of Leiden, The Netherlands; Former President of CASP, and AAS. Former Editor-in-Cheif of Archives of Suicide Research

**Gregory Luke Larkin** Professor of Surgery and Associate Chair at Department of Surgery, Section of Emergency Medicine, Yale University School of Medicine, New Haven, Connecticut, USA

**David Lester** Distinguished Professor of Psychology, The Richard Stockton College of New Jersey, Pomona, NJ, USA

**Jouko Lönnqvist** MD, PhD, Professor, Department of Mental Health and Substance Abuse Services, National Institute for Health and Welfare, Helsinki, Finland; Department of Psychiatry, University of Helsinki, Finland; President of IASR

**Ilkka Henrik Mäkinen** Associate Professor of Sociology, Stockholm Centre on Health of Societies in Transition (SCOHOST), School of Social Sciences, Södertörn University, Huddinge, Sweden

**Kevin Malone** MD, Professor of Psychiatry, Department of Psychiatry and Mental Health Research, University College Dublin, Dublin, Ireland

**John T Maltsberger** MD, Associate Clinical Professor of Psychiatry, Harvard Medical School, Boston, Massachusetts, USA; Faculty Member, Boston Psychoanalytic Society and Institute; Clinical Associate, McLean Hospital

**Donald J Mandell** PhD, MPH, Co-Director, International Center for Child Mental Health, National Center for Disaster Preparedness, Mailman School of Public Health, Columbia University; Research Scientist, New York State Psychiatric Institute, New York, New York, USA

**J John Mann** MD, The Paul Janssen Professor of Translational Neuroscience in Psychiatry and Radiology; Vice Chair for Research; Scientific Director, Kreitchman PET Center, Columbia University; Chief of Division of Molecular Imaging and Neuropathology, New York State Psychiatric Institute, New York, New York, USA

**Elizabeth Mårtensson** MA, Information Manager, National Swedish Prevention of Suicide and Mental Ill-Health (NASP) at Karolinska Institutet, Stockholm, Sweden

**Carlos Martínez** Licentiate in Psychology, Professor of Suicidology at Palermo University, Buenos Aires, Argentina; Former president and current Director General of Argentine Association of Suicide Prevention

**Andrej Marušič** MD, PhD, MRCPsych, MSc, BSc Professor of Psychiatry and Former Head of the Health Research Department, University of Primorska, Primorska Institute of Natural Sciences and Technology (UP PINT), Slovenia (Deceased)

**David McDaid** Senior Research Fellow in Health Policy and Health Economics at LSE Health and Social Care and European Observatory on Health Systems and Policies, London School of Economics and Political Science, London, UK

**Lars Mehlum** MD, PhD, Professor of Psychiatry and Suicidology, Director, National Centre for Suicide Research and Prevention, Institute of Psychiatry, University of Oslo, Norway; Senior Consultant Psychiatrist, Child and Adolescent Outpatient Clinic, Oslo University Hospital; Editor of the journal *Suicidologi*, Former President of IASP

**Duc Pham Thi Minh** MD, PhD, Professor and Head of Medical Education Department, Hanoi Medical University, Hanoi, Vietnam

**Milan Mirjanič** PhD-student and researcher, Health Research Department, University of Primorska, Primorska Institute of Natural Sciences and Technology (UP PINT), Koper, Slovenia

**Ellenor Mittendorfer Rutz** PhD, MSC, Department of Clinical Neuroscience Section of Personal Injury Prevention, Karolinska Institutet, Stockholm, Sweden; Board member of the Nordic Association of Psychiatric Epidemiology

**Alexander Mokhovikov** MD, PhD, Associate Professor, Department of Clinical Psychology, Odessa National University; Director of the Odessa Confidence Telephone Service (the Odessa Samaritans); President of the Ukrainian National Association of Telephone Counselors

**Hans-Jurgen Möller** MD, Professor of Psychiatry, Chairman of the Department of Psychiatry, University of Munich; President of EPA; Chair of the WPA Pharmacopsychiatry section; Chief Editor of the *World Journal of Biological Psychiatry*

**Véronique Narboni** MD, Guest researcher at the National Swedish Prevention of Suicide and Mental Ill-Health (NASP) at Karolinska Institutet, Stockholm, Sweden

**Arlette J Ngoubene-Atioky** PhD-student of Counseling Psychology, Lehigh University Bethlehem, USA

**Ana Nordenskiöld** Information Officer, National Swedish Prevention of Suicide and Mental Ill-Health (NASP) at Karolinska Institutet, Stockholm, Sweden

**Ahmed Okasha** Professor of Psychiatry, Director of the WHO Collaborating Centre for Training and Research in Mental Health, Institute of Psychiatry, Ain Shams University Cairo, Egypt; Former President, WPA; President of Egyptian Psychiatric Association

**Tarek Okasha** Professor of Psychiatry, Institute of Psychiatry, Ain Shams University Cairo, Egypt; Secretary for Scientific Meetings, WPA

**Maria A Oquendo** MD, Professor of Clinical Psychiatry, Division of Molecular Imaging and Neuropathology, New York State Psychiatric Institute, and Columbia University, New York, USA; Vice Chair for Education, Department of Psychiatry, Columbia University; Director of the Clinical Evaluation Core of the Silvio O Conte Center for the Neurobiology of Mental Disorders, Division of Molecular imaging and Neuropathology, New York State Psychiatric Institute, New York, USA

**Israel Orbach** PhD, Professor of Psychology, Bar-Ilan University, Department of Psychology, Ramat-Gan, Israel

**Emilio Ovuga** MD, Professor and Former Dean of Psychiatry, Faculty of Medicine, Gulu University, Gulu, Uganda

**Maria del Carmen Paparamborda** MD, PhD, Professor of Preventive Medicine and Epidemiology, School of Medicine, Montevideo, Uruguay; Director of Department at the Uruguayan Ministry of Public Health. Montevideo, Uruguay

**Ramin Parsey** MD, PhD, Associate Professor of Clinical Psychiatry, Director of the Brain Imaging Division, Department of Molecular Imaging and Neuropathology, New York State Psychiatric Institute; Co-Director of the PET Chemistry and Analysis Core, New York State Psychiatric Institute, USA

**Silvia Pelaez Remigio** MD, Clinical Psychiatrist, Former President of Association of suicidology for Latin America and the Carribbean (ASULAC); National Representative of Uruguay in IASP, AITS (International Association of Suicidology and Thanatology); National Representative in Uruguay of INSS; President of Scientific and Organizer Comittee of XXV World Congress IASP Montevideo, 2009

**Ana Petrović** BSc, Institute for Rehabilitation, Republic of Slovenia, Vocational Rehabilitation Center Ljubljana, Psychologist, Ljubljana, Slovenia

**Rossana Pettersén** Clinical Psychologist, PhD-student, Department of Clinical Neurosciences, Karolinska Institutet, Stockholm, Sweden

**Tim Pfeiffer-Gerschel** PhD, Psychologist, Competence Network 'Depression, Suicidality', Department of Psychiatry, University of Leipzig, Leipzig, Germany

**Michael R Phillips** MD, MA, MPH, Executive Director, WHO Collaborating Center for Research and Training in Suicide Prevention, Beijing Suicide Research and Prevention Centre, Beijing Hui Long Guan Hospital, China; Professor of Psychiatry and Epidemiology, Columbia University, USA

**Jane Pirkis** PhD, Associate Professor, School of Population Health, University of Melbourne, Australia; Chair of the IASP Task Force on Suicide and the Media

**Somparn Promta** PhD, Associate Professor of Buddhist Philosophy and Deputy Director of the Center for Buddhist Studies at Department of Philosophy and Center for Buddhist Studies, Chulalongkorn University, Bangkok, Thailand

**Aron Rabinowitz** Senior Lecturer in Clinical Psychology and School Psychology, Bar-Ilan University, Department of Psychology, Ramat-Gan, Israel

**Inga-Lill Ramberg** PhD, Senior researcher, National Swedish Prevention of Suicide and Mental Ill-Health (NASP) at Karolinska Institutet, Stockholm, Sweden

**Jerry Reed** MSW, PhD, Director of Suicide Prevention Resource Center Newton, Massachusetts, USA; Chair Council of Organizational Representatives International Association for Suicide Prevention (IASP)

**Nils Retterstøl** MD, PhD, Professor emeritus of Psychiatry, University of Oslo; Former Head of Gaustad Hospital, Oslo; Former Editor of European Archives of Psychiatry and Clinical Neurosciences; Honorary Member of AEP, IASP and the Swedish Psychiatric Association; Former President of IASP; Board member of AEP (presently known as EPA) (Deceased)

**Zoltán Rihmer** MD, PhD, DSc, Professor of Psychiatry and Director of Research; Faculty of Medicine, Department of Clinical and Theoretical Mental Health and Department of Psychiatry and Psychotherapy, Semmelweis University, Budapest, Hungary; Member of Executive Committee, European College of Neuropsychopharmacology

**Elsa Ronningstam** PhD, Associate Clinical Professor Harvard Medical School; Psychologist, McLean Hospital; Member of Boston Psychoanalytic Society and Institute; President of International Society for the Study of Personality Disorders, ISSPD

**Alec Roy** MD, PhD, Professor of psychiatry at New Jersey Medical School, New Jersey, USA

**Vsevolod Rozanov** MD, PhD, Professor of the department of Clinical Psychology, Odessa National University; Head of the Board of Human Ecological Health NGO, responsible for suicide research and prevention programs; Principal investigator, Odessa Center, WHO Pan-European Network on suicide prevention

**M David Rudd** PhD, ABPP, Professor and Chair of Psychology Department, Texas Tech University, Lubbock, USA

**Esther Ruf** PhD in Psychology and Master in Public Health, Institute of Epidemiology, Helmholtz Zentrum München, German Research Center for Environmental Health, München-Neuherberg, Germany

**Dan Rujescu** MD, PhD, University Professor and Head of Molecular and Clinical Neurobiology, Dept. of Psychiatry, University of Munich, Munich, Germany

**Wolfgang Rutz** MD, PhD, Professor of Social Psychiatry, Head of Unit for Psychiatry and Health Promotion, Division of Psychiatry, University Hospital, Uppsala, Sweden; Faculty of Social Sciences, University for Applied Sciences, Coburg/Germany; Vice Chair of the WPA Section for Psychiatry and Policy, Former Regional Advisor for Mental Health, WHO, European Region

**Paul Salkovskis** PhD, Professor of Clinical Psychology and Applied Science and Head of Graduate Studies (Research), Institute of Psychiatry, King's College London, UK; Clinical Director of the Maudsley Hospital Centre for Anxiety Disorders and Trauma, London, UK

**Benedetto Saraceno\*** MD, Doctor Honoris Causa, University of Lisbon and City University of Birmingham; Honorary Fellow of the Royal College of Psychiatry, UK and of the Spanish Society of Neuropsychiatry; Guest Faculty member of the Graduate Institute of International and Development Studies, Geneva, Switzerland; WHO Director of Department of Mental Health and Substance Abuse, World Health Organization, Geneva, Switzerland

**Marco Sarchiapone** MD, Professor of Psychiatry at the Health Department of University of Molise, Campobasso, Italy; Full Member of IASR; Member of IASP; Member of AAS; General Secretary of the WPA Section of Suicidology; Co-chair of the EPA Section of Suicidology and Sucidal Prevention

**Sylvia Schaller** PhD, Lecturer and Deputy Head of the Outpatient Clinic, Otto-Selz-Institut für Psychologie and the University of Mannheim, Germany

**Mark Schechter** MD, Chair of Department of Psychiatry, North Shore Medical Center; Instructor in Psychiatry, Harvard Medical School; Advanced Candidate, Boston Psychoanalytic Society and Institute

**Lourens Schlebusch** Professor and the Founder and Former Head of the Department of Behavioural Medicine, Nelson R. Mandela School of Medicine, University of KwaZulu-Natal, Durban, South Africa; Former Vice President of IASP

**Armin Schmidtke** PhD, Professor and Head of Clinical Psychology at the University of Würzburg, Department of Psychiatry, Germany; Foreign Adjunct Professor at the National Swedish Prevention of Suicide and Mental Ill-Health (NASP) at Karolinska Institutet, Stockholm, Sweden; Advisor on Suicide Prevention, WHO, EU; Former president of IASR; Principal Investigator MONSUE Pan-European Project (European Multicentre Study on Suicidal Behaviour and Suicide Prevention)

**Monique Séguin** PhD, Researcher at the McGill Group for Suicide Studies; Professor at the Department of Psychoeducation and Psychology, University of Québec in Outaouais, Quebec, Canada

**Menakshi Sharma** Msc, Researcher, Institute of Psychiatry, King's College London, UK

**Gal Shoval** MD, Child and Adolescent Psychiatry Division, Geha Mental Health Center and Tel Aviv University, Tel Aviv, Israel

**Xiao Shuiyuan** MD, Professor of Social Medicine and Psychiatry, Dean at the School of Public Health, as well as Director of the Clinical Psychological Center of Xiangya Hospital, Central South University, Changsha, Hunan, China; President, Chinese Mental Health Assocaition Subcommittee of Crisis Intervention

**Morton M Silverman** MD, Associate Professor of Clinical Psychiatry at The University of Colorado School of Medicine, Denver, Colorado, USA; Editor-in-Chief of the journal Suicide and Life-Threatening Behavior; National Representative for USA International Association for Suicide Prevention (IASP); Distinguished Fellow of the American Psychiatric Association (APA)

**Marcus Sokolowski** PhD, Researcher in the Genetic Investigation of Suicide Attempt and Suicide (GISS); Scientist and Teacher at the National Swedish Prevention of Suicide and Mental Ill-Health (NASP) at Karolinska Institutet, Stockholm, Sweden

**Jean-Pierre Soubrier** MD, Professor Emeritus of Psychiatry, Medical Collége of Paris, France; Former president IASP; Former Chairman WPA, Suicidology Section; Honorary member, executive board of WPA, Suicidology Section; WHO advisor; Vice President of UNPS (Union Nationale Prevention du Suicide)

**Anthony Spirito** PhD, Professor of Psychiatry and Human Behavior, Director of the Clinical psychology Training Consortium, and Associate Director of the Center for Alcohol and Addiction Studies at the Warren Alpert Medical School of Brown University, Providence, USA

**Flora von Spreti** Art Therapist, Technical University Munich, Psychiatric Clinic, Munich, Germany

**Barbara Stanley** PhD, Professor of Clinical Psychology, Department of Psychiatry, Columbia University College of Physicians and Surgeons, New York, USA; Research Scientist New York State Psychiatric Institute; Editor-in-Chief of the journal *Archives of Suicide Research*

**Egon Stenager** MD, PhD, Department of Neurology, Odense University Hospital, Odense, Denmark

**Elsebeth Stenager** MD, PhD and Lecturer, Institute of Clinical Research, Department of Psychiatry, Odense University, Odense, Denmark

---

\* This author is a staff member of the World Health Organization. He alone is responsible for the views expressed in this publication and they do not necessarily represent the decisions, policy or views of the World Health Organization.

**Sabrina Stefanello** MD, Faculty of Medical Sciences, State University of Campinas, Brazil

**Richard Stiliha** D. Min., Chaplain (Maj), US Army (Ret), Director of Education for suicide prevention and crisis intervention, International military community, Olive Branch International NGO, Virginia Beach, Virginia, USA

**Charlotta Sunnqvist** PhD-student Department of Clinical Sciences, Psychiatry, Lund University Hospital, Lund, Sweden

**Jerneja Svetičič** BSc, Australian Institute of Suicide Research and Prevention, Griffith University, Brisbane, Australia

**Prakarn Thomyangkoon** MD, Department of Psychiatry, Rajavithi Hospital, Department of Medical Services, Ministry of Public Health, Bangkok; Lecturer at Institute of Undergraduate Medical Education, Department of Medical Services, Rangsit University, Pathum Thani, Thailand

**Lars-Håkan Thorell** Associate Professor in Experimental Psychiatry, Department of Clinical and Experimental Medicine, Faculty of Health Sciences, Linköping University, Linköping, Sweden

**David Titelman** PhD, Associate Professor, Director of the Graduate and Post-Graduate Programs in Prevention of Suicide and Mental Ill Health at the National Swedish Prevention of Suicide and Mental Ill-Health (NASP) at Karolinska Institutet, Stockholm, Sweden

**Jan Toye** Founder and Chair of 'Go for Happiness' Foundation for Prevention of Depression and Suicide, Steenhuffel, Belgium

**Huong Tran Thi Thanh** MD, PhD, Coordinator for Prevention and Control of Non-communicable Diseases, Ministry of Health; Lecturer, Hanoi Medical University, Hanoi, Vietnam

**Lil Träskman-Bendz** MD, PhD, Professor of Psychiatry and Head, Department of Clinical Sciences, Psychiatry, Lund University, Lund, Sweden

**David RM Trotter** MA, Graduate Student in Clinical Psychology, Department of Psychology, Texas Tech University, Lubbock, USA; APA Student Member

**Gustavo Turecki** MD, PhD, William Dawson Chair and Director of the McGill Group for Suicide Studies; Associate Professor at Departments of Psychiatry and Human genetics, McGill University, Quebec, Canada; Head of Depressive Disorders Program at Douglas Mental Health Institute, McGill University

**Sam Tyano** MD, Professor Emeritus of Adult, Child and Adolescent Psychiatry, Tel Aviv University; Chairperson of the National Committee for Infant mental Health, Israel; Honorary President of the Israeli Child and Adolescent Psychiatric Association; Visiting Professor at Lille and Strasbourg Schools of medicine, France; Vice President of IACAPAP; President of the WPA Committee on Ethics

**Mark D Underwood** PhD, Professor of Clinical Neurosience and Director of Laboratory of Molecular Physiology, Division of Neurobiology, New York State Psychiatric Institute, Department of Psychiatry, Columbia University Medical Center, New York, New York, USA

**Herman M van Praag** MD, PhD, Professor Emeritus of Psychiatry, Department of Psychiatry and Neuropsychology, Academic Hospital, Maastricht University, The Netherlands; Chair of WPA Section, Religion, Spirituality and Psychiatry

**Airi Värnik** MD, Professor of Psychiatry and Mental Health at Tallinn University, Estonia. Director for Estonian-Swedish Mental Health and Suicidology Institute, Tallinn, Estonia; Visiting Professor at the National Swedish Prevention of Suicide and Mental Ill-Health (NASP) at Karolinska Institutet, Stockholm, Sweden; Full member of the International Academy for Suicide Reasearch; Member of Board for Estonian Centre of Behavioural and Health Sciences; Member of Scientific Council at Estonia National Institute for Health Development

**Freddy Vasquez** MD, Psychiatrist, Program for Suicide Prevention, National Institute of Mental Health, Lima, Peru

**Vladimir Voitsekh** MD, Professor of Psychiatry and Head of the Sucidology Department, Moscow Research Institute of Psychiatry, Moscow, Russia

**Naseema Vawda** PhD, King Edward VIII Hospital, Department of Behavioural Medicine, Nelson R Mandela School of Medicine, University of KwaZulu-Natal, Durban, South Africa

**Lakshmi Vijayakumar** MBBS, DPM, PhD, Professor and Head of Department of Psychiatry, Voluntary Health Services, Adyar Hospital, Chennai, India; Founder of SNEHA Suicide Prevention Center, Chennai, India; Former Vice President of IASP; Member of WHO International Network for Suicide Research and Prevention; Member of IASR

**Camilla Wasserman** MA in Anthropology; Scientific Project Director, Child Psychiatric Epidemiology, Department of Child and Adolescent Psychiatry, Columbia University and New York State Psychiatric Institute, New York, USA

**Danuta Wasserman** MD, PhD, Professor of Psychiatry and Suicidology, Founder and Head of the National Swedish Prevention of Suicide and Mental Ill-Health (NASP) at Karolinska Institutet and Chief of Clinical Services, NASP Karolinska University Hospital, Stockholm, Sweden; Director of the WHO Lead Collaborating Centre on Suicide Prevention; Chair of the WPA Suicidology Section; Board member of the EPA, Chair of the EPA Section of Suicidology and Suicide Prevention; Former President of the IASR; Former Vice President of IASP; Honorary President of ERSI; WHO, EU Mental Health Expert; Principal Investigator for GISS and SEYLE Projects

**Jerzy Wasserman** MD, PhD, Professor of Immunology; Scientific Field Director of the GISS Project (Genetic Investigation of Suicide and Suicidal Behaviours), National Swedish Prevention of Suicide and Mental Ill-Health (NASP) at Karolinska Institutet, Stockholm, Sweden

**Igor Weinberg** PhD, Instructor in Psychology, McLean Hospital, Department of Psychiatry, Harvard Medical School, Belmont, MA, USA

**Michael Westerlund** PhD, Lecturer, Department of Journalism, Media and Communication, University of Stockholm, Sweden; Lecturer, National Swedish Prevention of Suicide and Mental Ill-Health (NASP) at Karolinska Institutet, Stockholm, Sweden

**Ben Williams** MA, Graduate Student in Clinical Psychology, Department of Psychology, Texas Tech University; APA Student Member

**Lisa Wittenburg** MSW, Project Manager European Alliance Against Depression (EAAD), Department of Psychiatry, University of Leipzig, Leipzig, Germany

**Akiko Yamasaki**  Associate Professor of Psychiatry, Osaka University, Japan

**Wu Fei**  Professor of Philosophy and Religious Studies, Department of Philosophy, Peking University, Beijing, China

**Su Yin Yap**  Research Assistant, Department of Psychiatry and Mental Health Research, University College Dublin, Dublin, Ireland

**Paul Yip**  Professor of Social Work and Social Administration and Director of the Centre for Suicide Research and Prevention at the University of Hong Kong; National representative of the IASP; Fellow of IASR

**Gil Zalsman**  MD, Sackler School of Medicine, Tel Aviv University, Tel Aviv, Israel; Director of the Child and Adolescent Department of Geha Mental Health Center, Tel Aviv University; Member of the IASR; Board member of the EPA

**Maja Zorko**  PhD, Institute of Public Health of the Republic of Slovenia, Centre for Health Promotion, researcher, Ljubljana, Slovenia

# Acronyms and Abbreviations

| | | | | |
|---|---|---|---|---|
| 5-HIAA | 5-hydroxyindoleacetic acid | | BAC | Blood alcohol concentration |
| 5-HT | 5-hydroxytryptamine | | BD | Bipolar disorder |
| 5-HTTLPR | 5-HTT linked promoter region | | BDI | Beck Depression Inventory |
| 7-DHCR | 7-dehydrocholesterol reductase | | BDNF | Brain-derived neurotrophic factor |
| AAS | American Association of Suicidology | | BHS | Beck Hopelessness Scale |
| ABC | ATP-binding cassette | | BL-38 | *Beschwerden-Liste* (complaints schedule) |
| ABCDE | Activating event, Beliefs, Consequences, Disputing, Effect | | bp | Base pair |
| | | | BP | Binding potential |
| ACE | Angiotensin I-converting enzyme | | BPD | Borderline personality disorder |
| ACTH | Adrenocorticotropic hormone | | BPRS | Brief Psychiatric Rating Scale |
| ADHD | Attention-deficit hyperactivity disorder | | CARE | Care, Assess, Respond, Empower |
| ADIS | Association de Défense Contre l'Incitation au Suicide (France) | | CAST | Coping and support training |
| | | | CBA | Cost–benefit analysis |
| AEP | Association of European Psychiatrists | | CBF | Cerebral blood flow |
| AFSP | American Foundation for Suicide Prevention | | CBT | Cognitive behavioural therapy |
| AFSPP | United States Air Force Suicide Prevention Programme | | C-CASA | Columbia Classification Algorithm of Suicide Assessment |
| AHD | Anxiolytic–hypnotic drugs | | CDC | Centers for Disease Control and Prevention (USA) |
| AI | American Indian (USA) | | | |
| AIM | Awareness Intervention Methodology | | CDRS-R | Children's Depression Rating Scale-Revised |
| AIDS | Acquired immunodeficiency syndrome | | | |
| AN | Alaska Natives (USA) | | CeA | Central amygdala |
| AN | Anorexia nervosa | | CEA | Cost-effectiveness analysis |
| ANAES | Agence Nationale d'Accreditation et d'Evaluation de la Santé (France) | | CES-D | Center for Epidemiologic Studies Depression (scale) |
| apoE | Apolipoprotein E | | CFT | Category fluency test |
| ASA | Anti-Suicide Alliance (Romania) | | CGI | Clinical Global Impression (scale) |
| ASIST | Applied Suicide Intervention Skills Training (Scotland) | | CHDS | Christchurch Health and Development Study |
| ASQ | Affective States Questionnaire | | CHS | Columbia Health Screen |
| ASR | *Archives of Suicide Research* (journal of the IASR) | | CID | Clinical Interview for Depression |
| | | | CCK | Cholecystokinin |
| ASULAC | Asociación de Suicidología de Latinoamerica y el Caribe (South America) | | CME | Continuing Medical Education |

| | |
|---|---|
| CNS | Central nervous system |
| COGA | Collaborative Study on the Genetics of Alcoholism |
| COMT | Catechol-O-methyltransferase |
| CPRS | Comprehensive Psychopathological Rating Scale |
| CRH | Corticotropin-releasing hormone |
| CRHR1 | CRH receptor 1 |
| CSF | Cerebrospinal fluid |
| CCS | Columbia Suicide Screen |
| CUA | Cost-utility analysis |
| CV | Cardiovascular risk factors |
| D/ART | Depression/awareness, recognition, treatment |
| DA | Dopamine |
| DALY | Disability-adjusted life year |
| DASA | Defence Analytical Services Agency (United Kingdom) |
| DAT | Dopamine transporters |
| DBT | Dialectic behaviour therapy |
| DCIPS | Developing Centers on Interventions for the Prevention of Suicide (USA) |
| DDC | DOPA decarboxylase |
| DDD | Defined daily dose |
| DDS | Drawing Diagnostic Series |
| DHHS | Department of Health and Human Services (USA) |
| DIS | Diagnostic Interview Schedule |
| DPS | Durban Parasuicide Study |
| DR | Dorsal raphe |
| DRCR | Death Registry in Certain Regions (China) |
| DRN | Dorsal raphe nuclei |
| DSH | Deliberate self-harm |
| DSM | *Diagnostic and Statistic Manual of Mental Disorders* |
| DSP | Disease Surveillance Point system (China) |
| DST | Dexamethasone suppression test |
| DTI | Diffusion tensor imaging |
| DWMH | Deep white matter hyperintensity |
| DZ | Dizygotic |
| ECA | Epidemiological Catchments Area study |
| ECT | Electroconvulsive therapy |
| ECTS | European Credit Transfer and Accumulation System |
| EEAD | European Alliance Against Depression |
| EGCI | Empirically grounded clinical interventions |
| EMA | Estonian Medical Association |
| EPA | European Psychiatric Association |

| | |
|---|---|
| EPPIC | Early Psychosis Prevention and Intervention Centre (Australia) |
| EPS | Environment–person system |
| EPS | Extra-pyramidal symptoms |
| EPSIS | European Parasuicide Study Interview Schedule |
| ER | Emergency room |
| ERSI | Estonian–Swedish Mental Health and Suicidology Institute |
| EURODEP | European depression study |
| FDA | Food and Drug Administration (USA) |
| FL | Frontal lobe |
| fMRI | Functional magnetic resonance imaging |
| FVT | Fluid vulnerability theory |
| GABA | Gamma-aminobutyric acid |
| GAD | Generalized anxiety disorder |
| GAD | Glutamate decarboxylase |
| GAS | General adaptation syndrome |
| GBD | Global Burden of Disease |
| GDP | Gross domestic product |
| GDS | Geriatric Depression Scale |
| GEPS | Groupement d'Etude et de Prevention du Suicide (France) |
| GH | Growth hormone |
| GISS | Genetic Investigation of Suicide and Suicidal Behaviours |
| GP | General Practitioner |
| GP | Globus pallidus |
| GR | Glucocorticoid receptor |
| HAM-D | Hamilton Depression Scale |
| HC | Healthy controls |
| HHANES | Hispanic Health and Nutrition Epidemiological Survey (USA) |
| HIV | Human immunodeficiency virus |
| HMGCR | 3-hydroxy-3-methylglutarylCoenzyme reductase gene |
| HPA | Hypothalamic–pituitary–adrenal |
| HS | Hopelessness Scale |
| HSMF | Holy Spirit Mobile Forces (Uganda) |
| HVA | Homovanillic acid |
| IACAPAP | International Association of Child and Adolescent Psychiatry and Allied Professions |
| IASP | International Association for Suicide Prevention |
| IASR | International Academy of Suicide Research |
| ICD-10 | *International Classification of Diseases*, 10th edition |

| | | | |
|---|---|---|---|
| ICU | Intensive care unit | MEPS | Means–Ends Problem-Solving Procedure |
| IDDM | Insulin-dependent diabetes mellitus | MHPG | 3-methoxy-4-hydroxyphenylglycol |
| IDF | Israeli Defence Force | MINI | Mini International Neuropsychiatric Interview |
| IDP | Internally displaced persons (Uganda) | | |
| IFCS | Intergovernmental Forum on Chemical Safety | MMSE | Mini Mental State Examination |
| IFOTES | International Federation of Telephonic Emergency Services | MONSUE | Monitoring suicidal behaviour in Europe |
| | | MPFC | Medial prefrontal cortex |
| IMH | Institute of Mental Health (Singapore) | MR | Mineralocorticoid receptor |
| IMPACT | Improving Mood–Promoting Access to Collaborative Treatment | MRI | Magnetic resonance imaging |
| | | MRN | Medial raphe nuclei |
| IOM | Institute of Medicine, Washington DC | mRNA | Messenger ribonucleic acid |
| IPM | Institute for Psychosocial Medicine (Sweden) | MS | Multiple sclerosis |
| | | MSSI | Modified Scale for Suicidal Ideations |
| IPM | Integrated Pest Management | MST | Multisystemic therapy |
| IR | Immunoreactive | MZ | Monozygotic |
| ISO | Inventory of Suicide Orientations | NA | Noradrenaline |
| IPT-A | Interpersonal psychotherapy | NASH | Natural, accidental, suicide, and homicide |
| J-MISP | Japanese Multimodal Intervention Trials for Suicide Prevention | NASP | National Swedish Prevention of Suicide and Mental Ill-Health at Karolinska Institutet, Stockholm, Sweden |
| JNPS | Journée Nationale pour la Prévention du Suicide (France) | | |
| KI | Karolinska Institute (Sweden) | NaSPro | Nationales Suizidpräventionsprogramm (Germany) |
| KIRT | Karolinska Institute Research and Training | | |
| KIRT | Karolinska International Research and Training Committee | NATO | North Atlantic Treaty Organization |
| | | NEMESIS | Netherlands Mental Health Survey and Incidence Study |
| KT | Knowledge translation | | |
| LAMIC | Low- and middle-income countries | NGO | Non-governmental organization |
| LASPC | Los Angeles Suicide Prevention Center (USA) | NIDDM | Non-insulin dependent diabetes mellitus |
| | | NIMH | National Institute of Mental Health (USA) |
| LC | Locus coeruleus | NIMSS | National Injury Mortality Surveillance System (South Africa) |
| LDLR | Low-density lipoprotein receptor | | |
| LEAP | Life Events and Aging Project | NIR | Natural Increase Rate |
| LFT | Letter fluency test | NIST | National Implementation Support Team (Scotland) |
| LIFE | Living is For Everyone (Australia) | | |
| LMG | Lamotrigine | NLA | National Liberation Army (Uganda) |
| LOSS | Local Outreach to Suicide Survivors | NLMS | National Longitudinal Mortality Study |
| LOSS | Loving Outreach for Survivors of Suicide | NO HOPE | No framework for meaning, Overt change in clinical condition, Hostile interpersonal environment, Out of hospital recently, Predisposing personal factors, Excuses for dying are present and strongly believed |
| LPL | Lipoprotein lipase | | |
| LRA | Lord's Resistance Army (Uganda) | | |
| LTP | Long-term potentiation | | |
| MACT | Manual-Assisted Cognitive Behavioural Therapy | | |
| | | NREPP | National Registry of Evidence-Based Programs and Practices (USA) |
| MADRS | Montgomery–Åsberg Depression Rating Scale | | |
| MAO | Monoamine oxidase | NRI | Norepinephrine reuptake inhibitor |
| MAOA | Monoamine oxidase A | NSPL | National Suicide Prevention Lifeline (USA) |
| MDD | Major depressive disorder | NSSP | National Strategy for Suicide Prevention (USA) |
| MDE | Major depressive episode | | |
| MECA | Methodological Epidemiology of Children and Adolescents | OCD | Obsessive–compulsive disorder |
| | | OECD | Organization for Economic Co-operation and Development |

| | | | | |
|---|---|---|---|---|
| OFC | Olanzapine/fluoxetine combination | | SAD PERSONS | Sex, Age, Depression, Previous suicide attempt, Ethanol abuse, Rational thinking loss, Social support lacking, Organized plan (to commit suicide), No spouse, (somatic) Sickness (scale) |
| OFG | Orbitofrontal gyrus | | | |
| OGM | Over-generalized memories | | | |
| OIF-II | Operation Iraqi Freedom II | | | |
| OL | Occipital lobe | | SADS | Schedule for Affective Disorders and Schizophrenia |
| OPD | Outpatients department | | | |
| OPFC | Orbital prefrontal cortex | | SADS-C | Schedule for Affective Disorders and Schizophrenia-Change |
| OPHD | Oregon Public Health Division USA | | | |
| PAR | Population-attributable risk | | SAFER | Suicide Attempt, Follow-up, Education and Research Program (Canada) |
| PAS | Physician-assisted suicide | | | |
| PD | Panic disorder | | SAGE | Singapore Action Group for the Elderly |
| PD | Parkinson's disease | | SAMHSA | Substance Abuse and Mental Health Services Administration (USA) |
| PET | Positron emission tomography | | | |
| PFC | Prefrontal cortex | | SBQ | Suicide Behaviors Questionnaire |
| PFG | Prefrontal gyrus | | SBT | Skills-based therapy |
| pgACC | Pregenual anterior cingulate cortex | | SCH | Subcortical grey matter hyperintensity |
| PHC | Primary health care | | SCID-II | Structured Clinical Interview for DSM-IV Disorders Axis II |
| PL | Parietal lobe | | | |
| PMRs | Proportional mortality ratios | | SDH | Stress–diathesis–hopelessness |
| PMVA | Multisectorial programme with varied scope (Argentina) | | SDQ | Strengths and Difficulties Questionnaire |
| | | | SEAR | South East Asia WHO Region |
| POMC | Pro-opiomelanocortin | | SEM | Standard error of the mean |
| PRIME-MD | Primary Care Evaluation of Mental Disorders | | SERT | Serotonin transporter |
| PROSPECT | Prevention of Suicide in Primary Care Elderly: Collaborative Trial | | SEYLE | Saving and Empowering Young Lives in Europe |
| | | | sgACC | Subgenual anterior cingulate cortex |
| PST | Primary/secondary/tertiary (prevention model) | | SIM | Suicide intervention model |
| | | | SIREN | Suicide Information and Research Evidence Network (Scotland) |
| PSUD | Psychoactive substance abuse disorder | | | |
| PTSD | Post-traumatic stress disorder | | SMR | Standardized mortality ratio |
| PVH | Periventricular hyperintensity | | SMS | Short message service |
| PVN | Paraventricular nucleus | | SNP | Single nucleotide polymorphism |
| PYPLL | Premature years of potential life lost | | SOC | Sense of Coherence |
| QALY | Quality-adjusted life year | | SOLVE | Select a problem, Options, Likely outcomes, Very best option, Evaluates |
| QPR | Question Persuade and Refer | | | |
| rCBF | Regional cerebral blood flow | | SOS | Samaritan of Singapore |
| rCMRglu | Regional cerebral glucose utilization | | SOS | Signs of Suicide (US organization) |
| RCTs | Randomized controlled trials | | SOVRN | Suicides and Open Verdicts on the Railway Network |
| RFLP | Restriction fragment length polymorphism | | | |
| RISC | Recognizing an Imminent Suicide Crisis | | SPAN | Suicide Prevention Action Network (USA) |
| ROI | Regions of interest | | SPECT | Single photon emission computed tomography |
| RR | Relative risk | | | |
| RT-PCR | Reverse transcription polymerase chain reaction | | SPI | Suicide Prevention International |
| | | | SPM | Statistical parametric mapping |
| RY | Reconnecting Youth | | SPRC | Suicide Prevention Resource Center (USA) |
| SA | Suicide attempters | | SRT | Supportive relationship therapy |

| | | | |
|---|---|---|---|
| SRU | Suicide Research Unit (Sweden) | UPDA | Uganda People's Democratic Army |
| SSI | Scale for Suicide Ideation | USAF | United States Air Force |
| SSRIs | Selective serotonin reuptake inhibitors | USI | Universal/selective/indicated (prevention model) |
| STEP-BD | Systematic Treatment Enhancement Program for Bipolar Disorder | USSR | Union of Soviet Socialist Republics |
| SUAS | Suicide Assessment Scale | VA | Veterans Affairs |
| SUD | Substance use disorders | VAMP4 | Vesicle-associated membrane protein 4 gene |
| SUPRE | The WHO worldwide initiative for the prevention of suicidal behaviours | VHs | Village helpers (Uganda) |
| SUPRE-MISS | The WHO Multisite Intervention Study on Suicidal Behaviours | VM | Ventromedial |
| | | VNTR | Variable number tandem repeat |
| TADS | Treatment of Adolescent Depression Study | VOI | Voxel of interest |
| TAU | Treatment as usual | VYPLL | Valued years of potential life lost |
| TCA | Tricyclic antidepressant | WHO | World Health Organization |
| TGF | Train à Grande Vitesse | WHO-5 | WHO-Five Well-Being Index |
| TGOLNA2 | Trans-golgi network protein 2 gene | WISQARS | Web-based Injury Statistics Query and Reporting System (USA) |
| TH | Tyrosine hydroxylase | WM | White matter |
| TL | Temporal lobe | WPA | World Psychiatric Association |
| TPBs | Trauma-producing behaviours | WYPLL | Working years of potential life lost |
| TPH | Tryptophan hydroxylase | YRBS | Youth Risk Behavior Survey (USA) |
| TWB | Towards Well-being (New Zealand) | YST-1 | Youth-nominated support team |
| UN | United Nations | | |
| UNPS | Union Nationale pour la Prévention du Suicide (France) | | |

# PART 1

# Suicide in a Religious and Cross-cultural Perspective

# CHAPTER 1

# Suicide

## Considering religion and culture

Camilla Wasserman

Believing with Max Weber, that man is an animal
suspended in webs of significance that he himself has spun,
I take culture to be those webs, and the analysis of it to be
therefore not an experimental science in search of law but
an interpretive one in search of meaning.

C. Geertz (1973, p. 5)

The parallels between natural and social sciences are numerous: in each, both field and laboratory studies may include qualitative and quantitative tasks, and in part of the book the researchers combine their expertise in a cross-disciplinary fashion. Studies in suicidology in general aim to prevent suicides. Suicidology is interconnected with social change initiatives, and accordingly, as researchers of applied sciences, suicidologists need pay close attention to the relations between the phenomenon studied and wider arenas of social action. Ahead lies great work, directing attention to ways of experiencing the everyday world that is tied into processes of ruling and rules of thoughts. This includes consideration of the multiplicity of religious expressions and the interplay of religion, history and politics on international as well as local levels. The local is not just a site of meanings and practices, but also a node within an extended set of social relations: as such it can never be studied as separate from larger religious institutional structures.

Themes related to suicide in some of the major religions worldwide are here considered alongside customs, myths, practices and attitudes related to suicide and the risk of suicide. The chapters that follow provide insight into the multiple intrinsically linked factors that influence the decision to commit suicide and the ways such deaths are perceived in and by society, offering tools to link such attitudes to religion. The emphasis of each chapter differs, yet they speak to each other, at times through their contradictions but often through the many similarities found in religions worldwide regarding the issue of suicide. By and large, the focus is on the religious and cultural influences on discourses on suicide as well as manifestations and articulations of such discourses in religious practices, scriptures and historically. Discourse is here understood to be a system of thought defining and producing the object of our knowledge providing us with a language to talk about something.

Accordingly discourse is linked to power, assuming the authority and construction of 'truth' (Foucault 1969).

When reading the chapters, concepts such as religion, culture and tradition surface. Working closely with the contributors in contextualizing these complex notions, an effort was made to move away from rigid and essential notions of cultural territories, regional identities and a static view of customs. Attempting to bypass the rigidity of these issues, the chapters encourage a more flexible view of a world in movement characterized by detachments and attachments (Appadurai 2001). Such cultural analysis should be carefully extended to, and contextualized in, a historical framework (Cooper 2005; Spivak 2006). Yet, the confused narrative of origin found in many theoretical discussions on culture, often linking it to colonialism, should not lead to dismissal of the very real and everyday experiences of culture (Dirks 1992; Sahlins 2000). These theoretical and lengthy discussions can be followed elsewhere: here we will only bear these efforts in mind in order to make contextually appropriate use of them by absorbing what can be considered the fundamentals of this debate. Let us consider culture, religion and tradition in their widest possible form: mobile yet historically specific, tied to authority and power structures yet open to negotiation and flexibility.

In Chapter 12, 'Maya religion and traditions: influencing suicide prevention in contemporary Mexico', Gaspar Baquedano calls for a composed 'psycho anthropological perspective' aimed at better understanding of the wider socio-economic and cultural contexts of suicides. Here, much like anthropologists, the suicidologist is not simply a recorder of material: some might argue that the suicidologist's interpersonal and/or cross-cultural encounter with the people and practices they describe produces the data in the first place. Hence a suicidologist cannot remain neutral, but must be aware of her own beliefs and values influencing the encounters themselves alongside the analysis of practices.

The contributors share knowledge acquired as clinical practitioners, psychologists or psychiatrists across the world. They are for the most part not religious or historical scholars or anthropologists; rather, they can be described as first-hand experts of the cultural connections and practices tied to the religious histories, myths, laws and belief systems described. Instead of performing shorter, or longer, periods of field work as anthropologists do, the authors have—as members of society and suicidologists equally—their everyday work and life, come into contact with the religious representations and notions that they bring to light. Years of experience and encounters with suicide attempters, hospital staff, family members, the public and the media is here connected to and coupled with religious themes. Who has better insight in the emotive and controversial subject of suicide, often surrounded by stigma, than the practitioners themselves? Personal encounters and clinical experience have led the authors to consider specific religious expressions instead of others, consequently providing this section with certain elasticity.

In Chapter 2, 'The role of religion in suicide prevention', H M van Praag directs attention to the scarcity of data on religion and suicide and associates this to early psychiatry's underestimation of such a linkage, ultimately grounded in its fixation with atheism. He writes that the secularisation of the Western world concerns religious institutions and not religiosity and spirituality as such. In suicidology, loss of religious affiliation is frequently referred to as a suicide risk. Ahmed and Tarek Okasha in 'Suicide and Islam' (Chapter 8) and Nils Retterstøl and Øivind Ekeberg in 'Christianity and suicide' (Chapter 9) concurrently point to the faith factor in suicide prevention, demonstrating this with lower suicide rates in more religiously active Muslim and Christian societies. The relationship is complicated, however, with varied rates among Orthodox countries as well as between Catholic and Protestant countries. Yet, it has been argued that supportive religious networks greatly benefit suicide prevention efforts (Pescolido and Georgianna 1989, Pescolido 1990). In Japan, Shintoism offers a sense of belonging, moral support and a reinforced sense of community nationwide. The contribution of such valuing of human life to suicide prevention is discussed in Chapter 6, 'The Shinto religion and suicide in Japan', by Yoshihiro Kaneko, Akiko Yamasaki and Kiminori Arai.

Nonetheless, identifying what factors may lead to an increase in suicide through the breakdown of religious affiliation in categories of attachments or detachments may prove to be a Sisyphean task. Lost, diminished or altered religious affiliation is for the most part inseparable from larger sociopolitical, economic and cultural contexts (Asad 2003). Norms and attitudes emanating from religious beliefs are intrinsically linked to cultural expressions and often to power-laden societal structures, and vice versa. Politics and religion are intertwined in a complex manner, and legal issues with regard to dying and death are often linked. Legal definitions of the right to die and the prohibition of suicide cannot be separated from questions of religion, especially in the case of state religion (Nowenstein and Hennette-Vauchez 2007). Retterstøl and Ekeberg mention the relevance of the late adaptation of legal responses in Ireland. Most European countries formally decriminalized suicide in the eighteenth and nineteenth centuries, however Ireland did not do so until 1993. In many countries across the world, suicide is considered a crime to this day. Moreover, despite official decriminalization, suicide remains an indignity across the world. Religion can be a source of fear and guilt, possibly leading to lower rates of suicide, but throughout history, religious institutions have, more or less worldwide, played a part in obfuscating statistics about suicide. Stigma and taboos surrounding suicide also have very real consequences on under-reporting and individuals suffering in silence.

However, the association between religion, public opinion and suicide goes well beyond the sphere of the law. Religions are systems of thoughts composed of ideas, attitudes, courses of action, beliefs and practices. Philosophies of dying and death are often the foundation stones of religions, and contemplation and grounds for justifying and condoning death take multiple forms (Lambek 2008). In the ensuing chapters, concepts of after life and reincarnation and their influence on the dying, theologies of death, death rituals, morally accepted suicides, the ambivalence surrounding suicide and more is discussed.

In Chapter 3, 'Cultural and religious traditions in China: the influence of Confucianism on suicide prevention', Wu Fei tells us that suicide does not have an independent moral significance in Confucianism. He describes suicide as an acceptable way to resist and protect one's dignity, although it is never considered the best way to do so. Such contradictions are mentioned by many of the contributors, and are in fact the reality of everyday expressions of religion. Israel Orbach and Aron Rabinowitz, in 'Suicide in the Jewish scriptures' (Chapter 7), draw on the prohibition of suicide in these texts while emphasizing the narrowness of the definition of suicide. Condemnation of self-destructive behaviour is coupled with a call for an empathic state of mind in understanding the reasons for a suicide.

Ahmed and Tarek Okasha discuss Islamic scholars and philosophers who have sought to demonstrate that in spite of the condemnation of suicide by Islam, when life becomes too burdensome, physically or mentally, suicide may be a legitimate option. Lakshmi Vijayakumar explores the individual's decision over, his/her life and how religious suicides are not condemned in 'Hindu religion and suicide in India' (Chapter 4). According to Somparn Promta and Prakarn Thomyangkoon suicide is in some cases morally acceptable for Buddhists, as described in Chapter 5, 'A Buddhist perspective on suicide'. Representations of death and dying are abundant in religious myths, and the cultural and historical contingency of the acceptance and intolerance of suicide as well as the methods of taking one's life surface in these chapters. Wu Fei discusses historical idolization of female suicides for the sake of chastity in China, and Vijayakumar describes traditional practices of self-immolation among women in India for reasons linked to chastity and dignity. According to Baquedano, hanging is a common suicide method in some parts of Mexico, closely linked to pre-Hispanic Mayan traditions.

In 'Suicide prevention and religious traditions on the African continent' (Chapter 10), Lourens Schlebusch, Stephanie Burrows and Naseema Vawda correlate the rise in suicide to social changes and long-term strife. They underscore the importance of political stability and social health care systems, the obstacles of lack of infrastructure, funds, scarcity of data and the need for cross-national research. These difficulties are by no means unique to the African continent—but exist worldwide. The above-mentioned authors, alongside Gaspar Baquedano, and Emilio Ovuga with Jed Boardman, in Chapter 11, 'The role of religion in suicide prevention work in Uganda', all locate the development of customs in an historically ambiguous context of conquest. So-called traditional religion is not separated from Christianity in Uganda or Mexico, attention should instead be directed to the ambivalence and contradictions found in customs and practices. In effect, religious ideas and the everyday activities and thoughts related to religion are not bounded and demarcated. Promta and Thomyangkoon underscore the importance of exceptions, identifying different Buddhist schools, interpretations and customs cross-nationally and also within Thailand.

The contributors each offer different takes on the study of religion and its influence on suicide ideation, completion and societal opinion. Inviting the reader to further contemplation of the multiple facets behind suicide, this part of the book is a thought-provoking forum for further debate. Reasons, motivations and causes for suicide are sought for on a number of interconnected levels. The diverse nature of the knowledge at hand renders it a useful tool in further understanding of the cultural religious expressions of suicide and more effective suicide prevention.

In the study of religious expressions and practices, one can find the means to formulate people's attitudes towards, and representations of, a phenomenon such as suicide. Suicide triggers profound feelings and expressions of human beings' existential and social conditions. To many, suicide violates the drive to live and consequently the act provokes much controversy. The role of hope, penitence and forgiveness are all imperative in the understanding of suicide. Cultural acceptance of suicide in specific contexts does not exclude pain and grief; it simply accentuates the importance of contextualizing such a response. Some of the authors touch on the important issue of bereavement and models of grief. The place that grief counselling and grief therapy take, as well as rites and sites of remembrance, are revealing. It is also vital to raise important questions about the broader institutional processes of management, administration, and knowledge production, such as processes of 'ruling' and power at play, to which social worlds and practices are unavoidably linked. In forthcoming studies it would be interesting to examine critically the role of religion in the development of attitudes and forms of social organization that coordinate local worlds and suicide preventive practices.

I will leave you with these final thoughts about the complexity of culture as expressed by Edward Said (1994). This statement may prove a valuable analogy when coupled with religion, religiosity and secularism.

> Far from being unitary or monolithic autonomous things, cultures actually assume more 'foreign' elements, alterities, differences, than they consciously exclude. Who in India or Algeria can confidently separate out the British or French component of the past from present actualities, and who in Britain or France can draw a clear circle around British London or French Paris that would exclude the impact of India and Algeria upon those two imperial cities?
>
> Said (1994, p. 15)

## References

Appadurai A (2001). *Globalization*. University Press, London.

Asad T (2003). *Formations of the Secular: Christianity, Islam, Modernity*. Stanford University Press, Stanford.

Cooper F (2005). *Colonialism in Question; Theory, Knowledge, History*. University of California Press, Berkeley.

Dirks N (1992). Introduction: colonialism and culture. In N Dirks and A Arbor, eds, *Colonialism and Culture*, pp. 1–26. The University of Michigan Press, Michigan.

Foucault M (1969). *L'archéologie du savoir* (English title: *Archaeology of Knowledge*). Gallimard, Paris.

Geertz C (1973). *The Interpretation of Culture*. New York, Basic Books.

Lambek M (ed.) (2008). *A Reader in the Anthropology of Religion*. Blackwell Anthologies in Social and Cultural Anthropology. Wiley-Blackwell, Oxford.

Nowenstein G and Hennette-Vauchez S (2007) The return of the living-dead? Law, medicine, and definitions of death in the 20th century. Paper presented at the annual meeting of The Law and Society Association, 25 July, Berlin.

Pescosolido BA (1990). The social context of religious integration and suicide: pursuing the network explanation. *Sociological Quarterly*, **31**, 337–357.

Pescosolido BA and Georgianna S (1989). Durkheim, suicide, and religion. *American Sociological Review*, **54**, 33–48.

Sahlins M (2000). Sentimental pessimism. In D Larraine, ed., *Biographies of Scientific Objects*, pp. 158–202. The University of Chicago Press, Chicago.

Said E (1994). *Culture and Imperialism*. Vintage, New York.

Spivak GC (2006). *In Other Worlds: Essays in Cultural Politics*. Routledge, New York.

# CHAPTER 2

# The role of religion in suicide prevention

Herman M van Praag

## Abstract

In psychiatry, man's connection with religion and religiosity is underestimated. In the wake of Freud's *The future of an illusion* (1975), a wave of atheism inundated psychiatry. Both phenomena were considered to be atavisms: remnants of the past; manifestations of a lack of independence; to be treated, rather than to be cherished. This development disregards the human urge to provide meaning to one's life through a spiritual dimension, as well as the inclination to search for values that exceed one's material needs. In this context, religion is central: contrary to Freud, Emile Durkheim states that religion is not only 'true', but also 'real' (Durkheim 2001). A believer is not stuck in an illusion: their exaltation at the belief of a moral power beyond themselves is quite real to them, these are forces external to the individual and part of society as a whole.

Studies show that if religiosity is experienced as a source of hope and confidence, it reduces the risk of depression in times of mounting stress, facilitates recovery and diminishes suicide risk. Religiosity experienced as a source of guilt and fear probably has the opposite effects. Social bonding and confidence in God are a modus operandi.

The psychiatrist cannot and should not ignore or reject religion, irrespective of personal beliefs. In the interest of the evolution of the practice and for the best of their patients, psychiatrists need to reorient towards matters of spirituality, religion and meaning. Taking into account the present state of the discipline, the data on religion and suicide are relatively scarce.

## Religion, the impasse of psychiatry

Substantial parts of the Western world are presently highly secularized. This is true as far as the formal aspects of religion are concerned, such as membership in a congregation, church visits, and rituals as they are practiced in churches and synagogues. However, this is a limited analysis, disregarding religion as a state of mind, as openness to an imagined world beyond the horizon, governed by a metaphysical agency, conceived as a metaphor for morality, compassion and righteousness. That component of the human experiential repertoire is very much alive, and will presumably never quench, as it meets an emotional need.

## Theoretical perspectives on religion and religiosity

Durkheim suggested that the scientific study of religion itself presupposed that the various religions we compare are all species of the same class, and thus, possess certain elements in common. I define *religion* as the ideology that has developed around the assumed existence of supernatural authority. An authority not sensorially perceptible, impervious to empirical studies, that yet exercises a fundamental influence on individuals and on the society in which they live. This authority often goes under the name of God. The God-figure is experienced either anthropomorphically as a person with human features, or rather as an abstraction, as an impersonal, elusive, inconceivable field of force—'an uncaused cause'. Out of awe for the Godhead, arose a ritualized system of worship.

Affinity with the religious root idea I call religiosity, or preferably *religious receptivity*. I prefer the latter term, because it expresses more pointedly that religious belief is not an all-or-nothing quality, but one that occurs in various degrees of intensity. The construct of religious receptivity includes three elements: first, receptiveness—emotionally and intellectually—for the concept of God and the transcendent reality it represents; secondly, the affinity with worship and rituals associated with the concept of God; and finally, the acceptance, at least in the broad sense of the concept of man and the world view the religion in question champions.

What follows is the theoretical underpinnings of my line of reasoning. Religiosity is considered a normal constituent of the human behavioural repertoire, and as Durkheim has stated: 'it is far from being true that the notion of the religious coincides with that of the extraordinary or the unforeseen'. The concept of God—the very centre of religious life—is not an ingenious mental construct to come to terms with the many things in this world we do not understand, but a powerful metaphor for absolute morality and sublime, unlimited creativity.

Based on the following grounds, I qualify religious receptivity as a normal phenomenon, normal experientially, but also normal intellectually, as a conceptualization of the need to elevate from meaninglessness and the purely accidental.

## Frequency and utility of religion

In the studies below, religiosity in its different forms is expressed at a high frequency in various industrialized nations. In a Gallup poll carried out in 2000, 8 out of 10 Americans assented to the statement that 'the Bible still speaks to us today, and could even solve most or all of life's problems' (Podhoretz 2002); 71 per cent expressed that they had never doubted the existence of God, while 67 per cent believed in the after life and the reality of heaven (Shremer 2000). The UK National Opinion Poll Survey (1985) found that 72 per cent of a random sample had maintained belief in God. A recent study carried out in the Netherlands—regarded as one of the most secularized countries in the world—concluded that approximately 50 per cent of a random sample from the population reported that religious belief played an important role in their lives (Neeleman personal communication). A North American survey, carried out among natural scientists (biologists, physicists, mathematicians) found that 40 per cent expressed belief in a personal God (Larson and Witham 1997). According to a *Newsweek* poll, 78 per cent of Americans believe that Jesus rose from death (Meacham 2005). Religious paraphernalia had lost much of its former significance, yet many maintained belief in a divine power. When a particular phenomenon occurs in a majority of people it is unlikely to be a psychic anomaly.

One should not forget the utilitarian side of religiosity. It may provide one with a *sense of meaning*. The quest for meaningful goals is central to humankind. A desire to live a life that matters—and for spiritual values that surpass the satisfaction of physical needs—is to be found. Those two concerns are interconnected: meaningful goals are usually found on a spiritual level, i.e. in intangible assets, such as care for others, social involvement, creative activity, or less lofty but no less noble, in the desire to just do a good job—in one's family, in the community, in the workplace, in club-life—or in the urge to improve oneself intellectually, emotionally and culturally. Preoccupation with values of this kind can be experienced as immanent, as originating in one's inner self, or as transcendent, as prompted, inspired, or even dictated by an agency superior to the human species, eventually determining its weal and woe. Here, one touches on religion, and at a postulated, supernatural authority named God. God has expectations, and makes demands. Fulfilling these is for the believer both a commission and a source of satisfaction: for them, God is the sublime and ultimate source of meaning.

Religiosity may also satisfy the need of *emotional response*. Intense emotions—for instance sorrow, guilt, shame, joy, confrontation with death, thankfulness, qualms with life—invoke the need of another; someone who cares to respond. If such a soundboard is lacking, or if the other is unable to respond, an intense feeling of dissatisfaction or solitude may set in. One tends to seek refuge 'higher up', to turn to a metaphysical, compassionate resource: God. However, it should not be forgotten that in non-secularized environments, one does not choose to 'enter a religion'. In these environments, it exists in every sphere of life, although at times and in certain circumstances, it may be more relevant. In order to further explain this, two examples will be discussed.

## Sorrow

One loses part of what one considers to be the *raison d'être* of one's existence—partner or child, job, prestige, power, wealth—and feels in need of support, consolation, of someone who can somehow relativize the trauma, without minimalizing it. One does not find a human comforter and seeks contact with a super-human authority with God as a consoler. The opposite reaction too may, despite its appearance, actually draw God closer. God becomes a scapegoat. Why did He do this to me? Why did He, ostensibly almighty, not prevent this tragedy?

## Confrontation with death

The unexpected tiding that death is approaching is shattering. Seldom is all hope abandoned. The hope that a medical intervention exists that may turn one's condition for the better: 'God grant that something can be done.' This is a universal supplication: death is a faithful servant to God.

Furthermore, religiosity may meet someone's *dependency needs*. The relationship of a religious person to God is one of dependency. Relationships based on dependency, I consider, to be manifestations of maturity, at least if it concerns mutual dependency. The one helps out when the other is in need and vice versa. The unwillingness or inability to establish such alliances render a person lonely, unfulfilled. Is the relationship of man to God one of mutual dependency? It can be conceived as such. For a religious person, in Judeo-Christian religions, God is both guide and protector. God presents both the archetypical father—and the archetypical mother—figure. The concept of God, on the other hand, is carried by humans. 'The human soul is God's lamp' states one of the Proverbs (20:27). If it were not for human beings, God would not exist; or without man, there would be no one to be aware of Him; no one to testify to His presence. The relationship of man to God is thus one of reciprocal dependency. Owing to this, I qualify this bond as a normal one.

Finally, religiosity offers a mode of expression for one's *amazement*: in essence, amazement about the fact that there is life at all, and not a void. It is in this context that God is introduced as the symbol of ultimate creativity.

## Depression

Depression is a common disorder, and the largest single cause of non-fatal disease burden (Murray and Lopez 1996). Its frequency however is uncertain. The reported data are highly variable. Waraich *et al.* (2004) reported a lifetime risk of ever having a major depression of 6.7%, whereas Kruijshaar *et al.* (2005) estimated that risk to be 40 per cent in women and 30 per cent in men. Lifetime risk for major depression also varies from country to country, being for instance 3 per cent in Japan and 16.9 per cent in the USA (Andrade *et al.* 2003). A major reason for that disparity is, I believe, the fact that the border between distress (worrying) and depression is not clearly marked. Hence, the reported frequency of depression will vary with the number of worriers inadvertently included in the study. Furthermore, cultural factors may play a role in these results, i.e. what is the cultural acceptance of dejection and of depression? (Wasserman 2006).

Depression is a treatable disorder. Results concerning the efficacy of antidepressants state that they are fairly, but not highly effective (Khan *et al.* 2002), and according to others, hardly even efficient at all (Moncrieff and Kirsch 2005). The modest effect size is possibly due to the inaccuracy of our diagnostic system. The categories of major depression and dysthymia are repositories of many syndromes. Possible syndromal specificity of a certain antidepressant will thus be masked.

## Religion and depression

Depression is a major suicide precursor, therefore the first question to be answered in the given context is: are religion and depression interconnected? And if that is the case, how? While there probably is a connection, there is uncertainty surrounding it, which is based on three considerations:

1　The number of relevant studies is small;

2　It is still difficult to dissect the complex construct of religiosity into components relevant to the posited question; and

3　To measure them adequately.

Having said that, the available data indicate that religiosity may indeed reduce the risk of depressive symptoms and depression in stressful circumstances, and improve the therapeutic yield of antidepressive interventions.

Kendler and colleagues (1997, 1999) interviewed 1902 twin pairs, including questions reflecting a range of religious behaviours and beliefs. The number of stressful life events in the two months prior to the interview was measured, as well as current psychiatric symptoms. They found first that low levels of depressive symptoms were related to high levels of personal devotion. The latter construct is a measure of personalized and internalized religiosity. The number of stressful life events was positively associated with the number of depressive symptoms. High levels of personal devotion were associated with less of a response to the depressogenic effects of stressful life events. In other words, religious beliefs may serve as a stress-buffering state of mind.

In another sample, extracted from the general population, similar observations were made. In a group of 4000 individuals, aged 65 and over, a negative relationship was established between church attendance and the prevalence of depressive symptoms (Koenig *et al.* 1997). Several other authors have arrived at similar conclusions (e.g. Williams *et al.* 1991).

Levin (2002) studied mood state in primary care patients in association with 'religious love'. The latter construct was introduced by Sorokin (1954) and defined as a two-way loving relationship with God; giving love to God or the Absolute and receiving it in return. It was assessed with a unidimensional scale comprising eight items. Examples are: 'God's love never fails' and 'when I experience God's love, I feel perfect contentment'. Each item was scored on a 5-point scale. Mood was measured with the General Well-being Scale. A strong inverse relationship was found between depressive affect and 'religious love'.

Grief after the death of an important other may lead to a state of mind almost indistinguishable from pathological depression. Walsh *et al.* (2002) demonstrated that grief resolves more rapidly in those with strong spiritual beliefs than in dis-believers and religious sceptics. The Royal Free Interview for Religious and Spiritual Beliefs (King *et al.* 1995) was used to assess the nature and strength of spiritual beliefs and practices.

In depression, too, religiosity has been shown to provide a degree of protection against the occurrence of depression and to further remission, in particular in elderly patients with few social contacts and little self-confidence (Braam *et al.* 1997b; Koenig 1997; Braam *et al.* 1998; Koenig *et al.* 1998; Koenig 1999; Braam *et al.* 2000, Koenig 2001). Religiosity was measured on two levels: extrinsically, registering frequency of church visits and regularity of praying, and intrinsically, trying to gauge the genuineness of religious feelings

and the importance they have in someone's life relative to other concerns, such as earning a good income, building a satisfactory family life, enjoying good health and having risen to a high post. It appeared to be the plenitude of inner religious life rather than the more formal aspects of religiosity that correlated negatively with the risk of depression and its prognosis.

Koenig *et al.* (1998), for instance, studied patients 60 years or over admitted to medical inpatient's services. They were screened for depressive symptoms. Those meeting criteria for case depression (N = 111), were treated accordingly, and followed up after discharge. It appeared that greater religiosity independently predicted shorter time to remission. In accordance with these findings, Miller *et al.* (1997) reported that intrinsic religiosity protected against recurrence among severely depressed patients, younger than those in the study of Koenig *et al.* (1998), and not from the Bible Belt, but predominantly from working class areas in New Haven, Connecticut. They concluded that these data suggest 'that religiosity may be broadly protective in the course of depression, buffering against the full life course of negative events in patients with varying depression histories' (Miller *et al.* 1997).

In a community survey of elderly people in The Netherlands, Braam *et al.* (1997a) found that religiosity—defined as salience of religion, relative to the salience of other aspects of life—showed a relatively strong association with improvement of depression in the year after the first assessment. This association was most prominent in subjects with poor physical health. This latter observation was not confirmed in a later study (Braam 2002).

In a large epidemiological European depression study (EURODEP) (Copeland 1999), the association between religion and depression in elderly people living in several European countries was studied. The main religious variable studied was not salience of religion or intrinsic religiosity, but regularity of church attendance. Religious practice appeared to be associated with less depression, both on the individual and the national level (Braam *et al.* 2001).

In conclusion, the available evidence indicates that several indices of religiosity exert stress-buffering effects, diminishing risk of depression and further remission.

## Religiosity as a stress- and depression-buffering structure

Religiosity may exert a stress-buffering, anti-depressogenic effect. Religious life generally revolves around a community of like-minded people who mutually care and will provide support in times of spiritual hardship. Religion, moreover, if internalized and practised in freedom and not out of fear, fosters hope, repose and patience. It acts as a counterpoise to loneliness, despair and feelings of superfluity, states of mind that are known to undermine the ability to withstand adversity.

Negative, i.e. stress-producing life events, are much more frequent prior to depression than in the general population, but do they have causal significance? Proof for a causal relationship would require the demonstration that stress can cause brain alteration, which supposedly plays a role in the pathogenesis of (certain types of) depression. Several data sets suggest that this might indeed be the case (van Praag *et al.* 2004). In certain types of depression, the serotonin 5-hydroxytryptamine (5-HT) system in the brain is disturbed. Its synthesis is reduced and certain 5-HT receptors are hypoactive due to decreased sensitivity or to decreased production. This is particularly true for the 5-HTIA and the 5-HTID receptor. In addition, the corticotropin-releasing hormone (CRH)/adreno-corticotropic hormone (ACTH)/cortisol system is disinhibited. This leads to overactivity in CRH-mediated neuronal systems in the brain. Excess cortisol in the brain contributes to reduction in the synthesis of 5-HT and 5-HTIA receptors. Lowering of 5-HT activity in the brain, particularly in the 5-HTIA receptor-mediated systems, and increased brain activity of CRH are associated with increase of anxiety and aggression. These behavioural disruptions may eventually lead to disturbances in mood regulation, resulting in depression.

Sustained stress leads to neurobiological changes similar to those found in (certain types of) depression: reduced production of 5-HT, of 5-HTIA receptors and CRH/ACTH/ cortisol overdrive.

It seems likely, therefore, that in certain forms of depression, stress is indeed of causal significance (Van Praag *et al.* 2004). If so, goal-directed treatment of such types of depressions would imply increasing 5-HT, and in particular 5-HTIA receptor-mediated activity, inhibiting the CRH/cortisol system, in combination with psychological interventions aimed at stress reduction and increase of coping skills. In that latter context, religiosity may play a therapeutic and preventative role.

## Suicide and religion

Depression is considered to be one of the major suicide precursors. Suicidal behaviour occurs in approximately 75 per cent of patients ever having suffered from depression (Neeleman *et al.* 2004). Depression, however, hold no monopoly position over suicidal behaviour: it is nosologically non-specific. It also occurs in relation to other diagnoses, such as various personality disorders, schizophrenia, substance abuse and alcoholism (Hawton *et al.* 2002). Comorbidity of personality disorders with major depression increases the suicide risk (Soloff *et al.* 2000; Hansen *et al.* 2003; Dumais *et al.* 2005). Finally, in many somatic illnesses, the suicide rate is also increased, mostly in conjunction with depressive symptoms (Cooper-Patrick *et al.* 1994).

Taking into account the beneficial effects of religiosity on stress and depression vulnerability, one might expect religiosity to reduce suicide risk. Several studies show that this is indeed the case. Rates of completed suicide have been shown to be lower in countries considered to be more religious than in secular ones (Breault 1986; Neeleman *et al.* 1997; Neeleman and Lewis 1999). The negative association between religion and suicidal behaviour was also found on the individual level. In a study carried out in 19 Western countries comprising 28,085 individuals, the following variables were studied in face-to-face interviews (Neeleman *et al.* 1997; Neeleman and Lewis 1999): tolerance of suicide—'Do you think suicide can be justified?'—and personal religious beliefs, items such as 'Do you believe in God?' 'How important is God in your life?' 'How religious do you consider yourself?'. Stronger religious beliefs were associated with lower tolerance of suicide. Aggregate levels of suicide tolerance and suicide rates correlated positively, aggregate levels of religiousness and suicide risk correlated negatively.

Hasselback *et al.* (1991) and Stack (2001) reported that in 261 Canadian census divisions, a 10 per cent change in the proportion of the population with no religious affiliation—an index of low religious commitment—was associated with a 3.2 per cent

increase in suicide rate. It has furthermore been suggested that the alarming rise of suicide rate in Ireland in the last part of the twentieth century might be related to the decline in religious practices (Malone *et al.* 2000). Studying suicide rates in 71 countries, a negative association was found between suicide rates and a nation's percentage of Muslims, who traditionally have low suicide rates (Simpson and Conklin 1989). Finally, it has been demonstrated that both religious affiliation and the depth and authenticity of religious beliefs (intrinsic religiosity) are correlated with lower levels of aggressivity and hostility (Storch and Storch 2002).

Durkheim (1951) has argued that it is particularly because of social cohesion and social support of congregants that religion protects against suicide. Several authors found a negative association between religious integration and suicide rate (e.g. Breault and Barkley 1982). A study of Neeleman *et al.* (1997), however, demonstrated that suicide rates are more strongly related to religiousness and suicide tolerance than to church attendance and membership. In a later study, Neeleman and Lewis (1999) reported that the negative association of male suicide rates with religiosity was particularly apparent in the least religious countries. Associations between religiosity and female suicide rates did not vary across countries. A possible explanation could be that religiousness is generally stronger in females than in males and less culture-dependent. Comparable data were obtained in the Netherlands, which as we have noted is considered to be among the most secularised countries in the world (Neeleman 1998). Religious beliefs and religious affiliation turned out to be predictors of lower suicide acceptance in individuals, and of lower rates of completed suicide in the provinces.

Non-lethal suicidal behaviour, too, is inversely linked to various religious variables. In a community-based twin study in Australia, in which the participants were interviewed by telephone, it was shown that the prevalence of serious suicide attempts varied as a function of religious affiliation (Statham *et al.* 1998). Individuals reporting religious affiliation were less likely to report a serious suicide attempt. An inverse relationship has also been reported between religious belief and suicidal gestures (Nelson 1977), and suicidal ideation (Stack and Lester 1991).

Dervic *et al.* (2004) studied lifetime suicide attempts in depressed inpatients, comparing those reporting to belong to one specific religion with those describing themselves as having no religious affiliation. Religiously affiliated subjects were less likely to have a history of suicide attempts, and showed greater moral objections to suicide. Moral attitude towards suicide was measured with the Reasons for Living Inventory (Linehan and Nielsen 1983), an instrument including such items as 'I believe only God has the right to end a life' and 'my religious beliefs forbid it'. It was hypothesized that moral objections to suicide mediate the protective effect of religious affiliation against suicidal behaviour. Moreover, individuals with a religious affiliation reported less suicidal ideation at the time of evaluation, despite comparable severity of depression. The authors conclude that religion may provide a force counteracting suicidal ideation in the face of depression, hopelessness and stressful life events. No association was established between a specific religion and suicidal behaviour. They are of the opinion that social factors can explain religiousness' protective power. Religiously affiliated subjects reported a more family oriented social network, reflected in more time spent with first-degree relatives. Most unaffiliated subjects reported more non-familial relationships.

Stronger feelings of responsibility towards family members were inversely related to acting on suicidal thoughts. It is worth noting that most religions emphasize the importance of family bonds, and keeping families together.

In conclusion, the available evidence suggests that religiosity may suppress suicidal ideation as well as the acting out of it. Both social factors (the mutual care of congregational members), ethical considerations (man is generally not allowed to take his life in its own hand) and fear (for God's wrath) are involved in the protective effects of religiosity.

## Conclusive remarks

### God as consoler

Religious commitment—religiosity, and to a somewhat lesser extent religious affiliation—is associated with less suicidal behaviour. A variety of factors may explain this relationship. Active membership of a religious congregation may provide one with a support group ready to help, to assist, to console, to encourage if a fellow member worries or is in trouble. Social bonds are important to overcome misery and feelings of hopelessness. Religious congregations can serve as a kind of extended family. One belongs, feels accepted, appreciated, safe in the midst of like-minded people. If issues of a moral or ethical nature arise, a good pastor will serve as an advisor. A well-functioning congregation is a safe haven to its members. In addition, religion in its own right may offer relief and hope in times of stress. For the believer, God is the supreme consoler. As Job says (40:4):

> Behold, I am of small amount; what shall I answer Thee?
> I lay my hand upon my mouth.

In addition, fear may act as a barrier to suicidal behaviour. Judaism considers life as a personal gift of God: 'and surely your blood of your lives will I require'(Gen 9:5), an injunction which Rabbis took literally, and based on it the prohibition of suicide. Christianity adopted the same attitude based on the sixth commandment: 'Thou shall not kill' (Koch 2005). The same holds for Islam. Suicide is condemned. 'Don't cast yourself into perdition'. It is God who gave life and He alone is entitled to take it (Murthy 2000). The faithful are fearful of God's wrath and possible retribution in the here and now or in the after life.

The protective effects of religiosity on suicide attest that this spiritual commodity is still meaningful to many. The dechristianization of the Western world seems to concern the Church as an institution, much less religiosity as such.

### God as a tyrant

It seems conceivable that religiosity might influence mental health in the reverse direction: undermining rather than improving coping abilities. God may be experienced as a threatening, punishing authority. Religion might act as a straitjacket, thwarting spiritual growth, inducing guilt, fear, insecurity and leading to emotionally 'empty' preoccupation with religious precepts. Instead of lightening and illuminating life, religion becomes a burden, a source of worry. Religious beliefs may shrink to remorseful waiting until death arrives. Such spiritual climates could be considered as stress provoking and pre-depressive. This assumption is beared out by available data. In a meta-analysis of 147 studies (N = 98,975), Smith *et al.* (2003) confirmed that greater religiousness was mildly associated with fewer depressive symptoms. The effect was small but robust, and restricted to those for whom religiosity was associated with positive emotions, who experienced God as a benevolent deity. When the reverse was the case, religiosity was associated with higher levels of depressive symptoms: if it is experienced and practised in a sphere of fear and guilt, religiosity can be expected to generate suicidal ideas and to facilitate suicidal behaviour. Those ideas, however, may be counteracted by deep-rooted fears for God's assumed anger. The outcome of these two opposing forces is not known. Systematic studies on the influence of hyperorthodoxy on suicide rates are lacking.

### Consequences

As has been stated in this chapter, religion and suicide are interconnected. Consequently, religiosity should be taken into account in the examination of suicidal patients and in the design of preventative programmes. Expanding collaborations between clinicians and psychiatrists and members and representatives of religious communities will help and hasten this process. The fields of expertise need to be shared, and training programmes across the spheres are needed (van Praag 2007). The bonds between religion and psychiatry need to be tightened. Neglecting the interrelatedness of the two is detrimental to both realms, but most of all to the patients concerned.

### References

Andrade L, Caraveo-Anduaga JJ, Berglund P *et al.* (2003). The epidemiology of major depressive episodes: results from the International Consortium of Psychiatric Epidemiology (ICPE) Surveys. *International Journal of Methods of Psychiatric Research*, **12**, 3–21.

Braam AW (2002). *Religion and Depression in Later Life: An Empirical Study*. Amsterdam, Rozenberg Publishers.

Braam AW, Beekman AT, Deeg DJ *et al.* (1997a). Religiosity as a protective or prognostic factor of depression in later life; results from a community survey in The Netherlands. *Acta Psychiatrica Scandinavica*, **96**, 199–205.

Braam AW, Beekman AT, Knipscheer CP *et al.* (1998). Religious denomination and depression in older Dutch citizens: patterns and models. *Journal of Aging and Health*, **10**, 483–503.

Braam AW, Beekman AT, van Tilburg TG *et al.* (1997b). Religious involvement and depression in older Dutch citizens. *Social Psychiatry and Psychiatric Epidemiology*, **32**, 284–291.

Braam AW, Sonnenberg CM, Beekman AT *et al.* (2000). Religious denomination as a symptom-formation factor of depression in older Dutch citizens. *International Journal of Geriatric Psychiatry*, **15**, 458–466.

Braam AW, Van den Eeden P, Prince MJ *et al.* (2001). Religion as a cross-cultural determinant of depression in elderly Europeans: results from the EURODEP collaboration. *Psychological Medicine*, **31**, 803–814.

Breault KD (1986). Suicide in America: a test of Durkheim's theory of religious and family integration, 1933–1980. *American Journal of Sociology*, **92**, 628–656.

Breault KD and Barkley K (1982). A comparative analysis of Durkheim's theory of religious family integration. *Sociology Quarterly*, **23**, 321–331.

Cooper-Patrick L, Crum RM, Ford DE (1994). Identifying suicidal ideation in general medical patients. *JAMA*, **272**, 1757–1762.

Copeland JR (1999). Depression of older age. Origins of the study. *British Journal of Psychiatry*, **174**, 304–306.

Dervic K, Oquendo MA, Grunebaum MF *et al.* (2004). Religious affiliation and suicide attempt. *American Journal of Psychiatry*, **161**, 2303–2308.

Dumais A, Lesage AD, Alda M *et al.* (2005). Risk factors for suicide completion in major depression: a case-control study of impulsive and aggressive behaviours in men. *American Journal of Psychiatry*, **162**, 2116–2124.

Durkheim É (1951). *Suicide.* New York, Free Press.

Durkheim É (2001). *The Elementary forms of Religious Life.* Oxford, Oxford University Press.

Freud S (1975). *The Future of an Illusion.* New York, Norton.

Hansen PE, Wang AG, Stage KB *et al.* (2003). Comorbid personality disorder predicts suicide after major depression: a 10-year follow-up. *Acta Psychiatrica Scandanavica*, **107**, 436–440.

Hasselback P, Lee KI, Mao Y *et al.* (1991). The relationship of suicide rates to sociodemographic factors in Canadian census divisions. *Canadian Journal of Psychiatry*, **36**, 655–659.

Hawton K, Haw C, Houston K *et al.* (2002). Family history of suicidal behaviour: prevalence and significance in deliberate self-harm patients. *Acta Psychiatrica Scandanavica*, **106**, 387–393.

Kendler KS, Gardner CO, Prescott CA (1997). Religion, psychopathology, and substance use and abuse; a multimeasure, genetic-epidemiologic study. *American Journal of Psychiatry*, **154**, 322–329.

Kendler KS, Gardner CO, Prescott CA (1999). Clarifying the relationship between religiosity and psychiatric illness: the impact of covariates and the specificity of buffering effects. *Twin Research*, **2**, 137–144.

Khan A, Leventhal RM, Khan SR *et al.* (2002). Severity of depression and response to antidepressants and placebo: an analysis of the Food and Drug Administration database. *Journal of Clinical Psychopharmacology*, **22**, 40–45.

King M, Speck P, Thomas A (1995). The Royal Free interview for religious and spiritual beliefs: development and standardization. *Psychological Medicine*, **25**, 1125–1134.

Koch HJ (2005). Suicides and suicide ideation in the Bible: an empirical survey. *Acta Psychiatrica Scandanavica*, **112**, 167–172.

Koenig HG (1997). *Is Religion Good for Your Health?* Binghampton, Haworth Pastoral Press.

Koenig HG (1999). How does religious faith contribute to recovery from depression? *Harvard Mental Health Letter*, **15**, 8.

Koenig HG (2001). *Handbook of Religion and Health: A Century of Research Reviewed.* New York, Oxford University Press.

Koenig HG, George LK, Peterson BL (1998). Religiosity and remission of depression in medically ill older patients. *American Journal of Psychiatry*, **155**, 536–542.

Koenig HG, Hays JC, George LK *et al.* (1997). Modeling the cross-sectional relationships between religion, physical health, social support, and depressive symptoms. *American Journal of Geriatric Psychiatry*, **5**, 131–144.

Kruijshaar ME, Barendregt J, Vos T *et al.* (2005). Lifetime prevalence estimates of major depression: an indirect estimation method and a quantification of recall bias. *European Journal of Epidemiology*, **20**, 103–111.

Larson E and Witham L (1997). Scientists are still keeping face. *Nature*, **386**, 435–436.

Levin J (2002). Is depressed affect a function of one's relationship with God? Findings from a study of primary care patients. *International Journal of Psychiatry Medicine*, **32**, 379–393.

Linehan MM and Nielsen SL (1983). Social desirability: its relevance to the measurement of hopelessness and suicidal behaviour. *Journal of Consulting and Clinical Psychology*, **51**, 141–143.

Malone KM, Oquendo MA, Haas GL *et al.* (2000). Protective factors against suicidal acts in major depression: reasons for living. *American Journal of Psychiatry*, **157**, 1084–1088.

Meacham J (2005). From Jesus to Christ. *Newsweek*, 23 March.

Miller L, Warner V, Wickramaratne P *et al.* (1997). Religiosity and depression: ten-year follow-up of depressed mothers and offspring. *Journal of the American Academy of Child and Adolescent Psychiatry*, **36**, 1416–1425.

Moncrieff J and Kirsch I (2005). Efficacy of antidepressants in adults. *BMJ*, **331**, 155–157.

Murray CJ and Lopez AD (1996). *The Global Burden of Disease.* Geneva, World Health Organization.

Murthy RS (2000). Approaches to suicide prevention in Asia and the Far East. In K Hawton and K van Heeringen, eds, *The International Handbook of Suicide and Attempted Suicide*, pp. 631–643. Chichester, John Wiley.

National Opinion Poll (1985). *National Opinion Poll UK Survey.* London, HMSO.

Neeleman J (1998). Regional suicide rates in the Netherlands: does religion still play a role? *International Journal of Epidemiology*, **27**, 466–472.

Neeleman J, de Graaf R, Vollebergh W (2004). The suicidal process; prospective comparison between early and later stages. *Journal of Affective Disorders*, **82**, 43–52.

Neeleman J, Halpern D, Leon D *et al.* (1997). Tolerance of suicide, religion and suicide rates: an ecological and individual study in 19 Western countries. *Psychological Medicine*, **27**, 1165–1171.

Neeleman J and Lewis G (1999). Suicide, religion, and socioeconomic conditions. An ecological study in 26 countries, 1990. *Journal of Epidemiology and Community Health*, **53**, 204–210.

Nelson FL (1977). Religiosity and self-destructive crises in the institutionalized elderly. *Suicide and Life-Threatening Behaviour*, **7**, 67–74.

Podhoretz N (2002). *The Prophets.* New York, The Free Press.

Shremer M (2000). *How we Believe. The Search for God in an Age of Science.* New York, Freeman.

Simpson ME and Conklin GH (1989). Socio-economic development, suicide and religion: a test of Durkheim's theory of religion and suicide *Social Forces*, **67**, 945–964.

Smith TB, McCullough ME, Poll J (2003). Religiousness and depression: evidence for a main effect and the moderating influence of stressful life events. *Psychological Bulletin*, **129**, 614–636.

Soloff H, Lynch KG, Keller T *et al.* (2000). Characteristics of suicide attempter of patients with major depressive episode and borderline personality disorder: a comparative study. *American Journla of Psychiatry*, **157**, 601–608.

Sorokin PA (1954). *The Ways and Power of Love: Types, Factor and Techniques of Moral Transformation.* Boston, The Beacon Press.

Stack S (2001). Sociological research into suicide. In D Lester, ed., *Suicide Prevention. Resources for the Millenium*, pp. 17–30. Philadelphia, Brunner and Routledge.

Stack S and Lester D (1991). The effect of religion on suicide ideation. *Social Psychiatry and Psychiatric Epidemiology*, **26**, 168–170.

Statham DJ, Heath AC, Madden PA *et al.* (1998). Suicidal behaviour: an epidemiological and genetic study. *Psychological Medicine*, **28**, 839–855.

Storch EA and Storch JB (2002). Intrinsic religiosity and aggression in a sample of intercollegiate athletes. *Psychological Reports*, **91**, 1041–1042.

Walsh K, King M, Jones L *et al.* (2002). Spiritual beliefs may affect outcome of bereavement: prospective study. *BMJ*, **324**, 1551.

van Praag H, de Kloet R, van Os J (2004). *Stress, the Brain and Depression.* Cambridge, Cambridge University Press.

van Praag HM (2007). Psychiatry and religion. An unconsummated marriage. In G Glas, HM Spero, P Verhagen *et al.*, eds, *Hearing Visions and Seeing Voices, Psychological Aspects of Biblical Concepts and Personalities*, pp. 9–19. New York, Kluwer Academic Publishers.

Waraich P, Goldner EM, Somers JM *et al.* (2004). Prevalence and incidence studies of mood disorders: a systematic review of the literature. *Canadian Journal of Psychiatry*, **49**, 124–138.

Wasserman D (2006). *Depression: The Facts.* Oxford, Oxford University Press.

Williams DR, Larson DB, Buckler RE *et al.* (1991). Religion and psychological distress in a community sample. *Social Science and Medicine*, **32**, 1257–1262.

# CHAPTER 3

# Cultural and religious traditions in China

## The influence of Confucianism on suicide prevention

Wu Fei

## Abstract

In this chapter, we examine ideas about suicide in Confucianism and Taoism in China. In Confucianism, suicide is thought of as an acceptable way to protect one's dignity and virtue: in late imperial China, suicide was required for intellectuals who had survived their emperor and for women who had been raped. Nevertheless, most Confucian intellectuals do not consider suicide the best way to pursue human virtue. Although Qu Yuan—the great poet and the person responsible for the most famous suicide in Chinese history—is often praised for his loyalty and virtues, he is also criticised for being narrow-minded. According to the Taoist teachings of Zhuangzi, one should not be too concerned about worldly affairs, including life and death. Although the two cultural religious traditions are apparently different, there are similarities in their ideas about a good life and suicide. Examining ideas on life and death found in Confucianism and Taoism will provide a deeper cultural understanding of possible underlying motives for committing suicide. This knowledge can contribute to more effective suicide prevention.

## Confucius on suicide

Unlike Western culture, suicide does not have an independent moral significance in the classic culture in China, but is usually discussed along with other important issues. Seen as a spirited resistance against something bad, and a passionate protection of one's honor or integrity (Wu Fei 2005a, b), suicide is viewed positively when it is committed for a good purpose, and negatively when committed for a bad purpose.

People sometimes cite the famous maxim of filial piety to illustrate the Confucian attitude toward suicide: 'our bodies—from a single hair to a bit of skin—are derived from our parents, we must not in the least injure or wound them'. This saying is the first principle of filial piety (Zeng Shen 1993). Although this is a well-known idea in Confucianism, it is most likely not directly related to the issue of suicide. When Confucius says this to Zeng Zi (one of his famous students), he is explaining the principles of filial piety; but

Confucius and his disciples seldom advance this idea to prevent one from committing suicide. We cannot relate this idea to suicide simply because it shows some similarity to the Platonic idea that one cannot commit suicide because one's life belongs to the gods (Plato 1975, 62a 1–7).

Confucius expressed further philosophical ideas when involved in two famous debates about suicide. The first one concerns Shuqi and Boyi, who committed suicide in the beginning of the Zhou dynasty. The second is about Guan Zhong, who refused to commit suicide when his master was killed.

Boyi and Shuqi were two brothers who saw the transition from the Shang dynasty (c.1766–c.1100 BC) to the Zhou dynasty (c.1100–256 BC). Although they realized that the king of the Shang dynasty was an extraordinary tyrant, they insisted on being faithful to him and attempted to prevent the Zhou army from overthrowing the king. When the revolution finally succeeded and the Zhou dynasty was established, Boyi and Shuqi still identified themselves as subjects of the Shang dynasty and refused to possess anything awarded by the king of the Zhou Court. Since it was presumed that all the grain belonged to the king, they refused to eat and starved themselves to death (Sima Qian 2005, Chapter 61). Both were widely admired as models of virtuous men in ancient China. As to whether they should have committed suicide for such a bad king, there is much debate. Confucius agrees that Boyi and Shuqi were virtuous people because they neither debased (gave up) their ideas or brought shame to themselves. Yet, after praising them he said: 'However, I am different from them. I have neither favourable nor unfavourable situations' (Confucius 1997, Chapter 18.8). By this he meant: 'I would not have stubbornly insisted on doing something or not doing something.' Although Boyi and Shuqi are seen as virtuous people, Confucius does not think suicide is their best choice.

We can see Confucius's attitude about suicide more clearly in Guan Zhong's case. When Duke Xiang of Qi (a state of the Zhou dynasty, occupying half of today's Shandong province) was dead, Prince Xiaobai and Prince Jiu were both entitled to be the next duke. Although Guan Zhong, who belonged to Prince Jiu's fraction, almost killed Prince Xiaobai, when Jiu finally failed and was killed, Xiaobai became Duke Huan of Qi. A loyal official is supposed to commit suicide, but Guan Zhong did not do so and swore allegiance to the new duke. With the help of Guan Zhong, Duke Huan became the most powerful duke in China and defeated foreign invasions several times. Guan Zhong became a famous statesman, but he was always criticised for not being loyal to Prince Jiu, his former master (Zuo Qiuming 2000, p. 84; Sima Qian 2005, Chapters 32 and 62). Although Confucius sometimes criticises Guan Zhong for other issues, he does not think Guan Zhong should be condemned for not having committed suicide. One of his disciples asks him whether Guan Zhong is not humane for not committing suicide, and Confucius responds:

> Duke Huan nine times assembled the various princes without using war chariots. It was all due to Guan Zhong's capability. Who can compare with him in humanity? Who can compare with him in humanity!

Confucius (1997, Chapter 14.16)

He answers the same question to another student:

> Guan Zhong helped Duke Huan become overlord of the various princes and set everything right in the empire. The people to this day benefit from his favours. But for Guan Zhong, we would be wearing our hair loose with our garments fastened on the left. How could we expect him to be obstinately truthful like a common man or a common woman and hang himself in a gully without anyone knowing about it?

Confucius (1997, Chapter 14.17)

Comparing Confucius's attitudes toward Boyi, Shuqi, and Guan Zhong, we can form an idea of his views on suicide. For him, it is an acceptable choice to protect one's virtue and integrity, but it is never the best choice. In order to obtain the highest spiritual perfection, i.e., humaneness, one should be not only virtuous, loyal, and righteous, but also wise and prudent. Although Guan Zhong did not protect his personal virtue by committing suicide, he was still regarded as a cultivated human being because he contributed to the benefit of human happiness on a larger scale.

## Suicide and humaneness

Mencius, who puts more emphasis on virtue and self-cultivation, inclines to encourage people to forsake their lives to protect their virtue, because virtue is more important than life (Mencius 1993, Chapter 11.10). Xun Zi, another famous Confucian thinker, openly declares that Shentu Di, who drowned himself in a river, was not fully humane because suicide is at odds with the political order (Xun Zi 1988, Chapter 3). On one hand, personal virtue and honour are central to self-cultivation in Confucian thought; on the other hand, political harmony is also an important Confucian idea. A virtuous person is supposed to be both personally virtuous and beneficial to the empire.

Shentu Di's story is recorded in different books; as for when and why he committed suicide, we have very different versions. According to some books, he was a righteous person who lived at the end of the Xia dynasty. Because the first king of the Shang Court wanted to concede the kingdom to him, he was ashamed and committed suicide (Zheng Qiao 1987, p. 458). In *Zhuang Zi*, however, it is said that he committed suicide only because he heard that the king wanted to concede the kingdom to someone else (Zhuang Zhou 2002, Chapter 26). Yet, another chapter in

the same book refers to him as living at the end of the Shang Dynasty (Zhuang Zhou 2002, Chapter 29); because his suggestion could not be accepted by the tyrant, he committed suicide. According to *Han's Commentary on the Classics of Poetry* (Han Ying 1980, p. 26), *Huai Nan Zi* (Liu An 1989, Chapter 16), *History of the Han Dynasty* (Ban Gu 2004, Chapter 62), and *New Introduction* (Liu Xiang 1985, Chapter 7), he lived in transition between the Shang dynasty and the Zhou dynasty, and committed suicide because of misanthropy.

All of these accounts agree that he committed suicide in order to show his righteousness in contrast to the prevalent corruption. In *Han's Commentary on the Classics of Poetry*, a famous book composed in the early Han dynasty (202BC–8AD), the story of Shentu Di is commented on in detail. Here, Shentu Di is still seen as humane, but his humaneness is of the lowest rank. The author lists four types of humaneness: sacred, wise, moral, and pure. A sacredly humane person has knowledge about heaven, the earth, and human beings, and can make people happy; a wisely humane person also understands the three, and can make people feel free; a morally humane person is tolerant, trusted by the people, and does not sacrifice principles for a contingent matter; a purely humane person, however, is honest, righteous, courageous, and worried about the social disorder and corruption. He is uneasy wherever he is, and steadfastly insists on his way of making friends and earning benefits. He would take his own life when necessary. Of the four types of humaneness, pure humaneness is the lowest; yet it is still a type of humaneness, because it helps correct social disorder and benefits the people (Han Ying 1980, pp. 25–27).

In the Confucian tradition, humaneness is the highest virtue. It is not an idea independent from human beings as it is in Platonism, but is intrinsic to human behaviourur. People cannot be perfectly humane unless they behave in a moral, good and proper way and make themselves virtuous, righteous, dignified and happy persons. People who commit suicide often show some degree of courage, honour and righteousness. They are not condemned as evil in Chinese culture, but are seen as imperfectly humane. On the one hand, although there are many suicides that are greatly praised and admired, they are not seen as perfect. On the other hand, although many thinkers criticise those who commit suicide, they only see suicide as improper, and do not regard it as evil or sinful. In other words, what those who commit suicide aim at is usually good, but they should not seek that good by committing suicide.

Qu Yuan is perhaps the most famous suicide in Chinese history, and is often paralleled with Cato of ancient Rome (Lin 1990). Qu Yuan was a great poet and high official of the kingdom of Chu during the Warring States period. Deceived by a messenger from the Kingdom of Qin, the major enemy of Chu, the king of Chu banished Qu Yuan. As the king could not follow his good advice, Qu Yuan lived in sorrow and wrote many poems. Soon after the Qin army captured the capital of Chu, Qu Yuan jumped into a river and died (Sima Qian 2005, Chapter 84). In order to keep fish and turtles away from the corpse of this great poet and patriot, people threw food into the river to feed the animals. This has since become a festival that is celebrated annually on the day that Qu Yuan committed suicide (Zong Lin 1985, p. 92).

In addition to Qu Yuan's own poetry, the main historical source for Qu Yuan's story is his biography in Sima Qian's *Records of the History*, where the author shows great admiration for him (Sima Qian 2005, Chapter 84). In writing about Qu Yuan and other ancient heroes, Sima Qian states a very famous maxim: 'although everyone must die, death can be either weightier than Mount Tai or lighter than a feather' (Sima Qian 2004). Contemporary writers often quote this to illustrate the attitude toward suicide in Chinese intellectual tradition (Lin 1990). It is true that Sima Qian considers Qu Yuan's death weightier than Mount Tai, but after he contemplates the stories of Qu Yuan and others, he decides not to commit suicide himself.

As a historian and an official of the Han dynasty (202 BC–220 AD), Sima Qian was unjustly castrated when he offended the emperor. He saw this as the most shameful punishment one can suffer and wants to commit suicide on several occasions to resist the emperor. But when he contemplated the sufferings of Qu Yuan and other famous people, he decided to live (Ban Gu 2004, Chapter 74). In a letter to his friend Ren An, Sima Qian says:

> If I die now, it is no different than nine cows losing a hair, and I would have died like an ant. People would not see me as one of those who die an honourable death, but would see me as an evil and shameful criminal who has no idea how to avoid a worse punishment and hence takes my own life.
>
> Sima Qian (2004)

Obviously, Sima Qian does not see suicide as always honorable or weightier than Mount Tai. Qu Yuan's suicide is honorable, but Sima Qian's own suicide would be valueless. What makes such a big difference? Further explaining his idea, Sima Qian says: 'Why? Because the achievements are different. Although everyone must die, death can be either weightier than Mount Tai or lighter than a feather, because the context and aim are different.' His suicide would be shameful because he had already suffered a shameful punishment. Qu Yuan's suicide was honourable because he had achieved much and was seen as unjustly banished. The act of suicide itself hardly makes little difference: the reason and aim of the suicide are the key issues. After contemplation, Sima Qian decided to become a great historian and finally finished his famous book (Sima Qian 2004, 2005, Chapter 130).

Yang Xiong, another poet in the Han dynasty, is very critical of Qu Yuan and thinks his suicide is valueless. He composed a long poem in Qu Yuan's style and called it 'Anti-Li Sao' ('Li Sao' is Qu Yuan's major poem [Qu Yuan 1979]). He mocked Qu Yuan and attacked him as too unwise to survive hardship (Yang Xiong 1979). This is perhaps the most vehement critique against Qu Yuan in Chinese intellectual history. In his commentary to Qu Yuan's poetry, to which Yang Xiong's poem is appended, Zhu Xi, the famous philosopher in the Song dynasty, remarks that although Qu Yuan's suicide does not make him the perfect saint, Yang Xiong, who was not a loyal official when Wang Mang usurped the throne, was not entitled to criticise him at all (Zhu Xi 1979).

As the major figure in Neo-Confucianism that flourished in late imperial China, Zhu Xi's judgement shows the standard attitude toward Qu Yuan in Chinese cultural tradition. Not the perfect saint, he has done what a righteous intellectual is supposed to do, protecting virtuous integrity, showing arduous patriotism, and preserving his dignity and honour.

## Suicide and Taoism

Although Taoism does not say much about suicide, we can also see its attitude toward it in a detail of Qu Yuan's story.

When Qu Yuan was about to jump into the river, a fisherman came and asked him, 'Were you not a noble official? Why have you become like this?' Qu Yuan said, 'The whole world has been polluted but I am pure; everyone else is drunk but I am awake. That is why I am exiled.' The fisherman said, 'If the whole world is polluted, why don't you enjoy their rubbish? If everyone is drunk, why don't you enjoy drinking with them?' Qu Yuan answered, 'I have heard that everyone wants to wear clean clothes after a bath. How can I have my pure body bear dirty rubbish? How can I have my beautiful fame corrupted why their dirt?' The fisherman smiled and left him, singing, 'If the river is clean, I can wash my hat in it; if the river is dirty, I can wash my feet in it' (Qu Yuan 1979, pp. 116–117).

The anonymous fisherman's attitude is a typical Taoist one. He does not want to be too concerned about mundane affairs and would never commit suicide for such affairs. Zhuangzi, the leading Taoist thinker in the Warring State period, talks a lot about this idea, though not directly about suicide. According to him, one cannot be truly happy unless released from all concerns and restraints in the world, including the concern about one's life.

Zhuangzi does not think life is always better than death: what concerns him is not whether life is good, but whether one insists on something too much. In order to explain this, he tells a story of a young girl. When that girl is about to marry a duke she has never seen, she is very sad, as if she is going to hell. After she is married, however, she finds it is very enjoyable to be the duke's wife and regrets having mourned this. Zhuangzi compares the girl to a dying person: 'How can we know that a dead person would not regret being reluctant to die?' (Zhuang Zhou 2002, Chapter 3).

This does not mean that he encourages people to commit suicide. What he really wants to teach is that one should live a happy life peacefully, as exemplified in the fisherman's criticism of Qu Yuan. Although Zhuangzi does not think life is always better, he would not approve of suicide, which would be a sign of over-insistence on a single idea.

Taoism and Confucianism are not as different from each other as they sometimes seem to be. Although Confucianism emphasizes duty more than Taoism does, a perfect life in the Confucian sense is not very different from the Taoist one. When Confucius says, 'I have neither favourable nor unfavourable situations,' he is expressing something very similar to the fisherman's idea.

## Loyal intellectuals and chaste women

Although most major Confucian intellectuals judge suicide as improper, it is very difficult for an individual to tell a proper survival from a cowardly one. For instance, upon the collapse of the Yuan dynasty (1279–1368) and the establishment of the Ming dynasty (1368–1644), Wei Su, an official loyal to the Yuan Court, wanted to jump into a well. A friend stopped him and told him that he should do something better for the Yuan dynasty. Following Sima Qian's example, Wei Su survived and helped compose the history of the Yuan dynasty (Zhang Tingyu 2004, Chapter 285). Many people, however, despised Wei Su because he could not commit suicide for his emperor, but served the conquerors. Even the emperor of the Ming dynasty regarded him as a cowardly traitor. Once the emperor heard someone walking in the court and asked who it is. Wei Su said, 'It is me.' The emperor responded, 'Oh, it is you. I thought it was Wen Tianxiang' (Wen Tianxiang was a famous hero who died upon the collapse of the Song dynasty) (Tuotuo 2004, Chapter 418). The emperor was mocking Wei Su, who could not die for the Yuan dynasty. Having heard that, Wei Su became very depressed and was soon dead, although not from suicide (Wang Shizhen 1986, Chapter 6).

In late imperial China, although suicide was not seen as the best path of spiritual cultivation, it was more or less required for all the intellectuals upon the collapse of a dynasty. Anyone who did not commit suicide or even surrendered to the enemies was vehemently criticised.

Similarly, the best choice for women in this patriarchal culture who had been raped was also to commit suicide. Cheng Yi, another important philosopher in Neo-Confucianism, wrote a famous maxim: 'To starve to death is a minor thing; to lose one's chastity is a great thing' (Cheng Hao and Cheng Yi 2004, p. 301). The state encouraged women to commit suicide by erecting monuments for such suicides (Sommer 2000). Some intellectuals, including Dai Zhen in the Qing Dynasty (Dai Zhen 1982, p. 10) and Lu Xun in the Republican era (Lu Xun 1981), criticised this practice as being too cruel to the women. This critical attitude only arose in more recent times: for most of the period, women were not compelled to commit suicide but saw it as an honourable behaviour to preserve their chastity. In poetry (Fong 2001) and fiction (Zamperini 2001), female suicide is even seen as aesthetically beautiful (Carlitz 2001). It is true that encouraging this type of suicide was beneficial to the imperial state (Theiss 2001), but the empire never forced any woman to commit suicide if she did not want to.

Although we often read about female suicide in fiction and poetry of this period, it is probably less frequent than people have imagined. After examining cases in the legal archives of the Qing dynasty, Wang Yuesheng shows that not every woman who was praised by the empire committed suicide to protect her chastity. Some women committed suicide for a minor reason—due to a misunderstanding or another error which had nothing to do with chastity—but the state also made them chaste women and wholeheartedly praised them (Wang 2003, pp. 225–226). This was of course very helpful for promoting the Confucian ideology of the empire. The fact that the empire praised women who had committed suicide to protect chastity (whether it was genuine or not) does not mean that the empire compelled women who had been raped to commit suicide. To commit suicide is seen as embodying a high moral standard, but it is not required for every ordinary woman.

There are some famously influential stories about female suicide. For instance, Du Shiniang, a famous courtesan in the Ming dynasty, is deeply in love with Li Jia, a playboy who promised to marry her. When Du realizes that Li Jia has given up this idea and even plans to sell her to another man, Du Shiniang drowns herself in a river (Feng Menglong 2003, Chapter 32): what Du Shiniang protests is not a moral duty, but her dignity and true love.

Another story is that of Guo Liu, an ordinary wife whose husband is compelled by a great famine to beg in a faraway place. In order to serve her parents-in-law in this famine, Guo Liu prostitutes herself and has earned a lot of money by prostitution when her husband comes back. Guo Liu tells her husband that she cannot stay as his wife since she is not chaste any more, but she has accumulated sufficient money for him to marry another girl. She has even found a pretty girl for him. After telling her husband this, Guo Liu commits suicide, but although she is dead, she refuses to close her eyes. Only after her parents-in-law acknowledge that she is a chaste and good wife does she close her eyes (Ji Yun 1998, pp. 46–47).

In this story Guo Liu is in an impossibly difficult situation. She cannot be a good wife unless she feeds her parents-in-law in the famine; but practically she cannot do that without losing her chastity. She wants to be both a good and a chaste wife. In theory, her parents-in-law understand her situation, she cannot be regarded as a chaste woman unless she commits suicide.

The logic behind the suicide of intellectuals and female suicide is quite similar. In both cases, suicide is seen as a passionate and spirited behaviourur to protect one's dignity, honour or integrity. These suicides are praised because they are aimed at virtues. The suicide of loyal intellectuals and passionate women are two major types of honourable suicide. Suicide for other reasons is usually viewed negatively. This is best seen in another significant story in Ji Yun's *Notes in the Cottage of Observing the Subtle*.

A young man, as the story goes, meets a Buddhist monk when traveling. Since it is already very late, the young man has no choice but to stay with that monk, who is a ghost who has died from hanging. It is said in Chinese folklore that ghosts who commit suicide, especially those who die from hanging, usually entice other people to hang themselves too, so that they can soon be reborn as human beings; otherwise they would stay in the netherworld forever. This is called 'to seek a replacement', implying that such a ghost cannot be reincarnated without another ghost to replace him or her. There are also some such ghosts, however, who can be reincarnated without enticing other people. The young man realizes that the monk is not trying to entice him and boldly asks him why there is such a big difference between different ghosts. The monk explained:

> God weighs people's lives and does not want one to take his/her own life. When a loyal official commits suicide for the integrity of his virtue, or a passionate woman commits suicide to protect her chastity, he or she is not different than people who die a normal death. Hence they do not need someone to replace them. When someone is compelled in a really difficult situation, and suicide becomes the only choice, he or she can also be reincarnated as other people do. If someone commits suicide when there is still hope to survive, when someone simply cannot endure some offence, or when one wants to embarrass other people by committing suicide, that will be at odds with God's mercy, and the deceased has to seek someone to replace him/her by committing suicide. In some cases, they cannot find one until one hundred years later.
>
> Ji Yun (1998, pp. 57–58)

This story explains vividly how suicide was generally viewed in late imperial China. When suicide is necessary for one to protect his or her virtue, it is greatly praised; when it is committed without any moral significance, it is condemned. Although suicide is viewed differently across contexts, both 'good' and 'bad' suicides are seen as expressing pride, anger and spiritedness. For instance, one might commit suicide when done wrong, shamed or criticised. If the person in question is too angry to endure the wrongness, shame or criticism they might commit suicide to protect their pride, dignity or honour. The cause for such a suicide is not as morally powerful as that of loyal intellectuals or chaste women, but they may experience the same psychodynamics as these exemplars. They are not praised because they have chosen the wrong objective for their anger or resistance.

## Suicide in a new era

In the Ming and Qing dynasties (1368–1911), suicide of ordinary people often appears in fiction and poems. In the famous novel *Jin Ping Mei*, Song Huilian, a woman who has sexual affairs with several men and is anything but chaste, commits suicide when she learns that Ximen Qing, her master and lover, has killed her husband. The author obviously has a highly positive regard for Song Huilian's suicide, although she is by no means a chaste woman (Xiaoxiaosheng 1985, Chapter 26). In *A Dream in the Red Chamber*, another classic novel, several ordinary women commit suicide. Significant among them is that of You Erjie. As a concubine of Jia Lian, she cannot endure the harsh attitude of her husband's other wives and commits suicide (Cao Xueqin 1998, Chapter 69).

If the monk in Ji Yun's book judged these women, obviously he would see them as unworthy suicides who must seek replacements; but the authors of these stories show that there are deep reasons behind the suicides of these ordinary women. Toward the end of the imperial period, intellectuals became increasingly concerned about the happiness and suffering of those ordinary women. On the one hand, they still regarded suicide as a spirited resistance against injustice and a protection of virtues; on the other hand, they did not see loyalty or chastity as the only virtues that can be protected by suicide. The transformation of moral concepts reflects a new era in the intellectual history of suicide in China; but it is nonetheless consistent with the classical ideas about suicide in some crucial aspects.

This new idea gradually becomes evident in the last years of the Qing dynasty. In the New Cultural Movement of the early twentieth century, it finally became the mainstream idea about suicide. There were many debates about suicide at that time. The most significant one was about the suicide of Zhao Wuzhen, a young woman who cut her own throat in a bridal chair during her marriage ceremony. Zhao was betrothed to a man and was happy with it at first. A little before the wedding, however, she became reluctant. Her suicide provoked a hot debate. Among many young authors, Mao Zedong, who was only 26 years old, published at least nine articles about this event (Witke 1967). His main ideas can be summarized as:

1 Zhao Wuzhen was forced to commit suicide by the traditional family system and marriage system (Mao 1992a, c, d, e);

2 Zhao's suicide is a spirited resistance against the traditional society to attain her free will and personality (Mao 1992b):

3 Yet suicide is not the best way to do that (Mao 1992f);

4 The only way is to change the old systems through a social revolution (Mao 1992g, h, i).

Although Mao's terms are different to traditional views of suicide, it seems to me that he inherits the main idea about suicide. Suicide is seen as a spirited resistance against the evil and a protection of one's virtue (or personality in Mao's term); but it is not the perfect way to attain true happiness. What has been changed is the specific meaning of virtue and happiness: the significance of suicide is the same.

## Suicide and suicide prevention in contemporary China

Although ideas about suicide have undergone changes over time, the strong influence of traditional cultural and religious Chinese principles are evident today (Phillips *et al.* 1999). Traditional Chinese culture differs significantly in beliefs about human nature and life from Western Judeo-Christian traditions (Wu Fei 2005a). While suicide has become a very serious issue in China, we believe

the most serious obstacle of suicide prevention is the neglect of a profound understanding of the traditional ideas about suicide. Suicide was never strictly prohibited or stigmatized in Chinese culture. Instead, it has traditionally been considered an acceptable way to resist and protect one's dignity, though it is not regarded as the best way to do so.

In the eyes of ordinary Chinese people, only suicides committed by 'normal people' are seen as typical suicides. If a person with serious mental illness commits suicide, this is not counted as a suicide, because it does not show any social significance or resistance. In such a case, the death of the person in question is seen as no different from a death caused by another person or an accident. This does not mean that mentally ill people are treated positively. On the contrary, they are often seriously stigmatized and not considered as 'whole' persons. When a 'normal' person commits suicide, his or her family members are usually stigmatized. Even if people around the family know nothing about the reasons for the suicide, the thought that other members in the family have done something wrong to the deceased is widespread. For instance, if an old man commits suicide, his children must have treated him badly; if a young wife commits suicide, people usually show sympathy with her and imagine that her husband must have mistreated her. The connection to the immediate family, even after suicide, is further expressed in the burial rites: if a single person commits suicide, he or she is not to be buried in the main cemetery of the family, not because of the suicide, but because they died without being married. However, if a married person commits suicide, they will be buried in a normal way.

## Conclusion

The first step in suicide prevention is to understand the underlying motives of the people who commit suicide, but not to identify with them as patients or judge them as sinners. It is only when we understand all the motives behind a suicide, here focusing on the cultural religious ones, that we can take further action of prevention and suggest alternatives. This is the main lesson that we learn from the Chinese ideas about suicide. I believe that if we can take these ideas seriously, it will contribute to a more effective response to this extreme form of human suffering.

## References

Ban Gu (2004). *History of the Han Dynasty* (汉书). Han Yu Da Ci Dian Chu Ban She, Shanghai.

Cao Xueqin (1998). *Hong Lou Meng* (红楼梦). Shanghai Gu Ji Chu Ban She, Shanghai.

Carlitz C (2001). The daughter, the single-girl, and the seduction of suicide. *NAN NU – Men, Women and Gender in Early and Imperial China*, **3**, 22–46.

Cheng Hao and Cheng Yi (2004). *Collections of the Two Chengs* (二程集). Zhong Hua Shu Ju, Beijing.

Confucius (1997). *The Analects of Confucius* (论语). translated by Chiching Huang. Oxford University Press, Oxford.

Dai Zhen (1982). *A Literary Commentary on Mencius* (孟子字义疏证). Zhong Hua Shu Ju, Beijing.

Durkheim E (1951). *Suicide: A Study in Sociology*. Free Press, New York.

Feng Menglong (2003). *Jing Shi Tong Yan* (警世通言). Yue Lu Shu She, Changsha.

Fong, Grace (2001). Signifying bodies: the cultural significance of suicide writings by women in Ming–Qing China. *NAN NU – Men, Women & Gender in Early & Imperial China*, **3**, 105–142.

Han Ying (1980). *Interpretations of Han's Commentary on the Classics of Poetry* (韩诗外传集释). Zhong Hua Shu Ju, Beijing.

Ji Yun (1998). *Notes in the Cottage of Observing the Subtle* (阅微草堂笔记). Shanghai Gu Ji Chu Ban She, Shanghai.

Lin Yuan-Yuei (1990). The weight of Mount Tai. Ph.D. dissertation. Wisconsin University at Madison.

Liu An (1989). *Huai Nan Zi* (淮南子). Shanghai Gu Ji Chu Ban She, Shanghai.

Liu Xiang (1985). *New Introduction* (新序). Zhong Hua Shu Ju, Beijing.

Lu Xun (1981). The New Year Sacrifice. In *Wandering* (彷徨), translated by Yang Xianyi and Gladys Yang. Foreign Languages Press, Beijing.

Mao Zedong (1992a). Commentary on the suicide of miss Zhao, *Da Gong Bao*, 16 November, 1919, in *Mao's Road to Power (Vol. 1)*. Edited by Stuart Shram, Sharpe, Armonk, New York.

Mao Zedong (1992b). The question of miss Zhao's personality, *Da Gong Bao*, 18 November, 1919, in *Mao's Road to Power (Vol. 1)*. Edited by Stuart Shram, Sharpe, Armonk, New York.

Mao Zedong (1992c). The marriage question—an admonition to young men and women, *Da Gong Bao*, 19 November, 1919, in *Mao's Road to Power (Vol. 1)*. Edited by Stuart Shram, Sharpe, Armonk, New York.

Mao Zedong (1992d). The question of reforming the marriage, *Da Gong Bao*, 19 November, 1919, in *Mao's Road to Power (Vol. 1)*. Edited by Stuart Shram, Sharpe, Armonk, New York.

Mao Zedong (1992e). The evils of society and miss Zhao, *Da Gong Bao*, 21 November, 1919, in *Mao's Road to Power (Vol. 1)*. Edited by Stuart Shram, Sharpe, Armonk, New York.

Mao Zedong (1992f). Against suicide, *Da Gong Bao*, 23 November, 1919, in *Mao's Road to Power (Vol. 1)* Edited by Stuart Shram, Sharpe, Armonk, New York.

Mao Zedong (1992g). The question of love—young people and old people, *Da Gong Bao*, 25 November, 1919, in *Mao's Road to Power (Vol. 1)*. Edited by Stuart Shram, Sharpe, Armonk, New York.

Mao Zedong (1992h). Smash the matchmaker system, *Da Gong Bao*, 27 November, 1919, in *Mao's Road to Power (Vol 1)*. Edited by Stuart Shram, Sharpe, Armonk, New York.

Mao Zedong (1992i). The problem of superstition in marriage, *Da Gong Bao*, 28 November, 1919, in *Mao's Road to Power (Vol. 1)*. Edited by Stuart Shram, Sharpe, Armonk, New York.

Mencius (1993). *Mencius* (孟子), translated by Zheng Xunzuo. Shandong Friendship Press, Jinan.

Phillips M, Huaqing Liu, Yanping Zhang (1999). Suicide and social change in China. *Culture, Medicine and Psychiatry*, **23**, 25–50.

Plato (1975). *Phaedo*, translated by David Gallop. Clarendon University Press, Oxford.

Qu Yuan (1979). *Commentaries on the Songs of the South* (楚辞集注). Shanghai Gu Ji Chu Ban She, Shanghai.

Sima Qian (2004). pistle to Ren An (报任少卿书). In Ban Gu, *The Biography of Sima Qian*, Chapter 74 of *History of the Han Dynasty* (汉书·司马迁传). Han Yu Da Ci Dian Chu Ban She, Shanghai.

Sima Qian (2005). *Records of History* (史记). Han Yu Da Ci Dian Chu Ban She, Shanghai.

Sommer M (2000). *Sex, Law, and Society in Late Imperial China*. Stanford University Press, Stanford.

Theiss J (2001). Managing martyrdom: female suicide and statecraft in mid-Qing China. *NAN NU – Men, Women & Gender in Early & Imperial China*, **3**, 47–76.

Tuotuo (2004). *History of the Song Dynasty* (宋史). Han Yu Da Ci Dian Chu Ban She, Shanghai.

Wang Shizhen (1986). *Yi Yuan Zhi Yan* (艺苑卮言). Zhong Hua Shu Ju, Beijing.

Wang Yuesheng (2003). *Analyses of Conjugal Conflicts in the Middle Period of the Qing Dynasty* (清代中期婚姻冲突透析). She Ke Wen Xian Chu Ban She, Beijing.

Witke R (1967). Mao Tse-tung, women and suicide in the May Fourth era. *The China Quarterly*, No. 31.

Wu Fei (2005a). Elegy for luck: suicide in a county of north China. Ph.D. Dissertation, Harvard University.

Wu Fei (2005b). Gambling for qi: suicide and family politics in a north China rural county. *The China Journal*, **54**, 7–27.

Xiaoxiaosheng (1985). *Jin Ping Mei Ci Hua* (金瓶梅词话). Tian Yi Chu Ban She, Taipei.

Xun Zi (1988). *Commentary on Xun Zi* (荀子集解). Zhong Hua Shu Ju, Beijing.

Yang Xiong (1979). Anti-Li Sao (反离骚). In *Commentaries on the Songs of the South* (楚辞集注), pp. 236–241. Shanghai Gu Ji Chu Ban She, Shanghai.

Zamperini P (2001). Untamed hearts: Eros and suicide in late imperial Chinese fiction. *NAN NU – Men, Women & Gender in Early & Imperial China*, **3**, 77–104.

Zeng Shen (1993). *The Classic of Filial Piety* (孝经), translated by Liu Ruixiang and Lin Zhihe. Shandong Friendship Press, Jinan.

Zhang Tingyu (2004). *History of the Ming Dynasty* (明史). Han Yu Da Ci Dian Chu Ban She, Shanghai.

Zheng Qiao (1987). *Tong Zhi* (通志), volume 1. Zhong Hua Shu Ju, Beijing.

Zhu Xi (1979). Commentary on Anti-Li Sao. In *Commentaries on the Songs of the South* (楚辞集注), pp. 242–243. Shanghai Gu Ji Chu Ban She, Shanghai.

Zhuang Zhou (2002). *Zhuang Zi* (庄子). Shanghai Gu Ji Chu Ban She, Shanghai.

Zong Lin (1985). *Seasonal Festivals of South China* (荆楚岁时记译注). Hubei Ren Min Chu Ban She, Wuhan.

Zuo Qiuming (2000). *The Tso Chuen* (左传), Volume 4 of *The Chinese Classics,* translated by James Legge. SMC Publishing Inc., Taipei.

# CHAPTER 4

# Hindu religion and suicide in India

Lakshmi Vijayakumar

## Abstract

Hinduism is one of the oldest religions in the world. It is estimated that there are approximately 965 million Hindus in the world, of which, 909 million are in India.

As early as 3000 BC, suicides were generally condemned, but religious suicides were condoned. The practice of sati (self-immolation) and jauhar (mass suicide) was also prevalent among the Hindus. Suicide by self-immolation often occurs in Hindus, particularly among young women: the dowry system and arranged marriages are prevalent amongst Hindus and sometimes lead to suicides. Suicidal behaviour was higher among Hindus than that of the native population in the countries to which Hindus had migrated.

A case control study in India found that strong faith in Hinduism is a significant protective factor against suicide: odds ratio (OR) 6.83, confidence interval (CI) 2.88–19.69. Belief in karma and reincarnation probably make a Hindu more concerned that they should have a dignified death: in Hinduism it is ultimately the individual's decision as to how they live and die.

## Hindu religion and suicide

The term Hindu is a Persian and Arabic label given in ancient times to people living east of Sindu or the Indus River. It is difficult to define Hinduism or a Hindu: Hinduism is perceived as a way of life and is neither a monotheistic religion nor a unitary concept. Hinduism has no human founder or universal doctrine (Bhugra 2004). The Vedas are the original scriptures of the Hindus, and the oldest source of all wisdom about Hinduism: whoever believes in the authority of Vedas and/or worships any of the thousands of gods and goddesses can be considered a Hindu. Of the four Vedas—Rigveda, Yajur, Sama and Atharva—Rigveda is said to be the oldest (3000–1700 BC). The other three date from 2000–1100 BC. They were handed down through oral tradition and only recently written down comparatively. In the latter part of the Vedic period, the Upanishad group was formed. While Vedic writers analysed and admired nature, the Upanishidic (800–600 BC) were philosophers who turned their eyes inwards to understand 'Man – the Unknown' (Rao 2006).

The beliefs, morals and philosophy of a Hindu are based on the Vedas, Upanishads, and epics such as Ramayana, Mahabharatha, and other scriptures. The concepts of atman, karma and dharma, described below, are important dimensions in Hinduism. Hindus believe that all living forms have a soul or *atman*. Each atman is eternal; it is never created, will never perish and is characterized as unchanging truth, consciousness and bliss. The atman passes through infinite cycles of births and deaths based on its karmas, until it realizes the ultimate, and attains moksha or brahman (the ultimate reality). *Karma* literally means deed or act, but more broadly, describes the principle of cause and effect. Karma is a theory that states that every mental, emotional and physical act, no matter how insignificant, is projected out into the psychic mind substance and eventually returns to the individual with equal impact.

There are three categories of karma. The first is sanchita, which is the sum total of karmas yet to be resolved; secondly, there is the prarabdha karma, which is that portion of the karma being experienced in the present life. The third is kriyamana, the type of karma that one is creating in the present life. Though prarabdha and sanchita karma are experienced in the present life, they are different. Those experiences which we undergo in the present life, due to the karma of previous birth, are prarabhdha karma. The acts in our present life, which will have a bearing on our future, are called sanchita karma. Karma is often misunderstood as fate, destiny or predetermination. If one lives life righteously with good thought and deed—*dharma* (dharma means to live) and compassion, one can reduce the negative karma of the past and create positive karma for the future. In essence, we create our own experiences. Karma helps explain the disparities that occur in human population, such as, poverty, prosperity, happiness, misery, ability, disability, health and illness (The Himalayan Academy 2006). Reincarnation is the phenomenon through which the immortal soul is continuously born and reborn in any of the life forms until it attains moksha or truth. The atman is unchanging truth, consciousness and bliss. Just as a person casts off worn-out clothes for new ones, the embodied soul leaves worn-out bodies and enters into new ones, based on its karma, until it reaches moksha. In Hinduism, the basis of a man's search is himself. Chandogya Upanishad where sage Uddlaha answers his son Svetaketu's questions about the Creator and the origin of man with the now famous quote 'tat tvam asi'—you are that which is God—is considered the essence of Hinduism. Dharma is the social and ethical code of behaviour.

## Death in Hinduism

In Hinduism, to die well one must live well. When a person dies, their soul, along with some residual consciousness, leaves the body and goes to another astral plane. The *Bhagavad Gita*, a form of dialogue between the warrior Arjuna and Lord Krishna in the battlefield, states that life is like a running thread, interrupted by beads of births and deaths succeeding one another like day and night. (The *Bhagavad Gita* is also known as the celestial song. It has 18 chapters and 700-odd verses and it is dated to around the 3rd and 4th century BC.) As death is inevitable for one who is born so birth, too, is inevitable for one who dies. Though the inevitability of death is imprinted on the Hindu mind, there is great concern about having a good death. A good death is supposed to happen when all actions are selfless, without any thought for its fruits and motivated only by the love of any God.

Death is described by several terms:

◆ Panchatvam (death as a dissolution of five elements);

◆ Mrityu (natural death);

◆ Prayopavesha (self-willed death by fasting);

◆ Marana (unnatural death);

◆ Mahaparasthana (The Great Journey);

◆ Samadhimarana (dying consciously in a state of meditation); and

◆ Mahasamadi (the Great Merger or departure of an enlightened soul).

Hindus are usually cremated, but occasionally, some who are considered as enlightened are buried. In Hinduism, death is a very complex idea, encompassing visions of how the soul will be affected, how will your death affect society and finally, how will it affect future reincarnations? In the *Lancet* article on the Hindu view of the end of life, Firth urges that the Hindu good death provides a valuable model on how death can be approached positively and without apprehension (Firth 2005).

## Suicide in ancient Hinduism

It is difficult to find a particular term signifying individual suicides in Hinduism, though the most often used nomenclature is 'atmaghataka'. Thakur's 1963 book *The history of suicide in India* has been the source of much of the information presented here. The oral tradition indicates that suicides were prevalent even during Vedic times. Contemporary Vedic scholars are divided on the subject of whether Vedic injunctions allowed self-destruction, or if it was simply a symbolic ritual. The Upanishad categorically condemned suicide. The Isavasya Upanishad states 'he who takes his self, reaches, after death, the sunless region covered by impenetrable darkness'. Kautilya (also known as Chanakya) was a minister to the Mauryan Emperor Chandragupta and wrote *Arthashastra* (250 BC), which strongly condemns those who commit, or cause to commit, suicide by means of rope, arms or poison under infatuation of love, anger or other sinful passion. According to him, they should be dragged by rope on a public road, and funeral rites should not be performed. He had also instituted Kantakasodhana, a procedure for determination of death by suicide or homicide, which was performed by commissioners who examined the bodies, ascertained the circumstances, and tried to find the cause of death. The scripture Yama smriti (6–7th century AD) suggests that if

a person commits suicide, his body should be smeared with impure things: if he lives, he should be fined two hundred panas, and his friends and sons should be fined one pana each.

The writings of *Dharmashastra* (the Hindu book of code, conduct and ethics, 900–700 BC), make it clear that suicide, and attempted suicide, were to be condemned as great sins. However, there is a separate section, 'Allowable suicides', in which suicides were accepted in the following situations: a person was allowed to commit suicide to expiate sins committed by him, for example, the murder of a Brahmin or incest. Moreover, a hermit starting on the Great Journey (mahaparasthana), suffering from an incurable disease, and thus unable to perform the duties of his order, as well as old men, or one who cannot observe the rules of bodily purifications, e.g. someone who cannot control their bodily functions, or who is so ill that they are beyond medical help, is sanctioned to commit suicide. Furthermore, a housekeeper (a person living with the family) may resort to suicide if their life's work is over, if they have no desire for the pleasures of life and do not desire to live any longer. This person has to be convinced of the ephemeral nature of life, and then may kill themself by fasting in the Himalayas. Religious suicides are allowed, as is sati, a form of suicide performed by women and described below (Kane 1941).

## Religious suicides

The permitted religious suicide was mahaparasthana or the Great Journey. In this type of suicide, the person walks to the north-east towards Kailash, the abode of Siva, subsisting only on water and air, until his body sinks to rest. Even today, Hindu crematoriums are located in a north-easterly direction.

Certain places and rivers have a special significance in Hinduism. It is believed that if one ends one's life in these places, one is relieved of the cycle of births and deaths, thereby avoiding reincarnation. Ever since ancient times, Kasi or Varanasi in Uttar Pradesh, India, has been the most sacred of the places of pilgrimages. Death at Kasi was considered as the ultimate good death. Numerous pilgrims, both in good-health and ill, from all over the country, flock to Kasi. It is popularly believed that Lord Siva himself ensures the salvation of everyone who dies in Kasi, by whispering into the right ear of the dying person. Prayag, at the confluence of the three rivers—Ganga, Yamuna and the invisible Saraswathi—is another place where people choose to commit suicide. Historical examples of suicides such as those of the kings Karnadeva, Candella, Dhangadev and Chalukya Someswara at Prayag (Uttar Pradesh) and Tungabhadra (Andhra Pradesh), have reinforced the desirability of dying in these holy places. The scripture Kurma Purana asserted that 'he who abandons life in this sacred place in some way or other does not incur the sin of suicide': thus, suicides at Prayag were not considered as suicides. However, one is not allowed to commit suicide at Prayag after abandoning one's elderly parents, young wife or children who require support. A woman who is pregnant or who has young children or who had no permission from her husband was forbidden to take her life (Kane 1974). It was also believed that if one jumped from the sacred banyan tree (akshayavata) in Gaya in Allahabad and died, one would be reborn as a great king. Many commit suicide in this way at this location due to the belief that the Moghul Emperor Akbar (1555–1605 AD) had committed such a suicide in a past birth and was rewarded by becoming Emperor in the next birth.

At the Jagannath temple in Puri, in Orissa, the deity was taken out in the temple car, pulled by hundreds of people, once a year. People threw themselves under the wheels of the car, in the belief that by doing so, they would attain moksha, or salvation. In 1802, legislation was passed to prevent people from committing suicide in such a manner (Leenaars *et al.* 2001). In addition to religious and other kinds of suicides, Brahmins often resorted to suicide to avenge an injury or injustice: it was believed that their spirits would then harass or prosecute the offender.

## Sati (Suttee)

Sati or self-immolation was a form of suicide customary among Hindu women in India. There are two types: sahamarana or sahagamana, in which the widow ascended the funeral pyre of her husband and was burnt along with the corpse, and anumarana, in which the widow decided to die after the cremation of her husband, and so prepared a funeral pyre and killed herself (Vijayakumar 2004). Theologians still argue about the ambiguity of verse X 18.7 in the Rig Veda, with regard to sati. The custom was not common in the early Vedic period, when the widow was allowed to marry her husband's brother or any near kinsman upon his death. The earliest recorded historical instance of sati in India is that of the wife of the Hindu General Keteus, who died in 316 BC while fighting Antigonas of Greece (Thakur 1963).

In third century before Christ, sati was committed out of love for the husband. It was a period when bravery was highly esteemed, and women considered sati an act of bravery and a sign of their abundant love for their husband. Originally, sati was confined to a few queens and wives of nobles, and was a rare occurrence. Gradually, those who died by sati were idolised and treated as goddesses. Temples were constructed, prayers offered and memorial stones of sati were installed. During the Vedic period, throughout which women enjoyed equal status and were involved in religious and social life, sati was practically unheard of. Gradually, the patriarchal system prevailed. Women were subservient in the domestic sphere and were excluded from social and economic activities of the community. Polygamy was also prevalent. This period witnessed the widespread practice of sati.

One can distinguish psychological, social and economic factors in relation to the increase of satis. Psychologically the widow was extremely vulnerable emotionally soon after her husband's death, particularly in a society where the wife was entirely dependent on the husband for her self-esteem. By committing sati, the woman proves to the world that she is the most chaste and virtuous of all women. Widows had no social status, were prohibited from marrying again, had to shave their heads, could only wear white or brown saris, were not allowed to wear ornaments, were not included in any social activity, and their presence in religious activity or festivity was considered a bad omen. In the poem Purananuru (2 AD), there is a verse which is attributed to Perungopendu, wife of Bhuda Pandian, before she commits sati. The verse describes the arduous, demoralizing life she has to lead as a widow (eating food from the floor, sleeping on the ground, wearing worn out clothes, etc.). Rather than lead a life like that, she compares that the burning pyre to a lotus pond.

Sati was one of few acts of bravery a woman could show, and the only time she would receive public acclaim and appreciation. She was considered a martyr, and by her selfless sacrifice was supposed to have benefited the family for three generations. People valued the blessing of a woman who was on her way to the funeral pyre highly (Bhugra 2005). Economic factors also had an impact on sati. It was widely prevalent in the state of Bengal: between 1815 and 1827 there were 5388 immolations (Roy 1987). In the rest of India, the widows, as members in a Hindu joint family, were only entitled to maintenance allowance and had no other rights over the property of the family. In Bengal, the Dayabhaga law prevailed, in which a widow was entitled to almost the same rights over joint family property as her deceased husband would have had. This law could induce the surviving members to get rid of the widow, by reminding her of the significance of her devotion and love for her husband. Unsurprisingly, sati was more prevalent in Bengal than in the rest of India (Roy 1987). In Malabar (Kerala), on the other hand, a matriarchal system prevailed. Women had economic power, status and even polyandry was accepted. There is no instance of sati in Malabar, which clearly demonstrates that both religious and socio-economic factors played a part in this practice.

Pregnant women, women with young children and women menstruating were not allowed to commit suicide. Sati was not confined to widows: there were also instances in which following a king's death, his wife (or wives), ministers, soldiers and servants were supposed to die with him. Rajaram Mohan Roy from Bengal called for a complete prohibition of polygamy and sati. Lord Bentinck, the then Governor General of India, put forth a law in December 1829, in which sati was considered a culpable homicide, and banned. Despite this abolition, there were stray incidents, and people continued to worship at the sati Devi temples.

## Jauhar

Jauhar was a type of mass suicide prevalent among the Rajputs, and was committed by the community when faced with defeat. At the loss of a battle or the capture of a city, in order to prevent captivity and its horrors, which were considered worse than death, and to avoid intolerable shame, rape and torture, a huge pyre was built, and all the women and children jumped into it. Sometimes, an entire tribe died by jauhar. This occurred several times among the Rajputs when the Muslim rulers invaded Rajasthan. When Ala-ud-Din Khilji, the ruler from Delhi, invaded Chittore, Rajasthan in 1303 AD to capture Queen Padmini, some nineteen thousand women committed jauhar. Akbar's invasion of Marwar in 1568 also led jauhar to eight thousand women, men and children committing jauhar as a spontaneous outburst of violent reaction against the barbaric atrocities of the conquerors. With the fall of Muslim rule, there were no more invasions, and with the end of the Rajput supremacy, jauhar became extinct.

## Sallekhana (facing death by starvation)

Jainism was founded by Mahavira around 600 BC. Today, the majority of the five million Jains live in India, and practise self denial and non-violence. They are vegetarians and will not even eat tubers, like potatoes and onions, because the plants are killed in the process. The monks cover their nostrils and mouth to avoid inadvertent inhalation leading to the killing of insects. In Jainism, sallekhana means facing death by starvation. According to Jainism, life should be preserved as long as possible, but in old age, if suffering from an incurable disease or during severe famine, sallekhana can be considered. Sallekhana cannot be done impulsively, but only by careful planning, and is a slow process. The ascetic or the householder should give up food and consume only liquids: they will then give up other liquids and consume only water, gradually stopping that too. During this period, the individual should eliminate fear, shame, anger, regret, grief, love, hate, prejudice, and passion and face death with equanimity of mind. Five transgressions should be avoided: wishing that death would come a little later, wishing for a faster death, fear of facing death, remembering friends and relatives at the time of death, and wishing for a reward as a result of this vow. Time should be spent reading, listening to or lecturing the scriptures, meditation and intense self-introspection (Tukol 1976). Sallekhana is sometimes observed amongst the Jain ascetics even today.

## The Hindu religion and suicide in contemporary India

Throughout its history, Hinduism has had conflicting views on suicide, condemning general suicides on one hand, and glorifying religious suicides on the other: this is true even in present times. For a majority of Hindus, religion is all-pervading, though the individual is not preoccupied with it. Since Hinduism is a way of life, and hence can be said to be practiced every day, it has a significant impact on attitudes to suicide and suicidal behaviour. In India, suicide is often viewed as a social problem, and the emphasis has been on social factors rather than individual psychopathology. Ettzersdorfer *et al.* (1998) studied attitudes towards suicides among medical students in India and Austria and found that mental disorder was not considered a significant factor in India. Suicide was considered as an impulsive and unworthy act.

Over 100,000 people commit suicide in India every year. The suicide rate in India was 10.5 in 2002 (National Crime Records Bureau 2002), and the suicide rate has increased by 64 per cent from 6.4 in 1982 to 10.5 in 2002. The suicide rate among women is lower than that of men, but by a small margin when compared to the global sex ratio. The male:female ratio has been consistently low at 1.5:1. Marital status is not a significant risk factor for suicide in India (Vijayakumar *et al.* 2005). The majority of suicides (38 per cent) are committed by persons below the age of 30 years. Below 14 years, more girls (N = 1574) commit suicide than boys (N = 1306). Between 15 and 29 years, a more or less equal number of men and women commit suicide. Clearly, women below the age of 30 are at more risk of suicide. The status of women in Hinduism is complex and conflicting. A woman is worshipped as shakthi (shakthi means power and valour), but also considered the property of the male (father/husband/son). Hindu gods and goddesses personify Hindu religious concepts and nature. Interestingly, goddesses rather than gods are most often used to represent abstract fundamental principles such as power, strength, education and wealth as well as natural phenomena such as the mountains, rivers etc. (Pollisi 2003). Hinduism personifies divine power and strength in the form of the female figure of shakthi. With the advent of the patriarchal system, probably in 3000 BC, women became subservient. The lower status of women, the consequent lowered self-esteem in women at a young age and limited coping skills could be the explanation for suicides in young women in India. The suicide rate in women decreases after the age of 30, probably signifying that once she has children to look after, and thus attains a higher status in the family, suicidal behaviour is reduced.

## Hinduism and self-immolation

Suicide by self-immolation is one of the most violent methods of committing suicide. It is highly lethal, and most of the attempts are fatal. The ratio of attempters to completers is 1:25, a reversal of that in other types of suicide (Rao *et al.* 1989). In India, 9.7 per cent of the suicides (N = 10655) are by self-immolation. This is the only method of suicide where women (69 per cent) outnumber men (31 per cent). In the state of Gujarat, 18.26 per cent of the suicides are by self-immolation: other states with a high percentage of suicides by self-immolation are Maharashtra (14.94 per cent), Tamil Nadu (14.91 per cent), Uttar Pradesh (14.71 per cent), Madhya Pradesh (13.22 per cent), Jharkhand (13.6 per cent) and Bihar (11.39 per cent), all states in which the Hindu religion is deeply rooted. In the states of Manipur, Meghalaya, Mizoram, Sikkim and Tripura, there were no suicides by self-immolation (National Criminal Rrecord Board 2002). All these states are in the northeast hilly region where there are many tribes and Hinduism has less of an impact. The fact that more females burn themselves than men has been well documented (Adityanyjee 1986; Bhatia and Khan 1987). Self-immolation is the preferred method of suicide for women of Indian origin even after migrating to the UK (Soni *et al.* 1990). I argue that the reasons for the high incidence of suicides by self-immolation among Indian women of Hindu origin can be traced to customs of the Hindu religion.

Fire plays an integral role in Hindu religion. Fire is worshipped and it sanctifies birth, marriage, and death; furthermore, Hindus are cremated after death. The two great epics in Hinduism are Ramayana and Mahabharatha. In Ramayana, Sita, the wife of Rama, is kidnapped and taken to Sri Lanka. Rama gathers an army and rescues her. On their return, Rama overhears aspersions cast on Sita's character, so she walks through fire to demonstrate her purity and support for her husband. Hence, ending one's life in purifying, sanctifying fire was ritualized and practised by Indian women.

The practice of sati and jauhar, prevalent in the medieval period, are also important factors. There were stray occurrences even after its abolition. There were about 40 cases of sati after the independence of India in 1947, of which 28 occurred in the state of Rajasthan. In September 1987, in Rajasthan, Roop Kanwar, an 18-year-old, newly married woman, immolated herself in the funeral pyre of her husband. This caused a huge furore in the country, and there were raging protests from women activists, which were countered by traditionalists: it eventually became a political issue. After her death, Roop was elevated to the status of a goddess, and within a fortnight, over seven hundred thousand people had made pilgrimage to the pyre in which she died. The incident shook the whole country. Woman activists and an alarmed public pressed the government to promulgate the Sati Prevention Act 1987. According to the Act, anyone who attempts sati will be imprisoned for a year, with or without a fine, anyone who assists in a sati, either directly or indirectly, faces death or imprisonment for life. A person who glorifies sati will be imprisoned for 7 years and has to pay a fine. The Act also empowered the state government to remove any statue/temples constructed in the last 20 years to commemorate sati, and also to seize funds and donations collected in the name of sati. Since the introduction of the Act, there have been instances of sati.

Sati remains an unusual example of a cultural form of suicide, which is tolerated and, in some cases, even encouraged (Bhugra 2005). The contemporary explanatory factor for self-immolation in Hindu women could be the easy availability and accessibility of the means to suicide. Kerosene (paraffin) is the fuel used for cooking in many homes: to commit suicide, the woman pours kerosene on herself and sets herself alight. The means are easily procured, stored at home, used daily and readily available at the moment of suicidal impulse. Both religious context and the easy accessibility are the likely reasons for the high prevalence of suicide by self-immolation among Hindu women.

## Political self-immolation

Self immolation as a form of 'fiery' protest evolved in India in recent times, but can be traced to more ancient times. The state of Tamil Nadu is known for its political self-immolations, which began in 1965, when the Hindi language was made mandatory and the Tamils resisted it. Chinnasamy, a worker in a political party, committed suicide through self-immolation, protesting against the imposition of Hindi, and there was an outbreak of self-immolations following this. Those who died were considered martyrs.

What started as a protest among the political underclass in the 1960s turned into a ghastly expression of political loyalty in the 1980s. After the death of MGR, a famous actor who became an iconic leader of Tamil Nadu, over 100 people attempted self-immolation, and 31 died (*The Hindu* 2002). Successive governments and the respective political parties extol those who die as martyrs, and compensate them monetarily. In 2002, three persons committed self-immolation in the government offices in Chennai in an attempt to bring their plight to the notice of the authorities. People flocked to the Secretariat with bundles of petitions, poisons and petrol. The government started a support centre within the premises to counsel them.

In August 1990, V.P. Singh, the then Prime Minister of India, announced that his government would implement the recommendations of the Mandal Commission to reserve 27 per cent of the jobs in the government for lower classes as an affirmative action to uplift the backward classes. This created uproar and unrest, especially in the student community (Vijayakumar 2004). A student from an upper class, protesting against 'the reverse discrimination', committed suicide through self-immolation, and this was widely publicized, after which, around 75 youths killed themselves through self-immolation around the country. The public outcry which followed was considered as one of the reasons for the fall of the government.

Suicide by fasting was considered as one of the ways for an ascetic to end his life, and sometimes fasting unto death was undertaken as an act of revenge and to inflict guilt. Brahmins used this method to secure the attention of the King to redress their grievances. In one instance, a king usurped the land of a Brahmin, who then fasted at the palace gates until he died (Thakur 1963). This practice was clearly in vogue at the time as there was special officer—the superintendent of suicides by fast (Prayopavesha adhikrita)—to deal with these matters. Gandhi went on a fast unto death on four occasions in India's struggle for independence. After independence, Potti Sriramulu fasted unto death demanding a separate state for people speaking the Telugu language. Acharya Vinoba Bhave, a great leader and reformer, fasted unto death in November 1982.

Political leaders go on a fast unto death protest even today, to focus on a particular issue or redress a grievance: it has become a political tool to achieve one's objective. Moreover, suicide by drowning, at religiously revered places like Varanasi and Allahabad, is still prevalent today in India.

## Arranged marriages

The caste system is pervasive, and intertwined in Hindu belief. A caste is a social class to which a person belongs at birth. There are four loosely grouped castes, in hierarchical order:

♦ Brahmins (scholars and priests);

♦ Kshatriyas (warriors and rulers);

♦ Vaisyas (traders, farmers, merchants); and

♦ Sudras (daily labourers, artisans etc.).

Currently, they do not correspond to the professions, and one can find all castes in any profession. There are many hundreds of castes and subcastes, which vary in different regions and communities. The importance of caste has declined, but has not disappeared altogether. It always surfaces at the time of marriage, as generally people marry within their own caste. The majority of marriages in India are arranged marriages and they have been part of the Indian culture since the fourth century. Marriage is treated as an alliance between two families rather than as a union of two people. A marriage where partners choose each other is termed as a 'love marriage' (Kamat's Potpourri 2006). Usually the parents, friends and family arrange the marriage. In choosing a partner, the first criterion is belonging to the same caste; then education, physical attributes, family background and economic factors are taken into consideration in finding a suitable match. It has now become less rigid in that people marry outside their subcaste, their language and province, but still within the same caste. Increasingly, the bride and groom do have a role in the decision-making process in arranged marriages, in that they can either accept or reject a marriage proposal brought forward by the family. The families do not opt for an alliance from outside their own caste. Young persons who love each other, but whose families' disapprove of their relationship, consider suicide, either together or alone, as the prospect of marrying each other often means defying and severing ties with the family. In India, 2.81 per cent of suicides are due to love affairs or the failure of a love affair.

A major reason for parental anxiety is the inability to arrange their offspring's marriage, especially a daughter's marriage. After a particular age, the daughter also feels that she is a burden to her parents. It is also a major social stigma when a marriage, which had been arranged, has to be cancelled. Cancellation or non-settlement of marriage accounts for almost a thousand suicides a year in India. An important aspect of arranged marriages is dowry. Dowry is a continuing series of gifts, endowed before or after marriage, often by the bride's parents to the bridegroom. When dowry expectations are not met, the young bride is harassed and sometimes commits suicide by self-immolation. To curtail the dowry menace, the Indian government has enacted a law in which, if a woman dies within 7 years of marriage, the husband is considered guilty, and he is held responsible until he proves his innocence. However, there has always been a large gap between laws and reality

(Tousignast *et al*. 1998). In the year 2002, dowry-related issues were the reason for 2.18 per cent of all suicides, 98.7 per cent of which were committed by women.

Mass suicides and suicide pacts are also common in Hindu mythology. In Ramayana, Rama's brother Lakshmana drowned in the river Sarayu. Rama, having already lost his wife and mother, also drowns himself in the river with his other brothers. This prompted the people of Ayodya (his kingdom) to commit mass suicide by drowning. In a study of 148 pacts, it was found that women outnumber men in pacts, and that pacts were primarily due to social reasons rather than individual psychopathology. It can be considered a form of protest against archaic societal and religious norms (Vijayakujmar and Thilothamma 1993). Over a thousand persons died in suicide pacts in India in the year 2002. Some important reasons cited are love failure, and pacts by sisters due to worry about the inability to provide a dowry.

## Suicide in the Hindu diaspora

During the British colonization, large communities of people from India, with Hindu faith, settled in Malaysia, Mauritius, Fiji, Trinidad Guyana, Suriname, UK, Canada and other places. Studies on suicidal behaviour from these countries reveal that the suicide rate among persons of Indian origin (particularly that of young women), was much higher than among the native population. Hutchinson *et al*. (1999) report that 89 per cent of the suicides in Trinidad and Tobago were by people of east-Indian origin. Maharajah (1998) suggests that religious and cultural factors contribute to increased suicidal behaviour among Hindus. In Fiji, Haynes (1987) found that high rates of suicide were closely associated with Indian descent and Hindu faith. Maniam (1988), from a study in Malaysia, found that although Indians formed only 28 per cent of the population, they constituted 89 per cent of suicides and 78 per cent of the attempted suicides, and attributed the phenomenon to the ambivalent attitude to suicide among the Hindus, caste differences and arranged marriages. Bhugra (2004) also stated that in London, the rates of attempted suicide in South Asian women were 1.5 times higher than those in white women.

## Hindu religion as a protective factor

All the above information can be interpreted to suggest that being a Hindu places a person at a higher risk of suicide. However, a strong faith in Hinduism acts as protective factor. The Hindu belief in karma fosters a sense of acceptance of the vicissitudes of life with equanimity, and the belief in the cycle of births and deaths renders suicide meaningless, as one's soul continues after death. Their religious beliefs make Hindus tolerate and accept hardships and calamities stoically.

In Hinduism, looking after old parents is considered a major duty of the children, especially the sons. The common type of family structure is the extended family, with the parents living with their sons and sometimes even daughters. The elderly are generally not lonely, and are taken care of. Hindu religion also states that there are four stages of life, and in the last stage (usually after 60 years), one is supposed to detach oneself from worldly pleasures, and lead a life of simplicity, prayers and meditation. This policy provides a cultural support to the elderly, to tackle the problems associated with old age, and the emotional support that living with

children brings. The suicide rate for those above 60 years in India, is 9.7/100,000 (M = 12.4 and F = 7), lower than that of all age groups (above 14 years).

Whether it is individual faith that protects one against suicide or the social network associated with religion, that is, a protective factor, has been the focus of debate among suicidologists. In the Hindu religion, one does not belong to any temple. Anyone can go to any temple and pray to any God. The priests do not have social or community responsibilities, and their duties are confined to the temple. Hence, it can be surmised that in Hinduism, individual faith rather than a religious network plays a crucial role in reducing suicidality. A population-based psychological autopsy study in Chennai found significant differences in religiosity between those who committed suicide and those who live (Vijayakumar and Rajkumar 2003). Persons who committed suicide, had less belief in any God ($\chi^2$ 28.0, p < 0.001), had changed their religious affiliation (p <0.03), and rarely visited places of worship ($\chi^2$ 25.57, p < 0.001). The odds ratio for lack of belief in God was OR 6.83 (CI 2.88–19.69). In another case control study in Bangalore, Gururaj *et al*. (2004) also found that lack of religious belief was a risk factor for suicide (OR 19.18 CI 4.17–30.37).

Suicide in the Hindu religion can be conflicting and confusing. In India, attempted suicide is still a punishable offence according to the Indian Penal Code 309. The attitude is one of rejection when a suicidal behaviour is attributed to individual needs rather than family or societal needs. Religious suicides were accepted and tolerated. Sati, jauhar, sallekhana and mahaparasthana echo in present times, in the form of self-immolation of young women and fast until death protests. Hindu religious beliefs and the caste system are associated with arranged marriages and the system of dowry. Hence, marriages which are not sanctioned by the families (love marriages) and unmet dowry demands often lead to suicides by young women. These entrenched beliefs, which are culturally tolerated, are an impediment in preventing family suicides, dowry deaths and suicides due to love failures. However, a strong faith in Hindu religion is also a suicidal-counter. The ingrained belief in karma and rebirth increases the tolerance threshold, and there is greater acceptance of the vagaries of life. Externalization of traumas, failures and difficulties to karma makes it easier to cope with individual negative cognition and emotions. At the same time, hope is also extended: one can always hope for a better life or future if one leads a good life. The respect given to the elderly in the Hindu community and the Hindu philosophy of detaching oneself from the worldly pleasures as age advances, along with the fact that the majority of the elderly are taken care of by their children in Hindu families, lead to the uniquely low rates of suicide rates among the elderly. Hinduism is more a way of life than following a set of doctrines, and hence can be interpreted in many different ways. Suicide in Hinduism is interpreted according to the situation, the person and the reason for suicide. Generally suicides are condemned, but there are many instances where suicides have been celebrated. This ambiguity is reflected in contemporary India. In some situations, the Hindu religion acts as a protective factor; at other times it may increase the risk of suicide. It is important to understand these different nuances in the Hindu religion in formulating a suitable and culturally appropriate suicide prevention strategy. Ultimately, according to Hinduism, it is up to the individual to lead the life they wish to lead and to die correspondingly.

# References

Adityanjee DR (1986). Suicide attempts and suicides in India. Cross-cultural aspects. *International Journal of Social Psychiatry*, **32**, 64–73.

Bhatia SC and Khan MM (1987). High-risk suicide factors across cultures. *International Journal of Social Psychiatry*, **33**, 226–236.

Bhugra D (2004). *Culture and Self Harm. Attempted Suicide in South Asians in London*, pp. 8–40. (Maudsley monograph). Psychology Press, London.

Bhugra D (2005). Sati—a type of non-psychiatric suicide. *Crisis*, **26**, 73–77.

Etzersdorfer E, Vijayakumar L, Schony W *et al.* (1998). Attitude towards suicide among medical students—a comparison between Madras (India) and Vienna (Austria). *Social Psychiatry and Psychiatry Epidemiology*, **33**, 104–110.

Firth S (2005). End of life—a Hindu view. *The Lancet*, **366**, 682–686.

Gururaj G, Isaac MK, Subbakrishna DK *et al.* (2004). Risk factors for completed suicide: a case control study from Bangalore, India. *Injury Control and Safety Promotion*, **11**, 183–191.

Haynes R (1987). Suicide and social response in Fiji. *British Journal of Psychiatry*, **145**, 433–438.

Hutchinson G, Daisley H, Simson D *et al.* (1999). High rates of paraquat-induced suicide in southern Trinidad. *Suicide and Life-Threatening Behaviour*, **29**, 186–191.

Kamat's potpourri (2006). *Sati and Jauhar*. Retrieved 16 January 2006 from http://www.Kamat.com.

Kane PV (1941). *History of Dharmashastra*, v 2. pp. 925–927. Bhandarkar Oriental Research Institute, Pune.

Kane PV (1974). *The History of Dharmashastra*, pp. 6001–628. Bhandarkar Oriental Research Institute, Pune.

Leenaars A, Connolly J, Cantor C (2001). Suicide, assisted suicide and euthanasia—international perspectives. *The Irish Journal of Psychological Medicine*, **18**, 66–37.

Maharajh H (1998). Transgenerational cultural conflicts and suicide among Hindu girls in Trinidad. *Caribbean Medical Journal*, **60**, 16–15.

Maniam T (1988). Suicide and parasuicide in a hill resort in Malaysia. *British Journal of Psychiatry*, **153**, 222–225.

National Crime Records Bureau (2002). *Accidental deaths and suicides in India*. Ministry of Home Affairs, Government of India.

Pollisi C (2003). Universal rights and cultural relations. Hinduism and Islam deconstructed. *The Bologna Center Journal of International Affairs* Online edition, Spring, 2003. Retrieved 21 January 2006.

Rao AV (2006). *The Consolation of Psychiatry*, pp. 3–20. Compiled by Dr Parvathi Devi. Indian Psychiatric Society, Mumbai.

Rao AV, Mahendran N, Gopalakrishnan C *et al.* (1989). One hundred female burns cases: a study in suicidology. *Indian Journal of Psychiatry*, **31**, 43–50.

Roy BB (1987). *Socioeconomic Impact of Sati in Bengal*. Naya Prakash Publishers, Calcutta.

Soni RV, Bulusu L, Balarajan R (1990). Suicide among immigrants from the Indian subcontinent. *British Journal of Psychiatry*, **156**, 46–50.

Thakur U (1963). *The History of Suicide in India*, pp. 45–125. Oriental Publishers, New Delhi.

*The Hindu* (2002). Attempted self-immolation in government secretariat, Madras, India. Available at http://www.thehindu.com, accessed 2 January 2002.

TheHimalayan Academy (2006). *Hinduism*. Retrieved 20 January 2006 from http://www.Himalayanacademy.com.

Tousignant M, Seshadri S, Raj A (1988). Gender and suicide in India. *Suicide and Life-Threatening Behaviour*, **28**, 50–61.

Tukol TK (1976). *Sallekhana is not suicide*, pp. 11–112. Shivlal Jesalpura Swati Printing Press, LD Institute of Technology, Ahmedabad.

Vijayakumar L (2004). Altruistic suicide in India. *Archives of Suicide Research*, **8**, 73–80.

Vijayakumar L and Rajkumar S (2003). Psychosocial risk factors for suicide in India. In LVijayakumar, ed., *Suicide Prevention—Meeting the Challenge Together*, pp. 148–160. Orient Longman, Chennai, India.

Vijayakumar L and Thilothammal N (1993). Suicide pacts in India. *Crisis*, **14**, 43–46.

Vijayakumar L, John S, Pirkis J *et al.* (2005). Suicide in developing countries (2) Risk factors. *Crisis*, **26**, 112–119.

# CHAPTER 5

# A Buddhist perspective on suicide

## Somparn Promta and Prakarn Thomyangkoon

## Abstract

The basic morality of Buddhism is based on the content of the five precepts: killing is an evil; stealing is an evil; sexual misconduct is an evil; lying is an evil; and taking intoxicants is an evil.

Buddhism does not consider killing merely in its form but in its origin, and judges whether or not it is immoral case by case, according to its complicated and contextual factors. Suicide is a type of killing, and the moral rules applying to all types of killing, apply also to suicide. All of the precepts in Buddhism are written in general form, meaning that there is considerable room for interpretation. This chapter discusses interpretations of cases when suicide may be considered as morally wrong and when it can be morally acceptable. Generally speaking, suicide is not necessarily an evil in the Buddhist perspective: some are morally acceptable. All sects of Buddhism agree that death is just a transformation of life, and that we live to die and we die to live again. Therefore, suicide is viewed differently from other religions, which do not believe in life after death or reincarnation.

The chapter concludes with epidemiological data concerning suicide in different Buddhist countries in Asia, which show a range of 6/100,000 in Thailand to 35/100,000 in Sri Lanka. In accordance with the statistics, the Buddhist religion may impact the suicide rate differently depending on the national context.

## Suicide in Buddhist texts

### Killing in a Buddhist perspective

The first statement of the *Five Precepts* (*Pañca Sila*) found in the *Pali Canon* states that 'killing is an evil'. The content of the Five Precepts is:

1 Killing is an evil;

2 Stealing is an evil;

3 Sexual misconduct is an evil;

4 Lying is an evil; and

5 Taking intoxicants is an evil.

The Pali Canon is a collection of Buddha's teachings that were written down in the ancient Indian language Pali after his death (in Buddhist countries such as Thailand, the Pali Canon is usually called the Pali Tipitaka). The Pali Canon is very important for Buddhists: the Buddha said that after his death there would be no single master of Buddhism, instead his teachings would reign. Each of the 45 volumes contains about 500 pages and it is quite rare for monks to read all of it. There is a commentary to the Pali Canon written some 1000 years after Buddha's death, with interpretations and explanations of some unclear statements in Canon. These commentaries are contested by Buddhist university scholars.

Concerning the first of the Five Precepts, it is generally believed among Buddhists that the subjects concerned in this statement are both people and animals. Thus, according to the first precept, killing people or animals is morally wrong according to Buddhism. A brief introduction to the classification of present-day Buddhism follows. One common way to classify Buddhists is by dividing them into mahayana and theravada Buddhists. The mahayana are found mostly in China, Japan, Korea and Vietnam, and the theravada in Thailand, Burma, Sri Lanka, Laos and Cambodia. Some basic beliefs are shared by both groups, usually those concerned with the nature of Man and the universe. However, they hold different views about the nature of the Buddha: theravadans believe that the Buddha is a human being, while mahayanans believe that he is beyond humankind. Accordingly, there are at least two interpretations concerning killing: positive and negative. Generally, the mahayana Buddhists believe that the first precept covers both positive and negative forms of killing (Suzuki 1973), while the theravada Buddhists believe that it covers only the positive form (The Commentary to the Pali Canon 2003a). Positive killing means an action that leads directly to the death of a person or animal. For example, a person kills a dog with a knife—this is a positive killing. Negative killing is an action that leads to the death of a person or an animal indirectly. For example, a doctor lets a patient who is suffering greatly from some kind of incurable sickness dies by not giving further medical support. Such an action falls under the category of negative killing. The difference between the interpretations of the word 'killing' in theravada and mahayana leads to the two main different understandings of the first precept in Buddhism. For theravada Buddhists, this pertains only to direct killing; it does not cover indirect killing or letting someone die. In mahayana Buddhism, both positive and negative killings are intended in the first precept. As meat eating is considered by mahayana as a kind of negative killing, vegetarianism is widely practised among the mahayanists, but not by the theravada Buddhists. Although these two main factions of Buddhism have differing views on the meaning of killing, both agree that the killing stated in the first precept does not cover suicide. In the commentary to the Pali Canon of the theravada tradition, it is explicitly stated that killing under the first precept is the killing of another and not oneself (The Vimativinodani).

The commentary to the Pali Canon (2003b) says:

1   The Five Precepts is the moral standard for Buddhists, thus a person who commits suicide is at the outset *not* considered to be violating the moral standard taught in Buddhism.

2   However, suicide can originate from either bad or good motives.

There are three major forms of bad motives in Buddhist teaching: greed, hatred and ignorance. Among these three motives, it is believed that the last one, ignorance, plays an important role in relation to suicide. Ignorance takes many different expressions and forms. In those cases, where suicide is deemed to originate from bad motivations, the person who commits suicide could be viewed as doing an evil. However, such an evil is something placed outside the moral standard of Buddhism. This standard refers to the minimum requirement that sustains the moral life of the community and the individual. Without it, neither the individual nor the community can lead a good life. However, higher moral levels exist, and according to them, suicide because of bad motives is considered to be against such moral qualities. In brief, Buddhism does not consider a person who commits suicide as culpable as a person who kills another person, steals, commits sexual misconduct, lies or takes intoxicants. When a person violates the moral standard, he or she is considered a *bad person*, but if a person commits suicide, even if the suicide is performed as a result of bad reasons, they are simply deemed an *ignorant person*.

## The grounds for blaming a person in terms of morality

This view of suicide cannot be considered separately from the notion of how a person is to be blamed in terms of morality. The content of the Five Precepts suggests that a person should be held morally responsible when they harm another person or themselves. The first four precepts are concerned with harm toward another being and the fifth with harm toward oneself. Suicide is not included in the last precept, meaning that Buddhism does not consider a person who commits suicide as *necessarily* harming themselves. The use of intoxicants is an action that leads to the destruction of one's mental and physical health, and the devastating effect intoxicants have on people is often a long process. Intoxicants refers to alcohol, but the modern day interpretation would include other drugs such as heroin and cocaine. Suicide, however, is considered differently, and in some cases as discussed below, is considered as a better option than accepting the pains of life. Accordingly, suicide is not necessarily a sort of self-harm. For this reason, it is not included in any of the Five Precepts.

One of the basic assumptions of Buddhist ethics is that an individual can be morally blamed for an action that harms others or oneself. This broad moral criterion is of use in many circumstances. For example, if an action can be proved as not harming others or oneself it must be allowed, even though some Buddhists may be inclined to judge it as immoral from a common sense perspective or by religious feeling. In Thailand, for example, people generally think that suicide is an evil according to Buddhism, customarily judging it without knowing what the Buddhist teachings have to say about suicide. Even the monks have generally adopted the same view. Few Buddhists who know that such verdicts on suicide are not in accordance with the Buddhist teaching and stories in the Pali Canon.

## Suicide in the Pali Canon

Many cases of suicide appear in the Pali Canon. In this chapter, we will consider some of them in order to provide a broader perspective on the Buddhist outlook on suicide. Before plunging into the stories, it may be useful to define the term 'suicide'. Suicide can be considered both in form and content. Considered in its form, any action performed by a person that leads to his or her own death can be called a suicide. Considering its content, suicide can originate from various motives and objectives. An example can be a young man whose heart is broken who commits suicide. The motivation that leads to his suicide can be interpreted as an extremely demoralized state of mind: the boy is overwhelmed by the feeling that his love is meaningless in the eyes of the girl. The objective of his suicide could simply be to set himself free from the oppression of mind, or to take revenge on the girl by announcing his death as a result of his denied love. There is a difference between such suicides and those committed by a person whose main motivation and objective are to fight against something for public interest. In Thailand, a state official whose responsibility was to protect the wild life in the deep Thai forest decided to commit suicide in order to direct the public's attention to the great corruption among the policy-makers and managers of forest preservation programmes. This famous case is considered a suicide for the benefit of society. Suicide can be triggered by very different emotions and objectives but with the same result, the taking of one's own life.

In some cases, defining the taking of one's life as suicide is complicated. Imagine a mother and her children confronted with a tiger; the mother sees no other choice but to sacrifice her own life in order to save her children. She gives her life to the tiger and her children safely run away. Is this a suicide? Using the definition given above, this will count as suicide. In short, suicide is mainly considered in its form. If a person does something that leads to his or her death, it will be considered a suicide.

The following instances of suicide as defined above are found in the Pali Canon.

## Buddha's sermon

Once before a personal retreat, the Buddha gave a sermon to a large group of monks. In the sermon, the analysis of life as something empty of essence was considered. After hearing the sermon, some monks felt that life was a meaningless and sad state, and consequently committed suicide. Some monks could not commit suicide by themselves and thus asked other monks to kill them instead. No one reported this event to the Buddha as he was known to prefer solitude during his retreats. The two-week retreat passed, and the Buddha discovered that the number of his disciples was greatly reduced. After hearing what happened, the Buddha commanded the monks in the monastery to hold a gathering. During the assembly, the Buddha did not mention anything about the monks who themselves committed suicide. He only brought up the monks who killed other monks at request and said: 'This cannot be done. A monk must not kill even upon request.'

It should be noted that the above event led to the setting up of the *Third Defeat Rule* (*Tatiyaparajika*). A Buddhist monk must not violate the four defeat rules:

1 Sexual intercourse;

2 Stealing;

3 Killing a human being; and

4 Claiming to possess higher moral qualities which do not exist (The Pali Canon 2003a).

Why did the Buddha not set up a rule prohibiting suicide? This question is very important. The following story from the Pali Canon about a monk who committed suicide may provide us with a deeper understanding of the question.

## The dukkatam

The Pali Canon tells the story of a monk who was seriously demoralized by the desire that had taken over his mind. The monk was not happy with his life and inner voices suggested that he give up his life as a monk; leading to constant inner conflict for him. After trying to overcome this unwanted desire in every possible way, he deemed himself defeated, decided to commit suicide and threw himself from a cliff. Inadvertently, he fell on a man below, causing the man's death. The monk was unsure as to whether or not he had violated the *Third Defeat Rule*. Upon asking the Buddha for advice, Buddha questioned him about his state of mind and intentions when he threw himself off the cliff. The monk replied that he did not mean to harm anybody; he just wanted to die. The Buddha said, 'You do not violate the third defeat rule as you did not kill this man intentionally.' The story ends with the Buddha's statement that no monk should throw himself from a cliff to commit suicide, and he sets up a new monastic rule that if any monk violates this rule he will be given an offence (a punishment) called '*dukkatam*'. The monastic rule set up by the Buddha as a result of this event simply states that no monk should throw himself from a high place. The reason for such a prohibition is the safety of others, not in order to prohibit suicide: the rule is the result of one monk's carelessness and a protective measure to save people from the harm of others. If a monk transgresses the preceding monastic rule he is given a very small offence, '*dukkatam*', which is in fact the term used in the Buddhist monastic rules that refers to the smallest offence (The Pali Canon 2003b). Once again, we see that suicide is overlooked by the Buddha.

## Irreproachable suicide

The story of the senior monk Channa is the best known one among scholars of Buddhism. Once Channa was seriously ill and his illness made it impossible for him to perform his religious duties. He told his fellow senior monks that his illness was so strong that he thought it was useless to live and said 'I will commit suicide. But don't worry; I will commit suicide *in such a way that no one can fault me*.' Other senior monks asked him to reconsider the

decision to commit suicide. However, Channa insisted and finally committed suicide. His fellow senior monks asked the Buddha what he thought about Channa's deed. The Buddha said:

> Channa said before his death that he would commit suicide in a way that no one could reproach him. If a man thinks that after death he will leave his unwanted body and take another one which is more desirable and then commits suicide, then this action should be condemned. However, Channa did not do this and committed suicide in an irreproachable way.

In this story, the Buddha gives his opinion on suicide, but his opinion is in relation to a specific event. This event cannot be used as a general conclusion to Buddha's view on suicide. However, this example is useful in order to understand Buddhism's general standpoint on suicide. Channa is a senior follower of Buddha and thus understands the teaching of Buddha well. He knows that illness is one of the sufferings taught in Buddhism. Before committing suicide, other senior monks spoke with him, and his devotion to the understanding of Buddhism are unmistakable. Channa's suicide is based on at least two important factors: first, he commits suicide as Buddha's follower, aware of what the essence of Buddhism is; second, the motivation that leads to his suicide can be viewed as an act of natural self-defence. Channa knows well that illness is a fact of life, yet his illness is special. Normally, the human body's defence system will cease to work after a certain point of unbearable pain, and we die. The illness confronted by Channa reaches an insupportable point, but he does not die. Furthermore, the Pali Canon tells us that Channa has experienced this painful illness for a long time. This leads Channa to think that his life in that state is not worth anything. He knows that sickness is a natural event in life, but his specific sickness makes his life useless both for himself and others, and decides to commit suicide to free himself from the old useless body and take a new one in the next life by which he can do good things (The Pali Canon 2003c). What Channa does can be compared to getting out of a car that is stuck in traffic and then getting into another one in order to move ahead, and this is a natural process for Buddhists.

## Buddha's self-sacrifice

This story is from the *Jataka*. It is said that one time, a long time ago, the Buddha was born as a rabbit and lived in the forest with three animal friends. One day a Brahmin came to that forest. Other animals offered food to the Brahmin, but the rabbit had no food. So he jumped into the fire to give himself up as food for the Brahmin (The Pali Canon 2003d). As defined above, any action leading to one's own death is counted as suicide; hence, the rabbit's action could be considered as a suicide of the sort that is praised by Buddhism.

## Interpretations of the texts

The issue of Buddhism's view on suicide is controversial and interpreted quite differently by various Buddhist scholars. The following interpretations are those by the authors of this chapter, and are mainly based on the above stories.

### The general view on good and evil

A discussion concerning the Buddhist perspective on suicide cannot take place without considering the core ethical thoughts of Buddhism itself. The question of what human life is plays an important role in determining how people of different religious backgrounds think about suicide. For example, if you believe that your life is created by God, and that there is a life after this one, suicide seems to be an immoral as well as irrational action. It is irrational because even though you are suffering in life, only as long as you still live can you get something out of life. Despite this, if you think that there is nothing left for you to live for and that life is unbearable, suicide is an option. The options are getting something and getting nothing, and the former seems preferable. If you believe in a heaven with better conditions than on earth and that entry into this heaven is dependent on your acceptance of life despite your sufferings, then suicide is sinful. In contrast, if you believe that your life originates from nature, and that you will be reborn again and again, suicide is not as serious for you.

Buddhism teaches us that human life is created by nature and that we will be reborn after what is elsewhere considered as death. Buddhists do not believe in an almighty God, but believe that human life and the world are governed by natural laws. Five major laws of nature regulate the universe. Among these five laws, the law of karma deems actions performed by human beings as evil or good actions. In brief, the law of karma states that if something is evil, it is because you render it evil, hence you are ultimately responsible for it. An example of something that is considered as an evil in Buddhism is poison. If you consume a poison without knowing that it is in fact a poison, you are nevertheless responsible for your actions. According to the ethics of Buddhism, learning is a process through which you learn to distinguish between good and evil; similarly to how one distinguishes between what is good and what is bad for health in medical science. Knowledge is very important in Buddhist ethics. Knowledge in this context means the ability to be able to reason what should be considered as good and bad.

In the case of suicide, there are a large amount of conditions that give rise to a variety of suicides. It is possible that the Buddha considers suicide a question to be examined individually and hence does not give any fixed criterion to judge such an act. In Buddhism, any statement concerning morality can be examined deeply, and by doing this we may find that after a process of analysis what we consider as bad may not be as bad as we think. For example, killing is an evil according to the first precept. However, all the precepts in Buddhism are written in general forms, meaning that interpretations of these precepts may lead to different outcomes. Thus, euthanasia in some cases can be accepted by Buddhist ethics. In short, the core ethics of Buddhism are based on self-judgement and choice.

## Values of life and death

In Buddhism, death is treated in an interesting manner. First, death is not considered as a problem in the course of human life. Buddhism distinguishes between the facts and the problems of life: death is a fact of life while fear of death is a problem. In general, Buddhism considers three forms of desires as the problems of human life: desire for sensual pleasures, desire for existence, and desire for non-existence. Desire for existence basically means having the desire to achieve importance in the eyes of others. A need to be respected by others is the basic form of desire for existence. However, this kind of desire has more subtle forms, such as the self-preservation instinct. Fear of death is used by humans and animals to protect their lives in every possible way and is thus a sort of desire for existence. If we had no fears, we would lead shorter lives. Desires, in Buddhist teaching, are found deep inside of us and we

are unable to observe them directly. The third form of desire can be related to some kinds of suicide. A young boy asks his parents to allow him to go to a party. His parents do not let him go and he subsequently commits suicide. According to Buddhism, the action of the boy could be explained as related to the three forms of desire. First, he wants to go to the party, directed by his desire for sensual pleasures. When he is denied, his mind is oppressed, which is controlled by a desire for existence. Buddhism explains that desire for existence functions in pushing us to do anything to make us meaningful in the eyes of others. Not allowing the boy to go to the party is an event that is contradictory to his wishes, and by extension, his desire for existence. The unsatisfied existence leads to an oppressed state of mind. According to Buddhism, there are two possible outcomes of this state of mind. Either the desire for non-existence will kick in, or wisdom will turn things around for the better. In the case of the boy, the first thing happens, an unwise desire for non-existence leads him to consider and later commit suicide. The difference between the two states is that the desire for non-existence is irrational, while the state of wisdom is insightful and rational. Hence, to commit suicide in this case is a blind and irrational way out because it is governed by desire for non-existence.

In the case of suicides thought to originate from desires, they are not considered whether they lead to death or not. The immorality in such an action is considered from the origin of its desires. In other words, Buddhist ethics stress the means and not the ends. Killing is bad because it originates from hatred, which is a form of desire. Certainly, killing leads to death but that is not the main point. The Buddha says, 'I said, O monks, intention is action' (The Pali Canon 2003e). If our intentions are good, that makes our action good: if we have bad intentions, our action is bad. The suicide of the boy described above is bad because it originates from what is considered flawed intentions.

Even though death is not a problem in human life, this does not mean that Buddhism endorses death. In the *Dhammapada*, the Buddha said that a short life that knows truth is preferred over a long life filled with ignorance (The Pali Canon 2003f). This means that Buddhism does not consider the values of life in terms of longevity, but through its contents. Death usually affects our life in terms of time and not quality, so ultimately death does not affect human life greatly. In the Pali Canon, the Buddha says that the most powerful enemy of human beings is the mind that is wrongly trained, and not death (The Pali Canon 2003g). Buddhism teaches us to look at death as a friend. In the Tibetan Buddhist tradition, death is viewed as something beautiful (Thurman 1994). Generally, all factions of Buddhism agree that death is just a transformation of life. When we talk about life in its fullest meaning, we must talk about both living and dying. The living life is compared to a day, while life, in a state of death, is compared to a night. Both days, and nights are equally important. We live to die and we die to live again. Consequently, death is similar to a dream. After a dream, we will be awakened again. However, as Buddhism believes in karma, the state of mind before death has some importance. A person with good bodily and mental health usually has good dreams. Similarly, a person who accumulates good karma before dying usually dies with a peaceful mind and that peaceful mind will lead to a good state in the life after death. Suicide performed by a broken-down mind will lead to a bad state in the life after death: if suicide is performed by a pure mind, the state of life after death will be good. The case of Channa is an example of this kind of suicide.

The view of suicide performed by a pure mind raises serious issues among the scholars of Buddhism who believe that it is paradoxical to have a pure mind and commit suicide. For them, the senior monk Channa's suicide is problematic alongside the fact that he is well aware of the deceitfulness of the three forms of desire. Channa's mind is not governed by ignorance. Before committing suicide, there is no evidence showing that Channa is an *arahanta* (a totally liberated person in Buddhist teaching). The commentary to the Tipitaka notes that during the short process of committing suicide, Channa has a quick insight resulting from the pain, and that insight liberates him into a state of *arahanta* (The Commentary to the Pali Canon 2003c). According to the commentary, Channa becomes a liberated person, so there can not be anything wrong with his actions, hence Buddha's reasoning that 'Channa commits suicide in an irreproachable way.'

We do not know exactly what happened during the short period of Channa's dying, yet the commentary gives us the most reasonable argument for Buddha's judgement of Channa's case. However, there are other ways to explain this event. One is that Channa's suicide has nothing to do with the three forms of desire; it is governed purely by natural command. Consider this example: when we get sick we take medicine. It is believed that a liberated person who gets ill will do the same thing as we do. Taking medication against an illness is considered to be an activity governed by natural command; it is no different from eating when hungry or drinking when thirsty. Suppose the illness cannot be cured by any medicine in the world and the only way to stop it is to die? Some Buddhists would in this situation consider suicide. The question is: suppose a liberated person gets such an illness, would this person then choose to commit suicide? In some cases, stopping incurable suffering by ending one's life can be viewed as an extension of using medication. The Buddha himself does not mention this; but in a famous Buddhist text named *The Question of King Milinda*, there is a passage that could be interpreted that it is in fact impossible for an enlightened person to commit suicide (The Milindapañha 2003). However, the context discussed in *The Question of King Milinda* is quite different from the one discussed above. In that text, King Milinda asks 'As Nirvana is believed to be the highest peace, why does the enlightened person whose body is governed by natural sufferings, such as sickness, not commit suicide to enter Nirvana?' The sufferings denoted by the king are normal ones, such as old age, sickness and other natural physical demands such as hunger: even ordinary people who undergo such sufferings generally do not commit suicide, much less *arahantas*. The king does not understand why a liberated person who is not experiencing actual sufferings yet, but who may, like everyone else, one day have to confront potential sufferings, does not leave his body in order to avoid such bodily sufferings and enter Nirvana straight away. According to the text it is not in the nature of a liberated person to commit suicide in order to leave this life for Nirvana. Yet with pain such as that affecting Channa, even persons with deep knowledge of Buddhist teachings may choose to commit suicide. Consequently, we have reason to believe that worldly persons would do the same thing.

## A rational approach to life

Even though life is a valuable thing, this does not mean that the value of life can be considered separately from its conditions. Buddhism teaches us that our body possesses values so that we can use it to do good things; however, the body can be used to do bad things as well.

In the Buddhist *abhidhamma*, the body is morally neutral like other physical objects in the world (Thepwisutthimethi *et al.* 1989). In one sense, the body can be viewed as an instrument used by the mind to do valuable and good things, but it differs from other instruments in that it sometimes causes pain. The pain caused by the body are of great variety, yet we can distinguish between normal pain and abnormal pain. Normal pain is that which can be cured by medicine or medical practice; it does not affect us to the extent that we cannot use the body any more—a normal headache is as an example of this kind of pain. Abnormal pain cannot be cured and hinders the person from using their body. The pain occurring in Channa's case can be cited as an example of this kind of pain.

The significance of 'the body cannot be used any more' is not necessarily strict. In the case of Channa, the pain does not make him lose his mental ability to think, but it does make him unable to do what should be done as a Buddhist monk. We can imagine other cases in which pain hinders a person from doing what has been the main meaning of his or her life. The pianist who loses her finger control, suffers greatly from the pain in her hands and cannot accomplish her tasks as a pianist, is a person who is confronted with an abnormal pain. For this kind of person, it seems there is a possibility of *rational* suicide. Human life, according to Buddhist teaching, is much associated with rationality. Rationality in philosophy means several things; but in Buddhism it means 'doing what is proper to a specific situation'. Yet Buddhism does not teach situational ethics. It believes in some unchanged moral standards, but also says that to attain the unchanged goodness there can be several ways suitable for different persons and different situations. For example, one of the basic teachings of Buddhism is carefulness of mind (*appamada*). When a person drives with carefulness, it means driving in a way that is safest for them in that situation. The doctrine of carefulness does not teach that you must drive at a certain speed at all times. Rather, rationality in Buddhism suggests doing what is appropriate for a specific situation; which means that we can and should modify things to fit changing situations.

A rational approach sometimes means thinking 'why do I do what I do?'. The great Buddhist thinker of Thailand, Buddhadasa Bhikkhu, said that according to Buddhism, to be born as a human being entails questioning 'Why am I born?' (The Pali Canon 2003h). A person who never questions this should not be counted as a human being even though he or she possesses human DNA. In other words, living without questioning why I live is being alive without rationality—it is merely living by instinct. With the help of rationality, we will know how to distinguish between two or more things occurring in our life at the same time and know which one is the better. Suppose a man is seriously ill and suffers very much from that illness, he thinks: 'There are two things I can do now. The first is to live and the second to die. Between these two things, which one is the best for me?' According to Buddhism, the man is using rationality to decide about his life. As Buddhism believes that no one can set up the rules of living for another person, he himself is the best one to know how to do the best thing for him. Rationality in living thus depends on personal wisdom. In the case of Channa, we see that no one except Channa himself is the best person to know how to deal with his suffering. The Buddha always said that he is merely a guide; to walk along the right way is the duty and responsibility of each follower, the Buddha cannot choose which way to go or what thing to do for his followers (Keown 1996). During a journey on the same road to Nirvana, a person has their personal pattern of life which differs from that of others: this personal difference found in each one makes it impossible for a person to make a decision solely on the grounds of religious dogmas. Certainly, Buddhism believes that as a Buddhist one has to follow some religious recommendations, but this does not mean that the person should not use their rationality. On the contrary, sometimes blindly following religious doctrines could harm even a faithful practitioner. Religious doctrines taught in Buddhism are given in general forms, meaning that normally a person should follow them but they can be modified if the person comes to the conclusion that it is more reasonable to do things other than stated in these religious dogmas.

Some scholars of Buddhism argue that between life and death, Buddhism values the former (The Commentary to the Pali Canon 2003d). This should be considered as a general view as noted above, meaning that, in general, Buddhism thinks that we should choose life, not death, yet in some cases, it is possible that choosing life seems unreasonable when compared with choosing death. In this case, the principle of rationality in Buddhism advises us to choose the best thing for ourselves.

### The separation of brain and mind

In the Buddhist perspective, the brain is included in what is considered the body. The brain and the mind however are not the same thing. In the Pali Canon, it is clearly stated that a person with some kind of mental illness is included in a group of people whose actions cannot be considered as morally right or wrong. When a person purely acts with the help of the brain, their condition is considered no different from that of a machine. Some mental illnesses prevents the mind from functioning, in which case a person cannot know who they are. Moral actions must originate from the mind and not from the brain. A person who can judge whether or not their body can be used is a person whose brain functions normally. One distinguishes between pains in the brain and disorders of the brain. A person who is in great pain, from a brain tumor for example, may feel that they cannot live anymore and consequently consider suicide. A person who is considered as not having a properly functioning mind and commits suicide will be judged differently. This person's suicide should not be judged in terms of morality.

## Suicide as private action

By and large, the basic moral teachings of Buddhism stress avoiding harming one another. All private actions are of importance according to the basic moral teachings. Human actions that can be interpreted as negative moral qualities are classified into two categories. The first is an act that harms another person and the second is an act that harms only the doer. The person who commits the first kind of action is called 'a bad person'. Hence, if you kill another person you are a *bad* person. You can hate and harm others but you cannot hate and harm yourself intentionally. Consequently, one can only be a bad person in relation to someone other than oneself. A person who does harmful things to themself merely acts out of ignorance. It is believed that no one would do a bad thing to themself if they know that it is a bad thing. Buddhism distinguishes between being a bad person and being a fool. According to the Buddhist teachings concerning human action, the act of suicide should be thought of as originating from self-love and not self-hatred. However, there are two kinds of self-love: right and not right. The one that may be deemed as not right is the one that is governed by ignorance.

When applying these criteria to suicide, it is considered a personal choice performed by a person and affecting only that person according to the principle of karma; consequently, the person who commits suicide is not a bad person in terms of morality. Certainly, such a person could be considered a fool, or someone who does not think before acting. Not thinking before acting is not unusual, and the moral responsibility of a foolish person or for a foolish act is not the same as the reprimand or blame a *bad person* receives. It is of course possible that the suicide of a person may affect the family they leave behind. However, if the person has no intention of creating suffering for the people around them, their action is not deemed as bad karma. This does not mean that Buddhism thinks that a person should not think of others before deciding to commit suicide. On the contrary, Buddhism stresses that you must not think of yourself only, an objective reached through attained wisdom. Considering the case of Channa, as a monk he has been trained to think of himself as a member of a big family which is the community or the whole world. Buddhism thinks that the process of thinking of others may finally result in deciding to commit suicide, as we will see in the case of the commentary to the Vinaya. Regarding the so-called survivors of a suicide, they are advised to consider the person's position and ignorance, and to understand them. Perhaps this understanding might help people to come to terms with such a loss. In the Pali Canon, the monks ask Buddha what Channa's family thought about his suicide. The answer from the Buddha was that the family should understand him.

The burial rites for those who commit suicide are no different than for those who die a natural death. However, at the funeral of important or notable people in Thailand, it is common to ask the king to be present, but this is not done if the person has committed suicide. Recently, a very famous person in Bangkok was believed to have committed suicide. Normally, the king would be present at his funeral, but his family did not ask him as they were not sure that he died a natural death. This is not a Buddhist tradition, however, and may be a result of other cultural traditions, perhaps stemming from Hinduism, as they have been interpreted by the Thai royal family.

## Thoughts on suicide and Buddhism

As discussed in the text above, the Buddhist texts do not view suicide as something morally bad in itself. The reasons are as follows:

1   Suicide is a private action.

2   A person is advised to use the principles of rationality, meaning that to choose between living and dying is up to each and every person. In some cases, living is considered the reasonable choice, and a person should not commit suicide. Yet, in some cases, death could be more reasonable, thus committing suicide could be deemed appropriate. In the theravadan commentary to the *Vinaya* one of the three major parts of the Pali Canon, it is clearly stated that if a monk is seriously ill, but medicine and other monks to take care of him are available, staying alive is preferable. However, even if medicine and other monks to take care of him are available, if the sick monk sees that his illness causes burden to the other monks,

considering giving up the medication and dying is the proper thing to do. The commentary also says that if the sick monk considers that his illness could make him lose the spiritual heights he has attained, considering giving up food and dying is deemed a proper action. The advice from the commentary above can be cited as the example of using the principle of rationality practised in the community of Buddhist monks. In general, there is no difference between theravadans and mahayanans concerning suicide. This paper mainly explores suicide from the theravdada perspective because it is the original and most conservative form of Buddhism. In both theravada and mahayana Buddhism, suicide is accepted in the form of self-sacrifice for the benefits of others, but mahayana seems to stress this view more than theravada. In mahayana texts, statements saying that self-sacrifice is a good thing are frequent, while in theravada texts there are fewer statements of this kind. Theoretically, lay persons are thought to have lesser moral qualities than the monks, so it will be difficult to find someone committing a suicide similar to Channa's. Consequently, most suicides committed by lay persons could be viewed as wrong by Buddhism, except the ones performed for the love of family or society.

3 In some situations suicide can be viewed as a just and rational act. The advice in the commentary to the *Vinaya* is based on the belief that if we find that committing suicide leads to the well-being or utility of other persons involved, such a suicide is done on the grounds of good intentions and is consequently not bad. Likewise, in the case that suicide is not for another person's best interests but for one's own, when protecting something more valuable than just living, such as the jhana, considering committing suicide is accepted. Jhana is a meditative state of profound stillness and concentration in which the mind becomes fully immersed and absorbed in the chosen object of attention. Jhana is temporary, meaning that it may be attained and lost again, for example because of physical ill-health. At the time of the Buddha, some monks who had attained jhana but later lost it because of bad health, committed suicide when they had recovered and regained the state of jhana. They did this in order to die when their minds were in jhana; a way to defend the most valuable thing in a person's life which can be destroyed by a serious illness.

4 Suicide in the Buddhist perspective cannot be considered separately from the Buddhist belief in rebirth. There are two forms of rebirth: the first is good and the second bad. Before death, a person will know to which one they are heading, depending on the kind of life they have led. Suicide performed by a person with an unworthy existence and for irrational reasons will lead to a bad rebirth. Conversely, a justified suicide will lead to a good rebirth. Some monks, described in the Pali Canon, commit suicide thinking that if they die during the state of jhana they will be reborn in the world of Brahma. It happens that a person who has led a good life according to the Buddhist ethics considers taking their life if seriously ill: 'I am serious ill, but previously I led a good life, if I die now, my rebirth would be a good one. Why do I live to suffer from this illness? This is irrational.' In such a case, it seems as though this person cannot be held accountable by Buddhist ethics.

5 Even though there are some cases in which suicide is not deemed as sinful in a Buddhist perspective, it is generally believed that most people commit suicide because of a 'bad mind'. Suicide in this meaning is a wrong action. However, its wrongness differs greatly from the immorality found in actions that harm another person. Society should view a person who commits suicide differently from a person who kills another person. It is possible that those who commit suicide and kill others do such things because of similar reasons, but as suicide is a private action that harms only the karma of the person who commits the act, this person must be treated differently from a person who harms others in society.

## Thoughts on Buddhism and biomedical ethics

The view of Buddhism on possible rational suicide may be useful in terms of biomedical ethics. Suppose we accept that a person has a strong reason to die, then asking for a doctor-assisted suicide is possible. There is one important teaching widely practised in any sect of Buddhism, which is the preparation for death. In Tibetan Buddhism, there is a kind of literature dealing specifically with the preparation for dying. It seems that one major meaning of the preparation for death is that we should know when to die. Sometimes a proper time to die is before we lose the mental ability to judge what is good and what is bad. Serious illness in some situations leads us to such a state. Hence, the question arises as to why we should not end life before our mental abilities deteriorate completely.

## Suicide in Buddhist society

Most of the Buddhist countries are in Asia. China has the largest Buddhist population in the world, while Mongolia has the highest population percentage of Buddhists in the world, about 98 per cent. Over 90 per cent of the population in Thailand, Bhutan, Japan, Taiwan and Hong Kong are Buddhist.

Table 5.1 shows the suicide rate and percentage of Buddhists in Asian countries. We have not included Vietnam where a large number of Buddhists live, as there are no official statistics from Vietnam. Statistically, it seems that there is no exact correlation between the percentage of Buddhists and the countries' respective suicide rates. By this we mean that high rates can be found in countries with different percentages of Buddhists in the

**Table 5.1** Suicide rates within the Buddhist population in Asian countries

| Country | Suicide rate (per 100,000 population) | % of Buddhists |
|---|---|---|
| Thailand | 7.3 | 95 |
| China, Hong Kong SAR | 15.3 | 93 |
| China | 20.8; 23.2 | 80 |
| Sri Lanka | 23.9 | 76.7 |
| Singapore | 9.9 | 61 |
| South Korea | 26.1 | 48 |

population, such as Sri Lanka where 76.7 per cent of the population are Buddhists, and the suicide rate is 23.9 per 100,000, whereas in South Korea, 48 per cent are Buddhists and the suicide rate is 26.1 per 100,000.

Most Asian Buddhist countries have suicide rates of two digits, disregarding whether they are considered developed or developing countries. The suicide rates in Table 5.1 lead us to the conclusion that there is no direct correlation between the percentage of Buddhists and the suicide rate (Department of Mental Health 2007; Hendin *et al.* 2008).

In Thailand, the ratio of male to female suicide rates was reported to be 3:1 (Thomyangkoon *et al.* 2005, Lotrakul 2006). The highest suicide rate was among young males aged 25–29 and 30–39 in 2001 and 2006 respectively. Hanging is the most common suicide method in Thailand and Japan, while jumping from a height is the most common method of suicide in Hong Kong and Singapore (Ojima *et al.* 2005; Yip and Tan 1998). As shown in Table 5.1, Thailand has the lowest suicide rate among the six Asian countries listed. The highest suicide rate recorded in Thailand was 8.6 per 100,000 in the year 1997 during a time of serious economic crisis.

## Buddhism in practice: north-eastern Thailand

Thailand has the lowest amount of suicides among the Buddhist countries. Thailand and Sri Lanka are well known as the countries where theravada Buddhism is common. However, the suicide rates differ greatly between these two countries. They are similar in that the academic study of Buddhism has been widely practised in both places, which means that theoretically, the Thai and Sri Lankan people learn and know the teachings of the Buddha in a similar way (Swearer and Promta 2000). Drawing on this we may assume first that Buddhism differs in theory and practice according to the specific cultural history of where it is practised, and second that knowing what Buddhism teaches does not qualify as a suicide prevention in itself. However, it is important to remember that suicide rates are a correlation of different elements in which religion cannot be separated from other socio-economic, cultural and historic factors. Furthermore, there is limited sociological data concerning suicide in Thailand and other Buddhist countries: these are comments on the data available today.

Among the Thai people, the north-eastern region has the lowest suicide rates. At present, Thailand has four major regions with a total of 60,617,200 inhabitants: the north-eastern is the biggest region with a population of 20,759,908. According to the report of the National Statistical Office of Thailand in 2003, 33.5 per cent of all Thai families work in the agricultural sector and live in villages. Among them, nearly half, 45.6 per cent live in the northeast (National Statistical Office 2003a). In the north-east part of Thailand, the practice of Buddhist teaching has been dominant for a long time and most of the Buddhist monks in Thailand are from the north-eastern part of the country. Furthermore, most of the great Buddhist saints in Thailand are north-eastern residents and of north-eastern origin. There is one major school of meditation among the most important meditation schools in Thailand created by these north-eastern Buddhist saints. The practice of Buddhist teaching of the north-eastern people has a unique element that is rarely found in other places. Every Buddhist holy day (a month has four Buddhist holy days), people in the village will stay together at the monastery all day and night. Consequently, the people in the community know each other. At night, the abbot of the monastery usually gives a friendly talk to the people (a formal talk about the teaching of Buddhism is held in the daytime). This time is a time for people with personal problems to talk with the senior monk. This tradition leads to close relationships between the villagers and diminishes feelings of loneliness, since people have something to do every day (normally people in the village have to go to the monastery at least two times a day to give alms to the monks at 08.00 and 11.00). Additionally, in cases where someone has personal problems, especially serious emotional difficulties, the community has already designated trustworthy persons to take care of such events (normally the abbot of the monastery, who is highly respected by the villagers, is the person to do this job).

Buddhism in the north-east of Thailand is practised on a daily basis with regard to a variety of different aspects of daily life. Buddhism here is not merely words in the Pali Canon or practised only by the monks, it could be called a *sociological morality*. By sociological morality we mean morality that is expressed in the way of life of people in the community. *Doctrinal morality* on the other hand is morality as it is written in the texts or spoken of by people. Sociological morality is often closely linked to doctrinal morality, and these concepts are difficult to separate in practice. When attempting to compare the comparatively low suicide rates of Thailand with those of other Buddhist countries, the concept of sociological morality proves helpful. It is possible that the low suicide rates found in Thailand, as compared to other countries with important Buddhist populations, are related to the practice of everyday Buddhism and the sense of community described above. If loneliness is a major cause of suicide, sociological morality seems to play a significant role in preventing people from committing suicide. Moreover, Table 5.1 reveals that generally the more economically developed Buddhist countries have higher rates of suicide than those considered as developing countries (with the exception of Sri Lanka). This might be related to what we refer to as sociological morality and the lack thereof in the growing urban centres of the more economically developed countries.

## Final thoughts on suicide in Thailand

To Buddhists, life is deemed as valuable, and death should be avoided if there is no reasonable argument against it. Thus, the approach to suicide prevention should be that of the moral responsibility of society as a whole. Ultimately, as Buddhism never blames a person who commits suicide in the same way it blames a person who harms another person, the view of the public towards a person who commits suicide should be different. It is not generally known that suicide is accepted in Buddhism, and from experience we know that many Buddhists in Thailand consider suicide as morally wrong. However, as discussed in the first part of this chapter, suicide is not a crime and can at worst be judged as a foolish alternative. Buddhism accepts that some sicknesses may devastate our lives entirely, and that in such a circumstance where death is the only way to end the suffering, it would be irrational not to end one's life.

By interviewing patients who attempted suicide, as well as their relatives, the first author of this chapter has come to understand that suicide is generally considered a sin. Most monks also believe and teach that committing suicide is a sin. The Department of

Mental Health and the Ministry of Public Health has launched a mental health programme to educate monks so that they can help with suicide prevention. During the economic crisis, a couple of years ago when the suicide rate was increasing, a famous monk, in a radio broadcasting campaign aimed at suicide prevention, said that animals do not commit suicide and why then should people who are considered superior creatures to animals do so. Another famous monk, Puttatas Bhiku, held a sermon at the same time, trying to calm people down and hinder them from taking their lives by emphasizing that you do not have any material possessions when you are born and likewise when you die—you can not take anything with you. It is quite common that people in times of suffering consult a monk in order to find the origin of one's suffering and the means to stop it. Practicing religious rituals and giving things to others is suggested as a way to relieve people from suffering. Becoming a monk for a short time is a way to avoid bad times for men, whilst women may wear white cloth, practice meditation and not break eight rules for a period of time. We believe that the Buddhist teachings of compassion lead Thai Buddhists to tolerate suicide, even though by common sense they think of it as wrong. A sense of compassion here means understanding or trying to understand why others act the way they do. In conclusion, it can be said that Buddhism has a direct and indirect influence on the views of people towards suicide.

## References

Department of Mental Health (2007). *Suicide report 1997–2006*. Ministry of Public Health of Thailand, Bangkok.

Hendin H, Phillips M, Vijayakumar L *et al* (eds). (2008). *Suicide and Suicide Prevention in Asia*. World Health Organization, Geneva.

Keown D (1996). Buddhism and suicide: the case of Channa. *The Journal of Buddhist Ethics*, **3**, 31.

Lotrakul M (2006). Suicide in Thailand during the period 1998–2003. *Psychiatry and Clinical Neuroscience*, **60**, 90–95.

National Statistical Office (2003a). *Agricultural census of Thailand and North-eastern region*. Bangkok, Thailand.

National Statistical Office (2003b). *The population of Thailand*. Bangkok, Thailand.

Ojima T, Nakamura Y, Detels R (2005). Comparative study about methods of suicide between Japan and the United States. *Journal of Epidemiology*, **14**, 187–192.

Suzuki DT, trans. (1973). *The Lankavatara Sutra*, chapter 8. Routledge and Kegan Paul, London.

Swearer DK, and Promta S (eds) (2000). *The state of Buddhist studies in the world, 1972–1997*. Center for Buddhist Studies, Chulalongkorn University, Bangkok.

The Commentary to the Pali Canon (2003a). *Syamarattha Version*, volume 4, p. 108. Mahamakut Buddhist University, Bangkok.

The Commentary to the Pali Canon (2003b). *Syamarattha Version*, volume 1. Tatiyaparajika Vannana. Mahamakut Buddhist University, Bangkok.

The Commentary to the Pali Canon (2003c). *Syamarattha Version*, volume 9, pp. 872–873. Mahamakut Buddhist University, Bangkok.

The Commentary to the Pali Canon (2003d). *Syamarattha Version*, volume 1. *Tatiyaparajika Vannana*. Mahamakut Buddhist University, Bangkok.

The Milindapañha (2003). *Syamarattha Version*, p. 39. Mahamakut Buddhist University, Bangkok.

The Pali Canon (2003a). *Syamarattha Version*, volume 1, sections 176–179. Mahamakut Buddhist University, Bangkok.

The Pali Canon (2003b). *Syamarattha Version*, volume 1, section 213. Mahamakut Buddhist University, Bangkok.

The Pali Canon (2003c). *Syamarattha Version*, volume 14, sections 741–753. Mahamakut Buddhist University, Bangkok.

The Pali Canon (2003d). *Syamarattha Version*, volume 27, section 565. Mahamakut Buddhist University, Bangkok.

The Pali Canon (2003e). *Syamarattha Version*, volume 22, section 334. Mahamakut Buddhist University, Bangkok.

The Pali Canon (2003f). *Syamarattha Version*, volume 25, section 18. *The Dhammapada*. Mahamakut Buddhist University, Bangkok.

The Pali Canon (2003g). *Syamarattha Version*, volume 25, section 92. *The Udana*. Mahamakut Buddhist University, Bangkok.

The Pali Canon (2003h). *Syamarattha Version*, volume 35, section 33. Mahamakut Buddhist University, Bangkok.

The Pali Canon (2003i). *Syamarattha Version*, volume 25, section 30. *The Dhammapada*. Mahamakut Buddhist University, Bangkok.

Thepwisutthimethi P, Bhikkhu B, Swearer DK, eds (1989). *Me and mine: selected essays of Bhikkhu Buddhadasa*. State University of New York Press, New York.

The Vimativinodani (2002). *Chattha Sangayana Version*, section 174. Vipassana Research Institute, New Delhi.

Thomyangkoon P, Leenaars A, Wasserman D (2005). Suicide in Thailand, 1977 to 2002. *Archives of Suicide Research*, **9**, 361–368.

Thurman RAF, trans. (1994). *The Tibetan Book of the dead*. Bantam Books, New York.

Yip PS, and Tan RC (1998). Suicides in Hong Kong and Singapore: a tale of two cities. *The International Journal of Social Psychiatry*, **44**, 267–279.

# CHAPTER 6

# The Shinto religion and suicide in Japan

Yoshihiro Kaneko, Akiko Yamasaki and Kiminori Arai

## Abstract

The Shinto religion profoundly influences many Japanese. It is their emotional mainstay, although it has neither common commandments nor scriptures. Over time, the Shinto religion became involved in the state activities, which led to the development of shrines where the gods are worshipped.

Shinto coexists with Buddhism and a mixed practice of these two religions is common. According to Shinto, human beings are part of nature and can live only because nature is our parent. Mankind should live in the 'way of the gods'. The worship of ancestors is an important value in Shinto.

The Shinto attitude towards suicide is somewhat ambivalent. Shinto believes that humans return to nature after death, suicide does not constitute an exception, and suicide as a sacrificial act is condoned. On the other hand, believing that life is given by nature and ancestors implies that suicide is wrong.

The increasing number of suicides during recent years, mainly for socio-economic reasons, has deeply affected Japanese society and also its attitudes towards suicide. This has resulted in many suicide-prevention activities in which religion can also play an important role.

## Introduction

Since 1998, more than 30,000 people have killed themselves every year in Japan. An international comparison of suicide rates (per 100,000 people) by the World Health Organization ranked Japan 6th concerning suicide rates for females, at 12.8 in 2007, and 11th for males, at 35.6. The Japanese government established a joint committee comprising officials from government ministries and agencies with the aim of devising 'comprehensive measures' to promote suicide prevention. The Japanese Government now regards suicide as something society as a whole must deal with, rather than an individual problem alone.

Society as a whole is influenced by historical, economical, political and socio-psychological elements. One of the important factors that should be considered in suicide prevention is the interaction between the prevailing influence of religion and personal feelings related to individuals' mental health. In this chapter, we will describe the characteristics and history of Shinto, and examine Shinto's potential role in preventing suicide in Japan.

Shinto is a religious culture that influences many Japanese. It is their emotional mainstay, although it has neither common commandments nor scriptures like other religions, such as Buddhism, Christianity and Islam. Perhaps the reason Shinto has neither commandments nor scriptures may be due to the conscious gratitude of the Japanese, since ancient times, for the blessings of nature. This meant that Shinto began as a custom for worshipping many gods related to the origins of the community (e.g. villages and nations) in the area where people lived. It served as a way for individuals to appreciate the blessings of nature and the history of the community, and at the same time, to provide discipline in their lives so that peace could prevail in community life. In other words, Shinto has provided moral support to the Japanese: it gave them shared living norms, a sense of belonging, and a desire to contribute to the community, which were taught and passed on to new generations (Kamata 2000; Sonoda 2005; Takemitsu 2006).

While Shinto is characterized as a religious culture, it is also known to have a religious organization or national network of shrines formed to serve as places where people can visit and express religious feelings. Shrines have been erected since ancient times for the worship of objects that were the source of this moral support. Examples may be seen in the mountains and rivers, where water was sourced for the fields; in sacred places and objects that existed in nature, such as large trees symbolizing longevity; and in sacred places for the worship of noble ancestors who ploughed fields or founded, protected and guided the country (Inoue 2006; Mihashi 2007).

Shinto has religious cultural aspects symbolized by shrine events, as well as living norms to provide discipline for people's emotions. However, since it has neither commandments nor scriptures, it has never indoctrinated the people except during the period when State Shinto was promoted, from the Meiji period (1868–1912) to the end of the Second World War. In fact, Shinto coexisted with Buddhism in Japan as can be seen from the mixed practice of Shintoism and Buddhism, with some Confucian ideas introduced as well. Since the post-Second World War period, under the guarantee for freedom of religion in the Constitution of Japan, shrines across the country have maintained a loose network under a national organization called the Association of Shinto Shrines, and Shinto has provided moral support to many Japanese people while coexisting with other religions such as Buddhism, Christianity and Islam.

According to the Statistical Survey on Religion of the Cultural Affairs Department, Agency for Cultural Affairs of Japan, there are as many as 80,000 shrines in Japan, including the Meiji shrine, visited by three million worshippers in the first three days of the new year, and many small regional shrines. Owing to the mixed practice of Shintoism and Buddhism, the difference in number between the shrines of Shintoism and the temples of Buddhism are fairly small. The total number of Shinto and Buddhism adherents exceeds the total population of Japan, because many people observe both religions. Nevertheless, according to the official data on adherents from the Statistical Survey on Religion in 2005, Shintoists, Buddhists and Christians make up 50.8, 43.2, and 1.3 per cent of the population respectively.

Shinto has an influence on a high proportion of Japanese people, as we have seen. Although Shinto is a religious culture, and objects of worship are regarded with reverence, the shrines do not necessarily serve to propagate religious beliefs, but rather act as venues for people to express their faith, including participation in annual events. As a result, under the present situation, no particular influence or organizational measures based on Shinto exist for suicide prevention.

Based on such a viewpoint, this chapter provides an overview of the history and characteristics of norms of Shinto in Japan, clarifying the reasons why Shinto values human life, and also examines the relationship between Shinto and suicide prevention.

## The origin and history of Shinto

### From ancient times until the establishment of the Yamato Imperial Court (c. seventh century)

In the ancient Japanese language of *Yamato Kotoba*, 'god' (神: *kami*) had the same meaning as 'up' or 'top' (上: *kami*). In other words, any power or work that surpassed human knowledge or any being superior to man was considered to be *kami*. These gods would sometimes cause an extraordinary natural phenomenon or a plague, but they were essentially considered to bring natural blessings and good luck. Because everyone wishes to avoid trouble, people worshipped gods to try to appease their wrath and enjoy their blessings.

In Shinto, spirits that inspired appreciation or awe and were worshipped all became *kami* (god). In other words, only what one decided to worship became a god in Shinto. This is why Shinto researchers take the view that the relationship between god and man in Shinto is similar to human relationships, in which we associate with those we like and are helped by them if an opportunity arises. It explains the great variety or *yaoyorozu* of gods in Japan.

The gods that exist in large numbers in Japan are categorized in two main groups: *amatsukami* (god of heaven) and *kunitsukami* (god of Earth). According to the *Engi Shiki* (Procedures of the Engi era), compiled during the Heian period, *amatsukami* are gods above the clouds: *kunitsukami* are gods who settled in the clouds and mists in the mountains on Earth. According to the Japanese myths described in *Kojiki* (Records of ancient matters) and *Nihon shoki* (Chronicles of Japan), these two main lines originated with the God Susano-o, who is famous for killing Yamata no Orochi (the eight-forked serpent). Susano-o was ordered to descend to Earth shortly after his birth, because he rebelled against his parent god Izanagi and elder sister Amaterasu, and threw *Takama-no-hara* (the high plain of heaven) into confusion. According to this myth,

the gods were classified into two categories after Susano-o assumed the quality of a *kunitsukami*. It may be said that *amatsukami* are gods in the high plain of heaven, while *kunitsukami* are descendants of Susano-o.

In addition to the classifications of kami, based on the Japanese myths, the Yamato Imperial Court divided the gods into two categories, for the purpose of the regime subject to the influence of Confucianism that was introduced into Japan in the late fifth century. The Imperial court worshipped a god called *Ohomenonushi*, who was considered equal in rank to the gods worshipped by regional ruling clans, which were subordinate to the Imperial Court. The Imperial family could not assert their authority under this situation. The Yamato Imperial Court therefore introduced the Confucian idea of *tenjinchigi*, according to which the gods of heaven (*tenjin*) are positioned higher than the gods of Earth (*chigi*). Based on this idea, the gods worshipped by regional ruling clans became *chigi*, and gods of heaven, such as *Amaterasu-oomi-kami*, were positioned higher, which allowed the Imperial family to take precedence over other regional ruling clans in the religion.

## Formation and development of shrines

As the Shinto religion became more deeply involved in activities to govern the country, events to worship gods were organized and conducted on a regular basis. Since ancient times, a shrine has been referred to as the garden of god's house. Simple buildings were erected for each festival to welcome the god, and removed after the festival. After a while, when the state and the regional territories it governed organized Shinto events, permanent sanctuaries were built at locations where religious rites and festivals were held repeatedly. As Buddhism was introduced, and many Buddhist temples were built, Shinto responded by constructing shrines, mostly principal sanctuaries. Consequently, shrine precincts were formed in various parts of the country.

In ancient times, shrines were distinguished merely as *amatsu yashiro*—shrines for the worship of gods of heaven, and *kunitsu yashiro*—shrines for the worship of gods of Earth. By the time the country was governed in accordance with the *ritsuryo* (legal codes) system in the eighth century, shrines were maintained by the state, and eventually categorized into large and small national shrines and prefectural shrines. A provincial governor appointed by the Imperial Court visited a series of historic shrines in the territory as part of a ritual. Because a provincial governor had to gain support from the people in his territory, he visited shrines, mainly in the order of the length of each shrine's history. The shrines were thus called *ichinomiya* (first shrine), *ninomiya* (second shrine), *sannomiya* (third shrine), and so on, in the order in which they were visited. This led to the *ichinomiya* system that named the shrine and the area of the shrine precinct *ichinomiya*, *ninomiya*, etc.

By the eleventh and twelfth centuries, more and more aristocrats appointed as provincial governors did not follow the order to visit shrines in their territories, and instead, powerful warriors residing in the country began to engage in administration. Because it was time-consuming to visit many shrines as a local feudal lord, the influential warriors simplified the visits by ordering each region to divide the spirits of such an important shrine where their visit was strategically indispensable, and bring them to a combined shrine for worshipping different gods. After this kind of combined shrine system was introduced, the influential warrior's visit to *honsha* (the head shrine) was regarded as visiting all shrines from which the spirits were brought to *honsha*, which clarified his piety to all those shrines that the people in his territory believe in. This was the beginning of the combined shrine system that laid out *honsha* (head shrine), *sessha* (subordinate shrine), and *massha* (branch shrine of the subordinate shrine) at the combined shrine. Shrines were ranked so until the early twentieth century, just before the Second World War.

### From the Meiji period to the pre-Second World War period

During the modernization period in Japan after the Meiji Restoration, the Shinto–Buddhism separation policy was strongly enforced in the first year of Meiji (1868) and into the following year, and Shinto was separated from the Buddhist culture. In 1870, in order to strengthen its sovereignty, the Meiji government revived and promoted the blending of religion and politics, mainly around the concept of *kami* (god). Those ancient festivals that the Yamato Court observed were revived, and the Office of Shinto Worship, which once supervised shrines when the country was governed in accordance with the *ritsuryo* (legal codes) system, was reinstated. All shrines were ordered to belong to the Office.

While there was no governmental control over the systematization of Buddhism, Christianity and other religions, the shrines were given preferential treatment as government subsidies. At the same time, they came under strict supervision as State rites were subject to restrictions, and lost their local colour. In principle, the shrines had to devote themselves to observing the services according to guidelines issued by the government. Nevertheless, the Meiji government permitted the religious activities of those groups that established a new *kami* belief, or the so-called Shinto-derived religion, during the Meiji period. As a result, thirteen sects—Fusokyo, Izumo Taishakyo, Jikkokyo, Konkokyo, Kurozumikyo, Misogikyo, Ontakekyo, Shinrikyo, Shinshukyo, Shinto-Honkyoku, Shinto Shusei-ha, Taiseikyo, and Tenrikyo—formed Sect Shinto after 1882. Other sects (such as Oomotokyo) were later derived from these thirteen.

### From the Second World War to the present day

During the Second World War, State Shinto, functioning as State rites, organized local residents as 'family children', or 'parishioners', in each region, and the military used this system for suppressing freedom of thought. The General Headquarters of the Allied Powers (GHQ) carried out a reform to separate religion from politics, and abolished State Shinto in 1945, after Japan's defeat in the Second World War. GHQ ordered the Japanese government to separate shrines from the state under the Shinto Directive. Based on this order, all shrine-related laws and regulations that had been established in many different forms since the Meiji period were abolished in the following year. The Constitution of Japan then guaranteed freedom of religion, and all religions now abided by the same laws. In other words, separation of religion from politics and also freedom of religion were ensured both in name and in reality. Shrines were no longer under government protection, and served simply as elements of a religion (Yasumaru and Miyachi 1998). The Religious Corporations Ordinance, which was revised in 1946, opened the way for shrines to become religious corporations for the first time. Subsequently, the three shrine-related organizations—Kotenko Kokyusho, Dai-Nihon Jingikai and Jingu Hosaikai—founded Jinja Honcho (the Association of Shinto Shrines) a loose network of almost all shrines, in 1946.

Because Shinto is a religious culture based on natural worship, and the ancestor worship that originated in the people's old manners and customs, it includes a great variety of beliefs and manners towards the gods. In order to keep a balance between these varieties in Shinto, and the management of the network of shrines, it was necessary for the Association of Shinto Shrines to establish the minimum principles that could be shared by all of the shrines. In 1956, the Association of Shinto Shrines therefore announced the General Principles of Pious Shinto Life as principles to be put into practice, based on those ancient traditions, such as ancestor worship and observing the services. Because the principles were to be shared by numerous shrines with independent history, the General Principles are kept to three minimum articles, which are as follows:

1 We wish to express our gratitude for God's grace and our ancestors' kindnesses, and to honour God with feelings of the utmost sincerity by worshipping the God diligently both at the household altar and at the shrine.

2 We wish to serve not only one person but the whole world, and make the world better by being a person who follows the Way of God.

3 We wish to have a generous mind and faith, live harmoniously and peacefully, and pray for prosperity in the country as well as in the live-and-let-live world.

### Syncretism (multiple beliefs) and ancestor worship in Shinto

From ancient times through to the Edo period, the Shinto religion, which allowed people to select a number of gods to worship, did not conflict with religions introduced into the country as part of exchanges between continental and Japanese cultures. Rather, the religious culture of Shinto was seen as blending in harmony with such religions. Meanwhile, Christianity was introduced and propagated during the Warring States period (1467–1568). It was then prohibited in the Edo period under the Tokugawa Shogunate's national isolation policy. By the Meiji period, however, Christianity was reintroduced, and the characteristics of the religious culture of Shinto, essentially blending in harmony and not conflicting with other religions, persisted even after the Meiji period.

In fact, the Japanese have adopted not only Shinto and Buddhist customs, but also various Christian and Confucian customs. Christmas, the new year's visit to a shrine and reciting sutra at funerals are all derived from different religions.

This idea of having multiple religious beliefs is called syncretism. Shinto had a significant influence on the formation of a unique syncretism in Japan. Since ancient times, many new beliefs, including Confucianism, Buddhism and Taoism, have been introduced from the mainland into Japan. However, Shinto was not submerged by these religions; nor did it disappear: it changed these other religions into a form that suited Japan.

## Characteristics of religious norms in Shinto

### Living norms in Shinto

The ancient people recognized spirits in many different natural phenomena and called them *tama*. The ancient people of Japan saw two spirits or tama in one kami or god. That is, they saw both violent—*arami-tama*—and peaceful—*nigimi-tama*—tamas. The violent tama represented the rough aspects of gods that brought about divine punishment and extraordinary natural phenomena. What people did to pacify this violent tama became the origins of festivals.

In Shinto, holding religious rites was thought to calm the mysterious power of the violent tama, and change it into a peaceful one. This peaceful tama is filled with God's love. In Shinto, people pray to the peaceful tama for happiness. A peaceful tama is further divided into happiness—*sachimi-tama*— which offers happiness through *kushimi-tama*, which makes luck and wonders, and directly performs God's miracles. These four tama are among myriads of divinities, and they are worshipped separately at shrines.

Awareness that man is a part of nature (= God the parent), and is able to live because nature is our parent, is also related to the concept of ancestor worship. The way of the Gods, which Shinto has continuously passed down through the years, is to coexist with nature, to teach us all how to live happily and value our conscience.

Because Shinto has no holy scripture, written commandments do not exist. Unlike Buddhism and Christianity, no clear doctrine on how to live exists in Shinto. There could be 100 different ways for 100 different people.

Kamata (2000) points out that the interpretation of the 'Way of the Gods' became one of the important subjects in analysing Shinto among the foreign researchers after the Meiji period.

### Sense of sin in Shinto

The most important aspect of discipline in Shinto life is being pure, because this leads to tranquillity. Therefore *kegare* (impurity) is feared more than anything else. This impurity brings sin, and committing a sin became the most serious taboo.

Sin is mainly divided into two types: *amatsu tsumi* (sins of heaven) and *kunitsu tsumi* (sins of Earth). The sins of heaven are said to have been those committed by Susano-o in heaven before being banished from it, and are mainly related to farming. There are eight sins, which include damaging ridges between rice fields and filling up ditches in rice fields. These sins were considered to be the most serious because they obstruct rice farming, which is essential to the Japanese, who rely on the blessings of nature and crops.

The sins of Earth relate mainly to adultery. There are thirteen such sins, which include cutting a person's skin and incest. Natural calamities and diseases were considered to be punishments caused by sins.

### Death as taboo

Words associated with impurity or bad luck, such as death or blood, were considered taboo and their meaning was expressed by the use of other words (Masahiko 1989).

Death, which distinguished ancestors from those who were still alive, was originally thought of as *kegare* (impurity, i.e. drying-up or exhaustion of vitality) and was taboo and disliked. However, the ancient Japanese people believed that worshipping and appeasing the spirit of a dead person could change it into a purified spirit of an ancestor. In a country blessed with natural riches, the Japanese people believed they were able to live by sharing god's spirits that resided in nature. After living with God, and when it was time to die, a person's spirit was guided by *ubusunagami* (the tutelary kami

of one's birthplace) and returned to the world of ancestral spirits. The purified spirit became a kami, watched over the descendants from the world of ancestral spirits, and from time to time returned to where the descendants resided. So the descendants held festivals for the spirits to welcome these ancestral spirits returning to their homes. Owing to syncretism, which after the introduction of Buddhism, this ancestor worship in Shinto was passed down in various forms in religious culture. As a result, many events held to pay respect to ancestors, starting with the Bon festival, which are still celebrated in Japan to this day.

## How life and suicide are perceived in Shinto

The view that death and blood are regarded as *kegare* (impurity), and considering them as taboo and disliking them, might also apply to suicide. On the other hand, when visiting a shrine and experiencing the tutelary forest, people are reminded to respect nature and pay respect to the ancestors and historical persons who have achieved distinction. This gives a chain of association or unity between man and nature, leading to the conclusion that man will return to nature after all kinds of death, which in all likelihood also includes suicide.

Conversely, if people believe that their lives are nature-given, and recognize the need to value the lives given to them by respecting nature, it would suggest disapproval of suicide. In addition, an important norm in respecting ancestors is to value life that has been given to a person by one's ancestor. This, too, would imply that suicide is wrong.

This view of life as nature's blessing, bestowed on us by our ancestors, was a common interpretation of Shinto during the Edo period, and by scholars of Japanese classics called *kokugakusha* (thinkers on the desirable structure of the state), who identified a relationship between how people should live and how the country should be based on Shinto. The Shinto researcher Masahiko Asoya points out that this might serve as a basis for Shinto to play some kind of role in preventing suicide today (Masahiko 2006). Asoya says that, first of all, the four thinkers (Kadano Azumaro, Kamono Mabushi, Norinaga Motoori, and Hirata Atsutane) had a common conception of a child as a gift from god, which in turn implies that people are born as a result of god's intervention. Another common idea based on this thinking would be that the purpose of life or the meaning of life in Shinto would be the fulfilment of god's order in this world.

## Shinto religion and suicide in Japan

In the medieval and early modern periods in Japan, according to the Shinto religion and other elements of Japanese culture, suicide was considered as a permissible act of honour. Although there is no formal doctrine within the Shinto religion condoning suicide, there is evidence that the self-harming act for harmonious purposes was accepted. The Shinto religion has a long-standing history of allowing suicide for motivational purposes, such as patriotism, philosophy, romance and despair.

However, although the religion did endorse certain suicidal acts as honourable, the tradition of exhibitionist suicide was condemned (Barry 1994). Shinto religion and, incidentally, Japanese culture as a whole emphasize the importance not of individuals (as Western cultures do), but rather of society as a whole (Range *et al.* 1999). For this reason, an individual suicide for the greater good of society is often viewed as a self-sacrificing act. To a large extent, suicide for means of harmony is rooted in Shinto religious history, and still lingers today. Therefore, in the Shinto religion, those who commit suicide are not punished, and are still granted traditional Shinto burials.

## Characteristics of suicide in Japan

The variations of suicide in traditional Japan to acknowledge honour are well engraved in the Shinto religion and Japanese culture. From the medieval to the early modern age in Japan, suicide in such forms as seppuku or hara-kiri, kamakizi, and jigai were often emphasized as admirable acts.

*Seppuku*, a form of ritual suicide by disembowelment, was originally reserved for samurai alone. Part of the samurai code of honour, it was used by these warriors in order, for example, to die with honour rather than fall into enemy hands. The most famous form of *seppuku* is also colloquially known as *hara-kiri*. This form, consisting of a deep knife stab in the abdomen followed by a stab in the head, was a ceremonial act committed by warriors for displaying failure (in which death was preferred to bringing disgrace on the Emperor). *Jigai* is a suicidal method consisting of cutting of the jugular vein, used by females for penitence of sins. More recently, there has been *kamakizi* (the intentional suicide mission), the well-known method employed by Japanese soldiers and pilots during the Second World War (McDowell and Stewart 1992; Barry 1994; Ueno 2005), which can also be seen as reflecting cultural attitudes: suicide rather than surrender was the honourable act of the Japanese soldier.

To a great extent, suicide in contemporary Japan utilizes such methods, and society has transformed the honorary aspect of suicide during medieval and modern times into a more personal one. In fact, a study conducted by Takahashi *et al.* (1998) found that suicide methods in Japan mirror that of Western cultures, with hanging as the principal method used in suicide, followed by jumping, drowning, poisoning, $CO_2$ intoxication, burning and firearms, although firearms accounted for only 0.2 per cent given the strict gun laws in Japan.

There are other aspects of suicide in contemporary Japan which distinguish it from what occurs in Western cultures. The term *shinju* refers to a suicide committed among intimate persons, essentially among commoners. The forms of *shinju*, classified as familial suicides, are known in the Japanese culture as *oyako-shinju* (parent–child suicide), which classifies as *boshi-shinjyu* (mother–child suicide), *fushi-shinju* (father–child suicide) and *ikka-shinju* (complete family suicide) (Takahashi *et al.* 1998; Ueno 2005). Conversely, new forms of suicide are increasing in modern Japan, owing to the rapid modernization of the country. The term *karojisatsu* (work-related suicide) has attracted more attention by researchers, as elucidated in a study by Amagasa *et al.* (2005), which indicated long working hours and increased stress as factors related to *karojisatsu*.

## Mental disorders and suicide stigmatization in Japan

Mental disorders are a huge public health problem in Japan, as in the whole world. Stigmatization of mental disorders often prevents individuals from seeking help, thus worsening their condition. The idea of mental illness is a difficult concept in Japan. Mental disorders are highly stigmatized in Japanese culture, because they are seldom viewed as being illness, but rather a 'weakness of the

will' (Young 2002). Numerous studies have verified this claim, and compared with other countries, the Japanese tend not to seek help outside the family for mental disorders; believe that the disorder is the individual's fault; do not see it as a 'real' illness, but rather as a self-control problem; and view it as a weakness of character (Desapriya and Nobutada 2002; Young 2002; Nakane *et al.* 2005; Jorm *et al.* 2005; Griffiths *et al.* 2006). Owing to traditional values and Shinto religious beliefs, society acts collectively as a unit, and not as if it consisted of individuals.

In early Japanese culture, suicide was acknowledged as an honourable act, and was therefore portrayed not as a negative element in society but rather as a harmonious gesture. In contemporary Japan, however, a stigma of suicide is emerging, and now exists as in Western cultures (Takahashi 1997). However, Takahashi *et al.* (1998) highlight the fact that most Japanese people do not consider suicide as abnormal behaviour, and relate that those who commit *oyako-shinju* (parent–child suicide) are not severely condemned, but rather shown significant compassion. Young (2002) argues that although there is a cultural acceptance of suicide, it is a moral issue in Japan which affects society as a whole, not individuals as in Western civilization. Collectively through society, the moral act of suicide therefore has a redemptive quality. Traditionally, the ultimate act of suicide is regarded as the highest form of self-sacrifice (Young 2002). A person who fails in committing the ultimate act (suicide attempt) is viewed not as honourable or redemptive, but rather as stigmatized, and the individual and family members become alienated from society. Thus, the stigma against suicide attempters and their family members is considerable. They incur shame and disgrace, and are often met with negative overtones (Young 2002).

# The possibility of Shinto preventing suicide

In recent years, there has been a remarkable increase in suicide, mainly for socio-economic reasons in connection with the recession that has affected Japanese society profoundly. The authorities are engaged in suicide-prevention activities on different levels. However, this activity meets many obstacles owing to the enduring connotations of suicide both in the Shinto religion and in Japanese culture. Research in suicidology is developing increasingly, and more prevention programmes that allow for cultural and religious aspects are implemented.

The Shinto perception of life, based on the concept that one must value one's life as a means of respecting one's ancestors, can help prevent suicide.

Shrine-affiliated organizations have started addressing environmental issues based on the concept of nature worship by playing down religious aspects, and proposing exchanges of academic research and opinions.

As part of these non-political and voluntary efforts by shrines, important activities have been started at many locations. These may lead to suicide prevention, especially among the elderly, in workplaces and schools.

## Elderly

When elderly people feel isolated and useless, their situation is known to trigger suicide in some cases. Using shrines as places for the elderly to get together is helping to prevent suicide among them. In other words, in annual events at shrines, local elderly people have more occasions, although not constant, to cooperate with people in other age groups in organizing events. Furthermore, some of these shrines are working with local nursing care services to provide opportunities for the elderly to interact with one other, so that they can experience more occasions to lead a more fulfilling life and avoid becoming isolated, and these occasions can be used to watch over and listen to them.

## Workplaces and schools

To prevent suicide among working people and young people, it is hoped that causal factors can be reduced in workplaces through Shinto living norms. The suicide of an employee who had been verbally denied his existence by his superior in the company is still fresh in our memories. If a person could respect living norms, such as 'embracing the merciful mind of kami by leading a harmonious life' or 'praying for peaceful coexistence and prosperity of the entire world', then he would understand that harassment based on power that ends up denying a subordinate's existence is unacceptable. Friendly interpersonal relations at work and in schools would relieve the subordinate's stress and reduce the risk of depression caused by stress and other mental health-related problems, which would eventually help to prevent suicide.

Moreover, if we value the idea of offering service for the good of the world and the good of the people, volunteer work related to suicide prevention could be promoted.

# Conclusion

Because Shinto in Japan lacks commandments and scriptures, its influence may be weaker than other religions in terms of educating people about the value of life. In addition, the separation of religion from politics is strictly enforced today, and it is therefore difficult to include Shinto norms directly in school education, labour policy, or welfare policy for the elderly. However, even without indoctrination or legislation, Shinto has an important impact on everyday life, as 110 million adherents visit 80,000 shrines or possibly more. This fact may certainly contribute to the prevention of suicide in Japan.

## References

### In Japanese

Inoue H (2006). *Kamisama to Jinja* (God and shrine). Shodensha
Kamata T (2000). *Shinto Towa Nanika: Shizen no Reisei wo Kanjite Ikiru* (What is Shinto: living with the feeling of natural spirits).

Masahiko A (1989). *Shinto no Seishikan—Shinto Shiso to shi no Mondai* (Shinto's view of life and death—Shinto philosophy and the issue of death).
Masahiko A (2006). *Jisatsu ni Tsuite Shinto no Tachiba Kara Kangaeru* (A study on suicide from the perspective of Shinto).
Mihashi T (2007). *Jinja no Yurai ga Wakaru Shojiten* (Small dictionary on the origin of shrines). PHP Institute
Sonoda M (2005). *Bunka toshiteno Shinto* (Shinto as a culture). Kobundou
Takemitsu M (2006). *Shinto Nyumon* (Introduction to Shinto). Gentosha
Yasumaru Y and Miyachi M (1998). *Shukyo to Kokka* (Religion and the State). Iwanami Shoten

### In English

Amagasa T, Nakayama T, Takahashi Y (2005). *Karojisatsu* in Japan: characteristics of 22 cases of work-related suicide. *Journal of Occupational Health*, **4**, 157–164.
Barry R (1994). *Breaking the Thread of Life: On Rational Suicide*, pp. 57–61. Transaction Publishers, New Jersey.
Desapriya EBR and Nobutada I (2002). Stigma of mental illness in Japan. *The Lancet*, **359**, 1866.
Griffiths KM, Nakane Y, Christensen H *et al.* (2006). Stigma in response to mental disorders: a comparison study of Australia and Japan. *BMC Psychiatry*, **6**, 21.
Jorm AF, Nakane Y, Christensen H *et al.* (2005). Public beliefs about treatment and outcome of mental disorders: a comparison of Australia and Japan. *BMC Medicine*, **3**, 12.
Masahiko A (2006). *Jisatsu ni Tsuite Shinto no Tachiba Kara Kangaeru* (A study on suicide from the perspective of Shinto, peace and religion'). Niwano Peace Foudation, Tokyo, No.24.
Masahiko A (1989). *Shinto no Seishikan—Shinto Shiso to Shi no Mondai* (Shinto's view of life and death—Shinto philosophy and the issue of death)' Pelican Publishing Company, Tokyo.
McDowell J and Stewart D (1992). *Handbook of Today's Religions.* Thomas Nelson, Tennessee.
Nakane Y, Jorm AF, Yoshioka K *et al.* (2005). Public beliefs about causes and risk factors for mental disorders: a comparison of Japan and Australia. *BMC Psychiatry*, **5**, 33.
Range LM, Leach MM, McIntyre D *et al.* (1999). Multicultural perspectives on suicide. *Aggression and Violent Behavior*, **4**, 413–430.
Takahashi Y (1997). Culture and suicide: from a psychiatrist's perspective. In AA Leenaars, RW Maris, Y Takahashi, eds, *Suicide: Individual, Cultural, International Perspective*, p. 137. Guilford Publications, New York.
Takahashi Y, Hirasawa H, Koyama K *et al.* (1998). Suicide in Japan: present state and future directions for prevention. *Transcultural Psychiatry*, **35**, 271.
Ueno K (2005). Suicide as Japan's major export? A note on Japanese suicide culture. *Revista Espaco Academico*, **44**,1. ISSN: 1519.6186.
Young J (2002). Morals, suicide, and psychiatry: a view from Japan. *Bioethics*, **16**, 412–424.

# CHAPTER 7

# Suicide in the Jewish scriptures

Israel Orbach and Aron Rabinowitz

## Abstract

The Jewish scriptures and the commentaries of the scriptures throughout history present a very complex approach toward suicide. There is a categorical prohibition against suicide, but also an obligation to submit to death when there is an external coercion to transgress Jewish laws that pertain to the essence of the faith. Talmudic sages have shown a psychological and empathic understanding of the suicidal state of mind, but they have harshly condemned suicide and punished it by omissions of certain religious rituals for the dead. Yet, Jewish law defines suicide in a very minimalistic way, so it is very rare that a death is defined as a suicide. Inherent in this approach is the attempt to avoid further suffering by the family, to show respect for the frailty of the human being, but at the same time, to condemn self-destructive behaviour.

## Introduction: the Jewish scriptures and their interpretation

The Jewish religious laws and ethics are based on several sources: the Old Testament or the *Bible,* which consists of the *Torah, Prophets* and *Writings*; the *Talmud,* which contains the commentaries on the Bible and deduction of written and oral laws from it; the *Midrash,* a homilitical literature consisting of legal and non-legal discourse on the Bible by means of tales and maxims of prominent sages; and the *Shulchan Aruch,* the final and authoritative codification of the rabbinic law, or the *halacha,* which was completed in the sixteenth century. The *Shulchan Aruch* also serves as the fountain of knowledge, and provides the principles that are applied to new situations. New problems and issues arise as a result of changing conditions, technological advances, etc. Some of the important halachic decisions have been summarized and recorded at times in special volumes, or as part of the commentaries on the *Shulchan Aruch.* The halachic laws and opinions presented in this chapter are based upon the above-mentioned sources, and serve as the raw material from which Jewish attitudes towards suicide can be understood.

## Suicide in the scriptures

The Torah lists murder as one of the first of the ten commandments, thus sending a clear, severe, and unambiguous message about the taking of another person's life. The Torah also makes direct statements about the sanctity of life: 'See I have put before you today life and death, blessing and curse, and you shall choose life so that you and your seed shall live' (Deuteronomy 30:19). However, on the practical issue of suicide, the murder of the self, the Torah makes no direct reference to the topic. In fact, in the three sections of the Old Testament (Torah, Prophets, and Writings) there is no verb, noun, or adjective to denote suicide. The one singular reference to the prohibition of suicide is: 'And surely your blood I will require at the hand of every beast will I require it; and at the hand of man' (Genesis 9:5). Talmudic sages later understood these words literally, i.e. as 'your life blood', and the prohibition of suicide is based on this verse.

Although suicide is prohibited, suicidal wishes are not stifled in the Bible, and are in fact mentioned in the text and addressed by God. These include Rebecca's exclamation, 'I am weary of my life … what good should my life do to me'(Genesis 27:46); Moses' statement, 'If thou deal thus with me, kill me' (Numbers 11:14); Elijah's request, 'and he requested for himself that he might die … and said it is enough, now O Lord take my life' (Kings I, 19:4); Job's statement, 'So that my soul chooseth strangling and death rather than these bones' (Job 7:15); and Jonah, 'Therefore now, O lord, take, I beseech thee, my life from me for it is better for me to die than to live' (Jonah 4:3–4). According to Kaplen and Schwartz (1993), in all the instances where people expressed a wish to die, there was no condemnation of the wish; rather God has implemented a suicide-preventative approach of warmth and sympathy.

The first documentation of suicide in the prophets is the one committed by Avimelech in the book of Judges. Avimelech was one of the most brutal rulers (Judges) of Israel. During a battle in the city of Tabatz, a woman standing on the fortress of the city threw a stone on his head and broke his skull. The idea of being killed by a woman was too humiliating for Avimelech so he asked his carrier to make the final blow, since his condition did not allow him to kill himself. The servant obeyed without hesitation, and stabbed Avimelech to death (see Judges 9:25–31). Avimelech's act of suicide was not condoned. His name and image remained a symbol of shun and humiliation of his efforts to hide his shame and preserve his dignity after death (Samuel 11:21). He was remembered as a humiliated figure. Further, the Bible makes it very clear that Avimelech's death was actually a punishment by God for his bad deeds (see Judges 9:56–57 and Kaplan and Schwartz 1993).

Samson's suicide is the second mentioned in the prophets. His suicide was unique in that it was actually assisted by God. Samson was one of the greatest defenders and leaders of Israel. His heroism was made prominent in his victories over the Philistine army; his tragedy came about in his caveat to his Philistine lover, to whom he disclosed the secrets of his powers. Samson was captured, blinded, and publicly mocked by the Philistines. Faced with torture and death, he asked God for the strength to kill himself and to take as many of his enemies with him as possible. Samson asked God to assist him in the act of suicide: 'Let me die with the Philistines' (Judges 16:30). God granted his wish, and gave Samson the power to pull down the central pillars of the temple of Dagon, killing thousands in one blow.

Samson's suicide is clearly motivated, not only by a desire for revenge, but also by his sense of duty to complete his obligations to his people. His purpose was not self-annihilation, despite the grim reality that he was facing, but rather the carrying out of his divinely ordained mission to free Israel from the Philistines (Kaplan and Schwartz 1993). The scriptures state that his suicide was followed by a long period of peace for the Israelites. (Judges 16:23–31, and Kaplan and Schwartz 1993). According to Shneidman's theory (1984), one might say that the description of Samson's fate leaves room for the interpretation that his suicide was aimed at achieving a purpose, as opposed to the escape from pain. What is clear is that Samson's suicide is not condemned either in the Bible or by later commentators. On the contrary, he became a symbol of heroism (Shemesh 2003), and this is confirmed by the description of the respect that he received during his burial. Samson's birth and death both occurred with the direct involvement of God (Shemesh 2003).

The third suicide mentioned is that of King Saul, the first king of Israel. King Saul launched a war against the Philistines. He realized that he was losing the war: he was badly wounded, three of his sons and many of his soldiers were killed. Saul knew that he was going to be taken prisoner, and subsequently tortured and humiliated at the hands of his enemies.

In despair, Saul turns to his carrier and says: 'Draw thy sword and thrust me through therewith; lest these uncircumcised come and make a mock out of me.' He was, in a sense, requesting an assisted suicide. However, his servant refuses to obey. 'Therefore, Saul took his sword and fell upon it' (Samuel I, 31:1–4). Soon after Saul fell on his sword, his servant killed himself in, what seems to be an act of solidarity (Shamesh 2003).

Nowhere in the description of Saul's suicide is his act condemned. The tone of the narrative seems to even be one of sympathy towards Saul. The people of Yavesh Gilaad, a nearby village to the battle field, provided a dignified burial for Saul and his sons and mourned his death for seven days (see Samuel I, 3:11–13). While this may appear as simply a documentation of events, there is a meta-analytic fact involved, in that the scriptures do not choose to transpose their own attitude upon the story of the act committed. The absence of this message is, in itself, provoking.

The fourth suicide in the bible was committed by Ahitopel (Samuel I, 17:23) Ahitopel attained his reputation as one of the most wise and respected advisors of his times, serving as an advisor to King David. Ahitopel left King David and aligned himself with David's son Avshalom in a rebellion against the king. However, this new alliance was soon foolishly betrayed by Avshalom. Ahitopel was made aware that Avshalom was tricked by another advisor into

following a foolhardy plan certain to lead to David's victory and to the failure of Avshalom rebellion. In response, Ahitopel set his house in order, makes final arrangements for his family, and strangles himself (Samuel I, 17:23, see also Kaplan and Schwartz 1993).

While it is clear that Ahitopel's suicide was a response to the events described before it, his exact motives are left unclear. Commentators have suggested numerous post-mortem interpretations: that Ahitopel was overcome with disappointment in his own lack of judgement in aligning himself with Avshalom rather than David; that Ahitopel was deeply humiliated by Avshalom's preference for advice from another. A third view is that Ahitopel feared David's vengeance (Shemesh 2003). One Talmudic explanation is that the motive was a utilitarian one

The fifth suicide in the Book of Prophets is that one committed by Zimri, a high-ranking officer in the army who killed Elah the king of Israel, and took over the kingdom. However, Omri, another high-ranking officer, then lead the army to siege Zimri's palace. Zimri realized that he would not be able to overcome the siege and chose to commit suicide rather than be murdered, by setting fire to his palace (Kings I, 16:18). As in the case of Samson, there is an element of revenge by burning the palace, although his main motive was to escape being murdered. While Zimri's fate of being brought to suicide is described in the scriptures as a punishment for his wrong deeds, Zimri's decision to commit the suicidal act is not, in itself, addressed.

In reviewing all the suicides and death wishes that are described in the scripture, it seems that in no single case is there a condemnation of the suicidal act or death wishes. In most cases, the reputation of the figures that committed suicide seems undamaged by the act; the wicked are remembered for their wickedness, and the heroes remain remembered for their heroics. Even more puzzling is the case of Samson, whose suicide is assisted by God.

## Suicide in the Talmud and the Midrash

The Talmudic and the Midrashic approach to the issue of suicide are far more complicated than the one that is present in the Bible. The Talmud addresses the issue of suicide in three ways: (1) through discussion and interpretation of the suicides described in the Bible; (2) through Midrash stories of suicides that occurred at the time of the Talmud; (3) and finally, by drawing Halachic conclusions regarding suicide. From a purely Halachic perspective, the sages of the Talmud take a strong stand against suicide and determine decisively that suicide is prohibited and punishable by preventing burial honours from the suicide completers, such as rending of the mourner's garments, delivering of the memorial address (Semachot 2:1; Yoreh Deáh 345). Warnings against suicide also include punishment in the hereafter. At the same time, the Talmud and Midrash reflect ambivalence and present contradictions with regard to the issue of suicide. However, these actually serve to elucidate that defining suicide and determining its consequences is a complex matter. For example, the Midrash Raba (on Genesis 9:5) concludes that the suicide of Saul should not be considered a prohibited suicide. How was Saul's suicide not a suicide? Several reasons are mentioned for this exclusion: he was afraid of the torture that would be imminent if he were to be captured; he was afraid that he would be forced to worship idols; he did not want to cause a desecration of God's name by being captured and by committing suicide he saved many of his fighters' lives (Shemesh 2003). Thus, the Talmudic interpretation of Saul's suicide says that there are certain conditions under which taking one's own life may not be considered a sin.

There is a Talmudic story about Rabbi Hanina ben Tardion, who was bound to a Torah scroll and burned to death with it by the Romans. His students pleaded with him: 'Open then thy mouth… so that the fire enter into thee.' However, he refused to take even a slight active part in his own imminent death, despite his great suffering: 'Let Him who gave me [my soul] take it away, but no one should injure oneself.' The Roman executioner offered to end Hanina's torture by removing the wet sponge that was placed upon his heart to artificially prolong his torture. Rabbi Hanina agreed to this, and both he and the executioner were promised a place in heaven (Avoda Zara 18a). From this tale, it appears that no active role may be taken, even under intolerable pain, but a passive participation in suicide under such circumstances was acceptable. However, the Talmud also cites suicide stories with an embedded lesson that active suicide is permitted under certain circumstances. One example of this in the story that relates the suicide of 400 boys and girls who were captured by the Romans, and were to be condemned to a life of prostitution in Rome (Gittin 57b). They turned to the eldest among them and asked him if under such conditions suicide is considered a sin. The elder gave permission to commit suicide based on his interpretation of a verse in Psalms. The children leaped into the sea and died. They feared lest idol worshippers force them to sin and they preferred death, not out of fear of torture or personal reasons, but for purely religious reasons. The children's suicide is clearly condoned in the Talmud. There is also an account of a number of suicides of young Cohanim (priests who served in the Temple) who killed themselves when Romans set fire to the Temple (Taanit 29a). The Talmud justifies these suicides as an act aimed at sanctifying God's Holy name. The common thread to these stories, according to the Talmud, is that there are instances in which one is required to give up one's life rather than to transgress. Such instances include when one is forced to commit incest, murder, or idolatry. The Talmud determines that in these circumstances one should give up one's life passively, that is let oneself be killed, but not actively commit suicide (Sanhedrin 74a).

What of suicide because of personally unbearable emotional pain? One such suicide story involves a student whose name was falsely besmirched by a prostitute, and he killed himself out of sinless shame (Berachot 23a). The Talmud does not condemn his suicide.

The Talmud also discusses the case of Tzidkiyahu, a king who was captured and tortured by the Babylonians. The Babylonian king ordered that Tzidkiyahu's children be slaughtered before his eyes and then his eyes would be poked out. Rabbi Yehuda—a Talmudic sage—wondered why Tzidkiyahu did not, in this situation, smash his head against the wall in order to kill himself (Midrash Raba on Aicha, Chapter A, 59). Such a question obviously reflects the belief that under certain unbearable emotional distress, suicide can be considered as a logical conclusion.

In the Talmud, suicide is recognized as a social issue worthy of sensitivity. There are several stories reflecting this sensitivity, for example, there are two suicides of young children described in the Talmud (Semachot, Chapters 2 and 5). One child ran away from school, and the father was about to punish him. The child committed suicide as an escape from the punishment. Another child broke a bottle on the Sabbath (this is considered a transgression of the Sabbath observation). The child, similar to the previous case, also took his life out of the fear of being punished by his father. Neither of these cases was defined as being intentional suicides (Kaplan and Schwartz 1993). In relating these stories, the sages of the Talmud warn that educational strategies should not include unduly harsh punishment.

## Suicide in the rabbinic-halachic codex

The rabbinic codex that was established throughout the years after the Talmud was edited has strict rules against suicide. However, in order to obey these rules, the definition of suicide must first be clarified. The definition and examples, as well as the rules governing mourning are based on the *Shulchan Aruch* (Yoreh Deah, Chapter 355). It must be established without a doubt that the person was seen in an agitated state, and, indeed, intend to complete suicide. If, however, they did not declare intent, or the person was not actually seen before or during the act, the death cannot be proclaimed a suicide. There must be a clear connection between a declaration of intent and the actual deed. Otherwise, if, for example, a person declared intent but was not actually seen ascending or falling, the stated intent is attributed to exaggeration, and conjecture that they may have accidentally fallen or even have been pushed by another person. The following illustrations are even examples of the tendency to mitigate the humiliation and anguish associated with suicide whenever possible. Even if a person is found dead with the lethal weapon nearby; the rabbi may declare that the person was murdered. If a letter that obviously was composed in a clear state of mind is found, in the event that a long time has elapsed since it was composed, the possibility is raised that the writer may have changed their mind, and the death was perhaps accidental or executed when they were in a deranged state of mind. The following example adds another dimension to our understanding of the halacha concerning suicide. A person, after having declared their intent to end their life, jumps into a river. It seems obvious that this is a clear-cut case of suicide, nevertheless, if the possibility exists that perhaps the drowning person had second thoughts while struggling in the water, it is not declared a suicide. The examples and discussion clearly demonstrate that rabbinic authorities sought to minimize labelling death as suicide even when doing so seemed far-fetched. Their motives for doing so stem from the fact that the Talmud propounded the principle that when controversy exists in issues related to mourning, the lenient position takes precedence. The psychological meaning inherent in this principle is that it is proper to minimize the anguish of family members. It also shows a marked respect for the frailty of humans, engendering empathy, although it does not condone the act itself.

## Suicides in Jewish history

The renowned story about the heroism of the fighters of Mesada has become a mythological legend. However, documentation of the events lack clarification. No reference can be found in the writings of the sages on this topic, even though, given the period, one would expect reference to it. Perhaps the lack of attention indicates that the sages were not comfortable with this topic. We have no sound and reliable historical evidence about the event. Our knowledge is based upon the book, *The War of the Jews*, written by Josephus Falvius in 73 AD, which includes the speech of Eliezer ben Yair, the commander who led the others in slaughtering their wives and children, and then each other until they were all dead (pp. 600–601). If we chose to rely upon his speech as it appears in *Wars of the Jews* (some claim that it is fabricated, and content-wise seems to belong to Josephus, see Kaplan and Schwartz [1993]), the cause of suicide of ben Yair and his people was their refusal to live a life of slavery. We do not have sufficient information about the conditions of Roman captivity, and the threat that these individuals were facing if they were to surrender. In any event, it is clear that the sages did not find it justifiable to end one's life rather than be enslaved.

Josephus also documents the suicides of the fighters of Gamla, who held onto their wives and children and jumped into a pit with them. There is a critical tone in Josephus' writings in regards to the act:

> And the things occurred that the wrath of the Romans was revealed as more subtle than madness itself, because these [the Romans] killed only four thousand people, while these who threw themselves down were more than five thousand.
>
> *Wars of the Jews* (pp. 324–328)

During the Crusades between the years 1099 to 1204, in most of the European countries, entire communities were faced with the cruel decision: conversion or death. Some chose a superficial conversion to Christianity, they were the first *Anusim* (forced ones). However, most chose death. The testimonies left behind indicate that they did not wait for the Romans to kill them, but took the matter into their own hands. Many songs were written about that period in time to commemorate the martyrs: four of them were made part of the yearly prayers of the day of the destruction of the Temple, so that their memory is evoked with the memory of the destruction of the Temple. This seems to reflect the positive attitude of the sages towards their decision to kill themselves, rather than waiting for the crusaders to come and kill them.

## The philosophical perspective

Maimonides, a master, rabbi, and philosopher from the twelfth century, makes a distinction between murder and suicide (Nezikin, Chapter 2). The logical conclusion to his reasoning, it seems, is that suicide, notwithstanding the gravity of the sin, is not to be equated with murder. The act does not deprive a fellow human of their most prized possession—their life. It also is not as disruptive to society as murder, which negates the law and order of a civilized society. Suicide, unlike murder, does not unravel the fabric of society.

We are now faced with the question why, if suicide does not involve another human being and is not a major disruption of society, is it considered a grave transgression? The solution to this dilemma touches upon some of Judaism's cardinal beliefs. One's life and one's soul are, unlike one's possessions, not one's property. Life is not an object to dispense with whenever one chooses to do so. The sages (Pirkei Avot, *Ethics of the Fathers*, Chapter 4) teach that a person does not choose to be born, to live, or to die, and stand on judgment. Maimonides emphasizes that man is created in God's image [in a spiritual sense], hence the prohibition to obliterate it (Laws of Murder, Chapter 1, Halacha 4). Death is, in a spiritual sense, a cleansing force. This means that God deems one's difficulties and misfortunes, including one's demise, when judging the individual. This does not hold in the case of suicide, the rationale being that, if someone chooses to take their own life, death cannot be viewed as a cleansing force. On the contrary, the very act of dying by suicide is a sin.

An additional philosophical perspective on suicide can be deducted from the book of Job (Orbach 1994). The biblical story of Job is a story of a man's quest for meaning in the relationship between man and God in face of unbearable and unjust human suffering. The book of Job also sends a clear message against suicide. The incomprehensible, drastic, traumatic, and painful events occurring to Job may lead us, modern researchers of suicidal behaviour, to expect Job to put an end to his unjust suffering by suicide, just as his wife suggests to him. Nevertheless, for Job, this is out of the question. On the contrary, despite his sufferings, he seems to gain unexplained strength and emerges as a powerful personality with inner mental resources that enable him to sustain his tragic existential situation. Job is suffering from the sudden collapse of his secure environment, reduced status and health, loss of his beloved children, and the love of his friends. Yet, the crisis in his belief in God and his struggle to gain meaning from a religious standpoint is the most important paradigm that he faces. Job's lack of comprehension for God's leadership of the world constitutes a loss of meaning in life. This has a tremendous emotional impact. He is shaken by anxiety, fear, depression, and loss of direction.

What then prevented Job from killing himself? Why didn't he listen to his wife's advice to curse God and die? The scripture lends itself to two types of possible explanations, a psychological and a theological. The most potent motivational force against suicide in Job can be attributed to his unwillingness to give up the search for meaning in life in spite of his unfortunate destiny; a powerful life-enhancing motivation. Was it attitudes of self-righteousness, the stubborn search for meaning, holding onto hope in order to find meaning can constitute protective factors against suicide? The book of Job also uses a special literary device to convey the theological stance that suicide, as an option for solving problems and escaping pain, is forbidden. The author of Job portrays a protagonist struggling with extreme circumstances which may lead to suicide, but he stops short of committing this act, as though telling the reader that from a religious point of view, suicide is unacceptable. Although, there are several cases of suicide throughout the Bible, the Book of Job opposes suicide on personal and psychological grounds.

## Treatment and prevention as offered by the scriptures

Kaplan and Schwartz (1993) eloquently delineate therapeutic and preventive principles offered through biblical stories to respond to the suicidal thoughts or wishes expressed by various biblical heroes. The authors note several therapeutic interventions by God as examples of how suicidal urges should be approached therapeutically. These include protective regression, nurturance, support, guidance, practical advice, providing meaning and renewal of faith and relationships as well as encouragement to face difficulties.

Jonah, for example, not only expresses a wish to die, but also asks the sailors of the sinking ship to throw him overboard. God sends a whale to swallow him into the warmth and safety of the womb, a symbol of protective regression. Later on, Jonah sits under the hot sun and God shields him from the sun with a gourd. After the symbiotic protection, there is a drive toward an individuation, but still under a protective shield. Finally, God helps Jonah to find meaning in life by teaching him the value of mercy—to help others without being absorbed by them. Similar therapeutic interventions are taken by God when Alijah, Moses, David, and Rebecca express suicidal wishes (see Kaplan and Schwartz 1993).

The Talmudic sages, and later commentators of the Talmud and the Bible, emphasize the need for social support, warm relationships, and lenient educational measures for children; no harsh punishments, and if punishment is needed it should be carried out close to the transgressive act and not later in time. The most important preventative principle advocated by Jewish communities throughout history is support through a rich network of social relationships that promotes cohesiveness and a sense of belongingness and mutual support. The scriptures and rabbinic law demand mutual responsibility and involvement for the welfare of the other. This requires taking an active involvement when the other is in need of help. These psychological principles are absorbed, not only among orthodox Jews, but can be found throughout Jewish communities.

Religious authorities today are making strong efforts to clear the stigma of psychological and psychiatric problems. They encourage psychological and psychiatric help when needed, in addition to their own effort and the comfort to be found in religion. One example is an organization called Retorno (Return), an inpatient rehabilitation centre run by religious and professional authorities, geared at rehabilitating teens and adults with various self-destructive behaviours, including suicidal behaviours, using clinical methods with a religious orientation, including individual and group therapy, spiritual guidance, religious studies and practices. They place a strong emphasis on mutual support within the group and from as well as to the community outside the centre. Communal living, social support, advancement of social cohesion, and providing meaning to life by helping others, as well as warm and authoritative guidance and advice are some of the practical approaches applied in religious therapeutic centres for troubled youth.

Social support is not the only preventative measure implied in the Jewish approach to prevention of suicide. Although, the Biblical, Talmudic and Rabbinic views are complex, the message is very clear: suicide for personal reasons is categorically forbidden. Prohibition of suicide and its taboo is also reflected in the burial and mourning rituals. When a person dies of natural causes or an involuntary death, there are special burial rituals as well as mourning rituals for the first seven days, the first month and the first year after the death. These include, among others, the purification of the deceased body, the ritualistic tearing of the cloths by the blood relatives, funeral oration, saying the Kaddish prayer, barefoot sitting for seven days in mourning (Shiva), and the consoling of the relatives by the community members. In case of suicide, the Talmud determines that there should be no ritual tearing, no barefoot sitting and no mourning. Later, some rabbinic authorities added that people who have committed suicide will not receive the ritualistic purification and will be buried in a separate and distant section of the cemeteries (Liechtenstein 1991).

These omissions of the rituals were meant to warn the person who intends to commit suicide that their 'Post Self Image' (Shneidman 1985) intends will be damaged, thus, preventing the self-destructive behaviour.

In actuality, such omissions are very rarely implemented. As discussed earlier, the Jewish approach reflects an empathic understanding of human suffering and of the suicidal state of mind. It also offers a very minimalist definition of what is considered to be a suicide in an attempt to respect and avoid further suffering by the family.

## Suicide in Israel today

Israel has a relatively low rate of suicide. The latest figures that were released show that in the year 2005, the rates for the general population was 8.6/100,000 (Central Bureau of Statistics, Israel 2007). Although, Israel can be considered a secular state, where religious manners and views are held by a substantial majority of Israelis, and this is probably an important factor in the relatively low rate of suicide. The rates for those who were observant of religious laws cannot be determined, as no such information appears in any official statistics; but Levav, Magnes, Aisenberg and Rosenbaum (1988) have found that suicidal behaviour and suicidal ideation is far less prevalent among religious observers as compared to non-observers; the more the religiosity, the less the suicidality. These findings resonate with the general impression of very low suicide rates among observant people in Israel. This was also found to be true for other religions (Stack 1992). Apparently, any religious faith constitutes a first-degree protective factor against suicide.

## References

Central Bureau of Statistics (2007). *Annual Report*. Government Publications, Jerusalem.

Josephus, F (1981). *The Jewish Wars*, translated by GA Williamson. Penguin, New York.

Kaplan K and Schwartz M (1993). *The Psychology of Hope*. Praeger Publishers, Westport.

Levav I, Magnes J, Aisenberg E *et al.* (1988). Sociodemographic correlates of suicidal ideation and reported attempts. *Israel Journal of Psychiatry and Related Sciences*, **25**, 38–45.

Liechtenstein Y (1991). The prohibition of suicide in Jewish law. Masters thesis. Department of Talmud. Bar-Ilan University, Israel.

Orbach I (1994). Job—a biblical message about suicide. *Journal Of Psychology and Judaism*, 18, 241–247.

Shemesh Y (2003). Suicide in the Bible. Available at http://www.biu.ac.il/JSIJ/2–2003/shemesh.pdf.

Shneidman E (1984). *Definition of Suicide*. John Wiley and Sons, New York.

Stack S (1992). Religiosity, depression, and suicide. In JFE Schumaker, ed., *Religion and Mental Health*, pp. 87–97. Oxford University Press, New York.

# CHAPTER 8

# Suicide and Islam

Ahmed Okasha and Tarek Okasha

## Abstract

This chapter will discuss the historical and philosophical aspects of suicide in Islam. Influences of Islamic culture on the phenomena of suicide and attempted suicide will be emphasized, focusing chiefly on attitudes in Egypt. All studies show that suicide is less prevalent in Islamic societies compared to countries associated with other religions. Here, the reasons for suicide in different Islamic and Arabic countries are evaluated in relation to the sociocultural context.

The cognitive schemata of Muslims follow the phrases of the Koran that humans were created for the main reason of worshipping God, and that life and death issues should be controlled by God and not by self-destruction. This faith can be a factor in preventing suicide attempts, especially in those practising their religious rituals. The phenomenology of psychiatric disorders in Islamic culture is characterized and dominated in its content, whether hallucinations or delusions by religious themes.

## Historical and religious perspectives

Nor take life which Allah has made sacred except for just cause. And if any one is slain wrongfully, we have given his heir authority to demand Qisas or to forgive, but let him not exceed bounds in the matter of taking life, for his helped (by God).

The Holy Koran (Surat Al Isra'a 33)

Take not life, which Allah has made sacred, except by way of justice and law. Thus does he command you that you may learn wisdom.

The Holy Koran (Surat Al Ana'am 151)

## Introduction

In ancient Egypt, suicide was a disaster for both the body and the soul. By destroying the body, instead of having it embalmed, the soul would lose its home, as the soul must return every night to the body to be reborn, and the following morning at sunrise in order to live eternally. Not only the soul, but the whole body is under the responsibility of the Gods. The subject of eternal reprobation and whether suicide was sinful is irrelevant: it makes no difference whether one reaches death by suicide or by waiting for it. Suicide was not an issue in ancient Egypt (Ebbel 1937), except in the case of Cleopatra, who was originally Greek.

## Religion and suicide

Suicide is one of those issues that exist in a twilight zone between religion and psychiatry. Historically, there was always an overlap between those who provided the spiritual and the health needs of people, mostly represented by the clergy. This overlap, although separated throughout the ages, has in some cultures still left its imprint on the medical profession. In many Islamic cultures, a doctor is still referred to as 'Hakim', which means 'the wise man'. When health concerns are psychological rather than physical ailments, the boundaries between medical and spiritual/religious healing may become even more blurred.

Few authors have investigated the influence of religion on suicide from a medical and suicidological perspective. Bertolote and Fleischmann (2002) discussed the importance of the religious context and the prevalence of a religion in a country as major cultural factors in the determination of suicide. There are some indications that the religiousness of a person might serve as a protective factor against suicide. The data collected in the WHO SUPRE-MISS community study investigated the religious denomination of the respondents and their religiousness (Bertolote et al. 2005). Whereas there was one predominant religion (i.e. religious denomination) in many of the sites, this was not always reflected in the perceived religiousness of the respondents, who were asked whether they considered themselves to be a religious person. In Campinas, Brazil and Chennai, India, the respondents were predominantly Christian and Hindu respectively; they also considered themselves to be religious persons. In Colombo, Sri Lanka, there was a mixture of several religions and the respondents considered themselves as religious persons. Durban, South Africa also had a variety of religious denominations; however, the perceived religiousness was lower. In Tallinn, Estonia, there was a mixture of Christian and no religion, and the religiousness was even lower. In Karaj, Iran, Islam was predominant at 100 per cent, however, not everyone thought of themselves as a religious person. In Hanoi, Vietnam, the large majority did not have a religious denomination; however, a number of people considered themselves as being religious (Table 8.1).

Methodological deliberations aside, the results are nevertheless confronted with cultural influences, and the subject of suicide as value laden. Some of the differences across sites were probably affected by differences in the willingness of respondents

**Table 8.1** Health burden due to suicide expressed in DALY (%)

| Region | 1998 | 1999 | 2000 | 2001 | 2002 |
|--------|------|------|------|------|------|
| Africa | 0.2 | 1.0 | 0.2 | 0.2 | 0.2 |
| America | 1.2 | 1.7 | 1.1 | 1.1 | 1.0 |
| EMRO* | 1.0 | 0.9 | 0.5 | 0.7 | 0.7 |
| Europe | 2.2 | 2.9 | 2.5 | 2.3 | 2.3 |
| SE Asia | 1.3 | 1.3 | 1.2 | 1.6 | 1.7 |
| W Pacific | 3.6 | 3.3 | 2.8 | 2.5 | 2.6 |
| World | 1.6 | 1.7 | 1.3 | 1.4 | 1.4 |

* EMRO is the east Mediterranean region comprising 22 countries, all of which have a majority Muslim population, except for Lebanon, and all of them speak the Arabic language except for Iran and Pakistan.

from different cultures to report suicidal thoughts, suicide plans, and attempts. Different levels of perceived stigmatization may also have affected responses to questions about physical illness, mental illness, and alcohol use in the SUPRE-MISS study (WHO 2002), and thus, explain some of the observed differences across the sites. The way mental illness is understood in different cultures, and the particular difficulty of grasping such perceptions despite culture-specific adaptations of the instrument of analysis should also be taken into account. The overall results of the SUPRE-MISS need to be further explored in a careful analysis of the complete questionnaire.

There might be differences, not only in openly discussing suicidal behaviours, but also in the general awareness of such questions. Religious families assess quality of life according to adherence to religious rituals, regardless of symptomatology. Negative symptoms (withdrawal, alogia and avolition) may be perceived by a group of Islamic followers as piousness, and hence deeper contemplation about God considered virtuous. Positive symptoms, like auditory and visual hallucinatory experiences and delusions related to religious matters, are sometimes perceived as gifts from God by extraordinary perception, and thus, considered singular. The comparison of Egyptian, Indian and British depressive patients revealed that Egyptians have a significant increase in suicidal tendencies, but not in actual suicide or attempted suicide (Okasha 2000).

## Suicide in Islam

Islam means submitting to God. This submission entails that at the end it is God who decides everything. It follows that everything that happens carries with it a certain wisdom or rationale. Even if the individual fails to grasp that wisdom, Islam demands that a Muslim believe in their presence and in God's final judgment. Suicide is prohibited by Islam. It is *haram*—forbidden. The logic behind the prohibition is that it is an act that manipulates something, in this case life itself, which is meant to be only God's concern. Furthermore, it indicates lack of trust in God who is capable of making things better. However, haram also means acting in a way that is unjust to self and to others.

The Arab social historian Ibn Khaldoun (1332–1406) was the first author to give a clear description of the relationship between mental health and culture. He described the effects of urbanization on Islamic tribe warriors when they moved from nomadic life to live in towns. The movement was associated with an increase in the prevalence of psychological ailments, namely jealousy, suspiciousness, self-indulgence, and fear of others. He viewed this behaviour as a reaction to the change of social structure. In his view, the tribal system failed to adjust to the process of urbanization. Such failure was, in Ibn Khaldoun's view, at the origin of decline of Islamic civilization. The prevailing concept of mental illness at a particular state in the Islamic world depends on the dominance of development or deterioration of genuine Islamic issues. For instance, during periods of deterioration, the negative concepts of the insane as being possessed by evil spirits dominates, whereas during periods of enlightenment and creative epochs, the disharmony concept dominates, and so forth (Okasha 1999).

In the West, an individual is brought up from an early age to appreciate separateness, freedom, and self-responsibility. Life, even within the family, is focused clearly on give and take, and dependence is not tolerated for long. The extended family has almost disappeared except among the very affluent, and the nuclear family is under serious challenge from a high rate of marriage breakdown. The individual is presumably left to fend for themself with a make it or break it philosophy. These general statements are often compounded in individuals who are less endowed or disabled in one or more ways. Society tends to impose a subtle form of isolation on those with physical illness, the elderly and the mentally ill, among others, creating a state of defeat and alienation that becomes self-perpetuating and malignant towards the end. Research shows that in many traditional societies the social structure is different. The family retains a presence in the individual's life, and anomie is probably less frequently encountered or recognized.

## Suicide in the Koran

Islam bans self-destructive behaviour as an act of violation of the will of God in taking away life. Even the widely debated issue of suicide bombing, it is denounced by high-ranking religious authorities in the region, refusing to describe the actors as martyrs. Those who contemplate suicide know of never-ending graphic descriptions of torture in hell awaiting the person who takes their own life. A depressed believer would argue when questioned that they have been unhappy in this life and would not want to suffer eternally as well after death. Suffering in our common life is taken by believers as a test from God that should be endured, and promises even greater happiness in the after life. Suicidal behaviour drops markedly in frequency during the holy month of Ramadan (Bensmail *et al.* 1989; Al-Ansari *et al.* 1990). Ramadan is considered as a holy month because the Koran was revealed during this month: it is a time of fasting and it is dominated by religious rituals.

## Attitudes towards mental problems, suicide and stigma

It is generally accepted in Western countries that suicide is under-reported, hence this is to be expected in Islamic societies to a larger extent, because suicide is considered a major sin and shameful event for the family. Under-reporting of both suicide and attempted suicide is prevalent, especially in the case of female suicides, which are usually taken to be associated with the breaking of moral codes. The Egyptian spheres of authority and power have traditionally been dominated by men, however, female resistance and influence has always been widespread, and more so recently. When a female attempts or commits suicide, the blame and guilt are laid on the family as having failed to provide security and faith. The male is supposed to be more autonomous in his decisions.

It is worthy of note that the Coptic Orthodox Church, also known as the Egyptian Orthodox Church of Alexandria, does not offer any prayers for those who have committed suicide. In Islam, the suicidal individual is considered to have violated God's decisions, but the death prayers are still performed in the Mosque for him. In both religions, the individual who committed suicide is buried according to the social customs in Egypt.

Symptoms of mental illness are perceived very differently across the Islamic world; ranging from scientific beliefs of alterations in brain functions to a state of possession by Jinni and evil spirits. However, in all situations they are considered as God's will and a lesson for the worshipper to repent. For religious Muslims, death is sometimes looked upon as a blessing and a way to be near God. It is accepted as a continuation of life dependent on the individual's deeds. In Islam, mental symptoms are not taboo, the stigma exists that these may be a curse or a test from God, and good Muslims should accept the will of God. Thus, there is a stigma, but its interpretation is different. Suicide is dishonoured because it connotes a lack of belief in God's creation and a lack of adherence to the codes of Islam. Lack of awareness of an underlying psychopathology is one major element that contributes to the moral judgement of suicide. The concept of depression and mania is overlooked. Depression is attributed to being lazy, to a weak personality, lack of faith and attributed to God's will for redemption. Mania is described as crazy, possessed by Jinni or evil spirits, and the individual is perceived as irresponsible.

The following hypothetical reactions of the different members of a Muslim family to the attempted suicide of a family member reflect various permissive and aggressive attitudes that are frequent. A senior female family member usually adopts the permissive attitude by alleviating the guilt feelings and shame in the family, regarding the failure of its members to provide enough faith to prevent self-destruction. A male family member, usually the family head, adopts the aggressive attitude by ostracizing the family member who shamed the family by their suicide attempt. Long prospective follow-up studies of parasuicide (attempted suicide) with blind assessments could highlight the prognostic correlates of the permissive, aggressive and combined family attitudes (Suleiman *et al.* 1989).

Table 8.2 shows that the WHO Eastern Regional Mediterranean office, which covers a region comprising 22 countries who are predominantly Islamic, has the lowest rate of suicide expressed in disability-adjusted life years (DALYs) percentages: it was 0.7% for the east Mediterranean region in 2002. It is only the African region which shows lower percentage measured in DALYs.

Table 8.3 shows the low reported suicide rates in some Islamic countries over different years. The lack of reporting of suicide suggests that these figures cannot be taken as representative of reality. However, in other Islamic countries, namely those which separated from the former Soviet Union. For example Turkmenistan, Uzbekistan and Bosnia, the percentage is rather high compared to the Middle East.

Personal and family problems can be said to constitute the main trigger for suicide and attempted suicide in traditional societies. In intergenerational conflict, the disagreement between members of the young generation and their elders was found to involve their attitudes towards family relationships, marriage and emancipation of women. Arab Gulf communities have undergone rapid social change in these spheres (El-Assra 1989). The rapid growth of mass media, tourism, secular education and new occupational opportunities associated with oil wealth have influenced social change. Members of the young generation prefer equal authority, and responsibility for all family members instead of family relationships that favour the older and male children; they prefer marriage based on love rather than arranged by the family and a multi-role as opposed to a mono-role for women. Such changes have influenced psychiatric disorders, with intergenerational strife stated as the reasons for parasuicide (attempted suicide) in 57 per cent of cases (El-Islam 1974, 1976, 1979).

In a cohort of 157 Egyptian depressive outpatients, El-Islam (1969) reported that 62.7 per cent presented guilt feelings. However, the definition of guilt was broad. It involved self-reproach, death wishes, and attempted suicide. The experience of self-reproach in the sample ranged over a wide spectrum of behaviour, e.g. being irritable, imagined inadequacy at work, neglect of family affairs, letting down friends, or minor transgressions in which the patient had caused harm. Guilt feelings were not found to correlate statistically with religion in this culture. There was no significant difference between Christians and Muslims. However, anecdotal reports seem to indicate that guilt feelings are more common in Christian

**Table 8.2** Religious variables in the WHO SUPRE-MISS Community survey study (2005)

| Religion | Campinas | Chennai | Colombo | Durban | Hanoi | Karaj | Tallinn | Yuncheng |
|---|---|---|---|---|---|---|---|---|
| | N 516 | N 500 | N 683 | N 497 | N 2277 | N 504 | N 498 | N 503 |
| Christian | 86 | 3 | 13 | 40 | 3 | 0 | 47 | 1 |
| Muslim | 0 | 5 | 24 | 3 | 0 | 100 | 0 | 0 |
| Hindu | 0 | 92 | 18 | 13 | 0 | 0 | 0 | 0 |
| Buddhist | 0 | 0 | 44 | 0 | 6 | 0 | 0 | 1 |
| Other | 5 | 0 | 1 | 28 | 1 | 0 | 3 | 0 |
| None | 8 | 0 | 0 | 17 | 91 | 0 | 49 | 98 |
| **Religiousness** | | | | | | | | |
| | N 514 | N 499 | N 659 | N 484 | N 2106 | N 502 | N 492 | N 503 |
| Yes | 01 | 92 | 96 | 51 | 34 | 80 | 37 | No data |

Source: Bertolote JM, Fleischmann A, de Leo L (2005). Suicide attempts, plans, and ideation in culturally diverse sites: the WHO SUPRE-MISS community survey. *Psychological Medicine*, **35**, 1457–1465. Reproduced with kind permission from Cambridge University Press.

**Table 8.3** Reported suicide in some Islamic countries (WHO 2007)

|  | Year | Males | Females |
|---|---|---|---|
| Bahrain | 1988 | 4.9 | 0.5 |
| Egypt | 1987 | 0.1 | 0 |
| Iran | 1991 | 0.3 | 0.1 |
| Kuwait | 2001 | 2.5 | 1.4 |
| Syria | 1985 | 0.2 | 0 |
| Jordan | 1979 | 0 | 0 |
| Bosnia | 1991 | 20.3 | 3.3 |
| Turkmenistan | 1998 | 13.8 | 3.5 |
| Uzbekistan | 2003 | 8.1 | 3 |

depressed patients in Egypt. Guilt feelings were over-represented in the literate and psychotic groups of patients.

## Attempted suicide in Egypt

Feelings of hopelessness and the intention to kill oneself are rare among Muslim depressed patients, where losing hope in God's relief and self-inflicted death are considered blasphemous and punishable by eternal hell fire in the after life. However, the rates of suicidal attempts (parasuicide) as cries for help had no significant associations with religiosity among Muslims. Although, the wish to die is not uncommon among Muslim depressives, it usually remains at the level of wishing that God would terminate their life and does not progress to the wish to kill themselves (Okasha and Lotaif 1979).

An Egyptian investigation and a descriptive study of parasuicide in Cairo comprised 200 cases from a total of 1155 patients who attempted suicide in 1975 and were admitted to the casualty department of Ain Shams University Hospital in Cairo, with a catchment area comprising approximately 3 million people (Okasha *et al.* 1988). A crude rate of suicide attempts in Cairo was 38.5/100,000. There was a high percentage of attempted suicide among the 15–44 age group, with no major difference between the two sexes. Single patients represented 53 per cent of the total, with students showing the highest risk (40 per cent). Depressive illnesses, hysterical reactions, and the situational disorders, in that order of frequency, were the main causes of the attempt. Overdose by tablet ingestion was the most common method used (80 per cent). Official government reports are misleading and do not represent the true rate.

Another study of a sample of 91 persons who were admitted for attempted suicide to the casualty department of three hospitals in Cairo during the year 1981–1982, showed that a large majority of the attempters were young women (age range 15–34 years) belonging to large overcrowded families. They showed a higher tendency to be single, literate and unemployed than the corresponding age group in the general population. Drug overdose was the most common method used. The majority made their attempts at home when there was somebody nearby, and 31 per cent had previous non-serious attempts. Dysthymic disorders, adjustment, affective and personality disorders were the most common diagnoses encountered. Attempters scored higher in neuroticism, extraversion, and

psychoticism and they tended to be more flexible. There was a high percentage among the 15–44 age group. Rates were higher among students, followed by the unemployed. Individuals whose education stopped after secondary education constituted one-third of the group, coinciding with the population category showing the highest rate of unemployment. Single men and married women attempted suicide more frequently than married men, for single and widowed women, however, there was no significant difference. Suicide attempts showed a peak in the months April–June, which not only coincides with the seasonal transition, but also with a time of examinations in Egyptian schools and universities, a period that has been described as one of national stress. Single patients represented 53 per cent of the total, with students showing the highest risk (40 per cent). Depressive illnesses, hysterical reactions, and situational disorders, in that order of frequency, were the main causes of the attempts. Analysis of the attempts revealed a low prevalence of suicidal feelings and intent for a period before the attempt, indicating the impulsivity thereof. The majority had threatened to attempt suicide and had history of previous attempts, all of which had taken place in the residence of the individual where they would most likely be saved by a family member: 97 per cent of the sample had expressed feelings of social isolation, and their attempts can be taken as a cry for help (Okasha 1984).

A recent study attempting to find out the current prevalence of attempted suicide by ingestion in a representative Egyptian sample showed interesting results. The prevalence of suicide attempts by ingesting drugs/toxins was 0.066/6 months in contrast to official records showing only 0.0002/6 months. In this sample, 85.3 per cent were serious suicidal attempts and 14.7 per cent were cries for help. 43.9 per cent of the attempters below the age of 20 years had socio-familial difficulties, while 49.2 per cent between the ages of 20 and 40 years had financial difficulties; 6.9 per cent were above 40 years old, and again gave reasons of socio-familial problems as the direct cause of their attempts. Regarding sex, 64.2 per cent of the sample were females with emotional problems, while males attempted suicide because of studies/work problems. As for the occupational status, 38.6 per cent of the attempters were students with emotional problems and 27 per cent were unemployed. The commonest drugs/toxins used were organophosphorous compounds (54.1 per cent) used by female students below age 20, followed by cardiopulmonary drugs (13 per cent) used mainly by unemployed females with ages ranging between 20 and 40 years. Underlying psychiatric disorders were distributed as follows: 30.5 per cent mood disorders, 17 per cent personality disorders, 9.8 per cent anxiety disorders, and 5.3 per cent other psychotic disorders. 37 per cent of the attempters had no psychiatric morbidity and attempted suicide for socio-familial difficulties (Okasha *et al.* 2006).

## Attempted suicide in Islamic communties across the Middle East and Turkey

Studies of Muslim depressed patients suggest that symptom frequencies and expressions used in depressed Arab patients differ considerably from Western-derived definitions (El Islam *et al.* 1988; Hamdi *et al.* 1997). The Hamilton Depression Rating Scale was used in different Muslim communities (Pfieffer 1968; El Islam *et al.* 1988; Hamdi *et al.* 1997), and there was a higher incidence of retardation, somatic anxiety, and hypochondriasis, and a lower incidence of morning worsening of symptoms, suicide, guilt, and delayed insomnia. Our recent research suggests that Muslim countries are moving in the direction of the West; thus acquiring its ailments, including an increasing rate of suicide attempts (Okasha 2000).

Results of the WHO–EURO Multicentre Study on Suicidal Behavior in Turkey (Ozguven and Sayio 2003) investigated the rate and method of attempted suicides in all hospitals in the catchment area. The results were screened to identify suicide attempts for four years between 1 January 1998 and 31 December 2001. In the four-year period, 737 individuals attempted suicide (514 women and 223 men). The mean annual rate per 100,000 was 46.89 for men and 112.89 for women. The parasuicide rate increased by 93.59 per cent between 1998 and 2001. The most frequent method used by both men and women was self-poisoning. Compared with the results from other European research centres, attempted suicide rates in Turkey were relatively low. However, the increase in rates was striking. This upward trend may be related to the intense economic difficulties, increasing unemployment, and rapid social change experienced in Turkey in recent years. The risk groups appeared to be younger and female.

There is considerable confusion between the concepts of suicidal behaviour and deliberate self-harm. They overlap with evident suicidal intent at one end and acts of self-mutilation at the other. In Muslim countries, recent studies refer to the rise of parasuicide and probably failed suicide. In a study from Kuwait, attempted suicide constituted more than one quarter of 219 consecutive liaison referrals from all general hospitals (Al-Ansari *et al.* 1990). Another study from Kuwait on 208 inpatient referrals reported that attempted suicide constituted half the cases (Fido and Al-Munghaiseeb 1989). Daradkeh and Al-Zayer (1988) estimated the population attempting self-harm rate in the Eastern province of Saudi Arabia as 20/100,000, i.e. well below the 100–200/100,000 noticed in Western countries. In Egypt, Okasha (1984) estimated the rate of suicide attempts to be 38/100,000 of the population, well below European rates. The profiles of parasuicide are similar in that the majority is female; the ratio varies between 1.3–2 to 1 in Jordan (Daradkeh 1988) and 2.8:1 in UAE (Hamdi *et al.* 1989, 1991). In both studies, the act of deliberate self-harm followed acute stress reaction associated with interpersonal strains and frustration. The majority have low or medium intent as measured by the Beck Suicidal Intent Scale. Depressive disorders were diagnosed in one third of the patients. Low suicidal intent correlated with the ideo-affective states of frustration and anger. Serious suicidal intent correlated with antecedent feelings of hopelessness, helplessness, and being cut off and isolated. This is quite similar to very recent studies from the US (Soloff *et al.* 2000). In Kuwait, around 1.1 per cent of suicide attempters eventually killed themselves (Kuey and Gulec 1989). Around 20 per cent repeated suicide attempts in Dubai and Kuwait, a percentage not far removed from that reported in Western studies. The majority of suicide attempts, around 90 per cent, take the form of an overdose, usually of analgesics (Hamdi *et al.* 1991).

## Suicide across the Middle East

In a study of suicide from 1980 through 1985 in Jordan, there were 219 suicides with an annual suicide rate of 2.1 per 100,000. The peak suicide rate was found to be among the 15–34 age group. Nearly two-thirds of males that committed suicide were single, and unemployed. Females were married and suffering sociocultural problems. Nearly two-thirds of the total population that committed suicide had undergone previous psychiatric treatment. Violent methods of suicide were most frequent (Daradkeh 1989).

The suicide rate for the entire population in Saudi Arabia averaged 1.1/100,000 population per annum. The male to female ratio was 4.5:1. The highest suicide rate was among the 30–39 age group (44.3%). Immigrants formed 77% of the cases, and of these, Asians accounted for 70% of the overall cases, and Indians showed the highest suicidal rates (43%). The most common means of suicide chosen was hanging (63%), followed by jumping from heights (12%), and gunshot injuries (9%); death from poisoning accounted for only 6% of cases. Causes for suicide revolved around health and family related stressors (El-Fawal and Awad 1994).

Radovanovic (1994) studied the mortality patterns in Kuwait and concluded that there is a high likelihood of non-reporting of unnatural causes of death, including suicide, in death certificates. Still, this would not compensate for the repeated findings that completed suicide is much more frequent in non-Muslim countries. The difference is striking in that it probably is the most salient feature of cultural influence on mental illness and its complications. Two explanations have been invoked; namely the persisting influence of Islam compared to the declining presence of Christianity in the West, and a different social fabric allowing cohesiveness, and reinforcing belonging rather than individuality and social alienation in the West. A third explanation is closely related to religion, namely the marked prevalence of alcohol use in Western cultures compared to Islamic countries. In the UK, alcohol and drug use is involved in almost 15% of suicides in persons in contact with mental health services (Appleby *et al.* 1999).

## Disclosure about suicidality in Muslim countries

Degrees of suicidal behaviour are described by Waziri in Afghani depressive patients (Waziri 1973). In this Islamic culture, 54% expressed death wishes or prayed for God to take their life away: 20% admitted to passing thoughts of suicide but had banished these by thinking of the great sin they would be committing; 14% admitted having had suicidal intentions, and only 2.7% had actually attempted suicide by cutting their throats. The spectrum of suicidal behaviour in this study involves a wide range of degrees of suicidality. Religion seems to suppress the suicidal actions but not the suicidal thoughts. This observation may be supported by the findings that suicidal thoughts were elicited in 58% of depressive patients in Kuwait and only 11% had attempted suicide (Leff 1986). Similarly, the comparison of Egyptian, Indian and British depressive patients revealed that Egyptians have a significant increase in suicidal tendencies, but not in actual suicide or attempted suicide (Arafa 1978).

In a cross-cultural study, El-Rashidi (1992) compared suicidal thoughts, tendencies, acts and histories in Egyptian and French psychiatric inpatients. In 45% of the cases, Egyptian patients reported suicidal thoughts, whereas their French counterparts declared having suicide thoughts in 15% of the cases. With regards to actual attempts, the picture is reversed, with French patients having 2.5 times more histories of suicide attempts, and a tendency to use violent methods.

Muslim patients frequently answer direct questions about suicidal actions negatively. With open-ended questions, the picture is different. In some cases, the disclosure of suicidal ideation may appear in an indirect way, e.g. a depressive patient who was an officer in the army parachute regiment denied feeling suicidal at the beginning, and then spontaneously revealed in a different context that he suggested to his supervisor he would like to jump from the airplane with the spare parachute. Keegstra (1986) reported that suicidal thoughts were never revealed spontaneously during the assessment of Ethiopian depressives. He commented that suicidal plans or ideas were common in 71% of depressed patients. In 19% of the patients, specified plans or previous attempts had been made.

## The role of Islam in preventing suicide

Both 'psychiatry' and 'religion' are institutions developed over the course of cultural evolution to address and provide some relief for the inevitable problems that occur in the course of family and social interactions. Psychiatry and religion are parallel and complementary frames of reference for understanding and describing the human experience and human behaviour. All religions offer some type of explanation of how the universe was created, how life is maintained, and what happens when life ceases to exist. Religions attempt to give their followers explanations for life's meaning, including rationales for the reality of human suffering. They can, therefore, be an asset to enable religious individuals and groups to deal with painful conditions of existence.

It is deeply imbedded in the Islamic culture that life and death are God's will. The practice of religious duties, rituals, and the visits to the mosque reinforce the attribution of every deed to God. It is very interesting to note that believers in Islam, when they become depressed, lose interest in all aspects of life, but the last to disappear is their ablution rituals and their prayers to God. In Islamic code, humans were created primarily to worship God; this is followed by all other duties. Muslims' cognitive schema are geared day and night to remembering God's will. This has a strong protective value against suicide in that our lives do not belong to us, but to God.

The psychiatrist's knowledge about the religious background of the patient, and the careful evaluation and follow-up to observe symptom progression and effect on functioning and decision-making can be the keys to successful management. Religious belief systems may provide understandable explanations for traumatic life events or provide meaning for survival.

## References

Al-Ansari EA, El-Hilu MA, Hassan KI (1990). Patterns of psychiatric consultations in Kuwait general hospitals. *General Hospital Psychiatry*, **12**, 257–263.

Appleby I, Shaw J, Amos T (1999). Suicide within 12 months of contact with mental health services: national clinical survey. *BMJ*, **318**, 1235–1239.

Arafa M (1978). A clinical study of depression in Egyptian patients with cross-national comparisons. Masters thesis, Cairo university, Cairo.

Bensmail B, Merdji Y, Touari M (1989). Reflections on detection and intervention in depression in Algeria. *Psicopatologia*, **9**, 211–214.

Bertolote JM and Fleischmann A (2002). A global perspective in the epidemiology of suicide. *Suicidologi*, **2**, 6–8.

Bertolote JM, Fleischmann A, de Leo L (2005). Suicide attempts, plans, and ideation in culturally diverse sites: the WHO SUPRE-MISS community survey. *Psychological Medicine*, **35**, 1457–1465.

Daradkeh TK (1988). Reported parasuicide in Jordan 1980–1985: calls for urgent reorganisation of psychiatric service. *Dirasat*, **15**, 45–58.

Daradkeh TK (1989). Suicide in Jordan 1980–1985. *Acta Psychiatrica Scandinavica*, **79**, 241–244.

Daradkeh TK and Al-Zayer N (1988). Parasuicide in an arab industrial community: the Arabian-American oil company experience, Saudi Arabia. *Acta Psychiatrica Scandinavica*, **77**, 707–711.

Ebbel B (1937). *The Papyrus Ebers*. Levin and Munksgaard, Copenhagen.

El-Assra A (1989). The complaint of 'tightness' in the Saudi population. Paper read in the VIIIth World Congress of Psychiatry, Athens.

El-Fawal MA and Awad OA (1994). Deaths from hanging in the eastern province of Saudi Arabia. *Medical Science and Law*, **34**, 307–312.

El-Islam MF (1969). Depression and guilt. *Social Psychiatry*, **41**, 56–58.

El-Islam MF (1974). Hospital referred parasuicide in Qatar. *Egyptian Journal of Mental Health*, **15**, 101–112.

El-Islam MF (1976). Intergenerational conflict and the young Qatari neurotic. *Ethos*, **4**, 45–56.

El-Islam MF (1979). A better outlook for schizophrenics living in extended families. *British Journal of Psychiatry*, **135**, 343–347.

El-Islam MF, Moussa MAA, Malasi TH *et al.* (1988). Assessment of depression in Kuwait by principal component analysis. *Journal of Affective Disorders*, **14**, 109–114.

El-Rashidi A (1992). Suicidal behaviour in French and Egyptian patients admitted to a psychiatric hospital. *Egyptian Journal of Psychiatry*, **15**, 201–207.

Fido AA and Al-Munghaiseeb A (1989). Consultation liaison psychiatry in Kuwaiti general hospital. *International Journal of Social Psychiatry*, **35**, 274–279.

Hamdi E, Amin Y, Abou-Saleh MT (1997). Problems in validating endogenous depression in the arab culture by contemporary diagnostic criteria. *Journal of Affective Disorders*, **44**, 131–143.

Hamdi E, Amin Y, Mattar T (1989). Deliberate self-harm in the UAE: demographic and clinical correlates. *Egyptian Journal of Psychiatry*, **12**, 33–45.

Hamdi E, Amin Y, Mattar T (1991). Clinical correlates of intent in attempted suicide. *Acta Psychiatrica Scandinavica*, **83**, 406–411.

Holy Koran (1979). *The English translation of the meaning and commmentary*. The King Fahd Holy Koran. AL Madina Al Monawara, Saudi Arabia.

Keegstra HJ (1986). Depressive disorders in Ethiopia: a standardised assessment using the SADD schedule. *Acta Psychiatrica Scandinavica*, **73**, 658–664.

Kuey L and Gulec C (1989). Depression in Turkey in the 1980s: epidemiological and clinical approaches. *Clinical Psychopharmacology*, **12**, 1–12.

Leff JP (1986). The epidemiology of mental illness across cultures. In JL Cox, ed., *Transcultural Psychiatry*, pp. 25–39. Croom Helm, London.

Okasha A (1984). Depression and suicide in Egypt. *Egyptian Journal of Psychiatry*, **7**, 33–45.

Okasha A (1999). Mental health in the Middle East: an Egyptian perspective. *Clinical Psychology Review*, **19**, 917–933.

Okasha A (2000). Global burden of depression. Presented at the meeting on Globalization of psychiatry, international perspectives, Cairo.

Okasha A and Lotaif F (1979). Attempted suicide: an Egyptian investigation. *Acta Psychiatrica Scandninavica*, **60**, 69–75.

Okasha A, Bassim R, Okasha T (2008). Epidemiology and psychiatric morbidity in suicide attempters at the Poison Control Center. *Current Psychiatry*, **15**, 231–238.

Okasha A, Khalil AH, El-Fiky MR *et al.* (1988). Prevalence of depressive disorders in a sample of rural and urban egyptian communities. *Egyptian Journal of Psychiatry*, **11**, 167–181.

Ozguven HD and Sayio I (2003). Suicide attempts in turkey: results of the WHO–Euro multicentre study on suicidal behavior. *Canadian Journal of Psychiatry*, **48**, 324–329.

Pfieffer W (1968). The symptomatology of depression viewed transculturally. *Transcultural Psychiatric Research Review*, **5**, 121–123.

Radovanovic Z (1994). Mortality patterns in Kuwait: inferences from death certificate data. *European Journal of Epidemiology*, **10**, 733–736.

Soloff PH, Lynch KG, Kelly TM *et al.* (2000). Characteristics of suicide attempts of patients with major depressive episodes and borderline personality disorder: a comparative study. *American Journal of Psychiatry*, **157**, 601–608.

Suleiman MA, Moussa MA, El-Islam MF (1989). The profile of parasuicide repeaters in Kuwait. *International Journal of Social Psychiatry*, **35**, 146–155.

Waziri R (1973). Symptomatology of depressive illness in Afghanistan. *American Journal of Psychiatry*, **130**, 213–217.

WHO (2002). *Multisite Intervention Study on Suicidal Behaviors. SUPRE-MISS: Protocol of SUPRE-MISS*. World Health Organization, Geneva.

WHO (2005). *Suicide Rates per 100,000 by Country, Year and Sex*. World Health Organization, Geneva.

# CHAPTER 9

# Christianity and suicide

Nils Retterstøl and Øivind Ekeberg

## Abstract

First, the views on suicide as found in the Old and New Testament are presented. In the early Christian period, suicide does not seem to be prohibited. St Augustine (350–430 AD), however, considered it a sin, violating the fifth commandment, 'Thou shall not kill'. Later, synods of the Church gave strong regulation as to how the suicidee should be buried. The same negative attitudes were expressed throughout most of the Middle Ages across Europe.

The European Enlightenment movement brought about moderated views on suicide, challenging former Christian condemnations. From about 1800, psychiatry was established, stating that most people who committed suicide were mentally ill.

Contemporary official Christian attitudes are presented with special reference to the Roman, Greek and Russian Orthodox Church, as well as the Protestant Church.

The viewpoints on euthanasia are presented briefly. Finally, we discuss how Christian traditions influence suicide prevention today.

## Suicide in the Bible

In order to provide a broad presentation of the theme of suicide in Christian European history, we will map out traditions found in the Old and New Testament, present long-standing manuscripts as regards to customary beliefs, and finally, discuss the contemporary diverse states of custom and practice within the different churches and secular communities.

Among Jews, suicide was rare. In the Old Testament, life was considered to be sacred (Jacobs 1995): it was a personal divine gift which man had to protect. A Jew was allowed to break religious laws to save his life, but he must not commit murder, deny God, or practice incest. Suicide was regarded as a wrongful and unworthy act. A suicidal act was punished: the victim and the victim's family was denied the usual burial and mourning rituals (Jacobs 1995). It was considered a sin of unforgivable nature. In extreme circumstances, however, suicide was accepted. This was the case, for example, if disgrace could be avoided through suicide in the event of captivity or torture. The Jewish religious laws engendered a sort of heroic martyrdom (Mayer 1980).

There are four suicides that are the most well-known in the Old Testament (Farberow 1975): Samson, Saul, Abimelech and Ahitophael. Samson killed himself and the Philistines by breaking down the pillars of the temple. He was a former judge of the people of Israel, who had been taken prisoner and had been humiliated in the temple by the Philistine people. He received the appropriate postmortem honours (Koch 2005). King Saul killed himself after suffering defeat in battle, thus, avoiding the disgrace of surrender. According to Koch, King Saul seems to have had depressive periods in his life. Abimelech's skull was crushed by a woman during a battle, upon which he obliged his young armour-bearer to pierce him with a sword, as he did not want the disgrace of having been killed by a woman. Ahitophael hanged himself at home when he failed to betray David to Absalon (Koch 2005). In addition, Zimri may be mentioned, who burned the palace he was in when the capital of Israel was besieged and died in the flames, and finally, Eleazar who committed suicide with a sword to avoid being captured. An increasing number of suicides were considered in the Talmud with a distinct attitude of denunciation (Farberow 1975). A more detailed description of suicide in the Old Testament is found in Chapter 7 of this book.

In the New Testament, Judas Iscariot is the only person reported to have committed suicide. The best-known account of his suicide is by hanging (Matt. 27:4), but there is also a version of accidental death falling headlong and spilling out his bowels (Acts 1:18) (Koch 2005). However, Paul was not aware of the death of Judas, as he wrote of the 12 disciples who mourned after the death of Jesus (Koch 2005). The Bible gives the impression that Judas felt deep desperation when he became aware of the consequences of his betrayal, which he felt was a great sin. He threw the 30 silver coins he had received on the floor of the temple, and according to Matthew, committed suicide by hanging himself. The New Testament is markedly different from the Old in not condemning suicide. The issue of suicide was not examined systematically before the Synod in Arles in 452 AD.

## The early Christian period

In the early Christian period, acts of martyrdom were common, and the number of suicides increased during this period. There was a certain pessimistic attitude towards life, and a corresponding yearning for the values of eternity. Suicide was not prohibited in the first Christian period, but later. During the first centuries of Christianity, the fathers of the church developed a sceptical attitude in relation to suicide.

St Augustine's great work, *The City of God*, is the first codification of the Church's displeasure with and denunciation of the fact that suicide was spreading. In it, he states that life is a gift from God, and that breaking with life means committing an unavoidable sin against God and his dominion over life and death. It was a sin which violated the fifth commandment 'Thou shall not kill' (Augustine 1890). Augustine also denounced suicide committed by women after being raped; someone taking her life in this way was just as guilty as the man who had committed the injustice. Augustine's attitude was clear—suicide is murder. Only one exception can be allowed: if there is an absolute commandment from God. A true and noble soul will bear suffering, as Job did; he withstood terrible sufferings without depriving himself of life. A person committing suicide dies as the worst sinner. He is not only trying to escape the difficulties of life, but he also denies himself the possibility of absolution.

## Synods of the church after St Augustine

Suicide was denounced at the Synod in Arles, in 452 AD, on the basis that 'he who kills himself kills an innocent person and commits murder'. A strongly denunciatory attitude towards suicide gradually developed in Christianity. For a time, Judas Iscariot's betrayal of Christ was regarded as a lesser sin than his suicide. The noble soul will accept the sufferings of life; non-acceptance is an escape, which makes absolution impossible. At the Synod in Braga in 563 AD, it was decided that no religious rituals should be held after suicide, however, in practice, a situation gradually developed in which suicide was allowed under three circumstances: voluntary martyrdom, self-inflicted death through asceticism, and the suicide of the virgin and the married woman to preserve their virtue.

At the Synod of Antisidor, in 590 AD, a system of restrictions was established for the first time to condemn suicide. It was decided at the Synod, in Toledo 693 AD, that those who took their lives were to be excommunicated. At the Synod in Nîmes, 1096 AD, the resolution that those who committed suicide should be denied the right to be buried in consecrated soil was adopted. Gradually, the practice of burying the body of the person who had committed suicide outside the churchyard or alongside the churchyard wall developed. In many parts of Europe, the body was dragged through the streets and buried at crossroads, with a stake driven through it and with a stone placed over the face. Remarkable customs developed, such as in Danzig, where the body of a person who had committed suicide could not be taken out of the house through the door but had to be removed through the window. If there was no window, a hole had to be knocked through the wall. Such customs were possibly introduced to avoid the person who had committed suicide to haunt and become a ghost.

## The Middle Ages

The same negative attitudes were expressed throughout most of the Middle Ages across Europe. An exception was the kingdom of Charles the Great (768–814). This was a time marked by intellectual aristocracy and respect for the human mind in which the view that suicide might be a consequence of mental disorder was expressed. After Charles the Great, the old disapproving viewpoints reappeared. Mass suicides occurred in connection with persecution and suppression, such as among the persecuted Albigensians (Cathars) in southern France, where in 1218, more than five thousand killed

themselves when they were persecuted through their belief and identified as heretics. There were also pogroms against the Jews, not least in England, where the persecutions were extremely strong under Richard the Ist who is also known as Richard the Lionheart. Six hundred persons took their lives in York in 1190, rather than suffering suppression.

One of those who tried to commit suicide was Joan of Arc, who made an attempt while she was in prison. When she was brought before the court, the bishops used her attempted suicide as further proof of her alliance with the Devil, being a witch or sorceress. She was burnt at the market of Rouen in 1431 for witchcraft and sorcery, but the Pope declared the verdict null and void in 1456: she was beatified in 1909 and canonized in 1920. Today, the second Sunday of May is a French national holiday in honour of Joan of Arc, an enduring symbol of the country's unity.

In the thirteenth century, Thomas Aquinas (1224–1274), a noted scholastic theologian and philosopher, confirmed the antisuicidal attitude of the church (Aquinas 1991). Suicide was absolutely wrong because: 1) it was unnatural, 2) every person was a member of society, and suicide was therefore antisocial and 3) life was a gift from God and was not at man's disposal. Around this time (1307), Dante wrote the *Inferno*, in which light is shed on attitudes towards suicide. Dante was led through hell and purgatory to Paradise. The person who committed suicide was condemned to eternal unrest in the forests of self-destruction in the seventh hell, among heretics and murderers.

The Renaissance and the Reformation brought about a change of views regarding suicide. Luther's ideas cleared the way for a change from absolutism and subservience to personal decision and personal responsibility. Doubt was cast on what had previously been regarded as absolutes. The view gradually emerged that suicides had to be assessed individually. Calvinism appeared about that time, starting in Switzerland, spreading through France (the Huguenots) to England. Calvin exalted God and tended to remove Him and render of Him an inaccessible Superiority, in contrast to Luther's view. In his famous book, *Anatomy of Melancholy*, Burton (1621) broke emphatically with the church dogmas of the time, and questioned whether suicides were condemned for eternity. In the upper classes of society, suicide was gradually more accepted, but continued to be roundly condemned in the lower social classes.

## The Enlightenment and more tolerant times

The European philosophical movement called the Enlightenment brought about somewhat moderated views on suicide, thus, challenging former Christian condemnations.

Such views were expressed among others by Montesquieu (1721), who pointed out that man is part of nature, which he therefore has reason to modify. Montesquieu sharply criticised the official view of suicide, not least from the point of view of the survivors. Both Voltaire (1694–1778) and Rousseau (1712–1778) defended the individual's right to take their own life, and criticised the traditional attitude toward suicide.

David Hume, the Scottish writer, contradicted the doctrine by Aquinas and others that the overall (utilitarian) balance of suicide had to be negative in *Essay on Suicide and the Immortality of the Soul* (1783) (Hume 1929). According to Hume, logical conclusions of the theological arguments would generally call in question medical treatment and interventions. Hume's book was so radical that the publisher did not dare to publish it until after his death. Hume argues that it must be man's right to decide over his own death, if pain, illness, shame or poverty make life unbearable. Man does not do anything wrong by committing suicide, but stops doing well. He is fully entitled to avoid evil, including life. From the same century, yet, with radically different viewpoints, Immanuel Kant (1724–1804), considers that the categorical imperative must be followed: the principle of your actions have to follow a general law. Suicide is not acceptable from a moral viewpoint, since life is holy and must be preserved at whatever cost. Arthur Schopenhauer (1788–1860) was the leading writer on suicide in the nineteenth century and has been regarded incorrectly as a spokesman for suicide. According to him, suicide was neither a sin nor a criminal act, and he criticised the sanctions imposed by the church. The person who commits suicide does not seek death because he wants to die, but because he is not satisfied with the conditions under which he lives. Friedrich Nietzsche (1844–1900) was of the opinion that the individual has a complete moral right to take his own life, and used the expression *Freitod*, synonymous with suicide.

From about 1800, psychiatry was established as a medical specialty, and more scientific papers on suicide appeared. Jean-Etienne Esquirol (1772–1840) stated that most people who committed suicide were mentally ill (*maladie mentale*), while at the beginning of the twentieth century, Kraepelin (1856–1926) considered that about 30 per cent of the people who committed suicide had shown open symptoms of a psychosis (Kraepelin 1899). The association between religious/cultural beliefs and suicidality has been under debate since Emile Durkheim published his ecological studies of suicide in Europe at the end of the nineteenth century (Durkheim 1952). He demonstrated that Protestant provinces had higher suicide rates than Catholic provinces. Many studies have demonstrated that suicide rates, especially for men, tend to be lower in countries with religious or cultural belief systems that traditionally view suicide negatively, and higher in countries with belief systems which sanction it (Stack 1983; Lester 1996; Neeleman *et al.* 1997; Kelleher *et al.* 1998; Lester 1998; Neeleman 1998; Neeleman and Lewis 1999; Vijayakumar *et al.* 2005). Some caution should be exercised in interpreting these findings, as they may be an artefact of reduced reporting and recording of suicide in countries where it is taboo (Vijayakumar *et al.* 2005). Even if the figures were accurate, ecological fallacy may still be there; if deaths by suicide in predominantly Protestant countries were in fact most common in Catholics (Rothman and Greenland 1998).

## Contemporary official Christian attitudes

### The Roman Catholic church

*The Catechism of the Catholic Church*, second edition (Vatican 2008) is a basic source in the understanding of the morality of the Catholic Christianity. The issue of suicide is dealt with under article 5, The Fifth Commandment: *Thou shall not kill*.

The catechism says that suicide contradicts the natural inclination of the human being to preserve and perpetuate his life. It is gravely contrary to the just love of self. It likewise offends love of your neighbour, because it unjustly breaks the ties of solidarity with family, nation, and other human societies to which we continue to have obligations. Suicide is contrary to love for the living God. If suicide is committed with the intention of setting an example, especially to the young, it also takes on the gravity of scandal.

Voluntary cooperation in suicide is contrary to the moral law. Grave psychological disturbances, anguish, or grave fear of hardship, suffering, or torture can diminish the responsibility of the one committing suicide. We should not despair the eternal salvation of persons who have taken their own lives. By ways known to him alone, God can provide the opportunity for salutary repentance. The church prays for persons who have taken their own lives. Suicide is not only considered an individual act, but also a violation of solidarity with other people. The Catholic moral standpoint on suicide concerns suicide both as a direct act, when a person has the intention of causing their own death, as by inflicting a mortal wound or injury, or by omitting to do what is necessary to escape death, as by refusing to leave a burning house. From a moral standpoint, both the prohibition of positive suicide and the duty incumbent on man to preserve his life are addressed.

According to the Catholic church in England and Wales (2008) current guidelines, developed at a conference consecrated to the issue, suicide attempters are in a desperate situation and need help (Catholic Church of England and Wales 2008). Suicide should never be romanticized, promoted or encouraged. On the other hand, attempting suicide is considered an act of a desperate person, and it should be greeted with compassion rather than with blame. At the conference, it was underlined that this was the reason why the Suicide Act 1961 decriminalized suicide. It was underscored that the aim of the new law was by no means to encourage suicide, and that assisted suicide remained a serious crime. Suicide was thought of as a terrible act, but the help that suicidal people needed was seen as more easily given if those who survived the attempt were not treated like criminals. Most importantly, those who contemplate ending their life need to be given a sense of hope in life. This shows more respect and understanding of the suicide attempter than previous official positions of the Catholic church. The respect for those who suffer and the obligation to care for others is also outlined. A significant change in the understanding of suicidal behaviour is to be found in these texts. Suicide has traditionally been considered a sinful act leading to condemnation, however, presently an understanding of the suffering and despair that suicidal people experience is increasing. There is a frequent use of the terminology: 'suicide while of an unsound mind'. This is, in some measure, in accordance with the contemporary scientific understanding of the psychological, social and biological factors that are related to suicidal behaviour.

### The Greek Orthodox church

The Greek Orthodox church has, over the centuries, taught that we do not have the right to take our own lives, since life is a gift from God, which we are called upon to preserve and enhance (Harakas 2005). Hence, the Greek Orthodox church considers direct suicide to be the most serious kind of murder, because there is no opportunity for repentance. The canon and practice of the church thus prohibit a church burial to a person who has committed suicide. However, if it can be shown that the person who has committed suicide was not mentally sound, upon proper medical (certified by a doctor that the person has lost their sanity) and ecclesiastical certification, the burial can be conducted by the church. In cases where the deceased held a philosophical view affirming the right to suicide, or allowed despair to overcome good judgement, no such allowance can be made. Morally speaking, there is also the case of indirect suicide, in which people harm their health through abusive practices such as excessive smoking, excessive drinking of alcoholic beverages, and unnecessary risk-taking. The Orthodox church teaches that we are obligated to care for our health, so these kinds of practices are looked upon as immoral. However, they do not carry the same negative implications that the direct taking of one's own life has. Physician-assisted suicide is considered the same as suicide.

The Greek Orthodox church seems to be somewhat more negative to suicide than the Roman Catholic church. It is not clearly defined what criteria are necessary to classify a person who has lost his or her sanity. Is it a psychotic state, or is it a certain degree of depression? Even though most studies find that about 90 per cent of suiciders would fulfill the criteria for a psychiatric diagnosis, there is no doubt that a significant proportion of them had not lost their sanity. This is of particular relevance concerning adolescent suicide, where a psychiatric diagnosis is not made in about 1/4 of the cases (Grøholt *et al.* 1997). Farberow (1975) refers to a study of Roman and Greek priests in their parishes in Los Angeles, dealing with suicides and their survivors, indicating that burial was rarely denied, and neither was opprobrium attached to the family.

### The Russian Orthodox church

The Russian Orthodox Church is also clear about suicide not being permitted (Russian Orthodox Church of Three Saints 2000). If, however, a suicide is committed 'out of mind', that is, in a state of mental disease, the church prayer for the perpetrator, is allowed after the case has been investigated by the ruling bishop. At the same time, the Church says, it should be remembered that more often than not the blame for a suicide lies with the people around the perpetrator, proven incapable of effective compassion and mercy. The Russian Orthodox Church, thus, is not very different from the Greek. Suicide is basically considered a sin, but the bishop may give abolition if suicide is caused by mental illness.

### The Protestant church

The reasons that the Protestant church divided from the Catholic church during the Reformation had nothing to do with attitudes toward suicide, and in effect, the attitudes towards suicide in the two churches were rather similar. This was illustrated in the present day by the joint statement in 1996 by the Chairman of the German Catholic Bishops' conference and the Chairman of the Council of the Evangelical Church in Germany, both opposed to accepting mercy suicide (Evangelical Church of Germany 1996).

Suicide is by no means considered an act that is in accordance with the ethics that are the basic meaning of God. However, the concept of sin is not as strong as in the Catholic church. There are also various different branches of the Protestant church and no definite centre of the church such as the Vatican for Roman Catholics. Accordingly, it is not easy to agree on one particular ethical view. Generally, suicide is not condemned, and the basic attitude toward suicide attempters is to help and support them. It is not necessary to get permission from the bishop or other clergymen to be allowed a Christian funeral.

Generally, the Protestant church has condemned suicide as an offence against God's will, grace and judgement. The recent trend is to attribute suicide to insanity or to personal inadequacy viewed as a function of social disorganization (Ferm 1945).

## Euthanasia

Euthanasia has become an increasingly debated issue during the past decades, therefore, we will touch on the attitudes towards euthanasia among the Christian Churches. Euthanasia is the act of actively shortening life, e.g. by giving a lethal dose of a toxic agent. Assisted suicide means that someone facilitates a person in committing suicide. The different Christian churches on the whole have a similar outlook to such acts.

The Roman Catholic view on euthanasia is clearly outlined in the catechism (Vatican 2008). Euthanasia as an act of putting an end to the lives of handicapped, sick, or dying persons is considered morally unacceptable. The Church distinguishes between the active shortening of life and the discontinuing of medical procedures that are burdensome, dangerous, extraordinary, or disproportionate to the expected outcome. Here, one does not want to cause death; one's inability to impede it is merely accepted. Even if death is considered imminent, the ordinary care owed to a sick person cannot legitimately be interrupted. The use of painkillers to alleviate the sufferings of the dying, even at the risk of shortening their days, can be morally in conformity with human dignity. This requires that death is not willed as either an end or a means, but only foreseen and tolerated as inevitable. Palliative care is a special form of disinterested charity, and as such, it should be encouraged.

The current view of the Catholic church of England and Wales is that euthanasia is worse than suicide, for it involves the intentional killing of someone else, even if the person who dies may have asked to be killed (Catholic Church of England and Wales 2008). The Greek Orthodox church considers euthanasia as a form of suicide on the part of the individual, and a form of murder on the part of others who assist in this practice, both of which are regarded as sins. Thus, the Orthodox church, in the words of the 1976 Christmas, encyclical of former Archbishop Iakovos, considers 'euthanasia and abortion, along with homosexuality … a … moral alienation'. Modern medical practice, however, has affected another part of the church's perspective. The church does not expect that excessive and heroic means must be used at all costs to prolong dying, as has now become possible through technical medical advances. As current Orthodox theology expresses it:

> The Church distinguishes between euthanasia and the withholding of extraordinary means to prolong life. It affirms the sanctity of human life and man's God-given responsibility to preserve life. But it rejects an attitude which disregards the inevitability of physical death.
>
> http://www.goarch.org/ourfaith/ourfaith7101

According to the Russian Orthodox church, euthanasia is considered a form of homicide or suicide, depending on whether a patient participates in it or not. If he does, euthanasia comes under the canons, whereby, both the purposeful suicide and assistance to it are viewed as grave sins.

The Christian attitude towards suicide and euthanasia is generally strict, with focus on what is forbidden, particularly within the Catholic church. This view should be balanced with the church's view concerning the obligation to preserve life and growth. The catechism underlines that God considers life and physical health precious gifts entrusted to us. Concern for the health of its citizens requires that society helps in the attainment of living conditions that allow individuals to grow and reach maturity: food, clothing, housing, health care, basic education, employment, and social assistance. A basic level of nursing care is demanded by human solidarity. It must be recognized that leaving a patient cold, unclean, in pain or without human contact for significant periods of time would fall below a decent standard of care.

## Suicide in different countries according to Christian religion

It is generally accepted that religious faith is associated with lower suicide rates. It has also been suggested that the suicide rates vary according to the main religion in the country. Muslim countries, where suicide is strictly forbidden, generally report significantly lower suicide rates than Christian countries. Sainsbury and colleagues (1982) studied the relationship between stages in social conditions and changes in suicide rates after 1960 in 18 European countries in cooperation with WHO. An increased suicide rate was linked with five factors, of which, the decline in religious and church activities was one. A link between increased suicide rates, and a decline in religious commitment and church activities, probably reflecting a change in moral values and attitudes towards suicide, furthermore suggests declining social integration. The church has acted as a social network for people over centuries. Amongst Christian countries, most Catholic countries have lower suicide rates than the Protestant countries. Thus, the Catholic Mediterranean countries generally have lower rates than the Protestant countries in northern Europe. This has been attributed to the more restrictive attitude toward suicide in the Catholic church. The situation, however, is quite complicated, as suicide rates vary considerably among Orthodox countries. Greece has a low suicide rate, whereas many Russian Orthodox countries have very high suicide rates. Among the Baltic countries, which have the highest suicide rates in the world, Lithuania is Catholic, whereas Latvia and Estonia are Protestant. There are many different cultural and individual aspects that may explain different suicide rates. Even though a country has one main religion, the degree of religious attitude and practice may vary. In addition, socio-economic factors, health care system, the consumption of alcohol and drugs, and other factors have significant impacts on suicide rates. This was particularly evident in many former Soviet Union republics, where the suicide rates decreased by 32 per cent for males during perestroika and with a more restrictive alcohol policy (Varnik et al. 1998). There are many aspects concerning the relationship between suicide and religion that call for more studies.

## Laws on suicide in Norway

How have the views and laws of suicide developed in traditionally Christian countries? This, of course, varies in different cultures and geographical areas. What follows are illustrations of the current situation in Norway, on the whole, which is not very different from that in other Scandinavian countries (Retterstøl 1993; Retterstøl et al. 2002). In the period before Christianity was introduced in Norway, it appears that suicide could be accepted in order to avoid disgrace or painful illness, and also when bondsmen followed their master into death. The Gulating Law of western Norway (from the time when Norway became Christian) states:

> It is such that each person who dies shall be carried to the church and buried in sacred soil, apart from miscreants, those who betray the King, and murderers, thieves and those who take their own lives. Those who have just been named shall be buried in the tide, where the sea and the green turf meet.
>
> Den eldre Gulatingslova (1994)

There were exceptions: when the self-murderer had time to regret his deed and had confessed to the clergyman, or if he had a serious mental or physical disorder. In Magnus Lagabøter's National Law, which was in force from 1274 to 1688, suicide is mentioned as an irreparable deed (Keyser 1848).

The Norwegian Law of 1687, which also covered Iceland and the Faroe islands, was of a Christian foundation, and in it were clear rules that a self-murderer should not be buried in the church or the churchyard if they had not taken their life because of illness. The clergyman was not allowed to give a ceremony of funeral oration. Also, the descendents of the self-murderer should be punished: the heritage had to be given to the king, not the descendants. In Norway, those who committed suicide in the Middle Ages were often buried among executed criminals or in the forests. It was commonly believed that it would be particularly difficult for people who had taken their own life, or those of others, to find peace in the next world, and that they would therefore have to return as ghosts causing troubles for those of the living on whom they wanted to take revenge.

In 1842, it was stated that persons who commit suicide can not be buried in sacred earth, and that the heritage after a suicide should go to the king was abolished. The Law of Churches and Churchyards of 1897 allowed the clergyman to sprinkle earth on the coffin, and in 1902, funeral oration was allowed for people who had committed suicide.

At no time in Norway have there been sanctions against those who attempt suicide, seemingly because the attempter may take their life next time. In many other European countries, suicidal attempts were considered a crime, and the actor was punished accordingly: e.g. in England from 1745 to 1961, and in Ireland until 1994. Ireland was the last country in Europe to abolish punishment for suicidal attempts.

## How Christian traditions influence suicide prevention today

Throughout the centuries, Christian attitudes towards suicide have become less restrictive. The Catholic and the Orthodox churches consider suicide as an act that is not according to the intention of God. However, the previous practices of refusing to bury suicide victims and punishing suicide attempters have generally been abandoned. The understanding of the mental suffering of people with suicidal ideation has improved greatly. Accordingly, most churches now offer help for suicidal persons and for those who are left after a suicide. All the main churches focus on the fact that help should be offered to all who are suffering and in despair. They also highlight that suicide is not a restricted individual act, but that it also has a serious impact on family, friends, neighbours and colleagues. A restrictive attitude to suicide in a population may increase the threshold for such acts, as indicated by the lower suicide rates in more active religious societies. If the taboos are too strict, however, this may prevent suicidal people from seeking help. Suicidal behaviour is complicated and not only based on psychiatric problems. The individual suffering consists of mental suffering in relation to self conflicts, interpersonal or social problems, and not least religious and existential issues. Therefore, these issues should also be a focus of interest in suicide prevention.

## References

Aquinas T (1991). *Summa Theologica*. Translated by T McDermott Allen, 2nd and revised edn, 1920. Christian Classics, Texas.

Augustine St (1890). *The City of God*. In P Schaff, ed., and translated by Rev. M Dods. *A Select Library of the Nicene and Post-Nicene Fathers of the Christian Church*. Vol. II. Christian Literature Publishing, New York.

Burton R (1621). *The Anatomy of Melancholy*. Vintage, New York (reprinted 1977).

Catholic Church in England and Wales (2008). *Cherishing Life*. Retrieved on 9 June 2008 from http://www.catholicchurch.org.uk/

*Den eldre Gulatingslova* (1994). Norrøne tekster nr 6, Oslo Riksarkivet.

Durkheim E (1952). *Suicide: A Study in Suicidology*. Routledge and Kegan Paul, London.

Evangelical Church of Germany (1996). *EKD Bulletin 02/1996*. Retrieved 9 June 2008 from http://www.ekd.de/bulletin/index.html

Farberow NL (1975). Cultural history of suicide. In NL Farberow, ed., *Suicide in Different Cultures*, pp. 1–16. University Park Press, Baltimore.

Ferm V (1945). *An Encyclopedia of Religion*. Philosophical Library, New York.

Grøholt B, Ekeberg Ø, Wickstrøm L *et al.* (1997). Youth suicide in Norway 1990–1992. A comparison between children and adolescents completing suicide and age and gender matched controls. *Suicide and Life-Threatening Behavior*, **27**, 250–263.

Harakas S (2005). *The Stand of the Orthodox Church on Controversial Issues*. Retrieved 9 June 2008 from http://www.goarch.org/en/ourfaith/articles/article7101.asp

Hume D (1929). *An Essay on Suicide*. Kaho and company, Yellow Springs, Ohio.

Jacobs L (1995). *Concise Companion to the Jewish Religion*. Oxford University Press, Oxford.

Kelleher MJ, Chambers D, Corcoran P *et al.*(1998). Religious sanctions and rates of suicide worldwide. *Crisis*, **19**, 78–86.

Keyser R (1848). *Norges gamle love indtil 1387*. Chr. Gröndahl, Christiana.

Koch HJ (2005) Suicides and suicide ideation in the Bible: an empirical survey. *Acta Psychiatrica Scandinavica*, **112**, 167–172.

Kraepelin E (1899). *Psychiatrie: ein Lehrbuch für studierende und Ärzte*, 6th edn [Suicide: a personal and social problem]. Auflage, Barth, Leipzig.

Lester D (1996). Suicide in Indian states and religion. *Psychological Reports*, **79**, 342–342.

Lester D (1998). Ethnicity, religion and suicide in Swiss cantons. *Perceptual and Motor Skills*, **86**, 1210–1210.

Mayer R (1980). *Der Talmud*. [The Talmud.] Goldman Verlag, Munchen.

Neeleman J (1998). Regional suicide rate in the Netherlands: does religion still play a role? *International Journal of Epidemiology*, **27**, 466–472.

Neeleman J, Halpern D, Leon D, *et al.*(1997). Tolerance of suicide, religion and suicide rates: an ecological and individual study in 19 Western countries. *Psychological Medicine*, **27**, 1165–1171.

Neeleman J and Lewis G (1999). Suicide, religion, and socioeconomic conditions: an ecological study in 26 countries. *Journal of Epidemiology and Community Health*, **53**, 204–210.

Retterstøl N (1993). *Suicide. A European Perspective*. Cambridge University Press, Cambridge.

Retterstøl N, Ekeberg Ø, Mehlum L (2002). *Selvmord—et Personlig og Samfunnsmessig Problem*. Gyldendal Akademisk, Oslo.

Rothman KJ and Greenland S (1998). *Modern Epidemiology*. Lippincott-Raven Publishers, Philadelphia.

Russian Orthodox Church of Three Saints (2000). Bases of the social concept of the Russian Orthodox Church. Retrieved 9 June 2008 from http://www.3saints.com/ustav_mp_russ_english.html#4

Sainsbury P, Jenkins J, Levey A (1982). The social correlates of suicide in Europe. In R Farmer and S Hirsch, eds, *The Suicide Syndrome*, pp. 38–53. Croom Helm, London.

Stack S (1983). The effect of religious commitment on suicide: a cross-national analysis. *Journal of Health and Social Behaviour*, **24**, 362–374.

Varnik A, Wasserman D, Dankowicz M *et al.* (1998). Marked decrease in suicide among men and women in the former USSR during perestroika. *Acta Psychiatrica Scandinavica* (Supplement), **394**, 13–19.

Vatican (2008). *Catechism of the Catholic Church, 2nd edn*. Retrieved 9 June 2008 from http://www.vatican.va/archive/ccc_cssarchive/catechism.kat.

Vijayakumar L, John S, Pirkis J *et al.* (2005). Suicide in developing countries: 2. *Crisis*, **26**, 112–119.

# CHAPTER 10

# Suicide prevention and religious traditions on the African continent

Lourens Schlebusch, Stephanie Burrows and Naseema Vawda

## Abstract

Research on suicidal behaviour on the African continent has been limited. A number of sociopolitical and cultural reasons contribute to this situation, among them the political and economic instability that has characterized much of the continent for the last few decades; the lack of available infrastructure, funds and research expertise; and cultural and legal sanctions that contribute to under-reporting and misclassification of suicidal behaviour. In addition, the considerable diversity of cultures and religions in Africa make it difficult to give a comprehensive picture of the suicidal problem. Only certain trends are highlighted in this chapter. The African continent is characterized by its unique religious diversity, the mixture of traditional African beliefs with some of the world's major religions. Generally, suicide tends to be higher in countries in the east and south, compared to those in the north and west, and considerable gender and ethnic differences are apparent. Differing cultural and religious understandings of mental illness and suicidal behaviour contribute to divergent research results across and within various African countries. In the past, suicidal behaviour on the continent was thought to be rare, but more recent figures suggest it is a substantial public health burden. There is a growing need to focus on preventive efforts, with greater collaboration among African researchers and beyond being a key to this process.

## Introduction

Africa is not a cultural, ethnic or religious entity, and generalizations regarding the prevalence of suicidal behaviour and related research on the continent are difficult to make. Prevalence rates of suicidal behaviour not only vary across African countries, but also across regions and populations within countries. It has been suggested that generally a number of cultural and social factors influence suicide rates, including the effect of religious attitudes (LIFE 2000). Religion is a prominent and complex aspect of human culture (Kendler *et al*. 1997), and in some instances has been found to protect against suicide (Durkheim 1951; Stack 1983). In modern societies its effects are often more readily ascertained between individuals rather than between societies, and particularly in Western Europe it appears to be a major determinant of attitudes towards suicidal behaviour (Mäkinen and Wasserman 2001). Limited research in these areas has been conducted in Africa, yet awareness of the differences across various cultural and religious groups is important for prevention.

Differences in suicidal behaviour and psychiatric disorders between Africa and elsewhere in the world are frequently determined by cultural influences, predicted some three decades ago to reduce in importance as economic development on the African continent accelerates (German 1972). This is partially true, especially where acculturation is common (Schlebusch 1990). However, because considerable diversity remains, in this chapter we do not attempt to cover the entire spectrum of research related to suicidal behaviour in Africa, but rather to highlight certain trends. While there are some similarities to suicidal behaviour, psychiatric disorders and religious practices in other parts of the world (Schlebusch 2005), here we have tried to focus more on those aspects that are unique to the African continent.

## The African research context

In Africa, a good understanding of the full burden of suicidal behaviour is hampered by a lack of systematic data collection and good-quality research. Reasons are frequently sociopolitical and cultural in nature, and some discussion of these issues is important to understand the profile of suicidal behaviour on the continent. Political and socio-economic instability has characterized large areas of the continent for decades. This has affected the collection of accurate statistics on suicidal behaviour. Further, an investigation of suicide trends in many parts of Africa is complicated by a lack, *inter alia*, of research infrastructure and funds; limited death registers; a lack of expertise in suicide research; inadequate inter-African research collaboration, with research and prevention programmes often given a low priority; limited and outdated studies; a lack of standardized research designs and assessment instruments with most studies being descriptive in nature; an absence of follow-up studies; and a paucity of multi-centre studies (Kinyanda and Kigozi 2005, Schlebusch 2005).

## Reliability and validity issues

Suicidal behaviour in Africa is likely to be under-reported because of: the said research problems; sociocultural, religious or financial reasons; or misclassification, especially as 'undetermined' manner of death and accidental death (O'Carroll 1989; Jobes *et al.* 1991; Phillips and Ruth 1993). Problems with the reliability and validity of data are particularly pertinent for some African countries given their poor record of keeping statistics on suicidal behaviour, and because of religious, cultural and legal impediments that contribute to under-reporting. Several examples illustrate how sociopolitical factors influence this. In South Africa, vital statistics on suicidal behaviour from the apartheid years (legal segregation by ethnicity) have been shown to be questionable given the reported poor quality of mortality and population data for particular groups and regions during that time (Botha and Bradshaw 1985; Bradshaw *et al.* 1992). In Addis Ababa (Ethiopia), the decrease in suicides by hanging/strangulation and the concomitant increase in the percentage of 'unspecified/undetermined' suicides are argued to be due to a fall in the quality of police reports since 1991 (Bekry 1999).

Suicidal behaviour in most of the continent still carries negative cultural sanctions which distort reports of its occurrence (German 1987), and suicidal behaviour in some countries still remains a crime, thereby helping to perpetuate secrecy and non-reporting (Kinyanda and Kigozi 2005; Ovuga 2005). In Uganda some reports (Ovuga 2005) indicate that suicide victims do not receive a decent burial, that their families and the survivors of suicide attempts are shunned and that those who are employed do not have their terminal benefits paid to the surviving family members. In Ethiopia, suicidal behaviour was considered an offence although this is changing and it is now seen as a sign of psychological problems (Bekry 1999). Similarly, in Kenya, although non-fatal suicidal behaviour was an offence, the courts take a more liberal attitude towards people who engage in it, often placing them on probation (arap Mengench and Dhadpale 1984).

Few African studies have attempted to assess the extent to which suicidal behaviour is underestimated. Experience in Addis Ababa indicates that doubtful suicides are classified as 'undetermined' whether accidentally or purposefully inflicted, and suicidal behaviour (fatal and non-fatal) by poisoning is recorded as 'accidental poisoning' (Bekry 1999). Such procedures serve to underestimate rates of suicidal behaviour. In South Africa, although a standard approach to suicide certifications for an injury surveillance system is lacking, this does not seem to threaten the accuracy of the statistics in some areas (Burrows 2005) and variations in accuracy across sex, ethnic group and methods used are largely in line with international research (Warshauer and Monk 1978; Speechley and Stavraky 1991; Phillips and Ruth 1993; Cantor *et al.* 2001). However, suicides may still be underestimated given the challenge of tracing 'disguised' suicides, particularly those where there may be a low index of suspicion on the part of police and medical officers (such as poisonings, drowning, single vehicle crashes or pedestrian injuries) as also reported elsewhere (Phillips and Ruth 1993). The extent to which suicides are 'disguised' as other deaths may be strongly influenced by sociocultural factors. Similarly, non-fatal suicidal behaviour in the general population is generally under-reported (Schlebusch 2005), and we simply do not know the prevalence rates in remote rural areas. Likewise, hospital-based rates of attempted suicide are underestimated because many non-fatal attempts are not hospitalized unless critical. Among those who are admitted some present themselves as 'accidental' because of the stigma and possible legal problems associated with suicidal behaviour (Bekry 1999).

## Cultural and religious considerations

### Differences in magnitude

Early studies suggest that suicide was rare, for example, in Uganda (Orley 1970), Nigeria (Prince 1968) and Senegal (Collomb and Zwingelstein 1968). More recent research indicates that suicidal behaviour in a number of countries is not as infrequent as previously suggested (German 1987; Nwosu and Odesanmi 2001; Schlebusch 2005). Studies show that non-fatal suicidal behaviour is as prominent in South African black youth as in their peers in the West (Rosen 1985; Schlebusch 2005). A literature review indicated that suicidal behaviour in Sudan was very infrequent, yet an assessment of suicidal ideation in two groups of women revealed high levels, particularly in a displaced persons area; and the establishment of a Befrienders International volunteer service collated anecdotal evidence of substantial suicidal behaviour (Goldney *et al.* 1998). Recent hospital statistics in the Adjumani district of Uganda show suicide to be a major public health problem (Ovuga 2005).

Generally suicide seems to be lower in countries in the west and north of the continent, compared with those in the east and south (Kinyanda and Kigozi 2005). As found elsewhere in the world, suicide in Africa is more common in males than in females with the ratio varying between 1.75 in Egypt to a high of 9.00 in the island state of Seychelles (Kinyanda and Kigozi 2005, Schlebusch 2005). Similarly, non-fatal suicidal behaviour rates for southern and central Africa resemble what is seen in Western countries where young females predominate (Gelfand 1976; Schlebusch 2005; Williams and Buchan 1981) but in eastern and western Africa a mixed picture emerges. A reversal of the female preponderance is observed in regions such as Benin City and Ibadan (Nigeria) and Kampala (Uganda) (Eferakeya 1984; Odejide *et al.* 1986; Kinyanda *et al.* 2004). However, other studies from Uganda and from Ethiopia do not report marked gender differences (Cardozo and Mugerwa 1972; Kebede and Ketsela 1993; Kebede and Alem 1999), although a study from Gabon (Mboussou and Milebou-Aubusson 1989) and one from Ethiopia (Alem *et al.* 1999a) report a higher ratio of women compared to men.

Several studies have examined ethnic differences in suicidal behaviour. In Lusaka (Zambia) differences in the suicide rate between African and European residents, although large, were not statistically significant (Rwegellera 1978). Kebede and Alem (1999) found that ethnicity was not associated with suicidal ideation or non-fatal suicidal behaviour in Ethiopia. Compared to Nigerian Yoruban students, Zambian Lozi-speaking students viewed suicide more often as having clear motives (Lester and Akande 1998). A study conducted in north-eastern Nigeria found that among young burn patients, 1.4 per cent were suicide attempts by pregnant females (aged 11–15) protesting forced marriages, which the authors refer to as 'a cultural problem' (Gali *et al.* 2004a).

Since ethnicity has in the past been one of the major bases of division of South African life, it has frequently been considered a crucial sociodemographic variable in suicide outcome research in ethnic-specific groups (Burrows 2005; Schlebusch 2005). These ethnic groups are gross proxy measures of social groupings in South Africa and give no indication of intra-group diversity. Although there are dangers of presenting the data according to ethnic groups that have no anthropological or scientific validity (Bourne 1989; West and Boonzaier 1989), there remain important differences between ethnically defined groups in the share of ill-health, mediated by social and economic factors. In contrast to whites, who have fewer suicides among those aged 15–24 years compared to older groups, the other ethnic groups tend to have a concentration of suicides in those aged 15–34 years with fewer among the elderly (Burrows 2005). Several cultural factors have been offered to explain this (Wassenaar *et al.* 2000; Schlebusch *et al.* 2003). First, in traditional black and Asian cultures the elderly are respected and remain an integral part of the family and community and this is thought to be an important protective factor against self-destructive acts. Second, young people from traditional backgrounds in a multicultural South Africa, stressed by the conflict between traditional social roles and new roles offered by a more Western-oriented culture, could be more likely to engage in suicidal behaviour.

## Transformation

Over the past several decades, many African countries have undergone substantial sociopolitical changes, wars, political upheavals, and economic crises. Elsewhere, a number of studies examining the relationship between societal transformations and suicide have found the process of social, political and economic change to be paralleled by changes in suicide (Kaasik *et al.* 1998; Leon and Shkolnikov 1998; Värnik *et al.* 1998a, b; Mäkinen 2000; Rancans *et al.* 2001). Yet similar transformations do not necessarily produce the same suicide outcomes (Mäkinen 2000), nor are all social groups similarly affected by the transition. Studies in Eastern Europe have generally found males (Värnik *et al.* 1994, 1998a, b; Walberg *et al.* 1998; Rancans *et al.* 2001) and middle-aged individuals (Leon and Shkolnikov 1998; Värnik *et al.* 1998a; Walberg *et al.* 1998) to be most affected by sociopolitical changes. These differences both across and within countries, have led several researchers to point to the possible intermediate roles of culture in influencing the outcomes (Mäkinen 2000; Bjerregaard and Curtis 2002).

Chronic and acute stress (Schlebusch 1995, 2000; Wasserman 2001) are critical comorbid aetiological considerations in suicidal behaviour, and are of particular importance in many African societies. Gross human rights violations have not only severely traumatized citizens but in South Africa, for example, have left a heritage of stress-related psychological problems (Pillay and Schlebusch 1997; Schlebusch 2000) with potential suicidal implications. High prevalence rates of violence and trauma (McKendrick and Hoffman 1990; Suffla *et al.* 2004); personal outcome expectations which are not always realized following political and other transformation; acculturation; socio-economic difficulties including high unemployment levels; and economic pressures all combine to further produce a breeding ground for potential suicidality (Asuni 1962; Mboussou and Milebou-Aubusson 1989; Dong and Simon 2001; Schlebusch *et al.* 2003; Kinyanda and Kigozi 2005; Ovuga 2005; Schlebusch 2005).

In Addis Ababa, unusually high rates of non-fatal suicidal behaviour were observed in young and middle-aged males and older females during times of political, social and economic changes (Bekry 1999). In other instances, suicide rates have declined during times of war. For example, Bekry (1999) reports that in Ethiopia, there was a dramatic decline in suicide rates in both sexes following the civil war in the northern provinces (1985–1986) and the overthrow of the 'Derge' regime (1991–1992). There was also a minor decline coinciding with the evacuation of the military from the Tigray province and an aborted *coup d'état* in Addis Ababa (1988–1989). However, one can not exclude the lack of data during times of conflict and that suicides may be written off as conflict-related deaths in times of war. Trends in male and female suicide rates were similar except that male rates fluctuated within a wider range. Declines in suicide rates during wars may be a function of individuals' integration with a social group, the decline in value of individual life and the direction of aggressive feelings from the threatened self against the external enemy (Bekry 1999). In Addis Ababa, the mass mobilization of the youth to the war front and to the resettlement areas of drought victims may have reduced the vulnerable groups in the city, thereby decreasing suicide rates (Bekry 1999).

## Differing understandings of psychiatric disorders

Depressive disorders, a critical factor in the aetiology of suicidal behaviour, once thought to be rarer in Africa, are now recognized as fairly common, sometimes presenting a subtle form with features of somatization (Nwosu and Odesanmi 2001). Otote and Ohaeri (2000) argue that the difference in symptomology, found in their sample of Nigerian psychiatric patients, should not imply rarity of depression among Africans. In South Africa, despite reports of similarly high levels of depression in all ethnic groups (Schlebusch 2005), there is evidence that cultural factors modify the expression of depressive symptomatology in some groups, and this may result in an under-diagnosis. For example, according to some traditional beliefs symptoms of depression may be considered the result of the influences of ancestors or supernatural means (Schlebusch 2005). A mentally ill person may be thought of as being bewitched through black magic and when such a person 'has no strength' and commits suicide by hanging they become an evil spirit or a roaming ghost, thereby not entering into the realm of the ancestors (Oosthuizen 1988).

Differences in symptomology across cultures may result from differences in the conception of the illness (Jacobsson 1988) and in some regions there may be no specific words for diagnostic categories as specified in the DSM-IV or ICD-10. For example in Uganda (Ovuga 2005), occasionally the metaphor of the heart having fallen onto the foot or under the sole of the foot may be used to refer to a condition that is akin to major depressive illness. The individual will often use long winding descriptions to convey a sense of distress. Various communities attribute the causes of mental illness to the influences of evil spirits, the spirits of angry ancestors, or supernatural powers (gods of the land). A person manifesting features of *joki* (one mental health problem recognized by the Madi people), may meet the diagnostic criteria for major depressive disorder. During an episode of *joki* (a special form of possession state affecting both males and females), spirits who are not related to the spirit medium take control of the person in order to have a home to live in. Suicide is a special form of mental health problem, believed to run in families and resulting from a serious crime an ancestor committed generations back (Ovuga 2005).

## The scourge of HIV/AIDS

Countries in Africa are experiencing the quadruple burden of ill-health from the pre-transitional diseases (including communicable diseases, and those from maternal causes, perinatal conditions and nutritional deficiencies), the emerging chronic diseases, injuries and HIV/AIDS (Bradshaw *et al.* 2003). Data from the 1950s for Uganda suggest that physical diseases such as syphilis and leprosy, in an era before effective antibiotics become available, were important factors in suicide (Kinyanda and Kigozi 2005). The HIV/AIDS pandemic plaguing Africa has implications for suicidal behaviour (Schlebusch 2005). As for other chronic diseases, the link between HIV/AIDS and suicide has been under-researched in Africa, but studies coming from South Africa (Noor Mohamed and Karim 2000; Van Dyk 2001; Meel 2003; Schlebusch and Noor Mahomed 2004; 2005), Nigeria (Gali *et al.* 2004b) and Kenya (Sindiga and Lukhando 1993) have shown a link between HIV/AIDS and suicidal behaviour. Critical psychosocial stressors associated with HIV/AIDS include stigma, discrimination, isolation, lack of support from family and friends, and social devaluation—all of which contribute to an increased risk for suicidal behaviour.

## Religious understandings of suicidal behaviour

Africa is somewhat unique in that it represents most of the world's major religions in addition to the traditional African religions. For example in Durban and its immediate surroundings Christianity, Hinduism, Islam, Judaism, Buddhism, Jainism, Zoroastrianism, Confucianism, Taoism and other indigenous religions flourish (Oosthuizen 1988). This area is also where leading suicide research has been conducted for several decades (Schlebusch 2005).

Long-term studies on the relationship between religion and suicidal behaviour in Africa are lacking. As in other parts of the world (Lamm 1969; Cheng and Lee 2000), most religions as practised in Africa do not condone suicide (Mbiti 1975; Oosthuizen 1988; Ebrahim *et al.* 1995), based on the rationale that life is received from the Creator, and that the suicidal person has no right to destroy it. However, while contemporary religious views are often more tolerant than traditional ones, strong condemnation of suicidal behaviour is still evident in many instances. A study in Butajira, Ethiopia (Alem *et al.* 1999b) found that the attitudes of key respondents (consisting of both Muslims and Christians) towards suicidal behaviour were generally punitive and disapproving. In areas like western Ethiopia public opinion is not necessary unfavourable towards non-fatal suicidal behaviour, although the Coptic church and Islam condemn suicide (Jacobsson 1985).

Although most religious institutions are to a greater or lesser degree against suicide, exceptions are every so often seen in practice and suicide is accepted in the following circumstances among others: when a person is terminally ill; as a heroic deed; to destroy a person's enemies; to protect a person's fatherland; as martyrs for the sake of evoking faith; collective or mass suicides; and as in the case of the Rain Queen of the Venda people in South Africa, to make way for a successor (Oosthuizen 1988; Colt 1991; Schlebusch 2005).

From a traditional African perspective, religion forms part of the cultural heritage of the people which has had a powerful impact on shaping social, political and economic activities (Mbiti 1975). It is closely tied to the traditional African way of life, functioning more on a communal than individual basis. African religions evolved as people responded to and reflected upon their life situation and experience, rather than according to scriptures written in holy books. They are often described as pragmatic and realistic, and in the process the Creator is acknowledged to be God although there are many different African names and manners to denote such phenomena. African societies are sensitive to funeral rights and ceremonies when a death occurs, but when there is an abnormal death (such as a result of suicide) these may be affected (Mbiti 1975). Regarding cultural aspects of death in Zulu culture, there are broadly speaking two concepts of deaths, timely death—i.e., presupposed by family members who survived the deceased—and an untimely death which is regarded as a serious interference in the human life (Berglund 1976). Untimely death can be related to witchcraft and sorcery, anxiety and suspicion, and there is often a reluctance to talk about it (Berglund 1976).

With few exceptions assisted suicide, euthanasia or mercy killing have received little research publication interest in Africa. In South Africa the practices of suicide, euthanasia or mercy killing are illegal (Schlebusch 2005). Despite current debates on these issues, there is generally a strong belief that tolerating suicide, whether the act is carried out with assistance or whether it is self-imposed, lessens the value of life that society places on its members (Heuer 1988; Oosthuizen 1988; Schlebusch 2005). In a study among Sudanese doctors (92 per cent Muslim), the vast majority strongly opposed euthanasia and assisted suicide because of religious beliefs, inconsistency with the doctor's role, the presence of subtle pressures on patients, and the potential for misuse among the physically and mentally handicapped (Ahmed *et al.* 2001).

In certain parts of the world religious fundamentalism has been associated with suicide attacks, sometimes referred to as political suicides (Dingfelder 2004). These also have occurred in Africa. The sequelae can lead to direct or indirect trauma for survivors, resulting in trauma-producing behaviours (TPBs) (Schlebusch and Bosch 2002). Such TPBs often give rise to a range of different responses which can have significant implications for suicidal behaviour such as depression, anger, humiliation, emotional blunting, psychosocial problems, feelings of helplessness, and feelings of being dehumanized and alienated as a result of distrust in society (Schlebusch and Bosch 2002). TPBs are also often seen in surviving family members of murder-suicides or extended suicides where family members are murdered followed by the suicide of the perpetrator—an increasingly common phenomenon in, for example, South Africa (Schlebusch 2005).

## Suicide prevention today

The differential suicide outcomes across cultural and religious groups and geographic locations suggest that influences underlying them vary, or that in the face of common adverse influences different groups have varying expressions of protective factors (Gunnell *et al.* 2003; Garlow *et al.* 2005). Given this, investigations of the possible mechanisms that contribute to increased risk or protective factors are urgently needed to understand what drives outcome differences. Prevention efforts are likely then to be better designed and have greater effects.

The problem of suicidal behaviour has not been high on the policy agenda of many African countries in the past, being largely overshadowed by other numerous, and indeed pressing, health problems. Yet available figures for a number of countries suggest that suicidal behaviour is a cause for concern indicative of a substantial public health burden. Consequently, there is a growing need to focus on preventive efforts. It has been argued that to achieve the goal of access to mental health care for all Africans, such care needs to be included in primary health care programmes, regional postgraduate medical centres are needed, and a means of gathering statistics and funding research should be fostered (Odejide *et al.* 1989). Appropriately targeted prevention initiatives require ongoing and accurate information on suicidal behaviour to identify high-risk individuals and to monitor trends so that adequate interventions can be timeously established and evaluated (Burrows and Schlebusch 2006). The improvement of national data collection systems are, therefore, imperative and creating workable partnerships and alliances with professional groups, non-governmental organizations (NGOs), government sectors and the community are important.

As noted, a framework for a South African suicide prevention programme has been developed (Burrows and Schlebusch 2006) which can be adapted for use elsewhere on the continent. There is a need to extend this beyond South Africa's borders, and to develop collaborations among different African countries, as well as between countries in Africa and those elsewhere in the world. Much can be learnt from other international suicide prevention programmes providing that local African research is taken into consideration. These programmes, for example the National [Swedish] Council for Suicide Prevention 1996, Australian LIFE 2000, NHS Scotland 2002, and the International Association for Suicide Prevention (IASP) suggest that preventive efforts need to have a diversity of approaches, targeting the whole population, specific population subgroups and individuals at risk. They also should build on strengths, capacities and capabilities of individuals, families, and communities so that the activities are appropriate and responsive to the social, religious and cultural needs of the groups they serve. Finally, traditional healers and traditional beliefs are respected and integral parts of many African communities. They play a key role in dealing with disease and mental health issues in Africa (including in understanding suicide) and need to be involved in research, management and prevention (Schlebusch and Rugieri 1996; Freeman 2003; Mkize 2005; Ovuga 2005).

## Conclusion

With some notable exceptions, good-quality research and therefore, appropriately targeted preventive efforts are limited on the African continent for several reasons, including a lack of funding, infrastructure, expertise, cultural, sociopolitical, legal factors and others. Available evidence demonstrates that in some parts of Africa suicidal behaviour is more common than previously thought, but because of considerable intra-continental variations in prevalence rates data should be interpreted cautiously (Kiyanda and Kigozi 2005; Schlebusch 2005).

Any discussion on suicidal behaviour in Africa needs to look at the various religious and political approaches to this phenomenon. Although the religious treatment of those who engage in suicidal behaviour usually demands expert knowledge from religious leaders who have a definite pastoral task, limited research is done in this connection in Africa, despite pleas for a greater awareness of the issues involved (Heuer 1988; Oosthuizen 1988).

Integrated strategies to reduce suicidal behaviour in African countries need to be research-based and outcome-focused, with evaluation as an integral part. Studies suggest that such strategies should be appropriate and responsive to the religious, social and cultural needs of the populations they serve. Greater collaboration within Africa and beyond is required. We hope this chapter will go some way towards providing the foundation from which to answer the call made at the IASP 2005 Congress for suicidologists to play a more proactive role in spear heading intra-regional and cross-country research on the African continent.

## References

Ahmed AM, Kheir MM, Abdel Rahman A *et al.* (2001). Attitudes towards euthanasia and assisted suicide among Sudanese doctors. *East Mediterranean Health Journal*, **7**, 551–555.

Alem A, Jacobsson L, Kebede D *et al.* (1999b). Awareness and attitudes of a rural Ethiopian community toward suicidal behaviour. A key informant study in Butajira, Ethiopia. *Acta Psychiatrica Scandinavica*, **397**(Suppl.), 65–69.

Alem A, Kebede D, Jacobsson L *et al.* (1999a). Suicide attempts among adults in Butajira, Ethiopia. *Acta Psychiatrica Scandinavica*, **397**(Suppl.), 70–77.

arap Mengech HN and Dhadphale M (1984). Attempted suicide (parasuicide) in Nairobi, Kenya. *Acta Psychiatrica Scandinavica*, **69**, 416–419.

Asuni T (1962). Suicide in Western Nigeria. *British Medical Journal*, **2**, 1091–1097.

Bekry AA (1999). Trends in suicide, parasuicide and accidental poisoning in Addis Ababa, Ethiopia. *Ethiopian Journal of Health Development*, **13**, 247–62.

Berglund A-I (1976). *Zulu thought patterns and symbolism*. Hurst and Company, London.

Bjerregaard P and Curtis T (2002). Cultural change and mental health in Greenland: the association of childhood conditions, language and urbanization with mental health and suicidal thoughts among the Inuit of Greenland. *Social Science and Medicine*, **54**, 33–48.

Botha JL and Bradshaw D (1985). African vital statistics—a black hole? *South African Medical Journal*, **67**, 977–981.

Bourne DE (1989). Nomenclature in a pigmentocracy—a scientist's dilemma (Opinion). *South African Medical Journal*, **76**, 185.

Bradshaw D, Dorrington RE, Sitas F (1992). The level of mortality in South Africa in 1985—what does it tell us about health? *South African Medical Journal*, **82**, 237–240.

Bradshaw D, Groenewald P, Laubscher R *et al.* (2003). *Initial burden of disease estimates for South Africa, 2000*. South African Medical Research Council, Cape Town.

Burrows S (2005). Suicide mortality in the South African context: exploring the role of social status and environmental circumstances. Doctoral thesis. Department of Public Health Sciences, Karolinska Institutet, Stockholm.

Burrows S and Schlebusch L (2006). Priorities and prevention possibilities for reducing suicidal behaviour in South Africa. Medical Research Council–University of South Africa, Crime, Violence and Injury Lead Programme, Tygerberg.

Cantor C, McTaggart P, De Leo D (2001). Misclassification of suicide: the contribution of opiates. *Psychopathology*, **34**, 140–146.

Cardozo LJ and Mugerwa RD (1972). The pattern of acute poisoning in Uganda. *East African Medical Journal*, **49**, 983–988.

Cheng ATA and Lee CS (2000). Suicide in Asia and the Far East. In K Hawton and K van Heeringen, eds, *The International Handbook of Suicide and Attempted Suicide*, pp. 29–48. Wiley, Chichester.

Collomb H and Zwingelstein J (1968). Depressive states in an African community (Dakar). In T Lambo, ed., *First Pan-Africa Conference Report*, pp. 121–123. Abeokuta, Nigeria.

Colt GH (1991). *The Enigma of Suicide*. Simon and Schuster, New York.

Dingfelder SF (2004). Fatal friendships. *Monitor on Psychology*, **35**, 20–21.

Dong X and Simon MA (2001). The epidemiology of organophosphate poisoning in urban Zimbabwe from 1995 to 2000. *International Journal of Occupational and Environmental Health*, **7**, 333–338.

Durkheim E (1951). *Suicide*. Translated by JA Spaulding and G Simpson. Free Press, New York.

Ebrahim AFM, Hoosen GM, Hathout H (1995). *Death or dying: advising patients and family*. The Islamic Medical Association of South Africa, Durban (Qualbert).

Eferakeya AE (1984). Drugs and suicide attempts in Benin City, Nigeria. *British Journal of Psychiatry*, **145**, 70–73.

Freeman M (ed.) (2003). *Mental Health and HIV/AIDS: proceedings of the round-table meeting*. HSRC Publishers, Cape Town.

Gali BM, Madziga AG, Na'aya HU (2004a). Epidemiology of childhood burns in Maiduguri north-eastern Nigeria. *Nigerian Journal of Medicine*, **13**, 144–147.

Gali BM, Na'aya HU, Adamu S (2004b). Suicide attempts in HIV/AIDS patients: report of two cases presenting with penetrating abdominal injuries. *Nigerian Journal of Medicine*, **13**, 407–409.

Garlow SJ, Purselle D, Heninger M (2005). Ethnic differences in patterns of suicide across the lifestyle. *American Journal of Psychiatry*, **162**, 319–323.

Gelfand M (1976). Suicide and attempted suicide in the urban and rural African in Rhodesia. *The Central African Journal of Medicine*, **22**, 203–205.

German GA (1972). Aspects of clinical psychiatry in sub-Saharan Africa. *British Journal of Psychiatry*, **121**, 461–479.

German GA (1987). Mental health in Africa: II. The nature of mental disorder in Africa today. Some clinical observations. *British Journal of Psychiatry*, **151**, 440–6.

Goldney RD, Harris LC, Badri A *et al.* (1998). Suicidal ideation in Sudanese women. *Crisis*, **19**, 154–158.

Gunnell D, Middleton N, Whitley E *et al.* (2003). Why are suicide rates rising in young men but falling in the elderly? A time series analysis of trends in England and Wales 1950–1998. *Social Science and Medicine*, **57**, 595–611.

Heuer NAC (1988). The inside and outside of suicide: subjective and objective perspectives from pastoral analysis. In *Suicidal Behaviour: Proceedings of the First Southern African Conference on Suicidology*, pp. 69–86. Department of Medically Applied Psychology, Faculty of Medicine, University of Natal, Durban.

Jacobsson L (1985). Suicide and attempted suicide in a general hospital in Western Ethiopia. *Acta Psychiatrica Scandinavica*, **71**, 596–600.

Jacobsson L (1988). On the picture of depression and suicide in traditional societies. *Acta Psychiatrica Scandinavica*, **344**, 55–63.

Jobes DA, Casey JO, Berman AL *et al.* (1991). Empirical criteria for the determination of suicide manner of death. *Journal of Forensic Sciences*, **36**, 244–256.

Kaasik T, Andersson R, Hörte L (1998). The effects of political and economic transitions on health and safety in Estonia: an Estonian–Swedish comparative study. *Social Science and Medicine*, **47**, 1589–1599.

Kebede D and Alem A (1999). Suicide attempts and ideation among adults in Addis Ababa, Ethiopia. *Acta Psychiatrica Scandinavica*, **397**(Suppl.), 35–39.

Kebede D and Ketsela T (1993). Suicide attempts in Ethiopian adolescents in Addis Ababa high schools. *Ethiopian Medical Journal*, **31**, 83–90.

Kendler KS, Gardner CO, Prescott CA (1997). Religion, psychopathology, and substance use and abuse: a multimeasure, genetic–epidemiological study. *American Journal of Psychiatry*, **154**, 322–329.

Kinyanda E and Kigozi F (2005). Epidemiology of suicide in Africa. Paper presented at the XXIII World Congress of the International Association for Suicide Prevention, 13–16 September 2005, Durban, South Africa.

Kinyanda E, Hjelmeland H, Musisi S (2004). Deliberate self-harm as seen in Kampala, Uganda—a case-control study. *Social Psychiatry and Psychiatric Epidemiology*, **39**, 318–25.

Lamm M (1969). *The Jewish Way in Death and Mourning*. Jonathan David, New York.

Leon DA and Shkolnikov VM (1998). Social stress and the Russian mortality crisis (Editorial). *The Journal of the American Medical Association*, **279**, 790–791.

Lester D and Akande A (1998). Attitudes about suicide in Zambian and Nigerian students. *Perception and Motor Skills*, **87**, 690.

LIFE (Living Is For Everyone) (2000). *A Framework for Prevention of Suicide and Self-harm in Australia*. Commonwealth of Australia, Canberra.

Mäkinen IH (2000). Eastern European transition and suicide mortality. *Social Science Medicine*, **51**, 1405–1420.

Mäkinen IH and Wasserman D (2001). Some social dimensions in suicide. In D Wasserman, ed., *Suicide: An Unnecessary Death*, pp. 101–108. Martin Dunitz, London.

Mbiti JS (1975). *Introduction to African Religion*. Heinemann, London.

Mboussou M and Milebou-Aubusson L (1989). [Suicides and attempted suicides at the Jeanne Ebori Foundation, Libreville (Gabon)] [Article in French]. *Médecine Tropicale: revue du corps de santé colonial*, **49**, 259–264.

McKendrick B and Hoffman W (eds) (1990). *People and violence in South African*. Oxford University Press, Cape Town.

Meel BL (2003). Suicide in HIV/AIDS in Transkei, South Africa. *Anil Aggrawal's Internet Journal of Forensic Medicine and Toxicology*, **4**, 1–9.

Mkize DL (2005). Traditional healers and suicide in South Africa. Paper presented at the XXIII World Congress of the International Association for Suicide Prevention, 13–16 September 2005, Durban, South Africa.

National Council for Suicide Prevention (1996). *Support in Suicidal Crises: The Swedish National Programme to Develop Suicide Prevention*. National Council for Suicide Prevention, Stockholm.

NHS Scotland (National Health Service Scotland). (2002). *A National Programme to Improve the Mental Health and Well Being of the Scottish Population*. Paper (02)03: The suggested aims, objectives, principles and outcomes of the national programme. Retrieved 8 July 2004 from http://www.show.scot.nhs.uk/sehd/mentalwellbeing/Aims1.htm

Noor Mahomed SB and Karim E (2000). Suicidal ideation and suicide attempts in patients with HIV presenting at a general hospital. In L Schlebusch and BA Bosch, eds, *Suicidal Behaviour 4. Proceedings of the Fourth Southern African Conference on Suicidology*, pp. 38–48. Department of Medically Applied Psychology, University of Natal, Durban.

Nwosu SO and Odesanmi WO (2001). Pattern of suicides in Ile-Ife, Nigeria. *West African Journal of Medicine*, **20**, 259–262.

O'Carroll PW (1989). A consideration of the validity and reliability of suicide mortality data. *Suicide and Life-Threatening Behavior*, **19**, 1–16.

Odejide AO, Oyewunmi LK, Ohaeri JU (1989). Psychiatry in Africa: an overview. *American Journal of Psychiatry*, **146**, 708–716.

Odejide AO, Williams AO, Ohaeri JU *et al.* (1986). The epidemiology of deliberate self-harm. The Ibadan experience. *British Journal of Psychiatry*, **149**, 734–737.

Oosthuizen GC (1988). Suicide and religions. In L Schlebusch, ed., *Suicidal Behaviour: Proceedings of the First Southern African Conference on Suicidology*, pp. 61–68. Department of Medically Applied Psychology, Faculty of Medicine, University of Natal, Durban.

Orley J (1970). *Culture and Mental Illness*. East African Publishing House, Nairobi.

Otote DI and Ohaeri JU (2000). Depressive symptomatology and short-term stability at a Nigerian psychiatric care facility. *Psychopathology*, **33**, 314–323.

Ovuga E (2005). Depression and suicidal behaviour in Uganda: validating the Response Inventory for Stressful Life Events (RISLE) (Doctoral thesis). Karolinska University Press, Stockholm.

Phillips DP and Ruth TE (1993). Adequacy of official suicide statistics for scientific research and public policy. *Suicide and Life-Threatening Behavior*, **23**, 307–319.

Pillay BJ and Schlebusch L (1997). Psychological intervention to assist victims and others exposed to human rights violations in South Africa. *International Psychologist*, **37**, 94.

Prince R (1968). The changing picture of depressive syndromes in South Africa: is it a fact or diagnostic fashion? *Canadian Journal of African Studies*, **1**, 177–92.

Rancans E, Salander Renberg E, Jacobsson L (2001). Major demographic, social and economic factors associated to suicide rates in Latvia 1980–98. *Acta Psychiatrica Scandinavica*, **103**, 275–281.

Rosen EU (1985). The disease profile of hospitalized Third World urban black adolescents. *Journal of Adolescent Health Care*, **6**, 448–452.

Rwegellera GG (1978). Suicide rates in Lusaka, Zambia: preliminary observations. *Psychological Medicine*, **8**, 423–432.

Schlebusch L (1990). *Clinical Health Psychology: A Behavioural Medicine Perspective*. Southern Book Publishers, Halfway House, Johannesburg.

Schlebusch L (1995). Stress, analgesic abuse and suicidal behaviour. In L Schlebusch, ed., *Suicidal Behaviour 3. Proceedings of the Third Southern African Conference on Suicidology*, pp. 19–38. Department of Medically Applied Psychology, Faculty of Medicine, University of Natal, Durban.

Schlebusch L (2000). *Mind Shift: Stress Management and Your Health*. University of Natal Press, Pietermaritzburg.

Schlebusch L (2005). *Suicidal Behaviour in South Africa*. University of Kwa-Zulu Natal Press, Pietermaritzburg.

Schlebusch L and Bosch BA (2002). The emotional injuries of indirect trauma. In CE Scout, ed., *The Psychology of Terrorism: Clinical Aspects and Responses*, vol 2, pp. 133–141. Preager, Westport, Connecticut.

Schlebusch L and Noor Mahomed SB (2004). Suicidal behaviour in cancer and HIV/AIDS patients in South Africa. Paper presented at the tenth European Symposium on Suicide and Suicidal Behaviour, 23–28 August 2004, Copenhagen, Denmark.

Schlebusch L and Noor Mahomed SB (2005). Suicidal behaviour and HIV/AIDS prevention within the South African context. Paper presented at the XXIII World Congress of the International Association for Suicide Prevention, 13–16 September 2005, Durban, South Africa.

Schlebusch L and Ruggieri G (1996). Health beliefs of a sample of black patients attending a specialised medical facility. *South African Journal of Psychology*, **26**, 35–38.

Schlebusch L, Vawda N, Bosch BA (2003). Suicidal behaviour in black South Africans. *Crisis*, **24**, 24–28.

Sindiga I and Lukhando M (1993). Kenyan university students' views on AIDS. *East African Medical Journal*, **70**, 713–716.

Speechley M and Stavraky K (1991). The adequacy of suicide statistics for use in epidemiology and public health. *Canadian Journal of Public Health*, **82**, 38–42.

Stack S (1983). The effect of religious commitment on suicide: a cross-national analysis. *Journal of Health and Social Behavior*, **24**, 362–374.

Suffla S, Van Niekerk A, Duncan N (eds) (2004). *Crime, Violence and Injury Prevention in South Africa: Developments and Challenges*. Medical Research Council–University of South Africa, Crime, Violence and Injury Lead Programme, Tygerberg.

Van Dyk A (2001). *HIV-AIDS. Care and Counselling. A Multidisciplinary Approach*. Pearson Education, Cape Town.

Värnik A, Wasserman D, Dankowicz M *et al.* (1998a). Marked decrease in suicide among men and women in the former USSR during perestroika. *Acta Psychiatrica Scandinavia*, **98**(Suppl. 394), 13–19.

Värnik A, Wasserman D, Dankowicz M *et al.* (1998b). Age-specific suicide rates in the Slavic and Baltic regions of the former USSR during perestroika, in comparison with 22 European countries. *Acta Psychiatrica Scandinavia*, **98**(Suppl. 394), 20–25.

Värnik A, Wasserman D, Eklund G (1994). Suicides in the Baltic countries, 1968–90. *Scandinavian Journal of Social Medicine*, **22**, 166–169.

Walberg P, McKee M, Shkolnikov V *et al.* (1998). Economic change, crime, and mortality crisis in Russia: regional analysis. *BMJ*, **317**, 312–318.

Warshauer ME and Monk M (1978). Problems in suicide statistics for Blacks and Whites. *American Journal of Public Health*, **68**, 383–389.

Wassenaar DR, Pillay AL, Descoins S *et al.* (2000). Patterns of suicide in Pietermaritzburg 1982–1996: race, gender and seasonality. In L Schlebusch and BA Bosch, eds, *Suicidal Behaviour 4. Proceedings of the Fourth Southern African Conference on Suicidology*, pp. 97–111. Department of Medically Applied Psychology, Faculty of Medicine, University of Natal, Durban.

Wasserman D (ed.) (2001). *Suicide. An Unnecessary Death*. Martin Dunitz, London.

West ME and Boonzaier EA (1989). Population groups, politics and medical science (Opinion). *South African Medical Journal*, **76**, 185–186.

Williams H and Buchan T (1981). A preliminary investigation into parasuicide in Salisbury, Zimbabwe—1979/1980. *The Central African Journal of Medicine*, **27**, 129–135.

# CHAPTER 11

# The role of religion in suicide prevention work in Uganda

Emilio Ovuga and Jed Boardman

## Abstract

Central themes of traditional religious practice in Uganda have been the role of a creator, an understanding of life in an integral sense and maintenance of contact with the spirit world. Christianity was introduced to Uganda at the end of the nineteenth century and was associated with the colonial powers. Subsequent expressions of religious beliefs juxtaposed traditional and European beliefs. Present expressions of cosmology in everyday life mainly involve a strong sense of the collective and its responsibility, breakdown of which, and the subsequent loss of cohesion, plays a central role in suicide. Suicide has usually been seen as an uncommon occurrence in Uganda, but recent research suggests that this is no longer the case. The rise in suicide may be the result of substantial social changes and long-term strife affecting the population. Associated with this have been examples of mass suicide and internal wars, which have resulted in mass killings which may have their roots in traditional and non-traditional religious beliefs. An understanding and knowledge of the traditional world view of Ugandans may be helpful in developing strategies for the management and prevention of suicide in Uganda.

## Introduction

Contemporary Uganda is a predominantly Christian country, with a significant minority of Muslims. Traditional religions and practices dominate the private lives of many Ugandans, but are today often inseparable from Christian practices. Across the world, religion concomitantly serves social and political purposes as well as individual needs. In this chapter, we discuss the traditional religions, their evolution and social effects, which may assist in our understanding of the phenomenon and prevention of suicide. We then provide suggestions for research and suicide prevention that incorporates traditional notions of a meaningful, peaceful and worthwhile existence on earth.

## Traditional religion and Society in Uganda

### Life and death caught between traditional religion and Christianity

Traditional religious practices have varied across Uganda, but a central theme has been that life has been understood in a holistic or integral sense, with a creator giving knowledge about life; how to promote it, transmit it and heal it (Byaruhanga-Akiiki 1995). Human existence on earth is in constant touch with the spirit world; humans do not pass away in death, but proceed to new life in the spirit world where ancestors and the great God, who is responsible for all that happenings on earth, live (Oguejiofor 2003; Onah 2003), and along with ancestral spirits, are adored regularly through prayers (Ndoleriire 1995; Nyamiti 2005).

Christianity was introduced to Uganda by Europeans at the end of the nineteenth century, and Islam was ascertained in 1844. The first British explorers, Speke and Grant, visited Uganda in 1862, and were followed by Henry Morton Stanley, who attended the court of the King (Kabaka) of Buganda. Stanley took a letter from the Kabaka, which later appeared in the *Daily Telegraph*, back to England asking Queen Victoria to send missionaries to Buganda in order to teach the people about the Christian religion and 'Western knowledge'. This move to the British may have been prompted by the threat faced by the Kabaka from Egypt and from the neighbouring King of Bunyoro (Mutibwa 1992). The first Anglican missionaries arrived in 1877 and Catholics in 1879. Uganda became a British Protectorate in 1894, and remained so until independence in 1962. The early missionaries, and their respective African followers, were in conflict and this was fought out in the court of the Kabaka, giving it a political dimension, which resulted in civil wars in Buganda and the later dominance of the protestant faction. Protestantism became equated with the establishment and the colonial powers. In the colonial period, state and church were initially established as separate institutions: the Anglican church came to be associated with the Kingdom of Buganda, and the Catholic church with the democratic opposition in the rest of the country. After 1930, an African revivalist movement, the Balokole, arose and was critical of the established church hierarchies; subsequently establishing itself as the predominant church movement. The arrival of Christian missionaries transformed traditional beliefs and practices: out of the colonial invasion sprung transformed religious expressions juxtaposing indigenous beliefs with those from Europe (Behrend 1999).

An example of this transformation can be seen among the Acholi and Madi in northern Uganda. Spirits (Acholi—*jok*, plural *jogi*, in Madi *ori*) played a central role in the Acholi and Madi cosmology and religion (Behrend 1999). These *jogi* were mediated through mediums called *ajwaka* (Acholi) or *ojo* (Madi) and operated in the public or private arena. Traditionally, the *jogi* of chiefdoms and clans were responsible for the collective welfare of man and nature, and war as well. In addition, 'free jogi' could be used privately by ajwaka for good or bad purposes. With colonialism and consequent reduction in the power of the chiefdoms, these 'free jogi' predominated; often incorporating terms and forms taken from foreigners (Behrend 1999). External influences, such as the Christian belief of duality, of good versus evil, gradually altered the worldview of the Acholi and Madi, and produced a variety of spirits that could be used for witchcraft. The previous cultural system had ensured that all spirits lived in harmony with their relatives still on earth. The revivalist Balokole movement reinforced this, but introduced the ideas of salvation, which were previously unknown in Acholi and Madi religion. These newer ideas created the possibility of prophesy, which predicted the end of the world. Newer Christian spirits emerged in the 1970s and 1980s at a time of crisis and conflict for Uganda. The *tipu maleng* (holy spirits) and their mediums (*nebi*, the Alur ethnic group) were different in nature from the ori, jogi and ajwaka. These new spirits were unambiguously good; the nebi healed and did not bewitch or take revenge. These developments of prophesies and tipu maleng may have been influential in key movements in northern Uganda led by Alice Lakwena and Joseph Kony (see below). Both movements, like the Balokole movement, were concerned about evil and sin that threatened salvation and life after death; both movements sought to restore purity, hope and salvation from eternal destruction.

## Expressions of cosmology in daily life

In Uganda, it is widely believed that ancestral spirits, and the spirits of other dead relatives, live among the living and special shrines or huts are constructed for ancestors to live in. Among the Madi of north-western Uganda, every home has a guard post (*tumi*) for ancestral spirits to guard the entrance to the home of the living, protecting the residents against the intrusion of evil spirits and other malevolent forces. For the good health of the living, ancestral spirits are kept happy by timely offerings, paying homage and prayers, leading morally upright lives and strict observance of taboos by everyone. Clan and cultural leaders, and chiefs who represent the dead on earth, are supposed to lead exemplary lives. They are a source of inspiration in bad times, intercede with ancestors on behalf of the living in case of trouble, make rain, bless clan warriors in times of war, and provide treatment in case of ill-health. Elders at family level provide training in all spheres of life for the young, and ensure that the young shoulder the past burdens of the clan and family, and propagate and protect the past glories and successes of their ancestors. The roles of ordinary people are to respect chiefs, clan leaders and family elders; lead morally upright lives; meet personal obligations and responsibilities to the community and clan; take care of the needs of ancestral spirits at family level; provide for the welfare of the community and group; and protect the general interests of the clan and family.

The traditional cosmology of Ugandans may be summarized as a collective recognition of the universality of the human condition: what happens to one person will ultimately happen to the next. What happens in a person's life may be traced back to their own roots and past history, or may be due to the malevolent intentions of their enemies executed by evil spirits or through acts of witchcraft. Ill-health and other forms of personal or group misfortune may be understood in terms of personal or collective group failure.

People are expected to endure the human condition, seek help from the relevant agents, submit to group expectations and admit any acts of wrong-doing in reconciliation and repentance. In this way, people become rooted in the larger group, and experience the value and meaning of a full life in relationship to the value systems of the larger group. Individuals contribute to, and receive from, the larger group in a reciprocal manner, making life on earth worthwhile and making suicide, due to general psychosocial difficulties, irrelevant for most people. The occurrence of suicide has usually been observed in relation to individual or group failures in the observance of cultural norms, values, regulations, taboos and fulfilment of personal roles and obligations that severs interpersonal relations and makes susceptible individuals vulnerable to self-destructive behaviour. Interviews with various community groups and suicidal individuals reveal the significance of group cohesion and personal sense of belonging to the larger group, the recognition by group members of the value of each member in the group, and respect for each group member by members of the larger group. The sense of belonging is particularly strong among the elderly when they persistently express the wish to die and join the company of their dead colleagues whenever they face the challenges of social isolation in old age in contemporary society in rural Uganda. Suicidal women value the respect that their own offspring ought to accord them in old age, in recognition of their suffering and sacrifice in the upbringing of their offspring. Young women of active childbearing age derive tremendous value in being able to bear children and being able to fend for the children and their fathers. Children and adolescents become suicidal if their parents or guardians fail to educate them, and/or protect them from physical and psychological harm, as occurs in child abuse and neglect.

Cultural and traditional religious beliefs and practices, even when incorporated into Christian systems, are reflected in Ugandan social life in which collectivism predominates. Social networks are established using all available forms of social processes aimed to enlarge individuals' social support systems. Marriage between clan relatives is discouraged in order to widen and strengthen social networks, and equitably share wealth in the form of bride price. Homogeneity in religious affiliations is encouraged to strengthen social bondage between individuals. Alliances in political affiliation are sought after to strengthen the sense of belonging, social security and group dominance over others. What belongs to one person belongs to the group or family, community or clan on earth and to the spirits in the invisible world. Personal success, joy, possessions and other forms of wealth are shared, but so are all forms of loss, misery, sorrow and costs. Urban city dwellers, whether from the same clan or tribe, set up their own microcosmic worlds in order to retain their sense of social cohesion against potential adversity, and these in turn, keep in touch with their primary rural communities and keep their loyalties of extended family and village ties that hold them together (Leopold 2005). People frequently return to their villages from their residence in the cities to join members of their village community in solving family and clan issues, take part in funerals or celebrate important traditional rituals and cultural events like naming and christening a child, initiation, marriage ceremonies or other festivals. Elders from the countryside visit relatives in the city to discuss clan and family matters. City dwellers send financial assistance to their rural home communities to support various development projects or to pay for the education of children from financially less capable families. In this way, people of the same lineage provide support to one another at all times in the face of harsh conditions of living.

## Suicide in Uganda

Orley (1970) suggested that suicide was uncommon in Uganda, but more recent studies suggest that this is not the case (Ovuga *et al.* 2005a). Social changes over the past 100 years have altered traditional Ugandan society, and with endemic poverty, the advent of AIDS, perennial political strife and continued conflict leading to the internal displacement of more than 1.8 million people in northern Uganda alone and hundreds of thousands of refugees living in Uganda, the conditions are ripe for an increase in the rate of suicide. People struggle with little success in establishing new social alliances and groupings in which they might be able to fit and derive meaning for life. Poverty and unemployment levels are high. Alcohol abuse is common among the rural poor and other population groups resulting in significant social, economic and occupational impairment (Ovuga and Madrama 2006). People in some areas of Uganda currently have no ready access to the universal community support that individuals enjoyed during the first half of the twentieth century and earlier. Under such circumstances, people feel uprooted from the core of their existence, abandoned, and lack of meaning and purpose for existence. Life no longer seems worthwhile under the psychosocial strain that they might experience, paving the way to an escalation of suicide rates and the emergence of cult movements (Dein and Littlewood 2005). Sociopolitical and consequently economical changes, which could eventually have an effect on these phenomena, can hardly be foreseen in the future.

## Attitudes toward mental illness and suicide

In African cultures, mental illness is equated with madness. Less severe forms of psychological disorder may be labelled as 'stress' or a 'psychological problem' in an effort to grapple with the reality of emotional ill-health and its associated shame, stigma, fears and the eventual threat of discrimination. Mental illness can be conceptualized as a broad spectrum of ill-health, ranging from general symptoms of psychosocial distress to chronic psychotic behaviour that predisposes the affected person to social neglect and eventual death. Figure 11.1 illustrates a hierarchical concept of mental illness in Uganda. This figure is based on work carried out by the two authors using focus group discussions in two areas of Uganda, and field work in Adjumani and Gulu districts (Ovuga 2005; Ovuga *et al.* 2005a, b).

Mental ill-health occurring at the lower levels of the hierarchy may present with symptoms of dissociation or spirit possession (Ovuga 2005) for which therapy may be provided by a traditional healer. Symptoms of general psychosocial distress, including suicidal behaviour, may initially be handled by family, clan elders and close friends. Less severe forms of illness experience are explained and interpreted in terms of social cultural and existential experience and pain. Eighty per cent of traditional healers in one Ugandan district reported a personal history of mental illness (Ovuga *et al.* 1999) before they were trained as healers. In this context, African societies respect individuals who develop mental illness; affected persons who go on to become traditional healers enjoy high levels of respect, fame and prestige in their communities for having found favour to become mediums for ancestral and other spirits.

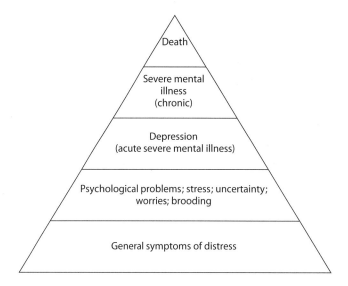

**Fig. 11.1** Hierarchical concepts in the evolution of mental illness in rural Uganda.

Once intercessions by recognized traditional healers fail the phenomena of social neglect, stigmatization and discrimination ensues as this signifies punishment from the spirit world. It is, however, important to recognize that African societies and cultures do not just neglect, stigmatize or discriminate against their kin who develop severe mental illness. This terminal phase in the evolution of mental illness to death signifies that the causes of the illness are simply too powerful for the family and traditional healer to tackle.

Problems in living, such as loss, disputes, unfulfilled rites of passage, problems of sexual unfaithfulness and poverty give rise to general symptoms of distress. Resulting cognitive evaluation of this paves way to the experience of 'stress' and fears over personal security safety and survival within an individual's cultural milieu. Persistence of distress leads to worries and brooding that result in 'depression' (equated with severe mental illness). When presented with vignettes depicting typical non-psychotic major depressive disorder, participants in Uganda interpret the symptoms as evidence of severe mental illness. Depression is invariably believed to lead to mental illness (seen as a form of chronic deteriorated psychotic illness) whose ultimate end is death. Depression as defined by existing diagnostic systems does not exist. Instead, this form of illness is explained within the context of social, cultural, and individual experience of real or imagined social adversity, crimes against social and cultural institutions, and the neglect of the welfare of the spirits of the dead. The spirits of relatives draw attention of the living to their welfare needs or anger over crimes committed by their relatives on earth by precipitating an episode of acute psychotic disorder. The spirits of the dead who have no living relatives may seek shelter from the family of an affected person through similar mechanism. Granting the wish of the spirit through the medium of a traditional healer leads to cure and the attainment of health for the affected person. Thus, African religion and ways of life foster harmony between the living and the dead, and the development of mental illness would suggest problems between the individual and the world of the dead, living and the gods. Health is restored with therapeutic strategies that seek to restore harmony between the affected individual, their family and the world of spirits.

Suicidal behaviour in Uganda is a crime and attracts shame, fear and avoidance, leaving behind a mark of impurity on the families of those who kill themselves. Attitudes toward suicidal behaviour are characterized by fear, shame, denial, stigma, avoidance behaviour, rejection and revulsion among friends and family. Suicide is a taboo subject liable to criminal prosecution and conviction. According to the Uganda constitution of 1995, suicide dehumanizes the individual, undermines the individual's dignity and right to life, robs the state of human capital and usurps the power of lawful killing from the state. The children's statute of 2003 criminalizes adult suicide on grounds that the suicidal person abdicates their responsibilities to provide for the needs and welfare of children under their care. Suicide is simply unlawful according to the Uganda Penal Code.

Suicide in Uganda is thought to arise from inheritance based on the observation that members from certain families seem to be at high risk for suicidal behaviour. It is believed that suicide behaviour may be the consequence of bad omen, witchcraft or the result of previous ancestral wrong-doings. Cultural explanations for suicide are similar to those for mental illness. Poverty, poor interpersonal relations and alcohol abuse have emerged as additional contributions to suicidal behaviour, particularly in the post-conflict of northern Uganda. Family, friends and clan elders provide initial counselling services to suicidal persons. The services of traditional healers are sought once the efforts of family and clan elders fail. Proximal factors that lead to suicidal behaviour include disputes in interpersonal relationships or the lack of material resources (poverty) necessary to support basic human needs and allay emotional distress.

Written accounts of traditional attitudes towards suicide are uncommon, and it remains unclear as to the influence of the colonial powers who introduced the laws on suicide. It would appear that suicide behaviour remains unaffected by the laws that seek to prevent them. Orley (1970), in his monograph of mental illness in Uganda, suggested that suicide was considered a 'most terrible act' among the Baganda. The body of a person who committed suicide was feared and suicide treated as contagious; no one of the same clan should touch the body as its ghost may enter him, causing the person to be tempted to kill himself (Orley 1970). Social responses to suicide include the performance of cultural rituals involving the sacrifice of animals. Among the Madi, rituals were performed to cast out the perceived evil for suicide and the tree from which a victim hanged was hewn down and burnt to ashes to prevent the act among surviving members of the victim's clan. The body of a suicide victim is hurriedly buried at the site of death without religious ceremonies or the enthronement of an heir. With the coming of newer religions, prayers and biblical teachings are used in the therapy and prevention of suicide behaviour.

## Mass suicide and rebel armies

On March 17, 2000, Ugandans woke to the news of the world's second largest cult suicide involving some 500 people, mainly women and children, burned to death in their chapel at Kanungu in the remote poor rural south-western Uganda district of Rukungiri. In the weeks that followed, 500 more bodies were discovered buried under the concrete floors of several houses belonging to cult leaders of the Restoration of the Ten Commandments, led by Joseph Kibwetere (Atuhaire 2003). Details of the cult remain obscure, and a planned government commission of inquiry to investigate it was never inaugurated to do its work, but its origins lay in the claim by a cult member of visions of the Virgin Mary and Jesus Christ. The cult prophesized that the cure for current hardships was the restoration of the 10 Commandments, and failure to do so would mean the end of a generation and the beginning of another one through a series of chastisements foretold by the Virgin Mary. They believed that only a quarter of the world would be saved. The power of this prophesy may be the mixture of the background context of a country afflicted by conflict, HIV/AIDS, poverty and the universal phenomenon of apparitions of the Virgin Mary, which may be seen to have a continuity with the older beliefs in the spirits.

On 2 January 1985, an Acholi woman, Alice Auma, was possessed by a Christian spirit, *Lakwena* (meaning 'messenger'), for which she became a medium (Behrend 1999). This later resulted in Alice Lakwena, as she became known, creating the Holy Spirit Movement and an army, the Holy Spirit Mobile Forces (HSMF), to wage war against evil. The movement purified Acholi soldiers returning after fighting with the National Liberation Army (NLA), the army of the new government, and took them into the HSMF. *Lakwena's* aims were essentially moral and peaceful, aiming to create 'new humankind' and 'a new society ... full of love and humility, all expressed in unity' (Behrend 1999). Other spirits possessed Alice, and the army that was created, had highly ritualized preparations for battle, including being sprinkled with water, 'loaded' with the Holy Spirit, and coated with shea butter oil to make them bulletproof. The HSMF won a series of battles with the government forces and marched from northern Uganda to Kampala, only being defeated at Jinja, not far from the capital. Joseph Kony, who founded and leads the Lord's Resistance Army (LRA), which was created out of the remnants of Lakwena's and the Uganda People's Democratic Army (UPDA) forces, has continued the war in northern Uganda for two decades. Kony claims to be a relative of Alice, and also acts as a medium for similar spirits.

These two examples of powerful figures leading fighting movements, the latter of particular brutality, combine aspects of examples of the dynamic bidirectional transition of traditional religious ideas into, and from, Christian beliefs in the setting of long-held cultural beliefs and continuous strife that has disrupted social relationships between the living and the dead, and promotes the potential for psychosocial distress, self-destructive behaviour and this particular type of war as an externalized equivalent of mass suicide. Like Alice Lakwena's HSMF, the LRA claimed that its mission was to create a new and pure Acholi society and to replace the impure, sinful and corrupt government of the day with one based on the teachings of the Old Testament. In an apparent attempt to fulfil its prophecy, the LRA set out to use brutal force to recruit personnel into its ranks, intimidate the populace and turn young abducted girls into wives to recreate a new Acholi society. Under the circumstances of war and violence, the communities were caught in between two opposing fighting forces with no protection from anywhere. Even though the government subsequently began moving whole communities into internally displaced persons' (IDP) camps, the populations initially resisted as this would undermine their cultural and traditional identities and ways of life. The communities in northern Uganda thus preferred to wait for every one of them to die in the course of the war, having surrendered into a state of helplessness and hopelessness.

## Implications for suicide prevention

Approaches to the management and prevention of suicide may need to be revised in order to incorporate the traditional world views of individuals and communities. In this way, the applications of scientific research will perhaps bear significant impact on suicide management and prevention in situations of chaos and helplessness. Current efforts in suicide prevention place too much reliance on biological, epidemiological and statistical data that bear no relevance to individuals' life circumstances or their evaluations of these (Onah 2003). For instance, the desire of an 80-year-old man in rural Uganda, without significant social support from his sons and daughters, to end his life by suicide in order to join the world of his peers who have long died may not be predicted solely by detecting traditional risk factors. It is necessary to additionally define his view of the world and quality of existence, in addition to an evaluation of risks for suicide in the usual clinical sense. Management might then require the provision of social services relevant to his situation.

The review of traditional religious practices in Uganda would seem to suggest the need to create social, political and health care systems that protect and strengthen traditional linkages within kinships, as a major collective contribution toward suicide prevention, by promoting overall health and social welfare. Concrete steps in creating this system, and which have proved effective in Adjumani district of Uganda, comprised training village representatives to recognize early warning signs of psychosocial distress, make thorough psychological assessments within the cultural belief systems of communities, provide opportunities for distressed persons and their families to narrate their difficulties in a therapeutic atmosphere, arrange for family group meetings to settle conflict issues, and to refer individuals with more complicated mental health problems to health care providers in the community. The training of village representatives, known in the context of Adjumani district as *village helpers* (VHs), was based on four culturally recognized common causes of psychosocial distress in the community: loss (most commonly in the form of bereavement), disputes (with fear of witchcraft), unfulfilled rites and poverty. Identified mental health problems are discussed based on an understanding of the emotional, cognitive, relational, and behavioural impacts of the causes of distress on an individual and the immediate members of their social group.

Following the institution of this approach in 2004, in Dzaipi, a subcounty in Adjumani district, the rates of completed suicide decreased from 206 per 100,000 in 2004 to 105 per 100,000 and 91 per 100,000 in 2006 for a base population of 18,612 inhabitants. Likewise, the rates of attempted suicide dropped from 452 per 100,000 in 2004 to 370 per 100,000 in 2005 and 270 per 100,000 in 2006. Thus, appropriate suicide preventive measures at population level might aim to improve social rootedness, and revitalize and sustain social and cultural practices that made life meaningful for the ordinary person in society. Advances in agricultural modernization, economic development, and democratic governance should aim to provide for the needs of individual members of society, as well as the protection and welfare needs of group entities within the national borders of individual countries. Research to develop interventions for the management and prevention of suicide from this perspective is recommended.

We recommend that the channels of communication be opened between biological and social sciences in the field of human health, with the aim of fostering close collaboration between the two groups. These disciplines have a vital input to make, and these contributions may be maximized through mutual respect for the understanding provided by the other in the field of suicide prevention and the promotion of health.

## Conclusion

Rates of suicide appear to have increased in Uganda in line with social changes and continued events that threaten the physical and emotional integrity of the population. An understanding of the traditional world view of Ugandans, and its adaptations in line with the introduction of Western religion, along with the known international literature on suicide, can help inform the management and prevention of suicide in Uganda. In particular, the emphasis placed on the collective nature of Ugandan society and the importance of kinship links can inform possible preventative approaches to suicide prevention as well as the treatment of the disorders underlying suicide.

## References

Atuhaire B (2003). *The Uganda Cult Tragedy. A Private Investigation.* Janus, London.

Behrend H (1999). *Alice Lakwena and the Holy Sprits.* War in Northern Uganda 1986–97, chapter 7. Fountain Publishers, Kampala.

Byaruhanga-Akiiki ABT (1995). Religious rehabilitation in Uganda. In PG Okoth, M Muranga and EO Ogwang, eds, *Uganda. A Century of Existence*, chapter 17. Fountain Publishers, Kampala.

Dein S and Littlewood R (2005). Apocalyptic suicide: from a pathological to an eschatological interpretation. *International Journal of Social Psychiatry*, **51**, 198–208.

Leopold M (2005). *Inside West Nile.* Fountain Publishers, Kampala.

Mutibwa P (1992). *Uganda Since Independence. A Story of Unfulfilled Hopes.* Fountain Publishers, Kampala.

Ndoleriire O (1995). *The Significance of Language and Worship in Kitoro Tradition.* In PG Okoth, M Muranga and EO Ogwang, eds, Uganda. A Century of Existence, chapter 18. Fountain Publishers, Kampala.

Nyamiti C (2005). *Ancestor veneration in Africa.* Accessed 4 February 2006 from http://www.afrikaworld.net/afrel/.

Oguejiofor JO (2003). *Resources for peace in African proverbs and myths.* Accessed 4 February 2006 from http://www.afrikaworld.net/afrel/.

Onah GI (2003). *The meaning of peace in African traditional religion and culture.* Accessed 4 February 2006 from http://www.afrikaworld.net/afrel/.

Orley JH (1970). *Culture and Mental Illness.* East African Publishing House, Nairobi.

Ovuga E (2005). Depression and suicidal behaviour in Uganda. Doctoral Dissertation, Karolinska Institute and Makerere University. Karolinska University Press, Stokholm.

Ovuga E and Madrama C (2006). The burden of alcohol use in the Uganda Police in Kampala district. *African Health Sciences*, **6**, 14–20.

Ovuga E, Boardman J, Oluka EGAO (1999). Traditional healers and mental illness in Uganda. *Psychiatric Bulletin*, **23**, 276–279.

Ovuga E, Boardman J, Wasserman D (2005a). Prevalence of suicide ideation in two districts of Uganda. *Archives of Suicide Research*, **9**, 321–332.

Ovuga E, Boardman J, Wasserman D (2005b). The prevalence of depression in two districts of Uganda. *Social Psychiatry and Psychiatric Epidemiology*, **40**, 439–445.

# CHAPTER 12

# Maya religion and traditions
## Influencing suicide prevention in contemporary Mexico

Gaspar Baquedano

## Abstract

Although suicide appears to be an individual act, this auto-destructive behaviour occurs in a wider context. Comprehension of this process can be improved through an analysis of its psychological, sociocultural and economic dimensions. Suicide occupies an important place in Maya religion and practices. In fact, it is the only pre-Hispanic culture strongly linked with suicide. For example, the Maya had a suicide goddess. The southeast region of Mexico, which geographically corresponds to the Maya area, where Maya worshippers lived, and still live, has the highest rate of suicide in the country today. What are the other factors behind suicide? There are many ways of exploring this question, and one of them could be a psycho-anthropological approach, elucidating attitudes and perceptions concerning life, death and suicide. In this chapter, an overview of Maya religion and traditions in regards to suicide are given.

## Introduction

The present chapter was developed from a psycho-anthropological perspective, and its central theme is religion and Maya traditions, specifically in Yucatan, Mexico. The psycho-anthropological approach towards suicide seems to be fruitful when added to other social, psychological or psychiatric models in suicide prevention. Suicide is a multifactorial problem that has an important cultural, religious and economic background. Any fragmented alternative approach makes interdisciplinary scientific work, and the perception of suicide prevention, very difficult.

The number of persons dying from suicide is increasing throughout the five continents. In particular, one observes high rates of suicide in societies which have similar cultural background, without knowing with certainty the reasons for these patterns (Bertolote 2001). Comprehension of this process can be improved through an analysis of its psychological and sociocultural dimensions (Heikkinen *et al.* 1995; Wasserman and Narboni 2001; Vijayakumar 2004). In spite of the fact that Emile Durkheim (Durkheim 1994), who was one of the pioneers for the study of suicide, was a sociologist, the scientific literature about this topic has largely been psychiatric and psychological for many years (Alonso 1981). Nevertheless, suicide is much more than a psychiatric or psychological issue: it is a complex multifactorial process that can be studied. (De Leo 2004; Silverman 2004; Soubrier 2004; Wasserman 2004).

The following chapter was developed from a psycho-anthropological perspective in Mesoamerica. Its central theme is religion and Maya traditions, and their present-day influence in some regions of Mexico.

## Origins

The presence of humans in what later would be called the American continent, is believed to have begun about 10,000 years ago (Quezada 2001). This chapter deals with the different cultures that flourished in what is now known as Mesoamerica, a relatively new term in anthropological terminology, and one which geographically covers a little more than one-half of the Mexican territory, including other Central American countries (Ruz 1991; López 1997; Lopez and Serrano 1997). Various cultures thrive in this area, and though local expressions are of importance, there is close interaction throughout the region (Piña 1972; Delgado 1993; Fernández *et al.* 2003). The Maya culture was greatly influenced by the Toltec, another Mesoamerican culture. This influence can be observed at the archaeological site of Chichen Itza, for example in the form of Toltec figures such as Kukulkan 'the feathered serpent', which left a significant mark in the life and religion of the Maya. Kukulkan symbolized water and vegetation, and this Toltec deity embodied a person who came to Yucatan approximately in the years 967 to 987 AD. The hero Kukulkan was a political and religious reformer whose teachings were appreciated by the Maya. The human sacrifices of the Maya, which made quite an impression on the Spanish priests, were probably of Toltec origin (Pijoan 1997). However, the Maya have other noticeable traditions justifying their presence in a suicide textbook, such as the important place suicide occupied in their practices. It is, in fact, the only pre-Hispanic culture (and probably the only in the world) with a suicide goddess.

At present, the highest suicide rates-in Mexico are to be found in the south-east region of Mexico and in the north parts of the Yucatan (Inegi 2002). This problem is also of concern in other Maya areas outside of Mexico, for example in Guatemala. To what extent does the influence of the Maya pre-Hispanic believes persist today? This is an important question when investigating suicide from a wider perspective, and as in this case, with a psycho-anthropological starting point.

## Overview: the pre-Hispanic Maya

According to Sylvanus Morley (Morley 1975), Maya history can be divided into three general periods: the Pre-classic, the classic and the post-classic. The glory of the Maya culture began in the classic period (317 AD to 889 AD), but after 900 AD it suddenly declined, and many cities with their magnificent ceremonial centres were left empty (Chase and Chase 1996). Eventually these centres, or pyramids, became covered by the jungle (Valdes 1996). The cause of this decline is uncertain. Some researchers hypothesize climatic changes, natural disasters or sicknesses were the reason for this collapse; others believe that the Maya abandoned their cities after there were rebellions by the masses against the economical abuses of the priest class (Sahloff 1998).

## Maya pre-Hispanic cosmogony

The existence of benevolent and evil deities that were opposing forces characterized the duality of the pre-Hispanic Maya religion. Life, death, health and sickness were interpreted through this religious duality (Román and Rodríguez 1997). According to the pre-Hispanic Maya, the universe consisted of three large areas from top to bottom vertically in space: the upper world, an intermediary plane and an underworld. The upper world was divided into 13 levels, which corresponds in present-day terminology to a Maya heaven. The middle area was earth, the centre of the universe and where man lived. The underworld was made up of nine levels, comparable to the Christian conception of hell. Within the concept of upper world and underworld, one can find similarities in the Aztec and Peruvian cosmogonies, something which points to Mesoamerican networking (Abilio 1997; Manzanilla 1997).

Surprisingly, the numbers 9 and 13, corresponding to the underworld and the upper world in Mayan cosmogony, are found in current beliefs related to health, sickness, life and death. The gods resided in the upper 13 levels, and the goddess of suicide, Ixtab, took those who hanged themselves there. Suicide, related in this way with the number 13, was not only permitted but associated with pleasure because the Maya paradise was an attractive place to rest, with abundant food and drink. An enormous tree that connected the upper world with the underworld reached up exactly through the centre of each. It was called the 'ceiba' tree (Ceiba Pentandra Gaertin), and was the sacred tree of the Maya (Freidel *et al.* 1993). Its roots brought their ancestors to the worlds, and the dead passed through its trunk and branches to the sky high above. This sacred tree, the ceiba, was the means to leave the pain of an earthly life and to reach the pleasures of the Maya heavens.

This tree, found in the fields of Yucatan, Mexico, has a special symbolism in the religion and traditions of the Maya: it is also surrounded by a halo of mystery, fear, death and sensuality. It is important to note that the method generally used to commit suicide in the Maya zone until recently was hanging, which occured often from a tree, in addition to other forms, for example, by firearms or drugs. This behaviour strongly suggests, in my view, a connection between contemporary suicides and pre-Hispanic traditions as symbolized by the ceiba tree.

## The conquest of the Yucatecan Maya

The Spanish invasion, with its imposition of a foreign conceptual model, was an event that had a profound impact on the Maya civilization. The ancient religion was prohibited and the Maya were obligated to practice Christianity (Reed 1964). They were constantly observed in order to not return to their polytheistic religion (Bretos 1983). The coercion of cultures wounded Mayan spirituality in a profound way; the new authority and laws represented fear, insecurity, illness and chaos (Feher 1976; Márquez 1996). The impact of this oppression, the anomie according to Durkheim, has left deep repercussions in Mayan culture (Alvira and Blanco 1998; Overrington 1998; Ramos 1998).

## Current religious attitudes toward death, suicide and mental illness

Religious beliefs toward death are an excellent observatory that permits one to delve into the attitudes of a culture. Death is much more than the cessation of biological functions, and from this perspective, which goes beyond the biological one, suicide and mental illness stand out as forms of death, because they include an intense emotional and sociocultural charge. The religion of the inhabitants of the Maya region in Yucatan is a mixture of polytheistic religion and Catholicism. As part the psycho-anthropological vision of this chapter, attitudes from inhabitants of the rural areas are described. The collection of viewpoints presented here by the author reveal a Mayan cultural framework, and could reflect the present-day Maya Christian attitudes toward death, suicide and mental illness (Baquedano 2004). Generally speaking, natural physical death is perceived as a rest, mitigation from the pain of daily living, and in the last instant, as the fulfilment of a divine will. On the other hand, a person who commits suicide is in a different situation since he gives in to the sudden reverses of life, and does not accept the suffering that God sends. When one dies a natural death, people speak of resting in peace, but when a suicide is committed, one speaks of escape, sin, punishment and diabolic occurrence.

On the one hand the attitudes observed in people from the rural zones, who were interviewed about suicide, are condemned; however, on the other hand it is also perceived as an option, an alternative, when faced with suffering, poverty and a loss of interest in life. One could say that in the conscious environment there is rejection, but that in the unconscious, there is a door that is halfway open and connected to self-destruction. That is, there is no strong opposition towards suicide, leaving it reserved implicitly for specific situations. This ambivalent attitude towards suicide could be the result of a crossing over of the permissiveness toward suicide of the old Maya religion, with the Christian prohibition imposed by the Spanish conquest.

Family members of those who commit suicide in most Maya towns today are the targets of stigma, because they are in some way or another held responsible for what happened. The house where a suicide has occurred is observed with fear and rejection, and in the community, that family is identified as the family of the 'one who hanged himself'. One interesting example that speaks of this stigma is what happens to the clothing of the person who committed suicide. No one will accept the clothing in fear of receiving some devilish influence—therefore the family habitually burns it. If the method used was hanging, the tree also must be burned because it is believed that the suicide was the work of the devil.

Wakes and funerals of those who commit suicide have a component of secrecy and fear, with a mixture of shame and guilt. People speak of compassion, but at the same time there is reproach. Nevertheless, the relationship to suicide is more complex than it first seems, and there is also a certain amount of curiosity and admiration. Habitually, the Catholic priests refuse to offer a mass, and the suicide victim is only permitted to be buried in the cemetery if the grave is not easily visible.

Generally, there is no concern about preventing future suicides in the current rural Maya communities, leaving this possibility available for the 'tired'. This term is used to describe those who commit suicide, and was registered by the Spanish chroniclers during the conquest in the sixteenth century. In fact, the term 'tired' persists today when one asks about the reasons for the suicide. Suicide is seen as a curse to which anyone can be exposed. It is not an activity that can be avoided through rational actions, and it is associated with the supernatural world. Perhaps this explains certain permissive attitudes, such as passivity toward its prevention, that have been observed.

The influence of Maya culture is not limited to those who inhabit the rural zone. Mayan culture is more apparent in these areas, but it is also present in the urban areas. Sorjonen interviewed university students and people from different social groups that live in the capital city: encountering among them a similar ambivalence, rejection, fear and passivity towards the idea of suicide prevention (Sorjonen 2003). It was left masked as an alternative. In other words, despite camouflage, one is essentially dealing with similar attitudes in the rural areas and the city.

In summary, in rural areas, mental illness and suicide are considered as having an evil origin. It is a manifestation of the devil under the disguise of a medical disorder, and even if it is treated with medicine, in the end it is connected to the supernatural world. Death, suicide and mental illness, sources of deep anguish, seem to share important cultural elements, which are observed in religious attitudes charged with fear, rejection, taboo, superstition, stigma and ambivalence.

## The Maya religion

Religion reflects the cosmology of a civilization in an important way (Fromm 1980). The principal sources of information about the ancient Maya religion can be divided into pre- and post-Hispanic. Most of the important Maya deities of the old pantheon have disappeared or have been transformed (Thompson 1982). Ixtab, the goddess of suicide, and her legacy lives on in a mutated form, even to this day.

### Pre-colonial and colonial beliefs combined in a contemporary legend

Ixtab, the suicide goddess, was portrayed with a rope tied around her neck, and for that reason, she is called the goddess of the hanged. Fray Diego de Landa wrote:

> They said that those that hanged themselves went to glory, and there were those who would do so when they were confronted with small occasions of sadness, work or illness, they went to rest in glory where they were received by the goddess called Ixtab.
>
> Landa (1938, p. 38)

Those who committed suicide, soldiers who died in battle, women who died in childbirth and priests went directly to the Maya paradise. This important pre-Hispanic Maya deity has been transformed in the contemporary legend of the Xtabay.

Stories and legends form a key part of the expressions of a culture, and are a privileged path to approach the interior of a group (Baqueiro 1981). The legend of the Xtabay, the goddess of suicide, was chosen from a large assortment, because it is one of the most popular in orally and written tradition in Yucatan Mexico today (Médiz 1974). The legend tells the story of a beautiful woman with Mayan physical characteristics who appears at the bottom of the ceiba tree (Maas 2000). Values related to sexuality, eroticism, sin, death and suicide are projected in this legend (Rosado and Rosado 2000). The Xtabay seduces her, oftentimes drunk male victims, who see a beautiful and sensual woman combing her hair under the ceiba tree and attempt to embrace her, upon which she transforms into a horrible creature. The men are ultimately torn by her nails and also by cacti thorns (Godelier 1981; Sosa 2000). If they live, they lose their mind, which in a psychosocial sense, is a form of death.

The Xtabay's origin is in the Maya goddess Ixtab, also associated with the ceiba tree: note the similarity in the two names. Xtabay pertains to the colonial and contemporary period, whilst Ixtab is of pre-Hispanic times. The benevolent goddess Ixtab has been transformed into the evil Xtabay, who no longer offers men the Maya paradise by means of suicide with a rope around their neck. This legend tries to lead men away from the tree of sin—the tree of suicide—and they are left to die in the Christian hell. This contemporary legend could be compared to an adaptation of the biblical story of the serpent and Adam, attempting to condemn a serious sin today, suicide. In this new version of Ixtab, developed by the Mayans during the colonial period, an evangelical tone is observed, that of the invader trying to lead the Maya away from the ceiba, the tree of temptations.

## Maya traditions and beliefs through time

### Attitudes toward death

Fear of death is probably a worldwide anxiety of the human being, and the exploration of this fear can be one way of exploring features of a culture (Abadi 1973). Although the Maya believed in immortality, death caused fear because it was related to evil (De la Garza 1997). This is found in the ancient Maya religion, which had a strong dualistic tendency in the eternal fight between good and bad influences over the destiny of humanity. Fear of death was associated with the destruction of man and the entire creation. In this duality, the benevolent Gods procured the rain, which would make the corn plentiful, this being an indispensable element for life. The evil gods caused the droughts, hurricanes and wars, which ruined the corn and caused hunger and death. In the twenty-first century, we can still find peasants of the remote Maya zones of Yucatán firing their rifles at the sky when a bolt of lightning falls. They believe that this is the way to calm the storm and the electrical charges. Lightning, which is frequent in these areas, is seen as a death threat and therefore something to attack.

Respect for immortality was expressed in former times through embalming and the preparation for necessities in the next life. For example, food would be needed, so the mouth might be filled with ground corn in the form of dough (Malvido 1997). Possibly, these ideas have been the reason behind the current day tradition of celebrating the Day of the Dead in Yucatan (Cuesta 2001). In order to illustrate some of the relevant Maya traditions, a few interviews on Mayan attitudes towards suicide today, as expressed through contemporary traditions and legends, were collected by the author in a typical rural Maya village as part of the fieldwork. Attitudes towards people who commit suicide observed on the Day of the Dead will be described. During this important Maya–Christian celebration, the souls of suicide victims are treated in almost the same way as the souls of other dead people. The types of food and drink, the different offerings, and the colour of the candles at the table are the same for all souls. There are no differences with respect to gender or age of the suicide victims.

Figuratively speaking, the souls of suicide victims sit down at the same table as deceased family or friends. No discrimination is apparent at first sight. However, one important consistent restriction exists: the name of 'the person who hanged himself' cannot be included in the Catholic prayers. Note here that the person is referred to as 'the person who hanged himself', a customary expression throughout the Maya zone. Interestingly, the Spanish chroniclers, and specifically Bishop Landa, wrote that the ancient Maya worshipped someone who they called the 'God of Hanging'. It appears that people in these communities still use the terms 'hanging' and 'suicide' synonymously.

Why is such ambivalence observed on the Day of the Dead? People who commit suicide are admitted but also censored. We can begin to reflect on the question if we understand that during this celebration dedicated to the dead, the fusion of the ancient Maya religion and Catholicism is explicitly manifested. Maya religious beliefs were oppressed during the Spanish colonization, with the objective of their complete eradication during the sixteenth century. Nevertheless, the resistance was considerable, because the danger of a Maya uprising could provoke a reinstallation of their deities. A change of strategy for social control was required, one which permitted a Christianity close to the existing polytheistic beliefs, but which venerated the victorious God, that is to say the Christian one. For this reason, the Christianity that was assimilated and transformed by the Maya is very different from the Roman Catholic version. The 'Mayanization' of the Christian ceremonies for the dead is particularly evident in the Day of the Dead celebrations. The Christianity observed on the altars of the Day of the Dead, as with the offerings in the fields before planting, is steeped in pre-Hispanic Mayan traditions. It is a way of saying that we observe a variant of polytheistic Christianity, which has clear boundaries marked by the Catholic Church, by means of ideas such as obedience to a one and only God and to his religious ministers.

Returning to the topic of the ambivalence, surrounding those who have committed suicide during the Day of the Dead celebration, the polytheistic Mayans accept them, but the Catholics censor them by prohibiting the mention of their name in prayers. The presence of the Christian cross is a strong one in a celebration in which one cannot include a suicide victim in the list of persons for whom you ask forgiveness and clemency before the Christian God.

## Attitudes towards suicide in a small community in the Maya area: two examples

Below, I have quoted fragments of two interviews that can be seen as representative in values and attitudes from a community studied. Here the undertaker and the medicine man speak about suicide. Don Santos, the undertaker, here speaks about a particular suicide that occurred in this town:

> Well, I believe that he committed suicide because he was old. He could not see well and he could not work or do anything and he was very poor. So it is better that he is dead since what is he good for? His name was Venancio and he was my cousin. He was obsessed with dying because he could not do anything any more. Those who commit suicide cannot go to glory, and worms devour them. They should not be in the cemetery either. They make problems for those that stay in this life. Those who suffer the most end up being those who stay, since the person who dies has the good life. Elderly people reach their limit and cannot give more. Men kill themselves more than women because they are more fucked up than women.

Don Hermenegildo, the medicine man in the same community:

> Well, the person who does these terrible things (suicide) is not received by God and instead is serving the bad angel. Evil is behind a person who hangs himself. Evil takes the soul of someone who commits suicide and converts him into his slave. In order to reach God they have to be put in fire, in boiling water and then they have to dry him. Then when he is clean he will go next to God.

### Comments about the two selected examples

As with the majority of those interviewed in this community, Don Santos sees suicide as both a rest from suffering and a complication for the surviving family. Suicide is perceived as advantageous, because all living beings suffer, but some decide to escape from their pain and cause problems for others. In this sense, suicide is imagined as an aggression towards others, as a problem for the living. In the interview with the undertaker, one can perceive a sentiment of hostility towards those who commit suicide: he says they do not have a right to Glory, nor should they be in the cemetery. Nevertheless, suicide is understood to some degree, as seen in his comments about Don Venancio: 'He could not work and so it is better that he is dead.' According to Don Santos and others interviewed in this community, suicide is perceived as the final escape in the case of loss of productivity and social roles. It is also seen in terms of gender: more men commit suicide because 'they are more fucked up', reflecting the economic and social pressure on them in these rural areas (Canetto and Sakinofsky 1998).

It is interesting to note that the degree of social damage present in the interview clearly exceeds the individualistic notion of suicide. Don Santos illustrates this in this sentence: 'Those who suffer the most end up being those who stay, since the person who dies has the good life.' Also, one should note that when he says that the person who commits suicide 'has the good life', suicide appears to be something other than death, rather a more pleasant way to exist than life. This suggests that he who commits suicide is not looking for death, but a better form of life than the present, coinciding with the ancient Maya conception of suicide. Perhaps this reflects a permissive attitude towards suicide in these poor areas on the periphery of modern society. The attitudes towards suicide, expressed by Dan Santos, are in some degree one of acceptance of suicide, especially when concerned with the elderly who 'reach their limit and cannot give more.' Nevertheless, this complacent attitude contrasts with his own punitive comments, which reflect the religious Christian influence present in this population. Don Santo further warns that those who commit suicide cannot enter the place of Glory, that they are judged, and that worms will devour them. They cannot be buried in the cemetery, and in this way, the process of living on the periphery of society that they had in life culminates when they are denied a place in the city of the dead.

In contrast, in the interview with the medicine man, one perceives an open rejection and even threats of eternal condemnation toward those who commit suicide. How can we explain these opposite attitudes, one which justifies and one which prohibits, represented in these two important figures in the community? One way might be to reflect on the social roles of both of them. The undertaker faces the cadaverous, skeletal way of death and the pain of the family. This is an important part of his social role. He pertains to a community with important economic needs, and perhaps in an unconscious way, he presents suicide as an option in cases of old age, sickness and poverty. That is to say that his direct contact with physical, emotional, social and economic death pushes him closer to the justification of suicide. In his personal account, he also expresses the perception of some members of his community.

The social role of the medicine man is to promote health, dealing with the fight against death, and hence he is probably bound to contest suicide. According to him, the person who commits suicide becomes a slave of the devil and one whose soul must be purified. Here, there is an element that cannot be overlooked, which is that the medicine man has a close relationship with the Catholic priest in the community. The latter gives help and advice so that the medicine man can perform better. The medicine man says that he has learned prayers in Latin (but admits he does not understand their meaning), which he thinks gives him power and status in comparison with other medicine men. In his healing, he mixes Maya, Spanish and Latin, giving us an image of something that resembles a Maya ceremony within a Catholic church. This appears to be a strategy of the Catholic church: instead of opposing almost pagan-like practices, the church mixes with them, trying to monopolize them. In this fusion of 'Mayachristian' interests, no ambivalent attitudes towards suicide are allowed and it is consequently condemned.

The significance of the previous interviews rests on two principal attitudes towards suicide. In the first interview, with the undertaker, we observed ambivalence, but some justification for suicide when the persons are elderly, sick, unable to work or with economic problems. The interview with the medicine man exposed prohibition, threats and punishment. Both attitudes will complicate any programme for the prevention of suicide in communities with this complex economic, social, religious and cultural framework.

## Suicide in Yucatan today

According to data by the National Institute of Statistics, the southeast region of Mexico, which corresponds to the Maya zone, has the highest rates of suicide in the country (Inegi 2002). Frequency of suicide is three times greater than the national average, which is 2.8 per 100,000 inhabitants. In the state of Yucatan, suicide is greater in the rural areas, a situation which prevails at the time of writing, and these zones are where people with a marked Maya heritage are living. The Yucatan state has 1.5 million inhabitants and an average of 12 suicides a month, representing three deaths by suicide a week: one suicide every second day, with the predominant method being hanging. Despite the elevated rates, there is no governmental programme in the country for the prevention of suicide. There exists a marked indifference by the government in promoting the investigation and prevention of suicide. There is opposition to community actions, and statistics are actively obscured. Nevertheless, in the state of Yucatan, the community has organized on its own, and in 1996, a programme for volunteers in the prevention of suicide was born (Let's Save a Life), and presently the only one of its kind in the country. Among other activities, the programme comprises visits to schools, a phone hotline, and a weekly radio show to broadcast messages of life.

Clearly, these actions are insufficient given the magnitude of the problem. University students, in particular, those of the social sciences, psychology and medicine, have shown increasing interest in the investigation of suicide. Within the local state university, the Faculty of Anthropology is known for its interest in this topic. The author works directly with both volunteers in the community and with university students interested in the investigation of suicide. Faced with governmental apathy, the community and the university have been the only ones to take action in response to the high rates of suicide.

## Discussion and final reflection

In Yucatan, only pieces of what once was the great Maya civilization remain. Aside from the archeological monuments that are silent witnesses to a savage destruction, what remains of the Maya civilization is a culture and language which have partly collapsed, economic and social marginalization of its people and the proliferation of alcohol, drugs, violence, unemployment, low education and a lack of basic services. This reality of economic and social deprivation collectively represents an increased suicide risk factor (Kendall 1983; Platt 1984; Wasserman 1989; Skog 1991; Yang and Lester 1994; Lester 1995; Stack 2000a, b; Botega and De Souza 2004). Today, as in former times, the anomie proposed by Durkheim is a useful tool to help comprehend suicide in chaotic psychosocial contexts (Besnard 1998). At the time of the conquest, we know that the Maya preferred to hang themselves rather than being forced to be Christianized. The Maya today live under another type of social control, by different state agencies and the Roman Catholic church. In a globalized world, one which reaches to the five continents, the economic destiny of Mexico is determined by industrialized countries, and there are few spaces or alternatives for the Maya population. The Maya is looked down on in Yucatan, and the population has developed strategies to be accepted and to survive in their own land. Many change their original Maya name for the Spanish equivalent, for example 'Ek' in Maya becomes 'Estrella' in Spanish ('Star' in English).

In the midst of anomie, poverty, drugs, ignorance and unhygienic conditions, the images of Ixtab emerge. Before the Spaniards arrived, she offered a Mayan paradise. Now a suffering and heroic Christ, who gave his life for others, offers a Christian paradise (Klopfer 1969). These two important pieces complete the puzzle that leads to the understanding of the current suicide behaviour in the Maya. Itzamna and Ixchel, the divine couple from the ancient Maya pantheon, have been replaced by Christ and the Catholic Virgin of Guadalupe. There are many indications that the current culture in the south-east region of Mexico is living in conflict with relation to suicide. Epidemiological data that support this affirmation are only the tip of the iceberg. What factors that are hidden below the surface? Of course, there are many ways of exploring these questions and one of them could be a psychoanthropological approach. When opting for this approach, one must also consider historical, social and cultural issues that can offer a longitudinal and transversal vision of the problem. For example, one can reflect on the devastating impact that the Spanish conquest had on the Maya civilization, imposing an ideology and a religion which conflicted violently with the ancient Maya beliefs. An essential part of this conflict with relation to suicide is that the ancient Maya religion permitted suicide, but the Christianity imposed in the sixteen century prohibited it. Is it sufficient to prohibit a conduct in order to abolish it? Both in anthropology and in psychoanalysis one can find many examples that demonstrate the results of censure. For example, cultures revert to strategies of survivorship in order to preserve a banned custom. Often this leads to violence or to clandestine behaviour. Similarly, on the psychological level, the subject reaffirms his neurotic symptoms before rigid, repressed and violent situations, reverting unconsciously to the ego-defence mechanism. In other words, before imposition and prohibition, individuals and groups tend to perpetuate or transform the censured conduct.

In our case, it would be simplistic to wait until the Christian prohibition towards suicide abolishes this practice. As with other observable customs in the present, pre-Hispanic permissiveness towards suicide may still be present today, particularity in groups where the influence of the Maya culture is the greatest, which is in groups where the Maya language is conserved as a first language, and where old traditions and beliefs are part of the daily life. The members of such groups often live in extremely bad conditions in rural areas, characterized by serious economic problems and the abuse of alcohol and other drugs. These are the groups of high suicide risk in Yucatan, Mexico, where prevention is complicated by the conflict between the unconscious permissiveness and the conscious prohibition. The prevention of suicide in Yucatan, as well as in societies in which there are more than one culture involved, is more complicated. For this reason, these areas require actions that bring historical beliefs and traditions and their reverberations to surface. In the case of Mayan culture, prevention must accentuate that there is a violent cultural message, which is not visible and considers suicide as an option for suffering and frustration. This message can block an individual from fighting for a better quality of life.

Becoming conscious of the influence of antagonistic cultural content, as well as the ambiguity in the management of aggression, should be a prominent objective in prevention programmes. This is particularly important in societies in which beliefs and traditions from two or more different cultures are superimposed, especially when one of them is introduced through coercion. The concept of Maya life and death has suffered many transformations over time, but it would not be exaggerating to say that in the past 500 years, the beliefs of the Maya transformed under the domain of power. The Mayan culture has been neglected as well as exploited for political purposes (Castillo and Castañeda 2004).

In reality, the image of a sad Christ as presented by Catholic religion has been superimposed on Ixtab for the purpose of efficient social control. This Christian image has a morbid message of suffering and auto sacrifice. This Christ that gave his life to save humanity (altruist suicide in Durkheim's categories) has been taken up with profound devotion by a culture which has incorporated this Catholic image of pain and resignation. All of this has been combined to build the contemporary attitude toward life and death. Ceremonies today, such as those used to ask ancient spirits for rain, or those used to pay homage to Christian saints, simultaneously reflect paganism and Christianity; they are the heart of a syncretism, a 'Mayachristianism' that we can observe in the rural Maya villages (Estrada 1978). The transformed influence of the pre-Hispanic goddess Ixtab is present in Yucatan today. Suicide by hanging is the most frequent method used, representing 90 per cent of the cases in the state. This is even more significant if we consider the fact that it is customary to have arms for hunting, and for protection in the rural villages. Why does the population prefer hanging to the use of a firearm in suicide? This emphasizes the importance of understanding the complexity of a cultural context before one tries to control the means and the method in prevention programmes. Current practice in at least one important local newspaper is to publish details of suicides: these news articles often include a sensationalist photograph and are printed in the police section. Why is news about suicides published in this section along with criminal and unlawful behaviour? The moral and condemned elements of suicide are present in this manner of reporting by the media, which suggests the need to increase the sensitivity of these professionals (Stack 1993; Schmidtke et al. 2001).

Today, it is difficult to find someone in a rural Maya area who will mention the goddess Ixtab, but I believe the Xtabay has taken her place. The legend is not only known in the villages, but has enormous popularity in the urban areas. The Maya influence beyond rural spheres is evident in Yucatan today. The presence of this chapter in a suicide textbook would be unjustified if we did not ask the next question. What influence could pre-Hispanic religious beliefs and traditions have on the attitudes toward suicide in present day Mexico? There are many ways to approach this question (one of which has maintained a low profile throughout this chapter). Two main paths are distinguished, the first a naive one and the second more complicated. The first would propose a forced correlation of the present day suicides in the region with the Maya goddess of the hanged. It is evident that this proposal is fragile and superficial. It is too simple, and it deals with the appearance of suicide and not with its essence. The other path is more complicated since it proposes an epistemological rupture (Bachelar 1948). It looks at suicides deeper than the surface level, and considers them a critical aspect of the life–death process. This leads to another question: if a marked Maya influence on the lifestyle in the south-east of Mexico exists, should there not be a marked Maya influence in the attitude toward death, and specifically suicide? Life and death are different aspects of one process and suicide develops in its contradictions.

The psycho-anthropological approach towards suicide seems to be fruitful when added to other social, psychological or psychiatric models in suicide prevention (Mishara 1996; Makinen 1997; Phillips 2004). Suicide is a multifactorial problem that has an important cultural, religious and economic background. Any fragmented alternative approach makes interdisciplinary scientific work, and the true perception of suicide prevention, very difficult.

## Conclusion

Due to the historical and anthropological complexity of the Maya culture of Yucatan, Mexico, a broad perspective, one which goes much further than biological, psychiatric and psychological, is required to understand the elevated rates of suicide in comparison with other regions of the country. It is necessary to consider the manner in which this culture has constructed the meaning of life and death. Within this ideological cultural mosaic, religion is a privileged path of entry to comprehend the pre-Hispanic Maya cosmogony, and to also explore current attitudes toward suicide.

The Maya were dominated by another culture, which violently imposed a different ideology and religion, causing the manner of explaining life and death to transform. It is possible to identify these manifestations in beliefs and traditions today. Within this process, suicide can be considered an indicator of change and also of permanence in the way of perceiving the life–death process.

That is why suicide prevention becomes complicated in this culture, as in those which have also had an aggressive imposition of ways of life through religion. If preventive strategies only focus on the biopsychic field, and do not include the social, anthropological and economic dimension in cultures that have suffered the impact of conquest, prevention actions will be fragmented. The psycho-anthropological perspective presented here can be an alternative for the global comprehension of the suicide process.

# References

Abadi M (1973). *La Fascinación de la Muerte*, p. 88. Editorial Paidós, Argentina.

Abilio C (1997). *El Cuerpo Humano y su Tratamiento Mortuorio*, pp. 51–53. Conaculta, México.

Alonso G (1981). *Algunas Ideas para el Estudio del Suicidio*, p. 9. Yucatan Historia y Economia, UADY, México.

Alvira F and Blanco F (1998). Estrategias y ténicas investigadoras en el suicidio, de Emile Durkheim. *Revista Española de Investigaciones Sociológicas*, **81**, 63–72.

Bachelar G (1948). *La Formación del Espíritu Científico*, pp. 7–22. Siglo Veintiuno, México.

Baquedano G (2004). Reflexiones sobre la muerte. Imágenes de Chumayel, Yucatán. Masters Dissertation, Social Anthropology. Faculty of Anthropological Sciences, University of Yucatán, México.

Baqueiro O (1981). *Magia, Mitos y Supersticiones entre los Mayas*, p. 31. Fondo Editorial de Yucatán, México.

Bertolote J (2001). Suicide in the world: an epidemiological overview 1959–2000. In D Wasserman, ed., *Suicide—An Unnecessary Death*, p. 6. Martin Dunitz, London.

Besnard P (1998). Anomia en la teoría de Durkheim. *Revista Española de Investigaciones Sociológicas*, **81**, 41–43.

Botega N and De Souza L (2004). Brasil: necesidad de prevención de la violencia (incluyendo el suicidio). *World Psychiatry*, **2**, 158.

Bretos M (1983). *Arquitectura y Arte Sacro en Yucatan*, p. 13. Editorial Dante, México.

Canetto S and Sakinofsky I (1998). The gender paradox in suicide. *Suicide and Life-Threatening Behavior*, **28,** 122.

Castillo J and Castañeda Q (2004). *Estrategias Identitarias. Educación y la Antropología Histórica en Yucatán*, pp. 264–268. Universidad Pedadógica Nacional, México.

Chase A and Chase D (1996). *Los Sistemas Mayas de Subsistencia y Patrón de Sentamiento: Pasado y Futuro. Los Mayas: el Esplendor de una Civilización*, pp. 39–48. Centro Cultural de la Villa, España.

Cuesta R (2001). *De la Tumba a la Vivienda*, p. 22. UADY, México.

De la Garza M (1997). *El Cuerpo Humano y su Tratamiento Mortuorio. Civilizados o Salvajes. Ideas Náhuas y Mayas Sobre la Muerte*, p. 17. Conaculta, México.

De Leo D (2004). La prevención del suicidio es mucho más que una cuestión psiquiátrica. *World Psychiatry*, **2**, 155.

Delgado G (1993). *Historia de México: Tomo I. Proceso de Gestación de un Pueblo*, p. 52. Editorial Alarubra Mexicana, México.

Durkheim, E (1994). *El Suicidio*, pp. 40–50. Ediciones Coyoacán, México.

Estrada R (1978). *Ceremonias y Leyendas Mayas*, p. 16. Fondo Editorial de Yucatán, México.

Feher E (1976). *El Choque de las Culturas Hispano— Indígenas*, p. 113. Ediciones Metropolitanas. México.

Fernández L et al. (2003) *Historia Prehispánica y Colonial Yucatán*.

Freidel D, Schele L, Parker J (1993). *Maya Cosmos. Three Thousand Years on the Shaman Path*, p. 394. Quill/William Morrow and Company, New York.

Fromm E (1980). *Psicoanálisis y Religión*, p. 48. Editorial Psique, Argentina.

Godelier M (1981). *Infraestructura, Sociedades, Historia*, p. 48. Cuicuilco, México.

Heikkinen M, Isometsa E, Marttunen M et al. (1995). Social factors in suicide. *British Journal of Psychiatry*, **167**, 747–753.

Inegi (2002). *Censo General de Población o Vivienda*, pp. 323–324. Informática Digital, México.

Kendall R (1983). Alcohol and suicide. *Substance and Alcohol Actions/Misuse*, **4**, 121–127.

Klopfer B (1969). *Estudio Sobre el Suicidio y su Prevención*, pp. 206–208. La Prensa Médica Mexicana, México.

Landa D (1938). *Relación de las Cosas de Yucatán*, pp. 38–39. Editorial Dante, México.

Lester D (1995). The association between alcohol consumption and suicide and homicide rates: a study of 13 nations. *Alcohol and Alcoholism*, **30**, 465–468.

López A (1997). *El Cuerpo Humano y su Tratamiento Mortuorio. De la Racionalidad de la Vida y de la Muerte*, p. 13. Conaculta, México.

López A and Serrano C (1997). *El Cuerpo Humano y su Tratamiento Mortuorio. Implicaciones Bioculturales del Tratamiento Mortuorio en la Necrópolis Maya de Jaina, Campeche*, p. 145, Conaculta, México.

Maas H (2000). *Leyendas Yucatecas*, p. 108. UADY, México.

Makinen I (1997). Are there social correlates to suicide? *Social Science and Medicine*, **44**, 1919–1920.

Malvido E (1997). *El Cuerpo Humano y su Tratamiento Mortuorio. Civilizados o Salvajes. Los Ritos al Cuerpo Humano en la Época Colonial*, p. 30. Conaculta, México.

Manzanilla L (1997). *El Cuerpo Humano y su Tratamiento Mortuorio. El Concepto de Inframundo en Teotihuacan*, pp. 127–132. Conaculta, México.

Márquez L (1996). Paleoepidemiología en las poblaciones prehispánicas mesoamericanas. *Arqueología Mexicana*, **IV**, 10.

Médiz A (1974). *La Tierra del Faisán y del Venado*, p. 113. B. Costa-Amic Editor, México.

Mishara B (1996). Commonalities and differences in perspectives on suicide from different cultures. *Omega*, **33**, 177–178.

Morley S (1975). *La civilización maya*, pp. 54–56. Fondo de Cultura Económica, México.

Overrington M (1998). Una apreciación retórica de un clásico sociológico: el suicidio, de Durkheim. *Revista Española de Investigaciones Sociológicas*, **81**, 102.

Phillips M (2004). Prevención del suicidio en países en vías de desarrollo: ¿dónde comenzar? *World Psychiatry*, **2**, 156.

Pijoan C (1997). *El cuerpo Humano y su Tratamiento Mortuorio. Evidencias de Sacrificio Humano, Modificación Ósea y Canibalismo en el México Prehispánico*, p. 193. Conaculta, México.

Piña R (1972). *Historia, Arqueología y Arte Prehispánico*, p. 104. Fondo de Cultura Económia, México.

Platt S (1984). Unemployment and suicide behavior: a review of the literature. *Social Science and Medicine*, **19**, 93–115.

Quezada S (2001). *Breve Historia de Yucatán*, pp. 17–19. Fondo de Cultura Económica, México.

Ramos R (1998). Un tótem frágil. Aproximación a la estructura teórica del suicidio. *Revista Española de Investigaciones Sociológicas*, **81**, 20.

Reed N (1964). *La Guerra de Castas*, pp. 16–17. Era, México.

Román J and Rodríguez M (1997). *El Cuerpo Humano y su Tratamiento Mortuorio. El Canibalismo Prehistórico en el Sureste de Estados Unidos*, p. 239. Conaculta, México.

Rosado G and Rosado C (2001). *Mujer Maya: Siglos Tejiendo una Identidad*, pp. 187–206. UADY, México.

Ruz A (1991). *La Civilización de los Antiguos Mayas*, p. 13. Fondo de Cultura Económica, México.

Sahloff J (1998). *La Civilización Maya en el Tiempo y en el Espacio*. Res libir/cnca-inah, Italia.

Schmidtke A, Schaller S, Wasserman D (2001). Suicide clusters and media coverage of suicide. In D Wasserman, ed., *Suicide—An Unnecessary Death*, pp. 265–267. Martin Dunitz, London.

Silverman M (2004). Prevención del suicidio: hay que tomar medidas. *World Psychiatry*, **2**, 152.

Skog O (1991). Alcohol and suicide, Durkheim revisited. *Acta Sociológica*, **34**, 193–206.

Slack S (2000a). Suicide: a 15-year review of the sociological literature. Part I. *The American Association of Suicidology*, **2**, 153–155.

Slack S (2000b). Suicide: a 15-year review of the sociological literature. Part II. Modernization and social integration perspectives. *The American Association of Suicidology*, **2**, 163–164.

Sorjonen K (2003). For whom is suicide accepted? Doctoral Dissertation. Department of Psychology, Stockholm University, Sweden.

Sosa R (2000). *La Xtabay*, p. 19. CIR-UADY, México.

Soubrier J (2004). Mirando hacia atrás y hacia delante. La suicidiología y la prevención del suicidio: ¿hay perspectivas? *World Psychiatry*, **2**, 160.

Stack S (1993). The media and suicide: a nonadditive model. *The American Association of Suicidology*, **23**, 65–66.

Thompson E (1982). *Historia y Religión de los Mayas*, p. 365. Siglo Veintiuno, México.

Valdes J (1996). Arqueología de la zona del río de la pasión, Guatemala. *Arqueología Mexicana*, **IV**, 51.

Vijayakumar L (2004). Altruistic suicide in India. *Archives of Suicide Research*, **1**, 73–80.

Wasserman D (2004). Evaluación de la prevención del suicidio: necesidad de enfoques diversos. *World Psychiatry*, **2**, 154.

Wasserman D and Narboni V (2001). Examples of suicide prevention in schools. In D Wasserman, ed., *Suicide—An Unnecessary Death*, pp. 269–275. Martin Dunitz, London.

Wasserman I (1989). The effects of war and alcohol consumption patterns on suicide: United States, 1910–1933. *Social Forces*, **68**, 513–530.

Yang B and Lester D (1994). Crime and unemployment. *Journal of Socio-Economics*, **23**, 215–222.

# PART 2

# The Magnitude and Implication of Suicide and Attempted Suicide

# CHAPTER 13

# Development of definitions of suicidal behaviours

## From suicidal thoughts to completed suicides

José M Bertolote and Danuta Wasserman

## Abstract

This chapter covers definitions of suicidal behaviours and how they vary over time, reflecting predominant philosophies and schools of thought. The limitations in the quality of information about suicide mortality, as a common feature affecting the whole vital registration system, are discussed. Coordinated efforts should be made to strengthen those systems, paying attention to the specificity of sociocultural factors' influence on defining, recording and reporting suicide as a cause of death.

## Introduction

### Causes of death

Mathers and colleagues (2005) assessed the global status of cause of death, based on the WHO Mortality Data Bank, which is composed with information provided since 1948 by WHO Member States, according to the WHO's Constitution. The data bank provides the cause of death by country, sex and age. Most of the global information used worldwide on mortality from any cause (including suicide) is based on that data bank; of course, individual countries, states, provinces, etc., may have additional and more detailed information that is *not* necessarily shared with the WHO.

According to Mathers *et al.* (2005), at the end of 2003, out of the 192 WHO member states (in 2008, there were 193 WHO member states), some information was available from 115 countries; although, for the years 1948–2003, it was complete for only 64 countries. As to the coverage of the information, it varies from nearly 100 per cent in European countries to less than 10 per cent in the African region. Ten per cent or less of deaths were attributed to ill-defined causes of death in less than 23 countries, according to ICD-9 or ICD-10. At the other extreme, there are 28 countries with less than 70 per cent data complete, and more than 20 per cent of deaths attributed to ill-defined causes.

In brief, using these and other criteria for assessing the quality of information on causes of death, Mathers *et al.* (2005) classified information as of high quality for 23 countries, of medium quality

for 55 countries, and of low quality for 28 countries. For the remaining 86, information is simply not available. This pattern follows the level, of development of countries closely; for instance, in more than 90 per cent of countries in Africa, there is no information on the cause of death after 1990.

### Quality of the mortality data

An important criterion used for assessing the quality of information for causes of death is the proportion of coverage, understood as the total number of deaths reported by a given country vital registration system divided by the total number of deaths estimated by WHO for that year for the total national population. It varies from 100 per cent, usually in developed countries (e.g. Germany, USA, or small populated countries as Luxembourg or Fiji), to less than 50 per cent (e.g. in China, India and most developing countries) with any information at all, and in some cases, this percentage can be as low as 10 per cent.

The smaller the coverage a country receives, the greater the probability of distortions, which adds to any previous distortions already flawing the data. It should be strongly emphasized that these shortcomings affect the system as a whole, and hence all causes of death. However, suicidologists seem to be much more punctilious about under-reporting of suicide, and the essential unreliability of this information, than experts dealing with mortality from other causes.

### The reliability of suicide mortality

It has become customary to hear, whenever suicide rates are mentioned, that 'they are underestimated'. This might well be true, but there is no systematic solid evidence on this, nor on its magnitude. Of course, it is known from several studies and surveys, which attempted to measure this underestimation/under-reporting, however, it is hard to generalize from them, given all the factors that impact it.

In the late 1960s, the WHO dedicated its attention to this issue and, in 1974, published a detailed report in its series, Public Health

Papers, in which factors affecting the reporting and recording of mortality related to suicide were reviewed and discussed, and a methodology to minimize it put forward (World Health Organization 1974).

On one hand, many factors distorting information about suicide also apply to other causes of death; on the other hand, distortions in recording/reporting on one single cause of death also distort other causes: we are dealing with a closed system, in which the total has to be 100 per cent, since there can be only one ultimate cause of death. Contributing/precipitating factors can also be recorded. Although it happens infrequently, WHO dedicates a lot of attention to this issue.

It is possible that the low magnitude of suicide rates compared with mortality due to cardiovascular diseases or cancer, for instance, and the development of sophisticated and detailed methods for assessing and ascertaining post-mortem factors specific for suicide—the so-called 'psychological autopsy'—has contributed to this specific interest: it both undermines the value of some of the research already done and forces a series of conceptual and methodological improvements in this field.

While striving for the improvement of the overall quality of countries' vital registration system, one should not miss the relativity of suicide as a cause of death, in relation to the total pool of causes of death: distortion in one component of the system is a distortion in the system as a whole.

## Suicide

Most contemporary definitions of suicide rely on two elements: a precise outcome (death) and a prerequisite (the intention or wish to die), as it can be seen in the operational definition proposed by the World Health Organization:

> For the act of killing oneself to class as suicide, it must be deliberately initiated and performed by the person concerned in the full knowledge, or expectation, of its fatal outcome.
>
> World Health Organization (1998)

In practice, however, there are more elements than dreams in our vain philosophy. More often rather than not, the classification of a death is based on exclusion principles—the so-called NASH system: Natural, Accidental, Suicide and Homicide— rarely on an affirmative basis. In most places, deaths from natural causes are usually certified by health personnel, without any involvement of police or justice agents. Once a natural cause of death is excluded, then the ascertainment of whether it was an accident, a suicide or a homicide is, in most instances, conducted by the participation of police or justice agents: in these cases, given legal and criminal implications, the procedure usually tries to rule out an accident, before considering suicide and homicide. Again, given the same implications, efforts will be directed towards ruling out (or confirming) a homicide; what is left is suicide, by exclusion of any other cause of death.

Ascertaining intentionality as post hoc evidence is sometimes very difficult, if not impossible. There are cases of concrete evidence (e.g. a 'suicidal note', to confirm it, or, of an act performed in circumstances in which help would be easily available to confirm it), however, in the majority of cases, such evidence simply does not exist, and intentionality is assumed rather than confirmed.

Suicide, as originally expressed in Latin by Thomas Browne in 1642 (Minois 1995), concerned mostly the agent that caused a death: *sui caedere*—to kill oneself—as distinct from *homo caedere*– to kill someone else. At its origin, this concept had a greater impact on philosophy and law than on medicine, although Browne was both a philosopher and a physician. The new word created by him made its way into several disciplines, and became firmly rooted in most Western languages, at least as an erudite term.

When, in 1964, Stengel proposed that suicide and suicide attempts referred to two distinct populations (Stengel 1964), he was, apparently, considering them as two distinct entities, reflecting the then predominant psychological and psychodynamic approach to understanding human acts. For him, intention, rather than outcome, was the discriminating decisive element. However, this does not prevent some acts of suicide performed with the intention of dying ending in survival due to improved health care—they will later be classified as a suicide *attempt*—while some suicide attempts without a true intention of dying may result in death, due to the lethality of the means utilized or lack of proper care—and classified as suicide.

## Attempted suicide

Stengel's concept had a major impact, one that led Kreitman and his colleagues (1969) to devise the term *parasuicide* to designate precisely those suicidal acts that did not carry an unquestionable wish or intention to die ('a cry for help'), but still preserving the connection to completed suicide. However, parasuicide soon came to be utilized in a variety of meanings (Bille-Brahe *et al.* 1994), so that eventually it fell from favour with most suicidologists. During a 25-year-long process, the WHO Multicentre Study on Parasuicide changed the terminology from parasuicide to *attempted suicide* (Bille-Brahe *et al.* 1994). The definition used in this study is:

> An act with nonfatal outcome, in which an individual deliberately initiates a non-habitual behaviour that, without intervention from others, will cause self-harm, or deliberately ingests a substance in excess of the prescribed or generally recognized therapeutic dosage, and which is aimed at realizing changes which the subject desired via the actual or expected physical consequences.
>
> Bille-Brahe *et al.* (1994, p. 7), Schmidtke *et al.* (2001, p. 7)

This definition is descriptive and does not take the person's intention into consideration, neither is the distinction between serious and non-serious suicidal attempts is applied. However, the evidence from the WHO Multi-centre Study on Parasuicide points towards the use of the terms parasuicide and attempted suicide in the same way, and that the term attempted suicide includes all intentional self-inflicted injuries and poisonings.

The term 'attempted suicide' is the subject of much definitional debate in the literature, the criticism being that it is used imprecisely (Linehan 1997). The argument centres around intent. Silverman and colleagues (2007a, b), for example, have argued that the term should be reserved for those behaviours that are perpetrated with the intent to cease life, distinguishing them from acts of self-harm that have the potential to be fatal, but which may or may not be undertaken with any intent to die. Specifically, they define a suicide attempt as 'a self-inflicted, potentially injurious behaviour with a non-fatal outcome for which there is evidence (either explicit or implicit) of intent to die' (Silverman *et al.* 2007b, p. 273).

Although, definitions like this are useful in theory, in practice they are difficult to operationalize because of the problems associated with measuring behavioural intent (Kerkhof 2000). A recent study by Posner *et al.* (2007) achieved some degree of success in this by using expert raters to classify suicidal events described in vignettes on the basis of intent and self-injury. The vignettes consisted of de-identified narratives derived from real-life case report forms and hospital records. Raters were relatively cautious in classifying events as 'suicide attempts', but achieved a high level of consistency in their assessments. It is unlikely that the same degree of precision regarding assessment of intent could be achieved from hospitalization data, or from population-based survey data, at least in the forms in which they are currently available.

In 1979, Morgan proposed the term 'deliberate self-harm' (DSH), once again stressing the volitional element, to which Hawton *et al.* (2002) added a distinction between fatal versus non-fatal, thus stressing outcome in addition to intention. Given the fundamental importance of outcomes from a public health perspective, this terminology had been adopted in 1992 by the *International Classification of Diseases, 10th edition* (ICD-10) (World Health Organization 1992), in the category 'Intentional self-harm', which includes 'purposefully self-inflicted poisoning or injury; and suicide (attempted)'.

It would be highly desirable to have comparable information on suicide attempts. However, the sad truth is that there is no national system recording and reporting on suicide attempts. At best, there are subsystems related to single hospital or catchment areas, usually as part of isolated or multi-site research initiatives (e.g. the WHO/EURO Multicentre Study on Suicidal Behaviour) (Schmidtke *et al.* 2001), and not as part of the broader and more comprehensive vital registration system.

## Suicidal process

An attempt to find a more common ground for definitions of suicide and suicide attempt leads to the concept of suicidal process proposed originally by Zubin (1974), who suggested that suicide does not just occur but is the end product of a process. That concept was further developed by several authors (Beskow 1979; Farberow 1980); Mann and colleagues proposed the 'stress–diathesis model' (Mann *et al.* 1999); and Wasserman a 'stress–vulnerability model' (Wasserman 2001).

Basically, what these models have in common are a sequence that goes from suicidal ideas (thoughts) to plans, then to attempts and, eventually to death, through a specific action or omission (Bertolote 2001; Wasserman 2001). The experience referred to by Farberow, as of most of those who followed him, was obtained in Western countries, mostly central and western European, and North-American countries. However, intellectually attractive this model might be, and however logical the sequence, in practice it can not always be demonstrated. Obviously, all pertinent research has demonstrated that there are more people entertaining ideas about suicide than people attempting suicide, and even more than those completing suicide; nevertheless, the relationships between these variables do not have the same magnitude everywhere on the five continents, and there is evidence of a disproportion of the magnitude of suicidal ideation in relation to suicide rates in some cross-countries comparisons, particularly between Asian, European and North American countries (Bertolote *et al.* 2005).

Experiences from Asian countries (Phillips *et al.* 2002) have presented a distinct suicidal process in almost every aspect, including predisposing and precipitating factors and timing of this process. The development of the suicidal process can also be gender-dependent, more female than male suicidal processes fade away from death wishes and suicidal ideation. The development of the suicidal process is also dependent on the access to health care services and skillfulness in recognizing suicidal communication and risk behaviours (Wasserman 2001).

## Suicidality

Finally, a few words about the concept of *suicidality*. This term has been proposed by Shneidman (1993) to designate an individual's risk level of danger to themselves. Nevertheless, suicidality is now used in diverse ways, distant from its original meaning, to indicate a variety of things related to suicides. Some use it to refer to suicidal ideation only (thoughts and plans), others include also suicide attempts, and still others also include suicide mortality under suicidality. Suicidality is not found in most English dictionaries; however, the *Oxford English Dictionary* has *suicidalism*, which is defined as 'in a suicidal manner; so as to bring destruction or ruin to the actor'—this term does not seem to be employed by suicidologists. Clearly, suicidality should be accompanied by an explanation of what it is meant to indicate.

## Conclusion

Whatever terms we might employ, the traditional distinction between 'suicide' and 'suicide attempt' has been eroded probably due to at least two main factors: (i) the growing use of lethal methods in suicide attempts, and (ii) the improvement of emergency care and of resuscitation methods.

The second factor is observed mostly in developed countries, and has not yet had any major impact for populations living in developing countries. The reason for this is that these countries are still largely rural, and an important number of deliberate self-harm acts take place in localities far away from the possibility of any reasonable emergency medical care; this increases the fatality rate of the acts that have a considerably lower fatality rate in developed countries. As a consequence, understanding the relationships between suicidal ideation and completed suicide has become more complex and difficult to grasp.

## References

Bertolote JM (2001). Suicide in the world: an epidemiological overview, 1995–2000. In D Wasserman, ed., *Suicide: An Unnecessary Death*, pp. 3–10. Martin Dunitz, London.

Bertolote J, Fleischmann A, De Leo D (2005). Suicide attempts, plans, and ideation in culturally diverse sites: the WHO SUPRE-MISS community survey. *Psychological Medicine*, **35**, 1457–1465.

Beskow J (1979). Suicide and mental disorder in Swedish men. *Acta Psychiatrica Scandinavica, Supplementum*, **277**, 1–138.

Bille-Brahe U, Schmidtke A, Kerkhof A *et al.* (1994). Background and introduction to the study. In AJFM Kerkhof, A Schmidtke, U Bille-Brahe *et al.*, eds, *Attempted Suicide in Europe. Findings from the Multicentre Study on Parasuicide by the WHO Regional Office for Europe*, pp. 3–15. DSWO Press, Leiden.

Farberow N (1980). *The Many Faces of Suicide*. McGraw-Hill, New York.

Hawton K, Rodham K, Evans E *et al.* (2002). Deliberate self-harm in adolescents: self-report survey in schools in England. *BMJ*, **325**, 1207–1211.

Kerkhof A (2000). Attempted suicide: patterns and trends. In K Hawton and K van Heeringen, eds, *The International Handbook of Suicide and Attempted Suicide*, pp. 49–64. John Wiley and Sons, New York.

Kreitman N, Philip AE, Greer S *et al.* (1969). Parasuicide. *British Journal of Psychiatry*, **115**, 746–747.

Linehan MM (1997). Behavioral treatments of suicidal behaviors: definitional obfuscation and treatment outcomes. *Annals of the New York Academy of Sciences*, **836**, 302–328.

Mann JJ, Waternaux C, Haas G *et al.* (1999). Toward a clinical model of suicidal behaviour in psychiatric patients. *American Journal of Psychiatry*, **156**, 181–189.

Mathers CD, Ma Fat D, Inoue M *et al.* (2005). Counting the dead and what they die from: an assessment of the global status of cause of death data. *Bulletin of the World Health Organization*, **85**, 171–180.

Minois G (1995). *Histoire du Suicide. La Société Occidentale Face à la Mort Volontaire*. Fayard, Paris.

Phillips M, Yang G, Zhang Y *et al.* (2002). Risk factors for suicide in China: a national case-control psychological autopsy study. *Lancet*, **360**, 1728–1736.

Posner K, Oquendo MA, Gould M *et al.* (2007). Columbia Classification Algorithm of Suicide Assessment (C-CASA): Classification of suicidal events in the FDA's pediatric suicidal risk analysis of antidepressants. *American Journal of Psychiatry*, **164**, 1035–1043.

Schmidtke A, Bille-Brahe U, De Leo D *et al.* (eds) (2001). *Suicidal Behaviour in Europe: Results from the WHO/EURO Multicentre Study on Suicidal Behaviour*. Hogrefe and Huber, Göttingen.

Shneidman ES (1993). *Suicide as Psychache: A Clinical Approach to Self-destructive Behaviour*. Jason Aronson Inc., Northvale.

Silverman MM, Berman AL, Sanddal ND *et al.* (2007a). Rebuilding the Tower of Babel: a revised nomenclature for the study of suicidal behaviors. Part 1: Background, rationale and methodology. *Suicide and Life-Threatening Behavior*, **37**, 248–263.

Silverman MM, Berman AL, Sanddal ND *et al.* (2007b). Rebuilding the Tower of Babel: a revised nomenclature for the study of suicidal behaviors. Part 2: Suicide-related ideations, communications and behaviors. *Suicide and Life-Threatening Behavior*, **37**, 264–277.

Stengel E (1964). *Suicide and Attempted Suicide*. Penguin Books, Baltimore.

Wasserman D (ed.) (2001). *Suicide: An Unnecessary Death*. Martin Dunitz, London.

World Health Organization (1974). *Suicide and Attempted Suicide*. Public Health Papers No. 58. World Health Organization, Geneva.

World Health Organization (1992). *International Statistical Classification of Diseases and Related Health Problems. Tenth Revision (ICD-10)*. World Health Organization, Geneva.

World Health Organization (1998). *Primary Prevention of Mental, Neurological and Psychosocial Disorders*. World Health Organization, Geneva.

Zubin J (1974). Observations on nosological issues in the classification of suicidal behavior. In A Beck, H Resnik, D Lettieri, eds, *The Prediction of Suicide*, pp. 3–25. Charles Press Publishers, Bowie, Maryland.

# CHAPTER 14

# A global perspective on the magnitude of suicide mortality

José M Bertolote and Alexandra Fleischmann

## Abstract

The lay press and clinical literature usually address suicide in terms of individual cases, whereas the epidemiological literature refers to rates, that is, the proportion of the sum of individual cases divided by a given population basis. Actually, both approaches have their place in a discussion on a worldwide perspective of suicide mortality; accordingly, in this chapter, both will be used, in order to better understand some of the implications of suicide. With a particular view to the prevention of suicide, it is important to use disaggregated rates, at least by gender and age, in order to identify specific groups at risk for suicide. In addition, information about the methods used for suicide is essential, as it has been demonstrated that the restriction of access to methods can reduce suicide.

## Sources of information

Shortly after its creation in 1948, the World Health Organization (WHO) started to compile and disseminate data on mortality reported by its Member States, according to its constitutional mandate. From 11 countries reporting data on mortality in 1950, the number of countries involved has increased to more than 120.

Suicide mortality is an integral part of the WHO mortality database. Although there have been modifications to the diagnostic categorization of suicide, through consecutive editions of the *International Classification of Diseases and Causes of Death* (ICD-6 to ICD-10), the instrument that is used by countries for the international reporting on mortality to the WHO has provided no evidence that this has significantly affected its reporting (Anderson *et al.* 2001).

## Reported data

Suicide deaths are reported in absolute numbers along with the mid-year population of a country. As very few children commit suicide, it would be of interest to present suicide rates for the population 15 years and older. However, this kind of data was not available for the authors. The most recent data available to the World Health Organization can be accessed through the WHO website (http://www.who.int), where they are presented by country, year, sex, and age group.

Data from developed countries (Europe, North America, and a few countries in the western Pacific Region) are received on a regular basis. Most developing countries (in Latin America, Asia and in the eastern Mediterranean region) report on a less regular basis, and very few countries in Africa report mortality regularly to the WHO.

Unfortunately, at present, some of the 70 least developed countries (mostly, in Africa, but also in South East Asia, and some of them quite populous countries) do not maintain vital registration systems due to the lack of means to collect and process data related to mortality in the general population. Some of the countries, however, collect only hospital-based mortality data, which is irrelevant for knowing the magnitude of the mortality related to suicide. Figures on suicide mortality made available to the WHO by its Member States are based on death certificates signed by legally authorized personnel, usually doctors and, to a lesser extent, police officers.

In contrast to data on completed suicide, few countries in the world have systematic data registration of attempted suicide (e.g. New Zealand), which makes it impossible to relate national trends of suicide to national trends of attempted suicide. In the absence of national data, one is forced to rely on local studies, which vary considerably, for instance, in terms of the operational definition of attempted suicide.

## Data on suicide mortality

Data presented and discussed in this section can be found at http://www.who.int/mental_health/prevention/suicide. Using both reported and estimated data (for countries that do not report to the WHO on mortality), the estimated number of individual cases of suicide in 2002 (the last year for which there are reliable reported data) was about 877,000 cases, of which 549,000 were males and 328,000 females, which gives a proportion of 1.7/1. The distribution of these cases (estimated) by countries is shown in Table 14.1. According to WHO estimates for the year 2020, approximately 1.53 million people will die from suicide (Bertolote 2001). As a reflection of the size of their population, almost one-third of all cases of suicide worldwide are found in China and India; the number of suicides in China alone are 30 per cent greater than the total number of suicides in the whole of Europe, and the number

**Table 14.1** Estimated total suicide deaths, in thousands (000), by WHO Member State, 2002

| Country | Estimated total deaths in 000s | Country | Estimated total deaths in 000s |
|---|---|---|---|
| Afghanistan | 1.5 | Czech Republic | 1.7 |
| Albania | 0.1 | Côte d'Ivoire | 1.8 |
| Algeria | 0.9 | Democratic People's Republic of Korea | 1.1 |
| Andorra | 0.0 | Democratic Republic of the Congo | 2.5 |
| Angola | 1.1 | Denmark | 0.7 |
| Antigua and Barbuda | 0.0 | Djibouti | 0.0 |
| Argentina | 3.9 | Dominica | 0.0 |
| Armenia | 0.1 | Dominican Republic | 0.2 |
| Australia | 2.2 | Ecuador | 0.8 |
| Austria | 1.5 | Egypt | 1.1 |
| Azerbaijan | 0.4 | El Salvador | 0.6 |
| Bahamas | 0.0 | Equatorial Guinea | 0.0 |
| Bahrain | 0.0 | Eritrea | 0.2 |
| Bangladesh | 17.5 | Estonia | 0.4 |
| Barbados | 0.0 | Ethiopia | 2.4 |
| Belarus | 3.8 | Fiji | 0.0 |
| Belgium | 2.1 | Finland | 1.2 |
| Belize | 0.0 | France | 9.5 |
| Benin | 0.3 | Gabon | 0.1 |
| Bhutan | 0.3 | Gambia | 0.1 |
| Bolivia | 0.2 | Georgia | 0.2 |
| Bosnia and Herzegovina | 0.6 | Germany | 11.4 |
| Botswana | 0.1 | Ghana | 0.8 |
| Brazil | 8.8 | Greece | 0.4 |
| Brunei Darussalam | 0.0 | Grenada | 0.0 |
| Bulgaria | 1.3 | Guatemala | 0.3 |
| Burkina Faso | 0.7 | Guinea | 0.4 |
| Burundi | 0.5 | Guinea-Bissau | 0.1 |
| Cambodia | 0.6 | Guyana | 0.2 |
| Cameroon | 0.7 | Haiti | 0.1 |
| Canada | 3.7 | Honduras | 0.6 |
| Cape Verde | 0.0 | Hungary | 2.8 |
| Central African Republic | 0.4 | Iceland | 0.0 |
| Chad | 0.4 | India | 182.4 |
| Chile | 1.7 | Indonesia | 24.6 |
| China | 272.6 | Iran (Islamic Republic of) | 5.6 |
| Colombia | 2.7 | Iraq | 1.7 |
| Comoros | 0.0 | Ireland | 0.5 |
| Congo | 0.2 | Israel | 0.3 |
| Cook Islands | 0.0 | Italy | 3.9 |
| Costa Rica | 0.3 | Jamaica | 0.0 |
| Croatia | 0.9 | Japan | 31.4 |
| Cuba | 1.7 | Jordan | 0.9 |
| Cyprus | 0.0 | Kazakhstan | 5.7 |

**Table 14.1** (Continued) Estimated total suicide deaths, in thousands (000), by WHO Member State, 2002

| Country | Estimated total deaths in 000s | Country | Estimated total deaths in 000s |
|---|---|---|---|
| Kenya | 1.9 | Philippines | 1.3 |
| Kiribati | 0.0 | Poland | 6.7 |
| Kuwait | 0.0 | Portugal | 0.7 |
| Kyrgyzstan | 0.7 | Qatar | 0.0 |
| Lao People's Democratic Republic | 1.2 | Republic of Korea | 8.6 |
| Latvia | 0.7 | Republic of Moldova | 0.8 |
| Lebanon | 0.2 | Romania | 2.8 |
| Lesotho | 0.1 | Russian Federation | 59.0 |
| Liberia | 0.2 | Rwanda | 0.6 |
| Libyan Arab Jamahiriya | 0.2 | Saint Kitts and Nevis | 0.0 |
| Lithuania | 1.6 | Saint Lucia | 0.0 |
| Luxembourg | 0.1 | Saint Vincent and the Grenadines | 0.0 |
| Madagascar | 0.7 | Samoa | 0.0 |
| Malawi | 0.8 | San Marino | 0.0 |
| Malaysia | 1.6 | Sao Tome and Principe | 0.0 |
| Maldives | 0.0 | Saudi Arabia | 1.4 |
| Mali | 0.6 | Senegal | 0.4 |
| Malta | 0.0 | Serbia and Montenegro | 1.6 |
| Marshall Islands | 0.0 | Seychelles | 0.0 |
| Mauritania | 0.2 | Sierra Leone | 0.5 |
| Mauritius | 0.1 | Singapore | 0.4 |
| Mexico | 4.0 | Slovakia | 0.7 |
| Micronesia (Federated States of) | 0.0 | Slovenia | 0.6 |
| Monaco | 0.0 | Solomon Islands | 0.0 |
| Mongolia | 0.3 | Somalia | 0.7 |
| Morocco | 0.7 | South Africa | 4.7 |
| Mozambique | 0.7 | Spain | 3.4 |
| Myanmar | 5.2 | Sri Lanka | 6.0 |
| Namibia | 0.1 | Sudan | 2.3 |
| Nauru | 0.0 | Suriname | 0.1 |
| Nepal | 2.5 | Swaziland | 0.0 |
| Netherlands | 1.4 | Sweden | 1.1 |
| New Zealand | 0.5 | Switzerland | 1.3 |
| Nicaragua | 0.6 | Syrian Arab Republic | 0.1 |
| Niger | 0.7 | Tajikistan | 0.3 |
| Nigeria | 6.0 | Thailand | 6.9 |
| Niue | 0.0 | The former Yugoslav Republic of Macedonia | 0.2 |
| Norway | 0.5 | Timor-Leste | 0.1 |
| Oman | 0.1 | Togo | 0.2 |
| Pakistan | 15.7 | Tonga | 0.0 |
| Palau | 0.0 | Trinidad and Tobago | 0.2 |
| Panama | 0.2 | Tunisia | 0.4 |
| Papua New Guinea | 0.6 | Turkey | 4.7 |
| Paraguay | 0.2 | Turkmenistan | 0.6 |
| Peru | 0.5 | Tuvalu | 0.0 |

**Table 14.1** (Continued) Estimated total suicide deaths, in thousands (000), by WHO Member State, 2002

| Country | Estimated total deaths in 000s | Country | Estimated total deaths in 000s |
|---|---|---|---|
| Uganda | 0.5 | Uzbekistan | 2.3 |
| Ukraine | 17.5 | Vanuatu | 0.0 |
| United Arab Emirates | 0.1 | Venezuela (Bolivarian Republic of) | 1.6 |
| United Kingdom | 5.0 | Vietam | 8.9 |
| United Republic of Tanzania | 0.8 | Yemen | 0.9 |
| United States of America | 30.1 | Zambia | 0.4 |
| Uruguay | 0.6 | Zimbabwe | 0.6 |

of suicides in India (the second highest) is equivalent to those in the four European countries with the highest number of suicides together (Russia, Germany, France, and Ukraine).

With regard to suicide rates, we have an estimated global rate of 14 suicides per 100,000 inhabitants, including 18 suicides per 100,000 for males and 11 suicides per 100,000 for females. Table 14.2 shows the distribution of rates per country. For both males and females, the highest suicide rates are found in Europe, predominantly in Eastern Europe, i.e. Lithuania, the Russian Federation, Belarus and, to a lesser extent, Finland, Hungary, and Latvia, a group of countries that share similar historical and socio-cultural characteristics. Nevertheless, some similarly high rates are found in countries that are quite distinct in relation to these characteristics, such as Cuba, Japan, and Sri Lanka. As a whole, the

**Table 14.2** Suicide rates (per 100,000 inhabitants), by country, year, and sex*

| Country | Year | Males | Females | Country | Year | Males | Females |
|---|---|---|---|---|---|---|---|
| Albania | 03 | 4.7 | 3.3 | Ecuador | 04 | 8.6 | 3.7 |
| Antigua and Barbuda | 95 | 0.0 | 0.0 | Egypt | 87 | 0.1 | 0.0 |
| Argentina | 03 | 14.1 | 3.5 | El Salvador | 03 | 12.2 | 4.2 |
| Armenia | 03 | 3.2 | 0.5 | Estonia | 05 | 35.5 | 7.3 |
| Australia | 03 | 17.1 | 4.7 | Finland | 04 | 31.7 | 9.4 |
| Austria | 05 | 26.1 | 8.2 | France | 03 | 27.5 | 9.1 |
| Azerbaijan | 02 | 1.8 | 0.5 | Georgia | 01 | 3.4 | 1.1 |
| Bahamas | 00 | 6.0 | 1.3 | Germany | 04 | 19.7 | 6.6 |
| Bahrain | 88 | 4.9 | 0.5 | Greece | 04 | 5.2 | 1.2 |
| Barbados | 01 | 1.4 | 0.0 | Guatemala | 03 | 3.4 | 0.9 |
| Belarus | 03 | 63.3 | 10.3 | Guyana | 03 | 42.5 | 12.1 |
| Belgium | 97 | 31.2 | 11.4 | Haiti | 03 | 0.0 | 0.0 |
| Belize | 01 | 13.4 | 1.6 | Honduras | 78 | 0.0 | 0.0 |
| Bosnia and Herzegovina | 91 | 20.3 | 3.3 | Hungary | 03 | 44.9 | 12.0 |
| Brazil | 02 | 6.8 | 1.9 | Iceland | 04 | 17.7 | 6.2 |
| Bulgaria | 04 | 19.7 | 6.7 | India | 98 | 12.2 | 9.1 |
| Canada | 02 | 18.3 | 5.0 | Iran | 91 | 0.3 | 0.1 |
| Chile | 03 | 17.8 | 3.1 | Ireland | 05 | 16.3 | 3.2 |
| China (selected rural and urban areas) | 99 | 13.0 | 14.8 | Israel | 03 | 10.4 | 2.1 |
| China (Hong Kong Special Administrative Region) | 04 | 25.2 | 12.4 | Italy | 02 | 11.4 | 3.1 |
| Colombia | 99 | 8.2 | 2.4 | Jamaica | 90 | 0.3 | 0.0 |
| Costa Rica | 04 | 12.1 | 1.6 | Japan | 04 | 35.6 | 12.8 |
| Croatia | 04 | 30.2 | 9.8 | Jordan | 79 | 0.0 | 0.0 |
| Cuba | 04 | 20.3 | 6.6 | Kazakhstan | 03 | 51.0 | 8.9 |
| Czech Republic | 04 | 25.9 | 5.7 | Kuwait | 02 | 2.5 | 1.4 |
| Denmark | 01 | 19.2 | 8.1 | Kyrgyzstan | 04 | 15.0 | 3.0 |
| Dominican Republic | 01 | 2.9 | 0.6 | Latvia | 04 | 42.9 | 8.5 |

**Table 14.2**  (Continued) Suicide rates (per 100,000 inhabitants), by country, year, and sex*

| Country | Year | Males | Females | Country | Year | Males | Females |
|---------|------|-------|---------|---------|------|-------|---------|
| Lithuania | 04 | 70.1 | 14.0 | Serbia and Montenegro | 02 | 28.8 | 10.4 |
| Luxembourg | 04 | 21.9 | 7.4 | Seychelles | 87 | 9.1 | 0.0 |
| Malta | 04 | 7.0 | 4.9 | Singapore | 03 | 12.5 | 7.6 |
| Mauritius | 04 | 12.7 | 3.6 | Slovakia | 02 | 23.6 | 3.6 |
| Mexico | 03 | 6.7 | 1.3 | Slovenia | 04 | 37.9 | 13.9 |
| Netherlands | 04 | 12.7 | 6.0 | Spain | 04 | 12.6 | 3.9 |
| New Zealand | 00 | 19.8 | 4.2 | Sri Lanka | 91 | 44.6 | 16.8 |
| Nicaragua | 03 | 11.0 | 3.7 | Suriname | 00 | 17.8 | 6.4 |
| Norway | 04 | 15.8 | 7.3 | Sweden | 02 | 19.5 | 7.1 |
| Panama | 03 | 11.1 | 1.4 | Switzerland | 04 | 23.7 | 11.3 |
| Paraguay | 03 | 4.5 | 1.6 | Syrian Arab Republic | 85 | 0.2 | 0.0 |
| Peru | 00 | 1.1 | 0.6 | Tajikistan | 01 | 2.9 | 2.3 |
| Philippines | 93 | 2.5 | 1.7 | Thailand | 02 | 12.0 | 3.8 |
| Poland | 04 | 27.9 | 4.6 | TFYR Macedonia | 03 | 9.5 | 4.0 |
| Portugal | 03 | 17.5 | 4.9 | Trinidad and Tobago | 00 | 20.9 | 4.9 |
| Puerto Rico | 02 | 10.9 | 1.8 | Turkmenistan | 98 | 13.8 | 3.5 |
| Republic of Korea | 04 | 32.5 | 15.0 | Ukraine | 04 | 43.0 | 7.3 |
| Republic of Moldova | 04 | 29.3 | 5.2 | United Kingdom | 04 | 10.8 | 3.3 |
| Romania | 04 | 21.5 | 4.0 | United States of America | 02 | 17.9 | 4.2 |
| Russian Federation | 04 | 61.6 | 10.7 | Uruguay | 01 | 24.5 | 6.4 |
| Saint Kitts and Nevis | 95 | 0.0 | 0.0 | Uzbekistan | 03 | 8.1 | 3.0 |
| Saint Lucia | 02 | 10.4 | 5.0 | Venezuela | 02 | 8.4 | 1.8 |
| Saint Vincent and the Grenadines | 03 | 6.8 | 0.0 | Zimbabwe | 90 | 10.6 | 5.2 |
| Sao Tome and Principe | 87 | 0.0 | 1.8 | | | | |

* Most recent year available. As of 2007.

Source: http://www.who.int/mental_health/prevention/suicide_rates/en/index.htm. Reproduced with kind permission from WHO.

**Table 14.3**  Ranking of the top 13 countries, number of suicides (estimated for the year 2000) and suicide rates (most recent year available)

| Country | Number of suicides | Rate per 100,000 | Ranking by suicide rate | Country | Number of suicides | Rate per 100,000 | Ranking by number of suicides |
|---------|--------------------|------------------|-------------------------|---------|--------------------|------------------|-------------------------------|
| China | 170,000 | 13.9 | 26 | Lithuania | 1500 | 42.1 | 28 |
| India | 105,000 | 10.7 | 38 | Russian Federation | 55,000 | 38.7 | 3 |
| Russian Federation | 55,000 | 38.7 | 2 | Belarus | 3500 | 35.1 | 16 |
| USA | 31,000 | 10.7 | 39 | Kazakhstan | 4500 | 28.8 | 14 |
| Japan | 30,000 | 23.8 | 11 | Slovenia | 600 | 28.1 | 44 |
| Ukraine | 13,000 | 26.1 | 9 | Hungary | 3000 | 27.7 | 18 |
| Germany | 11,000 | 13.5 | 27 | Estonia | 400 | 27.3 | 56 |
| France | 10,000 | 17.6 | 19 | Ukraine | 13,000 | 26.1 | 6 |
| Rep. Korea | 9000 | 17.9 | 18 | Latvia | 600 | 26.0 | 43 |
| Brazil | 7000 | 4.1 | 71 | Japan | 30,000 | 23.8 | 5 |
| Poland | 6000 | 15.5 | 22 | Sri Lanka | 5000 | 21.6 | 12 |
| Sri Lanka | 5000 | 21.6 | 11 | Belgium | 2000 | 21.1 | 24 |
| Thailand | 5000 | 7.8 | 52 | Finland | 1100 | 20.6 | 36 |

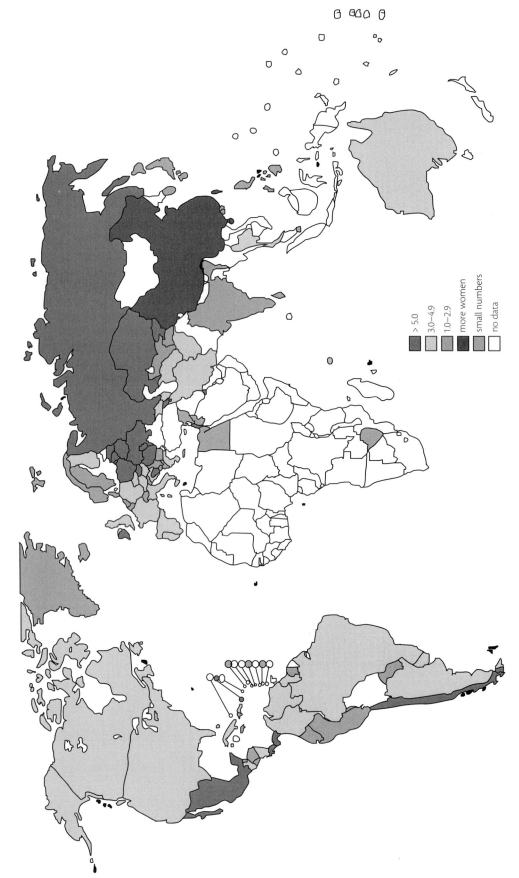

**Fig. 14.1** Proportion of suicide rates of men and women (most recent year available as of 2007: e.g. a proportion of three means that there are three times more men who commit suicide than women. Reproduced with permission from the WHO. (See also colour section.)

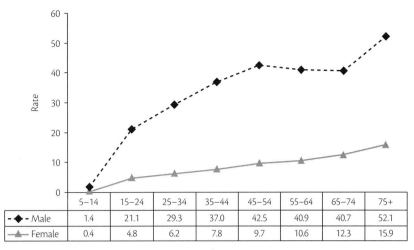

**Fig. 14.2** Distribution of suicide rates (per 10,000 inhabitants) by sex and age, 2000.

| | 5–14 | 15–24 | 25–34 | 35–44 | 45–54 | 55–64 | 65–74 | 75+ |
|---|---|---|---|---|---|---|---|---|
| Male | 1.4 | 21.1 | 29.3 | 37.0 | 42.5 | 40.9 | 40.7 | 52.1 |
| Female | 0.4 | 4.8 | 6.2 | 7.8 | 9.7 | 10.6 | 12.3 | 15.9 |

lowest rates are found in countries that primarily follow Islamic traditions, which is also true for some Central Asian republics that had formerly been integrated into the Soviet Union.

It is noticeable in Tables 14.2 and 14.3 that among those countries with the thirteen highest suicide numbers, only four (the Russian Federation, Ukraine, Japan, and Sri Lanka) are among the thirteen countries with the highest suicide rates.

As to gender distribution, Figure 14.1 shows the ratio male:female of suicide rates by country. Although it is not immediately clear from the map, there is a trend of higher ratios to be observed in more developed, mostly European countries, with smaller ratios being observed in developing, mostly Asian countries.

From a global perspective, there is a clear tendency for suicide rates to increase with age (Figure 14.2). In 2000, the male rates for specific age groups started at 1.4 (in the youngest age group) and gradually increase up to 52.1 (in the oldest age group, 75 years and older). The same growing trend is observed for females: from 0.4 per 100,000 (in the youngest age group 5–14 years) to 15.9 (in the oldest age group).

The age distribution shows relatively prominent differences when comparing rates to total numbers. Although suicide rates can be between six and eight times higher among the elderly as compared to young people, currently more young people die from suicide than elderly people, that is, on the global spectrum. Currently, more suicides (55 per cent) are committed by people aged 5–44 years than by people aged 45 years and older (Figure 14.3). Accordingly, the age group in which most suicides are currently completed is 35–44 years for both males and females.

This shift in the predominance of numbers of suicide occurring among the elderly than young people is a relatively new phenomenon that becomes even more significant when one considers the overall ageing of the total population. Furthermore, it is not the result of a divergent modification in suicide rates in these age groups; the suicide rate in young people is certainly increasing at a greater pace than it is in the elderly.

From a basic economic perspective in 1998, suicide represented 1.8 per cent of the global burden of disease, and it is expected to increase to 2.4 per cent by the year 2020. Suicide is presently among the ten leading causes of death for all ages in most countries where information is available; in some countries, it is among the top three causes of death for people aged 15–34 years.

## Reliability of the data

In spite of the seriousness with which health information systems are maintained, the trend towards under-reporting suicidal behaviours (both completed and attempted) occurring in some, although not in all places, is well known (Bertolote 2001; De Leo *et al.* 2002; Sakinofsky 2003; Andriessen 2006; Mäkinen 2006). In other words, the actual number of cases of suicides is higher than what is recorded or estimated. In most societies, suicide is perceived

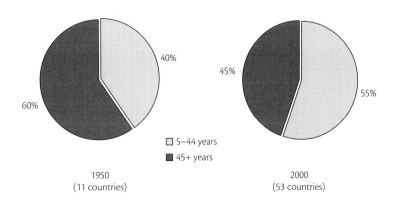

**Fig. 14.3** Changes in the age distribution of cases of suicide between 1950 and 2000.

□ 5–44 years
■ 45+ years

1950
(11 countries)

2000
(53 countries)

as 'inconvenient', due to reasons ranging from religious to legal and economic, for example insurance and compensation. In some instances (difficult to quantify), there is a collusion between families and death-certifying officers, whereby a case of suicide may be recorded as a death due to another cause: accidents, cardiac arrest, brain haemorrhage and undetermined cause of death are among the most frequently used diagnoses to conceal a case of suicide.

This practice, which distorts the whole health information system related to mortality, represents two major problems for public health. It reduces the real magnitude and importance of a cause of death (suicide) that otherwise could be better understood and prevented, and it artificially inflates statistics related to those substitute diagnoses, which can lead to unwarranted oversized programmes.

Every effort to improve the reliability of reporting on suicide related mortality will, in the end, benefit from the information on mortality and the overall health information system.

## Uses of data

As indicated in the previous section, suicide mortality data can be used for purely speculative and academic purposes or for monitoring societal trends, however, its greatest usefulness is perhaps related to preventive activities. In this respect, rates are more helpful than absolute numbers, and even more so than adjusted and disaggregated rates (at least by gender and age). This allows the identification of specific groups on which to focus preventive action, instead of a blanket overall action, which may hit at-risk groups but may also miss them, depending on the nature of the intervention.

In this respect, it is regrettable that reliable information is not available on methods used to commit suicide, on the same level as it is for number of suicide cases and suicide rates. Although the *International Classification of Diseases and Causes of Death* allows, recording the method employed in each case of suicide,

unfortunately, this is not always done. The importance of this information lies in the demonstrated effectiveness of reducing suicide, by restricting access to methods that are used in a significant proportion of suicide cases (Bertolote *et al.* 2006). This is the case in regions where, for instance, self-poisoning (by pesticides, carbon monoxide or medicines) or gunshot wounds are the predominant method of suicide (Gunnell *et al.* 2007).

Although a large amount of information on suicide mortality is already available, there is also room for improvement and refinement of this information, both at the level of national health information systems and individual research projects.

## References

Anderson RN, Miniño AM, Hoyert DL *et al.* (2001). *Comparability of Causes of Death Between ICD-9 and ICD-10: Preliminary Estimates.* National Vital Statistics Report, vol. 49, no. 2, National Center for Health Statistics, Hyattsville, Maryland.

Andriessen K (2006). Do we need to be cautious in evaluating suicide statistics? *European Journal of Public Health*, **16**, 445–447.

Bertolote JM (2001). Suicide in the world: an epidemiological overview, 1995–2000. In D Wasserman, ed., *Suicide: An Unnecessary Death*, pp. 3–10. Martin Dunitz, London.

Bertolote JM, Fleischmann A, Butchart A *et al.* (2006). Suicide, suicide attempts and pesticides: a major hidden public health problem. *Bulletin of the World Health Organization*, **84**, 260–261.

De Leo D, Bertolote JM, Lester D (2002). Self-directed violence. In E Krug, L Dahlberg, J Mercy *et al.*, eds, *World Report on Violence and Health*, pp. 183–212. World Health Organization, Geneva.

Gunnell D, Eddleston M, Phillips MR *et al.* (2007). The global distribution of fatal pesticide self-poisoning: systematic review. *BMC Public Health*, **7**, 357–395.

Mäkinen IH (2006). Suicide mortality of Eastern European regions before and after the Communist period. *Social Science and Medicine*, **63**, 307–319.

Sakinofsky I (2003). Suicide: the persisting challenge. *The Canadian Journal of Psychiatry*, **48**, 289–291.

# CHAPTER 15

# Suicidal thoughts, suicide plans and attempts in the general population on different continents

José M Bertolote, Alexandra Fleischmann, Diego De Leo and Danuta Wasserman

## Abstract

The concept of a suicidal process where the suicidal act is preceded by a plan, and that plan is preceded by suicidal thoughts or ideation, does not necessarily imply that every suicidal thought will end in a suicidal act. This chapter explores the relationship between different components of the suicidal spectrum by exam-ining different studies and the World Health Organization (WHO) Multisite Intervention Study on Suicidal Behaviours (SUPRE-MISS) in particular. In the case of suicidal ideation, the outlook with regard to its importance, and its validity as a predictor of other types of suicidal behaviour is uncertain. In addition, the strong cultural underpinning behind the whole spectrum of suicidal behaviours must be emphasized.

## Introduction

From a logical perspective, it makes sense to consider that a suicidal act is preceded by some sort of planning, and that planning is consequential to thinking about it. Clinical experience empirically confirms this. Moreover, the concept of a suicidal process, first proposed by Zubin (1974), follows these basic steps, usually conceived as suicidal thoughts or ideation—suicidal planning—suicidal act, whose outcome can be fatal or non-fatal.

This does not mean, however, that every suicidal idea will end in a suicidal act. The above-mentioned sequence reflects the clinical perspective and reconstructs the process backwards, a knowledge originated from clinical populations. The exploration of the sequence from the beginning is one way to confirm, or refute, the hypotheses of the suicidal process as that sequence. In other words, the fact that every suicidal act is eventually preceded by a suicidal idea/planning does not necessarily mean that every suicidal idea will be followed by a suicidal planning or act. One way of getting the information in its forward direction is to move away from clinical populations and survey general populations.

It should be kept in mind that there are major differences between data collected as part of a clinical interview and data collected in general population surveys. In relation to suicidal ideation, at least two elements might skew the information in one direction or another. The first one depends on the level of confidence the responder has on the interviewer, probably greater in the case of a patient and a clinician than in the case of a member of the community and a trained interviewer.

The second one refers to the timeframe. In a clinical interview, the clinician is likely to be more interested in that moment, or in the near past, whereas in community surveys the timeframe may vary from 'this moment' (rarely) to 'in your lifetime', with different time periods, depending on the scope of the survey.

A final introductory comment refers to the difficulty in comparing data across different studies and surveys. More often than not, each study/survey designs its own methodology and instrument according to its scope and needs, thus sometimes making it impossible to compare those data, which in any case, is not so abundant as to allow one to do a good selection.

## The Multisite Intervention Study on Suicidal Behaviours

As part of its global suicide prevention programme, the WHO launched SUPRE-MISS in 2002 (Bertolote *et al.* 2005; Fleischmann *et al.* 2005, 2008).

Although it was not intended to address the issue of the relationship among suicidal thoughts, suicide attempts and completed suicide specifically, data collected as part of SUPRE-MISS provided a good opportunity to explore the relationship between suicidal ideation and other components of the suicidal spectrum, namely suicide planning, suicide attempts and suicide mortality.

The community survey component of SUPRE-MISS (Bertolote *et al.* 2005), consisted of interviews conducted with subjects in the general population of nine cities/towns on the five continents:

- Brisbane (Australia);
- Campinas (Brazil);
- Chennai (India);
- Colombo (Sri Lanka);
- Durban (South Africa);
- Hanoi (Vietnam);
- Karaj (Iran);
- Tallinn (Estonia);
- Yuncheng (China).

Overall, some 20,000 subjects were interviewed, and the number of subjects per city varied from 500 to 13,810. All information was self-reported, and in most cases, interviews were conducted face-to-face (with the exception of Brisbane, where they were conducted over the telephone, and Colombo, where the questionnaire was mailed to respondents). Due to legal and technical reasons, all subjects were at least 15 years old.

All interviews were conducted by nurses, psychologists, medical students, medical doctors, family health workers, and public health professionals, previously trained in the use of the SUPRE-MISS survey instrument.

The instrument employed (World Health Organization 2002) was adapted from the European parasuicide study interview schedule (EPSIS) (Kerkhof *et al.* 1999), which had been applied in the WHO/EURO multi-centre study on suicidal behaviour. The key questions for assessing suicidal ideation, planning and attempts were quite simple and straightforward, and were stated as:

1 'Have you ever seriously thought about committing suicide?'

2 'Have you ever made a plan for committing suicide?'

3 'Have you ever attempted suicide?'

If the answer was 'yes' to any of these, further questions were asked according to the protocol. These concerned the age and how long ago this had happened.

The common survey instrument was translated into the local languages, and pilot tested by the research group, before the actual surveys were conducted. Essentially, it was more than a literal translation, given that the local principal investigators were asked to convey the questions in a meaningful and culturally relevant way (e.g. committing suicide/putting an end to your life/killing yourself).

## Suicidal thoughts, suicidal plans and suicide attempts

The proportion of subjects in the general population that admitted to having had suicidal thoughts in their lifetime varied from 25.4 per cent (Durban) to 2.6 per cent (Chennai). Those having planned a suicidal act varied from 15.2 per cent (Durban) to 1.1 per cent (Hanoi), whereas the proportion of suicide attempts ranged between 4.2 per cent (Brisbane and Karaj) and 0.4 per cent (Hanoi).

The factor of variation for these three variables was 9.8, 13.8 and 10.5, respectively. In other words, Durban had 9.8 times more subjects who had thoughts about suicide than Chennai; Durban had 13.8 times more subjects than Hanoi who had planned suicide; and lastly, Brisbane and Karaj had 10.5 times more subjects than Hanoi who had attempted suicide in their lifetime.

Figure 15.1 gives a graphic representation of these data. The only common feature for all sites is a decreasing gradient between ideation and planning, as well as between planning and attempts. However, among both, in terms of the magnitude of those percentages and of the slope of the decrease, there are important differences across sites.

In Figure 15.2, the rate of suicidal ideation (irrespective of its magnitude) was considered as 100 per cent, and the rates of

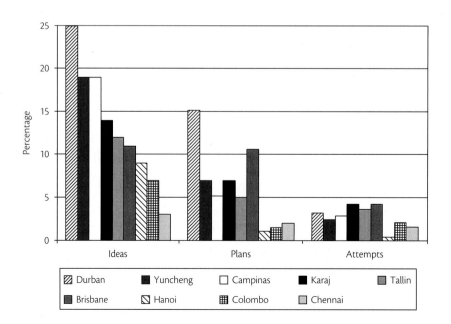

**Fig. 15.1** Suicidal ideation, plans and attempts 2004.

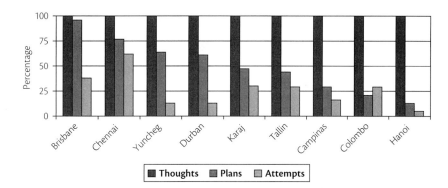

**Fig. 15.2** Proportion of suicidal plans and attempts relative to suicidal thoughts 2004.

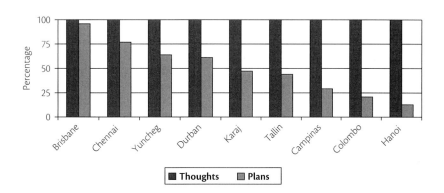

**Fig. 15.3** Proportion of suicidal plans relative to suicidal thoughts 2004.

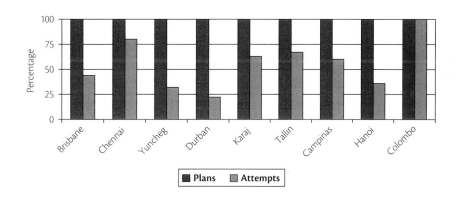

**Fig. 15.4** Proportion of suicide attempts relative to suicidal plans 2004.

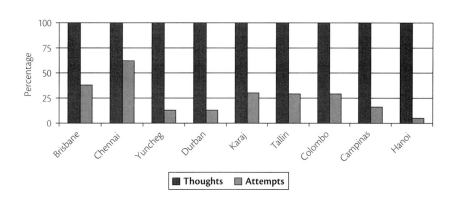

**Fig. 15.5** Proportion of suicide attempts relative to suicidal thoughts 2004.

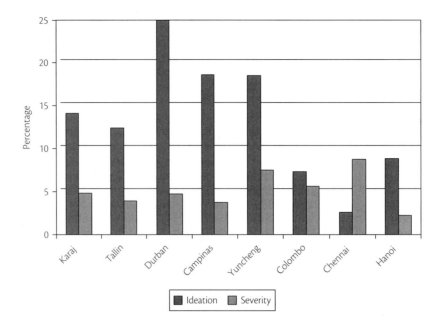

**Fig. 15.6** Suicidal ideation and
severity of suicide attempts 2004.

■ Ideation   ■ Severity

planning and attempting suicide were calculated as a percentage of the respective suicide ideation rate in each site.

It is remarkable to note the disparity across sites. For instance, in Brisbane, 96 per cent of those who thought about suicide also planned it and 38 per cent of those attempted it, whereas in Hanoi, the corresponding figures were 13 per cent and 5 per cent.

Looking separately at the comparisons between ideation versus planning and planning versus attempts gives us a clearer view of these relationships. If we compare suicidal ideation rates and suicidal planning rates in SUPRE-MISS sites (Figure 15.3), a huge discrepancy appears in the proportion between these two variables across sites, ranging from 96 per cent in Brisbane to 5 per cent in Hanoi (i.e. in Brisbane, 96 per cent of those who thought about suicide made a plan, compared to 5 per cent of those in Hanoi). In other words, moving from ideas into concrete plans is not as straightforward and immediate in Hanoi as it is in Brisbane.

The comparison of suicidal planning rates and suicide attempt rates (Figure 15.4) reveals a similar picture of discrepancy, however on a smaller scale, ranging from 80 per cent in Chennai to 22 per cent in Durban (i.e. in Chennai, 80 per cent of those who made a plan attempted suicide, and 22 per cent of those in Durban, accordingly).

However, it is perhaps the comparison of suicidal ideation rates and suicide attempt rates that gives us the most striking findings, particularly, in view of its importance for the timing of preventive interventions. Figure 15.5 shows the comparison of suicidal ideation rates to suicide attempt rates. An important discrepancy appears across countries, with the proportion between these two variables ranging from 62 per cent in Chennai to 5 per cent in Hanoi (i.e. in Chennai, 62 per cent of those who thought about it attempted suicide, and 5 per cent of those in Hanoi). In other words, in places like Chennai, very few people will attempt suicide without having thought about or planned it (almost two-thirds of those who ever considered suicide attempted it), whereas in a place like Hanoi, this proportion is only 5 per cent, which means that those who think about it or make a plan do not necessarily

attempt suicide. Clearly a universal preventive intervention based on suicidal ideation only will have quite distinct and different cost-effectiveness from place to place.

## The clinical severity of suicide attempts

A concluding element of information from the WHO SUPRE-MISS community survey, related to the importance of suicidal ideation, refers to the clinical severity of suicide attempts, measured in terms of the nature and intensity of medical attention required after the attempt. It is remarkable to see (Figure 15.6[1]) a virtual complete lack of relationship between these two variables; even a symmetrical and inverted relationship when comparing Chennai (very low ideation rate and very high severity of attempts) and Hanoi (moderate ideation rate and very low severity of attempts) with Durban (very high ideation rate and moderate severity of attempts). These findings are, in a way, confirmed by the analysis of the rate of suicide attempt as compared to its severity (Figure 15.7), at least for Chennai and Hanoi. Once again, one can observe a relatively low attempted suicide rate with very high clinical severity against a very low attempted suicide rate with a low clinical severity in Hanoi.

Another way of evaluating the importance of suicidal ideation is to compare its rates with those of suicide, to which a major methodological barrier exists. Most studies about suicidal ideation refer to limited population sets, whereas suicide mortality rates usually refer to a whole country. In the case of SUPRE-MISS, suicidal ideation rates were obtained from samples of the general adult population of some cities, for which no specific suicide mortality rates are available.

As with an experiment, and also as a suggestion for future studies, a comparison was tried between the suicidal ideation rates in the SUPRE-MISS sites and the respective national suicide mortality rate. The results of this can be seen in Figure 15.8. It is

---

[1] For this type of comparison unfortunately no data is available from Brisbane.

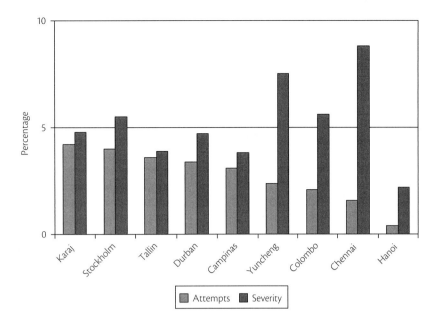

**Fig. 15.7** Suicide attempts and their clinical severity 2004.

clear from a mere visual inspection that no relation exists between these two variables.

## Other studies

There are not many studies on suicidal ideation that have been conducted in different places using a comparable methodology. In (1996), Weismann *et al.* published the results of a multisite survey conducted in several countries, such as Canada, Germany, France, New Zealand and the United States of America.

In Figure 15.9 overleaf, data from both SUPRE-MISS and Weismann's paper were displayed. No clear association between suicide ideation rates and suicide mortality rates emerges. This is even more evident for non-Western, non-industrialized countries.

## Conclusion

It is difficult to value the information concerning suicidal ideation, outside of clinical settings, particularly when looking at non-Western, non-industrialized countries.

Pirkis and colleagues (2001) have found that, in Australia, suicidal ideation in the general population is a good predictor of utilization of health services, but this might be a function of the quality of health services in Australia as much as of suicidal ideation. In fact, studying another Australian sample, Schweitzer and colleagues (1995) found that over half of those who attempted suicide did not use any type of mental health care services, and Goldney and colleagues (1990), studying yet another Australian population, raised doubts about the validity of suicidal ideation as a predictor of other types of suicidal behaviours. In the same paper, it was also reported that subjects who had previously acknowledged suicidal ideation denied it upon re-examination four years later. In this sense, suicidal ideation could be perceived as a sign of distress rather than one of long-term suicide outcome. Overall, there appears to be more of an obscure outlook than clearer points regarding the importance and value of suicidal ideation.

What seems clear, though, particularly from multi-site studies using a standardized methodology, such as the WHO SUPRE-MISS, is that there is a strong cultural underpinning behind the whole spectrum of suicidal behaviours. Without a clear understanding of the local meaning and implications of suicidal ideation, any further action, including prevention and care for suicidal people, becomes challenged.

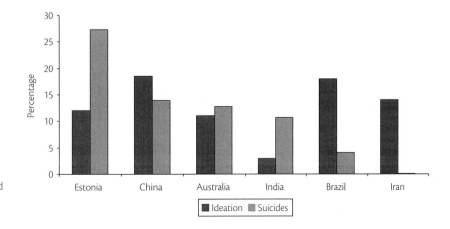

**Fig. 15.8** Suicidal ideation (in %) and suicide rates (in 100,000) in selected countries 2004.

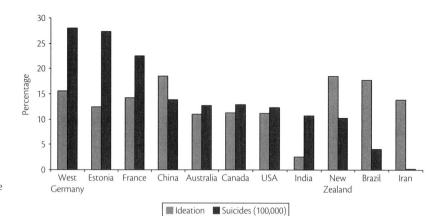

**Fig. 15.9** Suicidal ideation and suicide rates (in 100,000) in selected countries 2004.

## References

Bertolote JM, Fleischmann A, De Leo D *et al.* (2005). Suicide attempts, plans and ideation in culturally diverse sites: the WHO SUPRE-MISS community survey. *Psychological Medicine*, **35**, 1457–1465.

Fleischmann A, Bertolote JM, De Leo D *et al.* (2005). Characteristics of attempted suicides seen in emergency-care settings of general hospitals in eight low- and middle-income countries. *Psychological Medicine*, **35**, 1467–1474.

Fleischmann A, Bertolote JM, Wasserman D *et al.* (2008). Effectiveness of brief intervention and contact for suicide attempters: a randomized controlled trial in five countries. *Bulletin of the World Health Organization*, **86**, 703–709.

Goldney RD, Smith S, Winefield AH *et al.* (1990). Suicidal ideation: its enduring nature and associated morbidity. *Acta Psychiatrica Scandinavica*, **83**, 115–120.

Kerkhof A, Bernasco W, Bille-Brahe U *et al.* (1999). European Parasuicide Study Interview Schedule (EPSIS). In U Bille-Brahe, ed., *Facts and figures: WHO/EURO*. (EURO/ICP/PSF), pp. 1–4. World Health Organization Regional Office for Europe, Copenhagen.

Pirkis JE, Burgess PM, Meadows GN *et al.* (2001). Suicidal ideation and suicide attempts as predictors of mental health service users. *Medical Journal of Australia*, **175**, 542–545.

Schweitzer R, Klayich M, McLean J (1995). Suicidal ideation and behaviours among university students in Australia. *Australian and New Zealand Journal of Psychiatry*, **29**, 473–479.

Weismann MM, Bland RC, Canino GJ *et al.* (1996). Cross-national epidemiology of major depression and bipolar disorder. *Journal of the American Medical Association*, **276**, 293–299.

World Health Organization (2002). *Multisite intervention study on suicidal behaviours SUPRE-MISS: protocol of SUPRE-MISS*. World Health Organization, Geneva.

Zubin J (1974). Observations on nosological issues in the classification of suicidal behavior. In A Beck *et al.*, eds, *The Prediction of Suicide*, pp. 3–25. Charles Press Publishers, Bowie.

# CHAPTER 16

# Suicide attempts in Africa

Lourens Schlebusch and Stephanie Burrows

## Abstract

An understanding of the full burden of suicidal behaviour in many parts of Africa has been hampered by a lack of systematic data collection. Paucity of research, poor research designs and other influences have contributed to this situation. Given the resultant variability in the reliability of figures across countries, regions and population groups, prudence is needed when interpreting data. The figures discussed in this chapter are not representative of the entire non-fatal suicidal population in Africa and only salient features are highlighted. Figures that are available indicate that, in some areas, the situation is more serious than generally thought. Even more alarming is that known data most likely do not reflect the true extent of the problem. There are substantial variations across gender, age, and ethnic groups. Overdose (especially poisoning) is one of the most common methods of attempted suicide. Psychopathology (especially mood disorders) and substance abuse, HIV/AIDS, and family-related problems are strongly associated with increased risk of suicidal behaviour.

## Introduction

Early publications suggest that non-fatal suicidal behaviour on the African continent was rare, whereas more recent studies reported that, in a number of countries, it is not as infrequent as previously suggested (German 1987; Nwosu and Odesanmi 2001; Schlebusch 2004, 2005; Ovuga 2005; Ovuga et al. 2007). Nevertheless, the prevalence of non-fatal suicidal behaviour is not clear for several reasons. For example:

◆ With a few exceptions, many studies group fatal and non-fatal suicidal behaviours together;

◆ There has been a lack of systematic data collection, with information typically coming from small-scale ad hoc studies, often hospital-based;

◆ Attempted suicides are frequently not seen in hospitals or clinics unless the consequences are perceived as life-threatening and therefore known figures represent an underestimation;

◆ Studies have not always employed standardized assessment instruments and are mostly descriptive in nature, with an absence

of follow-up studies and epidemiological research making time trend analyses difficult;

◆ Suicidal behaviour is still a crime in some countries on the African continent and subject to negative cultural and religious sanctions (including secrecy), which further distort reports of its occurrence; and

◆ There is a hidden burden of suicidal behaviour, especially in the rural areas where little data is available (Pelser and Oberholzer 1987; Bekry 1999; Kinyanda and Kigozi 2005; Schlebusch 2005).

Given the resultant variations in the availability and reliability of data, caution should be exercised when making cross-national, cross-cultural and cross-regional comparisons. The figures discussed here are not representative of the entire non-fatal suicidal population in Africa: only salient features are highlighted. These, disturbingly, indicate that attempted suicide is an increasingly serious problem on the continent.

## Epidemiological aspects

### Estimates of the size of the problem

Hospital-based studies of attempted suicide have shown rates of 38.5/100,000 in Cairo (Egypt) in 1975 (Okasha and Lotaif 1979), and 49.8/100,000 in Addis Ababa (Ethiopia) between 1981/1982 and 1995/1996 (Bekry 1999). Community surveys showed that among Addis Ababa high school students aged 11–18 (1989–1990), a lifetime prevalence of attempted suicide was 14.3 per cent (Kebede and Ketsela 1993); while among a representative sample of adults in 1994 the prevalence was 0.9 per cent (Kebede and Alem 1999). A cross-sectional survey (Alem et al. 1999) in a rural and semi-urban community of Butajira, Ethiopia (1997), reported a lifetime attempted suicide prevalence of 3.2 per cent. Nigerian figures of 2.6/100,000 for Ibadan (Odejide et al. 1986) and 7.0/100,000 for Benin City have been reported (Eferakeya 1984), where the incidence did not increase over the four-year period 1978–1981. In north-west Uganda, a special programme has been instituted to empower local communities and train primary health care workers to prevent suicidal behaviours (Ovuga et al. 2007).

Considerably more South African research data on non-fatal suicidal behaviour is available, although as in the rest of Africa, divergent prevalence rates have been reported in the past (Schlebusch 2005). Several contemporary studies (Schlebusch *et al.* 2003; Ovuga 2005; Schlebusch 2005) dispel the myth that non-fatal suicidal behaviour is as rare in black South Africans as previously thought.

In South Africa, suicidal behaviour can be estimated using more readily available suicide data, which show a gradual increase in the overall figures. In 1999, suicides accounted for 8 per cent of a sample of non-natural deaths in South Africa (Butchart 2000), and in 2004 for 11.2 per cent (Matzopoulos 2005). Rates of 24.5 (for males) and 6.9 (for females) (Matzopoulos *et al.* 2004) and 17.2 to 19 (or higher) per 100,000 of the population have been reported, depending on when and how the sampling was done (Schlebusch 2005). For every fatal suicide, it is estimated that there are at least twenty (or more) non-fatal suicides (Schlebusch 2005), which is comparable to reported global ratios (Bertolote 2001).

### Distribution across sociodemographic groups

#### Gender differences

Suicide attempts in Africa vary considerably across gender, age and ethnicity. Studies suggest that southern and central Africa has a profile similar to that of Western countries, where young females predominate (Gelfand 1976; Williams and Buchan 1981; Bosch *et al.* 1995; Schlebusch 2005). In South Africa, generally, three times as many women as men engage in non-fatal suicidal behaviours (Schlebusch 2005). A mixed picture emerges from eastern, western and northern Africa. A study from Gabon reports a higher ratio of women compared to men, with three female attempts for every male (Mboussou and Milebou-Aubusson 1989), and a community study in Butajira found that 63 per cent of suicide attempts were female (Alem *et al.* 1999). Yet, studies from Uganda (Cardoza and Mugerwa 1972), Ethiopia (Kebede and Ketsela 1993; Kebede and Alem 1999) and Egypt (Okasha and Lotaif 1979) report no marked gender differences. Others show a reversal of the female preponderance. Male-to-female ratios have been reported as 2.9:1 in Addis Ababa (Bekry 1999), 1.7:1 in Kampala (Kinyanda *et al.* 2004), 1.4:1 in Ibadan (Odejide *et al.* 1986), and 1.2:1 in Benin City (Eferakeya 1984). In Addis Ababa (Bekry 1999), attempted suicide rates for males were consistently higher than those for females over a 15-year period (1981/1982–1995/1996). The average rate was 74.9 and 25.9 per 100,000 for males and females, respectively. There was a decline during the late 1980s with a substantial increase (more marked in males) beginning in 1991/1992, peaking at the end of the study period.

#### Age

All age groups are affected, but most studies report the young to be at particular risk for non-fatal suicidal behaviour. A community survey in Butajira found that attempted suicide was most frequent between the ages of 15 and 24 (Alem *et al.* 1999). Half of the victims in a study in Kampala (Kinyanda *et al.* 2004) and two-thirds of those in Addis Ababa (Kedebe and Alem 1999) were under 25 years old. More than three-quarters (76.9 per cent) of suicide attempts in general hospitals in Ibadan (Odejide *et al.* 1986) and 87 per cent in Benin City (Eferakeya 1984) occurred in those under 30 years (15–19 year olds constituted 39.4 per cent of the sample). Within an Ethiopian adolescent group, one study (Kebede and Ketsela 1993) found no significant association with age. Males aged 15–44 and 45–64, and females aged 45–64 contributed more to the steep rises in attempted suicides across time in Addis Ababa than in other age groups (Bekry 1999).

In South African, general hospital studies in Durban the peak age was the 20–29 age group followed by the 10–19 age group (Bosch *et al.* 1995, Schlebusch 2005). One study reported a mean age of 25 years for non-fatal suicidal behaviour in a Johannesburg general hospital sample involving mainly black patients (Deonarain and Pillay 2000). Several studies presented at South African suicide conferences have noted that during the last few decades, up to about one-third of all non-fatal suicidal behaviours involved children and adolescents (Schlebusch 2005). Other hospital-based studies reported that suicidal behaviour among the youth constituted about 10 per cent of referrals for psychological help (Mhlongo and Peltzer 1999), and that 24.5 per cent of the total sample of suicidal behaviour patients admitted were black youths aged 18 years and younger (Schlebusch *et al.* 2003).

#### Ethnic differences

As noted, contemporary studies show that non-fatal suicidal behaviour in blacks is more common than previously reported (Schlebusch 2005). For example, in South Africa a 1980s investigation in a catchment area near Pretoria indicated an attempted suicide rate of 11/100,000 among blacks (Pelser and Oberholzer 1987). More recently, between 10 per cent of black patients (Deonarain and Pillay 2000) and 12 per cent (Bosch *et al.* 1995) of patients of all ethnic groups (20.2 per cent white, 15.3 per cent coloured, 52 per cent Indian, 12.5 per cent black) who were referred for psychological/psychiatric help in general hospitals were suicide attempts. In a 1995 high school sample conducted amongst black youths in the eastern Cape region, up to 47 per cent of those surveyed had suicidal ideation (Mayekiso and Mkize 1995). A 1998 study among secondary high school pupils in the Limpopo province reported parasuicide rates of 17 per cent for boys and 13 per cent for girls (Peltzer and Cherian 1998). Another study (Madu and Matla 2003), in the same province, conducted among black secondary school adolescents (only 4.5 per cent were from other ethnic groups) reported that 37 per cent of the learners thought of taking their lives, 17 per cent had threatened to do so or had informed others about their suicidal intentions, 16 per cent had made plans to commit suicide, and 21 per cent had made attempts.

## Methods of choice in attempted suicide

Choice of method for all age groups is strongly influenced by factors such as accessibility to the method; knowledge or the lack of knowledge of the lethality of the method; experience and familiarity with the method; meaning, symbolism and cultural influence associated with the method; and the suicidal person's mental status (including the presence of a mental disorder) and the level of intent at the time (Schlebusch 2005).

In a study in Kampala (Kinyanda *et al.* 2004), the predominant method among non-fatal suicides was poisoning (mainly organophosphates). Hanging and poisoning were the most frequently reported methods of attempting suicide in Butajira, with men significantly more likely to use hanging to attempt suicide than women (Alem *et al.* 1999). Similarly, hanging was the preferred method for men and poisoning for women amongst adults in Addis Ababa (Kebede and Alem 1999). Among suicide attempters attending general hospitals in Ibadan, poisonings were most frequent, with 61.5 per cent of patients ingesting chemicals and 28.2 per cent ingesting psychotropic drugs (Odejide *et al.* 1986). In Benin City, ingestion of drugs (68 per cent) and chemicals

(20 per cent) were the predominant methods (Eferakeya 1984). In a Cairo study, the most common method was overdosing on tablets (Okasha and Lotaif 1979).

In South Africa, overdose predominates in attempted suicides, especially in young people (Schlebusch 2005). A wide variety of substances is ingested, but over-the-counter analgesics, benzodiazepines, antidepressants, household poisons and utility products are typically used. In one study (Pillay 1988), almost three-quarters of young self-poisoners used medicines belonging to family members in the same household. Other findings (Schlebusch et al. 2003) point to the common ingestion of household poisons such as paraffin, turpentine and insecticides. In a Johannesburg survey (largely amongst blacks), 61.9 per cent of patients overdosed on medication, 24.7 per cent ingested poisons, 4.2 per cent took detergents and 9.2 per cent tried other methods such as hanging, gassing, and cutting (Deonarain and Pillay 2000). The use of potentially lethal methods reported in many studies is disconcerting, not only because of the easy access to the methods, but also because they tend to confirm lethal intent in young people whose suicidal behaviour is often treated merely as a gesture (Schlebusch 2005).

# Clinical aspects of attempted suicide

## Psychopathology and substance abuse

Mental and addictive disorders are central risk factors for suicidal behaviour internationally, as also seen in Africa (Schlebusch 2005). A South African investigation reported that the diagnosis of mood disorders was applicable in nearly two-thirds (63.9 per cent) of suicide attempters, with other diagnoses including substance abuse, schizophrenia, and substance-induced psychosis (Schlebusch et al. 2003).

Mental illness was a predisposing factor in 32 per cent of attempted suicides in Benin City (Eferakeya 1984). In Butajira, mental distress and problem drinking were reported to be significant risk factors (Alem et al. 1999). Among Addis Ababa high school adolescents, suicide attempts were strongly associated with hopelessness, school grade, and alcohol intake (Kebede and Ketsela 1993). Depressive illnesses, hysterical reactions, and situational disorders, in that order of frequency, were the main precipitators of suicide attempts among patients seen in a Cairo hospital (Okasha and Lotaif 1979).

## HIV/AIDS

Africa is plagued by an HIV/AIDS pandemic that has implications for suicidal behaviour. Studies from South Africa (Meel 2003; Schlebusch 2005; Schlebusch and Noor Mahomed 2005), Nigeria (Gali et al. 2004) and Kenya (Sindiga and Lukhando 1993) have shown this link. The risk of suicidal behaviour may be higher at particular stages of the disease, e.g. within 3–6 months after diagnosis of infection with HIV and in later stages of the disease, which may be characterized by pain, various neurocognitive symptoms and dementia, and even after testing but before the results are known (Perry et al. 1990; Kelly et al. 1998; Schlebusch 2005). Pre-existing psychopathology and past suicidal behaviour tend to be associated with suicidal risk in HIV-infected individuals (Frierson and Lippmann 1988; Gala et al. 1992; Rundell et al. 1992; O'Dowd et al. 1993; Kelly et al. 1998; Schlebusch 2005).

The person's sociocultural context plays an important role in coping with the disease. For example, HIV/AIDS in partners and family members can produce relational problems that can trigger suicidal behaviour (Schlebusch 2005) and, in certain communities, infected individuals are discriminated against socially, in the workplace and even by health professionals. HIV/AIDS is conceptualized as a mystical force in some cultural groups and viewed as creating conditions of 'misfortune', 'disagreeableness' and 'repulsiveness', resulting in a dislike of the person by others. Such problems result in increased levels of stress, depression and subsequent suicidal behaviour (Schlebusch and Noor Mohamed 2005).

## Family dynamics and related issues

Many South African studies have noted the role of family problems and interpersonal conflicts in suicidal behaviour (Schlebusch 2005). Other risk factors commonly reported (Schlebusch 2005) are a history of repeated suicide attempts; financial and socio-economic pressures; academic-related problems; a history of suicidal behaviour in the family; exposure to family violence; child abuse and incest; chronic and acute stress; frequent exposure to violence; human rights violations; and difficulty in dealing with rapid transformation.

Although no significant differences were observed between suicide attempts and family history of suicide or parental educational levels among adolescents in Addis Ababa (Kebede and Ketsela 1993), disturbed interpersonal relationships (especially with parents) were found to have motivated suicide attempts among Ibadan hospital patients (Odejide et al. 1986). In Benin City, 24 per cent of attempters reported conflicts with parents as a predisposing factor (Eferakeya 1984). In Uganda, recent studies note the importance of psychosocial risk factors in suicidal behaviour such as financial difficulties, unemployment, poverty and feelings of loneliness (Kinyanda and Kigozi 2005), which indicate the urgency to respond to the population's psychosocial needs (Ovuga et al. 2007).

# Conclusions

As for many countries worldwide, the prevalence of attempted suicide is not clearly known for the African continent. Available figures in some parts of Africa indicate that the situation has reached more serious proportions than generally thought, and even more alarming is that they most likely do not reflect the true extent of the problem. Although, in South Africa, such programmes have been developed (Schlebusch 2005; Burrows and Schlebusch 2008), there is a pressing need for more research and the development of appropriate management and prevention programmes. For example, a comparative analysis can bring a fresh view, but obviously the size and demography of each country's population impact significantly on epidemiological trends of attempted suicide. This has important practical implications. Therefore, obtaining appropriate data is the first step towards public health strategies to reduce suicidal behaviour in Africa.

## References

Alem A, Kebede D, Jacobsson L et al. (1999). Suicide attempts among adults in Butajira, Ethiopia. *Acta Psychiatrica Scandinavica*, **397**, 70–76.

Bekry AA (1999). Trends in suicide, parasuicide and accidental poisoning in Addis Ababa, Ethiopia. *Ethiopian Journal of Health Development*, **13**, 247–62.

Bertolote JM (2001). Suicide in the world: an epidemiological overview 1959–2000. In D Wasserman, ed., *Suicide: An Unnecessary Death*, pp. 3–10. London, Martin Dunitz.

Bosch BA, McGill VR, Noor Mohamed SB (1995). Current trends in suicidal behaviour at a general hospital. In L Schlebusch, ed., *Suicidal Behaviour 3. Proceedings of the Third Southern African Conference on Suicidology*, pp. 71–94. Durban, Department of Medically Applied Psychology, Faculty of Medicine, University of Natal.

Burrows S and Schlebusch L (2008). Priorities and prevention possibilities for reducing suicidal behaviour. In A Van Niekerk, S Suffla and M Seedat, eds, *Crime, Violence & Injury Lead Programme in South Africa: Data to Action*, pp. 173–201. Tygerberg, Medical Research Council–University of South Africa.

Butchart A (ed.) (2000). *A Profile of Fatal Injuries in South Africa 1999: First Annual Report of the National Injury Mortality Surveillance System*. Johannesburg, Injury and Violence Surveillance Consortium.

Cardozo LJ and Mugerwa RD (1972). The pattern of acute poisoning in Uganda. *East African Medical Journal*, **49**, 983–988.

Deonarain M and Pillay BJ (2000). A study of parasuicide behaviour at the Chris Hani Baragwanath Hospital. In L Schlebusch and BA Bosch, eds, *Suicidal Behaviour 4. Proceedings of the Fourth Southern African Conference on Suicidology*, pp. 112–127. Durban, Department of Medically Applied Psychology, Faculty of Medicine, University of Natal.

Eferakeya AE (1984). Drugs and suicide attempts in Benin City, Nigeria. *British Journal of Psychiatry*, **145**, 70–73.

Frierson RL and Lippmann SB (1988). Suicide and AIDS. *Psychosomatics*, **29**, 226–229.

Gala C, Pergami A, Catalan J *et al.* (1992). Risk of deliberate self-harm and factors associated with suicidal behaviour among asymptomatic individuals with human immunodeficiency virus infection. *Acta Psychiatrica Scandinavica*, **86**, 70–75.

Gali BM, Na'aya HU, Adamu S (2004). Suicide attempts in HIV/AIDS patients: report of two cases presenting with penetrating abdominal injuries. *Nigerian Journal of Medicine*, **13**, 407–409.

Gelfand M (1976). Suicide and attempted suicide in the urban and rural African in Rhodesia. *The Central African Journal of Medicine*, **22**, 203–205.

German GA (1987). Mental health in Africa: II. The nature of mental disorder in Africa today. Some clinical observations. *British Journal of Psychiatry*, **151**, 440–446.

Kebede D and Alem A (1999). Suicide attempts and ideation among adults in Addis Ababa, Ethiopia. *Acta Psychiatrica Scandinavica*, **397**, 35–39.

Kebede D and Ketsela T (1993). Suicide attempts in Ethiopian adolescents in Addis Ababa high schools. *Ethiopian Medical Journal*, **31**, 83–90.

Kelly B, Raphael B, Judd F (1998). Suicidal ideation, suicide attempts and HIV intention. *Psychosomatics*, **39**, 405–415.

Kinyanda E, Hjelmeland H, Musisi S (2004). Deliberate self-harm as seen in Kampala, Uganda—a case-control study. *Social Psychiatry and Psychiatric Epidemiology*, **39**, 318–325.

Kinyanda E and Kigozi F (2005). Epidemiology of suicide in Africa. Paper presented at the XXIII World Congress of the International Association for Suicide Prevention, Durban, South Africa, 13–16 September 2005.

Madu SN and Matla MP (2003). The prevalence of suicidal behaviours amongst secondary school adolescents in the Limpopo Province, South Africa. *South African Journal of Psychology*, **133**, 126–132.

Matzopoulos R (ed.) (2005). *A Profile of Fatal Injuries in South Africa: Sixth Annual Report of the National Injury Mortality Surveillance System*. Tygerberg, Medical Research Council-University of South Africa, Crime, Violence and Injury Lead Programme.

Matzopoulos R, Norman R, Bradshaw D (2004). The burden of injury in South Africa: fatal injury trends and international comparisons. In S Suffla, A van Niekerk and N Duncan, eds, *Crime, Violence and Injury Prevention in South Africa: Developments and Challenges*, pp. 9–21. Tygerberg, Medical Research Council-University of South Africa, Crime, Violence and Injury Lead Programme.

Mayekiso TV and Mkize DL (1995). The relationship between self-punitive wishes and family background. In L Schlebusch, ed., *Suicidal Behaviour 3: Proceedings of the Third Southern African Conference on Suicidology*, pp. 95–103. Durban, Department of Medically Applied Psychology, Faculty of Medicine, University of Natal.

Mboussou M and Milebou-Aubusson L (1989). [Suicides and attempted suicides at the Jeanne Ebori Foundation, Libreville (Gabon)] [Article in French]. *Médecine Tropicale: revue du corps de santé colonial*, **49**, 259–264.

Meel BL (2003). Suicide in HIV/AIDS in Transkei, South Africa. *Anil Aggrawal's Internet Journal of Forensic Medicine and Toxicology*, **4**, 1–9.

Mhlongo T and Peltzer K (1999). Para-suicide among youth in a general hospital in South Africa. *Curationis*, **22**, 72–76.

Nwosu SO and Odesanmi WO (2001). Pattern of suicides in Ile-Ife, Nigeria. *West African Journal of Medicine*, **20**, 259–262.

Odejide AO, Williams AO, Ohaeri JU *et al.* (1986). The epidemiology of deliberate self-harm. The Ibadan experience. *British Journal of Psychiatry*, **149**, 734–737.

O'Dowd MA, Biderman DJ, McKegney FP (1993). Incidence of suicidality in AIDS and HIV-positive patients attending a psychiatry outpatient program. *Psychosomatics*, **34**, 33–40.

Okasha A and Lotaif E (1979). Attempted suicide. An Egyptian investigation. *Acta Psychiatrica Scandinavica*, **60**, 69–75.

Ovuga E (2005). Depression and suicidal behaviour in Uganda: validating the Response Inventory for Stressful Life Events (RISLE). PhD Thesis, Karolinska Institutet & Makerere University, Sweden.

Ovuga E, Boardman J, Wasserman D (2007). Integrating mental health into primary health care: local initiatives from Uganda. *World Psychiatry*, **6**, 60–61.

Peltzer K and Cherian VI (1998). Attitudes towards suicide among South African secondary school pupils. *Psychological Reports*, **83**, 259–265.

Pelser DJW and Oberholzer DJ (1987). Attempted suicide (parasuicide), Medunsa/Ga-Rankuwa Hospital, South Africa. *Psychotherapia*, **14**, 22–24.

Perry S, Jacobsberg L, Fishman B (1990). Suicidal ideation and HIV testing. *JAMA*, **263**, 679–682.

Pillay BJ (1988). Methods of self-destructive behaviour in adolescents and young adults. *Psychological Reports*, **63**, 552–554.

Rundell JR, Kyle KM, Brown GR (1992). Risk factors for suicide attempts: human immunodeficiency virus screening program. *Psychosomatics*, **33**, 24–27.

Schlebusch L (2004). Current perspectives on suicidal behaviour in South Africa. In S Suffla, A Van Niekerk and N Duncan, eds, *Crime, Violence and Injury Prevention in South Africa: Developments and Challenges*, pp. 88–113. Tygerberg, Medical Research Council-University of South Africa, Crime, Violence and Injury Lead Programme.

Schlebusch L (2005). *Suicidal Behaviour in South Africa*. Pietermaritzburg, University of KwaZulu-Natal Press.

Schlebusch L and Noor Mahomed SB (2005). Suicidal behaviour and HIV/AIDS within the South African context. Paper presented at the XXIII World Congress of the International Association for Suicide Prevention, 13–16 September 2005, Durban, South Africa.

Schlebusch L, Vawda N, Bosch BA (2003). Suicidal behaviour in black South Africans. *Crisis*, **24**, 24–28.

Sindiga I and Lukhando M (1993). Kenyan university students' views on AIDS. *East African Medical Journal*, **70**, 713–716.

Williams H and Buchan T (1981). A preliminary investigation into parasuicide in Salisbury, Zimbabwe—1979/1980. *The Central African Journal of Medicine*, **27**, 129–135.

# CHAPTER 17

# Suicide attempts in Asia

Guo-Xin Jiang and Qi Cheng

## Abstract

Data on the prevalence of attempted suicide are sparse in Asian countries, particularly data gathered from large, general population-based surveys. Rates of attempted suicide reported results in various target groups and different areas, sometimes with large variations. For example, the prevalence of suicide attempts could be as low as 0.4 per cent of a sample aged over years in Hanoi, Vietnam; and 7.0 per cent among adolescent students aged 12–18 years in a rural prefecture of China. However, the age and gender distribution of suicide attempts are similar in Asia to Western countries, with the highest being among females and young people. Self-poisoning by ingestion of various medications or pesticides is a common method in Asian countries, predominantly in the rural areas. In general, fewer suicide attempters in Asia have had a diagnosis of psychiatric illness before the attempt compared to Western countries. Large representative, population-based investigations on suicide behaviour with a well-designed epidemiological method are urgently needed in Asia.

## Introduction

How many people attempt suicide in Asia each year? Unfortunately, there is no exact answer to this question yet. In addition to those known difficulties regarding reliability and validity when obtaining statistical data for suicide attempts, for example, diagnostic criteria of a suicide attempt, confirmation of motivation to self-harm, availability of medical service for such patients, completeness and validity of data collection, etc., suicide behaviour is still taboo in many Asian countries, thus creating even more difficulties. Compared with other continents, data on suicide behaviour are generally rare in Asia, particularly population-based data.

We have made a literature search on this particular topic in Medline, and attempted to summarize general information about suicide, attempts in Asia on an epidemiological and clinical basis.

## The epidemiological aspect

### Rate or frequency of suicide attempts

Literature searches were conducted on Medline with words like 'suicide attempt' and 'rate', as well as the name of the desired country with a population over 10,000,000 in Asia: and relevant results published in English were only available for a few countries, such as Japan, China and Vietnam. Data presented here are as recent as possible, however, there may be nothing present for many countries in the past decade.

There is very little data on the prevalence of attempted suicide deriving from large population-based surveys in the general population, with a well-designed epidemiological method, in Asian countries. Reported information on the topic is usually restricted to a selected population with a specific age span, or hospital-based data with different settings (characteristics). Despite these limitations, the data are useful in explaining the situation as a public heath problem in Asia.

A self-administered questionnaire survey conducted in a rural prefecture of China, including 1,362 adolescent students aged 12–18 years, showed a suicide attempt rate of 7.0 per cent (Liu and Tein 2005). Negative life events were reported by suicide attempters during the past year more frequently than suicidal ideators and non-suicidal adolescents, and a significant dose–response relationship was observed between the number of life events and suicidal behaviour.

A face-to-face interview was conducted in a random and representative population sample of 2,219 Chinese people aged 15–59 years in Hong Kong, and 38 (1.7 per cent) respondents reported a suicide attempt within the past 12 months (Cheung et al. 2006). Results showed that approximately 40 per cent of suicidal ideation and attempts were attributable to depression and 20 per cent to hopelessness. Drug abuse and marital dissolution were also significant contributors to suicidality.

Among 2,148 inpatients admitted to the emergency department during a one-year period from February 2004 to January 2005, in the National Hospital Organization Disaster Medical Center located in the suburbs of Tokyo, 247 (11.5 per cent, 95 per cent CI: 10.2–12.9 per cent) had attempted suicide (Nishi et al. 2006).

Among 4,500 adolescent students from a cross-sectional school survey in Malaysia, 7 per cent had seriously considered attempting suicide, and 4.6 per cent had attempted suicide at least once during the 12 months preceding the survey (Chen et al. 2005).

According to the results from the WHO SUPRE-MISS (Multisite Intervention Study on Suicidal Behaviours) community survey, 0.4 per cent of a sample, including 2,267 people aged over 9 years in Hanoi, Vietnam responded with a 'yes' to the question 'Have you ever attempted suicide?'. This is the lowest rate in this 10-site survey, when compared with the rate of 1.6 per cent (population aged 14–65 years) from Chennai, India, 2.1 per cent (population aged over 11 years) from Colombo, Sri Lanka, 2.4 per cent (population aged over 17 years) from Yuncheng, China, and 4.2 per cent (population aged over 13 years) from Karaj, Iran (Bertolote *et al.* 2005).

## Age and gender distribution

Similarly to Western countries, suicide attempts in Asia regarding gender and age distribution show that females are dominant among suicide attempters, and the rate is also high among young people.

Among 14,771 suicide attempters treated in 24 general hospitals in northern China, the female-to-male ratio was 2.5 to 1, and the median age was 29 years (range: 10–97 years): the 15–34 age group accounted for two-thirds of all suicide attempters (CDC 2004).

Data presenting age-specific rates of suicide attempts in Hong Kong indicated a female-to-male ratio of 1.83, with rates peaking in the 20–29 age group (Pan and Lieh-Mak 1989).

Based on a questionnaire survey conducted among members of the Akita Prefectural Medical Association in Japan during the period July 2001–June 2002, there were 105 attempted-suicide cases. Among them, 62 were female (59.1 per cent) and 43 were male (41.0 per cent) with a female-to-male ratio of 1.44, and the mean age was 41.9 ± 19.7 years (male 44.4 ± 16.5 years; female 40.3 ± 21.6 years) (Fushimi *et al.* 2006).

Findings in Japan show that attempted suicides in females are rapidly increasing from two to five times that of completed suicides in females within the recent decades (1980–2000), while the ratios of attempted-to-completed suicide rate in males were stable, being nearly even at 1:1. Based on the information during two decades between 1980–2000 in Japan, the average attempted suicide rate was estimated at 29.5 for the total population, 23.3 for males and 35.2 for females, and 0.6:1 for their male-to-female ratio. The average completed suicide rate was 19.5 for the total population, 26.6 for males and 12.7 for females, with a male-to-female ratio of 2:1 (Yamamura *et al.* 2006). According to Yamamura and colleagues there is little difference in suicidal rate between males and females when one takes into consideration the sum of completed and attempted suicides.

## Methods used for suicide attempts

Regarding methods of attempting suicide, self-poisoning by ingestion of various types of medications and/or pesticides is common in Asian countries, particularly in rural areas. However, suicide attempts by firearm or other weapons are far fewer when compared with Western countries, which may be attributable to the strict control of weapons in most Asian countries. Similar characteristics of methods used for suicide attempt can be also observed for completed suicide in Asia (Phillips *et al.* 2002).

Among 14,771 suicide attempters treated in 24 general hospitals in northern China, approximately 90 per cent of the attempts were by self-poisoning; 54 per cent by ingestion of medications usually anti-anxiety agents or sleeping pills, 28 per cent by ingestion of pesticides, and 9 per cent by ingestion of other toxins, e.g. household cleaners. Ingestion of pesticides was four times more common among persons treated in rural hospitals (43 per cent) than those treated in urban hospitals (10 per cent) (p <0.01), and 66 per cent of the pesticide self-poisonings treated in rural hospitals were women (CDC 2004).

Data from consecutively sampled serious attempters of suicide (N = 74) from six hospitals, which had been randomly selected from approximately twenty in total, in Dalian, China, showed that pesticides were the most lethal means of suicidal behaviour, and familial or marital problems accounted for the majority of stressful life events in suicidal behaviours (Zhang *et al.* 2006).

In Sri Lanka, oleander seeds are the second most frequently used toxic poison for suicide attempts (Eddleston *et al.* 2006). Case fatality of pesticides, oleander, and medicinal poisoning was recognized to be 15 per cent, 8 per cent and <1 per cent, respectively. According to the authors, poisons for attempting suicide were chosen on the basis of availability, often at short notice, therefore restrictions on availability of highly toxic poisons must be very important in reducing self-poisoning deaths, particularly in rural communities in Asia.

In a recently published review of deliberate self-burning in various parts of the world, India had the highest absolute number of cases, the highest fatality rate, and the highest contribution of self-harm to burns admissions, while the highest reported incidence was from Sri Lanka. In Western countries, self-burning is relatively uncommon (Laloe 2004).

## Clinical aspects

### Physical and mental disorders

Six per cent of 509 suicide attempters admitted to Bach Mai General Hospital in Hanoi, Vietnam had a psychiatric illness diagnosed before the suicide attempt (Thanh *et al.* 2005).

Results from a study among Japanese cancer patients seen in a psychiatric consultation setting indicated that many suicidal cancer patients suffer from complicated physical and psychologicaldistress, such as impaired performance status, pain and/or psychiatric disorders and major depression (Akechi *et al.* 2002).

### Culture and psychopathology

A study was conducted to examine the characteristics of adolescents from Hong Kong and the United States by comparing suicide attempters with sex- and age-matched controls: the results indicated that depression, current and lifetime suicide ideation, hopelessness, poor interpersonal relationships, and exposure to suicide attempters and completers distinguished attempters from controls equally in the two cultures and in both genders (Stewart *et al.* 2006).

Wasserman and colleagues (2008) study aimed to explore thesuicidal process, suicidal communication and the psychosocial situation of 19 young suicide attempters aged 15–24, and was conducted in a rural community in Hanoi, Vietnam, with semi-structured interviews. Thirteen cases engaged in some form of suicidal communication before their attempt, although thecommunication was difficult for outsiders to interpret. Twelve cases were victims of regular physical abuse and sixteen had suffered psychological violence for at least one year before attempting suicide. None sought advice or consultation in the community despite long-standing psychosocial problems.

## Economic recession

A comparison of mental disorder distribution in suicide attempters was made between the period when an economic recession started (1992–1993), and the period when the recession became serious (2000) in Kanagawa, Japan. The percentages of subjects with depression, neurotic disorders or other disorders were higher in the latter than in the former group, while the percentage of subjects with schizophrenia was lower in the latter group than in the former group. However, it was not certain that this change of mental disorder distribution in suicide attempters was related to the economic recession and increased unemployment in Japan (Ichimura et al. 2005).

## Cathartic effect

Change of suicidal ideation just before and after a suicide attempt was studied in 88 suicide attempters in Kobe, Japan in order to test whether a cathartic effect (i.e. their suicidal ideation weakened transiently after a suicide attempt) exists. Results showed that scores, which ranked from 0 to 10 with 0 indicating no and 10 indicating the strongest suicidal ideation, decreased significantly after the suicide attempt in comparison with those just before the suicide attempt (p <0.0001). In addition, the results indicated that the cathartic effect induced by a suicide attempt is different among generations and psychiatric disorders. Significant decreases in scores of suicidal ideation after the suicide attempt were observed in suicide attempters of each generation under 60 years of age, but not in those over 60 years. Scores of suicidal ideation after the suicide attempt were significantly higher in the patients with diagnoses of neurotic, stress-related and somatoform disorders than those in patients with diagnoses of schizophrenia, and delusional disorders (Matsuishi et al. 2005).

## Other relevant issues

Suicide attempts are often impulsive. Among 594 medically serious suicide attempters treated in nine hospitals in northern China, 45 per cent (270) reported considering suicide for <10 minutes before their attempts (CDC 2004).

Among 1,025 Japanese homosexual, bisexual or other men questioning their sexual orientation, 154 (15 per cent) of the men reported a history of attempted suicide (Hidaka and Operario. 2006).

Results from a sample of 147 women suicide attempters under the age of 35 years and living in rural areas in China showed that the method used by 129 attempters (87.8 per cent) was poisoning with highly lethal insecticides, pesticides and fertilizers; family conflict accounted for around 60 per cent; and 62.6 per cent (87/139) of the sample showed no signs of formal psychiatric disturbance (Pearson et al. 2002).

Temporal variation of the incidence of parasuicide (attempted suicide) was examined in a Chinese community in Singapore between 1990 and 1994, and the results indicated that cases of parasuicide peaked on Mondays, while the lowest incidences occurred on Saturdays. The peak months were June, August and September with a dip in December and January (Ho et al. 1998).

## Conclusion

Quite large variation of reported attempted-suicide rates can be recognized from various reports, even from the same country. Differences in study subjects, methods and settings in the investigations of attempted-suicide prevalence make it difficult to evaluate the true situation in the general population, and to compare results between different studies. Even in the WHO SUPRE-MISS community survey (Bertolote et al. 2005), differences between study subjects were obvious regarding age and other aspects between different countries.

The population in Asia accounts for more than 60 per cent of the whole world, and suicide is recognized as a great public health problem on the continent. However, statistical data regarding suicidal behaviour are rare in many Asian countries, although such information is essential for organizing successful strategies for prevention of suicide in the population. Therefore, large population-based epidemiological investigations on suicidal behaviour are urgently needed.

## References

Akechi T, Nakano T, Akizuki N et al. (2002). Clinical factors associated with suicidality in cancer patients. Japanese Journal of Clinical Oncology, 32, 506–511.

Bertolote JM, Fleischmann A, De Leo D et al. (2005). Suicide attempts, plans, and ideation in culturally diverse sites: the WHO SUPRE-MISS community survey. Psychological Medicine, 35, 1457–1465.

CDC (Centers for Disease Control and Prevention) (2004). Suicide and attempted suicide—China, 1990–2002. Morbidity and Mortality Weekly Report, 53, 481–484.

Chen PC, Lee LK, Wong KC et al. (2005). Factors relating to adolescent suicidal behaviour: a cross-sectional Malaysian school survey. Journal of Adolescent Health, 37, 11–337.

Cheung YB, Law CK, Chan B et al. (2006). Suicidal ideation and suicide attempts in a population-based study of Chinese people: risk attributable to hopelessness, depression, and social factors. Journal of Affective Disorders, 90, 193–199.

Eddleston M, Karunaratne A, Weerakoon M et al. (2006). Choice of poison for intentional self-poisoning in rural Sri Lanka. Clinical Toxicology (Philaladelphia), 44, 283–286.

Fushimi M, Sugawara J, Saito S (2006). Comparison of completed and attempted suicide in Akita, Japan. Psychiatry and Clinical Neurosciences, 60, 289–295.

Hidaka Y and Operario D (2006). Attempted suicide, psychological health and exposure to harassment among Japanese homosexual, bisexual or other men questioning their sexual orientation recruited via the Internet. Journal of Epidemiological Community Health, 60, 962–967.

Ho BK, Kua EH, Hong C (1998). Temporal variation in parasuicide among Singaporean Chinese. Australia and New Zealand Journal of Psychiatry, 32, 500–503.

Ichimura A, Matsumoto H, Kimura T et al. (2005). Changes in mental disorder distribution among suicide attempters in mid-west area of Kanagawa. Psychiatry and Clinical Neurosciences, 59, 113–118.

Laloe V (2004). Patterns of deliberate self-burning in various parts of the world. A review. Burns, 30, 207–215.

Liu X and Tein JY (2005). Life events, psychopathology, and suicidal behaviour in Chinese adolescents. Journal of Affective Disorders, 86, 195–203.

Matsuishi K, Kitamura N, Sato M et al. (2005). Change of suicidal ideation induced by suicide attempt. Psychiatry Clinical Neuroscience, 59, 599–604.

Nishi D, Matsuoka Y, Kawase E et al. (2006). Mental health service requirements in a Japanese medical centre emergency department. Emergency Medicine Journal, 23, 468–469.

Pan PC and Lieh-Mak F (1989). A comparison between male and female parasuicides in Hong Kong. *Social Psychiatry and Psychiatric Epidemiology*, **24**, 253–257.

Pearson V, Phillips MR, He F *et al.* (2002). Attempted suicide among young rural women in the People's Republic of China: possibilities for prevention. *Suicide and Life-Threatening Behaviour*, **32**, 359–369.

Phillips MR, Yang G, Zhang Y *et al.* (2002). Risk factors for suicide in China: a national case–control psychological autopsy study. *Lancet*, **30**, 1728–1736.

Stewart SM, Felice E, Claassen C *et al.* (2006). Adolescent suicide attempters in Hong Kong and the United States. *Social Science andi Medicine*, **63**, 296–306.

Thanh HTT, Jiang GX, Van TN *et al.* (2005). Attempted suicide in Hanoi, Vietnam. *Social Psychiatry and Psychiatric Epidemiology*, **40**, 64–71.

Wasserman D, Thanh HTT, Minh DP *et al.* (2008). Suicidal process, suicidal communication and psychosocial situation of young suicide attempters in a rural Vietnamese community. *World Psychiatry*, **7**, 47–53.

Yamamura T, Kinoshita H, Nishiguchi M *et al.* (2006). A perspective in epidemiology of suicide in Japan. *Vojnosanit Pregl*, **63**, 575–583.

Zhang J, Jia S, Jiang C *et al.* (2006). Characteristics of Chinese suicide attempters: an emergency room study. *Death Studies*, **30**, 259–268.

# CHAPTER 18

# Suicide attempts in South and Central America

Neury J Botega and Sabrina Stefanello

## Abstract

Data on suicidal behaviour in Central and South America has derived from mortality statistics. Suicide rates in most countries of Central and South America are considerably lower than in North America and Europe. The recent increase in suicide rates particularly afflicts young people. An increase in suicide rates have also been reported among indigenous groups, and seem to be related to extreme pressure exerted by Western society, self-devaluation and alcohol misuse. A WHO worldwide initiative for the prevention of suicide (SUPRE-MISS) multi-centre study estimated the life prevalence of suicidal behaviour in a large Brazilian city at 17.1 per cent for suicidal ideation, 4.8 per cent for plans and 2.8 per cent for suicide attempts. Urban violence and high homicide rates have overshadowed the problem of suicidal behaviour in Latin American countries. It is only recently that awareness of suicidal behaviour among adolescents and young adults, as well as violence (including suicide) and prevention policies have received government attention. Apart from Brazil, most countries in that part of the world lack national suicide prevention programmes, however actions are underway in Chile and Argentina.

## Introduction

Central and South America are frequently denominated Latin America. There are several definitions of Latin America, however the most common view is that Latin America consists of territories in the Americas where Spanish or Portuguese prevail, e.g. Mexico, most of Central America, South America and the Caribbean. Around 90 per cent of the population is Catholic, but in recent decades, Protestant churches have increased in number. There is a great disparity of wealth and income across the countries, with the majority of people facing significant economic deprivation.

The political development of most Latin American countries after the Second World War has been similar, with the majority having gone through phases of populism (1940s–1950s) and military dictatorship (1960s–1970s). During the 1980s, with re-democratization, several changes occurred in the context of social and political movements, including the introduction of national mental health programmes (Larrobla and Botega 2001).

Latin America accounts for 29.2 per cent of the world's total burden of disease related to injuries caused by acts of violence.

Intentional injuries account for 12 per cent in this region. More than half (54.9 per cent) of health expenditures originate from the public sector. The majority of these countries, however, devote less than 2 per cent of their total health budget to mental health (Alarcón 2003).

## Suicide

The most continuous and comprehensive data on patterns of suicidal behaviour in Latin American countries derive from mortality statistics, therefore data is limited to completed suicides. Nonetheless, official rates tend to underestimate the true level of suicide mortality, as reported by a local study which assessed the quality of death certificates in cases due to external causes of death (Drumond et al. 1999).

Suicide rates in most South and Central America countries are considerably lower than in North America and Europe (Table 18.1). Rates tend to present a seasonal variation as they do in the northern hemisphere (Retamal and Humphreys 1998; Lawrynowicz and Baker 2005). The evaluation of 824 suicide autopsies in Bogota, capital city of Colombia, every five years from 1985 to 2000 indicated that physical or mental comorbidity, the use of psychoactive substances, access to lethal methods of injury, and the use of firearms were constant factors associated with suicide. At the same time, changes in some typologies were related to the presence of addiction in women and HIV/AIDS (Sanchez et al. 2004). A study that used the Brazilian Mortality Information System, from 1979 to 1998, for Rio de Janeiro State, showed that in both males and females, age-adjusted suicide rates had decreased until 1992, but have been on the rise since then (Rodrigues and Werneck 2005). The increase in suicide rates particularly afflicts young people (Sánchez et al. 2002; Souza et al. 2002; Serfaty et al. 2003).

In 1978, a mass suicide of 913 followers of the People's Temple Cult in Jonestown, Guyana, caught the world's attention (Nock and Marzuk 2002). Suicide epidemics have also been reported among indigenous groups in several Latin American countries (Oliveira and Lotufo Neto 2003). Under extreme pressure exerted by Western society, some Indian groups (especially younger individuals) may disassociate from the possibility of returning to their traditional way of living, thus leading to extreme self-devaluation, alcohol misuse and suicide (Morgado 1991).

**Table 18.1** Mortality rates due to external causes for selected South and Central American countries (2000–2005)

| Country | Mortality rate (per 100,000) | | |
|---|---|---|---|
| | **Suicide** | **Homicide** | **Road accidents** |
| Argentina | 8.2 | 7.0 | 8.9 |
| Brazil | 4.9 | 29.3 | 22.3 |
| Chile | 10.9 | 5.7 | 13.2 |
| Costa Rica | 6.7 | 6.7 | 18.1 |
| Colombia | 5.2 | 80.4 | 20.9 |
| Dominican Republic | 2.9 | 9.7 | 21.9 |
| Cuba | 15.9 | 5.8 | 13 |
| Ecuador | 5.9 | 21.2 | 13.4 |
| El Salvador | 11.5 | 50.5 | 30.2 |
| Guatemala | 1.9 | 22.8 | 4.1 |
| Guyana | 11.1 | 5.7 | 6.1 |
| Mexico | 4.1 | 11.3 | 11.9 |
| Nicaragua | 13.2 | 12.8 | 16.9 |
| Panama | 6.3 | 13.5 | 16.6 |
| Paraguay | 3.7 | 15.8 | 12.6 |
| Peru | 2.3 | 4.4 | 12.8 |
| Puerto Rico | 7.8 | 18.8 | 13.8 |
| Suriname | 11.5 | 3.0 | 13.7 |
| Trinidad and Tobago | 13.0 | 10.6 | 10.8 |
| Uruguay | 13.9 | 5.0 | 13.8 |
| Venezuela | 4.8 | 14.7 | 18.0 |

Source : Organización Panamericana de la Salud (OPS) 2004.

## Attempted suicide

There are no national registrations that reliably monitor the actual burden of suicide attempts. The information available comprises descriptive studies based on patient samples seen at health care services (Abbinante *et al.* 1995; Juarez-Aragon *et al.* 1999; Leveridge 1999; Trujillo *et al.* 1999; Borges *et al.* 2000; Freitas and Botega 2002; Rapeli and Botega 2005), and reports on specific methods of suicide attempt, such as self-poisoning with caustic substances (Mamede and De Mello Filho 2002; Andreollo *et al.* 2003). A study implemented in Montevideo (Uruguay) compared characteristics of those who have attempted suicide with those who committed suicide. Ninety per cent of the latter had psychiatric symptoms, and in 67 per cent of them, a psychiatric diagnosis could be made. The most frequent diagnoses were depression and alcoholism. Half of the suicides had previously attempted suicide. The group with suicide attempts were of younger age, and the most prevalent diagnoses were depression and personality disorder (Lucero *et al.* 2003).

Until recently, there has not been an in-depth investigation into suicidal behaviour in Latin America. The only exception was a community survey conducted in Puerto Rico in the 1980s, which was later used in a cross-national study. This cross-national comparison assessed the prevalence of suicide ideation and attempts among nine nations by standardizing random samples and assigning a design weight of 1.0 for each respondent. The results indicated that the overall prevalence of suicide ideation and attempts in

Puerto Rico was 9.51/100 and 5.93/100, respectively (Weissman *et al.* 1999). In the city of Leon, Nicaragua, a community-based study was conducted to identify factors associated with suicide attempts among young people (Rodriguez *et al.* 2006). From 352 randomly selected subjects aged 15–24 years, 278 individuals (145 males and 133 females) were interviewed. A suicide attempt in the past year was reported by 2.1 per cent of males and 1.5 per cent of females. There were no significant gender differences in reporting of separate types of suicidal expressions, except for death wishes, where females reported higher prevalence than males (33.8 per cent vs 20.7 per cent). Another community survey conducted among young people in Trinidad and Tobago, with a total of 45 respondents aged 14–20 years, found that significant social predictors of suicidal behaviour were: gender, higher suicidal ideation and attempts among females; attendance at a religious institution and prayer with the family were negatively associated with suicidal behaviour; family structure, respondents from reconstituted families had higher suicidal ideation compared to other family structures, while intact families had the lowest rate for suicide attempts; and alcohol abuse in the family was positively associated with suicidal behaviour (Ali and Maharajh 2005).

Brazil is the largest and most populous country in Latin America (2005 population estimate: 185 million). Regardless of the low suicide rate, the total number of suicides was 8550 in 2005, which places Brazil amongst the top ten countries with the highest number of suicide deaths in the world (Brasil—Ministério da Saúde 2007).

A research project organised by the World Health Organization, and conducted in eight developing countries, the Multisite Intervention Study of Suicide Behaviour—SUPRE-MISS (Bertolote *et al.* 2005), examined the estimated prevalence of suicidal behaviour in the city of Campinas, Brazil. Life prevalence rates were 17.1 per cent for suicidal ideation, 4.8 per cent for plans and 2.8 per cent for suicide attempts. Only one-third of those who had attempted suicide were seen in emergency care settings of general hospitals. The 12-month prevalence rates were 5.3 per cent, 1.9 per cent and 0.4 per cent, respectively. Suicidal ideation was reported more frequently among women (OR = 1.7), young adults aged 20–29 years (OR = 2.9) and 30–39 years (OR = 3.6) when compared to the 14–19 year age group, those living alone (OR = 4.2) and those presenting mental disorders (OR = 3.8). These figures are similar to those found in most studies carried out in other countries (Botega *et al.* 2005a).

## Violence

In several Latin America countries, homicides and road accidents greatly outnumber suicides (Krug *et al.* 2002; Organización Panamericana de la Salud 2004). Violence has traditionally been related to broader social problems, such as increasing urbanization, expansion of illegal drugs and firearms trafficking, a lengthy economic crisis, unemployment, and widening income inequality. On the one hand, urban violence and high homicide rates have overshadowed the problem of suicidal behaviour in many South American countries. However, on the other hand, the growing discussion about violence and economic problems, which takes place in several sectors of society, has brought about awareness of suicidal behaviour among adolescents and young adults, as well as violence (including suicide) and prevention policies (Aree 2002; Botega and Garcia 2003).

## Suicide prevention

Apart from Brazil, which launched a national plan for suicide prevention in 2006, Latin American countries lack national suicide prevention programmes. However, some recent initiatives in Chile and Argentina illustrate the first steps towards national suicide prevention strategies. Several violence prevention efforts have been developed. Non-governmental organizations have played an important role in promoting awareness about the risks of carrying firearms and supporting projects for violence prevention. Nevertheless, more severe legislation to inhibit illegal gun ownership is needed, as 70 per cent of homicides are committed with clandestine firearms. In Bogota, Colombia, after the implementation of a multifaceted set of violence prevention policies, including restrictions on the sale of alcohol and to bear firearms on weekends and special occasions, homicides have fallen substantially (Villaveces et al. 2000).

There is also an urge for additional control of other means of suicide like pesticides and insecticides. In rural areas, the intentional ingestion of pesticides reinforces the need for an epidemiological investigation to better evaluate and quantify these events among the rural population (Pires et al. 2005). In the city of Rio de Janeiro, a carbamate insecticide (aldicarb) illegally commercialized as a rat poison is frequently used in suicide attempts (Lima and Reis 1995). Effective measures by government authorities should be implemented to counteract the commercialization of such products.

Governmental and non-governmental special training and educational programmes for low-income young people are a growing priority. These are especially relevant to prevent violent acts, since both suicide and homicide victims around 18–24 years have a significant age/grade gap. In this age group, only 3.5 per cent of those who committed suicide were enrolled in university, and 49 per cent had only primary schooling, according to a study carried out in Brazil (Souza et al. 2002).

Academic interest in suicidology has been increasing. Recent papers have gone a step beyond the analysis of mortality data banks, or the report of patients seen at health care services, e.g. the development and evaluation of reliable research instruments (Werlang and Botega 2003; Botega et al. 2005b), attitude changes in nursing personnel after a training course on suicide prevention (Berlim et al. 2007; Botega et al. 2007), genetics (Correa et al. 2004, 2007), including findings which support Shneidman's hypothesis that psychache, general psychological and emotional pain that reaches intolerable intensity is an important suicide-related variable, and indeed, represents a source of suicidal behaviour (Berlim et al. 2003).

## Conclusion

Suicidal behaviour has only recently emerged as an important issue in the public health sector in Central and South America. There is a need to develop suicide prevention strategies based on data derived from local research studies, such as epidemiological information on those psychiatric disorders mostly associated with suicidal behaviour; early detection and appropriate treatment of psychiatric disorders and psychosocial conditions, which are significantly associated with suicide; suicide-prevention training of health care professionals; availability of medication for both mood and schizophrenic disorders; restriction of access to means of suicide such as firearms and pesticides; appropriate treatment after a suicide attempt; and the reduction of stigma towards the mentally ill and those who attempt suicide.

## References

Abbinante AF, Pasqualatto D, Paris V (1995). Incidencia de intentos de suicidio atendidos por el ciato durante el periodo 1984–1991 [Incidence of suicide attempts attended at the Ciato during 1984–1991]. Farmacia al Dia, 6, 194–195.

Alarcón RD (2003). Mental health and mental health care in Latin America. World Psychiatry, 2, 54–56.

Ali A and Maharajh HD (2005). Social predictors of suicidal behaviour in adolescents in Trinidad and Tobago. Social Psychiatry and Psychiatric Epidemiology, 40, 186–191.

Andreollo NA, Lopes LR, Tercioti V Jr et al. (2003). Barrett's esophagus associated to caustic stenosis of the esophagus. Arquivos de Gastroenterologia, 40, 148–151.

Arie S (2002). Teenage suicides double as the future crumbles. British Medical Journal, 324, 1238.

Berlim MT, Mattevi BS, Pavanello DP et al. (2003). Psychache and suicidality in adult mood disordered outpatients in Brazil. Suicide and Life-Threatening Behavior, 33, 242–248.

Berlim MT, Perizzolo J, Lejderman F et al. (2007). Does a brief training on suicide prevention among general hospital personnel impact their baseline attitudes towards suicidal behavior? Journal of Affective Disorders, 100, 233–239.

Bertolote JM, Fleischmann A, De Leo D et al. (2005). Suicide attempts, plans, and ideation in culturally diverse sites: the WHO SUPRE-MISS community survey. Psychological Medicine, 35, 1457–1465.

Borges G, Saltijeral MT, Bimbela A et al. (2000). Suicide attempts in a sample of patients from a general hospital. Archives of Medical Research, 31, 366–372.

Botega NJ and Garcia LSL (2004). Brazil: the need for violence (including suicide) prevention. World Psychiatry, 3, 157–158.

Botega NJ, Barros MBA, Oliveira HB et al. (2005a). Suicide behavior in the community: prevalence and factors associated to suicidal ideation. Revista Brasileira de Psiquiatria, 27, 45–53.

Botega NJ, Reginato DG, Silva SV et al. (2005b) Nursing personnel attitudes toward suicide: the development of a measure scale. Revista Brasileira de Psiquiatria, 27, 315–318.

Botega NJ, Silva SV, Reginato DG et al. (2007) Maintained attitudinal changes in nursing personnel after a brief training on suicide prevention. Suicide and Life-Threatening Behavior, 37, 145–153.

Brasil-Ministério da Saúde (2007). Informações de Saúde–Estatísticas Vitais [Information on health—vital statistics]. Sistema de Informações sobre Mortalidade/MS/SUS/DASIS. Available at: http://tabnet.datasus.gov.br Acessed January 2007.

Correa H, Campi-Azevedo AC, De Marco L et al. (2004). Familial suicide behaviour: association with probands suicide attempt characteristics and 5-HTTLPR polymorphism. Acta Psychiatrica Scandinavica, 110, 459–464.

Correa H, De Marco L, Boson W et al. (2007). Association study of T102C 5-HT(2A) polymorphism in schizophrenic patients: diagnosis, psychopathology, and suicidal behavior. Dialogues in Clinical Neurosciences, 9, 97–101.

Drumond M, Lira MM, Freitas M et al. (1999). Evaluation of the quality of mortality information by unspecified accidents and events of undetermined intent. Revista de Saude Publica, 33, 273–280.

Freitas GV and Botega NJ (2002). Prevalence of depression, anxiety and suicide ideation in pregnant adolescents. Revista da Associação Médica Brasileira, 48, 245–249.

Juarez-Aragon G, Castanon-Gonzalez JA, Perez-Morales AJ et al. (1999). Clinical and epidemiological characteristics of severe poisoning in an adult population admitted to an intensive care unit. *Gaceta Médica de México*, **135**, 669–675.

Krug EG, Dahlberg LL, Mercy JA *et al.* (eds) (2002). *World Report on Violence and Health*. World Health Organization, Geneva.

Larrobla C and Botega NJ (2001). Restructuring mental health: a South American survey. *Social Psychiatry and Psychiatric Epidemiology*, **36**, 256–259.

Lawrynowicz AE and Baker TD (2005). Suicide and latitude in Argentina: Durkheim upside-down. *American Journal of Psychiatry*, **162**, 1022.

Leveridge YR (1999). The pattern of poisoning in Costa Rica during 1997. *Veterinarian and Human Toxicology*, **41**, 100–102.

Lima JS and Reis CA (1995). Poisoning due to illegal use of carbamates as a rodenticide in Rio de Janeiro. *Journal of Toxicology—Clinical Toxicology*, **33**, 687–690.

Lucero R, Díaz N, Villalba L (2003). Caracterización clínica y epidemiológica de los suicidios en Montevideo y de los intentos de autoeliminación (IAE) en el Hospital de Clínicas en el período abril 2000–abril 2001 [Clinical and epidemiological characteristics of suicide cases in Montevideo and suicide attempts at the Hospital de Clínicas, April 2000–April 2001]. *Revista de Psiquiatría del Uruguay*, **67**, 5–20.

Mamede RC and De Mello Filho FV (2002). Treatment of caustic ingestion: an analysis of 239 cases. *Diseases of Esophagus*, **15**, 210–213.

Morgado AF (1991). The Guarani-Kaiwa suicide epidemic: investigating its causes and suggesting the 'impossible return' hypothesis. *Cadernos de Saúde Pública*, **7**, 585–598.

Nock MK and Marzuk PM (2002). Suicide and violence. In Hawton K and Heeringen K, eds, *The International Handbook of Suicide and Attempted Suicide*, pp. 437–456. Wiley, Chichester.

Oliveira CS and Lotufo Neto F (2003). Suicide among indigenous people: a Brazilian statistical view. *Revista de Psiquiatria Clínica*, **30**, 4–10.

Organización Panamericana de la Salud (2004). *Situación de la salud en las Americas, indicadores básicos* [Health conditions in the Americas: basic statistics]. OPS, Washington.

Pires DX, Caldas ED, Recena MC (2005). Pesticide use and suicide in the State of Mato Grosso do Sul, Brazil. *Cadernos de Saúde Pública*, **21**, 598–605.

Rapeli CB and Botega NJ (2005). Clinical profiles of serious suicide attempters consecutively admitted to a university-based hospital: a cluster analysis study. *Revista Brasileira de Psiquiatria*, **27**, 285–289.

Retamal P and Humphreys D (1998). Occurrence of suicide and seasonal variation. *Revista de Saúde Pública*, **32**, 408–412.

Rodríguez AH, Caldera T, Kullgren G *et al.* (2006). Suicidal expressions among young people in Nicaragua: a community-based study. *Social Psychiatry and Psychiatric Epidemiology*, **41**, 692–697.

Rodrigues NC and Werneck GL (2005). Age–period–cohort analysis of suicide rates in Rio de Janeiro, Brazil, 1979–1998. *Social Psychiatry and Psychiatric Epidemiology*, **40**, 192–196.

Sanchéz R, Orejarena S, Guzman Y (2004). Characteristics of suicides in Bogota, 1985–2000. *Revista de Salud Pública*, **6**, 217–234.

Sánchez R, Orejarena S, Guzmán Y *et al.* (2002). Suicidio en Bogotá: un fenómeno que aumenta en poblaciones jóvenes [Suicide in Bogota: an increasing phenomenon among youth]. *Biomédica*, **22**, 417–424.

Serfaty EM, Foglia L, Masautis A *et al.* (2003). Violent causes of death in young people of 10 to 24 years old. Argentina 1991–2000. *Vertex*, **14**, 40–48.

Souza E, Minayo M, Malaquias J (2002). Suicide among young people in selected Brazilian state capitals. *Cadernos de Saúde Pública*, **18**, 673–683.

Trujillo AH, Escudero GTR, Enamorado MCD *et al.* (1999). Influencia Del Medio Familiar en un Grupo de 5 a 19 Años con Riesgo Suicida [Family dynamics' influence on a group of suicidal teengers aged 5–19 years old]. *Revista Cubana de Medicina General Integral*, **15**, 372–377.

Villaveces A, Cummings P, Espitia VE *et al.* (2000). Effect of a ban on carrying firearms on homicides rates in two Colombian cities. *Journal of the American Medical Association*, **283**, 1205–1209.

Weissman MM, Bland RC, Canino GJ *et al.* (1999). Prevalence of suicide ideation and suicide attempts in nine countries. *Psychological Medicine*, **29**, 9–17.

Werlang BS and Botega NJ (2003). A semi-structured interview for psychological autopsy: an inter-rater reliability study. *Suicide and Life-Threatening Behavior*, **33**, 326–330.

# CHAPTER 19

# Suicide attempts in North America

Morton M Silverman

## Abstract

North America comprises Canada, the United States of America (USA), Mexico, and the Caribbean Island nations. North America covers 9,355,000 square miles (24,230,000 square kilometres). The two largest countries, Canada and the United States of America, have populations of approximately 33.4 million and 301.1 million respectively, and are home to multiple ethnic and racial groups, including Native Americans and immigrants from many other continents. The suicide rate in Canada has tended to be higher than that of the USA during the last two decades. There is virtually no reliable data on suicide and suicide attempt rates in North American countries other than Canada and the USA.

Suicide was the third leading cause of death for the age group 15–19 years in the USA during 2000. In Canada, suicide was the second leading cause of death for the age group 15–24 years, and the leading cause of death for men aged 25–29 and 40–44, together with women aged 30–34, and it is estimated that there are at least 100 attempts for every completed suicide. Furthermore, there are substantial variations across gender, age, and ethnic groups.

Suicide attempts in North America are a growing concern. Suicide attempts are known to be a primary risk factor for future suicidal behaviours, and those who have previously attempted suicide are at an increased risk of death by suicide. Brickman and Mintz (2003) claim that suicide attempt rates have more than doubled from 600 to 1600/100,000 from 1992–1999, with indications of continuously increasing. Therefore, more epidemiological research needs to be done in order to understand this problem.

This chapter examines published surveillance records and hospital records on the prevalence, trends, social and demographic factors of suicide attempts in North America.

## Epidemiology of suicide attempts in the USA

Data on suicide attempts in the USA are estimates at best, ranging from 600,000 to 1.8 million/year. Unfortunately, it is very difficult to get an exact number of suicide attempts given the percentages of misdiagnoses and lack of active monitoring systems (Claasen et al. 2006). Only one state in the USA systematically collects emergency department data on suicide attempts, and only for adolescents aged 17 and under. Furthermore, not everyone seeks medical treatment following a suicide attempt or self-injurious act. An obstacle to accurate surveillance is that there is no uniform definition for a suicide attempt (De Leo et al. 2006; Silverman et al. 2007), and there remains much confusion in the field regarding the appropriate use of terms such as deliberate self-harm, intentional self-injury, accidental self-harm, and suicide attempt when labeling self-injurious behaviours (Silverman 2006).

## Trends in suicide attempts in the USA

Annual data taken on attempted suicide rates in the USA were obtained by using CDC's Web-based Injury Statistics Query and Reporting System (WISQARS™ 2007). Hospitalizations due to intentional self-harm had increased over the 6-year span. In 2001–2002, self-harm rates were approximately 115/100,000, and then sharply increased to more than 140/100,000 in years 2003–04. Rates began to fall again in 2006 at approximately 135/100,000. However, there was an overall increase of self-harm rates of 20/100,000 from 2001 to 2006.

## Age-distributed suicide attempts in the USA

Suicide attempts among age-groups differ substantially in the USA. The highest suicide attempt rate is among the 15–24 age group. Adolescents have the highest ratio of non-fatal suicide attempts to suicide completions of all age groups (King 1997). Estimates of the ratio of attempts to completions in adolescence have ranged from about 100:1 to about 350:1. Extrapolating from the CDC's Youth Risk Behaviour Survey, a biannual survey of non-fatal suicidal behaviours among nationally representative samples of high school students in the USA, the ratio may be more than 800:1 for self-reported attempts and close to 300:1 for those requiring medical attention after the attempt. The typical youthful suicide attempter is a young female who ingests drugs at home in front of others.

In 2001, self-harm rates among the 15–24 age group were approximately 534/100,000, and then increased to its highest rate of 662/100,000 in 2004. In 2006, the self-harm rates for that age group levelled off at a rate of 609/100,000, having increased by a rate of 75/100,000 over the 6-year span (Figure 19.1).

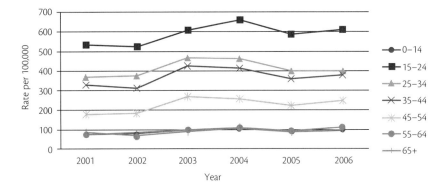

**Fig. 19.1** Crude rate per 100,000 for all self-harm injuries in US, distributed by age, 2001–2006. Source: WISQARS™ 2007. Based on information from the US Centers of Disease Control and Prevention.

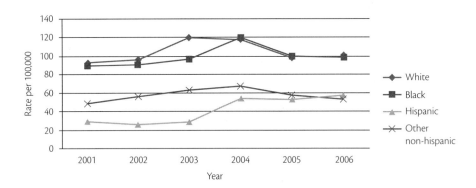

**Fig. 19.2** Crude rate per 100,000 for all self-harm injuries in US, distributed by ethnicity, 2001–2006. Source: WISQARS™ 2007. Based on information from the US Centers of Disease Control and Prevention.

## Suicide attempts in the USA distributed by gender

Intentional self-harm rates differ significantly between genders as well. Females have considerably higher rates than their male counterparts. This differential may be an artefact of surveillance, in as much as USA females seek health services at a much higher rate than males, and males are less likely to acknowledge self-injurious behaviours. There is, however, a similar trend expressed by both sexes over the 6-year span. Both sexes have had increased rates of self-harm; females were at 126/100,000 in 2001 and increased to 155/100,000 in 2006; and males were at 100/100,000 in 2001 and increased to 110/100,000 in 2006.

## Methods used in suicide attempts in USA

Poisoning was the number one choice of method for suicide attempts, with rates more than four times higher than the second most common method (cutting). The trend between 2001–2006 indicates that during 2002 there was a surge in the methodical use of poisoning for suicide attempts with rates rising from approximately 75 to 95/100,000, however, declined to just below 75/100,000 in 2006.

Nevertheless, studies have indicated that firearms are the number one method used in completed suicides in 2001, with 49 per cent in the 10–19 age group (CDC 2004). Given that firearms are often lethal, thus leading to death, firearms as a method have lower rates than other methods in suicide attempts.

## Ethnicity and suicide attempts in the USA

The trend for suicide attempts differs among ethnic groups, though similarities did occur in trends among whites and blacks. Figure 19.2 illustrates a rather similar pattern for suicide attempts among both whites and blacks from 2001–02, and in 2003, suicide attempt rates for blacks increased significantly, then levelled off and became similar to their white counterparts in 2006. Hispanics have shown a steady increase over the 6-year span reaching higher rates than other non-Hispanic groups in 2006.

Other studies have shown variations in suicide attempts among ethnic groups (YVPC 2003). Native Americans have the highest percentage of suicide attempts compared to their counterparts and nearly two times higher than Caucasians and nearly three times higher than African Americans. Unlike the data shown in Figure 19.2, this study showed that Hispanics had higher suicide attempts than both Caucasians and African Americans.

## Suicide attempts by state in the USA

Data published in the third edition of the State Injury Indicators Report illustrate considerable variations among states (Johnson *et al.* 2004). Wisconsin has the highest suicide attempt rate reaching nearly 90/100,000, followed by Arkansas at 74/100,000 and Utah at 72/100,000. Nebraska has the lowest rate with approximately 29/100,000.

## Epidemiology of suicide attempts in Canada

Data on hospitalizations due to intentional self-harm are limited in Canada, and therefore, often needs to be supplemented with other data sources for a clearer understanding of the problem (Health Canada 2002). Data from the National Trauma Registry at the Canadian Institute of Health Information and Canada's National Statistical Agency are utilized in this chapter.

## Trends in suicide attempts distributed by gender and age in Canada

In a report on mental illness in Canada, suicide trends among sexes differ substantially over the 13-year span of 1987/8 to 1999/2000 (Health Canada 2002). Figure 19.3 demonstrates that females had

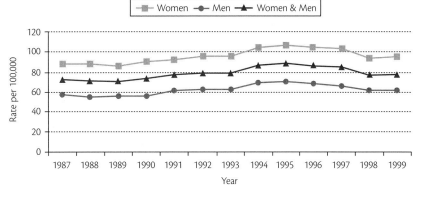

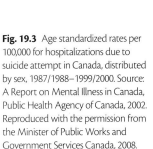

**Fig. 19.3** Age standardized rates per 100,000 for hospitalizations due to suicide attempt in Canada, distributed by sex, 1987/1988–1999/2000. Source: A Report on Mental Illness in Canada, Public Health Agency of Canada, 2002. Reproduced with the permission from the Minister of Public Works and Government Services Canada, 2008.

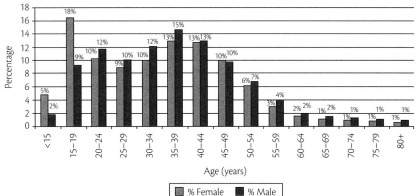

**Fig. 19.4** Hospitalizations due to suicide attempt in Canada, distributed by age and sex, 2001–2002. Source: Canadian Institute for Health Information (2004). Reproduced with kind permission.

much higher suicide attempt rates than their male counterparts. There was a peak for both sexes in 1995, then a decline into 1999. The overall trends for both genders follow similar patterns, with both having steady rates throughout this period.

Among all age groups, until 1995, the 15–24-year-olds had the highest suicide attempt rates. Conversely, from years 1995 to 2000, the 25–44 age group had the highest suicide attempt rates. In 1999/2000, the 25–44 age group had the highest rates, followed by 15–24 years and 45–64 years.

However, when the age groups are categorized in intervals of 5 years, the 15–19 and 35–39 groups have the highest percentages of suicide attempts, followed by the 40–44 age group.

According to Langlois and Morrison (2002), females in the 15–19 age group are more likely to make a suicide attempt than their male counterparts, with rates as high as 221/100,000 for females and 87/100,000 for males in 1999.

The CIHI report (2002) shows similar patterns for females aged 15–19 years (Figure 19.4). During 2001/02, females in this age group had the highest percentage of suicide attempts with 16 per cent and males 9 per cent, respectively. Females in this age group had nearly twice the percentage of suicide attempts than males. However, somewhat surprisingly, males aged 20 years and older have higher suicide attempts than females.

### Methods distributed by sex for suicide attempts in Canada

Similar to the United States, poisoning is the number one method used in a suicide attempt by both males and females. A total of 88 per cent of females were hospitalized for a suicide attempt due to poisoning of a solid/liquid, and 75 per cent of males. The second most commonly used method is cutting/piercing;

however, this method is higher among males (12 per cent) than females (8 per cent) (Figure 19.5).

Overall, the most common method used in completed suicide is suffocation—40 per cent males and 33.9 per cent females—however among females, the most common method was still poisoning at 41.3 per cent (Langlois and Morrison 2002)

### Ethnicity and suicide attempts in Canada

Studies have shown that suicide, suicide attempts and suicidal behaviour are much higher among aboriginal groups in Canada, especially those of the First Nation tribe (Inuit) (Kirmayer *et al.* 1996; Health Canada 2001).

There is little data reported on hospitalizations due to self-inflicted harm among Inuit communities, although Alberta statistics on emergency visits shows that during the year 2000, Members of the First Nation communities were hospitalized for attempted suicide were 6.74 times higher than those from non-First Nation populations (ACICR 2005).

### Suicide attempts distributed by province in Canada

The Territories had the highest suicide attempt rate at 19.3/10,000, followed by New Brunswick 9.6/10,000 and Saskatchewan 9.4/10,000. Quebec had the lowest suicide attempt rate at 4.6/10,000.

## Clinical aspects of suicide attempters

If there is one truism in evaluating risk for future behaviour, it is that the most significant predictor of future behaviour is past behaviour. About one-third of completed adolescent suicides have made a known prior attempt (Brent *et al.* 1999) with the

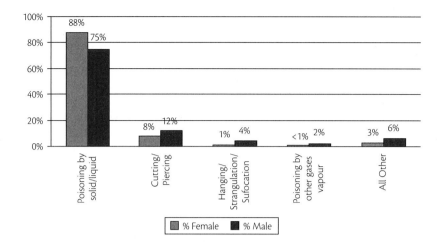

**Fig. 19.5** Cause of suicide attempt hospitalization in Canada, distributed by sex, 2001–2002. Source: Canadian Institute for Health Information (2004). Reproduced with kind permission.

prevalence of past attempts being more common among females. Once an attempt is made at any level of lethality, the risk for future and more serious attempts and completion increases significantly. Prior suicidal behaviour is more clinically significant to a current assessment when it was relatively recent, relatively lethal, or more death-intentioned; did not lead to a positive therapeutic experience or consequence; or was one of multiple, repetitive non-fatal attempts (Berman *et al.* 2006).

Reynolds and Eaton (1986) in Canada compared multiple suicide attempters with single attempters and found that repeaters had higher levels of depression, hopelessness, and substance abuse, as well as higher lethality ratings. Kessler *et al.* (1999) in the National Comorbidity Study conducted in the USA found that the risk for first suicide attempt related to being female, being previously married, having less than 12 years of education, and the presence of any mood disorder, non-affective psychosis, post-traumatic stress disorder, any substance abuse disorder, antisocial personality disorder, or generalized anxiety disorder.

In general population surveys, persons with a suicide attempt in their lifetime were 2.6 (Canada) and 8.4 (United States of America) times more likely to also have had a psychiatric disorder at some point in their lives (Tanney 2000). Plutchik (1995) listed 41 factors that were found to be correlated with the risk for suicide attempts, including psychiatric, psychological, situational, family, socio-economic, genetic, and historical variables.

In the USA National Comorbidity Study, the attempters reported that close to 40 per cent made a 'serious' life-threatening attempt, 13 per cent made a 'serious' attempt but did not use a 'foolproof' method, and 47 per cent made a 'cry for help' without the intent to die. Owens *et al.* (2002) found that following an episode of self-harm, 17 per cent will repeat within one year. Beautrais (2003) found that among her cohort of medically serious suicide attempters requiring hospitalization 8 per cent had died within 5 years (59 per cent by suicide). Hence, until proven otherwise, all suicide attempts must be taken very seriously.

In as much as there is a large overlap between the risk factors for suicide attempters and completers, the treatment for at risk suicide attempters does not differ from treatment approaches for at risk suicide completers. Once a suicide attempt has occurred, however, the focus is twofold: prevent the likelihood of any future suicidal behaviours and address the underlying

factors that precipitated the suicide attempt. Some key steps are to completely explore the events and thinking processes that lead up to the attempt, as well as understanding the consequences of the attempt for the individual. Stressful life events, as defined by the individual, often precipitate suicidal behaviour. Such stressful life events may include: relationship problems, interpersonal conflicts, problems with the law, recent humiliation and shaming events, and perceived acute losses. A strategic approach consists of exploring the problem, defining the problem, generating alternative solutions, testing hypotheses, and pursuing a resolution.

Suicide is rarely studied prospectively. Our theories, our hypotheses, and our assumptions are generally built on retrospective analyses of suicidal behaviours. Suicide attempters are our closest connection to the suicidal mind, and we need to work carefully with these individuals to better understand the mechanisms that lead to self-destructive behaviours.

## Conclusion

The annual rate and number of suicide attempts in Canada and the USA are a significant public health problem. Unfortunately, data provided on suicide attempts are merely estimates, and although these estimations give a reasonable view of the problem, they are far from accurate. Hospital and emergency department monitoring systems ought to be better implemented to get more accurate data on suicide attempts. Furthermore, we are lacking reliable surveillance data on suicide and suicide attempts from such countries as Mexico, Jamaica, Cuba, Trinidad and Tobago, and other Caribbean nations.

Nonetheless, the problem of suicide and suicidal behaviour continues to be a large public health problem and of great concern. More research is needed in identifying these behaviours, understanding their etiologies, and preventing them through collaborative efforts and interventions.

## References

Alberta Centre for Injury Control and Research (2005). *Injury-related Health Services use by First Nations in Alberta. Hospital Admissions, 2000 & Emergency Department Visits, 2000*. Alberta Centre for Injury Control and Research, Edmonton.

Anderson RN (2002). *Deaths: Leading causes for 2000. National Vital Statistics Reports, 50*. National Center for Health Statistics, Hyattsville.

Beautrais A (2003). Subsequent mortality in medically serious suicide attempts. A 5 year follow-up. *Australia and New Zealand Journal of Psychiatry*, **37**, 595–599.

Berman AL, Jobes DA, Silverman MM (2006). *Adolescent Suicide: Assessment and Intervention*. Washington, American Psychological Association,.

Brent DA, Baugher M, Bridge J, Chen J, Beery L (1999). Age and sex-related risk factors for adolescent suicide. *Journal of the American Academy of Child and Adolescent Psychiatry*, **38**, 1497–1505.

Brickman AL and Mintz DC (2003). US rates of self-inflicted injury and suicide. *Psychiatric Services*, **54**, 168.

Canadian Institute for Health Information (2004). *Hospitalizations Due to Suicide Attempts and Self-Inflicted Injury in Canada, 2001–2002*. National Trauma Registry Analytic Bulletin, Toronto (ON).

Canada Safety Council (2004). *Canada's Silent Tragedy*. Vol. XLVIII, No. 1. Retrieved 22 October 2007 at: http://www.safety-council.org/news/sc/2004/January.html.

Claassen CA, Trivedi MH, Shimizu I *et al.* (2006). Epidemiology of nonfatal deliberate self-harm in the United States as described in three medical databases. *Suicide and Life-Threatening Behaviour*, **36**, 192–212.

Centers for Disease Control and Prevention, National Center for Injury Prevention and Control (2007). *Web-based Injury Statistics Query and Reporting System (WISQARS)*. Retrieved 22 October 2007 at: http://www.cdc.gov/ncipc/wisqars.

Center for Disease Control and Prevention (2004). Methods of suicide among persons aged 10–19 years – United States, 1992–2001. *MMWR* **53**, 471–4.

De Leo D, Burgis S, Bertoote J *et al.* (2006). Definitions of suicidal behaviour: lessons learned from the WHO/EURO Multicentre Study. *Crisis*, **27**, 4–15.

Health Canada (2001). *Unintentional and Intentional Injury Profile for Aboriginal People in Canada*. Health Canada, Ottawa.

Health Canada (2002). *A Report on Mental Illness in Canada*. Ottawa: Retrieved on October 24, 2007 at: http://www.phac-aspc.gc.ca/publicat/miic-mmac/pdf/men_ill_e.pdf

Johnson RL, Thomas RG, Thomas KE *et al.* (2007). *State Injury Indicators Report, Third Edition — 2004 Data*. Centers for Disease Control and Prevention, National Center for Injury Prevention and Control, Atlanta.

Kessler RC, Borges G, Walters EE (1999). Prevalence of and risk factors for lifetime suicide attempts in the Natonal Comorbidity Survey. *Archives of General Psychiatry*, **56**, 617–626.

King CA (1997). Suicidal behaviour in adolescence. In RW Maris, MM Silverman, SS Canetto, eds, *Review of Suicidology*, pp. 61–95 Guilford Press, New York.

Kirmayer LJ, Malus M, Boothroyd LJ (1996). Suicide attempts among Inuit youth: a community survey of prevalence and risk factors. *Acta Psychiatrica Scandinavica*, **94**, 8–17.

Langlois S and Morrison P (2002). Suicide deaths and suicide attempts. *Health Reports*, **13**, 9–22.

Owens D, Horrocks J, House A (2002). Fatal and non-fatal repetition of self-harm. Systematic review. *British Journal of Psychiatry*, **181**, 193–199.

Plutchik R (1995). Outward and inward directed aggressiveness: the interaction between violence and suicidality. *Pharmacopsychiatry*, **28**, 47–57.

Reynolds P and Eaton P (1986). Multiple attempters of suicide presenting at an emergency department. *Canadian Journal of Psychiatry*, **31**, 328–330.

Silverman MM (2006). The language of suicidology. *Suicide and Life-Threatening Behaviour*, **36**, 519–532.

Silverman MM, Berman AL, Sanddal ND *et al.* (2007). Rebuilding the Tower of Babel: a revised nomenclature for the study of suicide and suicidal behaviours. Part 2: Suicide-related ideations, communications, and behaviours. *Suicide and Life-Threatening Behaviour*, **37**, 2864–277.

Suicide Information and Education Centre (2001). *A Suicide Attempt is Meaningful and Significant*. Retrieved 22 October 2007 at: http://www.suicideinfo.ca/csp/assets/alert45.pdf.

Tanney BL (2000). Psychiatric diagnosis and suicidal acts. In RW Maris, AL Berman, MM Silverman, *Comprehensive Textbook of Suicidology*, pp. 311–341. Guilford Press, New York.

Youth Violence Prevention Center (2003). *Under the Microscope: Asian and Pacific Islander Youth in Oakland*. API Youth Violence Prevention Center: National Council on Crime & Delinquency. Oakland, California. Retrieved 25 October 2007 at: http://www.api-center.org/documents/microscope_full_report.pdf.

# CHAPTER 20

# Suicide attempts in Europe

Ellenor Mittendorfer Rutz and Armin Schmidtke

## Abstract

The comparison of international statistics on suicide attempt across European countries is challenged by differences in definitions and the lack of compulsory registration of suicide attempts. The WHO/EURO multi-centre study on parasuicide has overcome these obstacles, and has provided comprehensive data on both the occurrence and background factors of suicide attempt in different European countries. This article summarizes findings from the WHO/EURO study as well as from various other clinical and community surveys carried out in the region. Peculiarities of the inter-European variation in patterns and trends of the phenomenon and various social and psychiatric determinants are described in detail. The WHO/EURO study is continued as the MONSUE (Monitoring suicidal behaviour in Europe) study, which will supply even more detailed data on specific risk groups. These can then be supported by tailor-made suicide prevention strategies.

## Introduction

Attempted suicide patients constitute a heterogeneous group with respect to evidence of planning, degree of medical damage, and choice of methods and intent, which can range from a cry for help, revenge, relief of anxiety and even to a clear intent to die. Differences in the definition of suicide attempt, and the lack of compulsory registration of deliberate self-inflicted injuries and poisonings in most European countries, make international comparison of clinical and epidemiological studies difficult.

Scandinavian countries have registers with national coverage on information of hospital admission after a suicide attempt. This data only records around 60 per cent of individuals attempting suicide, reflecting the actual size of the problem as being much bigger (Ramberg 2003). When interpreting the data on hospital admissions, one must keep in mind that this data is influenced by changes in accessibility and routines in health care services, as well as changes in the lethality of methods used.

### The WHO/Euro multi-centre study on attempted suicide

In order to overcome this lack of international comparable longitudinal data, the WHO/EURO multi-centre study on parasuicide (attempted suicide) was initiated in 1989, applying uniform methodology on studying suicide attempters who contact the health care system. The study collected longitudinal data from 16 European centres in 13 countries, with catchment areas, each approximately 200,000–300,000 inhabitants(Schmidtke et al. 1996) The study not only applied a uniform definition of suicideattempt, but also uniform definitions for a wide range of background factors, ranging from information on demographic, socio-economic, and psychosocial determinants to a detailed description of the methods utilized. The study is unique worldwide and contributes essential knowledge on prevalence of and risk groups for suicide attempts in Europe.

## The epidemiology of suicide attempts in Europe

Data obtained from this WHO/EURO monitoring study, based on hospital admission data, indicate a considerable variation of suicide attempt rates in Europe. The rates in the various entries ranged from 69/100,000 in Guipuzcoa, Spain to 462/100,000 in Cergy-Pontoise, France for females, and from 45/100,000 in Guipuzcoa to 314/100,000 in Helsinki, Finland for males (Schmidtke et al. 1996). Besides the accessibility and quality of mental health services, several cultural and socio-economic determinants influence the regional variations insuicidal behaviour. Cultural patterns may influence attitudestowards suicidal behaviour as well as help-seeking behaviour and the choice of methods used.

This international variability in the prevalence of suicideattempt is also reflected in data from community surveys: the prevalence of lifetime suicide attempts in the general population reached 2.6 per cent, 3.6 per cent, and 5.1 per cent in two Swedish studies and one Latvian study, respectively (Ramberg and Wasserman 2000; Salander Renberg et al. 2001; Rancans et al. 2003).

## Age and gender

In most European countries, females are more likely to attempt suicide than males. In the WHO/EURO study, the male:female ratio of attempted suicide of individuals over 15 years was 1:1.5 (Schmidtke et al. 1996). This ratio decreases with age to 1:1.1 in over 65-year-olds (De Leo et al. 2001). Finland seems to be the only exception with regard to gender differences in suicide attempt. The male:female ratio in Helsinki in the WHO/EURO study was

1:0.8, and the past year prevalence in a community based study was 0.9 per cent in women and 1.1 per cent in males (Hintikka J *et al.* 1998).

Suicide attempt rates typically decrease with increasing age, and the peak age for females tends to be lower than for males (Schmidtke *et al.* 1996). In nearly 50 per cent of the centres in the WHO/EURO study, the highest person-based rates were found in 15–24-year-old females (Schmidtke *et al.* 1996). Among males, the highest rates were in 25–34-year-olds in 10 of 15 centres.

The rates for 15–24-year-old girls reached 766/100,000 compared to 127/100,000 in women 55 years and older in Cergy-Pontoise, France. In community-based studies, the rates for adolescents were reported to reach 3.3 per cent for girls and 1.3 per cent for boys according to a Dutch study; and 3 per cent and 9 per cent for adolescents in a Swiss and Polish study, respectively (Kienhorst *et al.* 1990; Rey Gex *et al.* 1998; Gmitrowicz *et al.* 2003).

## Trends

In the WHO/EURO study on parasuicide during the period 1989–1992, the male suicide attempt rates decreased on average by 17 per cent and the female rates by 14 per cent, including data from 16 centres in Europe (Schmidtke *et al.* 1996). There is, however, evidence of recent increases reported for suicide attempts from countries with available data through national coverage or regional hospital admission data. The suicide attempt rate in the youngest age group, particularly among young girls, has been continuously increasing since the last 10 years in Sweden (Swedish National Board of Health and Welfare 2007). While the suicide attempt rate in 15–24-year-old girls was 190 per 100,000 in Sweden in 1990, it increased to 322 per 100,000 in 2004 (Swedish National Board of Health and Welfare 2007). Even evidence from regional hospital admission data at two different sites in England suggests a considerable increase in suicide attempts among other older age groups in young girls (Hawton *et al.* 2003b; O'Loughlin and Sherwood 2005). Reasons for this recent increase in suicide attempt rates, particularly among the young, are multifaceted, but may include an increase in mental disorders and substance abuse, changes among traditional family structures, increases in unemployment, and social isolation among others (Mittendorfer Rutz 2006).

## Methods for suicide attempts

The choice of methods for suicide attempt reflects the accessibility of means, the individual preference, cultural acceptability and the intent behind the behaviour. Non-violent methods (primarily self-poisoning) are most frequently found among suicide attempters, whereas violent or more lethal methods (hanging, shooting, jumping, drowning, and cutting) are often chosen for completed suicide. Males are more inclined to use more drastic violent methods than females, while women are over-represented among suicide attempters using poisoning. This gender difference in the chosen method is regarded as one of the reasons behind the gender paradox of suicidal behaviour. Violent suicide attempts can be regarded as having a stronger association with completed suicide, possibly reflecting a progress in the suicidal process often starting with non-violent suicidal behaviour (self-poisoning).

Based on data from the WHO/EURO multicentre study, 73 per cent of all events for men and 84 per cent for women consumed drugs, which were primarily psychotropic (Michel *et al.* 2000). Cutting and alcohol were the next most frequently used methods, with both being used in less than 17 per cent of episodes. The frequency of other methods was below 3 per cent. The choice of different methods for suicide attempt also varied considerably across regions in Europe. The highest rates for drug overdoses were found among female attempters in Oxford (347/100,000) Helsinki (238/100,000) and Stockholm (221/100,000). Guipuzcoa had the lowest rates (61/100,000) (Michel *et al.* 2000). The differences were most prominent in the 15–24 age group, with outstanding rates for women in Oxford (653/100,000), which was mainly due to the frequent use of analgesics.

Cutting, however, was particularly favoured by men (30 per cent of all events) in Wuerzburg, Germany and Innsbruck, Austria (Michel *et al.* 2000). Szeged, Hungary had exceptionally high rates of suicide attempt by pesticides and solvents, which comprised 20 and 15 per cent of all events in men and women respectively. In one quarter of all events, multiple methods were used, again showing considerable regional differences (Michel *et al.* 2000). This is not including multiple drug use, which is known to be common in suicide attempts (Michel *et al.* 1994, Neeleman and Wessely 1997).

## Socio-economic and marital status

The sociological approach, already postulated by Durkheim, mainly explains the variation in the frequency of suicidal behaviour by certain societal conditions, which increase or decrease the tendency to react to individual life difficulties. Low socio-economic status, e.g. low educational level, long-term unemployment, and social welfare receipts increase the risk of suicide attempt (Schmidtke *et al.* 1996; Christoffersen *et al.* 2003). According to data from the WHO/EURO multi-centre study, more than half of all suicide attempters have only a low level of education (Schmidtke *et al.* 1996). Furthermore, the proportion of unemployed and economically inactive people among the suicide attempters reached up to a fifth and a third respectively. A low socio-economic status seems to increase the risk of suicide attempt, independently of mental disorder, alcohol and drug abuse, or foster care during childhood (Christoffersen *et al.* 2003).

Single, widowed, and divorced individuals are typically over-represented in suicide attempters (Schmidtke *et al.* 1996; Hawton *et al.* 2003). As much as 18 per cent of suicide attempters were divorced or separated (Schmidtke *et al.* 1996). Males seem to be more vulnerable for separation and living alone (Hawton *et al.* 2003a).

## Psychopathology

Psychopathology clearly represents the strongest risk factor for suicide attempt. Up to 98 per cent of suicide attempters meet criteria for any psychiatric disorder, according to various European studies (Suiominen and Lonnqvist 1996; Persson *et al.* 1999; Balazs *et al.* 2003). Prior hospital admission due to any mental disorder is common in both young (26 per cent) and old (41 per cent) suicide attempters, and increases the risk by 30 to 33 times (Christoffersen *et al.* 2003; Mittendorfer Rutz 2005; Hawton and Harriss 2006).

The mental disorders which suicide attempters predominantly suffer from include substance abuse, affective and personality disorders (Suiominen and Lonnqvist 1996; Persson *et al.* 1999; Haw *et al.* 2001; Balazs *et al.* 2003; Mittendorfer Rutz 2005). Suicide attempts seem to be strongly associated with depressive disorders in females, and substance abuse disorders in males (Suiominen and Lonnqvist 1996; Wunderlich *et al.* 2001; Fekete *et al.* 2005). Substance abuse is common in suicide attempters. Up to 30 per cent of females abuse alcohol, according to a study carried out in Oxford (Hawton *et al.* 2003a). A high proportion (up to 80 per cent) of suicide attempters suffer from comorbid mental disorders, including comorbidity with personality disorders (Suiominen and Lonnqvist 1996; Haw *et al.* 2001; Hawton *et al.* 2003a).

## Repetition of attempted suicide

Recurrent suicidal behaviour places a great burden on the patients, on their relationships, and on the health care and welfare system. The risk of repetition of attempts was estimated to be 14 per cent, in a multi-centre study, during a 12-month follow-up period (Kapur *et al.* 2006). The tendency for repetitive self-destructive behaviour seems to increase with decreasing age as the 12-months-repletion risk reached 24 per cent in adolescents (Hulten *et al.* 2001). As many as 42 per cent and 45 per cent of male and female suicide attempters included in the WHO/EURO multi-centre study reported previous attempts respectively (Schmidtke *et al.* 1996). Several conditions increase the risk of repeating a suicide attempt, including the choice of violent method in earlier attempts, availability of psychiatric treatment, alcohol misuse, divorce, and unemployment (Schmidtke *et al.* 1996; Hulten *et al.* 2001; Kapur *et al.* 2006). The type of psychiatric diagnoses also seems to be different in repeaters when compared to 'first-ever' suicide attempters (Schmidtke *et al.* 1996). Addiction diagnoses, neuroses and personality disorders seem to be more frequent in male repeaters, while fewer males have had adjustment disorders and acute reaction to stress.

## Follow-up care of suicide attempters

Adequate follow-up care is crucial for effective treatment and prevention of further suicidality (Morgan *et al.* 1993; Dieserud *et al.* 2000; Motto and Bostrom 2001; Vaiva *et al.* 2006). However, large disparities with regard to the delivery and quality of follow-up care can be found across European countries, as well as within a particular country (Hulten *et al.* 2000; Suominen and Lonnqvist 2006). Results from the WHO monitoring study revealed that the proportion of young suicide attempters without follow-up can reach up to 56 per cent in some European countries (Hulten *et al.* 2000). However, both having previous attempted suicide and using violent methods were associated with an increased possibility of having recommended follow-up care (Hulten *et al.* 2000).

The type of after care most often recommended (53 per cent in males and 50 per cent in females) to suicide attempters was 'inpatient care' (Schmidtke *et al.* 1996). Several factors seem to predict the referral to inpatient care in a psychiatric hospital. Among those that ought to be mentioned are older age, psychotic and mood disorder, lack of alcohol consumption preceding the attempt, somatic disorder, suicide attempt on a weekday, and previous psychiatric treatment (Suominen and Lonnqvist 2006). 'Outpatient treatment' was recommended in 22 per cent and 19 per cent of female and male cases, respectively, followed by non-hospital based treatment (16 per cent and 14 per cent, respectively) (Schmidtke *et al.* 1996).

## Relation of suicide attempt to suicide

Suicide attempt and completion are two different phenomena with considerable overlap. They differ among other determinants with regard to their gender and age pattern, as well as in the intent and methods utilized for the act. A suicide attempt is by far the strongest risk factor for a completed suicide. Within nine years, 5 per cent of suicide attempters will eventually die by suicide (Owens *et al.* 2002). The correlation of suicide attempt and completed suicide is stronger for males than females (Hawton *et al.* 1998). The number of attempts for each completed suicide seems to decrease with increasing age as the proportion of suicide attempters with high suicide intent increases (Levinson *et al.* 2006, Hawton and Harriss 2006).

## Conclusion

Data derived from different clinical and epidemioligal studies throughout Europe supply a comprehensive picture of the international variability in the occurrence and in background factors of suicide attempt in Europe. In particular, the WHO/EURO multiicentre study contributed considerably to a more accurate picture of the situation. The study monitored suicide attempt in different centres in Europe, applying a uniform methodology since 1989. Known presently as the MONSUE study (Monitoring suicidal behaviour in Europe) it is funded by the EU and involves 38 research sites in 27 countries, covering approximately 9.5 million inhabitants in Europe. To date, it is the most extensive monitoring system of suicide attempts in Europe. The data obtained in this large-scale, international study is fundamental in proving an overall understanding of suicidal behaviour and, essentially, bestowing valuable knowledge for future suicide preventive interventions.

## References

Balazs J, Lecrubier Y, Csiszer N *et al.* (2003). Prevalence and comorbidity of affective disorders in persons making suicide attempts in Hungary: importance of the first depressive episodes and of bipolar II diagnoses. *Journal of Affective Disorders*, **76**, 113–119.

Christoffersen MN, Poulsen HD, Nielsen A (2003). Attempted suicide among young people: risk factors in a prospective register-based study of Danish children born in 1966. *Acta Psychiatrica Scandinavica*, **108**, 350–358.

De Leo, D Padoan, W Scocco P *et al.* (2001). Attempted and completed suicide in older subjects: results from the WHO/EURO Multicentre Study of Suicidal Behaviour. *International Journal of Geriatric Psychiatry*, **16**, 300–310.

Dieserud G, Loeb M, Ekeberg O (2000). Suicidal behavior in the municipality of Baerum Norway: a 12-year prospective study of parasuicide and suicide. *Suicide and Life-Threatening Behaviour*, **30**, 61–73.

Fekete S, Voros V, Osvath P (2005). Gender differences in suicide attempters in Hungary: retrospective epidemiological study. *Croatian Medical Journal*, **46**, 288–93.

Gmitrowicz A, Szymczak W, Kotlicka-Antczak M *et al.* (2003). Suicidal ideation and suicide attempt in Polish adolescents: is it a suicidal process? *International Journal of Adolescent Medicine and Health*, **15**, 113–24.

Haw C, Hawton K, Houston K *et al.* (2001). Psychiatric and personality disorders in deliberate self-harm patients. *British Journal of Psychiatry*, **178**, 48–54.

Hawton K, Arensman E, Wasserman D *et al.* (1998). Relation between attempted suicide and suicide rates among young people in Europe. *Journal of Epidemiology and Community Health*, **52**, 191–194.

Hawton K, Houston K, Haw C *et al.* (2003a). Comorbidity of axis I and axis II disorders in patients who attempted suicide. *Am J Psychiatry*, **160**, 1494–1500.

Hawton K, Harriss L, Hall S *et al.* (2003b) Deliberate self-harm in Oxford 1990–2000: a time of change in patient characteristics. *Psychological Medicine*, **33**, 987–995.

Hawton K and Harriss L (2006). Deliberate self-harm in people aged 60 years and over: characteristics and outcome of a 20-year cohort. *International Journal of Geriatric Psychiatry*, **21**, 572–581.

Hintikka J, Viinamaki H, Tanskanen A, Kontula O, Koskela K (1998). Suicidal ideation and parasuicide in the Finnish general population. *Acta Psychiatrica Scandinavica*, **98**, 23–27.

Hulten A, Wasserman D, Hawton K *et al.* (2000). Recommended care for young people (15–19 years) after suicide attempts in certain European countries. *European Child and Adolescent Psychiatry*, **9**, 100–108.

Hulten A, Jiang GX, Wasserman D *et al.* (2001). Repetition of attempted suicide among teenagers in Europe: frequency, timing and risk factors. *European Child and Adolescent Psychiatry*, **10**, 161–169.

Kapur N, Cooper J, King-Hele S *et al.* (2006). The repetition of suicidal behaviour: a multicentre cohort study. *Journal of Clinical Psychiatry*, **67**, 1599–1609.

Kienhorst CW, de Wilde EJ, van den Bout J *et al.* (1990). Self-reported suicidal behavior in Dutch secondary education students. *Suicide and Life-Threatening Behaviour*, **20**, 101–112.

Levinson D, Haklai Z, Stein N *et al.* (2006). Suicide attempts in Israel: age by gender analysis of a national emergency department database. *Suicide and Life-Threatening Behaviour*, **36**, 97–102.

Michel K, Waeber V, Valach L *et al.* (1994). A comparison of the drugs taken in fatal and non-fatal self-poisoning. *Acta Psychiatrica Scandinavica*, **90**, 184–189.

Michel K, Ballinari P, Bille-Brahe U *et al.* (2000). Methods used for parasuicide. Results of the WHO/EURO Multicentre Study on Parasuicide. *Social Psychiatry and Psychiatric Epidemiology*, **35**, 156–163.

Mittendorfer Rutz E (2005). Perinatal psychosocial and familial risk factors in youth suicidal behaviour. Doctoral thesis. Karolinska Institutet, Stockholm.

Mittendorfer Rutz E (2006). Trends in youth suicide in Europe during the 1980s and 1990s—gender differences and implications for prevention. *Journal of Men's Health and Gender*, **3**, 250–257.

Morgan HG, Jones EM, Owen JH (1993). Secondary prevention of non-fatal deliberate self-harm: the green card study. *British Journal of Psychiatry*, **163**, 111–112.

Motto JA and Bostrom AG (2001). A randomized controlled trial of post-crisis suicide prevention. *Psychiatric Services*, **52**, 828–833.

Neeleman J and Wessely S (1997). Drugs taken in fatal and non-fatal self-poisoning: a study in South London. *Acta Psychiatrica Scandinavica*, **95**, 283–287.

O'Loughlin S and Sherwood J (2005). A 20-year review of trends in deliberate self-harm in a Brittish town 1981–2000. *Social Psychiatry and Psychiatric Epidemiology*, **40**, 446–453.

Owens D, Horrocks J, House A (2002). Fatal and non-fatal repetition of self-harm. Systematic review. *British Journal of Psychiatry*, **181**, 193–199.

Persson ML, Runeson BS, Wasserman D (1999). Diagnoses, psychosocial stressors and adaptive functioning in attempted suicide. *Annals of Clinical Psychiatry*, **11**, 119–128.

Ramberg IL and Wasserman D (2000). Prevalence of reported suicidal behaviour in the general population and mental health care staff. *Psychological Medicine*, **30**, 1189–1196.

Ramberg IL (2003). Promoting suicide prevention. An evaluation of a programme for training trainers in psychiatric clinical work. Doctoral thesis, Karolinska Institutet, Stockholm.

Rancans E, Lapins J, Salander Renberg E *et al.* (2003). Self-reported suicidal and help-seeking behaviours in the general population in Latvia. *Social Psychiatry and Psychiatric Epidemiology*, **38**, 18–26.

Rey Gex C, Narring F, Ferron C *et al.* (1998). Suicide attempts among adolescents in Switzerland: prevalence associated factors and comorbidity. *Acta Psychiatrica Scandinavica*, **98**, 28–33.

Salander Renberg E (2001). Self-reported life-weariness death-wishes suicidal ideation suicidal plans and suicide attempts in general population surveys in the north of Sweden 1986 and 1996. *Soc Psychiatry Psychiatr Epidemiol*, **36**, 429–436.

Schmidtke A, Bille-Brahe U, DeLeo D *et al.* (1996). Attempted suicide in Europe: rates trends and sociodemographic characteristics of suicide attempters during the period 1989–1992. Results of the WHO/EURO Multicentre Study on Parasuicide. *Acta Psychiatrica Scandinavica*, **93**, 127–338.

Swedish National Board of Health and Welfare (2006). *Social Styrelsen Statistik*. Available at http://www.socialstyrelsen.se/Statistik/.

Suominen K and Lonnqvist J (2006). Determinants of psychiatric hospitalization after attempted suicide. *Gen Hosp Psychiatry*, **28**, 424–30.

Vaiva G, Ducrocq F, Meyer P *et al.* (2006). Effect of telephone contact on further suicide attempts in patients discharged from an emergency department: randomised controlled study. *BMJ*, **332**, 1241–1245.

Wunderlich U, Bronisch T, Wittchen HU *et al.* (2001). Gender differences in adolescents and young adults with suicidal behaviour. *Acta Psychiatrica Scandinavica*, **104**, 332–339.

# CHAPTER 21

# Suicide attempts in New Zealand and Australia

Jane Pirkis, Annette Beautrais and Tony Durkee

## Abstract

New Zealand and Australia both have national suicide prevention strategies in place. Initially, the prevention activities delivered through these strategies focused on completed suicide only. More recently, there has been an acknowledgement that suicidal behaviours occur on a gradient and attempted suicide is a significant problem in its own right. It is estimated that for every completed suicide, there are approximately fifty suicide attempts carried out by females and ten by males.

In both countries, suicide attempts are the highest among young people, however, national population-based surveys suggest that, overall, nearly 0.5 per cent of the adult population makes a suicide attempt in a given year. It is evident suicide attempts are a major public health problem and must be addressed accordingly. This chapter examines the epidemiology of suicide attempts in the two countries, drawing on hospitalization data and data from population-based surveys and commenting on how the findings can inform prevention activities.

## Hospitalization data on suicide attempts

New Zealand and Australia both routinely collect data on hospitalizations for suicide attempts. Crude (or age-specific) rates of hospitalization per 100,000 are presented for each country below. Age-standardized rates are also presented wherever relevant, in order to facilitate comparisons across time and across population groups. These have been calculated by direct standardization, using the World Health Organization standard population distribution (Ahmad *et al.* 2000).

New Zealand and Australian data have traditionally been collated by financial year (1 July to 30 June) and are presented this way below, beginning with 1995–1996 and ending with 2005–2006, the year for which the most recent data were available in both countries.

Between 1999–2000 and 2000–2001 there was a change in the coding system for morbidity and mortality statistics in both countries from ICD-9 to ICD-10. The now-obsolete ICD-9 codes represented 'Suicide and self-inflicted injury' and included E950 to E959; the current ICD-10 codes represent 'Intentional self-harm' and include X60–X84.

## Overall trends

A comparison of age-standardized rates of hospitalizations for suicide attempts between New Zealand and Australia illustrate noteworthy disparity in overall trends. The crude total rate in New Zealand has been fairly constant since 1995–1996 (sitting at between 90 and 100 per 100,000), but has begun to show a gradual decline in recent years, reaching a low of 80 per 100,000 in 2005–2006. The same pattern was evident for the age-standardized total rate, with the rates for the period generally being stable at around 115 per 100,000 but declining in recent times to a low of 98 per 100,000 in 2005–2006. Across time, the female:male rate ratio (both crude and age-standardized) has increased, sitting at around 1.5:1.0 early in the observation period and rising to closer to 2.0:1.0 later in the period.

The age-standardized rates of hospitalizations for suicide attempts for Australia have a distinct pattern, which differed from that of New Zealand, both in terms of overall magnitude and in terms of trends. Apart from an initial drop early in the observation period, the crude total rate was constant at about 115 per 100,000 until 1998–1999, rose to 162 per 100,000 over the next two years, and has remained fairly stable since then. The difference between the beginning of the period and the end of the period has sometimes been explained by the above-mentioned change from ICD-9 to ICD-10, but it is interesting to note that a commensurate pattern is not evident in New Zealand. The profile of the age-standardized total rate was similar, with the rate for the early period being around 135 per 100,000, and the rate for the later period being around 195 per 100,000. Compared with New Zealand, Australia's female:male rate ratio (crude and age-standardized) has remained more stable over time at around 1.5:1.00.

## Age-specific rates

Age-specific rates of hospitalization for suicide attempts in New Zealand among genders were also distinctive. For females, the highest rates were consistently experienced by 15–24-year-olds; for males this group had hospitalization rates that were similar to those of males aged 25–35. For both females and males, 15–24-year-olds demonstrated the most dramatic decline, with female rates dropping from 285 per 100,000 in 1995–1996 to 184 per 100,000 in 2005–2006, and male rates dropping from 161 per 100,000 to 88 per 100,000 in the same years. For both genders, the only age group to exhibit an increase in rates was the 45–54-year-old age group. Female rates for this group rose from 71 per 100,000 in 1995–1996 to 118 per 100,000 in 2005–2006; the pattern for males was not quite so linear, with the lowest rate being recorded in 1995–1996 (44 per 100,000) and the highest in 2003–2004 (70 per 100,000).

Age-specific rates of hospitalization for suicide attempts demonstrated an oscillating trend. For females, suicide attempts were most prevalent among 15–24-year-olds in all years (peaking at 455 per 100,000 in 2004–2005). For males, rates were consistently highest for 25–34-year-olds, reaching their maximum at 257 per 100,000 in 2000–2001. Early in the observation period, the next highest rates for males were experienced by 15–24-year-olds (peaking at 203 per 100,000 in 2000–2001). By the second half of the period, however, the rates for this group had converged with those of their peers in the 35–44-year-old age bracket, making them equal second.

## Rates for indigenous people

Hospitalization rates for suicide attempts for indigenous Maori in New Zealand were compared with rates for non-Maori. Rates that are included are from 1996–1997 onwards only, because this marked a change in how ethnicity was defined (from a biological definition to self-definition). The crude rates for Maori show greater fluctuation over time than those for non-Maori, but in general the former are higher than the latter. The age-standardized rates show a similar, albeit more exaggerated pattern.

Some caution should be exercised in interpreting these findings, since evidence from other quarters more consistently suggests that Maori may be at greater risk of suicide attempts than non-Maori (Ministry of Health 2006a). Some methodological issues may influence the findings. For example, Maori account for about 15 per cent of the total population of New Zealand, and their lower absolute numbers result in less reliable estimates of crude and age-standardized rates of hospitalization. In the case of age-standardized rates, some anomalies may result from the fact that the Maori population is younger than the WHO standard population and the non-Maori population is older than it (Robson et al. 2007). Over and above these methodological issues, there may be alternative explanations for the findings. For example, they may reflect differences in levels of access to services, such that non-Maori people may be more likely to be admitted to hospital following a suicide attempt than their Maori counterparts.

Data on trends in hospitalizations for suicide attempts by Aboriginal and Torres Strait Islander people are not readily available in Australia. Indigenous status is poorly recorded on the hospitalizations database, particularly going back in time, so trend data are unreliable (Australian Bureau of Statistics 2005). Ad hoc cross-sectional studies which have drawn on data from states and territories with more reliable recording of indigenous status, have consistently found overall rates for Aboriginal and Torres Strait Islander to be about twice as high than those for other Australians (Helps and Harrison 2006). The excess between rates for Aboriginal and Torres Strait Islander peoples and other Australians has been found for both females and males after the age of 15 (Helps and Harrison 2006).

## Population-based survey data on suicide attempts

New Zealand and Australia have both conducted mental health surveys with nationally representative samples of adults, and these surveys have gauged the 12-month community prevalence of suicide attempts via the following question: 'In the past 12 months, did you attempt suicide [have you attempted suicide]?' New Zealand's survey was administered between October 2003 and December 2004 to a sample of 12,992 participants aged 16 and over (Beautrais et al. 2006). Australia's survey was conducted between May and August 1997, and elicited responses from 10,641 individuals aged 18 and over (Pirkis et al. 2000). Australia has recently repeated its survey but data are not yet available.

Table 21.1 shows the 12-month prevalence of suicide attempts in New Zealand and Australia, as ascertained by the two surveys. The figures from the two surveys are very similar, and suggest that almost 0.5 per cent of the population make a suicide attempt in a given year. Both surveys found that the strongest correlate of making a suicide attempt was having a mental disorder—particularly a substance use disorder or a mood disorder, but also an anxiety disorder (Pirkis et al. 2000, Beautrais et al. 2006).

## Reconciling hospitalization data and population-based survey data on suicide attempts

The data on hospitalizations and the self-report data from population-based surveys clearly produce very different results. There are a number of fundamental reasons for this. First, they use quite different numerators. The hospitalizations data are enumerated as admissions for suicide attempts, and therefore count suicide attempts made in a given year (i.e., an event-based count). By contrast, the survey data quantify the number of individuals who have made at least one suicide attempt in a given year (i.e., a person-based count). Converting the hospitalization data to a person-based count would require a system of unique identifiers which allows hospitalizations to be reliably linked to individuals. New Zealand has such a system, and recent reports have begun to use this to count individuals rather than attempts (Ministry of Health 2006a, b). Australia has no such system. Converting the survey-based self-report data to an event-based

**Table 21.1** 12-month prevalence of suicide attempts (females, males, total): New Zealand and Australia

| 12-month prevalence (%, 95% CI): New Zealand | | | 12-month prevalence (%, 95% CI): Australia | | |
|---|---|---|---|---|---|
| Females | Males | Total | Females | Males | Total |
| 0.4 (0.3–0.6) | 0.4 (0.2–0.8) | 0.4 (0.3–0.6) | 0.4 (0.2–0.6) | 0.2 (0.1–0.3) | 0.3 (0.2–0.4) |

Sources: Beautrais et al. (2006); Pirkis et al. (2000).

count would require individual respondents who had made any attempt to be questioned further about the number of attempts they had made, but this information was not available from either of the surveys.

Even if both data sources readily permitted an event-based count and a person-based count, a second problem would arise. The New Zealand and Australian hospitalization data, by definition, consider only suicide attempts that have been deemed to require hospitalization. By contrast, the survey data from these two countries examine any suicide attempt, regardless of whether it resulted in a hospital admission. Rates drawn from the former source would therefore not be expected to correspond with those elicited

through the latter, but might rather be expected to be the most medically serious subset of them (Welch 2001). Of course, some suicide attempts that result in hospitalization will not be medically serious, and some that do not result in hospitalization will be medically serious, but it is reasonable to assume that, as a general rule, suicide attempts that require hospitalization are at the more severe end of the spectrum of all attempts.

If both of the above problems could be resolved, it would be possible to reconcile the data in a manner that would provide a much more complete picture of the suicide attempt rates in New Zealand and Australia. Figure 21.1 shows the information that would be available under these circumstances. Not only would

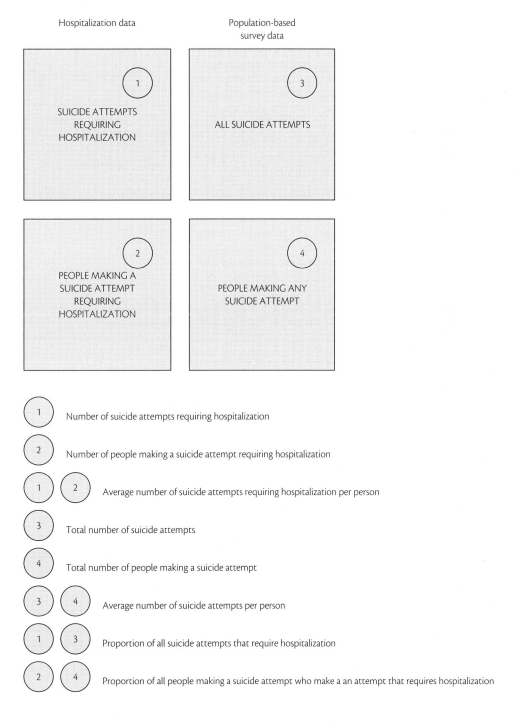

**Fig. 21.1** Reconciling hospitalization data and population-based survey data on suicide attempts.

it be possible to quantify the number of attempts requiring hospitalization and the total number of attempts, and the number of people making each kind of attempt, but it would also be possible to determine the average number of repetitions of each kind of attempt per person. In addition, it would be possible to calculate the proportion of all attempts that required hospitalization, and the proportion of all people making a suicide attempt who made one that required hospitalization.

# Using epidemiological data to inform preventive efforts in New Zealand and Australia

Although the above epidemiological profile of suicide attempts in New Zealand and Australia is not as comprehensive as it might be, it has still proved valuable in informing preventive efforts. Several initiatives have been, or are being, trialled in response to the finding that suicide attempt rates are particularly high among certain groups.

In Australia, Carter and colleagues evaluated a simple intervention with people aged 16 and older who had presented to the emergency department having deliberately ingested poison. Using a randomized controlled trial design, they examined repeat presentations for an intervention group (who received ongoing contact via postcards) and a control group (who received normal care). They found that although the proportions of repeat presenters did not differ between the groups, the average number of repeat episodes for those in the intervention group was lower (Carter et al. 2005). Robinson and colleagues are currently trialling a similar intervention with a group of young help-seekers presenting to a specialist early intervention service in Australia (Robinson et al. 2007) and Beautrais (personal communication) is also replicating and extending Carter et al.'s original study in New Zealand.

Hatcher and Sharon (2007) are currently conducting a randomized controlled trial of problem-solving therapy with suicide attempters in New Zealand. Those in the intervention group are being taught step-by-step strategies to rationally solve life's problems, with a view to equipping them with alternatives to future suicide attempts. It is too early to report definitive findings, but preliminary results are positive.

Also in New Zealand, Ellis and Smith have been trialling the Towards Well-Being (TWB) suicide monitoring programme (Ellis and Smith 2005). The programme is targeting young people under statutory supervision by the Child Youth and Family (Welfare) Service, whose suicide attempt rates are high. Social workers can refer at-risk members of this group to a specialized service which provides clinical advice to assist with the development and implementation of a management plan. The clinical advisers have no direct contact with the young people, but provide consultation–liaison support and assistance to the social workers. Although the suicide attempt rates for the young people associated with the programme have not decreased since its introduction, they have remained stable. This is in contrast to the rates for their counterparts who have not been referred to the programme, which have increased significantly.

# Summary and conclusions

Hosptialization data suggest that New Zealand and Australia have experienced somewhat different profiles of suicide attempts since the mid-1990s. New Zealand rates have been fairly constant until recently, and are now beginning to decline. By contrast, Australia's rates were constant until the beginning of the new millennium, rose at that point, and have remained relatively stable since. In New Zealand, the rate for females is now about twice that for males; in Australia the ratio is about 1.5:1.0. In both countries, the younger age groups account for the highest rates. National population-based surveys conducted in the two countries suggest that, overall, almost 0.5 per cent of the adult population make a suicide attempt in a given year. The figures from the two sources are difficult to reconcile because hospitalization data produce event-based rates and population surveys yield person-based rates, and the two sources are counting suicide attempts of differing levels of severity.

Despite some frustrations with the incompleteness of the epidemiological data available, it is clear that suicide attempts are a significant public health problem. According to the hospitalization data, for every completed suicide that occurs, there are around 50 suicide attempts by females and 10 by males (Australian Bureau of Statistics 2006). There is a clear imperative to ensure that efforts to reduce attempted suicide rates continue alongside efforts to reduce completed suicide rates. Some innovative approaches are being trialled in New Zealand and Australia, but there is scope for more to be done.

## References

Ahmad O, Boschi-Pinto C, Lopez A et al. (2000). *Age Standardization of Rates: A New WHO Standard.* GPE Discussion Paper Series No. 31. World Health Organization, Geneva.

Australian Bureau of Statistics (2005). *The Health and Welfare of Australia's Aboriginal and Torres Strait Islander Peoples*, ABS Catalogue No. 4704.0. Australian Bureau of Statistics, Canberra.

Australian Bureau of Statistics (2006). *Suicides, Australia.* Australian Bureau of Statistics, Canberra.

Beautrais AL, Wells JE, McGee MA et al. (2006). Suicidal behaviour in Te Rau Hinengaro: The New Zealand Mental Health Survey. *Australian and New Zealand Journal of Psychiatry*, **40**, 896–904.

Carter GL, Clover K, Whyte IM et al. (2005). Postcards from the EDge project: Randomized controlled trial of an intervention using postcards to reduce repetition of hospital treated deliberate self-poisoning. *British Medical Journal*, **331**, 805–807.

Ellis P and Smith D (2005). Evaluation of the Towards Well-Being suicide monitoring programme. *Australian and New Zealand Journal of Psychiatry*, **39**, A9.

Hatcher S and Sharon C (2007). A randomised trial of problem-solving therapy in self harm: preliminary three month results. International Association for Suicide Prevention XXIV World Congress: Preventing Suicide across the Life Span—Dreams and Realities. Killarney.

Helps Y and Harrison J (2006). *Hospitalised Injury of Australia's Aboriginal and Torres Strait Islander People*, AIHW Catalogue No. INJCAT 94. Australian Institute of Health and Welfare, Canberra.

Ministry of Health (2006a). *New Zealand Suicide Trends: Mortality 1921–2003, Hospitalisations for Intentional Self-Harm 1978–2004.* Monitoring Report No. 10. Ministry of Health, Wellington.

Ministry of Health (2006b). *Suicide Facts: 2004–2005 Data*. Ministry of Health, Wellington.

Pirkis J, Burgess P, Dunt D (2000). Suicidal ideation and suicide attempts among Australian adults. *Crisis*, **21**, 16–25.

Posner K, Oquendo MA, Gould M *et al.* (2007). Columbia Classification Algorithm of Suicide Assessment (C-CASA): Classification of suicidal events in the FDA's pediatric suicidal risk analysis of antidepressants. *American Journal of Psychiatry*, **164**, 1035–1043.

Robinson J, Gook S, Evans R *et al.* (2007). Baseline data from a randomised controlled trial designed to reduce suicide risk among young help seekers: The ORYGEN Postcard Study. International Association for Suicide Prevention XXIV World Congress: Preventing Suicide across the Life Span—Dreams and Realities. Killarney.

Robson B, Purdie G, Cram F *et al.* (2007). Age standardisation: an indigenous standard? *Emerging Themes in Epidemiology*, **4**, 4.

Welch SS (2001). A review of the literature on the epidemiology of parasuicide in the general population. *Psychiatric Services*, **52**, 368–375.

# CHAPTER 22

# Extended suicide

David Lester

## Abstract

Analyses of suicide committed by couples' suicide pacts and mercy killings and by groups of people in mass suicides are presented. Those involved appear to differ demographically and psychologically from suicides acting alone. In addition, examples of murderers who commit suicide after killing are presented, including mass murderers who have a high suicide rate and serial killers who have a much lower suicide rate than mass murderers. This chapter will examine these phenomena.

## Introduction

The majority of suicides involve just one individual who commits suicide, leaving behind relatively few survivors to mourn. Occasionally, however, suicide involves others in the act as partners in death, sometimes as suicides but sometimes as murder victims. Maris (1997) called these types of suicide 'social suicide' and included, in addition, suicide clusters, altruistic suicides such as those by soldiers, suicides that are witnessed by others, and even the death of an organization at the will of its director.

## Suicide in murderers

Some murderers commit suicide after their assault. The classic study on this behaviour was conducted in England by West (1966). He found that about one-third of murderers in England commit suicide after their act. These suicidal murderers were more often females, were older, more often killed close relatives, and used gas and shooting more than did the non-suicidal murderers. Their murders were, therefore, less brutal in that they did not use strangulation, stabbing or beating and they more often killed spouses and children. West did not find evidence that the suicidal murderers committed suicide out of guilt, but rather they killed themselves out of despair.

Wolfgang (1958a, b), in a study of murder in Philadelphia in the United States, also found that murderers who committed suicide more often killed close relatives or partners but, in his study, they were more often men and more often used brutal methods. Wolfgang suggested that perhaps the suicide was a result of a greater level of frustration and anger that is not dissipated after the murder and which is then turned inward upon the self. Since the murderers were more often men killing women, Wolfgang also suggested that guilt played a role. In his study of people killing their spouses, he found that about 20 per cent of husbands who killed wives committed suicide compared to about 2 per cent of wives who killed husbands. Wolfgang argued that husbands who are murdered are more likely to have precipitated their own murder, for example by physically abusing their wives than are wives who are murdered, and so wives who murder are less likely to experience guilt.

More recent studies confirm this pattern. In England, Milroy (1995) found that the typical murder-suicide was a man in his 30s, killing a spouse or lover after a breakdown in their relationship. The proportion of such murders, however, had declined to 5–10 per cent. In the United States, Aderibigbe (1997) also found that the typical murder-suicide was a man using a gun, murdering children (more often teenagers rather than younger children) or spouses/lovers, and a similar pattern has been reported in Japan (Kominato et al. 1997).

Berman (1996) described four types of murder followed by suicide.

1 In the erotic–aggressive type, a partner kills a lover or spouse when he or she threatens to sever the relationship.

2 In the unrequited love type, two lovers who are forbidden to marry kill themselves together.

3 In the dependent-protective type, the murderer sees the victim as dependent on him and, under financial or health stress, kills the dependent partner, a child, spouse or elderly parent out of mercy, pity or love.

4 In the symbiotic type, two people are enmeshed in a relationship and decide to die together.

Berman presented the case of twin brothers, both internationally known fertility specialists, who were abusing drugs, ignoring appointments, and refusing to submit insurance forms or pay bills. They committed suicide in a Manhattan apartment in July 1975 in an act which Berman saw as *folie à deux* and illustrative of the symbiotic type of dyadic death.

## Suicide in mass murderers and serial killers

Mass murderers, who kill three or more people in a period of a few hours, have a very high rate of suicide. Lester and colleagues (2005) studied 98 lone, rampage murderers in the United States in the period 1949–1999 who killed an average of 4.2 victims and wounded 4.7, and found that 34 committed suicide after the rampage. Those who committed suicide were often diagnosed with schizophrenia, were students killing fellow students and had experienced friction at work or school. Those mass murderers who committed suicide killed more victims than those who were captured or surrendered (4.8 versus 3.2 victims) but fewer than mass murderers killed by the police (8.1 victims).

White and Lester (2008) studied a sample of 594 serial killers who killed at least 3 people over a period of at least 3 months in the US from 1950 to 2002 and found that 26 (4.4 per cent) had committed suicide. Those committing suicide did not differ in sex, race, whether they were territorial or nomadic, whether they were killing for a personal cause or in their sadism. The suicides were more often engaged in criminal enterprises.

The reasons for the difference in the suicide rate of mass and serial murderers remain obscure, but the difference is consistent with Wolfgang's hypothesis of the greater amount of frustration and anger in some murderers resulting in self-directed aggression, a state which would seem to describe mass murderers more than serial killers. It may be also that mass murderers are experiencing more despair and hopelessness than serial murderers, but psychological data on these individuals are not available.

## Suicide pacts

Sometimes, partners decided to commit suicide together, most commonly in elderly couples where one or both are seriously ill. Fishbain and Aldrich (1985) found 20 suicide pacts, involving 40 individuals, in Dade County in Florida over a 25-year period, during which time there were 5895 suicides. Those involved in the suicide pacts were most often spouses, with the men unemployed, older with children grown up and gone from the home, and less often as a result of losses or financial problems. Fishbain and Aldrich found suicide pacts were more often between lovers in Japan, between friends in India, and between spouses in England and America. In all four nations, those dying in suicide pacts tended to use less violent methods for suicide.

In a study of 97 double suicides in the United States in the 1980s, Wickett (1989) found that two-thirds were mercy killings followed by the suicide of the remaining partner, and only one-third were double suicides. In mercy killings, typically the wife or both partners were suffering, and the husband was the instigator. The partners felt helpless and feared being institutionalized and separated. Brown and Barraclough (1997) found that suicide pacts accounted for 0.6 per cent of suicides in England, with the majority involving married couples and with little evidence for coercion from one partner to the other.

In rare cases, however, the husband decides to die and persuades the wife that she cannot live without him. Lester (1997) presented two famous cases, those of Arthur Koestler and his wife Cynthia in England and Stephan Zweig and his wife Lottie in Brazil, and argued that dominating (and perhaps abusive) husbands coerced their wives into dying with them for purely selfish motives.

Suicide pacts are becoming more common in adolescents, and Granboulin and colleagues (1997) reported several cases of such pacts in which the participants did not die. The adolescents in these pacts were most often same-sex friends and seemed to come from families with more dysfunction than the families of typical adolescent suicide attempters. Lester (1987) described the case of three teenagers in a small town in the US who committed suicide, and he identified the potential subcultural factors involved drug use, preference for heavy metal music, poor relations with parents, impaired self-esteem, and broken romantic relationships.

More recently, suicide pacts between two or more people are being formed by strangers using the Internet. People make contact online and then meet in a pre-arranged place where they die together. Using car exhaust is particularly common in Japan and South Korea (Samuels 2007) and, in these two countries, these suicide pacts now account for a sizeable proportion of all suicides.

## Mass suicide

There have been occasional instances where large groups of individuals have committed suicide together. Mancinelli and colleagues (2002) described two categories of mass suicide: (i) that by defeated and colonialized populations seeking to escape slaughter or a horrendous existence, and (ii) self-induced as a result of a distorted evaluation of reality. Type (i) suicides are more characteristic of historical times, such as that by the inhabitants of the Spanish city of Numance in 133 AD under siege by the Romans. Another famous example is that of the 936 Jewish members of the Sicarii sect who committed suicide at Masada in 73 AD to escape death at the hands of the Romans (Schwartz and Kaplan 1992).

An example of type (ii) is the mass suicide of several hundred people at Jonestown in Guyana in 1978, where coercion and perhaps murder played a role (Black 1990). These mass suicides illustrate the role of contagion in suicide (Lester 1987), as do suicide clusters of unrelated individuals, and appear to be especially common in cults, such as the suicides of 38 members of a group known as Heaven's Gate in 1997. In the Heaven's Gate episode, half of the suicides were women, a higher proportion than in the general population (Lester 2002). Type (ii) has become more common as in the French Alps in December 1995, when 16 members of the Ordre du Temple Solaire committed suicide in a star formation with their feet pointed toward the ashes of a fire. These sects were seen by Mancinelli and colleagues as helping the members, who are facing feelings of disorientation and isolation, solve existential issues by allying themselves with a charismatic and authoritarian leader who is often suffering from a chronic, paranoid delusional disorder.

Dein and Littlewood (2000) noted that there have been occasional studies of the leaders of suicidal cults, and these studies have noted characteristics such as an absent father from a young age, solitude in childhood, intolerance of criticism, and the presence of narcissistic and paranoid personality traits. There have been fewer studies of the followers of such leaders. Dein and Littlewood proposed four types of cult suicide:

1 Members of the group are disappointed when the divine millennium fails to materialize. The members of the Ordre du Temple Solaire, mentioned above, committed suicide when the new age promised by their leader failed to appear.

2  Members of the group believe that that they cannot live in the current world. The more than 900 members of the People's Temple who committed suicide in Guyana in 1978 preferred death to control by the US government.

3  Members of the group exit their bodies to go voluntarily to a better world. The 39 members of the Heaven's Gate cult who committed suicide in 1997 in San Diego in the United States believed that they would join a spaceship following the Hale-Bopp comet.

4  Members believe that they are immune from death and place themselves in situations that others would view as suicidal. Perhaps those who died during the attack by the FBI at Waco, Texas, fit this category, although they may also have fitted into category (2) above.

## Conclusion

Traditionally, suicide is the act of individuals acting alone, and social isolation is a common characteristic of these suicides. Increasingly today, people want company in death, and suicide pacts, even between strangers, are becoming more common. In other cases, murderous individuals commit suicide after murdering others, sometimes in mercy killings but often after murderous rampages. Suicide is increasingly moving from being a solitary act to becoming a social behaviour.

## References

Aderibigbe YA (1997). Violence in America. *Journal of Forensic Sciences*, **42**, 662–665.

Berman AL (1996). Dyadic death. *Suicide and Life-Threatening Behaviour*, **26**, 342–350.

Black A (1990). Jonestown—two faces of suicide. *Suicide and Life-Threatening Behaviour*, **20**, 285–306.

Brown M and Barracough BM (1997). Epidemiology of suicide pacts in England and Wales. *British Medical Journal*, **315**, 286–287.

Dein S and Littlewood R (2000). Apocalyptic suicide. *Mental Health, Religion and Culture*, **3**, 109–114.

Fishbain DA and Aldrich TE (1985). Suicide pacts. *Journal of Clinical Psychiatry*, **46**, 11–15.

Granboulan V, Zivi A, Basquin M (1997). Double suicide attempt among adolescents. *Journal of Adolescent Health*, **21**, 128–130.

Kominato Y, Shimada I, Hata N *et al.* (1997). Homicide patterns in the Toyama prefecture, Japan. *Medicine, Science and the Law*, **37**, 316–320.

Lester D (1987). *Suicide as a Learned Behaviour*. Charles C. Thomas, Springfield.

Lester D (1997). The sexual politics of double suicide. *Feminism and Psychology*, **7**, 148–154.

Lester D (2002). Cult suicide and physician-assisted suicide. *Psychological Reports*, **91**, 1194.

Lester D, Stack S, Schmidtke A *et al.* (2005). Mass homicide and suicide. *Crisis*, **26**, 184–187.

Mancinelli I, Comparelli A, Girardi P *et al.* (2002). Mass suicide. *Suicide and Life-Threatening Behaviour*, **32**, 91–100.

Maris RW (1997). Social suicide. *Suicide and Life-Threatening Behaviour*, **27**, 41–49.

Milroy CM (1995). Reasons for homicide and suicide in episodes by dyadic death in Yorkshire and Humberside. *Medicine, Science and the Law*, **35**, 213–217.

Samuels D (2007). Let's die together. *Atlantic Monthly*, **299**(4), 92–98.

Schwartz M and Kaplan KJ (1992). Judaism, Masada, and suicide. *Omega*, **25**, 127–132.

West DJ (1966). *Murder Followed by Suicide*. Cambridge, MA: Harvard University Press.

White J and Lester D (2008). Suicide and serial killers. *American Journal of Forensic Psychiatry*, **29**, 41–45.

Wickett A (1989). *Double Exit*. Hemlock Society, Eugene, Oregon.

Wolfgang ME (1958a). An analysis of homicide-suicide. *Journal of Clinical and Experimental Psychopathology*, **19**, 208–217.

Wolfgang ME (1958b). Husband-wife homicides. *Journal of Social Therapy*, **2**, 263–271.

# PART 3

# Theories of Suicidal Behaviour

# CHAPTER 23

# Social theories of suicide

Ilkka Henrik Mäkinen

## Abstract

In this chapter, some social theories in relation to suicide are presented together with examples from actual research. Although an individual act, suicide can be studied as a collective phenomenon, for example, as the relative number of cases that occur in different groups. Most social-scientific theories of suicide consider these not only as accumulations of individual observations, but also as results of social-level properties, events, and processes. The social environment in its different forms is thought to be connected with suicidal behaviour in multiple ways—the reasons for, the performance of, and the communication about the act all have strong social components. The currents in social research into suicide coincide largely with those in the social sciences more generally, with a preponderance, however, of structuralist studies following in the footsteps of Emile Durkheim.

## Social theories of suicide

In Lithuania, the country that currently leads the league of countries in terms of suicide, some 40 persons from each 100,000 take their own lives annually. In Greece, the corresponding figure is around four. If we knew which factors are responsible for this difference, would it be possible to reduce the number of suicides in Lithuania by 90 per cent? This question is a strong incentive for studying suicide from a collective point of view.

It is a common observation that the frequency of suicide varies between different social and demographic groups, between different locations and countries, and also over time. Many of its other properties such as, for example, its age distribution, vary on a group basis as well. This fact, along with our reflective understanding of the influence that the social environment wields over human behaviour, has inspired theories which assert in various ways that the collectivity in which one lives can make one more or less prone to commit suicide, other things being equal.

The hypothetical influence of the social environment on individual suicidality has many potential forms. It may consist of direct, personal oppression and discrimination, exclusion and isolation, or indifference shown in important relationships, of social norms and ideologies promoting suicide, and even in the tacit persuasion of certain persons to commit suicide. It may also be of a more indirect character such as, for example, the display of destructive role models or salient availability of information about ways to commit suicide. In most cases, however, the social environment is simply thought to produce circumstances that in one way or another make it psychologically more difficult for individuals to continue living, which enhance their suicidal impulses, should they exist in the personality, and/or strip away their defences against self-destruction.

This indirect influence can be of different types. Living in a social environment characterized by, for example, negative emotional communication and generally destructive ways of thinking, extreme individualism and a lack of common goals, difficult and rapidly changing social norms, roles and role systems, political oppression and persecution, and with suicides prominently visible in the media, may be thought to make individuals more prone to commit suicide than their counterparts in other kinds of environment. More developed social theories condense such circumstances into concepts such as 'anomie' or 'status incompatibility', and attempt to capture what the mechanism connecting the observable phenomena (for example, the overrepresentation of certain groups among suicides) is 'really' about.

## Theories and their use

A theory, in the empirical sciences, may be defined as an explicit formulation of determinate relations between a set of variables in terms of which a fairly extensive class of empirically ascertainable regularities can be explained (Schutz 1954). Its main function is the systematization of existing information by ordering, connecting, and abstractification, with the important related aim of thereby obtaining a better understanding of the phenomenon in question and its relations to a wider set of phenomena in order to create a more comprehensive model of reality. A theory is an important tool in turning information into knowledge.

A scientific work can be related to a theoretical perspective in several ways. It may be an *illustration* of a theory, seeking to show how its postulates manifest themselves in empirical facts. Emile Durkheim's (1992/1897) famous study of suicide served as an illustration of his basic contention of the existence and paramount importance of 'social facts' for human behaviour, while highlighting their independence from individual psychology. A study may also be designed to be a *test* of the predictive power of a theory, comparing the empirical results to the predictions made on its basis and, eventually, to those based on other theories. A good example of this is Stack's (1990) attempt to test Gibbs and Martin's (1964) theory of the effects of 'status integration' on suicide among divorced persons in comparison with the predictions arising from Durkheim's theory of anomie. Well-known theories may also be tentatively applied to new objects, such as suicide mortality (Rosenthal 1993). Finally, since the 'empirically ascertainable regularities' have to be located before their causes can be studied, some research is conducted in an *explorative* spirit, with more imprecise expectations. Mäkinen's (2000) analyses of some hypothetical causes of eastern European suicide mortality may serve as an example of this.

Theories provide explanations for the existence, nature, or behaviour of the phenomena at hand. On the basis of these, it should be possible to derive hypotheses and test their predictions against empirical data (Merton 1967). The causal distance, complexity, and level of abstraction of the hypothetical cause all affect the possibility of testing it.

## The nineteenth century and Emile Durkheim

The societal dimension of suicide became the theme of much passionate debate in the nineteenth century, as newly collected statistics on suicide showed a relentless increase in its frequency in Europe (Cavan 1928). This created a sense of urgency about the problem, and explanations were frequently connected to the ways in which the European (and other; see Drinot 2004) societies were moving towards modernity. Thomas Masaryk, in his *Suicide and the meaning of civilization* (1881) argued that the rise in suicide was a product of the spread of civilization and, in particular, due to increasing secularization: 'Suicide is the fruit of progress, of education, of civilization.'

The greatest name in the line of thinkers who turned their attention to this problem is undoubtedly Emile Durkheim, a French sociologist who in 1897 published *Suicide. A study in sociology*, the book that has had by far the largest impact on suicide research. He declared that his task was to explain the observed differences in the relative frequency of suicide between societies. He discarded the old theories of climate, and also the non-social causes of suicide, such as psychopathology and alcoholism, arguing that the distributions of these proposed causes, geographically or between different social groups, did not match those of suicide, and that therefore a causal relation was not likely.

Durkheim's basic view was that there are social structures ('social facts') that are external to, but nevertheless influence the lives of individuals. His main theory linked elevated suicide rates to the following circumstances:

◆ Deficient integration of society (*egoism* in Durkheim's words);

◆ Excessive integration of society (*altruism*);

◆ Deficient regulation of society (*anomie*);

◆ Excessive regulation of society (*fatalism*).

Durkheim supported his theory empirically by seeking to show that the variations in suicide rates between different groups and different time periods actually followed those in these defined states of society. For the first time he presented 'sociology's one law' (so termed by another sociologist, Robert Merton, in 1949), which stated that Protestants, due to the inherent individualism of their religious organization, always committed suicide more often than Catholics, whose religion was thought to be more collectively oriented and integrative. Anomie, a seminal concept created by Durkheim (1984/1893), depicted a state of society characterized by an imbalance between the need for stability and the insufficient or rapidly changing regulation of society. In *Suicide*, it was illustrated by the 'irregular' situations that emanated from economic change and divorce. Subsequent research has emphasized the elements critical to modern society and social change in general in Durkheim's research, as he also did himself. However, the less modern societies were in Durkheim's opinion plagued by altruistic and fatalistic types of suicide, which reflected the dependent position of individuals within them.

In spite of his basic thesis of the *sui generis* nature of the social, Durkheim also proceeded to speculate about the mechanisms through which the macrosocial factors influenced individuals, including the feelings they provoked in them. The anomie inherent in business life, for example, was thought to provoke feelings of insatiability, and, consequently, of violent disappointment when there were obstacles to obtaining gratification. This practice has subsequently been both adopted (Travis 1990; Hamlin and Brym 2006), and criticised (Lukes 1973; Gane 2005) by later researchers. Bericat Alastuey (2001) has recently interpreted Durkheim from an emotional–sociological perspective, postulating that integration is basically related to the intercommunicative dimension of the social order, and the feelings of shame and pride, while regulation relates to the interactive dimension and, hence, to anger and frustration.

## Durkheim's aftermath: structures and functions

In Durkheim's writings, it is possible to discern two important figures of thought which later formed an important part of twentieth-century sociology: structures and functions. Social structures can be generally defined as relatively enduring 'forms of social relations among a set of constituent social elements' (Heydebrand 2001, p. 15230). They are generally seen as being relatively independent and not reducible to individual actors or actions, constituting a *social* reality of their own. In this theoretical tradition, the identification of structures and their effects—indeed, understanding which phenomena are influenced by them—is the most important task of social analysis (Durkheim 1982/1895). This was also the core of *Le Suicide*.

The advantage of using these theoretical tools is that the complexity that is encountered when studying society 'as it is' is greatly reduced, hopefully in a manner that also leads to a better understanding of its development more generally. Structures may appear separately, or be connected with some hypothetical functions of society in models where they perform them, such as in Talcott Parsons's system-theoretic variant of 'structural functionalism', which dominated much of Western sociology in the 1940s–1960s (Parsons 1966; Luhmann 1984). Parsons's analytical model of society is based on the tasks which a society must perform in order to exist and survive, namely, physical adaptation, decision-making, social integration, and reproduction. Social structures are then formed to meet these needs. A smaller, modern variant of structural analysis is that of social networks, defined simply as the patterns of relations among a set of actors, the forms of which can be analysed in terms of their influence on the network members. They may also be conceived of as being determined by higher-level social structures (Berkman *et al.* 2000).

The application of structuralist theories to social suicide research consists most often of relating the frequency of suicide in society—or some other property of it—to some of the theoretical structures of society and, eventually, explaining its variations by their effects. In addition, a mechanism connecting the macro-level phenomena to individual behaviour may be provided. To take an example, is the weakening of the institution of marriage in Western societies causally associated with suicide? If there is a connection, is weakened social support for the individual the reason?

Following in the footsteps of Durkheim and attempting to refine his work, Maurice Halbwachs (1978/1930) constructed a theory which further simplifies the societal causes of suicide. It emphasizes the increasing *complexity* of the modern society, which causes breaks in social relations and leads to a sense of isolation that can ultimately lead to suicide. More recently, Travis (1990) has examined this theory in relation to Alaskan native suicide and found it valuable. Contemporaneously with Halbwachs, Ruth Cavan (1928) based her investigation of suicide in Chicago on the concept of social *disorganization*, which was thought to apply at both the collective (institutions and organizations) and individual levels.

At the beginning of the 1960s, Jack P Gibbs and Walter Martin attempted to construct a large-scale social theory of suicide in the Durkheimian tradition (Gibbs and Martin 1964). Their theory is based on the concept of role. It states that role statuses incompatible with each other produce an increasing number of role conflicts, which in turn damage social relationships and lead to suicidality. This theory has inspired studies of, for example, changes in the surplus risk of suicide among the divorced in times when divorce becomes more common, and thus more compatible with others' expectations (Stack 1990). The discussion and modification of Gibbs and Martin's theory continue to the present day.

Since the 1960s, there have been few social grand theories of suicide and none of them has had an influence comparable to the earlier ones, which are still used as points of reference. In his review of sociological suicide research in 1980–1995, Stack (2000) singles out the perspectives of modernization and societal integration. Both have their origins in Durkheim's work—the latter was his strongest thesis, and the former reflects the way in which the afterworld has interpreted his message. On a larger scale, modernization can also be regarded as the reverse of integration during a certain epoch.

## Modernization

Modernization is the shorthand used to describe the transition from an agricultural to an industrial mode of production in society, and the structural changes that characterize this process. Interpreted according to Durkheim's (1992/1897) theory, modernization during the twentieth century has undoubtedly resulted in more egoistic and anomic societies. However, the common indicators of modernization—industrialization, urbanization, and education—that so often seemed to covary with suicide in the nineteenth century no longer necessarily do so, at least when measured as processes over time (Fernquist and Cutright 1998; Otsu *et al.* 2004; McCall and Tittle 2007). Nevertheless, richer and more urbanized societies with higher average education levels often still have higher suicide rates than others (Allik and Realo 1997).

Stack (1997) has raised the possibility that the measures of modernization may have lost their value as indicators. This apparent loss of explanatory power may perhaps be helped by limiting the scope of the theory either to urban, industrial environments (Kowalski *et al.* 1987), or spatially or chronologically to the period of high modernization (Vijayakumar *et al.* 2005), after which relentless societal change may have become known and expected, and no longer suicide-provoking. However, there are also purely contrary findings: Moksony's (2001) analysis of 600 Hungarian villages showed that suicides are more common in the backward and isolated areas than in modernizing ones. Värnik and Wasserman described a similar situation in Estonia (Wasserman *et al.* 1998). Singh and Siahpush (2002) report a widening gap between rural and urban suicide rates in the USA, while Yip *et al.* (2005) find decreasing suicide rates in China during the period of hectic social and economic change in the 1990s.

It is also possible that the relationship between modernization and suicide has never been of a materially measureable nature, but that the cultural changes involved (individualization, secularization) have made it seem that way (Mäkinen 1997b). The central element in understanding the effects of modernization on suicide may lie in understanding its effects on personality. Girard's (1993) investigation of the different sex/age patterns of suicide mortality in different societies is a sociological study that bridges the individual and international levels, combining modernization theory with symbolic interactionist ideas of the self. It is based on the idea of 'self-concept', defined as 'an essential aspect of what a person believes to be his or her true self'.

Threats to one's self-concept are risky from the point of view of suicidality, because the desire for self-consistency resists the possibility of any change. Girard argues that suicide is a possible response to life-changing events that threaten the self-concept. In his opinion, the suicide risk is greatest for those persons whose self-concepts are performance-oriented. He points at the achievement-oriented lifestyle (or 'psychological career') as being the engine behind modern suicide. This vulnerability, replacement ability, and the probability of life-changing events happening are thought to vary according to sex, age, and the type of society one lives in. After locating the critical periods in both sexes' life cycles in both industrialized and 'traditional' societies, Girard proceeds to statistically study the sex/age patterns of suicide mortality in forty-nine societies, finding support for most of his hypotheses about the relative suicide frequencies at different ages in different types of societies.

Despite its relativization, the modernization perspective is kept alive by the suicidal crises occurring in many parts of the third (Mohanty 2005) and fourth (Bjerregaard and Lynge 2006; Hamlin and Brym 2006) 'worlds', which motivate further studies of the relationship between social change and suicide. These investigations do not stop at classic modernity—structural analyses may also be undertaken from a postmodern perspective, as Willis and colleagues (2002) interpretation of the societal background underpinning increasing suicide rates among African-American adolescent males shows.

## Integration

Integration, in a Durkheimian context, is considered as a characteristic of society rather than of individuals, although these are naturally interconnected. His rather vague definition of 'egoism' is '[the state] in which the individual ego asserts itself to excess in the face of the social ego and at its expense' (Durkheim 1992/1897). Durkheim considered integration in relation to different life spheres, mainly the family, religious community, and the larger society. This division has greatly influenced later research.

As regards familial integration, a number of studies have demonstrated that suicide rates are relatively low among the married, but that a surplus risk exists among the divorced (and often single and widowed persons as well)—at least for men (Stack 1990; Kposowa 2000; Stack 2000; Luoma and Pearson 2002; Yip and Thorburn 2004; Cutright *et al.* 2006). Even persons with a history of past family conflicts are clearly over-represented among suicides and suicide attempters (Dube *et al.* 2001). Having children has also been shown to have the protective effect that Durkheim's theory postulates (Qin and Mortensen 2003). At the collective level, there are generally more suicides in countries with modernized family patterns with many gainfully employed women, elder parents, less children, and more divorces; (Mäkinen 1997a; Stockard and O'Brien 2002; Neumayer 2003; O'Brien and Stockard 2006), although it is possible that this effect will, like the effects of other societal changes, diminish over time. However, Cutright and Fernquist (2000) maintain that no such adjustment can be found in relation to the impact of female labour force participation in the period 1955–1989.

When studying suicide in the United States over time, Stack (1985) found that religious and familial integration are very strongly interconnected. Burr *et al.* (1994) have argued that the Catholic religion in particular affects familial life by hindering divorce, and thus indirectly influences suicide rates. The relation between specific religious denominations and suicide, strongly postulated by Durkheim, has since largely disappeared (Neumayer 2003), although in some studies Islam has replaced Catholicism as the religion characterized by subordination and collective ritual—and low suicide rates (Simpson and Conklin 1989). The general suicide-protective influence of religiosity has, however, been repeatedly confirmed (Kelleher *et al.* 1999; Clarke 2003; Helliwell 2007).

Pescosolido and Georgianna (1989) have elaborated on the mechanisms underlying the relationship between religion and suicide by advancing the idea of the beneficial effects of supportive religious networks, irrespective of denomination. Their findings have, however, been relativized by van Tubergen *et al.* (2005) who used a large, historical, individual-level Dutch material to show how municipalities with higher proportions of believers had lower rates of suicide among members of *all* denominations— and even among those who did not belong to any denomination. They argue that since believers typically have more negative views on suicide than others, the norms in the communities with many believers will be more negative and prevent some acts from occurring. However, consistent differences in the suicide frequencies of different religious groups also surfaced in this study, with the re-reformed Protestants (who were the most ardent churchgoers) having the lowest rates.

Some other concepts that in many respects resemble integration (or a lack of it), such as social capital (Helliwell 2007), social fragmentation (Congdon 1996; Middleton *et al.* 2004, 2006), disorganization (Jarosz 1998; Mäkinen 2000), and social deviancy, have also been studied in relation to suicide mortality. According to social deviancy theory, those who deviate socially or culturally from the mass of the population experience more stress than others. Investigating this, Lester (1987a) found an inverse relationship between the proportion of the population belonging to a minority and the suicide rates among that minority. Pescosolido (1990), studying the proportions of different religious groups in 404 US counties in relation to suicide rates, found that the effect of the group size varied according to region, being strongest in the historical core areas. At the individual level, breaking the law is a sign of social deviancy, which in some cases may be so stigmatizing as to lead to suicide. Pritchard and King (2004), for example, have found extremely high suicide rates among men suspected of sexual abuse.

For Durkheim, integration and regulation were not only beneficial, but could also have negative consequences if they occurred excessively. In recent years, his concepts of altruism and fatalism, previously little used in relation to modern societies, have generated renewed interest from researchers utilizing them in new situations such as with the fatalism fostered by totalitarian political systems (Stack 1979; Straub 2000) or in connection to the situation of women in different societies (Kushner and Sterk 2005). Of course, fatalism is still thought to be relevant for suicide in traditionally oriented societies, and continues to be employed in that context (Acevedo 2005).

## The larger structures

Although much of Durkheim's theory can be condensed into the concepts of modernization and integration, they are only a part of it. Over the years, 'Durkheim's theory' has been repeatedly put to the test (van Poppel and Day 1996; Besnard 1997), but attempts to analyse his entire theory as a total, coherent system have not been numerous. In a study of 47 societies, Lester (1989) found that nations that had low levels of integration (or that were moderately integrated and little regulated) had the highest suicide rates. Stockard and O'Brien (2002), studying birth cohorts in fourteen Western countries, found that both low integration and low regulation had important effects on suicide. Fernquist and Cutright (1998) demonstrated that measures of domestic and religious integration, but not those of economic integration, had significant effects on suicide rates in twenty-one countries between 1955 and 1989. All these studies seem to support the notion that low integration is an important factor in shaping the differences in suicide mortality between societies.

However, Lester (1992a) did not find any relationship between integration, regulation and suicide in the 'primitive' societies that he investigated. Paradoxically, it would seem that Durkheim's theory, sometimes applied with success at the individual level, where persons with few familial, work-related, or religious ties seem to be at a greater risk for suicide, fails to fulfil its main purpose of explaining the variation in the suicide rates of societies. Finding relevant, high-quality social indicators is, however, a constant impediment for large-scale international studies.

Societies are also affected by the structures of the international community. Factors influencing the occurrence of suicide may spread between societies, which can be discerned in international increases and decreases in suicide rates, such as the generally rising youth suicide rates after World War II. Mäkinen (1997a) speculates about 'international waves', where suicide rates would change in a certain order, with the less modernized countries following the path of the more modernized, each at their own level of suicide mortality. Another possible consequence of this process of diffusion could be a long-term convergence of suicide rates, such as was found among the US states by Lester (1992b).

The mechanisms connecting the social structure to individual suicide in the contemporary approaches described above include broken or negative social relations, loss of status, frustration, insecurity, isolation, meaninglessness, and the disorientation brought about by rapid change in the environment, to which the notion of stress as the result of these or other social circumstances can be added. The protective mechanisms are less often considered in detail. Although very similar, Durkheim's explanatory hypotheses were, in comparison with these, more pointedly based on the needs of individuals—the necessity of living in a regulated social community was frustrated in egoistic or anomic social environments, with fatal consequences for some.

Is it possible to find stable social–structural determinants of suicide mortality? Sainsbury, Jenkins, and Levey (1980) found that the position of women in society, anomie, and socio-economic circumstances were connected with changes in the level of suicide mortality between the 1960s and the 1970s in eighteen European countries. However, Mäkinen's (1997a) replication of that study, with an identical design, but data from 16 years later, largely failed to reproduce the relationships. This may serve as an illustration of the problems connected with structuralist analyses: there are many indications of societal circumstances affecting suicidality in multiple and sometimes dramatic ways, yet it seems very difficult to define what exactly these circumstances are, since they seem to vary both across space and over time. There is, however, some later research (Cutright and Fernquist 2000; Neumayer 2003) that contests this opinion.

## Cultural theories

'Cultural theories' here denotes a mixture of different writings, whose common denominator is their use of the concept of culture as an important determinant of human behaviour and/or the existence and form of social institutions. There are literally hundreds of definitions of 'culture', but common to many of them is the notion that human mental structures, including ways of thinking and even cognition, are not unbiased but rather emerge in the course of the socialization and education that occur in the society and group that one is born into. This produces patterns where groups of people differ from each other in their outlook, interests, and way of life generationally, between social groups, and between larger cultures. Seen in this manner, culture can become an explanation of different phenomena in the same way that societal structures—or *other* societal structures—are in structuralist theories.

Suicide can be understood as a form of behaviour susceptible to cultural influence. Kral (1994, p. 245) expresses the basic idea laconically: 'suicide is caused by the idea of suicide and nothing else'. Once existing, the idea will soon have a meaning, the specific conceptualization of the act, revealing its 'nature' in the culture in question (Boldt 1988). The cultural influence is most obvious in culturally specific types of suicide, among which the traditional Indian *sati* and the Japanese *seppuku* are often cited. These tended to dominate traditional discussions of the role of culture in suicide. However, the notion that it is difficult to find stable structural correlates to the varying suicide rates between

societies (Mäkinen 1997a), together with the curious fact that there are occasions of even century-long continuities in the patterns of suicide rates internationally (Lester 1987b; Diekstra 1993), within single countries (Mäkinen *et al.* 2002), and within groups of people (Sainsbury and Barraclough 1968), point to the possibility that the cultural influences on suicide may be much more pervasive than has been previously thought.

In a Parsons-inspired theoretical analysis, Mäkinen (1997b, d) concludes that suicide, as a voluntary but non-rational act, is likely to be performed (or not) in modern societies according to cultural ideas concerning its relevance in the prevailing situation simply because there are few structural hindrances or incentives of other kinds affecting it. Suicide thus becomes an 'enactment of the cultural code' (Mäkinen 1997d, p. 31); moreover, 'social factors ... seem mainly to explain differences *within* the cultural units' while 'suicide mortality ... is ... likely to vary according to culture rather than to other macro-level phenomena' (Mäkinen 1997b, p. 37).

Culture is thought to influence suicide in multiple ways. Cultures have some pathogenetic effects, creating circumstances that may lead to more suicide; more importantly however, they also have *pathoselective* effects, which indicate that suicide is the best solution to the situation at hand (Tseng 2001; Colucci 2006). This is shown not least by the very different reactions of populations to roughly similar political-economic situations (Mäkinen 2000). Canetto (1997), for example, suggests that the connection between women's low status and suicide which is seen in only certain societies must be interpreted in the light of the cultural meanings attached to class, gender, and suicide. However, the changing, multifaceted, and multilevel nature of culture is likely to make its analysis a complex task.

Hamlin and Brym (2006), studying the South American Guarani-Kaiowá, complement a Durkheimian sociological analysis with the use of a cultural analysis, which assists in understanding the cultural–historical and psychosocial background, and also the preferred age and method of the suicides. Becoming an adult in Guarani-Kaiowá culture 'reveals all the difficulties of the Kaiowá mode of being that values dominance instead of submission, stubbornness instead of compliance, and nonconformity instead of conformity' (Hamlin and Brym 2006, p. 54). Ways of behaving, learned during one's socialization, become a cause of Kaiowá suicide—more exactly, of its relatively high frequency. In cultural comparisons, suicide may sometimes even become a matter of identity: the 'suicide is a white thing' attitude found both among African-Americans (Early 1992) and the South African Coloured (Laubscher 2003) is an example of this.

The problem of studying culture often lies in the form of the study—traditionally, cultural studies have been conducted in a descriptive manner, without attempts at systematic quantification, and this 'thick description', informative as it may be (Meng 2002; Laubscher 2003) is undoubtedly a problem when trying to establish causal relations between phenomena. However, there are international survey studies of emotions and values, the results of which can be related to the occurrence of suicide. Allik and Realo (1997) found that suicide rates correlated negatively with inequality and masculine values in a society, and positively with the value of individualism and the tendency to perceive an external locus of control. The three first-mentioned value-orientations explained 38% of the variation in the suicide rates of 41 countries.

However, suicide mortality also correlated positively with the level of certain aspects of subjective well-being. Interpreting a similar relationship, Inglehart (1990) argues that for unhappy persons, a happy environment can be worse than an unhappy one. His proposition is based on the notion of deviancy, however, deviancy in feeling (or cognition) rather than in group membership or some similar characteristic. This resembles Durkheim's (1992/1897) reasoning concerning one effect of social anomie on individuals—that high expectations do not tolerate restraint, and that in such a mental environment, shortcomings may be fatal. Seeing that the degree of men's satisfaction with finances and women's satisfaction with the family were positively connected with suicide rates, Allik and Realo interpret their results in a similar manner (cf. Girard 1993). However, Helliwell's (2007) investigation, using a larger body of material, found a clearly negative relationship between average life satisfaction and suicide mortality, and a very strong negative one between the amount of trust that is felt towards other people and suicide.

The conscious cognitive, emotional and evaluative background against which an act of suicide is committed in a certain social environment can be investigated with the help of studies of attitudes and attitude formation (Farber 1968; Bagley and Ramsay 1989; Stillion and Stillion 1998). Attitudes, in their turn, may be linked to the rate of suicide at the group level (Neeleman *et al.* 1997; Cutright and Fernquist 2005). In modern societies, cultural features are also directly documented in many shapes.

Law, the formal system of norms in society, also codifies cultural evaluations, but it has been little researched in relation to suicide. Suicide itself has been recently decriminalized in all of Europe and the USA. In a study of forty-two European legislations, which focused on the aiding and abetting of suicide, a relationship was found between the severity of punishments for these (in most European countries) crimes, folk attitudes towards suicide, and suicide rates (Mäkinen 1997c), indicating the existence of a relationship between norms, attitudes, and acts at a societal level.

Stack's innovative approach to the measurement of culture was to estimate the impact of certain American subcultures, differentiated by their musical tastes, as determined by the size of country music radio audiences (Stack and Gundlach 1992) and the number of subscriptions to heavy metal music magazines (Stack *et al.* 1994) in different cities. In our increasingly subculturalized world this type of analysis clearly points to future ways of research. The results from a recent historical study of suicide in Sweden (Mäkinen *et al.* 2002) show that differences in suicide mortality between ascriptive person categories, such as those based on sex, age, or place of birth, have tended to diminish during the last century, while those between categories of choice (marital status, for example) have remained. The authors hypothesise that the homogenization between ascriptive categories is a sign of their weakening hold on individual lives in modern society, and that future differences will increasingly be found between chosen subcultural lifestyles.

Finally, the importance of culture for studying suicide has been put into perspective by Neumayer (2003), who compared fixed- and random-effects analyses of the relation between certain social determinants and suicide across a large number of industrialized countries. This showed that taking 'suicide cultures' into account does not greatly affect the observed relation between social determinants and suicide rates. Consequently, cultural analysis can not replace social analysis. This conclusion brings to mind a model presented by Lester (1987b), in which cultural influences shape the background for personality, while structural influences affect the adult personality and its suicidal behaviour in a more direct fashion.

## Rational choice and economic theories

A rational-choice perspective on suicide can claim seniority as many historical sources discussing individual suicides tend to emphasize the element of choice made in the face of adverse circumstances. The Roman Emperor Otho is a prime example: after losing a decisive battle in 69 AD, he took his life with a dagger. Rational choice as a principle has traditionally been the base of economic and political-economic thinking, and it has been widely, if sometimes unconsciously, used in other social sciences as well. In the 1980s–1990s it experienced a renaissance in sociology, mainly due to the influential works of James Coleman. Problems where the outcomes of multiple and mutually dependent individual choices are at stake are often considered from this perspective, as it allows these outcomes to be calculated, assuming that they can be predicted because of their 'rationality'. The focus of the rational-choice perspective is on individual choice and strategy and the interplay of individual preferences.

In suicide research this perspective was revived in an economically inspired form by Hamermesh and Soss (1974), who contended that the utility of living could be calculated as the result of the possibility of consumption which increased it minus the cost of maintaining a minimum level of subsistence. When this utility reaches zero the individual would commit suicide. The authors successfully connected the expected average lifetime utilities of white working-age males in different age groups to their suicide rates in the USA between 1947 and 1967. They also showed that the marginal positive effect of consumption possibilities decreases with increasing income, as indeed it should in economic theory. The expected utility was psychologically biased towards current income, which was valued more highly than future income.

This approach has not had many followers, but it is nevertheless theoretically interesting because it goes against the current, prevailing since the nineteenth century, where the role of the individual is downplayed and the element of conscious decision-making in suicide depreciated. Dixit and Pindyck (1994), considering suicide as a kind of investment under uncertainty, claim that Hamermesh and Soss failed to take the 'option value of life' into account—which according to them would most probably lead to the postponement of suicide because of uncertainty, and only in irrational cases to suicide. In my opinion, this would probably result in stock market-like fluctuations in suicide rates, increasing when the environmental effects would make postponement seem hopeless, decreasing when waiting would seem to be worth the effort.

Yeh and Lester (1987), examining suicide decisions from a similar perspective, noted that the probability of suicide increases with the expected benefit from it, as indicated by the distress felt by the individual, but decreases when the cost of suicide, i.e. the multiple circumstances speaking against it, increases. Their interesting conclusion from this is that a suicidal situation is unstable and tends towards a polarization of action alternatives—and that outside intervention is needed if suicide is to be prevented. Rational choice or economic theories have also been applied to suicide attempts (Rosenthal 1993; Andrews 2006), life changes after suicide attempts (Marcotte 2003), and used in other contexts as well.

## The challenge of ethnomethodology

Ethnomethodology is a sociological approach that was initially developed in the USA in the 1960s. It can be briefly defined as 'the study of the practical methods of consensual reasoning used by members of society in the course of everyday life' (Clayman 2001, p. 4865), and its beginnings can be found in the works of Harold Garfinkel (1967) and Harvey Sacks, among others. It sees itself as a pre-scientific activity, since it studies, by way of experiment and close observation, the *processes* of making sense, rather than trying to make more sense of social life itself.

One of its main contentions is that sociology all too often uncritically absorbs the lay definitions of concepts, on the basis of which data are then collected. Not surprisingly, ethnomethodologically inspired works have strongly questioned the ways in which information on suicide is obtained. One of the most debated sociological works on suicide, Jack Douglas's *The social meanings of suicide* (1967), entirely denounced Durkheim's work and, implicitly, that of everyone else working with the help of official suicide statistics. According to Douglas, statistics are social constructs created by the rules of their classification, here, coroners' inconsistent interpretations of events and attempts at concealment on the part of the deceased.

Moreover, these statistics are not even consistent with the theoretical definitions of suicide. Douglas highlights how Durkheim, although being sceptical about the then published statistics concerning the motives of suicides, saw no problem in the fact that the classification of a case of death as suicide was made against the background of a more general appreciation of its possible motives. Douglas's book stimulated a 20-year-long debate on the validity of official suicide figures, and still constitutes a source for those who wish to delve deeper into the statistics upon which much research is based. Although empirical studies have provided varying results (Pescosolido and Mendelsohn 1986; Barraclough 1987; van Poppel and Day 1996, van Tubergen *et al.* 2005), the current consensus leans towards accepting the use of official statistics, while noting that administratively created categories do not always coincide with those that the scientist may wish to study.

As an alternative to the statistical study of groups, Douglas (1967, p. 231) suggested 'intensive observation, description, and analysis of individual cases of suicide' with a view to identifying the roles of both individual and shared meanings in these. This is consistent with the ethnomethodological contention that 'higher-level' social phenomena are nothing but aggregates of individual phenomena. However, Douglas did not undertake this task himself. Varty (2000) has pointed out that this form of analysis is actually independent of the quality of suicide statistics.

## Conclusions

This chapter has presented some types of social theories in relation to suicide. The feminist perspectives (Chapter 34 by Canetto), labour-market-related questions (Chapter 32 by Mäkinen and Wasserman), and those pertaining to religion and suicide (Part 1) are discussed elsewhere in this book.

Social theories are based on differing views of society, and are therefore not always capable of, nor used for, nor concerned with identical tasks. Adopting a particular theoretical perspective influences not only the manner of explanation, it also affects the choice of the research question and data collection in terms of what is thought to be interesting, and explicable, and at which level. Some theories lead almost automatically to the study of whole societies, while others are most often applied to small groups and local situations. Likewise, certain theories imply the use of statistical data, while others presuppose studying behaviour or the language used in social contexts.

For social studies, access to statistical data is important, and this, along with the necessity to conduct longitudinal studies, tends to delay the results. Many of the studies presented here make use of older data from the 1980s. The future will probably offer increasing amounts of data, possibly from places where they have previously not been collected. This in itself will act as a major incentive for the continuation and possible expansion of social research on suicide. At the same time, studies using more than one approach, and especially those connecting statistical studies with interpretations of meaning, are in short supply. Moreover, while there are examples of innovative quantification (Stack and Gundlach 1992), more creativity—and, at the same time, reflexivity—in how to quantify complex variables is needed. This is especially important as regards the impact of culture on suicide. Aspects of suicide other than the occurrence and number of completed suicides are still grossly under-researched. Finally, it should be noted that the theories presented above also have their consequences as regards the prevention of suicide.

## References

Acevedo GA (2005). Turning anomie on its head: fatalism as Durkheim's concealed and multidimensional alienation theory. *Sociological Theory*, **23**, 75–85.

Allik J and Realo A (1997). Psychological and cultural mechanisms of suicide. *Trames*, **1**, 306–321.

Andrews PW (2006). Parent–offspring conflict and cost–benefit analysis in adolescent suicidal behaviour—effects of birth order and dissatisfaction with mother on attempt incidence and severity. *Human Nature*, **17**, 190–211.

Bagley C and Ramsay R (1989). Attitudes towards suicide, religious values, and suicidal behaviour: evidence from a community survey. In RFW Diekstra, R Maris, S Platt *et al.*, eds, *Suicide and its Prevention: The Role of Attitude and Imitation*, pp. 78–90. E.J. Brill, Leiden.

Barraclough B (1987). *Suicide: Clinical and Epidemiological Studies*. Croom Helm, London.

Bericat Alastuey E (2001). El suicidio en Durkheim, o la modernidad de la trista figura (The suicide in Durkheim, or the modernity of the sad figure). *Revista Internacional de Sociología*, **28**, 69–104.

Berkman LF, Glass T, Brissette I, Seeman TE (2000). From social integration to health: Durkheim in the new millennium. *Social Science and Medicine*, **51**, 843–857.

Besnard P (1997). Mariage et suicide: la théorie durkheimienne de la régulation conjugale à l'épreuve d'un siècle (Marriage and suicide: Durkheim's theory of martial regurgitation in a hundred-year test). *Revue francaise de sociologie*, **38**, 735–758.

Bjerregaard P and Lynge I (2006). Suicide—a challenge in modern Greenland. *Archives of Suicide Research*, **10**, 209–220.

Boldt M (1988). The meaning of suicide: implications for research. *Crisis*, **9**, 93–108.

Burr JA, McCall PL, Powel-Griner E (1994). Catholic religion and suicide: the mediating effect of divorce. *Social Science Quarterly*, **75**, 300–318.

Canetto SS (1997). Gender and suicidal behaviour: theories and evidence. In RW Maris, SS Canetto, MM Silverman, eds, *Review of Suicidology*, pp. 138–167. Guilford, New York.

Cavan RS (1928). *Suicide*. Chicago University Press, Chicago.

Clarke CS (2003). Suicide and religiosity—Masaryk's theory revisited. *Social Psychiatry and Psychiatric Epidemiology*, **38**, 502–506.

Clayman SE (2001). General ethnomethodology. In N Smelser and P Baltes P, eds, *International Encyclopedia of the Social and Behavioural Sciences*, pp. 4865–4870. Elsevier Science, Oxford.

Colucci E (2006). The cultural facet of suicidal behaviour: its importance and neglect. *Australian e-Journal for the Advancement of Mental Health*, **5**, 1–13.

Congdon P (1996). Suicide and parasuicide in London: a small-area study. *Urban Studies*, **33**, 137–158.

Cutright P and Fernquist RM (2000). Effects of societal integration, period, region, and culture on male age-specific suicide rates: 20 developed countries, 1955–1989. *Social Science Research*, **29**, 148–172.

Cutright P and Fernquist RM (2005). Marital status integration, psychological well-being, and suicide acceptability as predictors of marital status differentials in suicide rates. *Social Science Research*, **34**, 570–590.

Cutright P, Stack S, Fernquist RM (2006). The age structures and marital status differences of married and not married male suicide rates: 12 developed countries. *Archives of Suicide Research*, **10**, 365–382.

Diekstra RFW (1993). The epidemiology of suicide and parasuicide. *Acta Psychiatrica Scandinavica*, **371**, S9–20.

Dixit AK and Pindyck RS (1994). *Investment Under Uncertainty*. Princeton University Press, Princeton.

Douglas J (1967). *The Social Meanings of Suicide*. Princeton University Press, Princeton.

Drinot P (2004). Madness, neurasthenia, and 'modernity': medico-legal and popular interpretations of suicide in early twentieth-century Lima. *Latin American Research Review*, **39**, 89–113.

Dube SR, Anda RF, Felitti VJ *et al.* (2001). Childhood abuse, household dysfunction, and the risk of attempted suicide throughout the life span: findings from the Adverse Childhood Experiences Study. *Journal of American Medical Association*, **286**, 3089–3096.

Durkheim E (1982/1895). *The Rules of Sociological Method and Selected Texts on Sociology and its Method*. Macmillan, London.

Durkheim E (1984/1893). *The Division of Labour in Society*. Macmillan, London.

Durkheim E (1992/1897). *Suicide. A Study in Sociology*. Routledge, London.

Early K (1992). *Religion and Suicide in the African American Community*. Greenwood Press, Westport.

Farber ML (1968). *Theory of Suicide*. Funk and Wagnalls, New York.

Fernquist RM and Cutright P (1998). Societal integration and age-standardized suicide rates in 21 developed countries, 1955–1989. *Social Science Research*, **27**, 109–127.

Gane M (2005). Durkheim's scenography of suicide. *Economy and Society*, **34**, 223–240.

Garfinkel H (1967). *Studies in Ethnomethodology*. Prentice-Hall, Englewood Cliffs.

Gibbs JP and Martin W (1964). *Status Integration and Suicide*. University of Oregon Press, Eugene.

Girard C (1993). Age, gender, and suicide: a cross-national analysis. *American Sociological Review*, **58**, 553–574.

Halbwachs M (1978/1930). *The Causes of Suicide*. Routledge and Kegan, London.

Hamermesh DS and Soss NM (1974). An economic theory of suicide. *Journal of Political Economy*, **82**, 83–98.

Hamlin CL and Brym RJ (2006). The return of the native: a cultural and social-psychological critique of Durkheim's Suicide based on the Guarani-Kaiowa of southwestern Brazil. *Sociological Theory*, **24**, 42–57.

Helliwell JF (2007). Well-being and social capital: does suicide pose a puzzle? *Social Indicators Research*, **81**, 455–496.

Heydebrand WV (2001). Theories of structuralism. In N Smelser and P Baltes, eds, *International Encyclopedia of the Social and Behavioural Sciences*, pp. 15230–15233. Elsevier Science, Oxford.

Inglehart R (1990). *Culture Shift in Advanced Industrial Society*. Princeton University Press, Princeton.

Jarosz M (1998). *Suicide*. Institute of Political Studies at Polish Academy of Sciences, Warsaw.

Kelleher MJ, Chambers D, Corcoran P (1999). Suicide and religion in Ireland: an investigation of Thomas Masaryk's theory of suicide. *Archives of Suicide Research*, **5**, 173–180.

Kowalski GS, Faupel C, Starr PD (1987). Urbanism and suicide: a study of American counties. *Social Forces*, **66**, 85–101.

Kposowa AJ (2000). Marital status and suicide in the National Longitudinal Mortality Study. *Journal of Epidemiology and Community Health*, **54**, 254–261.

Kral MJ (1994). Suicide as social logic. *Suicide and Life-Threatening Behaviour*, **24**, 245–255.

Kushner HI and Sterk CE (2005). The limits of social capital: Durkheim, suicide, and social cohesion. *American Journal of Public Health*, **95**, 1139–1143.

Laubscher LR (2003). Suicide in a South African town: a cultural psychological investigation. *South African Journal of Psychology*, **33**, 133–143.

Lester D (1987a). Social deviancy and suicidal behaviour. *Journal of Social Psychology*, **127**, 339–340.

Lester D (1987b). *Suicide from a Sociological Perspective*. Charles C Thomas, Springfield.

Lester D (1989). A test of Durkheim's theory of suicide using data from modern nations. *International Journal of Comparative Sociology*, **30**, 235–238.

Lester D (1992a). A test of Durkheim's theory of suicide in primitive societies. *Suicide and Life-Threatening Behaviour*, **22**, 388–395.

Lester D (1992b). The stability and variability of suicide rates in the states of the USA. *Perceptual and Motor Skills*, **75**, 494.

Lester D (1997a). *Making Sense of Suicide: An In-depth Look at why People Kill Themselves*. Charles Press, Philadelphia.

Luhmann N (1984). *Soziale Systeme. Grundriss einer allgemeinen Theorie*. Suhrkamp, Frankfurt am Main.

Lukes S (1973). *Emile Durkheim, his Life and Work: A Historical and Critical Study*. Penguin Books, London.

Luoma J and Pearson J (2002). Suicide and marital status in the United States 1991–1996: is widowhood a risk factor? *American Journal of Public Health*, **92**, 1518–1522.

Mäkinen I and Wasserman D (1997). Suicide prevention and cultural resistance: stability in European countries' suicide ranking, 1970–1988. *Italian Journal of Suicidology*, **7**, 73–85.

Mäkinen IH (1997a). Are there social correlates of suicide? *Social Science and Medicine*, **44**, 1919–1929.

Mäkinen IH (1997b). The importance of culture for suicide mortality. A discussion of Durkheim and Parsons. In IH Mäkinen, *On Suicide in European Countries. Some Theoretical, Legal and Historical Perspectives on Suicide and its Concomitants*. Almqvist and Wiksell, Stockholm.

Mäkinen IH (1997c). Suicide-related crimes in contemporary European criminal laws. *Crisis*, **18**, 35–48.

Mäkinen IH (1997d). *On Suicide in European Countries. Some Theoretical, Legal and Historical Perspectives on Suicide and its Concomitants*. Almqvist and Wiksell, Stockholm.

Mäkinen IH (2000). Suicide mortality in Eastern European transition. *Social Science and Medicine*, **51**, 1411–1420.

Mäkinen IH, Beskow J, Jansson A *et al.* (2002). Historical perspectives on suicide and suicide prevention in Sweden. *Archives of Suicide Research*, **6**, 269–284.

Marcotte DE (2003). The economics of suicide, revisited. *Economic Journal*, **69**, 628–643.

Masaryk TG (1970/1881). *Suicide and the Meaning of Civilization*. The University of Chicago Press, Chicago.

McCall PL and Tittle CG (2007). Population size and suicide in US cities: a static and dynamic exploration. *Suicide and Life-Threatening Behaviour*, **37**, 553–564.

Meng L (2002). Rebellion and revenge: the meaning of suicide of women in rural China. *International Journal of Social Welfare*, **11**, 300–309.

Merton RK (1949). *Social Theory and Social Structure*. Free Press, New York.

Merton RK (1967). *On Theoretical Sociology*. Free Press, New York.

Middleton N, Sterne J, Gunnell D (2006). The geography of despair among 15–44-year-old men in England and Wales: putting suicide on the map. *Journal of Epidemiology and Community Health*, **60**, 1040–1047.

Middleton N, Whitley E, Frankel S *et al.* (2004). Suicide risk in small areas in England and Wales, 1991–1993. *Social Psychiatry and Psychiatric Epidemiology*, **39**, 45–52.

Mohanty BB (2005). 'We are like the living dead': farmer suicides in Maharashtra, Western India. *The Journal of Peasant Studies*, **32**, 243–276.

Moksony F (2001). Victims of change or victims of backwardness? Suicide in rural Hungary. In G Lengyel and Z Rostoványi, eds, *The Small Transformation. Society, Economy, and Politics in Hungary and the New European Architecture*, pp. 366–376. Akadémiai Kiadó, Budapest.

Neeleman J, Halpern D, Leon D *et al.* (1997). Tolerance of suicide, religion, and suicide rates: an ecological and individual study in 19 Western countries. *Psychological Medicine*, **27**, 1165–1171.

Neumayer E (2003). Are socioeconomic factors valid determinants of suicide? Controlling for national cultures of suicide with fixed-effects estimation. *Cross-Cultural Research*, **37**, 307–329.

O'Brien RM and Stockard J (2002). A common explanation for the changing age distributions of suicide and homicide in the United States, 1930 to 2000. *Social Forces*, **84**, 1539–1557.

Otsu A, Araki S, Sakai R *et al.* (2004). Effects of urbanization, economic development, and migration of workers on suicide mortality in Japan. *Social Science and Medicine*, **58**, 1137–1146.

Parsons T (1966). *Societies. Evolutionary and Comparative Perspectives*. Prentice Hall, Englewood Cliffs.

Pescosolido BA (1990). The social context of religious integration and suicide: pursuing the network explanation. *Sociological Quarterly*, **31**, 337–357.

Pescosolido BA and Georgianna S (1989). Durkheim, suicide, and religion. *American Sociological Review*, **54**, 33–48.

Pescosolido BA and Mendelsohn R (1986). Social causation or social construction of suicide? *American Sociological Review*, **39**, 340–354.

Poppel F van and Day LH (1996). A test of Durkheim's theory of suicide—without committing the 'ecological fallacy'. *American Sociological Review*, **61**, 500–507.

Pritchard C and King E (2004). A comparison of child-sex-abuse-related and mental-disorder-related suicide in a six-year cohort of regional suicides: the importance of the child protection–psychiatric interface. *British Journal of Social Work*, **34**, 181–198.

Qin P and Mortensen PB (2003). The impact of parental status on the risk of completed suicide. *Archives of General Psychiatry*, **60**, 797–802.

Rosenthal RW (1993). Suicide attempts and signalling games. *Mathematical Social Sciences*, **26**, 25–33.

Sainsbury P and Barraclough B (1968). Differences between suicide rates. *Nature*, **220**, 1252.

Sainsbury P, Jenkins J, Levey A (1980). The social correlates of suicide in Europe. In R Farmer and S Hirsch, eds, *The Suicide Syndrome*, pp. 38–53. Croom Helm, London.

Schutz A (1954). Concept and theory formation in the social sciences. *The Journal of Philosophy*, **51**, 257–273.

Simpson M and Conklin G (1989). Socio-economic development, suicide, and religion: a test of Durkheim's theory of religion and suicide. *Social Forces*, **67**, 945–964.

Singh GK and Siahpush M (2002). Increasing rural–urban gradients in US suicide mortality, 1970–1997. *American Journal of Public Health*, **92**, 1161–1167.

Stack S (1979). Durkheim's theory of fatalistic suicide: a cross-national approach. *Journal of Social Psychology*, **107**, 161–168.

Stack S (1985). The effect of domestic/religious individualism on suicide, 1954–1978. *Journal of Marriage and the Family*, **47**, 431–447.

Stack S (1990). New micro-level data on the impact of divorce on suicide. *Journal of Marriage and the Family*, **52**, 119–127.

Stack S (1997). Modernization and suicide: a comment on 'An empirical examination of Thomas Masaryk's theory of suicide'. *Archives of Suicide Research*, **3**, 133–135.

Stack S (2000). Suicide: a 15-year review of the sociological literature. Part II: modernization and social integration perspectives. *Suicide and Life-Threatening Behaviour*, **30**, 163–176.

Stack S and Gundlach J (1992). The effect of country music on suicide. *Social Forces*, **71**, 211–218.

Stack S, Gundlach J, Reeves J (1994). The heavy metal subculture and suicide. *Suicide and Life-Threatening Behaviour*, **24**, 15–23.

Stillion JM and Stillion BD (1998). Attitudes towards suicide: past, present, and future. *Omega*, **38**, 77–97.

Stockard J and O'Brien RM (2002). Cohort effects on suicide rates: international variations. *American Sociological Review*, **67**, 854–872.

Straub S (2000). Der Suizid und die 'Wende' in der DDR (Suicide and "die Wende" in the GDR). *System Familie*, **13**, 59–69.

Travis R (1990). Halbwachs and Durkheim: a test of two theories of suicide. *The British Journal of Sociology*, **41**, 225–243.

Tseng WS (2001). *Handbook of Cultural Psychiatry*. Academic Press, San Diego.

Tubergen F van, Grotenhuis M te, Ultee W (2005). Denomination, religious context, and suicide: Neo-Durkheimian multilevel explanations tested with individual and contextual data. *American Journal of Sociology*, **111**, 797–823.

Varty J (2000). Suicide, statistics and sociology: assessing Douglas' critique of Durkheim. In WSF Pickering, ed., *Durkheim's Suicide: A Century of Research and Debate*, pp. 53–65. Routledge, London.

Vijayakumar L, Nagaraj K, Pirkis J *et al.* (2005). Suicide in developing countries (1): frequency, distribution, and association with socioeconomic indicators. *Crisis*, **26**, 104–111.

Wasserman D, Värnik A, Dankowicz M (1998). Regional differences in the distribution of suicide in the former Soviet Union during *perestroika*, 1984–1990. *Acta Psychiatrica Scandinavica*, **98**, 5–12.

Willis LA, Coombs DW, Cockerham WC *et al.* (2002). Ready to die: a postmodern interpretation of the increase of African-American adolescent male suicide. *Social Science and Medicine*, **55**, 907–920.

Yeh BY and Lester D (1987). An economic model for suicide. In Lester D, ed., *Suicide as a Learned Behaviour*, pp. 51–57. Charles Thomas, Springfield.

Yip PS and Thorburn J (2004). Marital status and the risk of suicide: experience from England and Wales, 1982–1996. *Psychological Reports*, **94**, 401–407.

Yip PSF, Liu KY, Hu JP *et al.* (2005). Suicide rates in China during a decade of rapid social changes. *Social Psychiatry and Psychiatric Epidemiology*, **40**, 792–798.

# CHAPTER 24

# Psychoanalytic theories of suicide

## Historical overview and empirical evidence

Elsa Ronningstam, Igor Weinberg
and John T Maltsberger

## Abstract

Psychoanalytic theories and studies have influenced the explorations of suicide over the past hundred years. Freud's first observations of self-objectification in melancholic depression were followed by contributions from object relation theorists and self-psychologists, highlighting foremost the role of narcissistic rage and structural vulnerability. Several of the central clinical concepts that unfolded have more recently been subject to empirical testing. This chapter provides an overview and discussion of the different psychoanalytic formulations applied to suicide. Empirical studies of several assumptions and constructs related to emotions, defences, and structural deficits and vulnerabilities verify their association to or explanation of chronic and acute suicidality. Further conceptualizations and research, especially on subtypes of suicide and individual experiences leading up to and dominating suicidal states, are called for.

## Early psychoanalytic theories of suicide

Although somewhat peripheral in recent years, the understanding of suicide has been an aim of psychoanalysis since its beginning. As early as in 1910 the Vienna Psychoanalytic Society held a meeting to discuss suicide, where Adler, Sadger, Stekel, and Freud himself exchanged views. The meeting ended inconclusively: Freud suggested only when further clinical observations accumulated would a psychoanalytic theory of suicide become possible (Friedman 1967).

Seven years later Freud published 'Mourning and melancholia' (1917), a paper in which he formulated dynamics of melancholic depression and of suicide. At the heart of that remarkable paper lies a clinical observation. Freud wrote:

> If one listens patiently to the melancholic's many and various self-accusations, one cannot in the end avoid the impression that often the most violent of them are hardly at all applicable to the patient himself, but that with insignificant modifications they do fit someone

else, someone whom the patient loves or has loved or should love. Every time one examines the facts this conjecture is confirmed.
>
> Freud (1917, p. 248)

Then he moved on to the critical inference:

> So we find the key to the clinical picture: we perceive that the self-reproaches are reproaches against a loved object which have been shifted away from it on to the patient's own ego.
>
> Freud (1917, p. 248)

These few lines stand out as the central insight that has dominated our understanding of suicidal phenomena ever since: suicide depends, from whichever perspective one examines it, on the capacity to stand aside from oneself, to objectify oneself, and to feel and act upon oneself as though one were someone else.

Freud acknowledged a paradox in suicide. He wrote that the ego's self love is so immense that the ego's consenting to its own self-destruction is inconceivable (Freud 1917). While relating suicide to melancholy, Freud tried to resolve the paradox by connecting suicide to narcissistic identification with a lost and ambivalently loved and hated object. A suicidal person is prone to narcissistic object choice and tends to ambivalence toward those whom he loves. In other words, he tends to experience love and hate concurrently towards his objects and to vacillate between these feelings without any resolution. Loss plays major role in the dynamics of melancholy and, consequently, of suicide. Loss of the object increases ambivalence, and the hostile side of the loving and hating acts like emotional glue, hampering the ability to give up investment in the object, to grieve, and to become invested in new objects. Consequently, the melancholically disposed patient is likely to regress from object relatedness with the lost object to identification with the object. The object becomes part of the ego and the sadism experienced towards the internalized object turns against the self: 'the shadow of the object falls upon the ego' (Freud 1917, p. 249). From the structural point of view, the superego uses all the available sadistic energy to fuel self-denigration (Freud 1923). Sadistic attacks of the superego drive the ego to suicide.

Yet another formulation of suicide was suggested by Freud in the same article (Freud 1923), namely, that the superego withdraws libidinal cathexis from the ego and the ego, feeling abandoned by its protective forces, surrenders and dies. These two formulations explain suicide as a result of self-attack as opposed to suicide due to withdrawal of self-love.

Menninger (1938) took up Freud's later elaboration of the death instinct and tried to explain suicide in terms of it. According to his theory, physical and mental health depend on fusion between the life and death instincts. Fusing ensures a balanced state of neutralization of the death instinct by life instinct. While various degrees of instinctual defusion manifest themselves in various forms of physical and mental illness, suicide constitutes the most extreme manifestation of death instinct and instinctual defusion. Suicide stems from combination of three wishes, he believed: the wish to kill, the wish to be killed, and the wish to die.

1  *The wish to kill* includes desires to attack, destroy or retaliate against another. These desires are not neutralized by positive feelings toward the other.

2  *The wish to be killed* is associated with masochistic tendencies, related to the desire to experience pain and suffering as well as submission to a destructive attack by the other. This wish is also associated with a desire to expiate guilt through suffering and self-inflicted punishment.

3  *The wish to die* includes the longing to die, which gives rise to preoccupations about the essence of death and dying.

## Object relations theories

After Freud's contributions, the next significant development in psychoanalytic study of suicide arose from the work of Melanie Klein (1935, 1946), who in many respects might be called the first 'object relations' theorist. Her understanding of suicide followed from her distinction between the 'paranoid–schizoid' and 'depressive' positions. The paranoid–schizoid position is characterized by the tendency to project hatred onto the object, giving it a persecutory and omnipotent colour in the mind of the projecting child. This provokes annhilatory anxiety (fear of self-disintegration and loss of sense of self) as well as fear of loss of the good object due to destructiveness of the bad object. One tends to attack the bad object to protect oneself from annihilation or in order to protect the good object. In some cases (e.g. hypochondria or body dysmorphic disorder), the bad object is projected into one's own body. In such an instance, to attack the body is to assault the seat of the bad object.

In the depressive position, where we encounter increased ability for integrative perception of the object and oneself, the ego experiences the good and bad objects as centring in the same object. This leads to depressive anxiety; loss of the object is feared, and guilt arises over the sadistic fantasies and wishes towards the object. The guilt feelings demand reparation and attempts to undo real or imaginary consequences of aggressive fantasies. However, in more pathological cases, guilt can lead to feelings of badness and beliefs about being destructive towards others in general and toward the good object in particular. Suicide might follow as an attempt to cleanse the world and prevent its destruction.

## Narcissism and the suicidal state

Any mental operation involved in the maintenance of the structural cohesion of the self, in protecting the temporal continuity of the self, or in maintaining a positive affective colouration of the self, is considered narcissistic. This understanding of the term is somewhat different, however, from the way in which some of the followers of Melanie Klein have used it.

Klein's assertion (1957) that early primitive envy represents a malignant and severe form of innate aggression (derivative of the death instinct) provided a base for connecting suicide to narcissism. Rosenfeld (1971) broadened the meaning of the term narcissism by expanding on this idea, somewhat idiosyncratically including in it destructive and aggressive elements. Rosenfeld believed that narcissistic character structure is a defence against envy and dependency inasmuch as dependency on an object recognized as good invites envy. In his view, narcissism involves both a libidinal and a destructive aspect—the destructive being the idealization of the omnipotent and destructive parts of the self, which often remain split off. However, in states of predominant destructiveness Rosenfeld observed that envy is more violent and associated with a wish to destroy the objects the patient depends upon, such as the analyst, but also to destroy or harm the self, i.e, one's own progress, success, and relationships. Rosenfeld also noted that 'Some of these patients become suicidal and the desire to die, to disappear into oblivion, is expressed quite openly and death is idealized as a solution to all problems' (1971, p. 173). This state, which evokes Freud's description of the death instinct, arises from the destructive, envious parts of the self. Rosenfeld continued:

> The whole self becomes temporarily identified with the destructive self, which aims to triumph over life and creativity … [and] ... these patients have dealt with the struggle between their destructive and libidinal impulses by trying to get rid of their concern and love for their objects by killing their loving dependent self and identifying themselves almost entirely with the destructive narcissistic part of the self which provides them with a sense of superiority and self-admiration.
>
> Rosenfeld (1971, pp. 173–174)

Of importance for the following theoretical accounts on suicide are Rosenfeld's notes of both the destructive aspect of suicide and the idealized view of death.

Influenced by Klein and Rosenfeld, Otto Kernberg (1984, 1992) asserted that an extreme form of hatred is expressed in suicide. 'The self is identified with the hated object and self-elimination is the only way to destroy the object as well' (1992, p. 23). He used the term 'malignant narcissism' (Kernberg 1992, 1998) to indicate a more severe level of superego dysfunction, characterized by antisocial behaviour, ego-syntonic sadism, and paranoid orientation. In patients with malignant narcissism, chronic suicidal preoccupation may be accompanied by cold, sadistic, vengeful satisfactions, and the development of secret means for exercising power and control over the clinician. The transference of these patients often reflects identification with primitive sadistic object representations, i.e, internalized negative and punitive early experiences of others, which are enacted for purposes of revenge and control. These patients may grow more suicidal when they feel that the therapist has been helpful (i.e. negative therapeutic reaction) (Kernberg 2001). It seems that the patients Kernberg has described as suffering from 'malignant narcissism' lie in a fixed, characterological position on a worsening continuum, stopping short of full psychotic fragmentation. Such patients turn life into an omnipotent operation in which cruelty drives out love and pleasure is only to be found in the domination and destruction of others.

Representing another perspective on suicide Lewin (1950) and Maltsberger (1997) suggested that self-execution can serve as a retreat to the archaic grandiose self, or the pathological grandiose self. In other words, the thought and act of suicide may relate to an idealized state of self and actually serve to increase self-esteem. The relatively common omnipotent fantasy of destroying all reality through suicide was put into poetry by A E Housman (1936, p. 185):

> Good creatures, do you love your lives
> And have you ears for sense?
> Here is a knife like other knives,
> That cost me eighteen pence.
> I need but stick it in my heart
> And down will come the sky,
> And earth's foundations will depart
> And all you folk will die.

The everyday psychopathology of a psychiatric unit yields many such examples. Consider the patient who kills herself with the conviction she will rejoin a dead sister in the world beyond the grave. Many persons kill themselves to escape the sufferings of this world in full confidence that they will pass over into a better life. Obviously this fantasy, which it is fair to call delusional, is grandiose. In suicide the ordinary rules of reality, its painful limitations, are denied, and, conquering limitations, the transfigured dying patient soars above them all. Some suicidal patients fondly believe that in death they will experience a body metamorphosis so that physical limitations will be overcome and they will re-emerge as golden, athletic gods. Sylvia Plath, the North American poet who died of suicide some years ago, filled her last writings with omnipotent and aggressive images of flying and destructive she-demons (1992).

Suicides that serve to protect honour, such as hara-kiri, do not appear to arise from depression. Euphoria, heightened self-esteem, and sexual arousal may be associated with the ritual preparations. Yukio Mishima, the Japanese writer, incorporated such themes in his writings before he died in this way. Hara-kiri suicides would sometimes appear to have a manic colouration (Piven 2001).

Suicidal breakdown sometimes represents a final and desperate operation by the failing ego to save itself. Object attachments are abandoned in these states, omnipotent narcissistic fantasies take their places, and the primitive operations of malignant envy and destructiveness come into play as the mad self attempts to assert its control over the whole world (Maltsberger 2004).

Chronic suicidal *preoccupation* (as opposed to bona fide suicide attempts) may help preserve an individual's self-esteem, sense of dignity, autonomy and internal control. It may even be useful for preserving a sense of connection to others, and provide a sense that it is worth staying alive. Lewin and Schulz (1992) contended that chronic suicidal preoccupation gives a sense of autonomy, control, and a grandiose sense of victory over the therapist; it covers feelings of emptiness and loss, reverses sense of helplessness or spoils the therapeutic progress. Rothstein (1980) suggested that in some patients the idea of suicide can represent an illusion of turning passive humiliation into active mastery. Other authors comment that awareness of the ability to end one's life can have an organizing and structuring effect, occasionally making life liveable and even enjoyable (Lewin 1992; Gabbard 2003).

## Self psychology

Although Kohut did not particularly concern himself with suicide, he penned a footnote in 1971 connecting shame, envy, ego-ideal and narcissistic rage to suicide (Kohut 1971). This minor comment has had major impact on more recent theoretical conceptualizations and approaches to treatment. Kohut wrote:

> This state of shame and envy may ultimately be followed by self-destructive impulses. These, too, are to be understood not as attacks of the superego on the ego but as attempts of the suffering ego to do away with the self in order to wipe out the offending, disappointing reality of failure. In other words, the self-destructive impulses are to be understood here not as analogous to the suicidal impulses of a depressed patient but as the expression of narcissistic rage.
>
> Kohut (1971, p. 181)

He believed that individuals who need absolute control of their environment to maintain self-esteem and self-cohesion depend upon the unconditional availability of a mirroring, admiring self-object. Deprived of it, they are prone to the most intense experiences of shame and violent forms of narcissistic rage (Kohut 1972). It is notable that Kohut introduced a distinction between suicide caused by the ego attacking the failing self as opposite to suicide caused by the cruel superego attack on the self (as in Freud's melancholic model). Kohut consequently differentiated suicide in the context of depression from suicide caused by narcissistic rage.

Based on self-psychological theory several new explanations of suicide have been introduced, addressing additional self-states, such as endangerment, narcissistic depletion, and vulnerability, as possible contributors to suicidal ideations and acts (see Table 24.1; Reiser 1992).

## Vulnerability to suicide

Several recent studies of suicide suggest particular personality aspects that may lead to suicide. The vulnerability model suggests that certain psychological traits and deficits specifically predispose to suicide. Such a theoretical model invites a more integrative approach to the understanding of the dynamics in suicidal states, and attends to more complex relationships between several possible contributing factors to suicide, including developmental, psychodynamic and internal subjective experiences of the suicidal person.

Beyond self-directed aggression and emergency operations to shore up crumbling self-esteem, the vulnerability studies attend to flaws in self-organization which predispose patients to structural fracture. The German psychoanalyst Heinz Henseler (Henseler, 1974, 1981; Etzersdorfer, 2001) has addressed the role of narcissistic vulnerability and compromised self-esteem regulation. Suicide, he suggests, is an extreme form of reaction to injury to the sense of self-worth. Departing from Freud's 'Mourning and melancholia' (1917) and the central role of depression in suicide, he assumes that the suicidal individual gives up his individuality by fusing with a primary object in order to gain safety. In other words, in suicide, the patient acts to save self-feeling or self-regard.

Buie and Maltsberger (1989) identified two aspects of suicide vulnerability, loss of the psychological self through mental

**Table 24.1** Suicidal dynamics according to the self psychology

| Self-experience | Formulation | Suicidal dynamics |
| --- | --- | --- |
| The endangered self | The self is organized at a primitive level. It is torn among the longing for closeness, threat of engulfment in the other, and annihilatory experience that stems from that. Therefore, the person avoids close relationships and retreats into isolation, restriction, and compulsive lifestyle. | Suicide represents coping with breakdown of this defence and with the threat of annihilation. |
| The enraged self | The person has a negative self-image due to identification with the negative introjects that had been projected into him by his parents. The person experience himself as a victim, as starved or attacked and tends to idealize the abusers. He tends to choose self-objects that maintain the childhood abusive experiences. Therefore, closeness evokes tremendous rage. | Suicide stems from a combination of turning of the negative strivings of the abusive introjects against the child-self, and expression of the rage against these introjects. |
| The vulnerable self | The person feels empty, lack of self-fulfilment, and pervasive lack of satisfaction. He is sensitive to separations, prone to hypochondria, obesity, poor physical health, and avoids direct expression of anger. | Due to pervasive misery, the person is at risk of chronic suicide and repetitive suicide attempts. |
| The grandiose self | The grandiose self is critically dependent on self-objects that supply experiences of mirroring, admiration, perfect empathy, and allow idealization. Empathic failure of self-object leads to self-disintegration, catastrophic feelings, emptiness, and rage. | Suicide is an escape from painful feelings of self-disintegration, emptiness, and rage. |
| The mirroring self | High sensitivity to the feelings of others. He is willing to become self-object for others and seeks this role in an almost compulsive fashion. While he is directing his empathy to others, he is depriving himself of it and, as a result, experiences emptiness and depression (Miller 1979). | Due to unrelenting self-sacrifice, the person experiences increasing depression, loneliness, emptiness, disappointment, anger, and exhaustion. |

disintegration and overwhelming negative self-judgement. They noticed that suicidal people are vulnerable to both unbearable experiences of aloneness as well as to a deep sense of worthlessness and guilt.

Maltsberger (1986, 1993, 1998, 2004) further integrated the role of self-disintegration and dissociation in suicidal states. In his view, suicidal people suffer from structural deficits in self-representation, in internalizations of others, and in object constancy. Paucity of positive introjects limits the capacity for emotional and self-esteem regulation. It follows that pre-suicidal patients are critically dependent on external resources for self-regulation, i.e, sustaining resources (e.g. significant others, work, pets, etc.). Loss of exterior sustaining resources precipitates three deadly affects: aloneness, self-contempt, and murderous rage. Aloneness refers to the inability to evoke positive memories of significant others or positive interactions with them. This eerie experience of aloneness implies a profound, despairing sense that one has never been loved and never will be loved, ever. Patients caught up in a state of aloneness are apt to be overwhelmed by annihilatory anxiety; they may feel they are already dead, or even show the conviction that they are dead in fact. In addition to the experience of anguished aloneness, suicidal patients can suffer from intense self-contempt—an experience of extreme scorn, disgust, and denigration, blame, and hate—all turned on the self. Murderous rage can lead to suicide when the person turns it against themselves—either because of guilt feelings over the murderous wishes or feelings of hopelessness to change the situation.

Structural deficits and vulnerability to aloneness, self-contempt, and murderous rage affect the way suicidal states unfold. First, lack of the ability to evoke positive introjects and excessive reliance on receding external sustaining resources can lead to escalation of anguish. The patient must then struggle with a flux of negative affect; we may observe frantic attempts to get help to endure intolerable mental pain; we may see self-mutilation, dissociation (Maltsberger 2004), or substance use (Hendin *el al.* 2001). If the patient is unable to summon help or rescue from outside himself,

the third stage of the suicide breakdown will begin to unfold– disintegration of the self-representation (Maltsberger 2004). Self-break-up together with de-neutralization of the aggression that colours these representations lead to pitting some parts of the self against others. The superego becomes harsher and more sadistic, unleashing an attack against the ego. In this case suicide represents fulfilment of sadistic forces of the super ego as well as an attempt to put an end to painful self-awareness. A more regressive scenario consists of projection of the sadistic and persecutory part of the self-representation into ones body and attacking it in self-defence (Maltsberger 1998).

The last stage of self-break-up in suicide is marked by grandiose survival manoeuvres that operate outside the scope of reality testing. At this stage, reality testing having failed, patients entertain psychotic, grandiose beliefs and act on them without hindrance. Some patients imagine death as a continuation of life, rebirth, reunion with loved ones, or perhaps self-cleansing or self-transformation (Maltsberger and Buie 1980). Here one encounters concrete conviction that the bad aspects of oneself reside in one's body and that by attacking it one can be rid of it and survive in an imaginary sphere without it (Maltsberger 2004). Other patients deny the irreversibility of death and see suicide as a survivable scientific experiment (Ronningstam and Maltsberger 1998).

Smith and Eyman (1985) proposes that there are a number of characteristic defining the 'vulnerable personality'. They enumerate high self-expectations, a tendency to inhibit negative emotions, an ambivalent attitude toward death, lack of ability to grieve past losses, a tendency to develop overly dependent relationships, passivity and neediness. Other characteristics described by Smith and Eyman include cognitive rigidity, arrested sexual development, and over-investment in appearance or intellectual ability. In order to compensate for these vulnerabilities one develops a 'life dream' to help regulate the self. Disappointments and losses can smash life dreams. In the absence of capacity to grieve and to moderate unrealistic aspirations, suicide can occur.

## The role of shame and ego ideal

Lansky (1991) averred that shame is the most significant affect in suicidal patients; other suicide-related emotional experiences such as depression, guilt, psychic pain and anger he thought secondary to shame in driving suicide. Shame is the feeling associated with the failure to live up to ideals or to achieve important aspirations and goals. It is a response to feedback from others suggesting incompetence, inefficacy, and the inability to influence, predict, or comprehend an event, in the face of expectations that one should be able to control or understand (Broucek 1982). Shame in this sense would appear to arise from helplessness to master either inner or outer challenges, or sometimes, both (Bibring 1953). Shame may even be indistinguishable from helplessness. We further note, however, that shame is often associated primarily with exhibitionism and ambitious strivings that are unrelated to the ego ideal (Kohut 1972). Excessive primitive shame triggered by the experience of incompetence, inadequacy, or lack of control can provoke cognitive impairment, autonomic reactions and even self-disintegration. Lansky (1991) related shame to the loss or impossibility of a meaningful bonding. Shame can be evoked both by an actual rejection from others but also by inner characterological tendencies to distance, to detach from, to overreact to, or to destroy relationships.

Unattainable and incompatible ego ideals are both major causes of shame, and are also associated with suicide vulnerability. The development of the self ideal is essential for self-esteem regulation. Incoherent or incongruent deformations in the ego-ideal system can make it impossible for the self to approximate what is demanded. Awareness that the demands of the ego ideal, in its own contradictory structure incapable of approximation by the self, are beyond reach, may unleash self-critical attacks and self-shaming, and spur the patient into suicide. In certain situations, especially when aspirations are meant to repair or heal narcissistic wounds, some patients may face conflicting ideals or be caught in between incompatible self-demands and expectations (Morrison 1989, 1994, 2005; Orbach *et al.* 1998). The subjective experience of helplessness that aroused in such circumstances invites narcissistic collapse and suicidal acting out.

## Deficient capacity for mentalization

Mentalization, according to Fonagy (1999), refers to the ability to understand behaviours, thoughts, and feelings about oneself and others in terms of intentions and wishes. He suggested that the capacity for metacognitive control, reflective self-functioning and mentalization that can help protect against narcissistic injury has not developed in suicidal narcissistic patients. They are unable to think and reflect beyond immediate experience, and unable to use aggression as a protective shield against overwhelming thoughts and feelings. Furthermore, capacity to reflect and understand the consequences of aggressive and self-destructive actions is impaired. Fonagy (1993) noted that a boy's self-sabotaging behaviour could be deadly; 'his primitive reflective self did not see the death of his body as leading to the death of his mental self' (1993, p. 481).

## Psychoanalytic family approaches

Sharp increases in the suicide rate of adolescents occurred in the United States during the 1980s, alarming the general public as well as the mental health community. Pfeffer (1981) theorized that parents in conflict may project responsibility for their troubles onto their child, who identifies with a sense of badness and lack of resolution of the parental conflict. Suicide in such children represents an attempt to resolve the conflict and to avoid feelings of badness. Sabbath (1969) described families that suggest to a child that he is unwanted; suicide may then occur because it seems to the scapegoated child that this is what the parents want. Richman (1978, 1980) described weak boundaries, enmeshment, and conflictual messages around independence in families of suicidal adolescents. These families encourage independence but invite symbiotic clinging at the same time. Suicide in such circumstances reflects strivings to symbiosis and flight from it at the same time.

Further description of family dynamics of suicidal children and adolescents were provided by Fischman (1988) who related suicide attempts to extremely polarized, distant relationships coupled with enmeshment with the parents, giving rise to a sense of confusion; 'ideal families' which prohibit expression of weakness and, thus, generate feelings of shame and a counterdependent attitude; and emotionally distant families that generate a sense of rejection.

## Other hypotheses

Orgel (1974) suggested that identification with the victim role paves the way to suicide. Such identification can function as a way of consolidating an identity, a way of maintaining idealization of the object. It can also be an instance of identification with both the aggressor and the victim, as well as a manifestation of fear of and avoidance of retaliatory impulses. Singer (1977) observed that suicide attempts in borderline and narcissistic patients help preserve sense of self and help to avoid experiences of emptiness and deadness. Litman (1970) described suicidal states in terms of acting out of an autonomous ego state that encompasses suicidal potential: preoccupation with suicide, planning, integrative function of suicide, emotional regulatory function of suicide, as well as contribution of fantasies, wishes, memories, and identification with this ego state. Campbell (1995) emphasized the protective effect to identification with a good father—this strengthens reality testing and protects patients from primitive regressive pulls toward fusion with the primitive mother imago of early childhood. Suicide, according to Campbell, often represents for the patients a longing to sleep forever in the arms of the primal mother.

## Empirical support for theoretical positions

Most psychoanalytic clinical concepts are difficult to operationalize. Nevertheless, several of the basic assumptions of these formulations have been subjected to empirical testing. Below we review a number of studies which confirm that certain emotional phenomena are indeed implicated in suicide.

### Anger

Reports that anger is associated with increased suicide risk cross-sectionally (Horesh *et al.* 1997), but not longitudinally (Goldney *et al.* 1997), suggest such feelings are a specific characteristic of the suicidal state rather than of the personality of the suicidal individuals.

### Anger turned against oneself

Recklitis and colleagues (1992) found that suicide attempters had a significant increase in use of the defence mechanism of *turning against the self*, as compared to suicide ideators or non-suicidal patients. Increased self-directed anger was noted among suicide attempters (Kaslow *et al.* 2000) as well as among people with-suicidal ideation (Mihura *et al.* 2003). Rutstein and Goldberger (1973) noted that subliminal stimulation of aggressive impulses (e.g. exposure to such message as 'destroy mother') increased levels of depression among suicidal subjects, whereas among non-suicidal subjects the same message increased outwardly directed aggression, as measured by self-report questionnaire of depression and the Rorschach test.

## Shame

The association between suicidal tendencies and shame was confirmed by Lester (1998) in suicide ideators and Hendin *et al.* (2001) in suicide completers, but more definitive studies are needed.

## Defence mechanisms

According to psychoanalytic theory suicidal people overly rely on certain defence mechanisms and patterns (such as denial, projection), and minimize sublimation. These occur parallel to self-break-up (Maltsberger 2004). Repression and internalization, i.e, accompaniments to internalization of aggression and of bad objects (Klein 1935); and compensation, i.e, reflecting attempted repair of ego vulnerability (Smith 1985), have been empirically shown to correlate with suicidal states (see Table 24.2).

## Friable self-representation

Six studies confirmed the above mentioned pathologically flawed self-representation in suicidal patients.

### Identity confusion

Dingman and McGlashan (1986) found that a major proportion of patients who attempted suicide had identity confusion at the time of admission to Chestnut Lodge Hospital. Identity confusion also prospectively predicted suicide attempts and threats in patients diagnosed with borderline personality disorder (Yen *et al.* 2004). When compared to non-suicidal adolescents, those adolescents who attempted suicide had a more confused identity defined by the following parameters: stability, continuity, meaningfulness, social recognition, commitment, and sense of resilience (Bar-Joseph and Tzuriel 1990).

### Incongruent self-representations

Orbach *et al.* (1998) compared self-representations in suicidal and non-suicidal inpatients including real self (i.e, actual self representation of the person), ideal self (i.e, representation of whom the person wants to be), and ought self (i.e, representation of whom the person thinks he or she ought to or should be). Suicidal adolescents had a larger gap between the ideal and the ought to be self-representation, indicating a larger confusion between goals and standards of the self.

### Increased self-focus

Stirman and Pennebaker (2001) observed increased use of the first person pronoun 'I' in literary works of poets who committed suicide as compared to poets who lived during the same time period with similar education and country.

### Self-disintegration

Use of the word 'whirling' and similar words (that might indicate propensity for self-disintegration) in Rorschach protocols predicted

**Table 24.2** Defence mechanisms in suicide attempters

| Defence mechanism | Study | | | | |
|---|---|---|---|---|---|
| | **Apter *et al.* (1989)** | **Pfeffer *et al.* (1995)** | **Apter *et al.* (1997) Study 1** | **Apter *et al.* (1997) Study 2** | **Corruble *et al.* (2004)** |
| Regression | ↑ | ↑ | ↑ | ↑ | |
| Displacement | ↑ | | | ↑↑ | |
| Repression | ↑↑ | | ↑ | ↑ | |
| Projection | | ↑ | ↑ | | ↑ |
| Compensation | | ↑ | | ↑↑ | |
| Undoing | | | | | |
| Intellectualization | | | | | |
| Sublimation | | | ↓ | | |
| Reaction formation | | ↑ | | | |
| Denial | ↓ | | ↑ | ↑ | |
| Introjection | | | ↑↑ | | |
| Autistic fantasy | | | | | ↑ |
| Passive aggression | | | | | ↑ |
| Acting out | | | | | ↑ |
| Defence Mechanisms Measure | Lifestyle Index | Ego Defence Scales | Ego Defence scales | Lifestyle Index | Defence Style Questionnaire |
| Suicide attempts sample size | 30 | 25 | 55 | 55 | 60 |

↑, increased use; ↑↑, increased use that is specific to the suicide attempters group; ↓, decreased use.

suicide among medical students over the period of 20–35 years (Thomas and Duszynski 1985).

### Self and object confusion

The presence of confusion between the self and others, described by several authors (Roth and Blatt 1974; Maltsberger 1993), was supported by studies that used Rorschach measures of boundary confusion (Rydin *et al.* 1990, Fowler *et al.* 2001; Blatt and Ritzler 1974; Rierdan *et al.* 1978; Hansell *et al.* 1988).

### Object relations

Suicide attempters tend to have more primitive object relations, i.e, less complex object representations, more negative affect tone associated with object relations, and less complex understanding of social causality (Kaslow *et al.* 2000). Predominance of projective identification and repetition of rejecting relationships were specifically confirmed by Kullgren (1988), who noted that suicidal people tend to evoke more negative responses from others which increase risk for suicide. Lower level of separation–individuation was confirmed by Kaslow *et al.* (2000).

### Body experience

A series of studies by Orbach and colleagues showed suicide attempters have negative body perceptions. Depressed suicidal people had significantly increased negative attitudes toward their bodies when compared to both depressed non-suicidal and normal subjects. Suicidal people also showed a significantly higher discrepancy between the ideal perception of the body and the actual one (Orbach *et al.* 1995a). These findings also applied to suicidal patients diagnosed with schizophrenia and personality disorders (Orbach *et al.* 1997; see also Orbach *et al.* 1996a, b). Suicidal individuals manifested decreased investment in their body as indicated by negative feelings and attitudes toward the body, negative body images, decreased body care, less body protection, and less experiences of comfort when touched physically (Orbach and Mikulincer 1998). With regard to body perception, suicide attempters revealed more negative attitudes and feelings about their bodies, lower body protection and sense of control over the body, and more aberrant body perception (Orbach *et al.* 2001). Sheffer (2001) also found that suicide attempters demonstrated lower touch sensitivity, more negative experience of touch, and a higher tendency to avoid touch. All these studies indicate a close association between suicidal tendencies and negative body perception.

### Dissociation

A number of studies demonstrated that suicidal people, including those diagnosed with schizophrenia and personality disorders, utilize dissociation to a higher degree than non-suicidal people (Orbach *et al.* 1995b, 1996a, 1997; Orbach 1997). More specifically, suicidal tendencies were closely connected with dissociative tendencies (Orbach *et al.* 1995b). Suicidal people displayed more affective dissociation (feeling of changes in affective life), and more control dissociation (feeling of changes in control) (Orbach *et al.* 1995b). This relation between dissociation and suicidal tendencies has been further supported in other studies (Ensink 1992; Herman *et al.* 1989; Orbach *et al.* 1996b; Sheffer 2001).

### Death perception

The perception that death is desirable was correlated with suicide tendencies and suicide attempts in several studies (Orbach *et al.*

1983, 1984, 1985, 1991, 1993, 1995a, 1997, 2001; Guttierrez *et al.* 1996; Osman *et al.* 1994). Gothelf *et al.* (1998) reported higher preoccupation with death in suicidal patients. Suicidal children tend to attribute living qualities to the dead (Orbach and Glaubman 1979) and refer to life after death and resurrection (Orbach and Glaubman 1978). Neuringer (1968) observed an increase in negative perception of death during the recovery from a suicide attempt, suggesting that the death perception in suicide attempters is state dependent.

### Deficient reality testing and thought disorder

Studies confirmed deficient reality testing (Plutchik *et al.* 1995) and increased unusual thinking (Mendonca and Holden 1996) in otherwise non-psychotic suicide attempters. This is consistent with clinical formulations of suicidal states (Maltsberger 1999, 2004; Laufer 1995) describing transient psychotic phenomena contributing to suicidality.

### Ego vulnerability

Smith and Eyman (1985) developed a detailed Rorschach manual that operationalized the four areas of ego vulnerability (Smith 1985) mentioned above. They noted that serious suicide attempters had either over controlled or lively aggressive fantasies, high expectations of themselves, conflict around passivity and dependency, and ambivalent attitudes toward death. Male serious attempters showed more conflicts related to dependency and passivity while female serious suicide attempters manifested affective over control only. It seems that ego vulnerability is useful for prediction of suicide in males.

### Family approaches

The 'expendable child' hypothesis (Sabbath 1969) was confirmed in a study by Woznica and Shapiro (1990). Suicidal adolescents experience themselves as burdens, unwanted, not essential, not valued, yet responsible for the problems of others. Observations by Richman (1978, 1980) of controlling and symbiotic relationships in the families of suicidal adolescents were further verified by Kaplan and Maldaver (1993).

### Masochism and self-defeating behaviours

Weinberg (2005) confirmed that increased self-defeating processes in suicidal people, including guilt, rejection provocation, and intolerance of ambiguity, contribute to suicidal tendencies.

## Critique of the existing research

Methodological difficulties in many studies attempting to validate psychoanalytic constructs, or parts of them, cast shadows over much of the research to this date. Some of the problems are as follows.

### Measurement difficulties

Many psychoanalytic constructs are difficult to measure in a valid fashion. Most of the studies mentioned above relied on self-report measures or on various projective indices of the constructs. We think that use of validated experimental measures of the constructs will increase validity of the results and enrich the field.

### Sampling ambiguities

The distinction between suicide ideators (probands who entertain ideas of committing suicide), suicide attempters, and successful completers is often blurred in the research. Each of these classes of patients differ from each other in a variety of ways, not the least in the potential or actual lethality that mark them. When patients from these groups are conflated together, research results are muddied. Though the patients are alike in many respects, they differ from each other in important ways. Some studies do not distinguish between the categories making extrapolation from one subgroup to another problematic. Our ability to confirm psychoanalytic formulations for suicidal attempters and completers in studies based on samples of suicide ideators is therefore problematical.

### Flawed research designs

Most studies reviewed used cross-sectional designs. Consequently, the predictive validity of the reported characteristics found in the suicidal individuals is unclear. This fact limits the clinical relevance of the findings.

### Control for other variables

Most studies did not control for confounding variables such as psychiatric diagnosis.

Several aspects of suicide still remain unknown or sparsely investigated. Those include: *suicide subtypes* (e.g. superego conflict vs narcissistic rage vs shame); *self-experience* (Reiser 1992); development and validation of *measures of relevant constructs* (e.g. 'life-dream', over-reliance on external sustaining resources, emptiness); and studies of people's *experience during suicidal states* as compared to non-suicidal states. Such follow-up studies would inform about and differentiate state-dependent and characterologically related characteristics of suicide attempters.

# Conclusions

Although suicide for a long time remained relatively unexplored in psychoanalytic studies, several theoretical trends are now discernable. The emphasis on the role of the attacking as opposed to the protective superego, and the economy of the libido, suggests that depression plays a central role in suicidal states. This stand has gradually been complemented by the increasing awareness of the role of narcissism. Narcissistic rage and narcissistic vulnerability in suicide vulnerable persons are now at the centre of attention. Integration of self-psychological theory with observations of self-disintegration, shame and deformity in egoideal development suggest several possible avenues that lead to both acute suicidal collapse and chronic suicidality. Despite the challenges involved in the empirical measuring and validating of psychoanalytic constructs, a substantial number of empirical studies do verify several of the central assumptions and constructs such as dissociation, ego vulnerability, primitive object relations and deficient self-representations in driving suicide.

## References

Apter A, Gothelf D, Offer R et al. (1997). Suicidal adolescents and ego defence mechanisms. *Journal of American Academy of Child and Adolescent Psychiatry*, **36**, 1520–1527.

Apter A, Plutchik R, Sevy S et al. (1989). Defence mechanisms in risk of suicide and risk of violence. *American Journal of Psychiatry*, **146**, 1027–1031.

Bar-Joseph H and Tzuriel D (1991). Suicidal tendencies and ego identity in adolescence. *Adolescence*, **25**, 215–223.

Bibring E (1953) The mechanism of depression. In P Greenacre, ed., *Affective Disorders*, pp. 13–48. New York Universities Press, New York.

Blatt SJ and Ritzler BA (1974). Suicide and the representation of transparency cross-sections on the Rorschach. *Journal of Consulting and Clinical Psychology*, **42**, 280–287.

Broucek, F. (1982). Shame and its relationship to early narcissistic developments. *International Journal of Psycho-Analysis*, **63**, 369–378.

Buie D and Maltsberger JT (1989). The psychological vulnerability to suicide. In D Jacobs and HN Brown, eds, *Suicide, Understanding and Responding*, pp. 59–72. International Universities Press, Madison.

Campbell D (1995). The role of the father in a pre-suicide state. *International Journal of Psychoanalysis*, **76**, 315–323.

Corruble E, Bronnec M, Falissard B et al. (2004). Defence styles in depressed suicide attempters. *Psychiatry and Clinical Neuroscience*, **58**, 285–288.

Dingman CW and McGlashan TH (1986). Discriminating characteristics of suicides. Chestnut Lodge follow-up sample including patients with affective disorder, schizophrenia and schizoaffective disorder. *Acta Psychiatrica Scandinavica*, **74**, 91–9.

Ensink BJ (1992). *Confusing Realities: A Study on Childhood Sexual Abuse and Psychiatric Syndromes*. VU University Press, Amsterdam.

Etzersdorfer E (2001). The psychoanalytical positions on suicidality in German-speaking regions. Paper presented at the International Congress on Suicidality and Psychoanalysis, Hamburg, Germany, 2001.

Fischman HC (1988). *Treating Troubled Adolescents: A Family Therapy Approach*. Basic Books, New York.

Fonagy P (1999) Attachment, the development of the self and its pathology in personality disorders. In J Derksen, C Maffei and H Groen, eds, *Treatment of Personality Disorders*, pp. 53–68. Kluwer Academic/Plenum Publisher, New York.

Fonagy P. (1993) Aggression and the psychological self. *International Journal of Psychoanalysis*, **74**, 471–485.

Fowler JC, Hilsenroth MJ, Piers C (2001). An empirical study of seriously disturbed suicidal patients. *Journal of the American Psychoanalytic Association*, **49**, 161–186.

Freud S (1917). Mourning and melancholia. In J Strachey (ed. and trans.), *The Standard Edition of the Complete Psychological Works of Sigmund Freud*, Vol. 10. Hogarth Press, London.

Freud S (1923). The ego and the id. In J Strachey (ed. and trans.), *The Standard Edition of the Complete Psychological Works of Sigmund Freud*, Vol. 19. Hogarth Press, London.

Friedman P ed. (1967) *On Suicide, with Particular Reference to Suicide Among Young Students*. International Universities Press, New York.

Gabbard GO (2003). Miscarriages of psychoanalytic treatment with suicidal patients. *International Journal of Psychoanalysis*, **84**, 249–261.

Goldney R, Winefield A, Saebel J et al. (1997). Anger, suicidal ideation, and attempted suicide: a prospective study. *Comprehensive Psychiatry*, **38**, 264–268.

Hansell AG, Lerner HD, Milden RS et al. (1988). Single-sign Rorschach suicide indicators: a validity study using a depressed inpatient population. *Journal of Personality Assessment*, **52**, 658–669.

Hendin H, Maltsberger JT, Lipschitz A et al. (2001). Recognizing and responding to a suicide crisis. *Suicide and Life-Threatening Behaviors*, **31**, 115–128.

Henseler H (1974) *Narzisstische Krisen. Zur Psychodynamik des Selbstmordes*. Westdeutcher Verlag, Opladen, Germany.

Henseler H (1981). Psychoanalytische Theorien zur Suizidalitaet. In H Henseler and C Reimer, eds, *Selbstmordgefardung. Zur Psychodynamik und Psychotherapie*, pp. 113–135. Frommann-Holzboog, Stuttgart.

Herman JL, Perry JC, van der Kolk BA (1989). Childhood origins of self-destructive behavior. *American Journal of Psychiatry*, **146**, 490–495.

Horesh N, Rolnick T, Iancu I et al. (1997). Anger, impulsivity and suicide risk. *Psychotherapy and Psychosomatics*, **66**, 92–96.

Housman AE (1936) XXVI in *More Poems*. Reprinted in *The Collected Poems of A. E. Housman*, p. 185. Henry Holt and Co, New York.

Kaplan KJ and Maldaver M (1993). Parental marital style and completed adolescent suicide. *Omega*, **2**, 131–154.

Kaslow NJ, Reviere SL, Chance SE *et al.* (2000). An empirical study of the psychodynamics of suicide. *Journal of the American Psychoanalytic Association*, **46**, 777–795.

Kernberg OF (1984). *Severe Personality Disorders*. Yale University Press, New Haven.

Kernberg OF (1992). *Aggressions in Personality Disorders and Perversions*. Yale University Press, New Haven.

Kernberg OF (1998). Pathological narcissism and narcissistic personality disorder: theoretical background and diagnostic classification. In EF Ronningstam, ed., *Disorders of Narcissism: Diagnostic, Clinical and Empirical Implications*, pp. 29–51.0 American Psychiatric Press Inc., Washington.

Kernberg OF (2001) The suicidal risk in severe personality disorders: differential diagnosis and treatment. *Journal of Personality Disorder*, **15**, 195–208.

Klein M (1935). A contribution to the pathogenesis of manic-depressive states. In M Klein, *Love Guilt, and Reparation,* pp. 262–305. Virago Press Ltd, London.

Klein M (1946). Notes on some schizoid mechanisms. *International Journal of Psychoanalysis*, **27**, 99–110.

Klein M (1957). *Envy and Gratitude*. Basic Books, New York.

Kohut H (1971). *The Analysis of the Self*. International Universities Press, New York.

Kohut H (1972). Thoughts on narcissism and narcissistic rage. *The Psychoanalytic Study of the Child*, **27**, 360–400.

Kullgren G (1988). Factors associated with completed suicide in borderline personality disorder. *Journal of Nervous and Mental Disease*, **176**, 40–44.

Lansky M (1991). Shame and the problem of suicide: a family systems perspective. *British Journal of Psychotherapy*, **7**, 230–242.

Laufer M ed. (1995). *The Suicidal Adolescent*. Karnac Books, London.

Lester D (1998). The association of shame and guilt with suicidality. *Journal of Social Psychology*, **138**, 535–536.

Lewin BD (1950). *The Psychoanalysis of Elation*. W. W. Norton and Co, New York.

Lewin RA (1992). On chronic suicidality. *Psychiatry*, **55**, 16–27.

Lewin RA and Shultz C (1992). *Losing and Fusing*. Aronson, New York.

Litman RE (1970). Suicide as acting out. In ES Shneidman, NL Farberow and RE Litman, eds, *The Psychology of Suicide*, pp. 293–304. Jason Aronson Inc., New York.

Maltsberger J.T. (1986). *Suicide Risk: The Formulation of Clinical Judgment*. New York, New York University Press.

Maltsberger JT (1993). Confusion of the body, the self and others in suicidal states. In A Leenaars, ed., *Suicidology: Essays in Honor of Edwin S. Shneidman*, pp. 148–171. Jason Aronson Inc., Northvale.

Maltsberger JT (1997) Ecstatic suicide. *Archives of Suicide Research*, **3**, 283–301.

Maltsberger JT (1998). Pathological narcissism and self-regulatory processes in suicidal states. In E Ronningstam, ed., *Disorders of Narcissism— Diagnostic, Clinical and Empirical Implications,* pp. 327–344. American Psychiatric Press, Washington.

Maltsberger JT (1999). The psychodynamic understanding of suicide. In DL Jacobs, ed., *The Harvard Medical School Guide to Suicide Assessment and Intervention*, pp. 72–82. Jossey-Bass, Inc., San Francisco.

Maltsberger JT (2004).The descent into suicide. *International Journal of Psychoanalysis*, **85**, 653–668.

Maltsberger JT (August 2001). Psychoanalytic Studies of Suicide in English. Presented at the First International Congress on Suicidality and Psychoanalysis, Hamburg Germany.

Maltsberger JT and Buie DH Jr (1980). The devices of suicide: revenge, riddance, and rebirth. *International Review of Psychoanalysis*, **7**, 61–72.

Mendonca JD and Holden RR (1996). Are all suicidal ideas closely linked to hopelessness? *Acta Psychiatrica Scandinavica*, **93**, 246–251.

Menninger K (1938). *Man Against Himself*. Harcourt, Brace and Company, New York.

Mihura JL, Nathan-Montano E, Alperin R (2003). Rorschach measures of aggressive drive derivatives: a college student sample. *Journal of Personality Assessment*, **80**, 41–49.

Miller A (1979). *Prisoners of Childhood*. Basic Books, New York.

Morrison AP (2005). On ideals and idealization. Paper presented at the American Psychoanalytic Association Winter meeting, New York, January 2005.

Morrison AP (1989). *Shame, the Underside of Narcissism*. The Analytic Press, Hillsdale.

Morrison AP (1994). Breadth and boundaries of a self-psychological immersion in shame. A one-and-a-half-person perspective. *Psychoanalytic Dialogues*, **4**(1), 19–35.

Neuringer C (1968). Divergencies between attitudes towards life and death among suicidal, psychosomatic, and normal hospitalized patients. *Journal of Consulting and Clinical Psychology*, **32**, 59–63.

Orbach I (1997). A taxonomy of factors related to suicidal behavior. *Clinical Psychology: Science and Practice*, **4**, 208–224.

Orbach I and Glaubman H (1978). Suicidal, aggressive, and normal children's perception of personal and impersonal death. *Journal of Clinical Psychology*, **34**, 850–856.

Orbach I and Glaubman H (1979). Children's perception of death as a defensive process. *Journal of Abnormal Psychology*, **88**, 671–674.

Orbach I and Mikulincer M (1998). The body investment scale: construction and validation of a body experience scale. *Psychological Assessment*, **4**, 415–425.

Orbach I, Carlson G, Feshbach S *et al.* (1984). Attitudes toward life and death in suicidal, normal, and chronically ill children: an extended replication. *Journal of Consulting and Clinical Psychology*, **52**, 1020–1027.

Orbach I, Feshbach S, Carlson G *et al.* (1983). Attraction and repulsion by life and death in suicidal and in normal children. *Journal of Consulting and Clinical Psychology*, **51**, 661–670.

Orbach I, Gross Y, Glaubman H *et al.* (1985). Children's perception of death in humans and animals as a function of age, anxiety and cognitive ability. *Journal of Child Psychology and Psychiatry*, **26**, 453–463.

Orbach I, Kedem P, Gorchover O *et al.* (1993). Fears of death in suicidal and nonsuicidal adolescents. *Journal of Abnormal Psychology*, **102**, 553–558.

Orbach I, Lotem-Peleg M, Kedem P (1995a). Attitude toward the body in suicidal, depressed, and normal adolescents. *Suicide and Life Threatening Behavior*, **25**, 211–221.

Orbach I, Kedem P, Herman L *et al.* (1995b). Dissociative tendencies in suicidal, depressed, and normal adolescents. *Journal of Social and Clinical Psychology*, **14**, 393–408.

Orbach I, Mikulincer M, Cohen D *et al.* (1997). Thresholds and tolerance of physical pain in suicidal and non-suicidal adolescents. *Journal of Consulting and Clinical Psychology*, **65**, 646–652.

Orbach I, Mikulincer M, Stein D *et al.* (1998). Self-representation of suicidal adolescents. *Journal of Abnormal Psychology*, **107**, 435–439.

Orbach I, Milstein I, Har-Even D *et al.* (1991). A multi-attitude suicide tendency scale for adolescents. *Psychological Assessment*, **3**, 398–404.

Orbach I, Palgi Y, Stein D *et al.* (1996a). Tolerance of physical pain in suicidal individuals. *Death Studies*, **20**, 327–340.

Orbach I, Stein D, Palgi Y *et al.* (1996b). Perception of physical pain in accident and suicide attempt patients: self-preservation vs. self-destruction. *Journal of Psychiatric Research*, **30**, 307–320.

Orbach I, Stein D, Shani-Sela M *et al.* (2001). Body attitudes and body experiences in suicidal adolescents. *Suicide and Life-Threatening Behavior*, **31**, 237–249.

Orgel S (1974). Fusion with the victim and suicide. *International Journal of Psychoanalysis*, **55**, 531–541.

Osman A, Barrios FX, Panak WF *et al.* (1994). Validation of the Multi-Attitude Suicide Tendency scale in adolescent samples. *Journal of Clinical Psychology*, **50**, 847–855.

Pfeffer CM, Hurt SW, Peskin JR *et al.* (1995). Suicidal children grow up: ego functions associated with suicide attempts. *Journal of American Academy of Child and Adolescent Psychiatry*, **34**, 1318–1325.

Pfeffer RC (1981). Suicidal behavior in children: a review with implications for research and practice. *American Journal of Psychiatry*, **138**, 154–159.

Piven J (2001) Phallic narcissism, anal sadism, and oral discord: the case of Yukio Mishima, Part I. *Psychoanalytic Review*, **88**(6), 771–791.

Plath S (1992) *The Collected Poems*. T Hughes, ed. Harper Perennial, New York.

Plutchik R, Botsis AJ, van Praag HM (1995). Psychopathology, self-esteem, sexual and ego functions as correlates of suicide and violence risk. *Archives of Suicide Research*, **1**, 27–38.

Recklitis CJ, Noam GG, Borst SR (1992). Adolescent suicide and defensive style. *Suicide and Life-Threatening Behavior*, **22**, 375–387.

Reiser E (1992). Self psychology and the problem of suicide. In A Goldberg, ed., *Progress in Self Psychology*, Vol. 2, pp. 227–241. Guilford Press, New York.

Richman J (1978). Symbiosis, empathy, suicidal behavior, and the family. *Suicide and Life-Threatening Behavior*, **3**, 139–149.

Richman J (1980). Suicide and infantile fixations. *Suicide and Life-Threatening Behavior*, **10**, 3–9.

Rierdan J, Lang E, Eddy S (1978). Suicide and transparency responses on the Rorschach: a replication. *Journal of Consulting and Clinical Psychology*, **46**, 1162–1163.

Ronningstam E and Maltsberger JT (1998). Pathological narcissism and sudden suicide-related collapse. *Suicide and Life-Threatening Behavior*, **28**, 261–271.

Rosenfeld H (1971). A clinical approach to the psychoanalytic theory of the life and death instincts: an investigation into the aggressive aspects of narcissism. *International Journal of Psycho-Analysis*, **52**, 169–178.

Roth D and Blatt SJ (1974). Spatial representations of transparency and the suicide potential. *International Journal of Psychoanalysis*, **55**, 287–293.

Rothstein A (1980). *The Narcissistic Pursuit of Perfection*. International Universities Press, Inc., New York.

Rustein EH and Goldberger L (1973). The effect of aggressive stimulation on suicidal patients: an experimental study of the psychoanalytic theory of suicide. In EH Rubinstein, ed., *Psychoanalysis and Contemporary Sciences*, Vol 2, pp. 157–174. Macmillan, New York.

Rydin E, Asberg M, Edman G *et al.* (1990). Violent and non-violent suicide attempters—a controlled Rorschach study. *Acta Psychiatrica Scandinavica*, **82**, 30–39.

Sabbath JC (1969). The suicidal adolescent—the expendable child. In JT Maltsberger and MJ Goldblatt, eds, *Essential Papers on Suicide*, pp.. New York University Press, New York and London.

Sheffer A (2001). Touch experience in suicidal adolescences. Doctoral dissertation, Psychology Department, Bar Ilan University, Israel.

Singer M (1977). The experience of emptiness in narcissistic and borderline states: II the struggle for the sense of self and the potential for suicide. *International Review of Psychoanalysis*, **4**, 471–479.

Smith K (1985). Suicide assessment. *Bulletin of the Menninger Clinic*, **49**, 489–499.

Smith K and Eyman J (1985). Ego structure and object differentiation in suicidal patients. In H Lerner and P Lerner, eds, *Primitive Mental States*, pp. 175–202. International Universities Press, Madison.

Stirman SW and Pennebaker JW (2001). Word use in the poetry of suicidal and nonsuicidal poets. *Psychosomatic Medicine*, **63**, 517–522.

Thomas CB and Duszynski KR (1985). Are words of the Rorschach predictors of disease and death? A case of 'whirling'. *Psychosomatic Medicine*, **47**, 201–211.

Weinberg I (2005). Self-defeating behaviors and suicide: mechanisms, their classification and consequences. Doctoral Dissertation, Bar Ilan University, Israel.

Woznica JG and Shapiro JR (1990). An analysis of adolescent suicide attempts: the expendable child. *Journal of Pediatric Psychology*, **6**, 789–796.

Yen S, Shea MT, Sanislow CA *et al.* (2004). Borderline personality disorder criteria associated with prospectively observed suicidal behavior. *American Journal of Psychiatry*, **161**, 1296–1298.

# CHAPTER 25

# Psychological theories of suicidal behaviour

M David Rudd, David RM Trotter and Ben Williams

## Abstract

In this chapter a review of the most prominent and influential psychological theories of suicide and suicidal behaviour is presented. Most, if not all, of these theories have had direct and important implications for both the assessment and treatment of suicidality, with cognitive approaches at the forefront over the last decade. Many have been tied to treatment paradigms and programmes, with some emerging directly from therapeutic practice. As has been evidenced elsewhere in this text, the majority of more recent theoretical efforts have revolved around cognitively (and behaviourally) oriented approaches, with natural integration of social and related contextual elements.

## Introduction

Although originally described as 'sociological' in its focus, Durkheim's theory is inescapable as central and foundational to psychological approaches to understanding and treating suicidality. Accordingly, it is included here. An effort has been made to review only theories specific to suicidality, with broader theoretical approaches (e.g. social learning, social cognitive, behavioural) purposefully ignored if not targeting or applied to suicidality in a specific manner. Also, psychodynamic theory has not been included since it is discussed in full in Chapter 24. Clearly, these broader theories have been influential in the evolution of suicide-specific approaches, with identifiable common constructs and related elements. Those common elements are easily identified in the ummaries to follow, particularly social learning and social cognitive components.

## Durkheim's theory

One of the earliest and most influential theories of suicidal behaviour was offered by Durkheim (1897). Given consistent and converging scientific evidence that the vast majority of those that die by suicide suffer from a mental disorder at the time of death (Harris and Barraclough 1997), there has been a clear shift to predominantly psychological, biological-based or blended theories, with most being integrative and complimentary in nature. Nonetheless, Durkheim's original conceptualization has continued to have considerable influence on subsequent psychological approaches, emphasizing the critical role of social forces, support, and broader societal values, related beliefs and mores. Durkheim proposed that two social forces, social and moral integration, could result in suicide. More specifically, he suggested that limited social integration in society can result in egoistic suicide because individuals lack the vital connection to others (i.e. a connection to society). This connection transcends self and is critical for healthy individual functioning. This has been a prominent thread in many subsequent theories, integrating social support, networks and relationships as critical in understanding individual emotional health, related dysfunction, and ultimately suicidal desire and behaviour.

Durkheim also hypothesized that excess social integration can result in altruistic suicide because individuals will sacrifice themselves for society, purportedly for the greater good. The best and most practical examples are those in which there are limited resources in the system. Similarly, Durkheim speculated about the role of moral regulation, defined as the degree to which society regulates the beliefs and behaviours of individuals though societal norms and the legal system. The net result of too little moral regulation is anomic suicide, primarily secondary to economic disequilibrium and the inability of individuals to meet basic life needs. In this case, economic disequilibrium can lead to restricted access to basic survival needs (e.g. food, clothing, shelter) resulting in dysphoria and eventual death by suicide. Conversely, too much moral integration can lead to fatalistic suicide, with the classic example offered by Durkheim being suicide of those enslaved by society. (See Chapter 23.)

Although labelled as sociological in its perspective, Durkheim's theory has had enduring and significant impact on subsequent psychological theories, with almost universal recognition and integration of social factors, the most prominent being the availability and accessibility of support, including early attachments and intimate relationships, along with impact on one's self-image and sense of efficacy. The inescapable fingerprint of Durkheim is embedded in, arguably, all of the theories to follow. The connection between individual identify (broadly defined) and social context is consistent across all of the subsequent theories. Although Durkheim did not address individual experience and suffering from an intrapsychic perspective, he provided for an understanding of contextual and social factors, all clearly relevant to an accurate understanding of suicidality in individual cases.

As evidenced in the summaries that follow, those theories identified as 'psychological' in nature target, to a larger degree, the intrapsychic experience (drives, desires, wishes, goals, beliefs, etc.) that results in the emergence and persistence of suicidality. For the purposes of this chapter, suicidality includes the full spectrum ranging from suicidal thoughts to acts (attempts and death by suicide). As Durkheim speculated, social forces are critical to understanding the individual experience, most incorporate social elements, at least to some degree. The difference, though, is the focus is on individual perception and appraisal of social factors.

## Baumeister's escape theory

Baumeister (1990) argued that suicide and suicidal behaviour are an effort to escape from intense and potentially unbearable psychological pain. Baumeister's theory is sequential in nature, with a series of steps leading to the eventual emergence of suicidality. First, individuals have to experience a serious negative discrepancy between personal expectations and outcomes, that is, frustrated goals and personal failures. This is a noticeable similarity between Baumeister's approach and that of Shneidman (1993), with Shneidman noting that frustrated psychological needs are essential for suicide. As is evident, personal expectations and outcomes occur in social context, that is, in the midst of relationships, both casual and intimate. Additionally, Baumeister recognized that the experienced negative discrepancy between identified goals and perceived failures can (and likely will be) replete with distortion in the appraisal process.

The next step in the process is that the subsequent attribution is internal, with profound self-blame. More specifically, the individual attributes blame internally, interpreting the discrepancy or failure as a function of individual characteristics, qualities or skills. As is evident in all of the theories that follow, Baumeister also emphasizes the identity piece. The unique thing about personal characteristics, qualities and skills is that they are routinely believed to be enduring and more resistant to change, particularly in the face of failure and defeat. The net result is painful, negative and overwhelming affect, not dissimilar from Shneidman's notion of 'psychache'.

The final element of the escape theory is that the individual is compelled to 'escape' from the internal negative affect, something that is accomplished by a subsequent state of *cognitive deconstruction*. Clearly, what is evident in this effort to 'escape' is a deficient individual skill set, one that does not allow for adequate problem-solving and regulation of the associated affect. Characteristic features of this cognitive state ('deconstruction') include a focus on concrete sensations and movements, along with targeting only proximal goals of immediate importance (i.e. day to day and immediate needs). Of particular importance for understanding suicidality, cognitive deconstruction results in reduced behavioural inhibition, with resultant impulse control problems and the emergence of risk-taking behaviours (e.g. substance abuse), including suicidality. The decline in impulse control helps explain a host of related suicide risk factors, including substance abuse, self-harm, and related risky and potentially life-threatening behaviour (e.g. driving fast without taking precautions like wearing a seat belt). The net result, according to Baumeister's theory, is that cognitive deconstruction leads to constricted thinking (similar

to one of Shneidman's commonalities of suicide), difficulty in effective problem-solving, with escalating risk for death by suicide.

What is unique about Baumeister's theory is that reduced behavioural inhibition is a common element and characteristic of suicidal states, helping explain how an individual overcomes inherent 'survival instincts' in order to either attempt suicide or, ultimately, die by suicide. It is also of note that Baumeister's theory is consonant with data evidencing that the vast majority of those that die by suicide suffer a mental disorder at the time of death, with associated impairment in mental status and cognitive processing. The idea of *cognitive deconstruction* is similar, in some ways, to the construct of cognitive distortions (including maladaptive core beliefs) that is prominent in cognitive theories. It is also amenable to the integration of other cognitively oriented approaches emphasizing impaired problem-solving (Rudd Joiner and Rajab 2004). Understanding and targeting impaired mental status is essential in the treatment of suicidality, regardless of theoretical orientation.

## Shneidman's theory of psychache

In a variant of the escape theory approach, Shneidman (1993) puts forward the hypothesis that suicide is the consequence of overwhelming, unmanageable psychological pain, referred to as 'psychache' and defined as 'general psychological or emotional pain that reaches intolerable intensity' (Shneidman 1993, p. 13). Shneidman hypothesized that suicide occurs *when psychache is unbearable*. Similar to Baumeister, Shneidman hypothesized that psychache resulted from thwarted psychological needs, with reference to Murray's (1938) identified psychological or 'psychogenic' needs. Murray and Shneidman differentiated two types of needs, primary (based on biological demands) and secondary (generally psychological in nature). Psychogenic needs are further grouped across a number of domains including: ambition, materialistic, power, affection, and information. Although individual needs are certainly important, it is hypothesized that they are interrelated and, to some degree, interdependent. Of critical importance, though, Shneidman differentiated between *modal needs* and *vital needs*. Modal needs are those that help define an individual personality, that is, those characteristic of an individual's day to day relationships and general emotional functioning. In contrast, vital needs are those deemed essential for life, the frustration of which will lead to considering suicide as an option. The frustration or blocking of vital needs are most apparent during periods of acute stress, for example, the dissolution of a marriage or close relationship. Similar to Baumeister, Shneidman believes that you can identify vital needs by asking about critical *failures, losses, rejections or humiliations* in one's life.

The central factor in suicide, according to Shneidman, is the emergence and persistence of psychache secondary to frustrated vital needs. Shneidman acknowledged the importance of other risk factors, but their impact on experienced psychache is believed to be the most critical factor in understanding and anticipating suicide. Shneidman described suicide as *adjustive*, that is, it represents an effort to reduce psychache, not necessarily end life. As is a central element of Linehan's (1993) theory, Shneidman also argued that individuals have different thresholds for tolerating emotional upset, dependent on individual history and experience (i.e. the developmental context that determines modal and vital needs). As is evident, suicidality according to Shneidman is almost entirely a psychological construct, behaviour driven by frustrated or blocked emotional and/or psychological needs. Shneidman (2001) has so elegantly offered that *suicide is a drama in the mind, where the suicidal drama is almost always driven by psychological pain, the pain of negative emotions—called psychache.* Shneidman also speculated that the majority of suicide cases are secondary to frustrated needs that fall into one of four categories:

1 Thwarted love, acceptance or belonging.

2 Fractured control, excessive helplessness, and frustration (related primarily to the need for achievement).

3 Assaulted self-image and avoidance of shame, defeat, humiliation, and disgrace.

4 Ruptured key relationships and subsequent grief.

These themes originally identified by Shneidman emerge in different forms in the theories that follow, including Beck's cognitive theory, Rudd's elaboration, Linehan's emotion dysregulation theory, and Joiner's interpersonal-psychological theory.

According to Shneidman (1993), the central element in treatment is to *mollify* psychache, a uniquely individual experience based in the frustrated or thwarted need(s). Shneidman differentiated psychache from traditional constructs and diagnostic entities like depression and hopelessness, noting psychache captures the unique phenomenological nature of suicide. Suicide prevention is, accordingly, simple and straightforward. It is about understanding, identifying and reducing psychache.

## Linehan's dialectical behaviour therapy and emotion regulation theory

Linehan's (1993) dialectical behaviour therapy (DBT) is based on the critical role played by emotion regulation, and the pathological variant, emotion dysregulation. Linehan proposed that emotion dysregulation is central to understanding and altering suicidal behaviour. Although developed as a treatment, Linehan's approach has a solid theoretical and empirical base. Actually, its empirical base is easily the strongest of any single treatment targeting suicidality, with six randomized, controlled trials documenting treatment efficacy (see Chapter 58). Linehan (1993) identified a number of broad *distinctive defining features* of DBT, including the following:

◆ The importance of dialectics across many functional domains (e.g. vacillating between being motivated and optimistic for change and hopeless).

◆ Behavioural skill deficits (e.g. emotion regulation, interpersonal effectiveness, distress tolerance, core mindfulness, and self-management) are actively taught within a problem-solving and skill-training training paradigm.

◆ There is limited emphasis on cognitive modification, with the primary emphasis on skill building and subsequent behavioural change.

◆ There is a primary focus on validation and hopefulness for change embedded in an emphasis on the therapeutic relationship as essential for change.

These features differentiate Linehan's approach from more traditional cognitive or behavioural approaches. As is evident, Linehan's theory evolved from a treatment paradigm, but is one grounded in psychological theory, with a heavy dose of social learning theory.

Unlike some other psychologically based theories, Linehan (1993) acknowledged the importance of both biological and social factors, describing the *environment–person system* (EPS) as critical to understanding suicidality, emphasizing its transactional nature and differentiating her approach from traditional *diathesis–stress* models. Linehan differentiated the transactional nature of the model that provides the foundation for DBT as assuming that individual functioning and environmental conditions are *mutually and continuously interactive, reciprocal, and interdependent,* grounded in the basic principles of reciprocal determinism. At the heart of the theory is that individuals and the environment both continuously adapt to one another, and accordingly, influence and change one another. Hence the central role played by the therapeutic relationship in instilling hope and motivation for change. In addition to the transactional nature of the environment–person system, Linehan's approach also emphasizes that the system is constantly in flux, the genesis of the core construct of emotion dysregulation. The transactional approach is amenable to biological influences as well, that is, despite a supportive and nurturing environment psychopathology can still emerge as the result of underlying genetic influence. Someone with a heavy genetic loading can manifest psychopathology despite a supportive and nurturing environment.

She identified two critical subsystems, including the environmental subsystem and the behavioural subsystem. The environmental subsystem incorporates social support, life change, suicidal models and suicidal consequences (i.e. reinforcement of suicidal behaviour and related contingencies). The behavioural subsystem includes physiological/affective elements, the overt motor system, and the cognitive system. In contrast to more purely cognitive or psychological approaches, and consistent with the central role of emotion regulation, Linehan's approach acknowledges the importance of biological and physiological elements. Of particular relevance, an individual's response to stress and emotion regulation skill is determined, at least partially, by underlying biology and physiology. In particular, she stressed the importance of 'invalidating environments', that is, social contexts that result in punitive and erratic reinforcement of various manifestations of suicidality. Invalidating environments occur not just in the individual's day to day context, but can also occur in the process of treatment. The individual's underlying biology is characterized by sensitivity to negative stressors and sharp emotional reactions, coupled with poor skills to facilitate emotional recovery. According to Linehan, suicidal behaviour (and related self-injury and mutilation) emerge as an effort to cope or regulate affect, not necessarily because someone is genuinely motivated to die. This notion is not dissimilar from that of Baumeister and Shneidman, both of who noted that suicidal acts emerge secondary to an effort to quell suffering.

Linehan's theory is, arguably, integrative in many respects, with emphasis on underlying biology/physiology, social context, and individual skill level (variables that influence emotion regulation). There are clearly similarities across Baumeister's, Shneidman's and Linehan's theories, with the individual experience of emotional suffering as central to understanding and modifying suicidality. Each, however, does have its unique focus. In Linehan's case, the integration of social context in the form of invalidating environments has importance for understanding not only emotion regulation, but also social reinforcement, both in and out of treatment.

## Beck's cognitive theory and the central role of hopelessness

Central to cognitive theory is that the meaning that an individual assigns to various events and environmental context is critical to understanding the subsequent affective experience and associated behaviour (Beck 1967). The net result is that stressors and environmental events alone are not explanatory for suicidality; rather, our interpretation and perception are central to understanding emotional impact and behavioural responses, including suicidality. It can be argued that Beck (1990) has had more impact on current psychological thinking about suicidality than anyone else in recent history. Beck and colleagues (1990) emphasized cognitive aspects of psychological functioning in understanding suicidal behaviour, speculating that the central factor is the emergence of hopelessness, defined as negative future expectancies. Considerable empirical evidence has accumulated over the years supporting the role of hopelessness in cases of suicide and suicide attempts. Of importance, Beck speculated that hopelessness pervades all aspects of the cognitive triad, that is, beliefs about self, others and the future. Aish and Wasserman (2001) showed in a sample of suicide attempters the statement 'my future seems dark to me' seems to be a good measurement of hopelessness.

When talking about cognitive theory, it is important to recognize that cognitions (including maladaptive ones) are not random, but they are determined by our developmental histories, including the unique characteristics of our individual lives. In cases where suicide is an issue, negative schemas are particularly problematic. Clark and Beck (1999) defined schemas as *relatively enduring internal structures of stored generic or prototypical features of stimuli, ideas, or experiences that are used to organize new information in a meaningful way thereby determining how phenomena are perceived and conceptualized*. Negative schemas are secondary to psychological disturbance (e.g. depression and anxiety), with the net result being biased, distorted information-processing and related affective and behavioural symptoms.

Wenzel, Brown and Beck (2008) have proposed the presence of *suicide schemas*, that is, beliefs directly related to exacerbation of hopelessness and emergence of intent to die by suicide. Information-processing bias is a central tenet of cognitive theory. More specifically, negative schemas result in individuals attending to negative, maladaptive information at the expense of positive, productive information that could generate a sense of hope. Bias in information-processing is observable in two primary domains with suicidal individuals, including both attention and memory. Wenzel, Brown and Beck (2008) have speculated about the presence of *suicide-relevant attentional bias*, which results in the selective processing of suicide-relevant stimuli. Similarly, suicidal individuals also evidence impairment in memory processes, including an *over-general memory style* (Williams *et al.* 2006). It is believed that an over-general memory style exacerbates hopelessness during suicidal crisis since it is likely that suicidal person will have trouble recalling specific reasons for living or being hopeful about life. Suicidal individuals have been found to have marked difficulty remembering specific positive experiences that might offer some protection during periods of acute stress (Williams 1996).

Beck (1996) modified traditional, linear cognitive theory and proposed the presence of 'modes'. Modes are defined as structural/organizational unites that contain schemas. Modes are interconnected networks of cognitive, affective, motivational, physiological, and behavioural schemas that are activated simultaneously by relevant internal and external events. Beck has speculated that repeated activation of the modes lowers the threshold for future activation of the mode; that is, creating a sensitivity or vulnerability for future problems. Rudd, Joiner and Rajab (2004) applied the theory of modes specifically to suicide, proposing a 'suicidal mode', again characterized by hopelessness, described as a 'suicidal belief system'. Rudd (2006) subsequently extended the notion of the suicidal mode and offered 'fluid vulnerability theory' (FVT) to explain the emergence, subsequent resolution, and reemergence of suicidality over extended periods of time.

Wenzel, Brown and Beck (2008) recently expanded on the theory of modes in four important ways. First, they have clarified the nature of *suicidal cognitions*, differentiating between cognitions characterized by trait hopelessness and those characterized by *unbearability* (Joiner *et al.* 2005). Second, their recent modification has helped clarify the interplay between risk factors, psychiatric illness, activation of suicide cognitions, associated emotional distress, and related self-destructive behaviour, identifying variable cognitive pathways to suicidality. More specifically, different suicidal beliefs are associated with different stressors, risk factors, psychiatric symptoms. Of particular importance, the most recent expansion of cognitive theory is much more friendly and amenable to integration of problem-solving and related diathesis–stress approaches. Perhaps most importantly, though, the recent expansion allows for a detailed and precise conceptualization of the myriad variables involved in a suicidal crisis, allowing each to be recognized and targeted in treatment, not just the cognitive elements. A broad cognitive conceptualization, integrating affective, physiological, situational and behavioural elements, allows for the integration of constructs such as impulsivity, problem-solving deficits, perfectionism, and dysfunctional attitudes. Such an expanded model allows for easy integration of topics such as this with considerable empirical support. From a cognitive perspective, the importance of these other variables revolves around their impact on cognitive processing, to include over-general memory and attention bias mentioned earlier. In short, a range of dispositional factors heighten vulnerability and interact with life stressors to increase the likelihood that negative suicide-relevant schemas and associated cognitions (i.e. hopelessness) will be activated, along with related cognitive processes that increase risk for suicide (e.g. attentional bias).

One of the unique and attractive elements of Beck's approach and Rudd's subsequent elaboration is the integrative nature of the theory. Although cognitive process (i.e. the cognitive triad, related core beliefs, hopelessness, etc.) is central to understanding suicidality, the theory of modes integrates affective, motivational, physiological, and behavioural elements more precisely than some other psychologically based approaches. As a result, the theory is flexible and amenable to integration of social factors, relationships, skill-building (e.g. emotion regulation training), along with a host of others. Regardless, though, it is hypothesized that cognitive change, not just behavioural change, is central to effective treatment and lasting change. This is in sharp contrast to Linehan's approachm which hypothesizes that cognitive change is not essential to success in treatment and recovery.

## Rudd's fluid vulnerability theory

As mentioned above, Rudd (2006) offered an expansion and elaboration of Beck's (1996) cognitive theory, proposing FVT as a way to understand the emergence, resolution and reemergence of suicidality over time, providing a psychological groundwork to understanding variations in acute and chronic (i.e. enduring) suicide risk. FVT is embedded in the idea of the suicidal mode mentioned previously. At a fundamental level, FVT is guided by the assumption that suicidal crises and behaviour (i.e. activation of the suicidal mode) are time-limited. FVT hypothesizes that the suicidal state, the factors that trigger crises, and the elements that determine relative severity and duration are fluid and not static. This notion is not dissimilar from Linehan's idea of a transactional system. In short, an individual's vulnerability to suicide is variable, but ultimately identifiable and quantifiable. The suicidal mode can be activated and deactivated, with each successive suicidal episode increasing future vulnerability or 'priming' for subsequent episodes. As noted previously, the various components of the suicidal mode (cognitive, affective, physiological, and behavioural) are interdependent and interactive, and become sensitized to subsequent triggering, primarily because of the *suicidal belief system* (i.e., the cognitive component of the suicidal mode).

It is believed that the suicidal belief system has recognizable or *core* cognitive themes, including unlovability (*I don't deserve to live*), helplessness (*I can't fix this problem*), poor distress tolerance (*I can't stand this pain anymore*), and perceived burdensomeness (*Others would be better off if I were dead*). As is evident, the various core beliefs noted are also apparent in other psychological theories of suicide, including Linehan's (1993) notion of poor distress tolerance, Shneidman's idea of psychache and Joiner's perceived burdensomeness. Repeated episodes provide the 'cognitive scaffolding' to support the belief and prime the individual for subsequent triggering. Vulnerability of the suicidal mode for subsequent triggering (a low threshold for activation) and emergence of suicidal crises extend across all four domains of the suicidal mode including:

- Cognitive susceptibility (to include impaired problem-solving, attentional bias, over-general memory, cognitive rigidity, cognitive distortions and maladaptive core beliefs).

- Biological susceptibility (i.e. secondary to physiological and affective symptoms consistent with an Axis I disorder, including a *sensitive and reactive* system and one slow to recover).

- Behavioural susceptibility (e.g. deficient skills that cut across a number of areas including interpersonal, self-soothing, and general emotion regulation).

As mentioned previously, the *core* themes of the suicidal belief system include beliefs specific to each of the above elements. More specifically, they relate to hopelessness about self (unlovability), symptomatology (poor distress tolerance), and skill or ability level (helplessness and perceived burdensomeness).

It is hypothesized that all individuals have baseline levels of risk, that is, the susceptibility of the suicidal mode to get activated. For some, the risk level is non-existent; they would not consider suicide under any conditions and for others it is very low, meaning suicidal thoughts would emerge only under considerable stress. For others, the baseline risk level is quite high with considerable vulnerability to activation because of a prominent and sensitive suicidal belief system. The slightest provocation might activate the system (e.g. a mild interpersonal conflict perceived as a rejection). A low threshold for activation of the suicidal mode results in recurrent suicidal crises, with each episode increasing vulnerability and priming for future episodes. For example, a serious suicide attempt can be interpreted as *evidence* that an individual cannot cope effectively, is beyond hope, or simply a burden on loved ones.

As with Beck's approach, Rudd's FVT emphasizes the importance of cognitive change in the treatment and recovery process. In other words, without changes in beliefs about self and others, vulnerability and susceptibility continue, and potentially grow with each subsequent suicidal crisis.

## Williams' theory of over-general memory and the cry of pain model of suicide

As mentioned in the discussion of cognitive theory, Williams and colleagues (2006) has discussed the critical role of overgeneral memory in the suicidal process. They provided empirical evidence that those at risk for suicidal behaviour have impairment in autobiographical memory. More specifically, they have a deficit in the specificity of autobiographical memory, making it difficult to recall *reasons for living* and accessing other cognitive material that facilitates both hope and problem-solving (in varied forms). Of particular importance, it does not appear that over-general memory correlates with the severity of depression or related mood disturbance; rather it appears to be a relatively independent cognitive and psychological variable that elevates suicide risk. Williams has noted some uncertainty about specific mechanisms of action for over-general autobiographical memory, but reported convincing empirical evidence that links it to trauma, particularly that which appears during childhood and adolescence.

From a functional perspective, it is hypothesized that over-general memory helps blunt the impact (and potential psychological damage) of negative emotions, consistent with an *affective gating* mechanism and similar to Linehan's theory of emotion regulation and dysregulation. The complication of affective gating, though, is that over-general memory contributes to an escalation of risk for a suicidal crisis by limiting problem-solving and future-oriented thinking (i.e. hope). Although over-general memory, according to Williams, blunts immediate emotional distress and dysphoria, it comes at a considerable practical cost, one that increases the probability of a suicidal crisis. Williams has summarized empirical findings about the consequences of overgeneral memory in relation to suicidality:

1 Episodes of emotional upset endure for longer duration secondary to impaired problem-solving.

2 It impairs interpersonal problem-solving (social consequence).

3 It limits an individuals' ability to think in future terms and manifest hope.

The net outcome is increased risk for suicidality, broadly defined.

Williams and his colleagues (2006) have integrated overgeneral memory into the *cry of pain* model of suicide (Williams 2001). The original *cry of pain* model integrated both biological and cognitive elements, describing suicidal behaviour as a reaction to a situational stressor experienced as 'feeling trapped' without any escape. In some ways, this model is similar to Baumeister's escape theory, including feeling 'defeated' or 'humiliated' in life. If escape is believed unlikely or impossible, suicide emerges as an alternative. Williams emphasized two potential sources of individual entrapment: impaired problem-solving and hopelessness. With his recent findings on autobiographical memory, Williams offers a more refined and precise mechanism of action for impaired problem-solving and hopelessness leading to suicide, with overgeneral memory having the direct consequences summarized above. The implications for treatment are clear, particularly from a cognitive and problem-solving perspective.

## Joiner's theory: blending psychological and interpersonal elements

In contrast to cognitive purists, Joiner (2005) hypothesized that psychological factors converge with interpersonal ones to predict suicide, including both the desire to die and the capability to do so. Joiner's theory is parsimonious and specific, resulting in several important questions. What is the desire to die by suicide and are there identifiable elements? What is the ability to die by suicide and what is its developmental trajectory? The desire to die by suicide is believed to be the function of two interpersonal constructs, perceived burdensomeness (*feeling like a burden to friends and loved ones*) and thwarted belongingness (*a sense of low belongingness or social alienation*). Joiner defines thwarted belongingness as emerging secondary to an unmet need to belong. Perceived burdensomeness results from the inability to engage in meaningful, reciprocal relationships. The capability for suicide is defined as a *fearlessness of pain, injury, and death*. Joiner believes that individuals acquire the capability for suicide through a process of repeatedly experiencing painful and otherwise provocative events, such as self-injury, physical fights, accidental injury secondary to high-risk behaviour, and workplace exposure such as soldiers and physicians. Direct or vicarious exposure both can heighten the capability for suicide. The net outcome of repeated exposure to such events is the loss of the instinctual *fear of death* and what has often been described as the survival instinct or self-preservation motive.

It is the interaction of multiple factors in Joiner's theory that result in suicide. Suicidal desire alone is not sufficient. Suicidal desire must be coupled with acquired capability for lethal harm in order for the individual to die by suicide. In sum, suicide is the outcome of three intersecting elements, including thwarted belongingness, perceived burdensomeness, and acquired capability. There is a growing body of empirical support for Joiner's (2005) theory.

## Conclusions

As is evident, there is considerable overlap across the various psychological theories of suicidality. It is important to recognize, though, that each emphasizes the critical role of the individual's intrapsychic experience, recognizing that there is variation in individual experience of day to day events and stressors. Each of the theories summarized emphasizes a core element more than other factors, but all recognize the importance of social context. All of these theories have been tested to varying degrees, with empirical support emerging for each. Similarly, each of these theories is parsimonious in nature, lending themselves to clearly stated and testable hypotheses. The net result has been a growing body of treatment protocols, many tested in well-designed clinical trials (covered elsewhere in this text). As research continues and we learn more about the nature of suicidality, there will undoubtedly be additional variants of the models offered above.

## References

Aish AM and Wasserman D (2001). Does Beck's Hopelessness Scale really measure several components? *Psychological Medicine*, **31**, 367–372.

Baumeister RF (1990). Suicide as escape from self. *Psychological Review*, **97**, 90–113.

Beck AT (1967). *Depression: Causes and Treatment.* University of Pennsylvania Press, Philadelphia.

Beck AT (1996). Beyond belief: a theory of modes, personality and psychopathology. In P Salkovkis, ed., *Frontiers of Cognitive Therapy*, pp. 1–25, Guilford Press, New York.

Beck AT, Brown G, Berchick R *et al.* (1990). Relationship between hopelessness and ultimate suicide: a replication with psychiatric outpatients. *American Journal of Psychiatry*, **147**, 190–195.

Clark DA and Beck AT (1999). *Scientific Foundations of Cognitive Theory and Therapy of Depression.* John Wiley and Sons, New York.

Durkheim E (1897). *Le Suicide: Etude de socologie.* Alcan, Paris.

Harris EC and Barraclough B (1997). Suicide as an outcome for mental disorders. *British Journal of Psychiatry*, **170**, 205–228.

Joiner TE (2005). *Why People Die by Suicide.* Harvard University Press, Cambridge.

Joiner TE, Brown JS, Wingate LR (2005). The psychology and neurobiology of suicidal behaviour. *Annual Review of Psychology*, **56**, 287–314.

Linehan MM (1993). *Cognitive-Behavioural Treatment of Borderline Personality Disorder.* Guilford Press, New York.

Murray HA (1938). *Explorations in Personality.* Oxford University Press, New York.

Rudd MD (2006). Fluid vulnerability theory: a cognitive approach to understanding the process of acute and chronic suicide risk. In PT Ellis, ed., *Cognition and Suicide: Theory, Research, and Therapy*, pp. 355–368. American Psychological Association, Washington.

Rudd MD, Joiner TE, Rajab H (2004). *Treating Suicidal Behaviour.* Guilford Press, New York.

Shneidman ES (1993). *Definitions of Suicide.* Wiley, New York.

Shneidman ES (2001). *Comprehending Suicide.* American Psychological Association, Washington.

Wenzel A, Brown G, Beck AT (2008). *Cognitive Therapy for Suicidal Patients: Scientific and Clinical Applications.* American Psychological Association, Washington.

Williams JMG (1996). Depression and the specificity of autobiographical memory. In DC Rubin, ed., *Remembering our Past: Studies in Autobiographical Memory*, pp. 244–267. Cambridge University Press, New York.

Williams JMG (2001). *Suicide and Attempted Suicide.* Penguin, London.

Williams JMG, Barnhoffer T, Crane C *et al.* (2006). The role of overgeneral memory in suicidality. In TE Ellis, ed., *Cognition and Suicide: Theory, Research, and Therapy*, pp. 173–192. American Psychological Association, Washington.

# CHAPTER 26

# Neurobiology and the genetics of suicide

Danuta Wasserman, Marcus Sokolowski,
Jerzy Wasserman and Dan Rujescu

## Abstract

Besides serotonin dysfunction, which was the main focus for about three decades, many other aspects of brain neurobiology have now been shown to be involved in the causality of suicidal behaviour. This chapter attempts to provide a broad overview of the entire range of studies performed in the area of neurobiology of suicide. The investigated involvement of genetics in each presently known neurobiological alteration is likewise presented. Although, the complexities and challenges in this field may sometimes seem overwhelming, this overview shows that the knowledge in this area is constantly being increased and refined in its details, and small breakthroughs occur constantly. Thus, it appears that if sufficient time and resources are dedicated to this problem, a critical mass of understanding will be reached, enabling the development of entirely novel tools for prevention of suicide.

## Stress–vulnerability model of suicidality

The causes of suicide appear to be heterogeneous and complex, and no simple explanations of the phenomenon exists. Risk of suicide-related behaviour is considered to be determined by a complex interplay of sociocultural factors, traumatic life experiences, psychiatric history, personality traits and genetic vulnerability, as depicted in a stress–vulnerability model (Figure 26.1) (Mann and Arango 1992; Wasserman 2001; Carballo et al. 2008). Suicidal individuals show remarkable neurobiological alterations, which are often shared with other psychiatric conditions, depression, and other behaviours/traits, such as increased anger/hostility, impulsivity, anxiety and impaired behavioural inhibition. However, a substantial proportion of such individuals have likely never considered taking their own lives nor commit such an act. Therefore, it is further likely that suicidal individuals must carry some type of neurobiological alteration of these expressions, which specify the increasing vulnerability towards suicidal acts. Indeed, an intrinsic predisposition towards suicidal behaviour has been demonstrated by evidence for involvement of genetic components, by using family, adoption and twin studies. The progress in understanding the involvement of neurobiology and genetics in suicide has been reviewed elsewhere (Kamali et al. 2001; Wasserman 2001; Mann 2003; van Heeringen 2003; Balazic and Marusic 2005; Brent and Mann 2005; Bondy et al. 2006; Mann et al. 2006; Mann and Currier 2007; Rujescu et al. 2007; Voracek and Loibl 2007; Wasserman et al. 2007b; Brezo et al. 2008; Carballo et al. 2008; Currier and Mann 2008; and in the 1997 December issue, no. 29, volume 836, of the *Annals of the New York Academy of Sciences*).

Adoption, twin and family studies indicate that suicidal acts have a genetic contribution in terms of cause or diathesis, which is independent of the heritability of major psychiatric disorders (Schulsinger et al. 1979; Roy et al. 1991). Aggregation of the risk estimates from 21 family-study reports, with a total of nearly 25,000 suicidal subjects and close relatives (Baldessarini and Hennen 2004), showed that even a cautious estimate of the overall pooled risk ratio, based on a meta-analytic method, was 2.86.

Twin studies compare the concordance for suicidal behaviour in monozygotic twins, which share 100 per cent of their genes, and dizygotic twins, which share 50 per cent of their genes on average. This allows separating effects due to shared environment from genetic factors. Roy et al. (1991) examined 62 monozygotic and 114 dizygotic twin pairs, and reported concordance rates for suicide of 11.3 per cent and 1.8 per cent, respectively. A recent study, based on this data, suggested heritability for completed suicide of about 43 per cent by using a logistic regression model (McGuffin et al. 2001). Similar results have been found for suicide attempts. An Australian twin study with a total of nearly 6000 twins estimated that genetic factors account for approximately 45 per cent of the variance in suicidal thoughts and behaviour (Statham et al. 1998). The co-twin of monozygotic pairs, where the other twin had a history of suicide attempts, was shown to have an elevated risk

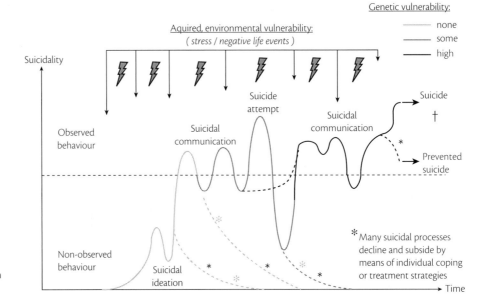

**Fig. 26.1** The stress–vulnerability model in suicidal behaviour. The different aspects of suicidality (ideation, attempted or completed/prevented suicide), and the relationships to acquired environmental exposure and the individual's genetic vulnerability, as depicted. (Modified from Wasserman 2001, p.20.)

for suicidal behaviour. Even after controlling for contributing risk factors like depression and other psychiatric disorders, the authors observed a highly significant 3.9-fold increased risk. A more recent review of twin-studies published between 1812 and 2006 (Voracek and Loibl 2007), confirmed the influence of genetic components (with heritability of 30–55 per cent) in suicide behaviour, largely independent of the inheritance of other psychiatric disorders.

Adoption studies are less commonly performed. Three classical studies used the same Danish health statistics register (Kety *et al.* 1971; Schulsinger *et al.* 1979; Wender *et al.* 1986). The investigation of Schulsinger *et al.* identified 57 suicide victims among early adopted Danish citizens and defined them as index cases. The biological relatives of these index cases showed a sixfold higher suicide rate (4.46 per cent) than the biological relatives of a matched, non-suicidal adoptee control group (0.74 per cent). Furthermore, there was no suicide among the adoptive relatives of the index cases.

For suicide-related behaviour, the number of susceptibility genes, the risk conferred by each gene, as well as the degree of interaction(s) between the genes is unknown. It is likely that a high degree of complexity exists (including redundant, complementing, silencing or augmenting effects/interactions), involving different genes, as well as interactions between genes and environment (stress, xenobiotics and drugs), which will further vary during the different developmental stages of the human being (Kendler 2005; Lin *et al.* 2007). Thus, finding genes that predispose to suicide-related behaviour presents a major challenge, given that the neuropathology of suicide, as well as neurobiological mechanisms in general, are far from being understood. The search for susceptibility genes of suicide is presently confronted by using two different strategies: either to look at all genes at once ('genome-wide') in a less detailed manner, or to directly perform detailed studies of biologically plausible 'candidate' genes, sometimes as a secondary follow-up of an indicative result from a genome-wide study. Candidate genes are usually identified following the experimental investigation of certain proteins in particular neurobiological pathways, studied in human subjects (by post mortem, brain scans or other means),

animal models (including use of transgenic animals) or tissue cultures (using various lineages of nerve cells).

In the population–genetic approaches, one may study the co-segregation of certain genetic variants/mutations with the trait/disorder of interest in families ('linkage' studies), or to investigate if there are differences in the occurrence of certain genetic variants between non-related groups of affected, suicidal individuals, in comparison to unaffected, healthy controls ('association' studies). However, the progress of many population–genetic studies is often hampered due the problems of phenotypic and genetic heterogeneity, as well as under-powered investigations caused by too small sample sizes, often resulting in inconsistencies, and even statistical artefacts. As these problems are being addressed, and complemented with experimental measures, a psychobiological understanding is emerging.

The inclusion and definition of the genetic components involved in suicidality are of great interest when specifying the individuals having the clinical manifestations of, for example, depression, increased anger, impulsivity, anxiety, and/or behavioural disinhibition, who may be at increased risk of performing suicidal acts. The suicide-specific neurobiological alterations involved are likely to be assessed by using 'endophenotypes', which involves any measurable neurobiological parameters whose outcome/state are more directly linked with any underlying genetic alterations, and which act on the pathway of development of suicidal vulnerability. Thus, the genetic variables must be determined as they form the basal layer of information, which could influence all secondary variables/endophenotypes, and the sum of these effects would shape the individual's susceptibility to suicidality. From a pharmacogenomic perspective, it is of importance to have knowledge about how the individual's genetic variation relates to a drug in question (e.g. SSRI, lithium or other drug treatments), in context to its functionality, enabling better evaluation of drug efficacy and development of diagnostic tools by, for example, explaining side-effects and treatment failures and by improving individualized drug treatments. In the future, knowledge about unfavourable/'dysfunctional' genetic variants will likely bring about new, highly specific treatment possibilities with, for example, inhibitory ribonucleic acid (RNA), so-called 'gene therapy' (Sah 2006).

# Search for the basis of specific components, at neurobiological and genetic levels, which may influence suicidal vulnerability

## Monoamine systems

### Serotonin (5-HT)

The serotonin system projects through many areas of the brain, and is considered to be important in mood and behaviour. Serotonin (5-hydroxytryptamine, or 5-HT) is the major monoaminergic neurotransmitter, first identified in blood in 1948 (Rapport et al. 1948). It is synthesized in cells from the precursor molecule L-tryptophan, an essential amino acid, catalyzed by enzymes tryptophan hydroxylase (TPH) and aromatic L-amino acid/DOPA decarboxylase (DDC). 5-HT has a long history of being widely implicated in the causality of depression, originating from the 'monoamine hypothesis', which proposed the involvement of a deficiency in monoamines, including 5-HT, in depression (Schildkraut 1965). There is also much evidence concerning the involvement of the 5-HT system in suicide, independently of other diagnoses. This line of research, which now spans over more than four decades, was initiated by the observations of lowered 5-HT and 5-HT metabolite (5-hydroxyindoleacetic acid—5-HIAA) levels in various brain regions of suicide victims (Shaw et al. 1967; Pare et al. 1969; Birkmayer and Riederer 1975), as well as lowered 5-HIAA in the cerebrospinal fluid (CSF) in relation to depression and violent suicide attempts (Åsberg et al. 1976a, b). Later, blunted prolactin response to fenfluramine (which acts by inducing serotonin release), altered binding/levels of serotonin receptors, and changes in the 5-HT transporter (5-HTT) were also observed (Åsberg 1997; Mann et al. 2001). Brain regions shown to be affected in relation to suicide and serotonin are mainly, among others, the brain stem (dorsal raphe nuclei)/limbic system and prefrontal cortex (PFC), with the former being related to stress responses and the latter with cognitive and behavioural restraint, with rich innervations in-between. These neurobiological observations relate well with the frequent occurrence of impulsive–aggressive behaviours among suicidal individuals, as suicide is often deemed to be an impulsive act and/or an aggression which is directed inwards. The field has then progressed further by dissecting the roles and involvement of the various components of the serotonergic system.

### 5-HT anabolism: tryptophan hydroxylase

Tryptophan is an essential amino acid and a rate-limiting source-molecule for serotonin synthesis. At the population level, it has been observed that a high intake diet of tryptophan, which may conteract any diet-induced serotonin deficiencies, is associated with lowered levels of suicide in the industrialized populations (Voracek and Tran 2007). Conversely, depletion of serotonin by a low-tryptophan diet, reverse the effects of antidepressant treatment with selective serotonin reuptake inhibitors (SSRIs) (Delgado et al. 1990). The enzyme tryptophan hydroxylase (TPH) is involved in the biosynthesis of serotonin, converting L-tryptophan, in a rate-limiting step, into 5-hydroxytryptophan, which is a substrate for subsequent conversion into serotonin by DDC. Inhibition of TPH by parachlorophenylalanine will, similarly to low-tryptophan diets, also result in serotonin depletion. Thus, available tryptophan and TPH are important for serotonergic function. To explain the inter-individual variations in the response to such treatments, in terms of effects on the serotonergic system, as well as in terms of psychopathology, polymorphisms in the TPH gene(s) have been studied.

Initially, many studies were focused on the gene *TPH1*, which was for a long time the only known TPH-encoding gene. An early meta-analysis by Lalovic and Turecki (2002), did not find an association of the commonly studied intron 7 A218C single nucleotide polymorphism (SNP) with suicidal behaviour. A further meta-analysis by Rujescu et al. (2003b) summarized the results of seven studies and found a higher frequency of the A218C allele in patients with suicidal behaviour, strongly suggesting that this TPH polymorphism is associated with suicidal behaviour among at least Caucasians. A subsequent meta-analysis included nine studies and confirmed the association between the A218C polymorphism and suicidal behaviour, using both the fixed effect method and the random effect method (Bellivier et al. 2004). The most recent meta-analysis included a total of 22 studies, and examined the involvement of the A779C, A218C and A6526G polymorphisms, employing several strategies to maintain the power and robustness in the analysis (Li and He 2006). This study, which investigated all reports published between 1997 and July 2005, revealed strong cumulative evidence of association for the A779C and A218C polymorphisms among international populations (Li and He 2006). The lessons learned for other genes/polymorphisms, which often show inconsistent findings in initial studies, may be that it takes considerable time before sufficient sample size is gathered (in the thousands to tens of thousands), which carry enough statistical power required for the detection of the weak, single-locus effects believed to be involved in suicidal behaviour, as have often been observed for other complex/somatic disorders.

Almost two decades after the initial identification of the *TPH1* gene (Grenett et al. 1987; Ledley et al. 1987), a second gene encoding for TPH (*TPH2*) was discovered in mice, and later in humans, which was shown to be highly restricted to the brain regions (Walther et al. 2003; Zhang et al. 2004). It suddenly appeared that some of the roles previously implicated for the *TPH1* gene in brain serotonin and psychiatric disorders, may have been of an artefactual nature, being e.g. secondary to *TPH2* activity, but recent studies demonstrate that there is actually a duality in the brain serotonin system, involving the two different TPH genes, with equal amounts of expression in regions such as the frontal cortex, hippocampus, hypothalamus and amygdala, and differential expression in the dorsal raphe (Nakamura et al. 2006; Zill et al. 2007; Abumaria et al. 2008). Nevertheless, attention has mostly shifted to *TPH2*, recently shown to have elevated expression levels in brainstem dorsal and median raphe nuclei of depressed suicides (Bach-Mizrachi et al. 2008), the region where most forebrain serotonin is being produced, which may reflect a homeostatic response to deficient serotonin levels. Breidenthal et al. (2004) screened the coding and exon-flanking intronic sequence of the *TPH2* gene and identified several genetic variants that might serve as markers for association studies. Zill et al. (2004) could find an association of SNPs and a haplotype with completed suicide, whereas De Luca *et al.* (2004) could not find any association. However, a comprehensive investigation performed a linkage analysis in 1798 subjects from four different populations, and detected significant haplotype linkage of *TPH2* to suicide attempt and major depression (Zhou *et al.* 2005). Another single marker and haplotype analysis was conducted in a large, family-based sample of patients with bipolar affective disorder. The authors detected significant association of a haplotype with both suicide attempts and bipolar affective disorder (Lopez *et al.* 2007). Interestingly, a new, truncated isoform of *TPH2* has recently been identified and characterized, along with genetic variants, which likely cause this structural alteration and were associated with suicide and depression (Haghighi *et al.* 2008). In summary, the results on *TPH2* are promising and further studies will better clarify the role of this gene in several facets of suicidal behaviour.

### Monoamine catabolism: monoamine oxidase

Besides the enzymes involved in serotonin synthesis (TPH and DDC), the main catabolic enzyme of serotonin (and noradrenaline, dopamine) was identified (Hare 1928), now called monoamine oxidase (MAO). MAO has been implicated in various forms of psychopathology, including suicidality, ever since the formulation of the monoamine hypothesis and the advent of MAO-inhibiting antidepressants (Schildkraut 1965). Early on, a twin study showed that inter-individual variation in the enzyme activity might be genetically determined, promoting the development of schizophrenia (Wyatt *et al.* 1973), and such differences were later suggested to be involved also in suicidality (Buchsbaum *et al.* 1977). Early knowledge about the biochemical characterization of two major MAO isoforms (A and B), likely helped to form the idea that heritable, genetic alterations might be causing the differences between the two isoforms, e.g. differences in substrate specificity, inhibitor sensitivity and tissue distribution, and that such alterations might be sufficient for causing psychobiological and behavioural consequences (Breakefield and Edelstein 1980; Murphy and Kalin 1980).

With the rapid development in DNA technologies, it was later possible to show that, as with TPH, there were two genes responsible for the major MAO isoforms (MAOA and MAOB), identified to be located on the X-chromosome (Breakefield and Edelstein 1980; Pintar *et al.* 1981; Ozelius *et al.* 1988; Sims *et al.* 1989) and to be expressed in the brain (Shih *et al.* 1990). Interestingly, loss of MAOA gene function is related to increased aggression (Brunner *et al.* 1993; Cases *et al.* 1995), a behaviour/trait which has long been considered to be of importance in explaining the suicide diathesis (i.e. the 'anger out—anger in' hypothesis), as well as in relation to an increased noradrenalin and cortisol levels, ideas originating from work previously done in the 1950s (Funkenstein *et al.* 1954; Schildkraut 1965; Ostroff *et al.* 1982). Curiously, the failures to demonstrate local/regional effects in the PFC in relation to MAO activity and suicidality (Mann and Stanley 1984), may have served as a stimuli for research on other serotonergic components.

The gene coding for the monoamine oxidase A (MAOA) has been shown to contain a variable number of tandem repeats (VNTR) polymorphism in the promoter region. The 30 base pair (bp) repeated sequence is present in 3, 3.5, 4 or 5 copies, and alleles with 3.5 or 4 copies are transcribed 2–10 times more efficiently than those with 3 or 5 copies (Sabol *et al.* 1998). Studies investigating the possible association of this MAOA–uVNTR polymorphism and suicidal behaviour have yielded inconsistent results. Several groups found no significant differences in genotype or allele distribution between subjects with suicidal behaviour and comparison groups (Kunugi *et al.* 1999; Ono *et al.* 2002; Huang *et al.* 2004b), whereas one investigation delivered a significant association (Ho *et al.* 2000). Ho and colleagues examined this VNTR and the Fnu4H1 polymorphism in a sample of patients suffering from bipolar affective disorder. They found the VNTR variant to be associated with a history of suicide attempts, especially in females. The Fnu4H1 restriction fragment length polymorphism (RFLP) only showed significant differences in allele frequencies for female subjects, but not in the total sample. Another study showed a strong association between the high activity-related EcoRV allele and depressed suicide in male subjects, but not in females or the total sample (Du *et al.* 2002). As discussed above, strong lines of evidence also indicate that the MAOA gene is involved in impulsive/aggressive behaviours (af Klinteberg *et al.* 1987; Klinteberg *et al.* 1987). In this context, Courtet *et al.* (2005a) showed that genetic variation was associated with violent methods of suicide attempt among men. The dimorphic nature of the results is not surprising, due to the location of the MAO genes on the X chromosome, and probably represents an important explanation of the higher incidence of completed suicide among men (Du *et al.* 2002). Gender differences may also be caused, because MAOA gene expression is controlled not only genetically, but also epigenetically in females, but not in males (Pinsonneault *et al.* 2006). Future studies will likely better clarify the role of genetic variation in relation to suicidality, probably in the context of other genes.

### 5-HT neurotransmission: transporter

The serotonin transporter (5-HTT, SLC6A4) is located on the presynaptic membrane of serotonergic neurons and is another key serotonergic regulator, which acts by removing the serotonin released into the synaptic cleft. Carrier-facilitated 5-HT transport into, and release from the pre-synaptic neuron, which are essential for the fine tuning of serotonergic neurotransmission, directing the magnitude and duration of postsynaptic neural responses. Alterations (reduction) of 5-HTT binding in suicidal individuals, appeared related mainly to the PFC, and were originally observed as a reduction of pre-synaptic binding of antidepressant imipramine (Stanley *et al.* 1982). Genetic variation in this gene has been, and continues to be, massively studied in the context of various forms of psychopathology (Serretti *et al.* 2006). The amounts of 5-HTT present at the pre-synaptic neuron is regulated in part at the transcriptional level, involving a now well-studied polymorphism in the promoter region, located about 1 kilobase upstream of the transcription start site, often termed as the 5-HTT linked promoter region (5-HTTLPR) (Heils *et al.* 1996). 5-HTTLPR is located in a repetitive sequence, which is polymorphic by insertion/deletion of 44 basepairs, resulting in short (S) and long (L) alleles, respectively, whereby the S-allele mediates reduced 5-HTT transcription (Heils *et al.* 1996). This results in reduced serotonin uptake and reduced serotonin responsivity at the nerve synapse, as well as reduced levels of 5-HIAA in the CSF.

A number of studies have been performed in relation to suicide and suicide-related characteristics, with some degree of inconsistency between the separate/independent studies (Courtet *et al.* 2005b; Currier and Mann 2008). The most studied polymorphism is 5-HTTLPR, which has been shown to affect emotional regulation in different contexts, e.g. in the presence of gene–gene interactions (Ebstein *et al.* 1998) and environmental stress factors (Caspi *et al.* 2003), which is likely to be of importance for the eminence of suicidal behaviour. An initial meta-analysis conducted by Anguelova *et al.* (2003) included 12 studies investigating the 5-HTT promoter polymorphism. The study sample contained 10 Caucasian populations, one US population and one Chinese sample. In the pooled sample, with a total number of 1168 suicide completers/attempters and 1371 controls, a significant association of the S allele with suicidal behaviour was found (Anguelova *et al.* 2003). A second meta-analysis, including 18 studies with 1521 suicide attempters or completers and 2429 controls, delivered different results (Lin and Tsai 2004). In contrast to the investigation of Anguelova *et al.* (2003), Lin and Tsai (2004) found no overall association of 5-HTTLPR alleles with suicidal behaviour in a subsequent meta-analysis. This was also true if only the 15 studies with subjects of Caucasian origin were examined. The authors also compared the allelic and genotype distribution between 190 violent suicide attempters or completers and 733 normal control subjects. Here, they did observe a significant association of the S allele with violent suicidal behaviour, mainly characterized by the use of highly lethal and violent methods, such as hanging or shooting, but not with non-violent suicide (Lin and Tsai 2004). Lin and Tsai concluded that violent suicidal subjects might be a relatively homogenous group, and that patients carrying the S allele are likely to act more impulsive and aggressive, which is the concept of fundamental theory in suicide research (Brent and Mann 2005), as also discussed above. Similarly, we have also showed a higher occurrence of the S allele among suicide attempters with a high medical damage score of ≥ 2, as evaluated by using the Medical Damage Rating Scale (Beck *et al.* 1975; Wasserman *et al.* 2007a). In a meta-analysis covering all 38 studies up to January 2006, with a total of 3096 cases and 5936 controls, the results showed consistent and strong associations, both among all studies as a whole and among subgrouped studies (Li and He 2007). The L allele was lowered in frequency among suicidal individuals at allelic and genotypic levels in European and Asian populations, but ethnicity possibly affected gender differences (a dichotomy used in only three studies). The results were no longer specifically confined to violent suicide attempters, and suicidality subgroups (i.e attempter and/or completers, compared with non-attempters and/or healthy individuals) did not bias the analysis significantly. Furthermore, the results supported the notion that the relation to suicide was independent of psychiatric diagnoses.

Interestingly, further allelic variation in 5-HTTLPR has now been identified, namely a SNP in the inserted L allele, whereby reduced 5-HTT transcription was also further linked with a (new) subvariant of the L allele ($L_G$), in addition to the S allele (Hu *et al.* 2006). Incorporation of this expanded level of information has been used for implicating a role for the 5-HTTLPR in childhood trauma-related suicidality (Roy *et al.* 2007), depression (Zalsman *et al.* 2006; Frodl *et al.* 2008) and childhood aggression (Beitchman *et al.* 2006). More studies will clarify how this additional variant of the 5-HTTLPR polymorphism relates to suicidal behaviour.

## 5-HT neurotransmission: receptors

5-HT receptor genes are also classical candidate genes for suicidal behaviour. All functions related to 5-HT on mood and behaviour, are exerted through action on the receptors. They represent an apparent target for local regulation of 5-HT neurotransmission at the specific synapse, by alterations in amounts of receptor sites, affinities and levels of intracellular signal propagation. Such functional variations could well be explained by genetic determinants, which may alter expression levels and receptor structure. While genes of the $5\text{-HTR}_{1A}$, $5\text{-HTR}_{1B}$, $5\text{-HTR}_{2A}$, $5\text{-HTR}_{1D}$, $5\text{-HTR}_{1E}$, $5\text{-HTR}_{1F}$, $5\text{-HTR}_{2C}$, $5\text{-HTR}_{5A}$ and $5\text{-HTR}_6$ have been studied genetically so far, there is a general lack of consistency in the findings to date (Bondy *et al.* 2006; Rujescu *et al.* 2007). Among these, the synaptic $5\text{-HTR}_{1A}$ and $5\text{-HTR}_{2A}$ receptors have shown the most extensive links to suicidality, based on a variety of neurobiological measurements (Albert and Lemonde 2004; Norton and Owen 2005), among which the post-synaptic $5\text{-HTR}_{2A}$ was the first to be implicated with suicide, by demonstration of increased binding in the PFC (Stanley and Mann 1983).

$5\text{-HTR}_{1A}$ is located on both pre- and post-synaptic sides of the synapses and has been shown to be involved in neurobiology of depression and anxiety. It performs major tasks in regulating the functions of 5-HT system (Albert and Lemonde 2004; Drago *et al.* 2007). When being pre-synaptic (autoreceptor), they mediate a short feedback regulation loop of importance in the raphe nuclei in controlling the release of brain 5-HT, involving also gamma-aminobutyric acid (GABAergic) cells, via $5\text{-HTR}_{2A/2C}$. Post-synaptic $5\text{-HTR}_{1A}$ is present in both limbic (hippocampal) and cortical medial prefrontal cortex (mPFC) regions, with a variety of roles in the coordinated functions of these brain regions (Albert and Lemonde 2004; Drago *et al.* 2007). In relation to suicide and the $5\text{-HT}_{1A}$ gene, Lemonde *et al.* (2003) examined a functional C-1019G SNP in the promoter region of the $5\text{-HT}_{1A}$ gene and found the G allele to be significantly over-represented in a depressed, suicide completer group. However, this type of relationship was not observed in a similarly designed study (Huang *et al.* 2004a), which nevertheless observed increased $5\text{-HT}_{1A}$-binding in PFC of suicides, and associations to other clinical diagnoses. More recently, we showed that the G allele was associated and linked among suicide attempters exposed to high levels of stressful life events, but not among suicide attempters in general, a finding which is congruent with possible action of a gene–environment interaction at this polymorphism (Wasserman *et al.* 2006b). Moreover, it was discussed, and to some degree shown, that the discrepant results among the three studies may have been expected due to the sample heterogeneities, a common problem in the comparisons between different population-based studies. The investigation of other $5\text{-HTR}_{1A}$ polymorphisms, Pro16Leu and Gly272Asp, revealed no association with suicidal behaviour in Japanese subjects (Nishiguchi *et al.* 2002). This lack of association with suicidality for the Pro16Leu polymorphism was replicated by a second Japanese group (Ohtani *et al.* 2004).

A second gene, the gene for the $5\text{-HTR}_{1B}$ receptor, was studied by New *et al.* (2001). They found an association of the G861C SNP with a history of suicide attempts in a subsample of 90 Caucasian patients with personality disorders, but this association did not reach statistical significance in the total sample of 145 patients (New *et al.* 2001). Ten other studies in different populations did not report any implication of gene variants of the $5\text{-HTR}_{1B}$

receptor in the susceptibility to suicidal behaviour (Huang *et al.* 1999; Nishiguchi *et al.* 2001; Arango *et al.* 2003; Huang *et al.* 2003; Pooley *et al.* 2003; Rujescu *et al.* 2003c; Turecki *et al.* 2003; Hong *et al.* 2004; Stefulj *et al.* 2004b; Tsai *et al.* 2004).

Most studies show that the $5\text{-HTR}_{2A}$ receptor binding sites are elevated in the PFC of suicide victims (Arango *et al.* 1997). This is also of interest in view of the functional interactions with $5\text{-HTR}_{1A}$, particularly this region. Interestingly, $5\text{-HTR}_{2A}$ was recently shown to have decreased signal transduction in violent suicide attempts (Malone *et al.* 2007). Most genetic studies investigated the common C102T SNP. A meta-analysis regarding this variant pooled nine studies with 596 suicide completers or attempters and 1003 healthy controls showed the lack of association of this particular $5\text{-HTR}_{2A}$ polymorphism with suicidal behaviour (Anguelova *et al.* 2003).

Turecki and colleagues examined variations in seven different 5-HTRs (1B, 1Dα, 1E, 1F, 2C, 5A and 6), in a sample of 106 suicide completers and 120 controls, and found no significant association for any of these receptors with suicide (Turecki *et al.* 2003). Two recent studies examined the 5-HTR2C polymorphism Cys23Ser and found no significant association between this variant and deliberate self-harm or suicidal behaviour, respectively (Pooley *et al.* 2003; Stefulj *et al.* 2004a). Overall, while these results do not provide evidence for a major effect of the examined 5-HT receptor variants on the susceptibility of suicidal behaviour, the studies also had small sample sizes, which may have carried insufficient power for detection of genetic effects, and at least 12 known 5-HT receptors remain to be tested.

In summary, the most interesting genes from a neurobiological point of view, remain $5\text{-HTR}_{1A}$ and $5\text{-HTR}_{2A}$. Future genetics studies should perhaps involve other genes involved in modulation of various function(s) of these receptors, and perhaps novel polymorphisms.

## Catecholaminergic monoamines

### Anabolism: tyrosine hydroxylase

Our present molecular understanding of neurotransmission emanates from the works which followed the discovery of adrenalin, about a hundred years ago (Bennett 2000). Tyrosine hydroxylase (TH) is the rate-limiting enzyme in the conversion of tyrosine, into the array of catecholamine neurotransmitters of dopamine (DA), noradrenaline (NA) and adrenaline, a biochemical subgroup of the monoamines (Levitt *et al.* 1965). The implication of TH in suicidality comes from the important roles of this entire system in responses to stress. Decreased NA in the brainstem and increased alpha2-adrenergic receptor densities were observed, indicative of a deficient NA system (Ordway *et al.* 1994). Various studies reported different observations concerning the alterations of TH-levels in the locus coeruleus (LC) of suicide victims. Biegon *et al.* (1992) described reduced TH immunoreactivity in the LC of suicide completers, while Ordway *et al.* (1994) reported elevated amounts of tyrosine hydroxylase in the LC of suicide victims, and Baumann *et al.* (1999) found unaltered levels in depressed suicide patients. Variable expression levels of TH may be controlled by polymorphic variants. Polymeropoulos *et al.* (1991) described a penta-allelic short tandem repeat in the first intron of the TH gene. We also examined the allelic distribution of this polymorphism and reported a tendency for a low incidence of the

TH-K1 allele among suicide attempters, compared to the controls (Persson *et al.* 1997). Furthermore, we found a significant association between the TH-K3 allele in a subgroup of patients with adjustment disorders and attempted suicide. Another study also observed tendencies for transmission distortion at several alleles in this polymorphism, in relation to severe suicide behaviour in bipolar disorder (De Luca *et al.* 2008). Interestingly, a previous study observed significantly lower levels of 3-methoxy-4-hydroxy-phenylglycol (MHPG), the main metabolite of NA, in TH-K3 allele carriers (Jönsson *et al.* 1996). In contrast, Giegling *et al.* (2008) instead investigated two SNPs in the TH-gene among 167 suicide completers, and found no significant associations (Giegling *et al.* 2008). However, this study was not comparable to the previous ones, since e.g. different polymorphisms were studied, and further clarification is needed.

### Catabolism: catechol-O-methyltransferase

The catechol-O-methyltransferase (COMT) is a major enzyme involved in the inactivation of the catecholamines dopamine and noradrenalin. Lachman *et al.* (1996) described a common functional polymorphism in the COMT gene, in which valine (Val) at codon 158 is replaced with methionine (Met). Homozygotes for 158Val (high-activity H allele) have three- to fourfold higher levels of enzyme activity than 158Met homozygotes (low-activity L allele). The Val/Met genotype results in an intermediate COMT activity (Weinshilboum *et al.* 1999).

Several studies investigated the relationship between the described COMT genotype and violent and/or suicidal behaviour. An initial study found no differences in allele distribution between schizophrenic patients and controls, but a subsample of extremely violent patients was found to be more often homozygous for the L allele (Strous *et al.* 1997). Other investigations replicated the association of the L allele with aggressive behaviours in schizophrenic patients (Kotler *et al.* 1999; Strous *et al.* 2003; Volavka *et al.* 2004). The association appeared to be expressed particularly among males (Lachman *et al.* 1998; Nolan *et al.* 2000), but this effect has not yet been systematically studied. However, other studies failed to show an association of this polymorphism with violent behaviour (Wei and Hemmings 1999; Liou *et al.* 2001; Zammit *et al.* 2004) or obtained contrary results (Jones *et al.* 2001). An investigation of this polymorphism in a sample of German suicide attempters and German control subjects without a lifetime history of psychiatric disorders, measured anger-related traits in both groups (Rujescu *et al.* 2003a). The genotype or allele frequencies did not differ significantly between controls and suicide attempters, but the L allele was over-represented in violent suicide attempters. In addition, a multivariate effect of the COMT genotype on anger-related traits was observed. LL-carriers expressed their anger more outwardly, whereas HH-carriers expressed it more inwardly and reported more state anger, as assessed by the self-report questionnaire. Nolan *et al.* (2000) examined the genotype distribution of the 158Val/Met polymorphism in a sample of Finnish and US schizophrenic and schizoaffective patients, and found the low-activity allele to be more frequent in male subjects with a history of violent suicide attempts, but not in females. Similar results have been reported in a Japanese sample (Ono *et al.* 2004). In this case, the high-activity Val/Val genotype occurred significantly less frequently in male suicide completers compared with male controls. The authors concluded that the Val/Val genotype may be a protective factor against suicide in males, which implies that the low-activity Met allele increases the suicide risk. One study failed to detect an association between suicidal behaviour and COMT genotype frequencies in patients who were considered to be at high risk of suicide versus controls, but the possible association was not analysed by gender in this investigation (Russ *et al.* 2000). The study of Ono *et al.* (2004) mentioned above also failed to show significant differences in genotype distribution if the results for both genders were combined. The observed sexual dimorphism could be a result of the modulation of neurotransmission and neuronal excitability of catecholaminergic systems by estrogen in females (Balthazart *et al.* 1996). The results with COMT are thus reminiscent of those observed with MAOA, and both genes are along the same biological pathway, since both COMT and MAO are needed for DA and NA catabolism.

### Dopaminergic system

The identification of dopamine (DA) as a neurotransmitter in the brain in the late 1950s, was followed by better understandings of the chemical synapse, the development of the first SSRI as well as treatment of Parkinson's disease with L-DOPA. The DA-system is abnormal in depression, and CSF studies have provided support for a possible involvement of the dopaminergic system in suicidal behaviour. Some investigations showed a correlation between low levels of the dopamine metabolite, homovanillic acid (HVA), and suicidal behaviour (Roy *et al.* 1986), although other groups failed to detect significant differences. Recently, an inverse correlation between mental energy and dopamine transporters (DAT) in the basal ganglia was observed among suicide attempters by brain imaging (Ryding *et al.* 2006). Furthermore, depressed patients with a history of suicide attempt showed a diminished growth hormone (GH) response to DA-agonist apomorphine, compared to depressed patients without such a history (Pitchot *et al.* 1992). This blunted response was also found in non-depressed male suicide attempters compared to non-depressed controls (Pitchot *et al.* 2001).

The genetic investigations have so far been focused on two of the DA-receptors. A SNP in the 3′-UTR of exon 8 (E8) in the DA-receptor D2 gene (*DRD2*) was investigated in alcoholics and non-alcoholic controls (Finckh *et al.* 1997). The E8 A/A genotype was found to be associated with an increased number of suicide attempts, and with increased anxiety and depression scores in the alcoholic group. The *DRD2* gene further contains a functionally relevant −141C insertion/deletion polymorphism upstream to exon 1. Ho *et al.* (2000) observed no association of this *DRD2* promoter polymorphism with a history of suicidal behaviour in a sample of unipolar and bipolar patients. Another group found the −141C deletion to be over-represented in alcoholics with suicidality compared to controls, although this association did not remain significant after Bonferroni correction (Johann *et al.* 2005). Two studies examined the association of a 48 bp repeat polymorphism in the DA-receptor D4 gene (*DRD4*) with suicide attempts (Persson *et al.* 1999; Zalsman *et al.* 2004). Both groups did not find any evidence for an implication of this DRD4 polymorphism in suicidal behaviour. More studies are required.

### Noradrenergic system

The observed increase of TH and alpha2-adrenergic receptor densities could be indicative of NA depletion, compensatory to increased NA release. This hypothesis is important with regard to the relation between the NA system and stress response, as severe anxiety or agitation are associated with NA over-activity, higher suicide risk and over-activity of the hypothalamic–pituitary–adrenal (HPA) axis (Ordway 1997; Mann 2003). Post-mortem studies reported fewer NA neurons in the LC (Arango *et al.* 1996), high NA and reduced alpha2-adrenergic receptor in the PFC (Arango *et al.* 1993) and increased brainstem levels of TH (Ordway *et al.* 1994). Furthermore, lowered levels of 3-methoxy-4-hydroxy-phenylglycol (MHPG, a metabolite of NA) has been observed in suicide attempters (Pandey and Dwivedi 2007). Besides these neurobiological abnormalities, the genetics of the NA system in suicide has not been studied to a large extent (Ordway 1997; Pandey and Dwivedi 2007). Sequeira *et al.* (2004) investigated four variants in the alpha 2A adrenergic receptor gene; three of them were located in the promoter region and showed no differences in allele or genotype distribution. The fourth polymorphism (N251K) was functional, leading to an asparagine to lysine amino acid change. The rare N251K allele was only present in three suicide cases, two homozygous and one heterozygous. The two N251K homozygous subjects were depressed, while no clinical information was available for the heterozygous individual. This result could suggest a possible implication of this variant in the susceptibility to suicide or depression (Sequeira *et al.* 2004). Further studies are required.

## Neurotrophins

The development of neurons in the growing, and adult nervous system and synaptic plasticity is controlled, in part, by members of the neurotrophin family. Neurotrophic factors are secreted by developing neuronal cells and protect them from apoptosis; those neurons that obtain sufficient amounts of neurotrophins survive. The neurotrophic hypothesis of depression suggests that stress increases the susceptibility to depressive illness via increased HPA axis activation, in turn decreasing neurotrophic factors that are required for hippocampal neuronal survival and function. It is also likely that such interruptions may contribute to the developing of vulnerability for suicide, maybe in relation to early childhood adversity. Indeed, levels of neurotrophins are lowered in suicide. Dwivedi *et al.* (2003) examined the post-mortem brains of 27 suicide victims and 21 non-psychiatric control subjects, and found a significant reduction of messenger ribonucleic acid (mRNA) levels of brain-derived neurotrophic factor (BDNF) and tyrosine kinase B, its receptor, in both PFC and hippocampus of suicide subjects. The reduction of BDNF mRNA expression was accompanied by a decrease in protein levels of BDNF, suggesting that this neurotrophin may play a role in the etiology of suicidal behaviour. In support of this finding, other studies have further indicated lowered BDNF in suicide, measured in serum, plasma and brain (Dawood *et al.* 2007; Deveci *et al.* 2007; Kim *et al.* 2007b). Less is known about the genetics. Hong *et al.* (2003) examined a functional BDNF Va166Met polymorphism in a Chinese sample, and found no association of this SNP with mood disorders, age at onset or suicidal behaviour. Interestingly, there is a study by Lang *et al.* (2005), which describes an association of this BDNF polymorphism with anxiety-related personality traits, in a sample of 343 unrelated subjects of German descent. A study by Perroud *et al.* (2008) showed further compelling evidence for a genetic effect of BNDF along the lines discussed, i.e. an interaction between BDNF Va166Met and childhood trauma, affecting violent suicide attempts in adulthood. Another genetic component of neurotrophins has also been examined, the low-affinity neurotrophin receptor p75NTR. Kunugi *et al.* (2004) studied a common missense S205L mutation in p75NTR, whereby the minor allele was under-represented among sucidal, depressed Japansese patients. However, this was subsequently not observed in a sample of suicide attempters with child-onset mood disorders in Canada (McGregor *et al.* 2007). In summary, neurotrophins represent an interesting new pathway in suicidal causality, which remains to be further explored.

## Cholesterol

There is evidence that low serum cholesterol levels are associated with a higher risk of violent and aggressive behaviour, although there are some contradictions (Golomb 1998). A disordered cholesterol metabolism may contribute to a serotonergic deficit in the central nervous system, and thus, increase the susceptibility for suicidal behaviour (Brunner and Bronisch 1999). Convincing evidence for the association of violence and low cholesterol levels comes from studies in non-human primates. In juvenile monkeys, dietary cholesterol lowering inhibits the central serotonergic activity (Kaplan *et al.* 1994). In addition, the low cholesterol-diet monkeys behave more aggressively. An investigation in humans reported a significant correlation between plasma serotonin and cholesterol levels, a population of 100 men with low cholesterol, although this was not observed in a reference population with normal cholesterol levels (Steegmans *et al.* 1996). Terao *et al.* (1997) found a significant positive correlation between serum cholesterol and prolactin response to the serotonin agonist *m*-chlorophenylpiperazine in ten healthy volunteers (Terao *et al.* 1997). The relationship between a depletion of brain serotonergic activity and impulsive, aggressive behaviour has been demonstrated repeatedly (Coccaro 1989; Lesch and Merschdorf 2000).

Cholesterol is a main component of the lipid bilayer of neural membranes, and experimental reduction of the level of membrane cholesterol was reported to decrease the activity of the serotonin transporter due to a loss of substrate affinity and a reduction of the maximal transport rate (Scanlon *et al.* 2001). Pucadyil and Chattopadhyay *et al.* (2004) showed that cholesterol modulates specific ligand binding and binding affinity of the $5\text{-HTR}_{1A}$ receptor from bovine hippocampus.

An association study of suicidal behaviour with polymorphisms of genes involved in the cholesterol biosynthesis or transport was conducted by Lalovic *et al.* (2004). The 3-hydroxy-3-methylglutaryl CoA reductase (HMGCR) and the 7-dehydrocholesterol reductase (7-DHCR) are enzymes catalyzing important steps in cholesterol biosynthesis. Mutations in the DHCR7 gene have been shown to cause the Smith–Lemli–Opitz syndrome. Patients affected by this autosomal recessive disorder have abnormal low levels of cholesterol, mental retardation and display aggressive, self-injurious behaviour (Tierney *et al.* 2001). Variants in the genes coding for the enzyme lipoprotein lipase (LPL) and the low-density lipoprotein receptor (LDLR) are associated with low levels of cholesterol (Gudnason *et al.* 1998; Nicklas *et al.* 2000). Apolipoprotein E (apoE) is involved in the transport of cholesterol and lipids throughout the circulation. Lalovic *et al.* (2004) investigated variants in these five genes in a sample of 305 Caucasian male subjects of French-Canadian origin, 145 suicide completers and 160 controls with no history of suicidal behaviour and no major psychiatric diagnoses. They found no differences in allele or genotype frequencies between the suicides and controls for the HMGCR, DHCR7, LPL and LDLR polymorphisms. The examination of the APOE gene by characterizing the allelic forms E2, E3 and E4, using nomenclature as described by Zannis *et al.* (1982), also showed no relationship between suicidal behaviour and allele or genotype distribution. The authors also tested the possible association of the polymorphisms examined and violent and impulsive behaviours. Measures of impulsive and aggressive behaviours were available for a subset of 42 suicide cases, and no significant relationship was found between these traits or any of the genes studied. The ATP-binding cassette (ABC) transporter is a less known component, which may be involved in human cholesterol homeostasis, and variants in its gene have been associated with the aggressive traits, but not suicide per se (Rujescu *et al.* 2000; Gietl *et al.* 2007). These genetic studies have not yet found evidence of a major role of the investigated polymorphism in the etiology of suicide, although this may very well be due to a lack of sufficient statistical power.

The implication of cholesterol in suicidal behaviour might be due to other factors, and the biological relationship remains puzzling. One clue into the causal pathway may come from the many interactions between blood lipids and RORalpha (orphan Rev-erb nuclear receptor), which has key roles in neuroendocrine homeostasis and circardian regulation (Ramakrishnan and Muscat 2006), and which is a biological target of lithium treatment (Yin *et al.* 2006). Furthermore, it is also interesting to note that cholesterol is the biochemical precursor for cortisol synthesis.

## The CRH system and the neuroendocrine hypothalamic–pituitary–adrenal axis—a systemic stress modulator

Hans Selye pioneered the scientific field of stress and hormones in the 1930s (Selye 1936), particularly that of corticosteroid effects on brain function (general adaptation syndrome—GAS), inspired by interaction with the works of Walther B Cannon on adrenal secretion of adrenalin in response to emotions, i.e. sympathetic systems adaptations, defining the terms 'fight or flight' response and 'homeostasis' (Cannon and de la Paz 1911). GAS was described to have three stages, namely an initial alarm phase (fight or flight), an adaptation phase, building resistance to the stress upon survival of the initial phase, and if the stress duration was sufficiently long/chronic, a third exhaustion stage similar to 'ageing' (Selye 1936). This pathway of stress-response and -modulation is nowadays defined as the hypothalamic–pituitary–adrenal (HPA) axis, being receptive to externally or internally perceived stress stimulation, by physical, psychological or inflammatory means, whereby the homeostasis of secreted steroids is altered, affecting e.g. behavioural, cognitive, autonomic, psychological and immunologic functions.

Upon affective or sensory input stimuli, the HPA-axis is activated in a sequential manner (Figure 26.2); (i) release of corticotropin-releasing hormone (CRH) from the paraventricular nucleus (PVN) of the hypothalamus, which is transported by portal vessels to the corticotrophs in the anterior pituitary; (ii) binding to CRH receptor 1 (CRHR1), resulting in preferential release of adrenocorticotropic hormone (ACTH), derived from the pro-opiomelanocortin (POMC)-prehormone, into blood circulation; (iii) stimulation of the adrenal gland cortex to secrete cortisol. Cortisol acts on two types

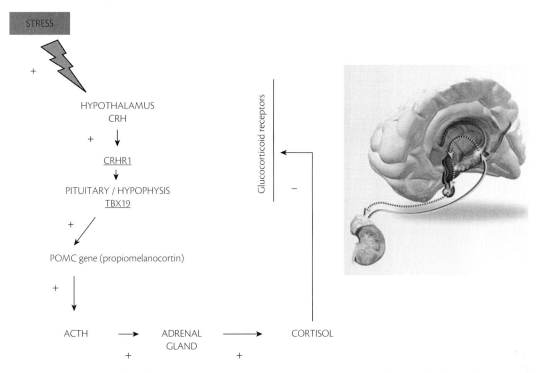

**Fig. 26.2** The hypothalamic–pituitary–adrenal (HPA) axis. Exposure to stress activates a biological signalling cascade, ultimately elevating the levels of the stress-hormone cortisol, which itself also acts in a negative feedback regulation loop on the axis, as depicted. Prolonged dysregulation in the HPA-axis results in a variety of pathologies.

of receptors, glucocorticoid (GR) and mineralocorticoid (MR), throughout many parts the brain, with GRs having the broadest effects, being distributed in the limbic system, frontal cortex, brainstem, pituitary and hypothalamus. A functional response in the feedback regulation at all levels, through the balanced activation of GRs and MRs by cortisol and on CRH-secretion from the PVN by ACTH, is essential for returning to a normal state. Furthermore, CRH itself acts heavily on other neurosystems, directly through hypothalamic–central amygdala connections (CeA), affecting e.g. all monoaminergic systems, in response to stressful situations, e.g. by suppression of 5-HTR$_{1A}$ in the dorsal raphe nuclei (Meijer and de Kloet 1998) or tryptophan-/5HT-depletion and neurotoxicity, due to activation of the indoleamine 2,3-dioxygenase pathway, as well as glutamatergic hyperfunction (Leonard 2005; Muller and Schwarz 2007). Thus, the HPA axis/CRH system may act as a central modulator of emotions (amygdala) and memory (hippocampus), with consequences for subsequent executive processing of, and behavioural response to, these parameters (PFC).

An overactive HPA axis is a consistent neurobiological indicator of depression (Roy *et al.* 1987; Hasler *et al.* 2004; Bale 2005; Nemeroff and Vale 2005; Swaab *et al.* 2005), and was the first biological risk factor to be implied in the causality of suicide (Bunney and Fawcett 1965). The HPA axis has been shown to be affected neurobiologically in relation to suicidality, at the level of CRH (Arato *et al.* 1989; Traskman-Bendz *et al.* 1992; Brunner *et al.* 2001; Austin *et al.* 2003; Merali *et al.* 2006) and its receptors (Nemeroff *et al.* 1988; Hiroi *et al.* 2001; Merali *et al.* 2004), or at the levels of other HPA components (Lopez *et al.* 1992; Pitchot *et al.* 1995; Dumser *et al.* 1998; Pitchot *et al.* 2005; Kozicz *et al.* 2008). Most studies have confirmed that an overactive HPA axis, manifested as e.g. hypercortisolism or failure to suppress cortisol after GR

stimulation in the dexamethasone suppression test (DST), often precedes suicide (Coryell and Schlesser 2001; Young 2005; Mann and Currier 2007). There is a high degree of prognostic value of predicting suicide among depressed, by using such measures of HPA responsiveness, particularly when combined with measures of 5-HT activity, i.e. CSF 5-HIAA or cholesterol (Mann *et al.* 2006; Coryell and Schlesser 2007; Mann and Currier 2007). However, there have also been observations of reductions in HPA axis activity among suicide attempters (Pfennig *et al.* 2005). As observed initially (Selye 1936), a prolonged state of HPA hyperactivity, e.g. by exposure to chronic stress, is pathological to brain development and function. Less well studied, but nevertheless of equal importance, is that prolonged HPA hypoactivity may have equally detrimental consequences (Raison and Miller 2003). In summary, the HPA axis is dysregulated in suicide (as well as in other psychopathologies), with consequences for cognition, emotions and memory, and a better understanding of these dysregulations will likely come from studying variation in (new/further) key participants of this system.

One such key component is the *CRHR1* gene, which is involved in both HPA activation and direct central effects in the CeA. Consequently, antagonists active against *CRHR1* are being developed as a novel type of antidepressants (Nielsen 2006), which are likely have applications in the treatment of suicidality. From a pharmacogenomic perspective, it is of importance to have access to the level of individual variation in this gene in context to its functionality, which can be needed for evaluation of treatment efficacy as well as being used in diagnostic tools. Knowledge about dysfunctional *CRHR1* variants may also bring about new, highly specific treatment possibilities with inhibitory RNAs (Sah 2006). Surprisingly, little is known about the influence of subtle, 'natural' genetic variations in the human *CRHR1* gene in these contexts, since only a few studies have been reported to date. Polymorphisms in human *CRHR1* have been shown to be associated with depression, treatment efficiency of depression and levels of alcohol intake, in the contexts of stressful life events (Licinio *et al.* 2004; Liu *et al.* 2006, 2007; Papiol *et al.* 2007; Bradley *et al.* 2008; Wasserman *et al.* 2008a). So far only our group has investigated the *CRHR1* gene in relation to suicide (Wasserman *et al.* 2008a). We demonstrated association and linkage of an SNP to suicide attempt, among whom most males were depressed. The finding was also confined to individuals who had been exposed to low levels of lifetime stress, and it was proposed that these individuals may carry variants of *CRHR1*, which were more likely to produce a dysregulated HPA/CRH system (Wasserman *et al.* 2008a). A subsequent follow-up investigation, with more SNPs in the *CRHR1* gene, confirmed and expanded these findings to several non-correlated SNPs (Wasserman *et al.* 2008b). Interestingly, these studies emanated after we had reported associations between genetic variants in the *TBX19* gene and neurotic personality traits. The transcription factor *TBX19* is along the same biological pathways as *CRHR1*, i.e. the HPA axis, since they are both involved in the activation of the POMC gene, of key importance for ACTH production, in the corticotrophs of the anterior pituitary (Wasserman *et al.* 2006a).

As indicated, the 5-HT system is highly intertwined with the HPA axis (Sullivan Hanley and Van de Kar 2003). Slight changes in one system affect the other, and these interactions will probably be more accounted for in future suicide research. It is interesting that cortisol deficiencies can cause antisocial aggression behaviour in rats upon stress exposure, with loss of the normal 5-HT-related aggression-control in mPFC (Kim and Haller 2007). It is likely that measurement of cortisol levels/HPA-responsiveness is a too crude measurement, towards understanding the full neurocognitive effects, as this also involves CeA and mPFC activities. One common pathological denominator of both HPA hyper- and hypoactivity is however the hippocampal processing of emotion and memories, as both conditions impede long-term potentiation (LTP)/plasticity, involving e.g. neurotrophins such as BDNF. Hippocampus, which is innervated with both CeA (fear) and medial PFC (behavioural inhibition), is highly affected by cortisol, being the part of the brain with highest amounts of GRs, and with biochemistry and gene expression altered in suicide brains (Sequeira *et al.* 2007). Furthermore, the stress-response related to traumatic memories, which often involves suicidality, has been studied by the investigation of hippocampal LTP processes, in relation to CeA, mPFC and HPA activity (Diamond *et al.* 2007). Such a systemic neurobiological model should also be implemented in studies of suicidality, in which the HPA axis is given a more central importance.

## Further genes/pathways being indicated with suicidality

### Genome-wide studies

*Genetic population studies.* As described, complex neural circuitry with many interacting neurotransmitters and their effectors, each involving polygenic influences, needs to be considered when delineating the genetics of the complex phenotype of suicidal behaviour. Ultimately, all genes expressed in the central nervous system (CNS) represent potential candidate genes

for suicidal behaviour, and ideally, identification of genetic vulnerability factors should involve a comprehensive survey of the entire human genome. One such attempt is by using 'genome-wide' approaches, whereby the goal is to look at all genetic variation in all genes at a time.

The first genome-wide linkage study of suicidal behaviour used the COGA (Collaborative Study on the Genetics of Alcoholism) sample of alcohol-dependent subjects and their biological relatives (Hesselbrock *et al.* 2004). Chromosome 2 showed a maximum LOD score of 4.2 for the qualitative phenotype 'ever tried suicide' near marker D2S1790. In addition, Hesselbrock *et al.* (2004) created a 'suicidality index' regarding lifetime suicidal thoughts and behaviour and examined this second phenotype. This investigation yielded modest evidence for linkage of suicidality to chromosomes 1 and 3, but these results did not reach statistical significance.

Zubenko *et al.* (2004) performed a genome-wide linkage survey for suicidal behaviour in 81 families with mood disorders. Significant evidence of linkage was found at cytogenetic location 8p22–p21 for all phenotypes. The marker DXS1047 at location Xq25–26.1 showed significant LOD scores for affected relative pairs with recurrent MDD. The cytogenetic locations for the other markers that reached genome-wide adjusted levels of significance are 2p12 (peak at marker D2S1777), 5q31–q33, 6q12 and 11q25 (Zubenko *et al.* 2004).

Interestingly, these two studies actually showed concordant signals for a region of chromosome 2, namely 2p12 (with markers being 6.5 mb apart), and this was replicated in a third, independent study of 162 bipolar pedigrees, including suicide attempt as a covariate (Willour *et al.* 2007). This region now needs to be dissected in a more detailed manner, in order to identify the gene(s) which influence suicidality. 2p12 contains 170 known genes, including the interesting candidates TACR1 (the substance P receptor) and TGOLN2 (a trans-golgi network protein), genes which have been experimentally implicated in depression/anxiety/aggression or completed suicide, respectively (De Felipe *et al.* 1998; McLean 2005; Sequeira *et al.* 2006).

The genome-wide approaches used so far only represent an approximation of full genome coverage, and the method has relied heavily on indirect associations between genetic variants through linkage disequilibrium, using e.g. 'tag-SNPs'. There is tremendous progress in this field, but it is also becoming clear, thanks to the efforts of the HapMap project, that much novel genetic variation remains to be included in the future analyses, in addition to the previous markers. Even when true genome-wide coverage will be available by cheap and fast DNA-sequencing of entire human genomes, the candidate genes approach will be viable due to the need of detailed and focused studies of subsets of genes and proteins. Nevertheless, despite the initial flaws, current genome-wide approaches still have huge potential in the primary indication of new, previously unknown neurobiological pathways, due to its screening/hypothesis-free nature. This approach is only likely to increase in importance, as a tool for progressing our understanding of psychobiological mechanisms in the future.

*Gene expression studies.* The use of microarray technology, has also made it possible to quantify the abundance of many different mRNAs at once. Once again, while the technology might not be entirely genome-wide in its coverage, it has potential to find complex multipoint patterns/changes in mRNA expression levels. It should also be noted that steady state levels of mRNA is quite a crude measurement, which may not always represent the actual levels of gene expression, due to a variety of other factors, e.g. expression control at levels of mRNA transport or mRNA translation. Furthermore, the tendency of RNA to be degraded easily, as well as with differential rates of decay, e.g. in post-mortem suicide brains (Gwadry et al. 2005), itself presents a technological challenge microarray studies.

Sibille et al. assayed the PFC of depressed suicide victims with an array of 22,000 annotated genes, but found no significant alterations in mRNA levels compared to matched, non-suicidal subjects (Sibille et al. 2004). A Japanese study showed increased levels of 14–3–3 epsilon gene brain expression, a protein implicated in neurogenesis, together with association results for three polymorphisms in this gene, among suicide victims (Yanagi et al. 2005). In one of the most extensive studies to date, differential expression was demonstrated among several genes in the cortical brain regions of suicide victims (Sequeira et al. 2006). Among these genes, detailed analysis was performed of the SSAT gene, with verification using reverse transcription polymerase chain reaction (RT-PCR), as well as by quantification of the protein product, with additional evidence of polymorphic association with suicide (Sequeira et al. 2006). Since the identified SSAT-gene has key roles in the metabolism of polyamines, potent neuromodulators of the stress-response linked to the HPA axis (Gilad and Gilad 2003), the results demonstrate the potential to identify new psychobiological pathways in the causality of suicidal behaviour. The research group further extended the study to the limbic system, which provided confirmatory evidence of a global alteration of GABAergic neurotransmission (Sequeira et al. 2007). Further on, Kim et al. (2007a) has evaluated post-mortem microarray data on the PFC, implicating differential expression among 70 genes in relation to suicide completion, among which, results with PLSCR4 and EMX2 seemed independent of other diagnoses, which may provide entry points for novel pathways. Tochigi et al. (2008) also studied differential gene expression in the PFC, and one of the comparisons found that suicide victims had differential expression of CAD and ATP1A3 genes, as was observed in relation to major depression. This summary shows that experimental gene expression screening at the level of the genome has already showed significant potential for future suicide research, and more is likely to follow, particularly as the methods of this study are being refined and improved (Ernst et al. 2008).

### Candidate gene studies

Many more systems are further implicated with suicidality, either directly or through correlated clinical measures.

Modulations of anxiety, as well as certain behaviour, e.g. motor activity and exploration, are the effects of cannabinoids, which is indicated as another pathway involved in suicide (Vinod and Hungund 2006). It involves activation of the HPA axis/CRH system, possibly by multiple routes, e.g. modulation of GABAergic/cholecystokinin (CCK)—containing neurons, glutamatergic transmission, opioid receptors and 5-HT/5-HTR$_{1A}$ (Viveros et al. 2005). Increased cannabinoid receptor (CB1) binding has been observed in the PFC of depressed suicide victims (Hungund et al.

2004). The genetics of the endocannabinoid system remain to be studied in the context of suicide.

Furthermore, neuropeptide CCK is, by itself, not only implicated in anxiety modulation, but also in suicide, as CCK was elevated in the PFC and CSF in relation to suicide (Harro et al. 1992; Bachus et al. 1997; Lofberg et al. 1998). Moreover, this may be influenced genetically, as promoter polymorphisms in CCK were associated with male suicide behaviour (Shindo and Yoshioka 2005).

Similarly, substantial evidence has accumulated for the involvement of gamma-aminobutyric acid (GABA) system, the principal inhibitory neurotransmitter, as well as the glutamatergic system, in depression and suicidality (Manchon et al. 1987; Pandey et al. 1997; Sundman-Eriksson and Allard 2002; Merali et al. 2004; Choudary et al. 2005; Marazziti et al. 2005; Zhu et al. 2006). GABA is synthesized from glutamate by enzyme glutamate decarboxylase (GAD), and upon release in the synapse, active on two receptors types, A and B. GABA is then catabolized after pre-synaptic reuptake, by GABA transaminase. This metabolic cycle thus involves a balance with glutamatergic transmission, which increases in depression, interactively with 5-HT system/HPA axis modulations (Muller and Schwarz 2007). The indicated components specific for suicidality have so far implicated GABA-A receptor subunits (Merali et al. 2004), but the further mechanisms and genetic involvements remain to be resolved.

The gender differences, related to both depression and suicide, are commonly hypothesized to be affected, in part, by the differential actions of HPA-secreted oestrogen (Fourestie et al. 1986; Leibenluft 1999). Interestingly, Tsai et al. (2003) found support for such possible involvement, by examination of the oestrogen alpha receptor (ESR1) gene in relation to suicide and depression. More studies in this context are expected.

Another psychobiological pathway involves the angiotensin I-converting enzyme (ACE), which is a peptidase involved in e.g. producing bioactive receptor-ligand angiotensin II, as well as in degrading substance P, a 5-HT modulator in the dorsal raphe. Reduced depression has been observed, both in relations to antagonists against ACE, or in ACE-deleted mice mutants. Inter-individual variations in this system have been observed in relation to psychopathologies (Arregui et al. 1980; Callreus et al. 2007), and polymorphic variation in the ACE gene has been associated with suicide in one study (Hishimoto et al. 2006), but not in another (Hong et al. 2002).

It has also been observed that among individuals with the Wolfram syndrome, who have homozygous (or are heterozygous carriers of) loss-of-function mutations in the WSF1 gene, often suffered from severe depression, anxiety, impulsive aggression and attempted suicide. Certain genetic variants within this gene may have involvement in suicide (Sequeira et al. 2003; Aluclu et al. 2006), whereas other may not (Crawford et al. 2002). Interestingly, novel mouse models will help to investigate this psychobiological pathway further (Kato et al. 2008).

Finally, preliminary data has further showed association and linkage of genetic variants of novel genes relevant for signal transduction, a sodium channel gene (SCN8A) and a gene for one of the vesicle-associated membrane proteins (VAMP4), in suicide attempter families (Wasserman et al. 2005). The role of these genes remains to be investigated further, with implications for possible cognitive/affective effects.

## Conclusions

More systemic approaches are needed when interpreting 'local' alterations, since e.g. the prefrontal cortex–hippocampus–central amygdala–HPA tend to function as one operational unit, by the effects of many functional interactions wherein each part contributes in its unique manner. Furthermore, more/novel (biological) endophenotypes, which better reflect these interactions, may be informative (novel, 'common denominators'), such as long-term potentiation in hippocampus/BDNF levels and other subreceptor intracellular processes. Novel psychobiological pathways identified may shed light on the interacting processes related to stress response, as identified by e.g. genome-wide approaches. The temporal aspects of stress exposure, i.e. duration and time point in development, are also of crucial importance in the shaping of the suicidal brain; therefore, this aspect of environmental exposure must be continuously included. In all this, the influence of the individual's genetic set-up must be determined at all stages of discovery, since it is of major importance for the function of all neurobiological process. To summarize, it seems that suicidal vulnerability appears through changes in the brain's neurobiology, which occur in its development, being influenced by environmental exposures and the genetic set-up of the individual, and that such changes may produce life-lasting psychobiological alterations of brain structure and function, by e.g. epigenetic mechanisms (McGowan *et al.* 2008). To this end, progress in the field is continuing to evolve rapidly and knowledge emanate with greater detail from the original discoveries described here, enabling the development of better tools for prevention, diagnosis and treatment of suicidality in the future.

## References

Abumaria N, Ribic A, Anacker C *et al.* (2008). Stress upregulates TPH1 but not TPH2 mRNA in the rat dorsal raphe nucleus: identification of two TPH2 mRNA splice variants. *Cellular and Molecular Neurobiology*, **28**, 331–342.

af Klinteberg B, Schalling D, Edman G *et al.* (1987). Personality correlates of platelet monoamine oxidase (MAO) activity in female and male subjects. *Neuropsychobiology*, **18**, 89–96.

Albert PR and Lemonde S (2004). 5-HT1A receptors, gene repression, and depression: guilt by association. *Neuroscientist*, **10**, 575–593.

Aluclu MU, Bahceci M, Tuzcu A *et al.* (2006). A new mutation in WFS1 gene (C.1522–1523delTA, Y508fsX421) may be responsible for early appearance of clinical features of Wolfram syndrome and suicidal behaviour. *Neuroendocrinology Letters*, **27**, 691–694.

Anguelova M, Benkelfat C, Turecki G (2003). A systematic review of association studies investigating genes coding for serotonin receptors and the serotonin transporter: II. Suicidal behavior. *Molecular Psychiatry*, **8**, 646–653.

Arango V, Ernsberger P, Sved AF *et al.* (1993). Quantitative autoradiography of alpha 1- and alpha 2-adrenergic receptors in the cerebral cortex of controls and suicide victims. *Brain Research*, **630**, 271–282.

Arango V, Huang YY, Underwood MD *et al.* (2003). Genetics of the serotonergic system in suicidal behavior. *Journal of Psychiatric Research*, **37**, 375–386.

Arango V, Underwood MD, Mann JJ (1996). Fewer pigmented locus coeruleus neurons in suicide victims: preliminary results. *Biological Psychiatry*, **39**, 112–120.

Arango V, Underwood MD, Mann JJ (1997). Post-mortem findings in suicide victims. Implications for *in vivo* imaging studies. *Annals of the New York Academy of Science*, **836**, 269–287.

Arato M, Banki CM, Bissette G *et al.* (1989). Elevated CSF CRF in suicide victims. *Biological Psychiatry*, **25**, 355–359.

Arregui A, Mackay AV, Spokes EG *et al.* (1980). Reduced activity of angiotensin-converting enzyme in basal ganglia in early onset schizophrenia. *Psychological Medicine*, **10**, 307–313.

Åsberg M (1997). Neurotransmitters and suicidal behavior. The evidence from cerebrospinal fluid studies. *Annals of the New York Academy of Science*, **836**, 158–181.

Åsberg M, Thoren P, Traskman L *et al.* (1976a). 'Serotonin depression'— a biochemical subgroup within the affective disorders? *Science*, **191**, 478–480.

Åsberg M, Träskman L, Thorén P (1976b). 5-HIAA in the cerebrospinal fluid: a biochemical suicide predictor? *Archives of General Psychiatry*, **33**, 1193–1197.

Austin MC, Janosky JE, Murphy HA (2003). Increased corticotropin-releasing hormone immunoreactivity in monoamine-containing pontine nuclei of depressed suicide men. *Molecular Psychiatry*, **8**, 324–332.

Bach-Mizrachi H, Underwood MD, Tin A *et al.* (2008). Elevated expression of tryptophan hydroxylase-2 mRNA at the neuronal level in the dorsal and median raphe nuclei of depressed suicides. *Molecular Psychiatry*, **13**, 507–513, 465.

Bachus SE, Hyde TM, Herman MM *et al.* (1997). Abnormal cholecystokinin mRNA levels in entorhinal cortex of schizophrenics. *Journal of Psychiatric Research*, **31**, 233–256.

Balazic J and Marusic A (2005). The completed suicide as interplay of genes and environment. *Forensic Science International*, **147**, S1–3.

Baldessarini R and Hennen J (2004). Genetics of suicide: an overview. *Harvard Review of Psychiatry*, **12**, 1–13.

Bale TL (2005). Sensitivity to stress: dysregulation of CRF pathways and disease development. *Hormones and Behaviour*, **48**, 1–10.

Balthazart J, Foidart A, Absil P *et al.* (1996). Effects of testosterone and its metabolites on aromatase-immunoreactive cells in the quail brain: relationship with the activation of male reproductive behavior. *Journal of Steroid Biochemistry and Molecular Biology*, **56**, 185–200.

Baumann B, Danos P, Diekmann S *et al.* (1999). Tyrosine hydroxylase immunoreactivity in the locus coeruleus is reduced in depressed non-suicidal patients but normal in depressed suicide patients. *European Archives of Psychiatry and Clinical Neuroscience*, **249**, 212–219.

Beck AT, Beck RA and Kovacs M (1975). Classification of suicidal behaviors: I. Quantifying intent and medical lethality. *American Journal of Psychiatry*, **132**, 285–287.

Beitchman JH, Baldassarra L, Mik H *et al.* (2006). Serotonin transporter polymorphisms and persistent, pervasive childhood aggression. *American Journal of Psychiatry*, **163**, 1103–1105.

Bellivier F, Chaste P, Malafosse A (2004). Association between the TPH gene A218C polymorphism and suicidal behavior: a meta-analysis. *American Journal of Medical Genetics B Neuropsychiatric Genetics*, **124**, 87–91.

Bennett MR (2000). The concept of transmitter receptors: 100 years on. *Neuropharmacology*, **39**, 523–546.

Biegon A and Fieldust S (1992). Reduced tyrosine hydroxylase immunoreactivity in locus coeruleus of suicide victims. *Synapse*, **10**, 79–82.

Birkmayer W and Riederer P (1975). Biochemical post-mortem findings in depressed patients. *Journal of Neural Transmission*, **37**, 95–109.

Bondy B, Buettner A, Zill P (2006). Genetics of suicide. *Molecular Psychiatry*, **11**, 336–351.

Bradley R, Binder E, Epstein M *et al.* (2008). Influence of child abuse on adult depression. *Archives of General Psychiatry*, **65**, 190–200.

Breakefield XO and Edelstein SB (1980). Inherited levels of A and B types of monoamine oxidase activity. *Schizophrenia Bulletin*, **6**, 282–288.

Breidenthal SE, White DJ, Glatt CE (2004). Identification of genetic variants in the neuronal form of tryptophan hydroxylase (TPH2). *Psychiatric Genetics*, **14**, 69–72.

Brent DA and Mann JJ (2005). Family genetic studies, suicide, and suicidal behavior. *American Journal of Human Genetics C Seminars in Medical Genetics*, **133**, 13–24.

Brezo J, Klempan T, Turecki G (2008). The genetics of suicide: a critical review of molecular studies. *Psychiatric Clinics of North America*, **31**, 179–203.

Brunner HG, Nelen M, Breakefield XO *et al.* (1993). Abnormal behavior associated with a point mutation in the structural gene for monoamine oxidase A. *Science*, **262**, 578–580.

Brunner J and Bronisch T (1999). Neurobiological correlates of suicidal behavior. *Fortschritte der Neurologie-Psychiatrie*, **67**, 391–412.

Brunner J, Stalla GK, Stalla J *et al.* (2001). Decreased corticotropin-releasing hormone (CRH) concentrations in the cerebrospinal fluid of eucortisolemic suicide attempters. *Journal of Psychiatric Research*, **35**, 1–9.

Buchsbaum MS, Haier RJ, Murphy DL (1977). Suicide attempts, platelet monoamine oxidase and the average evoked response. *Acta Psychiatrica Scandinavica*, **56**, 69–79.

Bunney WE Jr and Fawcett JA (1965). Possibility of a biochemical test for suicidal potential: an analysis of endocrine findings prior to three suicides. *Archives of General Psychiatry*, **13**, 232–239.

Callreus T, Agerskov Andersen U *et al.* (2007). Cardiovascular drugs and the risk of suicide: a nested case-control study. *European Journal of Clinical Pharmacology*, **63**, 591–596.

Cannon WB and de la Paz D (1911). Emotional stimulation of the adrenal secretion. *American Journal of Physiology*, **28**, 64–70.

Carballo JJ, Akamnonu CP, Oquendo MA (2008). Neurobiology of suicidal behavior. An integration of biological and clinical findings. *Archives of Suicide Research*, **12**, 93–110.

Cases O, Seif I, Grimsby J *et al.* (1995). Aggressive behavior and altered amounts of brain serotonin and norepinephrine in mice lacking MAOA. *Science*, **268**, 1763–1766.

Caspi A, Sugden K, Moffitt TE *et al.* (2003). Influence of life stress on depression: moderation by a polymorphism in the 5-HTT gene. *Science*, **301**, 386–389.

Choudary PV, Molnar M, Evans SJ *et al.* (2005). Altered cortical glutamatergic and GABAergic signal transmission with glial involvement in depression. *Proceedings of the National Academy of Sciences, USA*, **102**, 15653–15658.

Coccaro EF (1989). Central serotonin and impulsive aggression. *British Journal of Psychiatry*, S52–S62.

Coryell W and Schlesser M (2001). The dexamethasone suppression test and suicide prediction. *American Journal of Psychiatry*, **158**, 748–753.

Coryell W and Schlesser M (2007). Combined biological tests for suicide prediction. *Psychiatry Research*, **150**, 187–191.

Courtet P, Jollant F, Buresi C *et al.* (2005a). The monoamine oxidase A gene may influence the means used in suicide attempts. *Psychiatric Genetics*, **15**, 189–193.

Courtet P, Jollant F, Castelnau D, Buresi C, Malafosse A (2005b). Suicidal behavior: relationship between phenotype and serotonergic genotype. *American Journal of Medical Genetics C Seminars in Medical Genetics*, **133**, 25–33.

Crawford J, Zielinski MA, Fisher LJ, Sutherland GR, Goldney RD (2002). Is there a relationship between Wolfram syndrome carrier status and suicide? *American Journal of Medical Genetics*, **114**, 343–346.

Currier D and Mann JJ (2008). Stress, genes and the biology of suicidal behavior. *Psychiatric Clinics of North America*, **31**, 247–269.

Dawood T, Anderson J, Barton D *et al.* (2007). Reduced overflow of BDNF from the brain is linked with suicide risk in depressive illness. *Molecular Psychiatry*, **12**, 981–983.

De Felipe C, Herrero JF, O'Brien JA *et al.* (1998). Altered nociception, analgesia and aggression in mice lacking the receptor for substance P. *Nature*, **392**, 394–397.

De Luca V, Mueller D, Tharmalingam S *et al.* (2004). Analysis of the novel *TPH2* gene in bipolar disorder and suicidality. *Molecular Psychiatry*, **9**, 896–897.

De Luca V, Strauss J, Kennedy JL (2008). Power-based association analysis (PBAT) of serotonergic and noradrenergic polymorphisms in bipolar patients with suicidal behaviour. *Progess in Neuropsychopharmacology and Biological Psychiatry*, **32**, 197–203.

Delgado PL, Charney DS, Price LH *et al.* (1990). Serotonin function and the mechanism of antidepressant action. Reversal of antidepressant-induced remission by rapid depletion of plasma tryptophan. *Archives of General Psychiatry*, **47**, 411–418.

Deveci A, Aydemir O, Taskin O *et al.* (2007). Serum BDNF levels in suicide attempters related to psychosocial stressors: a comparative study with depression. *Neuropsychobiology*, **56**, 93–97.

Diamond DM, Campbell AM, Park CR *et al.* (2007). The temporal dynamics model of emotional memory processing: a synthesis on the neurobiological basis of stress-induced amnesia, flashbulb and traumatic memories, and the Yerkes–Dodson law. *Neural Plasticity*, **2007**, 60803.

Drago A, Ronchi DD, Serretti A (2007). 5-HT1A gene variants and psychiatric disorders: a review of current literature and selection of SNPs for future studies. *International Journal of Neuropsychopharmacol*, 1–21.

Du L, Faludi G, Palkovits M *et al.* (2002). High activity-related allele of MAO-A gene associated with depressed suicide in males. *Neuroreport*, **13**, 1195–1198.

Dumser T, Barocka A, Schubert E (1998). Weight of adrenal glands may be increased in persons who commit suicide. *American Journal of Forensic Medical Pathology*, **19**, 72–76.

Dwivedi Y, Rizavi HS, Conley RR *et al.* (2003). Altered gene expression of brain-derived neurotrophic factor and receptor tyrosine kinase B in post-mortem brain of suicide subjects. *Archives of General Psychiatry*, **60**, 804–815.

Ebstein RP, Levine J, Geller V *et al.* (1998). Dopamine D4 receptor and serotonin transporter promoter in the determination of neonatal temperament. *Molecular Psychiatry*, **3**, 238–246.

Ernst C, Bureau A, Turecki G (2008). Application of microarray outlier detection methodology to psychiatric research. *BMC Psychiatry*, **8**, 29.

Finckh U, Rommelspacher H, Kuhn S *et al.* (1997). Influence of the dopamine D2 receptor (DRD2) genotype on neuroadaptive effects of alcohol and the clinical outcome of alcoholism. *Pharmacogenetics*, **7**, 271–281.

Fourestie V, de Lignieres B, Roudot-Thoraval F *et al.* (1986). Suicide attempts in hypo-oestrogenic phases of the menstrual cycle. *Lancet*, **2**, 1357–1360.

Frodl T, Zill P, Baghai T *et al.* (2008). Reduced hippocampal volumes associated with the long variant of the tri- and diallelic serotonin transporter polymorphism in major depression. *American Journal of Medical Genetics B Neuropsychiatric Genetics*, **147B**, 1003–1007.

Funkenstein DH, King SH, Drolette M (1954). The direction of anger during a laboratory stress-inducing situation. *Psychosomatic Medicine*, **16**, 404–413.

Giegling I, Moreno-De-Luca D, Rujescu D *et al.* (2008). Dopa decarboxylase and tyrosine hydroxylase gene variants in suicidal behavior. *American Journal of Medical Genetics B Neuropsychiatric Genetics*, **147**, 308–315.

Gietl A, Giegling I, Hartmann AM, *et al.* (2007). ABCG1 gene variants in suicidal behavior and aggression-related traits. *European Neuropsychopharmacology*, **17**, 410–416.

Gilad GM and Gilad VH (2003). Overview of the brain polyamine stress response: regulation, development, and modulation by lithium and role in cell survival. *Cellular and Molecular Biology*, **23**, 637–649.

Golomb BA (1998). Cholesterol and violence: is there a connection? *Annals of Internal Medicine*, **128**, 478–487.

Grenett HE, Ledley FD, Reed LL *et al.* (1987). Full-length cDNA for rabbit tryptophan hydroxylase: functional domains and evolution of aromatic amino acid hydroxylases. *Proceedings of the National Academy of Sciences, USA*, **84**, 5530–5534.

Gudnason V, Zhou T, Thormar K *et al.* (1998). Detection of the low density lipoprotein receptor gene PvuII intron 15 polymorphism using the polymerase chain reaction: association with plasma lipid traits in healthy men and women. *Disease Markers*, **13**, 209–220.

Gwadry FG, Sequeira A, Hoke G *et al.* (2005). Molecular characterization of suicide by microarray analysis. *American Journal of Medical Genetics C Seminars in Medical Genetics*, **133C**, 48–56.

Haghighi F, Bach-Mizrachi H, Huang YY *et al.* (2008). Genetic architecture of the human tryptophan hydroxylase 2 gene: existence of neural isoforms and relevance for major depression. *Molecular Psychiatry*, **13**, 813–820.

Hare ML (1928). Tyramine oxidase: a new enzyme system in liver. *Biochemical Journal*, **22**, 968–979.

Harro J, Marcusson J, Oreland L (1992). Alterations in brain cholecystokinin receptors in suicide victims. *European Neuropsychopharmacologyy*, **2**, 57–63.

Hasler G, Drevets WC, Manji HK, Charney DS (2004). Discovering endophenotypes for major depression. *Neuropsychopharmacology*, **29**, 1765–1781.

Heils A, Teufel A, Petri S *et al.* (1996). Allelic variation of human serotonin transporter gene expression. *Journal of Neurochemistry*, **66**, 2621–2624.

Hesselbrock V, Dick D, Hesselbrock M *et al.* (2004). The search for genetic risk factors associated with suicidal behavior. *Alcoholism Clinical and Experimental Research*, **28**, 70S–76S.

Hiroi N, Wong ML, Licinio J *et al.* (2001). Expression of corticotropin releasing hormone receptors type I and type II mRNA in suicide victims and controls. *Molecular Psychiatry*, **6**, 540–546.

Hishimoto A, Shirakawa O, Nishiguchi N *et al.* (2006). Association between a functional polymorphism in the renin-angiotensin system and completed suicide. *Journal of Neural Transmission*, **113**, 1915–1920.

Ho LW, Furlong RA, Rubinsztein JS *et al.* (2000). Genetic associations with clinical characteristics in bipolar affective disorder and recurrent unipolar depressive disorder. *American Journal of Medical Genetics*, **96**, 36–42.

Hong CJ, Huo SJ, Yen FC *et al.* (2003). Association study of a brain-derived neurotrophic-factor genetic polymorphism and mood disorders, age of onset and suicidal behavior. *Neuropsychobiology*, **48**, 186–189.

Hong CJ, Pan GM, Tsai SJ (2004). Association study of onset age, attempted suicide, aggressive behavior, and schizophrenia with a serotonin 1B receptor (A-161T) genetic polymorphism. *Neuropsychobiology*, **49**, 39451.

Hong CJ, Wang YC, Tsai SJ (2002). Association study of angiotensin I-converting enzyme polymorphism and symptomatology and antidepressant response in major depressive disorders. *Journal of Neural Transmission*, **109**, 1209–1214.

Hu XZ, Lipsky RH, Zhu G *et al.* (2006). Serotonin transporter promoter gain-of-function genotypes are linked to obsessive-compulsive disorder. *American Journal of Human Genetics*, **78**, 815–826.

Huang YY, Battistuzzi C, Oquendo MA *et al.* (2004a). Human 5-HT1A receptor C(-1019)G polymorphism and psychopathology. *International Journal of Neuropsychopharmacology*, **7**, 441–451.

Huang YY, Cate SP, Battistuzzi C *et al.* (2004b). An association between a functional polymorphism in the monoamine oxidase a gene promoter, impulsive traits and early abuse experiences. *Neuropsychopharmacology*, **29**, 1498–1505.

Huang YY, Grailhe R, Arango V *et al.* (1999). Relationship of psychopathology to the human serotonin1B genotype and receptor binding kinetics in post-mortem brain tissue. *Neuropsychopharmacology*, **21**, 238–246.

Huang YY, Oquendo MA, Friedman JM *et al.* (2003). Substance abuse disorder and major depression are associated with the human 5-HT1B receptor gene (HTR1B) G861C polymorphism. *Neuropsychopharmacology*, **28**, 163–169.

Hungund BL, Vinod KY, Kassir SA *et al.* (2004). Upregulation of CB1 receptors and agonist-stimulated [35S] GTP gamma S binding in the prefrontal cortex of depressed suicide victims. *Molecular Psychiatry*, **9**, 184–190.

Johann M, Putzhammer A, Eichhammer P *et al.* (2005). Association of the -141C Del variant of the dopamine D2 receptor (DRD2) with positive family history and suicidality in German alcoholics. *American Journal of Medical Genetics B Neuropsychiatric Genetics*, **132**, 46–49.

Jones G, Zammit S, Norton N *et al.* (2001). Aggressive behavior in patients with schizophrenia is associated with catechol-O-methyltransferase genotype. *British Journal of Psychiatry*, **179**, 351–355.

Jönsson E, Sedvall G, Brené S *et al.* (1996). Dopamine-related genes and their relationships to monoamine metabolites in CSF. *Biological Psychiatry*, **40**, 1032–1043.

Kamali M, Oquendo MA, Mann JJ (2001). Understanding the neurobiology of suicidal behavior. *Depression and Anxiety*, **14**, 164–176.

Kaplan JR, Shively CA, Fontenot MB *et al.* (1994). Demonstration of an association among dietary cholesterol, central serotonergic activity, and social behavior in monkeys. *Psychosomatic Medicine*, **56**, 479–484.

Kato T, Ishiwata M, Yamada K *et al.* (2008). Behavioral and gene expression analyses of Wfs1 knockout mice as a possible animal model of mood disorder. *Neuroscience Research*, **61**, 143–158.

Kendler KS (2005). 'A gene for': the nature of gene action in psychiatric disorders. *American Journal of Psychiatry*, **162**, 1243–1252.

Kety SS, Rosenthal D, Wender PH *et al.* (1971). Mental illness in the biological and adoptive families of adpoted schizophrenics. *American Journal of Psychiatry*, **128**, 302–306.

Kim JJ and Haller J (2007). Glucocorticoid hyper- and hypofunction: stress effects on cognition and aggression. *Annals of the New York Academy of Science*, **1113**, 291–303.

Kim S, Choi KH, Baykiz AF *et al.* (2007a). Suicide candidate genes associated with bipolar disorder and schizophrenia: an exploratory gene expression profiling analysis of post-mortem prefrontal cortex. *BMC Genomics*, **8**, 413.

Kim YK, Lee HP, Won SD *et al.* (2007b). Low plasma BDNF is associated with suicidal behavior in major depression. *Progess in Neuropsychopharmacology and Biological Psychiatry*, **31**, 78–85.

Klinteberg B, Levander SE, Oreland L *et al.* (1987). Neuropsychological correlates of platelet monoamine oxidase (MAO) activity in female and male subjects. *Biological Psychology*, **24**, 237–252.

Kotler M, Barak P, Cohen H *et al.* (1999). Homicidal behavior in schizophrenia associated with a genetic polymorphism determining low catechol O-methyltransferase (COMT) activity. *American Journal of Medical Genetics*, **88**, 628–633.

Kozicz T, Tilburg-Ouwens D, Faludi G *et al.* (2008). Gender-related urocortin 1 and brain-derived neurotrophic factor expression in the adult human midbrain of suicide victims with major depression. *Neuroscience*, **152**, 1015–1023.

Kunugi H, Hashimoto R, Yoshida M *et al.* (2004). A missense polymorphism (S205L) of the low-affinity neurotrophin receptor p75NTR gene is associated with depressive disorder and attempted suicide. *American Journal of Medical Genetics*, **129B**, 44–46.

Kunugi H, Ishida S, Kato T *et al.* (1999). A functional polymorphism in the promoter region of monoamine oxidase-A gene and mood disorders. *Molecular Psychiatry*, **4**, 393–395.

Lachman HM, Nolan KA, Mohr P *et al.* (1998). Association between catechol O-methyltransferase genotype and violence in schizophrenia and schizoaffective disorder. *American Journal of Psychiatry*, **155**, 835–837.

Lachman HM, Papolos DF, Saito T *et al.* (1996). Human catechol-O-methyltransferase pharmacogenetics: description of a functional polymorphism and its potential application to neuropsychiatric disorders. *Pharmacogenetics*, **6**, 243–250.

Lalovic A and Turecki G (2002). Meta-analysis of the association between tryptophan hydroxylase and suicidal behavior. *American Journal of Medical Genetics*, **114**, 533–540.

Lalovic A, Sequeira A, DeGuzman R *et al.* (2004). Investigation of completed suicide and genes involved in cholesterol metabolism. *Journal of Affective Disorders*, **79**, 25–32.

Lang U, Hellweg R, Kalus P *et al.* (2005). Association of a functional BDNF polymorphism and anxiety-related personality traits. *Psychopharmacology (Berl)*.

Ledley FD, Grenett HE, Bartos DP *et al.* (1987). Assignment of human tryptophan hydroxylase locus to chromosome 11: gene duplication and translocation in evolution of aromatic amino acid hydroxylases. *Somatic Cell and Molecular Genetics*, **13**, 575–580.

Leibenluft E (ed.) (1999) *Gender Differences in Mood and Anxiety Disorders.* American Psychiatric Press, Washington.

Lemonde S, Turecki G, Bakish D *et al.* (2003). Impaired repression at a 5-hydroxytryptamine 1A receptor gene polymorphism associated with major depression and suicide. *J Neurosci*, **23**, 8788–8799.

Leonard BE (2005). The HPA and immune axes in stress: the involvement of the serotonergic system. *European Psychiatry*, **20**, S302–306.

Lesch K and Merschdorf U (2000). Impulsivity, aggression, and serotonin: a molecular psychobiological perspective. *Behavioural Sciences and the Law*, **18**, 581–604.

Levitt M, Spector S, Sjoerdsma A *et al.* (1965). Elucidation of the rate-limiting step in norepinephrine biosynthesis in the perfused guinea-pig heart. *Journal of Pharmacology and Experimental Therapeutics*, **148**, 39455.

Li D and He L (2006). Further clarification of the contribution of the tryptophan hydroxylase (TPH) gene to suicidal behavior using systematic allelic and genotypic meta-analyses. *Human Genetics*, **119**, 233–240.

Li D and He L (2007). Meta-analysis supports association between serotonin transporter (5-HTT) and suicidal behavior. *Molecular Psychiatry*, **12**, 47–54.

Licinio J, O'Kirwan F, Irizarry K *et al.* (2004). Association of a corticotropin-releasing hormone receptor 1 haplotype and antidepressant treatment response in Mexican-Americans. *Molecular Psychiatry*, **9**, 1075–1082.

Lin PI, Vance JM, Pericak-Vance MA *et al.* (2007). No gene is an island: the flip-flop phenomenon. *American Journal of Human Genetics*, **80**, 531–538.

Lin PY and Tsai G (2004). Association between serotonin transporter gene promoter polymorphism and suicide: results of a meta-analysis. *Biological Psychiatry*, **55**, 1023–1030.

Liou YJ, Tsai SJ, Hong CJ *et al.* (2001). Associa tion analysis of a functional catechol-o-methyltransferase gene polymorphism in schizophrenic patients in Taiwan. *Neuropsychobiology*, **43**, 39766.

Liu Z, Zhu F, Wang G *et al.* (2006). Association of corticotropin-releasing hormone receptor 1 gene SNP and haplotype with major depressi on. *Neuroscience Letters*, **404**, 358–362.

Liu Z, Zhu F, Wang G *et al.* (2007). Association study of corticotropin-releasing hormone receptor 1 gene polymorphisms and antidepressant response in major depressive disorders. *Neuroscience Letters*, **414**, 155–158.

Lofberg C, Agren H, Harro J *et al.* (1998). Cholecystokinin in CSF from depressed patients: possible relations to severity of depression and suicidal behaviour. *European Neuropsychopharmacologyy*, **8**, 153–157.

Lopez JF, Palkovits M, Arato M *et al.* (1992). Localization and quantification of pro-opiomelanocortin mRNA and glucocorticoid receptor mRNA in pituitaries of suicide victims. *Neuroendocrinology*, **56**, 491–501.

Lopez VA, Detera-Wadleigh S, Cardona I, Consortium NIoMHGIBD *et al.* (2007). Nested association between genetic variation in tryptophan hydroxylase II, bipolar affective disorder, and suicide attempts. *Biological Psychiatry*, **61**, 181–186.

Malone KM, Ellis SP, Currier D *et al.* (2007). Platelet 5-HT2A receptor subresponsivity and lethality of attempted suicide in depressed in-patients. *International Journal of Neuropsychopharmacology*, **10**, 335–343.

Manchon M, Kopp N, Rouzioux JJ *et al.* (1987). Benzodiazepine receptor and neurotransmitter studies in the brain of suicides. *Life Sciences*, **41**, 2623–2630.

Mann J (2003). The neurobiology of suicidal behavior. *Nature Reviews Genetics*, **4**, 819–828.

Mann JJ and Arango V (1992). Integration of neurobiology and psychopathology in a unified model of suicidal behavior. *Journal of Clinical Psychopharmacology*, **12**, 2S–7S.

Mann JJ and Currier D (2007). A review of prospective studies of biological predictors of suicidal behavior in mood disorders. *Archives of Suicide Research*, **11**, 3–16.

Mann JJ and Stanley M (1984). Post-mortem monoamine oxidase enzyme kinetics in the frontal cortex of suicide victims and controls. *Acta Psychiatrica Scandinavica*, **69**, 135–139.

Mann JJ, Brent DA, Arango V (2001). The neurobiology and genetics of suicide and attempted suicide: a focus on the serotonergic system. *Neuropsychopharmacology*, **24**, 467–477.

Mann JJ, Currier D, Stanley B *et al.* (2006). Can biological tests assist prediction of suicide in mood disorders? *International Journal of Neuropsychopharmacology*, **9**, 465–474.

Marazziti D, Dell'Osso B, Baroni S *et al.* (2005). Decreased density of peripheral benzodiazepine receptors in psychiatric patients after a suicide attempt. *Life Sciences*, **77**, 3268–3275.

McGowan PO, Sasaki A, Huang TC *et al.* (2008). Promoter-wide hypermethylation of the ribosomal RNA gene promoter in the suicide brain. *PLoS ONE*, **3**, e2085.

McGregor S, Strauss J, Bulgin N *et al.* (2007). p75(NTR) gene and suicide attempts in young adults with a history of childhood-onset mood disorder. *American Journal of Medical Genetics B Neuropsychiatric Genetics*, **144B**, 696–700.

McGuffin P, Marusic A, Farmer A (2001). What can psychiatric genetics offer suicidology? *Crisis*, **22**, 61–65.

McLean S (2005). Do substance P and the NK1 receptor have a role in depression and anxiety? *Current Pharmaceutical Design*, **11**, 1529–1547.

Meijer OC and de Kloet ER (1998). Corticosterone and serotonergic neurotransmission in the hippocampus: functional implications of central corticosteroid receptor diversity. *Critical Reviews in Neurobiology*, **12**, 1–20.

Merali Z, Du L, Hrdina P *et al.* (2004). Dysregulation in the suicide brain: mRNA expression of corticotropin-releasing hormone receptors and GABA(A) receptor subunits in frontal cortical brain region. *Journal of Neuroscience*, **24**, 1478–1485.

Merali Z, Kent P, Du L *et al.* (2006). Corticotropin-releasing hormone, arginine vasopressin, gastrin-releasing peptide, and neuromedin B alterations in stress-relevant brain regions of suicides and control subjects. *Biological Psychiatry*, **59**, 594–602.

Muller N and Schwarz MJ (2007). The immune-mediated alteration of serotonin and glutamate: towards an integrated view of depression. *Molecular Psychiatry*, **12**, 988–1000.

Murphy DL and Kalin NH (1980). Biological and behavioral consequences of alterations in monoamine oxidase activity. *Schizophrenia Bulletin*, **6**, 355–367.

Nakamura K, Sugawara Y, Sawabe K *et al.* (2006). Late developmental stage-specific role of tryptophan hydroxylase 1 in brain serotonin levels. *Journal of Neuroscience*, **26**, 530–534.

Nemeroff CB and Vale WW (2005). The neurobiology of depression: inroads to treatment and new drug discovery. *Journal of Clinical Psychiatry*, **66**, 5–13.

Nemeroff CB, Owens MJ, Bissette G *et al.* (1988). Reduced corticotropin releasing factor binding sites in the frontal cortex of suicide victims. *Archives of General Psychiatry*, **45**, 577–579.

New AS, Gelernter J, Goodman M *et al.* (2001). Suicide, impulsive aggression, and HTR1B genotype. *Biological Psychiatry*, **50**, 62–65.

Nicklas BJ, Ferrell RE, Rogus EM *et al.* (2000). Lipoprotein lipase gene variation is associated with adipose tissue lipoprotein lipase activity, and lipoprotein lipid and glucose concentrations in overweight postmenopausal women. *Human Genetics*, **106**, 420–424.

Nielsen DM (2006). Corticotropin-releasing factor type-1 receptor antagonists: the next class of antidepressants? *Life Sciences*, **78**, 909–919.

Nishiguchi N, Shirakawa O, Ono H *et al.* (2001). No evidence of an association between 5HT1B receptor gene polymorphism and suicide victims in a Japanese population. *American Journal of Medical Genetics*, **105**, 343–345.

Nishiguchi N, Shirakawa O, Ono H *et al.* (2002). Lack of an association between 5-HT1A receptor gene structural polymorphisms and suicide victims. *American Journal of Medical Genetics*, **114**, 423–425.

Nolan KA, Volavka J, Czobor P *et al.* (2000). Suicidal behavior in patients with schizophrenia is related to COMT polymorphism. *Psychiatric Genetics*, **10**, 117–124.

Norton N and Owen MJ (2005). HTR2A: association and expression studies in neuropsychiatric genetics. *Annals of Internal Medicine*, **37**, 121–129.

Ohtani M, Shindo S, Yoshioka N (2004). Polymorphisms of the tryptophan hydroxylase gene and serotonin 1A receptor gene in suicide victims among Japanese. *The Tohoku Journal of Experimental Medicine*, **202**, 123–133.

Ono H, Shirakawa O, Nishiguchi N *et al.* (2002). No evidence of an association between a functional monoamine oxidase a gene polymorphism and completed suicides. *American Journal of Medical Genetics*, **114**, 340–342.

Ono H, Shirakawa O, Nushida H *et al.* (2004). Association between catechol-O-methyltransferase functional polymorphism and male suicide completers. *Neuropsychopharmacology*, **29**, 1374–1377.

Ordway GA (1997). Pathophysiology of the locus coeruleus in suicide. *Annals of the New York Academy of Science*, **836**, 233–252.

Ordway GA, Smith KS, Haycock JW (1994). Elevated tyrosine hydroxylase in the locus coeruleus of suicide victims. *Journal of Neurochemistry*, **62**, 680–685.

Ostroff R, Giller E, Bonese K *et al.* (1982). Neuroendocrine risk factors of suicidal behavior. *American Journal of Psychiatry*, **139**, 1323–1325.

Ozelius L, Hsu YP, Bruns G *et al.* (1988). Human monoamine oxidase gene (MAOA): chromosome position (Xp21-p11) and DNA polymorphism. *Genomics*, **3**, 53–58.

Pandey GN and Dwivedi Y (2007). Noradrenergic function in suicide. *Archives of Suicide Research*, **11**, 235–246.

Pandey GN, Conley RR, Pandey SC *et al.* (1997). Benzodiazepine receptors in the post-mortem brain of suicide victims and schizophrenic subjects. *Psychiatry Research*, **71**, 137–149.

Papiol S, Arias B, Gasto C *et al.* (2007). Genetic variability at HPA axis in major depression and clinical response to antidepressant treatment. *Journal of Affective Disorders*, **104**, 83–90.

Pare CM, Yeung DP, Price K, Stacey RS (1969). 5-hydroxytryptamine, noradrenaline, and dopamine in brainstem, hypothalamus, and caudate nucleus of controls and of patients committing suicide by coal-gas poisoning. *Lancet*, **2**, 133–135.

Perroud N, Courtet P, Vincze I *et al.* (2008). Interaction between BDNF Va166Met and childhood trauma on adult's violent suicide attempt. *Genes, Brain and Behavior*, **7**, 314–322.

Persson ML, Geijer T, Wasserman D *et al.* (1999). Lack of association between suicide attempt and a polymorphism at the dopamine receptor D4 locus. *Psychiatric Genetics*, **9**, 97–100.

Persson M-L, Wasserman D, Geijer T *et al.* (1997). Tyrosine hydroxylase allelic distribution in suicide attempters. *Psychiatry Research*, **72**, 73–80.

Pfennig A, Kunzel HE, Kern N *et al.* (2005). Hypothalamus–pituitary–adrenal system regulation and suicidal behaviour in depression. *Biological Psychiatry*, **57**, 336–342.

Pinsonneault JK, Papp AC, Sadee W (2006). Allelic mRNA expression of X-linked monoamine oxidase a (MAOA) in human brain: dissection of epigenetic and genetic factors. *Human Molecular Genetics*, **15**, 2636–2649.

Pintar JE, Barbosa J, Francke U *et al.* (1981). Gene for monoamine oxidase type A assigned to the human X chromosome. *Journal of Neuroscience*, **1**, 166–175.

Pitchot W, Ansseau M, Gonzalez Moreno A *et al.* (1995). The flesinoxan 5-HT1A receptor challenge in major depression and suicidal behavior. *Pharmacopsychiatry*, **28**, 91–92.

Pitchot W, Hansenne M, Ansseau M (2001). Role of dopamine in non-depressed patients with a history of suicide attempts. *European Psychiatry*, **16**, 424–427.

Pitchot W, Hansenne M, Moreno AG *et al.* (1992). Suicidal behavior and growth hormone response to apomorphine test. *Biological Psychiatry*, **31**, 1213–1219.

Pitchot W, Hansenne M, Pinto E *et al.* M (2005). 5-hydroxytryptamine 1A receptors, major depression, and suicidal behavior. *Biological Psychiatry*, **58**, 854–858.

Polymeropoulos MH, Xiao H, Rath DS *et al.* (1991). Tetranucleotide repeat polymorphism at the human tyrosine hydroxylase gene (TH). *Nucleic Acids Research*, **19**, 3753.

Pooley EC, Houston K, Hawton K *et al.* (2003). Deliberate self-harm is associated with allelic variation in the tryptophan hydroxylase gene (TPH A779C), but not with polymorphisms in five other serotonergic genes. *Psychological Medicine*, **33**, 775–783.

Pucadyil TJ and Chattopadhyay A (2004). Cholesterol modulates ligand binding and G-protein coupling to serotonin (1A) receptors from bovine hippocampus. *Biochimica Biophysica Acta*, **1663**, 188–200.

Raison CL and Miller AH (2003). When not enough is too much: the role of insufficient glucocorticoid signaling in the pathophysiology of stress-related disorders. *American Journal of Psychiatry*, **160**, 1554–1565.

Ramakrishnan SN and Muscat GE (2006). The orphan Rev-erb nuclear receptors: a link between metabolism, circadian rhythm and inflammation? *Nuclear Receptor Signaling Atlas*, **4**, e009.

Rapport MM, Green AA, Page IH (1948). Crystalline serotonin. *Science*, **108**, 329–330.

Roy A, Agren H, Pickar D *et al.* (1986). Reduced CSF concentrations of homovanillic acid and homovanillic acid to 5-hydroxyindoleacetic acid ratios in depressed patients: relationship to suicidal behavior and dexamethasone nonsuppression. *American Journal of Psychiatry*, **143**, 1539–1545.

Roy A, Hu XZ, Janal MN *et al.* (2007). Interaction between childhood trauma and serotonin transporter gene variation in suicide. *Neuropsychopharmacology*, **32**, 2046–2052.

Roy A, Pickar D, Paul S *et al.* (1987). CSF corticotropin-releasing hormone in depressed patients and normal control subjects. *American Journal of Psychiatry*, **144**, 641–645.

Roy A, Segal NL, Centerwall BS *et al.* (1991). Suicide in twins. *Archives of General Psychiatry*, **48**, 29–32.

Rujescu D, Giegling I, Dahmen N *et al.* (2000). Association study of suicidal behavior and affective disorders with a genetic polymorphism in ABCG1, a positional candidate on chromosome 21q22.3. *Neuropsychobiology*, **42**, 22–25.

Rujescu D, Giegling I, Gietl A *et al.* (2003a). A functional single nucleotide polymorphism (V158M) in the COMT gene is associated with aggressive personality traits. *Biological Psychiatry*, **54**, 34–39.

Rujescu D, Giegling I, Sato T *et al.* (2003b). Genetic variations in tryptophan hydroxylase in suicidal behavior: analysis and meta-analysis. *Biological Psychiatry*, **54**, 465–473.

Rujescu D, Giegling I, Sato T *et al.* (2003c). Lack of association between serotonin 5-HT1B receptor gene polymorphism and suicidal behavior. *American Journal of Medical Genetics B Neuropsychiatric Genetics*, **116B**, 69–71.

Rujescu D, Thalmeier A, Moller HJ *et al.* (2007). Molecular genetic findings in suicidal behavior: what is beyond the serotonergic system? *Archives of Suicide Research*, **11**, 17–40.

Russ MJ, Lachman HM, Kashdan T *et al.* (2000). Analysis of catechol-O-methyltransferase and 5-hydroxytryptamine transporter polymorphisms in patients at risk for suicide. *Psychiatry Research*, **93**, 73–78.

Ryding E, Ahnlide JA, Lindstrom M *et al.* (2006). Regional brain serotonin and dopamine transporter binding capacity in suicide attempters relate to impulsiveness and mental energy. *Psychiatry Research*, **148**, 195–203.

Sabol SZ, Hu S, Hamer D (1998). A functional polymorphism in the monoamine oxidase A gene promoter. *Human Genetics*, **103**, 273–279.

Sah DW (2006). Therapeutic potential of RNA interference for neurological disorders. *Life Sciences*, **79**, 1773–1780.

Scanlon SM, Williams DC, Schloss P (2001). Membrane cholesterol modulates serotonin transporter activity. *Biochemistry*, **40**, 10507–10513.

Schildkraut JJ (1965). The catecholamine hypothesis of affective disorders: a review of supporting evidence. *American Journal of Psychiatry*, **122**, 509–522.

Schulsinger F, Kety SS, Rosenthal D *et al.* (1979). A family study of suicide. In M Schou and E Stromgren, eds, *Origin, Prevention and Treatment of Affective Disorders*, pp. 277–287. Academic Press, New York.

Selye H (1936). A syndrome produced by diverse nocuous agents. *Nature*, **138**, 32.

Sequeira A, Gwadry FG, Ffrench-Mullen JM *et al.* (2006). Implication of SSAT by gene expression and genetic variation in suicide and major depression. *Archives of General Psychiatry*, **63**, 35–48.

Sequeira A, Kim C, Seguin M *et al.* (2003). Wolfram syndrome and suicide: evidence for a role of WFS1 in suicidal and impulsive behavior. *American Journal of Medical Genetics B Neuropsychiatric Genetics*, **119B**, 108–113.

Sequeira A, Klempan T, Canetti L *et al.* (2007). Patterns of gene expression in the limbic system of suicides with and without major depression. *Molecular Psychiatry*, **12**, 640–655.

Sequeira A, Mamdani F, Lalovic A *et al.* (2004). Alpha 2A adrenergic receptor gene and suicide. *Psychiatry Research*, **125**, 87–93.

Serretti A, Calati R, Mandelli L *et al.* (2006). Serotonin transporter gene variants and behavior: a comprehensive review. *Current Drug Targets*, **7**, 1659–1669.

Shaw DM, Camps FE, Eccleston EG (1967). 5-Hydroxytryptamine in the hindbrain of depressive suicides. *British Journal of Psychiatry*, **113**, 1407–11.

Shih JC, Grimsby J, Chen K (1990). The expression of human MAO-A and B genes. *Journal of Neural Transmission Supplement*, **32**, 41–47.

Shindo S and Yoshioka N (2005). Polymorphisms of the cholecystokinin gene promoter region in suicide victims in Japan. *Forensic Science International*, **150**, 85–90.

Sibille E, Arango V, Galfalvy HC *et al.* (2004). Gene expression profiling of depression and suicide in human prefrontal cortex. *Neuropsychopharmacology*, **29**, 351–361.

Sims KB, de la Chapelle A, Norio R *et al.* (1989). Monoamine oxidase deficiency in males with an X chromosome deletion. *Neuron*, **2**, 1069–1076.

Stanley M and Mann JJ (1983). Increased serotonin-2 binding sites in frontal cortex of suicide victims. *Lancet*, **1**, 214–216.

Stanley M, Virgilio J, Gershon S (1982). Tritiated imipramine binding sites are decreased in the frontal cortex of suicides. *Science*, **216**, 1337–1339.

Statham DJ, Heath AC, Madden PA *et al.* (1998). Suicidal behavior: an epidemiological and genetic study. *Psychological Medicine*, **28**, 839–855.

Steegmans PH, Fekkes D, Hoes AW *et al.* (1996). Low serum cholesterol concentration and serotonin metabolism in men. *BMJ*, **312**, 221.

Stefulj J, Buttner A, Kubat M *et al.* (2004a). 5HT-2C receptor polymorphism in suicide victims. Association studies in German and Slavic populations. *European Archives of Psychiatry and Clinical Neuroscience*, **254**, 224–227.

Stefulj J, Buttner A, Skavic J *et al.* (2004b). Serotonin 1B (5HT-1B) receptor polymorphism (G861C) in suicide victims: association studies in German and Slavic population. *American Journal of Medical Genetics B Neuropsychiatric Genetics*, **127B**, 48–50.

Strous RD, Bark N, Parsia SS *et al.* (1997). Analysis of a functional catechol-O-methyltransferase gene polymorphism in schizophrenia: evidence for association with aggressive and antisocial behavior. *Psychiatry Research*, **69**, 71–77.

Strous RD, Nolan KA, Lapidus R *et al.* (2003). Aggressive behavior in schizophrenia is associated with the low enzyme activity COMT polymorphism: a replication study. *American Journal of Medical Genetics B Neuropsychiatric Genetics*, **120B**, 29–34.

Sullivan Hanley NR and Van de Kar LD (2003). Regulation of the hypothalamic–pituitary–adrenal axis in health and disease. *Vitamins and Hormones*, **66**, 189–255.

Sundman-Eriksson I and Allard P (2002). [(3)H]Tiagabine binding to GABA transporter-1 (GAT-1) in suicidal depression. *Journal of Affective Disorders*, **71**, 29–33.

Swaab DF, Bao AM, Lucasson PJ (2005). The stress system in the human brain in depression and neurogeneration. *Ageing Research Reviews*, **4**, 141–194.

Terao T, Yoshimura R, Ohmori O *et al.* (1997). Effect of serum cholesterol levels on meta-chlorophenylpiperazine-evoked neuroendocrine responses in healthy subjects. *Biological Psychiatry*, **41**, 974–978.

Tierney E, Nwokoro NA, Porter FD *et al.* (2001). Behavior phenotype in the RSH/Smith–Lemli–Opitz syndrome. *American Journal of Medical Genetics*, **98**, 191–200.

Tochigi M, Iwamoto K, Bundo M *et al.* (2008). Gene expression profiling of major depression and suicide in the prefrontal cortex of post-mortem brains. *Neuroscience Research*, **60**, 184–191.

Traskman-Bendz L, Ekman R, Regnell G *et al.* (1992). HPA-related CSF neuropeptides in suicide attempters. *European Neuropsychopharmacologyy*, **2**, 99–106.

Tsai SJ, Hong CJ, Yu YW *et al.* (2004). Association study of serotonin 1B receptor (A-161T) genetic polymorphism and suicidal behaviors and response to fluoxetine in major depressive disorder. *Neuropsychobiology*, **50**, 235–238.

Tsai SJ, Wang YC, Hong CJ *et al.* (2003). Association study of oestrogen receptor alpha gene polymorphism and suicidal behaviours in major depressive disorder. *Psychiatric Genetics*, **13**, 19–22.

The Neurobioloy of Suicide: From the Bench to the Clinic (1997). *Annals of the New York Academy of Sciences*. **836**(28): p. 1–364.

Turecki G, Sequeira A, Gingras Y *et al.* (2003). Suicide and serotonin: study of variation at seven serotonin receptor genes in suicide completers. *American Journal of Medical Genetics B Neuropsychiatric Genetics*, **118B**, 36–40.

van Heeringen K (2003). The neurobiology of suicide and suicidality. *Canadian Journal of Psychiatry*, **48**, 292–300.

Vinod KY and Hungund BL (2006). Role of the endocannabinoid system in depression and suicide. *Trends in Pharmacological Sciences*, **27**, 539–545.

Viveros MP, Marco EM, File SE (2005). Endocannabinoid system and stress and anxiety responses. *Pharmacology Biochemistry and Behavior*, **81**, 331–342.

Volavka J, Kennedy JL, Ni X *et al.* (2004). COMT158 polymorphism and hostility. *American Journal of Medical Genetics B Neuropsychiatric Genetics*, **127B**, 28–29.

Voracek M and Loibl LM (2007). Genetics of suicide: a systematic review of twin studies. *Wien Klin Wochenschr*, **119**, 463–475.

Voracek M and Tran US (2007). Dietary tryptophan intake and suicide rate in industrialized nations. *Journal of Affective Disorders*, **98**, 259–262.

Walther DJ, Peter J, Bashammakh S *et al.* (2003). Synthesis of serotonin by a second tryptophan hydroxylase isoform. *Science*, **299**, 76.

Wasserman D (2001). *Suicide—An Unnecessary Death*. Martin Dunitz, London.

Wasserman D, Geijer T, Rozanov V *et al.* (2005). Suicide attempt and basic mechanisms in neural conduction: relationships to the SCN8A and VAMP4 genes. *American Journal of Medical Genetics*, **133B**, 116–119.

Wasserman D, Geijer T, Sokolowski M *et al.* (2007a). Association of the serotonin transporter promotor polymorphism with suicide attempters with a high medical damage. *European Neuropsychopharmacologyy*, **17**, 230–233.

Wasserman D, Geijer T, Sokolowski M *et al.* (2006a). Genetic variation in the hypothalamic pituitary adrenocortical (HPA) axis regulatory factor, T-box19, and the angry/hostility personality trait. *Genes, Brain and Behavior*, **6**, 321–328.

Wasserman D, Geijer T, Sokolowski M *et al.* (2006b). The serotonin 1A receptor C(-1019)G polymorphism in relation to suicide attempt. *Behavioral and Brain Functions*, **2**, 14.

Wasserman D, Geijer T, Sokolowski M *et al.* (2007b). Nature and nurture in suicidal behavior, the role of genetics: some novel findings concerning personality traits and neural conduction. *Physiology and Behavior*, **92**, 245–249.

Wasserman D, Sokolowski M, Rozanov V *et al.* (2008a). The CRHR1 gene—a marker for suicidality in depressed males exposed to low stress. *Genes, Brain and Behavior*, **7**, 14–19.

Wasserman D, Wasserman J, Rozanov V *et al.* (2008b). Depression in suicidal males: genetic risk variants in the *CRHR1* gene. *Genes, Brain and Behavior*, in press.

Wei J and Hemmings GP (1999). Lack of evidence for association between the COMT locus and schizophrenia. *Psychiatric Genetics*, **9**, 183–186.

Weinshilboum RM, Otterness DM, Szumlanski CL (1999). Methylation pharmacogenetics: catechol O-methyltransferase, thiopurine methyltransferase, and histamine N-methyltransferase. *Annual Review of Pharmacology and Toxicology*, **39**, 19–52.

Wender PH, Kety SS, Rosenthal D *et al.* (1986). Psychiatric disorders in the biological and adoptive families of adopted individuals with affective disorders. *Archives of General Psychiatry*, **43**, 923–929.

Willour VL, Zandi PP, Badner JA *et al.* (2007). Attempted suicide in bipolar disorder pedigrees: evidence for linkage to 2p12. *Biological Psychiatry*, **61**, 725–727.

Wyatt RJ, Murphy DL, Belmaker R *et al.* (1973). Reduced monoamine oxidase activity in platelets: a possible genetic marker for vulnerability to schizophrenia. *Science*, **179**, 916–918.

Yanagi M, Shirakawa O, Kitamura N *et al.* (2005). Association of 14–3–3 epsilon gene haplotype with completed suicide in Japanese. *Journal of Human Genetics*, **50**, 210–216.

Yin L, Wang J, Klein PS *et al.* MA (2006). Nuclear receptor Rev-erbalpha is a critical lithium-sensitive component of the circadian clock. *Science*, **311**, 1002–1005.

Young EA (2005). Suicide and the hypothalamic–pituitary–adrenal axis. *The Lancet*, **366**, 959–960.

Zalsman G, Frisch A, Lewis R *et al.* (2004). DRD4 receptor gene exon III polymorphism in inpatient suicidal adolescents. *Journal of Neural Transmission*, **111**, 1593–1603.

Zalsman G, Huang YY, Oquendo MA *et al.* (2006). Association of a triallelic serotonin transporter gene promoter region (5-HTTLPR) polymorphism with stressful life events and severity of depression. *American Journal of Psychiatry*, **163**, 1588–1593.

Zammit S, Jones G, Jones SJ *et al.* (2004). Polymorphisms in the MAOA, MAOB, and COMT genes and aggressive behavior in schizophrenia. *American Journal of Medical Genetics*, **128B**, 19–20.

Zannis VI, Breslow JL, Utermann G *et al.* (1982). Proposed nomenclature of apoE isoproteins, apoE genotypes, and phenotypes. *Journal of Lipid Research*, **23**, 911–914.

Zhang X, Beaulieu JM, Sotnikova TD *et al.* (2004). Tryptophan hydroxylase-2 controls brain serotonin synthesis. *Science*, **305**, 217.

Zhou Z, Roy A, Lipsky R *et al.* (2005). Haplotype-based linkage of tryptophan hydroxylase 2 to suicide attempt, major depression, and cerebrospinal fluid 5-hydroxyindoleacetic acid in 4 populations. *Archives of General Psychiatry*, **62**, 1109–1118.

Zhu H, Karolewicz B, Nail E *et al.* (2006). Normal [3H]flunitrazepam binding to GABAA receptors in the locus coeruleus in major depression and suicide. *Brain Research*, **1125**, 138–146.

Zill P, Buttner A, Eisenmenger W *et al.* (2007). Analysis of tryptophan hydroxylase I and II mRNA expression in the human brain: a post-mortem study. *Journal of Psychiatric Research*, **41**, 168–173.

Zill P, Buttner A, Eisenmenger W *et al.* (2004). Single nucleotide polymorphism and haplotype analysis of a novel tryptophan hydroxylase isoform (TPH2) gene in suicide victims. *BiologicalPsychiatry*, **56**, 581–586.

Zubenko GS, Maher BS, Hughes HB *et al.* (2004). Genome-wide linkage survey for genetic loci that affect the risk of suicide attempts in families with recurrent, early-onset, major depression. *American Journal of Medical Genetics*, **129B**, 47–54.

# CHAPTER 27

# Interaction of hereditary and environmental factors in the psychiatric disorders associated with suicidal behaviour

Alec Roy and Marco Sarchiapone

## Abstract

Data from clinical, twin and adoption studies suggest that genetic factors may play a role as a distal risk factor in suicidal behaviour. The serotonin transporter gene, as a model for studies examining interaction between genes and environment, is discussed. Studies that report interaction between the serotonin transporter and stressful life events, in relation to the development of depression in both adults and adolescents and in relationship to suicidal behaviour, are reviewed. Relevant interaction studies in primates are also discussed.

## Introduction

Nobel Laureate James Watson considers Darwin to be the preeminent scientist in the history of mankind, because of his observation that evolution progressed due to the interaction of species variation with the environment—i.e. natural selection (Public Broadcasting Interview 2005). The observations of Watson and Crick on the structure of DNA are considered by many to be the second most important scientific discovery in the history of mankind, because it showed how species information is stored and transmitted (Public Broadcasting Interview 2005).

Suicidology is a young discipline with a history of just over 100 years. For most of that time, scientific enquiry about suicidal behaviour has been sociological, epidemiological, psychological and psychiatric. However, over the past two decades, accumulating data has strongly suggested that genetic factors also play a role in the multidetermined act of suicide (see Chapter 26).

## Distal risk factors for suicide

The current and most generally accepted model of suicide risk—the stress–diathesis risk factor model—includes hereditary factors. Risk factors may be either distal or proximal. Distal risk factors create a predisposing diathesis and determine an individual's response to a stressor. They include developmental, personality, biological, and genetic variables like childhood trauma, a family history of suicide, and impulsive, aggressive personality traits. They affect the threshold for suicide and increase an individual's risk when he or she experiences a proximal risk factor.

## Genetic distal risk factors

Data from clinical, twin, and adoption studies suggest that genetic factors play a role in suicidal behaviour. Clinical studies have shown that significantly more patients who have attempted or completed suicide have a first- or second-degree relative who has also exhibited suicidal behavior. Twin studies by the authors, and others, have shown that monozygotic (MZ) twins have a significantly higher concordance for both suicide and attempted suicide than dizygotic (DZ) twins (Roy et al. 2000). The authors pooled data from 399 twin pairs (129 MZ and 270 DZ) and found a higher concordance for suicide in MZ (13.2 per cent) than in DZ twins (0.7 per cent) (Roy et al. 2000). Adoption studies, using the Danish adoption and death registers, report that significantly more of the biological relatives of adoptees who committed suicide had themselves committed suicide in comparison with the biological relatives of control adoptees.

Recent genetic epidemiological studies have estimated that approximately 50 per cent of the variance in attempting suicide is due to genetic factors (Statham et al. 1998; Glowinski et al. 2001). For example, in a Veterans Affairs (VA) sample Fu et al. (2002) reported a twin study of genetic and environmental influences on suicidality in 3372 twin pairs from the VA Vietnam Era Twin Registry. They concluded that there may be a genetic susceptibility to suicidal behaviour, which is not explained by the inheritance of the common psychiatric disorders. The relevance of this genetic component to suicide is demonstrated by Preuss *et al.* 2003 in a 5-year follow up of 1237 alcoholics. They found that clinical factors alone contributed only 36.4 per cent of the variance for suicidal behaviour.

## Interaction of distal factors with proximal risk factors

Proximal, or trigger, factors are more closely related to the suicidal behavior and act as precipitants. They include life events, stress, acute episodes of mental illness, and acute alcohol or substance abuse. Suicidal individuals differ from non-suicidal individuals in distal risk factors, e.g. impulsivity and specific genetic factors, and may be moved toward suicidal behaviours by proximal risk factors.

## Molecular genetic studies

Biological studies of suicidal behaviour have, with notable exceptions, focused on serotonergic genes, because of the evidence that suicidal behaviour is associated with diminished serotonin functioning in the brain (Asberg 1997; Zhou *et al.* 2005. However, the results as found in genetic studies of other behaviours and psychiatric disorders have been inconsistent. In the past five years, studies have progressed in complexity by examining genetic variation and its interaction with the environment—akin to the observations of Darwin. As several of the studies, which are relevant to suicidal behaviour, have examined the serotonin transporter gene, they will be reviewed here as a model for future studies examining interaction between other genes and environment in relation to suicidal behaviour.

## The serotonin transporter promoter gene (5-HTTLPR gene) and adult depression

Post-mortem psychological autopsy studies of suicide victims have shown the close association of suicide with psychiatric disorder—particularly depression (Harris and Barraclough 1997). Caspi *et al* (2003) were the first to report a gene–environmental interaction in depression. They carried out a prospective longitudinal study of a birth cohort of 1037 Dunedin children assessed at regular intervals until the age of 26 years. They measured stressful life events occurring between the age of 21 and 26 years with a life history calendar. They also used the Diagnosis Interview Schedule to measure depressive symptoms over the years before 26. Subjects were genotyped. A gene–environment interaction was found. Individuals with an S allele, and with stressful life events after 21 years of age, had an increase in depressive symptoms whereas L/L homozygotes did not.

In addition, stressful life events predicted a diagnosis of major depression among individuals with an S allele, but not among L/L homozygotes. Furthermore, when Caspi *et al.* (2003) examined childhood maltreatment that occurred during the first ten years, a gene–environment interaction was again observed. Childhood trauma predicted depression as an adult only among individuals with the S allele, but not among L/L homozygotes.

Relevant to suicidal behaviour is that 3 per cent of the sample had attempted suicide in the past year or had recurrent thoughts of suicide. When examined, it was found that stressful life events predicted suicidal ideation or attempt among persons with an S allele, but not among L/L homozygotes.

Kendler *et al.* (2005) replicated the findings of Caspi *et al.* (2003) using a twin sample drawn from the Virginia Twin registry. Twin pairs were interviewed longitudinally at intervals from 1988 to 1997. They found that among 549 twins those with two S alleles were more sensitive to the depressogenic effects of life events than twins with one or two L alleles. They concluded, like Caspi *et al.* (2003), that 5-HTTLPR variation moderates the sensitivity of individuals to life events, with SS individuals having increased sensitivity to mildly stressful life events.

However, another twin study failed to replicate the findings of Caspi *et al.* (2003) and Kendler *et al.* (2005). Gillespie *et al.* (2005) examined 1206 twins from the Australian Twin Register. Although stressful life events were associated with the development of depression, there was no significant interrelation between 5-HTTLPR genotype and stressful life events in relation to depression. However, Gillespie *et al.* observed that theirs was an older sample than that of Caspi *et al.*, and wondered if this age difference might account for the different results in the two studies.

## Studies in depressed children and adolescents

Kaufman *et al.* (2004) set out to examine the role of 5-HTTLPR in the development of depression in maltreated children, as well as the potential modifying impact of social supports. They studied 57 children removed from their parents' care in the previous 6 months because of abuse or neglect. Controls were 44 community children with no history of childhood trauma. As expected, the maltreated children were found to be significantly more likely to meet criteria for a depressive disorder on diagnostic interview with the Schedule for Affective Disorder and Schizophrenia for School Age Children (Kaufman *et al.* 1997). The Arizona Social Supports Interview Schedule was used to assess children's social supports. Depressive symptoms were also measured.

There were no significant differences between the two groups for 5-HTTLPR allele frequency. Similarly, 5-HTTLPR genotype did not predict children's scores on a measure of social support.

Maltreated children did have significantly higher depression symptom scores and lower social supports. Maltreated children with L/L or L/S genotype had only minor increases in depressive symptoms compared with controls. However, maltreated children with the S/S genotype had depression scores twice as high as those of controls with S/S genotype. They also had depression scores higher than maltreated children with L/L or L/S genotypes.

Similar findings emerged when social supports were examined. Maltreated children with the S/S genotype and low social support had depression scores twice as high as those of maltreated children with the S/S genotype and high social support. The authors concluded that the risk for depression in children associated with the S allele and childhood trauma is moderated by the quality of social support. Thus, the risk for depression is influenced by both genetic and environmental factors, but is modified by social support promoting resiliency even in the presence of a predisposing genotype.

An English group examined 377 adolescents. Depressive symptoms and family environmental risk factors were measured, and the adolescents also gave a sample for DNA analysis (Eley *et al.* 2004). Several serotonergic genes were examined. The adolescents were divided into four groups—those with high or low depression scores and those with high or low environmental risks. The authors found significant interaction between 5-HTTLPR genotype and the environmental risk group in female subjects. Specifically, an increase in the number of S alleles increased the chance of being in the high depression group for adolescent girls in the high environmental risk group. Girls with two S alleles in the high environmental risk group had nearly twice the risks of being in the high depression group, in comparison to girls with the two S alleles, but in the low environment risk group.

## Relationship to stress

Stress and physical disorders are an important proximal risk factor for suicidal behaviour. Thus, a German study that set out to examine both mental and physical stress, in relation to the 5-HTTLPR gene, is of interest (Grabe *et al.* 2005). The Study of Health in Pomerania is a cross-sectional study of the population in western Pomerania. A self-report *Beschwerden-Liste* (complaints schedule) BL-38 scale measured psychological and somatic symptoms in 1005 subjects who were genotyped. There was no independent association between 5-HTTLPR genotype with mental or physical distress on the BL-38 scale (von Zerssen and Koeller 1976). However, there was a significant interaction between genotype, unemployment and chronic diseases in females in relation to BL-38 distress scores. The authors concluded that the presence of the S allele indicated increased mental vulnerability to social stressors and chronic diseases.

## 5-HTTLPR life event interaction and substance use

Patients with the diagnosis of substance dependence are another group at increased risk for suicidal behaviour (Harris and Barraclough 2007). Schuckit's group (Dick *et al.* 2007) reported a relationship between the 5-HTTLPR L allele and low level of response to alcohol, as well as to alcoholism in a prospectively studied cohort of Caucasian men, first evaluated approximately at age 20. Covault *et al.* (2007) showed that 5-HTTLPR genotype interacted with negative life events in relation to drug and drinking outcomes. They obtained daily reports of drinking and drug use in college students using a daily web-based survey. They also had self reports of past year negative life events. They found that individuals homozygous for the S allele who experienced multiple negative life events reported more frequent drinking and heavy drinking, stronger intentions to drink, and greater non-prescribed drug use. In individuals homozygous for the L allele, drinking and drug use were unaffected by life events in the previous year. Heterozygous individuals showed drinking outcomes that were intermediate to the two homozygous groups. The authors concluded that the S allele is associated with increased drinking and drug use among individuals who have experienced negative life events. The authors observed that the S-allele carriers may be at risk for a variety of adverse outcomes in response to stress.

## Post-traumatic stress disorder

Individuals who develop post-traumatic stress disorder (PTSD) symptoms in response to traumatic stress have also been noted to be at increased risk for suicidal behaviour. For example, Kessler *et al.* (2008) reported that among residents of the New Orleans area there were significant increases in PTSD symptoms and suicidal ideation and plans after Hurricane Katrina. Workers in Florida reported that, after a hurricane in Florida, it was particularly individuals with a low functioning 5-HTTLPR genotype and low social supports who were at increased risk of developing PTSD symptoms (Kilpatrick *et al.* 2007). They genotyped 589 adults who were interviewed about hurricane exposure, social support, post-hurricane PTSD and depression in thirty-eight Florida counties. It was found that the low expression variant of 5-HTTLPR increased the risk for post-hurricane PTSD, but only under conditions of high hurricane exposure and low social support. High-risk individuals with high hurricane exposure, low expressing genotype, low social support were at 4.5 times the risk of PTSD, compared with low risk individuals.

One of the main systems involved in the body's response to stress is the hypothalamic–pituitary–adrenal (HPA) axis. *FKBP5* is a gene involved in regulation of the HPA axis. Binder *et al.* (2008) administered the modified PTSD Symptom Scale and 28-item Childhood Trauma Questionnaire to 900 clinic patients who had blood drawn for genotyping. They found that four SNPs of the *FKBP5* gene interacted with severity of childhood abuse scores as a predictor of adult PTSD symptoms. There were no significant effects of the SNPs alone on PTSD symptoms, suggesting a potential gene–environment interaction for PTSD.

## The serotonin transporter and suicidal behavior

The many studies in psychiatric diagnostic groups of an association between functional polymorphism of the serotonin transporter gene promoter (5-HTTLPR) and suicidal behaviour were reviewed by Lin and Tsai (2004). They reviewed the eighteen studies that used a case–control design of 5-HTTLPR genotype in relation to suicidal behaviour. When they compared the total 1521 patients exhibiting suicidal behaviour with the total 2429 normal control subjects, they found no significant difference for 5-HTTLPR distribution between cases and controls. They noted that the limitation of case-control studies are that they are susceptible to bias, due to population stratification, but observed the same negative result in the fifteen studies with only Caucasian patients and controls were examined. Lin and Tsai also observed significantly heterogeneity among the odds ratios of the eighteen studies they reviewed. This led them to suggest the presence of some moderating variables that might account for the heterogeneity of odds ratios. The possibility exists that such moderating variables may include the environmental ones of childhood trauma and recent life events.

Childhood maltreatment is a developmental risk factor that may predispose an individual for later suicidal behaviour. Many general population and clinical studies have shown that childhood trauma like physical, sexual, emotional abuse—and neglect—are associated with attempting suicide as an adult.

## Suicidal behavior and substance dependence

As patients with substance dependence are at increased risk of both completed and attempted suicide, we genotyped a large group of abstinent substance dependent patients and controls. Patients completed a questionnaire about childhood trauma (Bernstein *et al.* 1994). Patients who had or had not attempted suicide and controls did not differ for 5-HTTLPR genotype. However, among patients, there was a significant interaction between childhood trauma and a low expression 5-HTTLPR genotype in relation to making a suicide attempt (Roy *et al.* 2007). Recently, a third functional polymorphism in the 5 regulatory promoter region was discovered, and we made use of this when constructing 5-HTTLPR genotypes (see Roy *et al.* 2007). Logistic regression showed an increase risk of a suicide attempt with increasing reports of childhood trauma scores. In addition, this increase was exaggerated among those with low expressing forms of the 5-HTTLPR genotype. Childhood trauma interacted with low expressing 5-HTTLPR genotype to increase the risk of suicidal behaviour.

## Serotonin transporter gene-environment interaction in primates

As low central serotonin is implicated in suicidal behaviour, the interaction between 5-HTTLPR genotype and early experience reported to affect central serotonin functioning in primates is of interest (Bennett *et al.* 2002). Bennett *et al.* compared monkeys reared with their mothers with monkeys separated from their mothers at birth and peer-reared. The measure of central serotonin function used was cisternal CSF 5-HIAA concentrations, which they and others had previously shown were influenced by both genetic and environmental factors (Higley *et al.* 1991, 1992, 1993; Rogers *et al.* 2004). They found that CSF5-HIAA concentrations were significantly influenced by genotype, but only in the peer-reared monkeys. Peer-reared heterozygous monkeys, with both the S and L 5-HTTLPR alleles, had significantly lower CSF 5-HIAA concentrations than homozygous monkeys with two L alleles. However, among the mother-reared monkeys, there was no difference for CSF 5-HIAA concentrations between monkeys with either the SL or LL 5-HTTLPR genotype. Thus, there was an interaction between early childhood trauma and 5-HTTLPR genotype on central serotonin functioning; in that only monkeys with early deleterious rearing experiences showed the difference in CSF 5-HIAA concentrations.

Also relevant, are earlier findings by Higley *et al.* and others, which showed that monkeys with low CF 5-HIAA concentrations were significantly more impulsive and aggressive than monkeys with CSF 5-HIAA concentrations within the normal range (Higley *et al.* 1992, 1996, 1998; Mehlman *et al.* 1994: Westergaard *et al.* 1999). This is relevant as the trait of impulsive–aggression is associated with low central serotonergic activity, and is thought to be an intermediate phenotype for suicidal behaviour in humans (Roy and Linnoila 1985; Highley and Linnoila 1997; Williams *et al.* 2003). In humans, we have shown that childhood trauma is associated with low CSF 5-HIAA (Roy 2002).

## Conclusion

Further studies of gene–environment interactions are necessary in order to shed light on this complex interplay involved in suicidal behaviours.

## References

Asberg M (1997). Neurotransmitters and suicidal behavior: the evidence from cerebrospinal fluid studies. In DM Stoff and JJ Mann JJ, eds, *The Neurobiology of Suicide. From the Bench to the Clinic*, pp 158–181. The New York Academy of Sciences, New York.

Bennett A, Lesch P, Heils A *et al.* (2002). Early experience and serotonin gene variation interact to influence primate CNS function. *Molecular Psychiatry*, **7**, 118–122.

Bernstein D, Fink L, Handelsman L *et al.* (1994). Initial reliability and validity of a new retrospective measure of childhood abuse and neglect. *American Journal of Psychiatry*, **151**, 1132–1136.

Binder E, Bradley R, Lin W *et al.* (2008). Association of FKBP5 polymorphisms and childhood abuse with risk of posttraumatic stress disorder symptoms in adults. *JAMA*, **299**, 1291–1305.

Caspi A, Sugden K, Moffit TE *et al* (2003). Influence of life stress on depression: moderation by a polymorphism in the 5-HTT gene. *Science*, **301**, 386–389.

Covault J, Tennen H, Armeli S *et al.* (2007). Interactive effects of the serotonin transporter 5-HTTLPR polymorphism and stressful life events on college student drinking and drug use. *Biological Psychiatry*, **61**, 609–616.

Dick DM, Plunkett J, Hamlin D *et al.* (2007). Association analyses of the serotonin transporter gene with lifetime depression and alcohol dependence in the Collaborative Study on the Genetics of Alcoholism (COGA) sample. *Psychiatr Genet*, **1**, 35–38.

Eley T, Sugden K, Gregory A *et al.* (2004). Gene–enviroment interaction analysis of serotonin system markers with alolescent depression. *Molecular Psychiatry*, **9**, 908–915.

Fu Q, Heath AC, Bucholz K *et al.* (2002). A twin study of genetic and environmental influences on suicidality in men. *Psychological Medicine*, **32**, 11–24.

Grabe H, Lange M, Wolff B *et al.* (2005). Mental and physical distreess is modulated by a polymorphism in the 5-HT transporter gene interacting with social stressors and chronic disease burden. *Molecular Psychiatry*, **10**, 220–224.

Gillespie N, Whifield J, Williams B *et al.* (2005). The relationship between stressful life events the serotonin transporter (5-HTTLPR) genotype and major depression. *Psychological Medicine*, **35**, 101–111.

Glowinski A, Bucholz K, Nelson E *et al.* (2001). Suicide attempts in an adolescent female twin sample. *Journal of the America Academy of Child and Adolescent Psychiatry*, **40**, 1300–1307.

Harris E and Barraclough B (1997). Suicide as an outcome for mental disorder: a meta-analysis. *British Journal of Psychiatry*, **170**, 205–228.

Higley D, Suomi SJ, Linnoila M (1991). CSF monoamine concentrations vary according to age, rearing and sex and are influenced by the stressor of social separation in rhesus monkeys. *Psychopharmacology*, **103**, 551–556.

Heils A, Teufel A, Petri S *et al.* (1996). Allelic variation of human serotonin transporter gene expression. *Journal of Neurochemistry*, **66**, 2621–2624.

Higley D, Suomi SJ, Linnoila M (1992). A longitudinal assessment of CSF monoamine metabolite and plasma cortisol concentrations in young rhesus monkeys. *Biological Psychiatry*, **32**, 127–145.

Higley D, King S, Hasert M *et al.* (1996). Stability of interindividual differences in serotonin function and its relationship to severe aggression and competent social behavior in rhesus macaque females. *Neuropsychopharmacology*, **14**, 67–76.

Higley D, Mehlman P, Poland R *et al.* (1998). CSF testosterone and 5HIAA correlate with different types of aggressive behaviors. *Biological Psychiatry*, **40**, 1067–1082.

Higley D, Thompson W, Champoux M *et al.* (1993). Paternal and maternal genetic and environmental contributions to cerebrospinal monoamine metabolites in rhesus monkeys (*Macaca mulatto*). *Archives of General Psychiatry*, **50**, 615–623.

Higley D and Linnoila M (1997). Low central nervous system serotonergic activity is trait-like and correlated with impulsive behavior. A non-human primate model investigating genetic and environmental influences on neurotransmission. In D Stoff and JJ Mann, eds, *Neurobiology of Suicide*. Annals of New York of New York Academy of Science. **836**, 39–56.

Kaufman J, Burmaher B, Brent D *et al.* (1997). Schedule for affective disorders and schizophrenia for school aged children. *Journal of American Academy of Child and Adolescent Psychiatry*, **36**, 980–988.

Kaufman J, Yang BZ, Douglas- Palumberi H *et al.* (2004). Social supports and serotonin tranportor gene moderate depression in maltreated children. *PANS*, **101**, 17316–17321.

Kendler K, Kuhn J, Vittum J *et al.* (2005). The interaction of stressful life event and serotonin transporter polymorphism in the prediction of episodes of major depression. A replication. *Archives of General Psychiatry*, **62**, 529–535.

Kessler K, Galea S, Gruber N *et al.* (2008). Trends in mental illness and suicidality after Hurricane Katrina. *Molecular Psychiatry*, **13**, 374–384.

Kilpatrick D, Koenen K, Ruggiero K *et al.* (2007). The serotonin transporter and social support and moderation of post traumatic stress disorder and depression in hurricane exposed adults. *American Journal of Psychiatry*, **164**, 1693–1699.

Lin PY and Tsai G (2004). Association between serotonin transporter gene promoter polymorphism and suicide: results of a meta-analysis. *Biological Psychiatry*, **55**, 1023–1030.

Mehlman P, Highley J, Faucher I *et al.* (1994). Low CSF 5-HIAA concentrations and severe aggression and impaired impulse control in nonhuman primates. *American Journal of Psychiatry*, **15**, 1485–1491.

Preuss U, Schuckit M, Smith T *et al.* (2003). Predictors and correlates of suicide attempts over 5 years in 1,237 alcohol dependent men and women.American. *Journal of Psychiatry*, **160**, 56–63.

Rogers J, Martin L, Comuzzie A *et al.* (2004). Genetics of monoamine metabolites in baboons: overlapping sets of genes influence levels of 5-hydroxyindoleacetic acid, 3-hydroxy-4-methoxyphenylglycol, and homovanillic acid. *Biological Psychiatry*, **55**, 739–744.

Roy A (2002). Self-reported emotional neglect in childhood and CSF 5-HIAA in adult cocaine patients: possible implications for suicidal behavior. *Psychiatry Research*, **112**, 69–75.

Roy A and Linnoila M (1985). Suicidal behavior, impulsiveness and serotonin. *Acta Psychiatrica Scandinavica*, **78**, 529–535.

Roy A, Nielsen D, Rylander G *et al.* (2000). The genetics of suicidal behavior. In K Hawton and Van Heeringen, eds, *The International Handbook of Suicide*, pp. 209–221. John Wiley, Chichester.

Roy A, Hu XZ, Janal M *et al.* (2007). Interaction between childhood trauma and serotonin gene variation in attempting suicide. *Neuropsychopharmacology*, **32**, 2046–2052.

Statham D, Heath A, Madden P *et al.* (1998) Suicidal behavior: an epidemiological and genetic study. *Psychological Medicine*, **28**, 839–855.

Von Zerssen D and Koeller D (1976). *Beschwerden-Liste* (Complaints Schedule). Beltz, Weinheim.

Westergaard G, Suomi S, Higley D *et al.* (1999). CSF 5-HIAAand aggression in female macaque monkeys: species and inter-individual differences. *Psychopharmacology*, **146**, 440–446.

Williams R, Marchuk D, Gadde K *et al.* (2003) Serotonin-related gene polymorphisms and central nervous system serotonin function. *Neuropsychopharmacology*, **28**, 533–541.

Zhou Z, Roy A, Lipsky R *et al.* (2005). Haplotype-based linkage of tryptophan hydroxylase 2 (TPH2) with suicide, major depression and CSF 5-HIAA in four populations. *Archives of General Psychiatry*, **62**, 1109–1118.

# PART 4

# Political Determinants of Suicide

# CHAPTER 28

# Suicide during transition in the former Soviet Republics

Airi Värnik and Alexander Mokhovikov

## Abstract

Significant social, political, and economic changes in the countries of the former Soviet Union present a good model for investigation of the impact of environment on suicide mortality during times of transition. During the period of perestroika (1985–1990), when promising social changes were rapid, a significant decrease of suicide mortality was observed for both genders in all fifteen republics of the USSR. One of the factors which contributed to the decrease was the strict anti-alcohol policy implemented in 1985 and suspended by 1989. However, times of spiritual liberation, the aspiration of democracy, social optimism and hopes for higher living standards could also have attributed to the causality of suicide decrease. In the years 1990–1994, after the disintegration of the Soviet Union, the suicide rates in post-Soviet countries increased, with the exception of prevailingly Muslim central Asiatic, and the Caucasus countries which have a traditionally low level of suicides. The transitional period called for high adaptation capacity and the necessity of developing suicide-prevention programmes to increase social support and re-education measures.

## Introduction

Knowledge about the reasons of suicide, its risk factors and trigger mechanisms are necessary for effective suicide prevention. To work out local suicide prevention programmes, the organizers must know the specific local features of suicidal behaviour in a certain country or region. Psychological and medical problems (Mokhovikov and Donets 1999; Kopp et al. 2000; Mokhovikov and Donets 2000; Durkheim 2002/1897; Kopp et al. 2004; Baud 2005; Khmaruk and Gorbatkova 2005), as well as 'genetic' and other biological factors (Rozanov et al. 1999; Baud 2005; Marušič 2005), predispose people to suicidal behaviour. External social and environmental factors can enhance or diminish suicidal tendencies in people (Värnik 1993; Sosedko and Pustovalov 1994; Wasserman and Värnik 1994; Värnik 1997; Rancans 2001; Rancans et al. 2001a, b; Leister et al. 2003; Värnik et al. 2005; Panchenko and Gladyshev 2004). Sudden social changes cause problems, and can provoke suicidal ideation and behaviour in people who cannot adjust to new circumstances. The countries of the former Soviet Union, which have experienced significant social, political and economical changes beginning in 1985, present a good model for the investigation of sudden social changes' influence on suicide rates. A number of researchers have carried out studies on the features of suicide in these countries (Värnik 1993; Chuprikov et al. 1996; Ester 1996; Mokhovikov and Donets 1996a, b; Lester and Yang 1998; Värnik et al. 1998; Chuprikov et al. 1999; Lester 1999; Anokhin and Boyko 2000; Mäkinen 2000; Stone 2000; Leister et al. 2003; Khmaruk et al. 2005; Smirnov 2005).

The purpose of this review is to sum up the statistics of suicides in the countries of the former Soviet Union, during the transition period and in the present. Moreover, an analysis of the social and psychological consequences of the transition processes will follow, as well as a discussion of the suicide prevention measures that are taken and planned in these countries.

## A short history of the Soviet Union and the transition period

The following historical sketch will stand as a background to the researched reviewed and it is based on these sources: the *Meyers Neues Lexicon* (1971–1977); Hosking (1985); *The Baltic States Reference Book* (1991); *The Encyclopedia Americana* (1991); *Estonia: A Reference Book* (1993); *The World Book Encyclopedia* (1994); Värnik (1997).

The first step in the formation of the Soviet Union was the Bolshevist coup d'tat in October 1917, following the collapse of the Tsarist regime in February 1917. As a result of the October Revolution, the huge Russian Empire was disintegrated and, after the Civil War that followed, a large part of Russia went under the control of the communist regime. The Baltic republics managed to use the weakening of Russia's military to obtain independence in the period between the first and Second World Wars. The October Revolution ignited the civil war, in which several foreign powers participated, as well as the fight for freedom of many nations of the former Russian Empire (Podhoretz 2002). The Civil War lasted from 1918 to 1922, ending with the establishment of the Union of Soviet Socialist Republics (USSR) comprising the Russian Federation, Belarusian SSR, Ukrainian SSR and Transcaucasian Soviet Federated Socialist Republic. In 1936, this latter republic was divided into three separate republics: Georgia, Armenia and Azerbaijan. In 1925, the territories of the present Central Asian countries, Kazakhstan, Uzbekistan, Tajikistan, Kirgizia and

Turkmenistan, were incorporated into the USSR. The Kazakh SSR and Kirgizian SSR were formed as separate republics in 1936.

The dictatorship of the Communist Party took shape throughout the 1920–1930s as the personality cult of Joseph Stalin was established. This cult was based on dictatorship and terror by a group of Communist Party leaders, and was executed by organs of state security such as the OGPU (United State Political Administration) and later by the NKVD (People's Commissariat of Internal Affairs). Between 1929–1932, compulsory collectivization of the rural economy was carried out, with all farmers forced to join collective farms (kolkhoz settlements). During the process of collectivization, 6–14 millions peasants were deported and imprisoned in labour or concentration camps in Siberia, constituting a large part of the so-called gulags (Solzhenitsyn 1974). The standard of living worsened significantly. Between 1932–1933, large territories were seized by famine and 3–7 million people died (Hosking 1985). At the same time, a heavy weapons industry was developed. Prisoner labour was largely used for the building of industrial and other grand strategic constructions (the Moscow–Volga Canal, White Sea–Baltic Sea Canal, Moscow underground). On a larger scale, massive repression of all classes of people, but especially many Communist Party members, intellectuals, army leaders and prosperous members of society, continued. Altogether, more than 42 million people died in Soviet concentration camps, between 1929–1953, according to Rummel (1995).

On the 23 August 1939, a non-aggression pact (known as the Molotow–Ribbentrop pact) was concluded with Nazi Germany. In a secret protocol attached to this pact, spheres of influence in Eastern and Central Europe were defined. After the beginning of the Second World War, in agreement with this pact, the Soviet Union assailed Finland, and occupied and annexed Estonia, Latvia, Lithuania, Bessarabia, Northern Bukovina and the eastern part of Poland. The People's Republic of Tannu Tuva was forcefully joined to the Soviet Union in 1944. In 1941, Germany attacked the Soviet Union, and during the war that continued until May 1945, the USSR lost 29.4 million people (Keegan 1989).

After the Second World War, the totalitarian political regime became even more severe. During the rebuilding of the economy, particular attention was paid to heavy industry. Political repressions were widespread in the USSR and especially heavy in the Baltic region. Intellectuals and leading persons were killed or deported to Siberia. A relatively large group from the Baltic countries escaped to the West. Immigration of Slavic people to the Baltic region was state-facilitated. Socialist realism was the only mode of art permitted during the Soviet times, glorifying the Communist Party and the Soviet Union. Both educational and other literature, as well as the press, was mainly written in Russian, with small regional exceptions (among others in the Baltic states). The Russian Cyrillic alphabet was forced upon many nations, which previously used other alphabets. Only after Stalin's death in 1953 did the situation begin to change.

Concomitantly, the USSR established satellite regimes that carried out similar modes of repression in practically all Eastern European Countries. The USA and most of the West European countries opposed this development and founded an antagonistic defence system, the North Atlantic Treaty Organization (NATO). The ensuing political antagonism and bilateral armament are known as the *Cold War*.

# The period of stagnation 1965/68–1984

After the Stalinist reign of terror, a certain degree of emancipation took place under Nikita Khrushchev from 1953, especially after the 20th Party Congress in 1956. However, the 23rd Party Congress confirmed the return to highly centralized politics in 1966, after Leonid Brezhnev became the general secretary of the Communist Party (1964–1982). In internal politics, this meant continuing isolation from other countries, with stricter censorship and curbs on creative freedom. The USSR's attitude towards its satellite states were illustrated by the military intervention in Czechoslovakia, following the 'Prague Spring' in 1968.

The consequences of this repression were manifold, leading to problems of identity crises, mistrust and a developed system for *double morality* (one truth to be kept to oneself, another—accepted in Moscow—to be uttered out loud) arose. Low standards of psychiatric treatment and ethics deterred people from seeking help. Attention to, and respect for, individual integrity were superseded by 'pan-collectivism' (Värnik 1991). The members of society responded in a variety of ways, with passive resistance and alcoholism being widespread. Alcohol consumption was facilitated by the state, which obtained very high profits from the sale of alcohol. Moreover, alcohol was considered to be an important tool to solve the problem of leisure time, and to withdraw people's attention from politics (Värnik 1997).

# The reform period from 1985
## Political and economic reforms

The stagnation period, which ended in 1984 after the short leadership of Jurij Andropov (1982–1984) and Konstantin Chernenko (1984–1985), was succeeded by what is known as the period of reforms. The reforms were first of political concern and later also economic, beginning when Gorbachov came to power on 10 March 1985, continuing to different extents until and after the disintegration of the USSR. This process implied society's successive release from the Soviet system, with rapid changes calling for a high adaptive capacity. The period from 1985 until the moment of the disintegration of the USSR in 1991 was called perestroika—the restructuring of society. It was a period of hope for positive changes, for more honesty in human relations, aspirations for democracy, spiritual liberation, social optimism and even euphoria, as well as hopes for higher living standards and a better economic situation. Later, some of these hopes turned out to be unrealistic. The totalitarian regime gained some features of democracy; the 'fresh wind' of change (a line from one of the popular songs of that period) ventilated the human minds. One transformation of that time is especially pertinent to our thesis: Gorbachev introduced strict restrictions on the production and sale of alcohol as well as on the use thereof (Wasserman et al. 1994; Värnik 1997; Wasserman et al. 1998a, c; Värnik et al. 2007).

The economic reforms implemented from 1989 and onward, especially in the later period (see below), necessitated new values, attitudes, professional expertise and completely different views of work and ethics. Gradually, after the disintegration of the USSR, a free market system was established, albeit lacking many essential controlling mechanisms, at least in most of the former Soviet republics. Forces of the free market imply a need for initiative taking, self-realization and responsibility, as well as the presence of sharp differences in income distribution. Controlling legislation as well as social security systems, expected to balance the forces of the free market, were not developed.

## Transition periods with rapid change requires psychological adaptation

The rapid changes in these societies in transition required a high capacity for psychological adaptation. People who were used to a passive lifestyle in the past found it difficult to integrate into the new political and socio-economic framework. Their previous education—especially that of the elderly and those in the rural areas—did not enable them to cope with the new demands. Many people had unrealistically high expectations of the free market system. This new situation may be said to have caused an adaptation shock.

Several psychologists and sociologists have tried to analyse the consequences of the changes which took place in the countries of the former Soviet Union (Wasserman and Värnik 1994; Sartorius 1995; Mokhovikov *et al.* 1996; Mokhovikov and Donets 1996b; Värnik 1997; Lester 1998; Wasserman *et al.* 1998b; Värnik *et al.* 1998; Lester 1999; Kopp *et al.* 2000; Mäkinen 2000; Stone 2000; Kopp *et al.* 2004; Smirnov 2005). Many positive changes in society took place, such as: spiritual (religious) and social liberation, political freedoms, openness of communication with foreigners, the possibility to travel freely, more openness inside society, freedom and independence of mass media and the right to express one's opinions. Unfortunately, there were also negative consequences, such as economical instability, unemployment (which barely existed in the former USSR), pronounced stratification (polarization) of society, with some people rapidly becoming extremely rich, while others quickly sank below the poverty level, a worsened criminal situation, including organized criminal activity, and a system of pseudo-information or vacuum of information as a vestige of the Soviet regime. Some investigators called this situation 'the general social disorganization' (Lester 1999; Stone 2000; Rancans 2001; Skrabski *et al.* 2003, 2005; Smirnov 2005). Many people, who have been strictly governed and guided by the Soviet regime during 50–70 years, depending on the region, found themselves helpless when initiative-taking was needed. For the Baltic countries, popularly referred to as the most 'Westernized' part of the Soviet Union, the period of socio-economic crisis was shorter, and nowadays, the market economy is flourishing (in Estonia for example economic growth is more than 10 per cent per year) accompanied by its negative and positive features.

This chapter will focus on the negative outcomes of the transition period in relation to suicidal behaviour.

> When Eastern Europeans gained their freedom people had high expectations that their lives would improve. For many, those hopes were dashed by bumpy transition to a market economy. Disillusionment led to stress and depression. And depression was a harbinger to death.
>
> Stone (2000, p. 1732)

Rapid changes require a high capacity for psychological adaptation from the populations at stake. Namely, a change of lifestyle from more passive to more active, a re-education process because the previous education often was not sufficient. Further, there was a need to cope with very high demands and unrealistic expectations. What were the psychological reactions to this situation, especially among those people who could not answer to these demands? Several researchers tried to describe the psychological reactions of the population to the transition phenomena. First of all, one should underscore that a large portion of the Soviet population had certain general psychological features, which had developed because of their life in a totalitarian society, and thus made them less flexible and ready to change and adjust. Mokhovikov and colleagues (1996) described the complexity of these features as the 'Soviet Syndrome', the signs of which include:

1 Identification of 'I' and 'We', and as a consequence insufficient acceptance of self, and/or low self-esteem.

2 Perception of the present as a point of intersection of a symmetrical past and future: thus, a life in the past full of fears and/or creating illusions about the future, whereas the present moment is tinted by passiveness and hypo-motivation.

3 Feeling of belonging to a people incapable of controlling its fate, impression of excommunication from civilization combined with envy.

4 Aiming at avoidance of misfortune or failure, instead striving to achieve positive results.

5 Constant anxiety or fear, absence of the feelings of safety and stability, 'identification confusion' causing suffering.

6 Split consciousness, a division of the social and personal ego, aggression and conformity, moral relativity.

7 Consciousness closed for empirical personal experience, uncritical trust in the collective mentality.

8 Transfer of the responsibility for failures to external factors, taking personal responsibility only for favourable results of one's activities, anarchic conduct towards the state and its laws.

9 Dogmatism, manipulative attitude and insufficient reflexive ability of consciousness, conservatism and rigidity of thinking together with low criticism of the results of one's activities (Mokhovikov *et al.* 1996a).

One can also add the factor of the lack (and prohibition) of spirituality and religious faith in the Soviet Union; atheism was propagated as the main 'religion' and world outlook.

In this situation of transitional crisis, the main psychological reactions of the people with the above described 'Soviet Syndrome' turned out to be:

◆ General pathogenic social *stress* (Mäkinen 2000);

◆ Feelings of *lack of control* over one's life and work situation (Kopp *et al.* 2000, 2004);

◆ Increased level of *depression* (Kopp *et al.* 2004);

◆ Loss of *life meaning* (Skrabski *et al.* 2005);

◆ Loss of trust in the support of society (Skrabski *et al.* 2003);

◆ Growing *anger and aggression* (Lester 1998);

◆ Suicidal *ideation and actions* (Sartorius 1995; Lester 1998; Lester 1999; Mäkinen 2000).

It is understandable that such negative responses caused an increase in premature health deterioration (morbidity), as well as the mortality rate during the phase of transition (Kopp *et al.* 2000; Skrabski *et al.* 2003; Kopp *et al.* 2004; Skrabski *et al.* 2005). They also influenced the rate of suicidal acts and attempts in these countries (Sartorius 1995; Lester 1998; Lester and Yang 1998; Wasserman *et al.* 1998b; Lester 1999; Värnik *et al.* 2005).

## Characteristics of the different regions of the former USSR

When discussing the statistics and specific features of suicide in the post-Soviet countries, one should take into consideration that these countries differ greatly in their geographic location, historical and cultural features, ethnicity, religion, etc. Because of this diversity, it would be inappropriate to give only the average suicide rates for all the republics together, merely due to the fact that some fourteen years ago they had belonged to one state—the USSR. The suicide rates in these countries differ significantly with respect to suici-dality. In some studies, the post-Soviet countries were divided into 'European' 'Asiatic', or 'Central Asiatic' (Lester 1999). In other works (Sartorius 1995), they are classified according to the level of the suicide rates. In this chapter, using as a tool common cultural features and geographic location, the post-Soviet countries are divided into the four following groups, according to the division of the republics used in the former Soviet Union:

1  The Slavonic countries and partly Moldova (prevailingly Eastern Orthodox);

2  The Baltic countries;

3  The Caucasus Region countries;

4  The Central Asiatic (prevailingly Muslim) countries (Värnik 1993; Wasserman *et al.* 1998b).

*The Slavonic countries* include Russia, Belarus and the Ukraine. The Republic of Moldova is close to them geographically and culturally, although the ethnic roots of the Moldovian people are lost to the Romanian group. All these countries are European, although a large part of Russia from the Ural Mountains east-ward is situated in Asia. The ethnic majority in Russia, Belarus and Ukraine are Slavonic people, and the prevailing religion in all these countries is Eastern Orthodox. Russia is the most multi-ethnic country in this group. It is a federation including autono-mous republics and regions, with populations of varied ethnic and cultural backgrounds. The culture of these countries has been formed by influences of their eastern and western (European) neighbours. In the Soviet period, their culture was subject to the enforcement of the communist culture ideology, for example, the so-called social realism in art and literature glorifying the Soviet Regime. Certain aspects of the Belarusian, Ukrainian and Moldovan culture have been lost due this policy and pronounced russification. The ethnic cultures of Russia were also suppressed and have lost some of their peculiar features.

*The Baltic countries* (Estonia, Latvia and Lithuania) have all had a rather smooth transition to a democratic society, and these coun-tries are respectively the most independent from the influence of their former neighbours, especially Russia, of all former Soviet states. Their economic structures were well-functioning before being incorporated into the Soviet Union in 1939, and they are cul-turally and politically close to the central and northern European

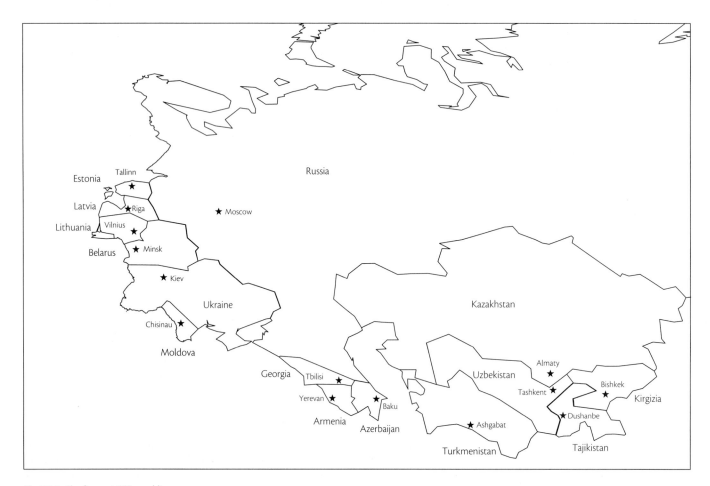

**Fig. 28.1** The former USSR republics.

countries, such as Germany, Finland and Sweden. All the Baltic countries refused to join the Commonwealth of Independent States created by Russia after the disintegration of the USSR and are now members of the EU. The economic level of their populations is higher than in other post-Soviet countries. The prevailing religion is Christianity, in particular, the Lutheran church in Estonia and Latvia and Catholicism in Lithuania. Significant parts of the populations do not belong to any church, for exception for Lithuania, primarily because of the religious persecution in the former USSR, and also because of the ongoing secularization across Europe.

*The Caucasian region* includes Armenia, Azerbaijan and Georgia, which in spite of differences in ethnic roots and religions have much in common. They all have a rich historical and cultural heritage and are traditionally multinational. Their location on the border between Europe and Asia make them transcontinental nations. Because of their strategic location, they are within both the Russian and Western spheres of influence. Armenia and Georgia were the first nations to adopt Christianity as a state religion, in 301 AD and 327 AD respectively. The prevailing religion in Azerbaijan is Islam. In spite of the persecution of religions and the USSR communist culture policy, the populations of these countries managed to preserve much of their former national identities and religious faiths.

*The Central Asiatic countries* including Kazakhstan, Kyrgyzstan, Tajikistan, Turkmenistan and Uzbekistan have more economical and political problems than the post-Soviet countries situated in Europe. All these states are republics, but they have governments with a strong autocratic presidency (e.g. Turkmenistan has a single-party system and was ruled by one president for life). The economy in all these countries is largely based on agriculture, although Kazakhstan and Turkmenistan possess major oil and gas fields, which are not exploited sufficiently due to the lack of adequate export routes for natural gas and oil. This in turn is caused by non-developed technology and international political rivalries. A large percentage of people live below the level of poverty, and there is a high level of unemployment. In all these countries, a large fraction of the population resides in rural areas. The prevailing religion in these countries is Islam. The people have largely preserved original national culture and customs, with roots in the Mongoloid ethnic group, with the exception of Tajikistan, which has an Indo-European population. In Kazakhstan, there is a very large proportion of Russians amounting to about 60 per cent of the whole population.

## Suicide statistics in the post-Soviet countries during the transition period

First, an effort will be made to analyse the dynamics of suicide rates during the decade, in which the social changes were especially fast, unpredictable and critical. Table 28.1 shows the average numbers of suicides per 100,000 of the total population between in the years 1985–1994, during perestroika, and directly after the disintegration of the USSR in 1991.

The suicide rates in the prevailing majority of the Soviet Union republics decreased during the perestroika period, the years with the lowest suicide rate being 1986–1988. This decrease was especially prominent in the republics with high suicide rates and high alcohol consumption as in the Slavonic and Baltic republics. One can assume that one of the factors that contributed to the decrease of suicides during the first years of perestroika was the strict anti-alcohol policy implemented in 1985 and ceased by 1989 (Wasserman *et al.* 1994, 1998a, c; Värnik *et al.* 2007). However, spiritual liberation, aspiration of democracy, social optimism and hope for higher living standards, all mentioned in the historical outline above, could also have influenced the causality of suicide decrease.

Age-specific differences in suicide rates observed in the Slavic and Baltic regions during perestroika (1985–1990) showed direct increase with age for women, and bimodal distribution for the 45–54 age groups and 75 and older for men. In 1990, suicide rates in the Slavic and Baltic regions ranged from 25.1 for the 15–24 age group to 86.9 for men 75 years and older, and from 6.0 to 29.8 for women, while suicide rates in Europe ranged from 13.0 to 64.8 for men and 3.6 to 18.7 for women (Värnik *et al.* 1998).

Several researchers (Stolyarov *et al.* 1990; Razvodovskiy 2003, 2004; Kõlves *et al.* 2006) have shown that alcohol consumption plays a negative role in suicidal behaviour. Alcohol intoxication precipitates suicidal tendencies, and may act as a factor in rendering behaviour more impulsive and less regulated by logic. Thus, the strict control of alcohol use in the USSR in 1980s had the following consequences:

◆ Significant decrease of suicide mortality for both genders in all fifteen republics of the USSR.

◆ Fall in suicide rates in men by 40 per cent in the years 1984–1986 in comparison with 3 per cent in twenty-two European countries studied during the same period.

◆ The decrease was largest in men in the workforce aged 25–54 years; possibly the age range during which one is most responsive to social changes as well as to alcohol policy.

◆ No corresponding decline in suicide rates for this age group (25–54 years) was noted in any other country in the twentieth century. Significant decrease of suicide mortality was observed in all fifteen republics of the former USSR (Wasserman *et al.* 1998a, b).

The preceding figures in Table 28.1 show that between the years 1990–1994, especially after the disintegration of the Soviet Union, suicide rates in the post-Soviet countries began to increase. The highest numbers of suicides could be observed in Russia and all the Baltic countries. Different authors explain these changes in relation to different political and social conditions. According to Sartorius (1995), suicide increased due to the stress caused by an unforeseeable future, economic decline and unemployment. These factors contributed greatly to increased alcohol consumption and depression. Lester (1998, 1999) lists the following explanatory factors among others: disappointment in the change of regime, lack of dictatorship to blame for misery, and economic decline. Both Sartorius and Lester mention shortage in health care leading to poor or lack of treatment of suicidal persons.

In some countries of the former USSR, the suicide rates did not increase or decrease after 1991 (Lester 1999). This concerns the prevailingly Muslim central Asiatic countries and the Caucasus region, as well as Moldova. The majority of these countries belong to regions with a traditionally low level of suicides, with the exception of Moldova, formerly a part of Romania, in which the level of suicides is above the average for Europe. Azerbaijan, Tajikistan, Turkmenistan and Uzbekistan are Muslim countries. These figures

**Table 28.1** Age-adjusted suicide rates (SDR) in the post-Soviet countries, the republics of the former USSR in the years of transition (per 100,000 of population)

| Country/republic | 1985 | 1986 | 1987 | 1988 | 1989 | 1990 | 1991 | 1992 | 1993 | 1994 |
|---|---|---|---|---|---|---|---|---|---|---|
| **Slavonic (prevailingly Orthodox) countries (republics)** | | | | | | | | | | |
| Belarus | 24.2 | 18.9 | 19.9 | 19.1 | 22.6 | 21.3 | 22.0 | 24.5 | 29.0 | 31.7 |
| Russia | 32.0 | 23.8 | 23.9 | 25.1 | 26.5 | 27.1 | 27.0 | 31.5 | 38.6 | 42.4 |
| Ukraine | 22.5 | 18.5 | 19.5 | 18.9 | 21.1 | 20.6 | 20.6 | 22.4 | 23.9 | 26.6 |
| Moldova | 23.3 | 21.1 | 19.1 | 19.1 | 19.2 | 16.8 | 18.9 | 17.9 | 18.7 | 20.6 |
| **Baltic countries (republics)** | | | | | | | | | | |
| Estonia | 31.4 | 28.1 | 25.8 | 24.8 | 26.1 | 27.4 | 27.1 | 32.6 | 38.8 | 41.7 |
| Latvia | 29.2 | 24.9 | 23.1 | 22.6 | 25.5 | 25.8 | 28.3 | 35.1 | 42.6 | 40.7 |
| Lithuania | 35.6 | 26.5 | 30.3 | 27.6 | 28.2 | 27.2 | 32.1 | 36.5 | 44.3 | 48.1 |
| **Caucasus region countries (republics)** | | | | | | | | | | |
| Armenia | 3.0 | 2.4 | 3.2 | 2.2 | 2.8 | 3.3 | 2.5 | 2.8 | 3.6 | 4.2 |
| Azerbaijan | 5.0 | 4.8 | 5.2 | 4.5 | 4.5 | 2.2 | 2.3 | 2.6 | 2.0 | 0.9 |
| Georgia | 5.0 | 4.9 | 4.6 | 4.6 | 4.9 | 3.8 | 3.4 | 4.5 | — | 3.5 |
| **Central Asia (prevailingly Muslim) countries (republics)** | | | | | | | | | | |
| Kazakhstan | 28.0 | 20.9 | 20.5 | 21.2 | 24.0 | 22.9 | 21.5 | 23.1 | 27.5 | 28.4 |
| Kyrgyzstan | 17.1 | 12.8 | 16.0 | 16.0 | 16.8 | 17.8 | 17.0 | 15.2 | 18.4 | 18.5 |
| Tajikistan | 9.4 | 8.0 | 6.3 | 6.0 | 7.1 | 7.0 | 6.0 | 5.8 | 4.1 | 5.7 |
| Turkmenistan | 10.5 | 13.1 | 12.6 | 11.3 | 10.3 | 11.4 | 10.3 | 8.9 | 8.6 | 8.2 |
| Uzbekistan | 12.1 | 10.8 | 10.1 | 9.3 | 11.0 | 10.3 | 9.7 | 8.4 | 8.6 | 9.0 |

Source: WHO (2007).

lead to the assumption that being part of a predominantly Muslim society is a protective factor against suicidal behaviour.

## Non- Slavonic nations in the Russian Federation

Multi-ethnic Russia has great diversity in suicide rates in different regions. The lowest suicide rates are observed in the northern Caucasus region (Ingushetia, Chechnya, North Ossetia and other districts), and the highest in north-western Siberia, where they exceed 150 per 100,000 of population (Polozhiy 2002, 2004; Nevmayatulin 2005). These differences are probably due to cultural, religious, demographic, economic and other factors.

However, according to Boris Polozhiy, suicide largely depends on the ethnic grouping of people (Polozhiy 2002, 2004). Analysing suicide rates in different countries, he concluded that three ethnic groups: the Finno-Ugric, the Baltic and the Germanic group belong to high suicide risk ethnicities. The Finno-Ugric group is composed of Finns, Hungarians, Estonians as well as the Finno-Ugric peoples of Russia: Mordvins, Udmurts, Permian-Komis, Maris, Karelians, Ostyaks, Voguls. Latvians and Lithuanians represent the Baltic ethnic group. Finally, Germans, Austrians, the German-speaking Swiss, Danes and Swedes represent the Germanic group. This theory seems to be rather speculative and based on static and conventional notions of ethnicity, not taking into account its fluctuating construction and cross-section with other identities, such as economic class, religion, gender, sexuality, social status, etc.

In fact, Polozhiy does not consider that people might not favour ethnic belonging over some of the above-mentioned distinctive identities. Moreover, no genetic research has been performed to sustain these findings.

Investigating the incidence of suicides in Russia, Polozhiy found the highest suicide rates in the Koryak autonomous area (suicide rate 133.6 per 100,000), the Komi-Permyak autonomous area (suicide rate 124.4), the Nenets autonomous area (suicide rate 95.7) and the Republic of Buryatia (suicide rate 87.6). Although the peoples of these areas belong to different ethnic groups, they have much in common, due to traditional beliefs of Shamanism, not viewing suicide negatively and even implying its admissibility, viewing human life as a series of sufferings. Polozhiy suggests a particular approach to suicide prevention taking ethnic belonging into account (Polozhiy 2002, 2004).

## Gender-specific and age-specific features of suicide rates in the post-Soviet countries

The gender distribution of suicide rates during the Perestroika period varied greatly between different regions, with suicide rates of men ranging from 4.9 in the Caucasian region to 45.9 in the Baltic, and suicide rates of women from 2.1 in Caucasus to 12.3 in the Baltic region (Wasserman *et al.* 1998b). The data from the WHO database presented in Table 28.2 show that the Slavonic countries have the highest suicide rates among the post-Soviet

**Table 28.2** Gender-specific suicide rates in the former USSR republics per 100,000

| Country | Year | Males | Females | Ratio M/F |
|---|---|---|---|---|
| **Slavonic and prevailingly Eastern Orthodox countries** | | | | |
| Belarus | 2003 | 63.3 | 10.3 | 6.1 |
| Russia | 2002 | 69.3 | 11.9 | 5.8 |
| Ukraine | 2002 | 46.7 | 8.4 | 5.6 |
| Moldova | 2003 | 30.6 | 4.8 | 6.4 |
| **Baltic countries** | | | | |
| Estonia | 2002 | 47.7 | 9.8 | 4.9 |
| Latvia | 2003 | 45.0 | 9.7 | 4.6 |
| Lithuania | 2003 | 74.3 | 13.9 | 5.3 |
| **Caucasus region countries** | | | | |
| Armenia | 2003 | 3.2 | 0.5 | 6.4 |
| Azerbaijan | 2002 | 1.8 | 0.5 | 3.6 |
| Georgia | 2001 | 3.4 | 1.1 | 3.1 |
| **Central Asia (prevailingly Muslim) countries** | | | | |
| Kazakhstan | 2002 | 50.2 | 8.8 | 5.7 |
| Kyrgyzstan | 2003 | 16.1 | 3.2 | 5.0 |
| Tajikistan | 2001 | 2.9 | 2.3 | 1.3 |
| Turkmenistan | 1998 | 13.8 | 3.5 | 3.9 |
| Uzbekistan | 2002 | 9.3 | 3.1 | 3.0 |

Source: WHO mortality database (2007).

countries, with male:female ratios also being high. Male and female suicide rates in Lithuania rank among the highest in the world.

Interestingly, the suicide rates for males and females in Kazakhstan approach the levels in the Slavonic countries, which one can assume is due to the large Slavonic population in Kazakhstan. Besides ethnicity, of course, one cannot exclude other reasons more specific to the Slavonic people living in Kazakhstan.

Research focusing on the transition period strongly suggests that negative social factors cause more stress reactions with increased suicidal tendencies in men rather than women. Males are more vulnerable in terms of unemployment and decreased income, as well as to the inequality of income and the loss of social status. Studies across the world show that men are less likely to seek psychological support than women, and have weaker trust in receiving help from official and private sources (Moller-Leimkuhler 2003; Skrabski et al. 2003). In addition, men in the former USSR countries consume more alcohol than women, and it has been demonstrated that alcohol abuse increases suicidal risk (Kõlves et al. 2006). All these circumstances make males more susceptible to suicidal risk than females in situations of sharp social change.

Moreover, there are some specific features in the age distribution of suicides. It was shown that in contrast to other age groups, the suicide rates in elderly people, 75 years and older, did not increase one year after the disintegration of the USSR, and in some regions even decreased, according to the division of the republics used in the former Soviet Union (Sartorius 1995). This decrease of suicide rates for the elderly, shortly after the disintegration of the USSR, is interpreted by Sartorius as giving them a sense of being needed: they are not as exposed to unemployment and job insecurity as younger people, they rarely abuse alcohol and are often religious, which may give them a sense of security. Finally, many of them had learned survival skills during the Second World War.

## Suicide prevention in post-Soviet countries

The increase of suicide rates in post-Soviet countries, after perestroika and the disintegration of the USSR, highlighted the necessity of developing suicide prevention programmes. In most cases, the initiative of developing such programmes did not come from governmental bodies, but rather from specialists in the health services. Individual foreign specialists, in particular, members of the WHO network on suicide prevention as well as other suicidological services of the European countries, rendered great help in organizing suicide prevention in the post-Soviet countries (Pilyagina 1998; Chuprikov and Pilyagina 2002; Panchenko and Gladyshev 2004; Panchenko et al. 2004).

Experiences from the former USSR, regarding suicide prevention during transition periods show that the focus should be on the male population. It is important to increase social support and re-education measures, to involve those with low educational achievement in new economic developments and allow them to benefit from economic changes, and also to be aware of the role of alcohol consumption on mental and physical health. It is also important to detect mental problems, especially depression, to bear in mind specific features of male depression (Wasserman 2006) and to promote modernized comprehensive health care systems equally accessible for all.

## Conclusions

The specific features of suicidal behaviour in the period of transition in post-Soviet countries lead us to numerous conclusions and questions for further research. The statistics and research performed illustrate a decrease of suicide rates during the 5-year period of perestroika, followed by a significant increase in the majority of the countries studied after the disintegration of the Soviet Union. Today, the distribution of suicide rates in the former USSR is extremely uneven, with the highest rates found in Lithuania and Russia, and the lowest in the countries of the Caucasus region. When analysing the general suicide rates in specific regions, it is important to keep in mind that multiple factors are at stake, the interaction of biological, hereditary and sociocultural features are closely related to political, socioeconomic, and other environmental circumstances. Suicide rates in the transition period have been strikingly gender-related: men being more vulnerable than women towards unfavourable social changes such as unemployment, relative income inequality and loss of social status.

In conclusion, the following aspects are important to focus on when implementing suicide prevention programmes during times of transition: the involvement of those with less education or no education at all in new economic development, and allowing them to benefit from economic changes. Further, an increased awareness of the role of alcohol consumption on health needs to be emphasized, alongside the early detection and treatment of mental problems, especially depression, and particularly in males.

# References

(1971–1977). *Meyers Neues Lexicon, band 1–18.* VEB Bibliographisches Institut, Leipzig.

(1991). *The Baltic States Reference Book,* Estonian Encyclopedia Publishers/ Latvian Encyclopedia Publishers/Lithuanian Encyclopedia Publishers, Tallinn/Riga/Vilnius.

(1992). *The Encyclopedia Americana, vol. 1–30.* Connecticut, Grolier Incorporated, Danbury.

(1993). *Estonia: A Reference Book.* Estonian Encyclopedia Publishers, Tallinn.

(1994). *The World Book Encyclopedia,* vols 1–22. World Book Inc, London.

Anokhin LV and Boyko IB (2000). Obschiye zakonomernosti razvitiya suitsidal'noy situatsiy v strane [General regularities of the suicidal situation in the country development]. *Zdravookhraneniye Rossiyskoy Federatsii,* **10,** 154–157.

Baud P (2005). Personality traits as intermediary phenotypes in suicidal behaviour: genetic issues. *American Journal of Medical Genetics,* **133,** 34–42.

Chuprikov AP, Mokhovikov AN, Donets OY (1996). Epidemiology of suicides in Ukraine. Suicide: Biopsychosocial Approaches, International Conference, Athens.

Chuprikov AP and Pilyagina GA (2002). K voprosu o neobkhodimosti organizatsii suitsidologicheskoy sluzhby v Ukraine. [On the necessity of creating a suicidological service in Ukraine]. *Ukrainskiy Vistnik Psikhonevrologii,* **10,** 154–157.

Chuprikov AP, Pilyagina GA, Nikiforuk RI (1999). Problema suitsidov v Ukraine [The problem of suicides in Ukraine]. *Mezhdunarodniy Meditsinskiy Zhurnal,* 1.

Durkheim E (2002/1897). *Suicide: A Study in Sociology.* Routledge, London and New York.

Hosking G (1985). *A History of the Soviet Union.* Collins/Fontana, London.

Keegan J (1989). *The Second World War.* Pimlico, London.

Khmaruk IN and Gorbatkova EA (2005). Motivatsionnyi konflikt kak faktor riska suitsidal'nogo povedeniya voennosluzhaschih po prizyvu [The motivational conflict as a risk factor of suicidal behaviour in the military servants]. All-Russian Scientific and Practical Conference with International Participation: 'Actual Problems of Clinical, Social and Military Psychiatry' Proceedings. St Petersburg.

Kõlves K, Värnik A, Tooding LM, Wasserman D (2006). The role of alcohol in suicide: a case–control psychological autopsy study. *Psychol Med,* **36,** 923–930.

Kopp MS, Csoboth CT, Rethelyi J (2004). Psychosocial determinants of premature health deterioration in a changing society: the case of Hungary. *Journal of Health Psychology,* **9,** 99–109.

Kopp MS, Skrabski A, Szedmak S (2000). Psychosocial risk factors, inequality and self-rated morbidity in a changing society. *Social Science & Medicine,* **51,** 1351–1361.

Leister MS, Varego D, Kunst AB (2003). Estonia in 1989–2000: enormous increase in mortality differences by education. *Population Health.*

Lester D (1998). Suicide and homicide after the fall of communist regimes. *European Psychiatry,* **13,** 98–100.

Lester D (1999). Suicide in post-Soviet Central Asia. *Central Asian Survey,* **18,** 121–124.

Lester D and Yang B (1998). *Suicide and homicide in the 20th century.* Commack, Nova Science, New York.

Marušič A (2005). History and geography of suicide: could genetic risk factors account for the variations in suicide rates? *American Journal of Medical Genetics,* **133,** 43–47.

Mokhovikov A and Donets OY (1999). Does psychache cause suicide? The experience of using ES Shneidman's Psychological Pain Assessment Scale. Twentieth Congress of the International Association for Suicide Prevention, Final Program and Abstract Book. Greece, Athens.

Mokhovikov A and Donets OY (2000). Psychological paradigm of existential pain and suicide. The fourth International Congress on Thanatology and Suicidology. Stockholm, Sweden, Final Program and Abstract Book.

Mokhovikov AN, Chuprikov AP, Donets OY (1996). Characteristics of suicidal behaviour in modern Ukraine. Tenth World Congress of Psychiatry; Satellite Symposium on Suicidal Behaviour: National Characteristics of Suicidal Behaviour. Hungary, Budapest.

Mokhovikov AN and Donets OY (1996a). Suicide in the Ukraine: epidemiology, knowledge and attitude of the population. *Crisis,* **17,** 128–134.

Mokhovikov AN and Donets OY (1996b) Self-destructive behaviour in the post-totalitarian society and adolescents. The fifth Biennial Conference of the European Asociation For Research on Adolescence, Liege, Belgium.

Moller-Leimkuhler AM (2003). The gender gap in suicide and premature death or: why are men so vulnerable? *European Archives Of Psychiatry And Clinical Neuroscience,* **253,** 1–8.

Mäkinen IH (2000). Eastern European transition and suicide mortality. *Social Science & Medicine,* **51,** 1405–1420.

Nevmayatulin A (2005). Analiz struktury i dinamiki samoubiistv v respublike Mariy El za 1984–2002 gody [The analysis of the structure and dynamics of suicides in the Mariy El Republic in 1984–2002]. The Sixth All-Russian Conference of Forensic Medicine: 'Perspectives of Development and Perfection of the Forensic Medicine Science and Practice', Tumen.

Panchenko EA and Gladyshev MV (2004). Analiz vliyaniya etnokul'tural'nyh faktorov na suitsidal'noe povedenie v Udmurtii [The analysis of the influence of ethic and cultural factors on the suicidal behaviour in Udmurtia]. The First National Congress on Social Psychology 'The Mental Health and Safety of the Society', Moscow.

Panchenko IE, Levinson AA, Solonenko AV, Demyanov AV (2004). K probleme autoagressii v armii [On the problem of auto-aggression in the army]. The First National Congress on Social Psychology 'The Mental Health and Safety of the Society', Moscow.

Pilyagina GY (1998). Aktual'nie problemy suitsidologii v Ukraine I puti ikh resheniy [Actual problems of suicidology in Ukraine and the ways of their solving]. *Jurnal Prakticheskogo Vracha,* **6,** 2–6.

Podhoretz N (2002). *The Prophets.* The Free Press, New York.

Polozhiy BS (2002). Suitsidy v kontekste etnokul'tural'noi psihiatrii [Suicides in the context of ethno-cultural psychiatry]. *Psihiatriya i psihofarmakoterapiya: zhurnal dlya psihiatrov i vrachei obschei praktiki,* **6,** 245–247.

Polozhiy BS (2004). Sotsial'no-ekonomicheskie i etno-kul'tural'nye determinanty rasprostranennosti suitsidov v Rossii [Social-economical and ethno-cultural determinants of suicides distribution in Russia]. The First National Congress on Social Psychology 'The Mental Health and Safety of the Society', Moscow.

Rancans E (2001). Suicidal behaviours in Latvia 1980–2000. Umea University medical dissertation. Umea, Umea University.

Rancans E, Alka I, Salander Renberg E *et al.* (2001a). Suicide attempts and serious suicide threats in the city of Riga and resulting contacts with medical services. *Nordic Journal of Psychiatry,* **55,** 279–286.

Rancans E, Salander Renberg E, Jacobsson L (2001b). Major demographic, social and economic factors associated to suicide rates in Latvia 1980–98. *Acta Psychiatrica Scandinavica,* **103,** 275–281.

Razvodovskiy YE (2003). Suitsidy I uroven' potrebleniya alkogolya. [Suicides and the level of alcohol consumption]. *Problemy Social'noy Gigiyeny, Zdravookhraneniya I Istorii Meditsiny,* **4,** 22–25.

Razvodovskiy YE (2004). Alkogol I suitsidy: populyatsionniy uroven' vzaimosvyazi. [Alcohol and suicides: population level of correlation.] *Jurnal Nevrologii I Psikhiatrii im SS Korsakova,* **2,** 48–52.

Rozanov VA, Mokhovikov AN, Wasserman D (1999). Neurobiologicheskiye osnovy suitsidal'nosti. [The neurobiological basis of suicidal tendencies.] *Ukrainskiy Medichniy Chasopis,* **6,** 5–15.

Rummel RJ (1995). Democracy, power, genocide and mass murder. *Journal of Conflict Resolution,* **1,** 3–26.

Sartorius N (1995). Recent changes in suicide rates in selected Eastern European and other European countries. *International Psychogeriatrics*, **7**, 301–308.

Skrabski A, Kopp M, Kawachi I (2003). Social capital in a changing society: cross-sectional associations with middle aged female and male mortality rates. *Journal of Epidemiology and Community Health*, **57**, 114–119.

Skrabski A, Kopp M, Rozsa S *et al.* (2005). Life meaning: an important correlate of health in the Hungarian population. *International Journal of Behavioural Medicine*, **12**, 78–85.

Smirnov F (2005). Gazety pishut o samoubiistvah v Rossii. [Newspapers write about the suicides in Russia.] *Meditsinskaya gazeta.* [The Medical Newspaper], October 26.

Solzhenitsyn A (1974). *The Gulag Archipelago.* Harper & Row, New York.

Sosedko YI and Pustovalov LV (1994). Profilaktika suitsidal'nikh proisshestviy sredi voennosluzhaschikh. [Prevention of suicidal incidents among the military servants.] *Voyenno-meditsinskiy Zhurnal*, **4**, 17–19.

Stolyarov AV, Borokhov AD, Zhamanbayev EK, Bedilbayeva GA (1990). Alkogol' kak provotsiruyuschiy faktor suitsidal'nikh deystviy. [Alcohol as a provoking factor of suicidal actions.] *Jurnal Nevrologii I Psikhiatrii im SS Korsakova*, **90**, 55–58.

Stone R (2000). Social science. Stress: the invisible hand in Eastern Europe's death rates. *Science*, **288**, 1732–1733.

Värnik A (1991). Suicide in Estonia. *Acta Psychiatrica Scandinavia*, **84**, 229–232.

Värnik A (1993). Suicide in Estonia and other former USSR republics. *Crisis*, **14**, 185–186.

Värnik A (1997). Suicide in the Baltic Countries and in the former republics of the USSR. Doctoral dissertation, Stockholm, Karolinska Institute.

Värnik A, Kõlves K, Wasserman D (2005). Suicide among Russians in Estonia: database study before and after independence. *British Medical Journal*, **330**, 176–177.

Värnik A, Kõlves K, Väli M *et al.* (2007). Do alcohol restrictions reduce suicide mortality? *Addiction*, **102**, 251–256.

Värnik A, Wasserman D, Dankowicz M *et al.* (1998). Age-specific suicide rates in the Slavic and Baltic regions of the former USSR during perestroika, in comparison with 22 European countries. *Acta Psychiatrica Scandinavica Supplementum*, **394**, 20–25.

Wasserman D (2006). *Depression: The Facts.* Oxford University Press, Oxford.

Wasserman D, Varnik A, Eklund G (1998a). Female suicides and alcohol consumption during perestroika in the former USSR. *Acta Psychiatrica Scandinavica Supplementum*, **394**, 26–33.

Wasserman D and Värnik A (1994). Increase in suicide among men in the Baltic countries. *Lancet*, **343**, 1504–1505.

Wasserman D, Värnik A, Dankowicz M (1998b). Regional differences in the distribution of suicide in the former Soviet Union during perestroika, 1984–1990. *Acta Psychiatrica Scandinavica Supplementum*, **394**, 5–12.

Wasserman D, Värnik A, Dankowicz M *et al.* (1998c). Suicide-preventive effects of perestroika in the former USSR: the role of alcohol restriction. *Acta Psychiatrica Scandinavica Supplementum*, **394**, 1–44.

Wasserman D, Värnik A, Eklund G (1994). Male suicides and alcohol consumption in the former USSR. *Acta Psychiatrica Scandinavica*, **89**, 306–313.

World Health Organization (2007). *Mortality Database.* Available at http://data.euro.who.int/hfamdb.

# CHAPTER 29

# Suicide among migrants

Menakshi Sharma and Dinesh Bhugra

## Abstract

Migration or mobility of individuals from one location to another is a frequent phenomenon and has been the case for millennia, although reasons for such movement of people have varied. Reasons for migration and the experiences an individual has when arriving at the new place are important, especially in terms of understanding the experiences and problems they may encounter. How well an individual adapts to the new country can be explained by factors of acculturation and how well this occurs may in turn affect the mental health of the person. Studies have shown that migration across the world is on the increase, as are the mental health problems amongst the migrant population; especially self-harm and suicide. Investigating the factors for this is important in order to develop strategies of prevention from a public health point of view. In this chapter we examine differences in the rates of suicide amongst the migrant groups across different countries and explore preventative methods from a public health perspective.

## Introduction

Migration is the process of social change whereby an individual moves from one cultural stetting to another for the purposes of settling down either permanently or for a prolonged period. This move can occur for a number of reasons, most commonly for economic, political or educational betterment (Bhugra and Jones 2001). Migration and its accompanying stressors affect migrating individuals and their families. The process of migration is not simple or straightforward (Bhugra 2004a). There needs to be a distinction between actual settlers and migrant workers. Rack (1982) defines reasons for migration to include both 'push' and 'pull' factors. Settlers as well as political exiles, asylum seekers and refugees, may have to deal with stringent legal procedures, which will test their psychological stamina. Factors like language spoken, skills, communication and social networks and knowledge of the culture that the individual is migrating to will play a role in the processes of dealing with initial adversity, settling down and assimilation. Research has found differences in suicide risk among different generations of immigrants, with higher rates for more recent immigrants (Neeleman et al. 1997; Bhugra et al. 1999; Kennedy et al. 2005).

The migratory process can be seen in three stages especially if migration is a planned process. The first, pre-migration, is when the individuals decide to migrate and plan the move. The second stage involves the process of migration itself and the physical transition from one place to another, involving all the necessary psychological and social steps. The third stage, post-migration, is when the individuals deal with the social and cultural frameworks of the new society, learn new roles and become interested in transforming their group. However, even though there are similar terms for describing migration, they do not explain the heterogeneity inherent within each setting. Not all migrants have the same experiences or even the same reasons for migration and certainly the new societies' responses are not likely to be similar either (Bhugra and Jones 2001).

Migrants make personal choices for economic or aspirational reasons and also the society they come from may force them to migrate. The nature of the pull or push factors will determine not only the migratory forces, but also the type of response in the individual as well as among those who are around the individual. Again the difference between forced and voluntary nature of migration must be remembered when trying to understand the impact of migration. The third factor, which may play a role in the genesis of stress related to migration, is that of the geographical distance traversed in the migratory process. It is likely that the longer the distance, the more reality change may well have to occur (Bhugra 2004a) although this may not always be the case. It is impossible to consider 'migrants' as a homogenous group concerning the risk for mental illness, due to differing ability to develop mediating structures; different legal residential status, as well as distance from the host culture (Carta et al. 2005). Migrating people's mental health and personal states should be assessed specifically in response to their circumstance and response to the environment.

## Migrant community and suicidal behaviours

### Suicidal ideation

Grube (2004) investigated the correlation of belonging to an ethnic cultural minority with non-fatal suicidal ideation and self-injurious behaviour in a group of 494 psychiatric inpatients at the time of admission. This research was conducted in Germany between German patients and Mediterranean immigrants. No significant difference was found between these groups in relation to suicide risk, choice of method and suicide intention.

Whilst investigating other ethnic groups, Nazroo (1997) was able to demonstrate that in the UK, 0.7 per cent of Caribbeans, 0.9 per cent of

Asians and 0.6 per cent of Pakistanis had expressed suicidal thoughts in comparison with 3.3 per cent in British born. For the British born Caribbeans, the rate was 4.9 per cent compared with 3.35 per cent for Indians and 4.4 per cent for Pakistanis, whereas the equivalent rate for Caucasians was 3.1 per cent. Those who were not fluent in English showed rates to be 1.2 per cent in Indians and 1.1 per cent in Pakistanis, but among those who were fluent, the rates were 2.2 per cent and 4.7 per cent respectively.

## Suicide attempts

The impact of the migration process, socio-economic status, and acculturation may underlie differences in major depression and suicide attempt rates across ethnic groups (Oquendo *et al.* 2004). Major depression is the most common psychiatric disorder in the US with up to 17 per cent lifetime prevalence in the general population (Kessler *et al.* 1994). The aim of the study was to investigate whether there is a variation among ethnic groups in the USA in lifetime rates of suicide attempts in relation to rates of depression. Data was obtained based on the Epidemiological Catchments Area Study (ECA) (1980–84) (Moscicki *et al.* 1987); in addition to the Hispanic Health and Nutrition Epidemiological Survey (HHANES). The HHANES study investigated respondents up to 74 years of age, in complex clusters, and stratified samples. Respondents living in institutions (psychiatric hospitals, nursing homes and prisons) and those living in the community across five different sites in the US were used in a clusters, two-staged, stratified sample; in the ECA study. Both surveys confirmed DSM-III diagnosis by using the Diagnostic Interview Schedule (DIS). Age distribution and sex of the population of persons of Hispanic origin in the USA were standardized with data from the two surveys and combined with lifetime rates of Major depressive Episode (MDE) and suicide attempt. The results indicate that 17–20% of participants reported a lifetime history of MDE across ethnic groups. These same participants had a history of suicide attempts. This was in all groups, except for the Puerto Ricans who regardless of whether they had made a suicide attempt had approximately twice the rate of MDE. The only group to have significantly higher rates of suicide attempts compared with Mexican Americans were the Puerto Rican group.

Monk and Warshauer (1974) found that rates of major depression and suicide vary across ethnic groups within the US. This may be true of suicide attempts. Puerto Ricans had higher suicide attempt rates compared with other groups. Suicide attempt rates ranged from 9.1% for Puerto Ricans to 1.9% for Cuban Americans; these results are reflective of what was found in the study by Oquendo *et al.* (2004). It is evident that the Puerto Ricans suffer from both high rate of depressive episodes as well as higher rates of suicide attempts. The study is demonstrating the differences between ethnic groups, however the major limitation is that the data is derived from two surveys taken in the early 1980s, which may make it out of date in response to today's times. The research did not distinguish between the various sub-Hispanic groups and did not take into account the response rates of the minority subgroup as they may have adapted differently according to their situation and circumstance.

In Germany, the frequency of attempted suicidal acts was significantly higher in the Mediterranean immigrant group (15.3%) compared to the German-born group (8.9%). The difference is significant, but suicide attempts rate covaried with the variables of being female and a young age. However, in the immigrant group, nonfatal suicidal acts also correlate with 'cultural conflict'(Grube 2004). This can be understood in the context of majority and minority cultural views at conflict with each other. For example parents may hold traditional views on various issues but the children, who mingle more readily with majority culture, may hold more modern views thus creating tension between parental and children's views (Bhugra 2004). Research suggests that other factors should be taken into account when assessing reasons for suicide risks amongst immigrant groups; apart from being female and young (Grube (2004)

## Suicide

Cross-cultural research has found that ethnic differences and cultural values influence suicide rates (Bhugra *et al.* 1999). Research has also found differences in suicide risk among different generations of immigrants, with higher rates for more recent immigrants (Neeleman *et al.* 1997).

Grube (2004) shows that immigrant psychiatric inpatients are involved in managing the additional stress, which results from their immigration. It may be that 'self-harm' is an insufficient but manageable way for the individuals to cope with the stress and makes them feel that they are 'in control' (Grube 2004).

Over three decades ago, Whitlock (1971) reported that among migrants to Australia, rates of suicide were higher in the British and Irish when compared with rates in their countries of origin. The rates among migrants from south European countries were reported to be lower than in their country of origin; suggesting that not all migrants will respond to stress caused by immigration in the same way. It may be possible that religion and other factors may play a protective role. Whitlock (1971) argues that these differences in rates may relate to pre-migration health checks, integration enjoyed or isolation experienced. He observed that south Europeans may enjoy more family cohesion which may affect reduction of rates.

Suicide rates were highest in the English, Germans and Indians in the recent immigrants (less than 10 years) to Australia. However, the results are not conclusive as another study shows that suicide rates were highest amongst Russians, Poles and New Zealanders who were immigrants and who had lived in Australia for longer than 10 years (Whitlock 1971).

Other factors linked to suicide among immigrants are age and social support. Immigrant suicides compared with suicide rates of Canadian born demonstrate that the immigrants were older, were more educated, had experienced more life events and had less mental illness in their families. There was no difference in employment rates or prior suicide attempts (Chandrasena *et al.* 1991). Higher suicide rates were found amongst the younger, Finnish immigrants to Sweden compared to the Swedish people (Ferrada-Noli *et al.* 1995) and Korean immigrants to New York City compared to the American whites (Stellman 1996). In Sweden, the reasons given for the higher rates were associated with being single, unemployed and foreign born, and with somatic disease.

Amongst Russian immigrants to Israel, suicide was associated with being non-married, having less social support, depression, distress and loneliness (Ponizovsky *et al.* 1997). Patel and Gaw (1996) report that young female immigrants from the Indian subcontinent had higher suicide rates than young immigrant men and women in the home nations. Rates of suicide were high amongst Hindus and violent methods were more common.

## Gender and suicidal behaviours in migrants

Monk and Warshauer's (1974) findings have been drawn from six studies conducted worldwide. The common recurring themes linked with the migrant community and extent of suicide indicates a connection with gender, with the female group portraying higher rates of self-harm.

There is considerable evidence that the rates of attempted suicide are much higher in women aged 18–24 amongst migrant population compared with white women although the rates among young Asian adolescents are not elevated (Thompson and Bhugra 2000; Bhugra et al. 2002). The rates of attempted suicide in Asian females are nearly seven times those of Asian males. The reasons for these differences are many and it has been suggested that when the individuation process starts the young women are probably being urged to comply with parental and familial pressures, and the act of deliberate self-harm offers 'time out' to the individual (Thompson and Bhugra 2000; Bhugra 2004b).

Research has shown there to be a difference between the genders at this age in term of mental health. Odegaard (1932) reported higher incidence of mental disorders in females than males. In other studies, rate of schizophrenia were shown to be higher amongst the older Asian females (Bhugra et al. 1997). Amongst the older generations reasons for migration may have been different between the genders. Murphy (1968) suggested that it may be the males who decide to migrate and the females simply followed them. If so, migrating may not have been a female choice, and dealing with any mental health problems may also be reflected in this. In the younger migrants, reasons for migration may be different between the genders.

Therefore, differences in mental health between the genders may be reflective on the reasons for migration.

Adding further evidence regarding difference in self-harm between the genders is a study conducted by Ponizovsky et al. (1997). Following recent adult immigrants from the former Soviet Union to Israel, an epidemiological survey of suicide ideation was carried out. Immigrants isolated from social and emotional support had the most frequent suicide ideation. For both sexes, the strongest predictor of suicide ideation was dependent on the level of psychological distress. However, the severity of depression predicted suicide in females and not males. These findings are consistent with the finding from Grube (2004). Being female is a recurring theme in the contributing factors for suicidal ideation. As a result such findings can be used to base and develop prevention programmes especially designed to be gender-specific, in order to assist the concerns and experiences of the specific sexes.

## Acculturation and suicidal behaviour

The process of migration involves a further process, that of acculturation. Acculturation has been defined as a 'phenomenon' which results when groups of individuals from different cultures come into continuous first-hand contact with subsequent changes in the original culture patterns of either one or both groups (Berry 1976). At an individual level, in terms of behaviour, six domains have been identified which can be linked with acculturation. These include language, clothing, religion, entertainment, food and shopping habits. Other areas which may be more difficult to identify and measure include cognitive style, behavioural patterns and attitudes. These concepts of acculturation are very closely linked to self-esteem and identity of the self (Bhugra 2004a).

As culture and personality are interlinked (Abbott et al. 1999), one's childhood and early experiences and socialization may also play a role. These behavioural patterns above all form an element of the culture and can then be reflected in the person's choice of what they choose to wear, eat, their main language, their religious practices and shopping habits. All of these are influenced by the environment they live in and the culture they are used to, which in turn may be affected during the process of acculturation.

Acculturation types may have a specific affect on how an individual adapts to the new environment: for some it can be positive and for others, negative. If there are conflicting issues, this can lead to suicide ideations or acts. Pressures associated by acculturation and its affects on suicide were investigated by Kennedy et al. (2005). This study was carried out in Canada where 1135 undergraduates were assessed using the Vancouver Index of Acculturation; this measured the extent of individuals identify with their heritage culture and the mainstream culture. The measure of suicide ideation and behaviours were based on three self-reports, with questions requiring yes/no answers. These questions assessed whether participants had ever experienced any suicidal thoughts, had ever attempted suicide and had ever made plans to commit suicide. It was found that lack of mainstream acculturation did not increase suicide ideation, plans and attempts for any of the ethnic groups studied, namely, European, Chinese and Indo-Asian. Nor did suicidal thoughts and behaviours vary among ethnic groups. Interestingly, the results showed that individuals who identified closely with their heritage culture were at an increased risk of suicidal thoughts but not for suicide plans or attempts (Kennedy et al. 2005). This is in contrast with the UK findings indicating that suicide attempters were more likely to hold more modern and less traditional beliefs compared with controls or parents (Bhugra 2004b).

The fact that ethnicity, generation level, or mainstream acculturation failed to predict differences in suicide ideation, plans, or attempts may suggest that interventions can be handled similarly for different ethnic groups (Kennedy et al. 2005). These authors also propose that young immigrants who live in traditional homes face added pressures due to culture clash' (Kennedy et al. 2005). Although this research adds support to the idea that migrants are at an increased risk of cultural conflict and in turn suicide ideation, this notion is still a modest one and may change if other psychological factors are taken into account. This research can be criticised for being only applicable to the specific group it was researching, nevertheless the results are still interesting and may stimulate production of local strategies for suicide prevention in specific environments.

The need for tailored suicide prevention measures are supported by Makinen and Wasserman (2003) who investigated the level of suicide trends (1982–92) among first- and second-generation immigrant Finnish Swedes. It was found that the level of suicide mortality among immigrant Finnish Swedes was very high and a significant increase was shown among women between 1982–1992. Most interestingly the level of suicide mortality among the quarter of a million immigrant Finnish Swedes was higher than that of any European nation during the period studied. Reasons that suicide rates may be high in the second generation immigrants are, amongst other factors, poor acculturation which calls for specific preventive measures.

## Socio-economic status, social support and suicidal behaviours in immigrants

The process of acculturation and the relevance of social support during the migratory process are key factors in determining the extent of suicide amongst the migrant community.

Social support is important especially amongst the migrating individuals, as arriving into a new environment can be very stressful; there is the issue of adapting to a new culture, way of living and language. If one is alone then dealing with these changes becomes even more stressful; however if there are other individuals who are going through the same transition or have dealt with the same situation then this can act as a buffer to stress, if experiences and difficulties can be shared and support given in this way.

Some issues have been highlighted, such as risk factors for suicidal behaviour in immigrants include marital functioning and specific aspects of emotional functioning (Dusovic *et al.* 2002), socio-economic status especially for men (Taylor *et al.* 1999) and cultural transitions, tensions and quality of life for women (Wassenaar *et al.* 1998). In the case of migration, an individual may develop poor coping strategies as a result of stress or cultural conflict, or conflict which is imposed by the family. Other reasons may be in response to other, wider environmental or social factors such as racism and economic difficulties. This may lead to a sense of hopelessness or feelings of being trapped, and the only way out may be self-harm.

Social support is an integral component of the migratory process and may facilitate a positive acculturation process, the result of which may help eliminate any depressive or suicidal outcomes. Hovey (1999) explored social support as a moderator in the relationship between depression and suicidal ideation in a sample of 104 immigrant Mexican-American adults. Spanish versions of the personal Resource Questionnaire—Part 2 (Weinert 1987) was administered. This measured the perceived effectiveness of social support. In addition, the Adult Suicidal Ideation Questionnaire (Reynolds 1991) and the Centre for Epidemiological Studies— Depression Scale (CES—Depression) (Reynolds 1991) were given to the participants to complete in a classroom setting. The results indicate a positive correlation between depression and suicidal ideation. Compared to the depressed individuals with adequate social support, those individuals who lacked effective social support reported possessing significantly more suicidal ideation. The author concludes that these findings are consistent with the theoretical notion that social support may help buffer against the risk for suicidal ideation during the acculturative process (Hovey 1999); thereby suggesting that social support may serve as a protective factor against suicidal ideation during the acculturation process. The notion of social support and loneliness is a recurring theme in the range of research covered across countries and cultures.

This is further enhanced by Sher (1990), who states that immigrants have higher rates of suicidal behaviour compared to those in their countries of origin and the population in the new host countries. 'Immigration is a stressful life event which may lead to depression and suicidal behaviour' (Sher 1990). However, the author suggests that most immigrants who exhibit suicidal behaviour in the new country may have had suicidal tendencies, and/or some degree of depression, and/or certain maladaptive personality traits before they left their countries of origin.

## Mental health of immigrants

As is evident from this review, there are links with migration and mental health, in particular with attempted suicide and self-harm. Particular attention should be paid to public health and the promotion of preventative measures agenda within communities.

The state of loneliness, which has been recognized as a public health problem in immigrants (Ponizovsky *et al.* 2004) requires the attention of not only clinicians and researchers, but also of public health professionals, both as a condition in itself and in its relation to other conditions. The authors examined the relationship between self-reported loneliness, psychological distress, and social support among immigrants. In particular when arriving and establishing oneself in a new country, migration is not only a very stressful time but may also be a period of immense loneliness, where there is a breakdown of social network and distance from friends and family. Depending on an individual's acculturation state, different support networks from agencies may help improve feelings of loneliness. Informing and educating individuals may be one preventative measure to be taken as a public health strategy. Information sheets and pamphlets can be provided, as was the case in the Bhugra and Hick's (2004) study described below.

Ahmad *et al.* (2004) carried out qualitative research aimed to elicit experiences and beliefs of recent South Asian immigrant women about their major health concerns after immigration. Twenty-four Hindi-speaking women who had lived less than five years in Canada participated in four focus groups. The main health concern was mental health covering three main themes, which included stress-inducing factors, coping strategies and appraisal of the mental burden (this included general susceptibility and extent of the burden). Many participants agreed that mental health did not become a concern to them until after immigration. Although specific reasons were not given for this the women identify stress-inducing factors as occurring due to climate, food changes, lack of social support, economic uncertainties, downward social mobility, mechanistic lifestyle and barriers in accessing health services. The participants made efforts to overcome these stressful encounters: these included being self-aware, and use of preventative health practices and efforts to socialize.

Migration, adaptation, acculturation, and settlement experiences impact on the health of refugees and are dependent on a number of barriers and enablers, both at a personal and societal level. These should be taken into account in the provision of health and social care services and in particular, services should be provided in a culturally competent manner. The same applies to undocumented immigrants and migrants, who are not registered and are without a status. Being excluded from the system and being unaware of any support faculties may affect the degree of their acculturation levels and in turn may influence their mental health and suicidal behaviours.

Although efforts have been made, further promotions are needed by health care professionals and agencies to develop methods to implement preventative measure and information for those individuals that may be prone to develop mental health problems due to their migration process, and a support network provided for such individuals.

Barry and Mizrahi (2005) examined the relationship between guarded self-disclosure, psychological distress, and willingness to use psychological services if distressed among 170 east Asian immigrants in the United States. Participants who endorsed overall guarded self-disclosure, self-concealment or conflict avoidance were significantly more likely to report psychological distress and were significantly less likely to report willingness to use psychological services. These findings point to the importance of assessing multiple factors in distressed immigrants, which appear to be associated with willingness to use psychological services.

## Educational suicide preventive intervention tailored for immigrants

Bhugra and Hicks (2004) sampled a total of 180 British south Asian women to test an educational pamphlet about depression and suicidality and to investigate its feasibility, acceptability and the effect on help-seeking attitudes. The pamphlet provided information about recognizing depression and the risk of suicide, preventing suicide, finding sources of help, and using various coping mechanisms (Bhugra 2004b). The aim of the pamphlet was to provide educational material as part of forming a preventative strategy to reduce depression and suicide attempts in Asian women; as well as aiming to increase community awareness of risk factors for depression and suicide in Asian women and to increase knowledge of available sources of help. The final aim was to train staff at accident and emergency departments to be aware of key risk factors which led to attempted suicide in Asian women (Bhugra 2004b).

The development of the pamphlet was conducted in three stages: stage one was the focus group study; which involved gathering preliminary, in-depth, descriptive data on causes of attempted suicide and conceptualizations of suicide and its risk factors from the perspectives of ten focus groups with forty-three Asian women living in the community. The second stage was the development of the educational pamphlet which was based on three sources of information; the results of the focus groups, the ethnography and participant observation in the London Asian community over previous years and findings from a previous study of British Asian women who had attempted suicide (Bhugra *et al.* 1999). The final stage was to pilot test intervention with the educational pamphlet (Bhugra 2004b).

Having read the pamphlets, significantly more women assessed themselves as willing to confide in their clinicians, friends and spouses if they felt depressed or suicidal rather than not telling anyone. In addition to being able to express their feelings, more women reported seeing the benefit of antidepressants having read the pamphlet, which may not have been the case before. The change in attitude persisted four to six weeks after the initial reading of the pamphlet (Bhugra and Hicks 2004). In particular, among recent immigrants (32 women), the pamphlet increased the reported acceptance of antidepressants by 28%. The pamphlet was also well received by professionals from general practitioner clinics and community organizations. Facilities adopted the pamphlet and its translations for general use and stated that it filled an important gap in south Asian public health. More than 90% of the participants themselves stated that they liked the pamphlet and thought that it was useful for increasing community awareness. This study demonstrates the need of various public health measures required in response to the rates of increased suicide amongst minority groups, in particular immigrants. This strategy is considered important as a preventative strategy to the increased rates of suicide and attempted suicide among south Asian women, in particular amongst the younger age group in UK (Hicks and Bhugra 2003). Male migrants bring double jeopardy issues of not only gender, but being a migrant as well as the perceived weaknesses in a migrants status—which have to be addressed in any strategy. Using approaches seen as males gender congruent, for example in HIV prevention in Hispanics in New York where Superman-type comics were used to educate men about the use of condoms, may help.

## National suicide preventive strategies and migrants

Over the last decade an increasing number of countries have established national strategies for suicide prevention.

Understanding various cultures and their attitudes to mental health is a good starting point in developing intervention programmes. Conrad *et al.* (2005) found that religious beliefs and social stigma attached to mental illness contributed to prolonged denial of the condition, difficulty in expressing emotional problems to professional caregivers, and delayed professional intervention. The traditional family hierarchy rooted in age and gender inequality interfered with help-seeking behaviours and heightened some family conflicts and hindered family adaptation after migration to the United States. Such examples demonstrate the significance of understanding ethnic diversity in relation to public health service and intervention programmes.

Papadopoulos *et al.* (2004) explored Ethiopian refugees' and asylum seekers' experiences of migration, adaptation and settlement in the UK and their health beliefs and practices. Many of the participants faced difficulties with the immigration system, housing and social services and felt socially isolated. A general belief was that happiness is a prerequisite to healthiness and also an indication of healthiness. Thus a majority believed that sickness is caused by disease and that mental illness is caused by both supernatural and psychosocial causes. Most of the participants sought the help of their GP in the first instance of illness, although some had experienced difficulties accessing health services due to language problems and poor understanding of the primary health care system. The participants also believed that the stress of adaptation and settlement affected their mental health and led to depression.

In collectivist cultures the concept of the self can be influenced with acculturation and individuals who have sociocentric traits may respond better to prevention strategies, which focus on communities rather than on individuals. However, we were unable to find such interventions in the literature. Attitudes of help givers to suicide will also play a key role in the development of preventative strategies.

The main problem of planning any suicide preventive strategy for migrants is often a lack of knowledge regarding the particular minority groups. Wider knowledge and research may be required to assess the issues experienced by such individuals (Carta *et al.* 2005).

In many European countries there are migrants who fall outside the existing health and social services, something which is particularly true for asylum seekers and undocumented immigrants. In order to address these deficiencies, it is necessary to provide with an adequate financing and a continuity of the grants for research into the multi-cultural health demand.

Carta *et al.* (2005)

## Conclusion

Migration occurs across cultures and across the world. Studies covered in this chapter include research from countries across the continents and look at studies of countries with an influx of communities from different part of the world.

Given the impact of socio-cultural aspects in the development and clinical manifestations of mental health problems it is necessary to know the demands of the immigrant population and to adjust current facilities for their care.

Ochoa *et al.* (2005)

The emerging issues are of developing policies being culturally specific and informative. The information pamphlet developed in England (Bhugra and Hicks 2004), aided in informing and encouraging immigrants and such straightforward procedure proved to be very effective.

Preventative strategies for migrants must make allowances for type of migration, reason for migration, culture-specific issues and social aspects. For example the strategies for migrants who are professional will differ from those who are white collar or blue-collar workers. In addition, if the migrant comes from collectivist cultures to individualist cultures (e.g. Mexicans to the USA, Turks to Germany, Greeks to Australia) they will require community involvement, perhaps using religious leaders more often. On the other hand if individualist migrants move to individualist cultures (e.g. from Germany to Switzerland, Finnish migrants to Sweden or Greenlanders to Denmark), the target will perhaps have to be the individual.

Investing time and money in research to further understand migrants would enable the development of specific suicide preventive programmes for immigrant groups on the five continents.

## References

Abbott MW, Wong S, Williams M *et al.* (1999). Chinese migrant's mental health and adjustment to life in New Zealand. *Australian and New Zealand Journal of Psychiatry*, **33**, 13–21.

Ahmad F, Shik A, Vanza R *et al.* (2004). Voices of south Asian women: immigration and mental health. *Women Health*, **40**, 113–30.

Barry DT and Mizrahi TC (2005). Guarded self-disclosure predicts psychological distress and willingness to use psychological services among East Asian immigrants in the United States. *Journal of Nervous and Mental Disease*, **193**, 35–39.

Berry JW (1976). *Human Ecology and Cognitive Style*. Sage, New York.

Bhugra D, Leff J, Mallett R *et al.* (1997). Incidence and outcome of schizophrenia in Whites, African Caribbeans and Asians in London. *Psychological Medicine* **27**, 791–798.

Bhugra D, Baldwin D, Desai M *et al.* (1999). Attempted suicide in west London II. Intergenerational comparisons. *Psychological Medicine*, **29**, 1131–139.

Bhugra D and Jones P (2001). Migration and mental illness. *Advances in Psychiatric Treatment*, **7**, 326–223.

Bhugra D, Singh J, Fellow-Smith E *et al.* (2002). Deliberate self-harm in adolescents: a case note study among two ethnic groups. *European Journal of Psychiatry*, **16**, 145–151.

Bhugra D (2004a). A Migration and mental health. *Acta Psychiatrica Scandinavica*, **109**, 243–258.

Bhugra D (2004b). *A Culture and Self-harm: Attempted Suicide in South Asians in London*. Psychology Press, London.

Bhugra D and Hicks MH (2004). Effect of an educational pamphlet on help-seeking attitudes for depression among British South Asian women. *Psychiatric Services*, **55**, 827–829.

Carta MG, Bernal M, Hardoy MC *et al.* (2005). The 'Report on the Mental Health in Europe' working group. Migration and mental health in Europe (the state of the mental health in Europe working group: appendix 1). *Clinical Practice and Epidemiology in Mental Health*, **31**, 1–13.

Chandrasena R, Beddage V, Ferrnando MLD (1991). Suicide among immigrant psychiatric patients in Canada. *British Journal of Psychiatry*, **159**, 707–709.

Conrad MM and Pacquiao DF (2005). Manifestation, attribution, and coping with depression among Asian Indians from the perspectives of health care practitioners. *Journal of Transcultural Nursing*, **16**, 32–40.

Dusovic N, Baume P, Malak A-E (2002). *Cross-cultural Suicide Prevention*. Transcultural Mental Health Centre, Sydney, Australia.

Ferrada-Noli M, Asberg M, Ormstad K *et al.* (1995). Definite and undetermined forensic diagnoses of suicide among immigrants in Sweden. *Acta Psychiatrica Scandinavica*, **91**, 130–135.

Grube M (2004). Nonfatal suicidal acts in a group of psychiatric inpatients: situation of Mediterranean immigrants *Nervenarz*, **75**, 681–687.

Hicks MH and Bhugra D (2003). Perceived causes of suicide attempts by UK South Asian women. *American Journal of Orthopsychiatry*, **7**, 455–462.

Hovey JD (1999). Moderating influence of social support on suicidal ideation in a sample of Mexican immigrants. *Psychological Reports*, **85**, 78–79.

Kennedy MA, Parhar KK, Samra J *et al.* (2005). Suicide ideation in different generations of immigrants. *Canadian Journal of Psychiatry*, **50**, 353–356.

Kessler RC, McGonagle KA, Zhao S *et al.* (1994). Lifetime and 12-month prevalence of DSM- III-R psychiatric disorders in the United States. *Archives of General Psychiatry*, **51**, 8–19.

Makinen IH and Wasserman D (2003). Suicide mortality among immigrant Finnish Swedes. *Archives of Suicide Research*, **7**, 93–106.

Monk M and Warshauer ME (1974). Completed and attempted suicide in three ethnic groups. *American Journal of Epidemiology*, **130**, 348–360.

Moscicki EK, Rae DS, Regier DA *et al.* (1987). The Hispanic Health and Nutrition Examination Survey: depression among Mexican Americans, Cuban Americans, and Puerto Ricans. In M Gaviria and J Arana, eds, *Health and Behaviour Research Agenda for Hispanics*, pp. 145–159. Research monograph no. 1, University of Illinois Press, Chicago.

Murphy HBM (1968). Socio-cultural factors in schizophrenia. In A Zubin and V Freyhan, eds, *Social Psychiatry*, pp. 74–92. Grune and Stratton, New York.

Nazroo J (1997). *Ethnicity and Mental Health*. Policy Studies Institute, London.

Neeleman J, Mak V, Wessely S (1997). Suicide by age, ethnic group, coroner's verdicts and country of birth. *British Journal of Psychiatry*, **171**, 463–467.

Ochoa Mangado E, Vicente Muelas N, Lozano Suarez M (2005). Depressive syndromes in the immigrant population. *Revista Clínica Española*, **3**, 116–118.

Odegaard O (1932). Emigration and insanity. *Acta Psychiatricia et Neurologica Supplementum*, **4**, 1–206.

Oquendo MA, Lizardi D, Greenwald S *et al.* (2004). Rates of lifetime suicide attempt and rates of lifetime major depression in different ethnic groups in the United States. *Acta Psychiatrica Scandinavica*, **110**, 446–451.

Papadopoulos I, Lees S, Lay M *et al.* (2004). Ethiopian refugees in the UK: migration, adaptation and settlement experiences and their relevance to health. *Ethnicity and Health*, **9**, 55–73.

Patel SP and Gaw AC (1996). Suicide among immigrants from the Indian subcontinent. *Psychiatric Services*, **47**, 517–521.

Ponizovsky AM and Ritsner MS (2004). Patterns of loneliness in an immigrant population. *Comprehensive Psychiatry*, **45**, 408–414.

Ponizovsky A, Safro S, Ginath Y *et al.* (1997). Suicide ideation among recent immigrants: an epidemiological study. *Israel Journal of Psychiatry and Related Sciences*, **34**, 139–148.

Rack P (1982). *Race, Culture and Mental Disorder.* Tavistock, London.

Reynolds WM (1991). *Adult Suicidal Ideation Questionnaire: Professional Manual.* Psychological Assessment Resources, Odessa.

Sher L (1999). On the role of neurobiological and genetic factors in the aetiology and pathogenesis of suicidal behaviour among immigrants. *Medical Hypotheses*, **53**, 110–111.

Stellman SD (1996). Proportional mortality ratios among Korean immigrants to New York City, 1986–1990. *Yonsei Medical Journal*, **37**, 31–37.

Taylor R, Morrell S, Slaytor E *et al.* (1999). Suicide in urban New South Wales. Australia 1984–1994: socio-economic and migrant interactions. *Social Science and Medicine*, **47**, 1677–1686.

Thompson N and Bhugra D (2000). Rates of deliberate self-harm in Asians: findings and models. *International Review of Psychiatry*, **12**, 37–43.

Wassenaar DR, Van Der Veen MBW, Pillay AL (1998). Women in cultural transition: suicidal behaviour in South African Indian women. *Suicide and Life-Threatening Behaviour*, **28**, 82–93.

Weinert C (1987). A social support measure: PRQ85. *Nursing Research*, **36**, 273–277.

Whitlock FA (1971). Migration and suicide. *Medical Journal of Australia*, **2**, 840–848.

# CHAPTER 30

# Suicide and attempted suicide among indigenous people

Danuta Wasserman, Tony Durkee and Gergö Hadlaczky

## Abstract

There are hundreds of indigenous groups and peoples around the world. Examples are the Australian Aborigines, the North American Indians (Native Americans) of the US and Canada, and the Maori of New Zealand. Such groups and peoples often have elevated suicide rates compared with the general population in their countries, and divergent epidemiological characteristics. Adoption of culture-specific prevention strategies in countries where indigenous peoples live is proposed and discussed.

## Introduction

There is no internationally accepted definition of 'indigenous peoples'. However, Sims and Kuhnlein (2003) cite several key characteristics used (but not adopted) by United Nations' bodies and other agencies to distinguish indigenous peoples:

◆ Residence within or attachment to geographically distinct traditional habitats, ancestral territories, and natural resources in these habitats and territories;

◆ Maintenance of cultural and social identities, and social, economic, cultural and political institutions separate from mainstream or dominant societies and cultures;

◆ Descent from population groups present in a given area, most frequently before modern states or territories were created and current borders defined;

◆ Self-identification as being part of a distinct indigenous cultural group, and the display of desire to preserve that cultural identity.

The hundreds of indigenous groups all over the world are often referred to by local and regional names. Examples are the Aborigines of Australia and the North American Indians (Native Americans and Canadians), or 'first peoples' and 'first nations' as they are also called, of the US and Canada. Although widely known as the world's 'first peoples', they nevertheless lack territorial, economic and political autonomy. Many people attribute this to colonization and ever accelerating modernization and cultural globalization (Ray 1996; Bartholomew 2004).

Indigenous people's physical and mental health and social indicators are often less favourable than those of other inhabitants of the same areas (Clelland *et al.* 2007). This may indicate a vulnerability to suicidal impulses. On the basis of data taken from the WHO, it was concluded that indigenous people are among the highest risk groups for suicide in the world today (WHO 2002; Leenars 2006).

Below, suicides and attempted suicides among selected indigenous groups around the world are reviewed. Risk and protective factors are described, as are the preventive measures being taken in these societies.

## Suicide and attempted-suicide rates among Inuits in Canada and Greenland

### Canada

Indigenous people in various parts of Canada comprise of the 'First Nations' or 'Inuits'. There were approximately 45,070 Inuits living in Canada in 2001. The majority live in remote communities spread across two provinces and two territories, in four distinct regions (Advisory Group on Suicide Prevention 2002):

◆ Nunatsiavut (Labrador);

◆ Nunavik (Northern Quebec);

◆ Nunavut Territory;

◆ Inuvialuit (Western Arctic).

As Figure 30.1 shows, Inuits from three distinctive regions had higher suicide rates than non-indigenous Canadians in 2002. Inuits from the Inuvialuit region were an exception, with a rate (18/100,000) that was very much lower than those of their counterparts in the other regions, and only slightly higher than that of non-indigenous Canadians (Advisory Group on Suicide Prevention 2002).

A study conducted by Chandler and Lalonde (1998) showed that suicide rates among Inuit tribes vary greatly. For some, suicide rates exceed 600/100,000; for others, it is as low as approximately 10/100,000. It may be useful to examine why some tribes have such

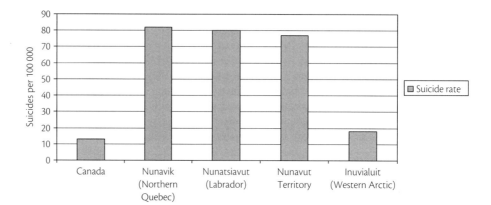

**Fig. 30.1** Suicide rates per 100,000 among Inuits and Canadians, 2002. Source: AGSP (2002).

extremely high suicide rates while others have rates as low as, or even lower than, Canada's mean national suicide rate.

Scant data on hospitalization due to self-inflicted harm in Inuit communities are reported. Statistics on emergency medical consultations in Alberta show that in the year 2000, the rate of hospitalization for attempted suicide among the First Nations was 6.74 times higher than that among other ethnic groups in the Canadian population (Alberta Centre for Injury Control and Research 2005).

### Greenland

Greenland has some of the highest suicide rates in the world (Leineweber *et al.* 2001). According to Leineweber (2000), people born in Greenland are regarded as 'Inuit' or 'Natives'. Of the country's 56,000 inhabitants, 89 per cent were born there, i.e. Inuits make up the vast majority of Greenland's inhabitants (Bjerregaard and Curtis 2002).

Suicide rates vary widely from one region of Greenland to another (Henderson 2003). Although suicide attempts are not well documented in Greenland, a study conducted by Grove and Lynge (1979) showed that the rate of attempted suicide among the Greenland Inuits was approximately 100/100,000. This does not differ substantially from rates in, for example, Europe or North America.

### Suicide and attempted suicide among North American Indians and Alaska Natives

Alaska has the highest percentage of indigenous people in the US (Barnhardt 2001). The ethnic group often referred to as 'Alaska Natives' includes the Inputiat, Yupik and Aluet people. Alaska Natives make up 16.4 per cent of the total Alaskan population; together, they and the American Indians account for 25 per cent (Barnhardt 2001).

Alaska Natives' suicide rates are some five to six times the overall US rate, and two to three times the Alaskan rate for all deaths by suicide. Although they make up only 16.4 per cent of the Alaskan population, Alaska Natives account for 39 per cent of suicides in the state (Alaska Injury Prevention Center 2006).

The regions in the north and west of Alaska—North Slope, Northwest Arctic, Nome and Yukon-Kuskokwim (Y-K) Delta—where the majority of the population are Inupiats ('Eskimos') have the state's highest suicide rates. In contrast, the

south-eastern regions, with an Aleutian majority, have the lowest rates (Alaska Injury Prevention Center 2006).

This relationship seems, however, to be age-dependent. Perkins (2005) reported that there were fewer suicide attempts among Alaska Natives than Caucasians in 2001–2002. This is true of suicide attempters aged 19 and over who were hospitalized for attempted suicide in Alaska: 40 per cent were Natives and 50 per cent were Caucasians. On the other hand, the corresponding figures for adolescent suicide attempters (aged 18 and below) were 55 per cent Native and 40 per cent Caucasian. Other statistics show that in 1994–99 too, the rate of attempted suicide among Alaska Natives aged below 19 was, at 157/100,000, far higher than their white counterparts' rate, which was 38/100,000 (Alaska Department of Health and Social Service 2003).

There are currently over 560 federally recognized American Indian (Native American) tribes living in urban and rural communities around the US (Olson and Wahab 2006). American Indians and Alaska Natives, the largest indigenous groups in the US, have the highest mortality rates. In Alaska, the Natives' mortality rates were 60 per cent higher than those in the US white population in 1989–1998. Alaska Natives had significantly elevated mortality rates due to cancer, cerebrovascular disease, diabetes, chronic obstructive pulmonary disease and suicide (Day and Lanier 2003).

The suicide rate for American Indians and Alaska Natives combined is 31/100,000, which is twice the rate in the non-Hispanic white population (15/100,000) and more than three times the rates of African Americans and Hispanics (National Adolescent Health Information Center 2006).

Metha and Webb (1996) report wide variation among the various tribes' suicide rates, ranging from a low of 6/100,000 among Chippewa Indians (mostly located in Minnesota, Wisconsin and Michigan) to a high of 130/100,000 among the Blackfeet (who are nomadic and dispersed across the United States).

The Navajo are the largest American Indian tribe in the US, with the majority of the population residing in New Mexico and Arizona. The Comanche live in Oklahoma and Texas, and Athabascans are the largest group, with some 12,000 members in Alaska (American Indian Heritage Foundation 2005). These tribes show considerable differences in suicide rates. The Athabascans in Alaska, for example, have a suicide rate of 41.9/100,000, while the Navajos in Arizona have a rate of 16/100,000, and the Comanche living in Oklahoma have a rate 11.9/100,000. The overall American Indian rate is 73 per cent higher than the US as a whole (Indian Health Service 2004; American Indian Heritage Foundation 2005).

Approximately 6.2 per cent of American Indian youth between the ages of 12 and 17 attempt suicide, compared with 3.7 per cent of Hispanics, 3.4 per cent of Caucasians, and 2.4 per cent of African Americans. The incidence of suicidal ideation for these age groups is 8.6 per cent for American Indian youth, 6.3 per cent for Hispanics, 8.1 per cent for Caucasians and 4.8 per cent for African Americans respectively (Youth Violence Prevention Center 2003).

## Suicide and attempted suicide among Aboriginal and Maori people

Indigenous people in Australia, known as 'Aborigines' (a term that includes both Aboriginal people and Torres Strait Islanders), make up 2.5 per cent of the country's population. Suicide was fairly rare in Aboriginal society until the late 1960s, and in the 1970s there was a noticeable increase in suicide and suicidal behaviour. Today, studies have shown that Aboriginals have a significantly higher rate of suicide and attempted suicide than non-Aboriginals in Australia (Elliot-Farrelly 2004).

The data demonstrate that suicide rates are much higher among Aboriginal males than non-Aboriginal males across all age groups, except 40–44 and 50–54. In the 40–44 age group, Aboriginal males have only half the suicide rate of non-Aboriginals, while the rate in the 50–54 age group is slightly lower than among non-Aboriginals. Aboriginal males aged 15–19 have a suicide rate some 4 times higher than non-Aboriginals (Harrison et al. 1997).

Data from the Australian Bureau of Statistic show that, in 1999–2003, there were twice as many suicides among Aboriginal males than among non-indigenous males in Australia, and the male rate was more than three times higher for the age groups below 34 years (Australian Institute for Health and Welfare 2005). Females below the age of 24 had a suicide rate 5 times higher than that of non-indigenous females. However, for those aged 35 years and over, Aboriginal females' rates were similar to, or even lower than, their non-indigenous female counterparts (Australian Institute for Health and Welfare 2005). One study showed that in the Northern Territory between 1981 and 2002, suicide rates rose in both the indigenous and the non-indigenous male population, by 800 per cent and 30 per cent, respectively (Measey et al. 2006).

Helps and Harrison (2006) report that, among males and females alike, suicide attempts are significantly more frequent among indigenous groups than among other Australians.

## Suicide and attempted suicide among the New Zealand Maori

In 2001, Maori people made up nearly 15 per cent of the total New Zealand population (Ministry of Health 2006). Suicide rates among Maori aged 15–24 years had risen since 1957, reaching 35.2/100,000 for men and 6.0/100,000 for women in 1987–91. These high rates were similar to those of young non-Maori New Zealanders (Skegg et al. 1995).

Of the various ethnic groups, the Maori had the highest suicide rate for all ages, at 17.8 per 100,000, in the years 2000–2003. Other ethnic groups, such as European, Pacific and Asian, had rates of 13.1, 10.4 and 8.8 respectively during this period (Ministry of Health 2006).

Over a 24-year span, the frequency of suicide attempts among Maori people has been consistently higher than among their compatriots of European, Pacific and Asian origin. At the end of 2003, Maori people had an attempted-suicide rate of more than 200/100,000, whereas Asians had the lowest rate, approximately 60/100,000 (Ministry of Health 2006). One study showed that suicidal ideation was greater among Maori than non-Maori people, but after adjustment for sociodemographic variables Maori and non-Maori people were found to have similar rates of suicidal ideation (Beautrais et al. 2006).

## Suicide and attempted suicide among indigenous groups in Brazil, Siberia and Taiwan

Little is known about indigenous groups and suicide in remote and restricted areas in Brazil, Siberia and Taiwan, for example.

### Brazil

The indigenous peoples in the state of Mato Grosso do Sul in the south-west corner of Brazil are known as 'Guaraní'. The Guaraní make up 2.6 per cent of the Mato Grosso do Sul's population (Coloma et al. 2006).

Coloma, Hoffman and Crosby (2006) conducted a longitudinal study on suicides in 2000–2005 among Guaraní clans in the state of Mato Grosso do Sul. Their findings showed that suicide rates among the Guaraní were 121.5/100,000 in 2000 and 113.2/100,000 in 2005 for males, and 63.7/100,000 and 59.1/100,000 respectively among females. In 2005 the overall suicide rate among the Guaraní was 86.3/100,000, which was approximately 10 times the overall rate in Mato Grosso do Sul and 19 times the Brazilian national rate. In the 20–29 age group in 2005, Guaraní suicide rates were 159.9/100,000, and people aged 30 years and under accounted for 85 per cent of the suicides.

### Siberia

Data on suicidal behaviour among the indigenous groups residing in Siberia are also somewhat limited. Two areas of eastern Siberia, the republic of Buryatia and the Chita region, had a suicide rate of approximately 60/100,000 in 2001, and Krasnoyarsk territory had a suicide rate of some 52/100,000 (Andreeva 2005). Lester (2006) reports that some indigenous groups, such as the Gilyak in south-east Siberia and the Chukchee, Koryak and Kamchadal in north-east Siberia, have relatively high suicide rates. The Chukchee and Gilyak have high suicide rates even in comparison with other indigenous groups around the world (Lester 2006).

### Taiwan

In Taiwan, there are nine indigenous tribes, with a combined population of approximately 330,000, accounting for 1.5 per cent of the total Taiwanese population (Wen et al. 2004). Very little is known about the indigenous peoples and suicide in this region. One study has found that suicide mortality among the indigenous population is two to three times greater than the general population in Taiwan. The disparity is even greater among females, whose suicide mortality is three to eight times higher than that of the general population. The study also shows that of the 212 female Aboriginals investigated, 20.3 per cent had suicidal ideation (Yang and Yang 2000).

## Risk and protective factors

Indigenous groups throughout the world appear to have higher suicide and attempted-suicide rates than the general population in their respective societies. Hunter and Harvey (2002) discuss colonization as a factor contributing to the elevated suicide rates. The process of colonization throughout the world pushed indigenous people out of their territories into remote areas where they now have less access to health care, social welfare and education.

Bjerregaard and Curtis (2002) discuss the role of rapid societal development caused by colonization and globalization; how people cope with loss or change of cultural identity; and how indigenous groups can become integrated in modern society.

### Risk factors

Studies have also revealed universal risk factors that can be detected in many indigenous groups. Examples are high poverty rates, low education, unemployment and substance abuse (Advisory Group on Suicide Prevention 2002).

Risk factors for suicide and attempted suicide among indigenous people, as in the general population, include substance abuse by individuals or their parents, depression, somatic diseases, physical or sexual abuse, family and relationship problems, emotional problems, gang involvement, gun availability and prior suicide attempts. These factors have been identified among American Indian and Alaska Native (Inupiat) groups (Borowsky et al. 1999; Wexler and Goodwin 2006).

Aboriginal people in Australia and Maori in New Zealand, too, show similar characteristics which boost the risk for suicide and attempted suicide: lack of a sense of purpose in life, a lack of recognized role models, disintegration of the family, lack of support networks, sexual assault, psychological distress, prior suicide attempts, socially and/or educationally disadvantaged backgrounds, substance abuse and alienation (Coupe 2001; Elliot-Farrelly 2004).

### Protective factors

Protective factors have also been studied, and have proved valuable as a basis for interventions and reducing risks for suicidal behaviour.

One study conducted on the First Nations in Canada (Advisory Group on Suicide Prevention 2002) identified the following protective factors: self-government and access to land, education, health care and cultural facilities.

Other studies have also identified certain protective factors that reduce risk for suicide and attempted suicide (Kirmayer et al. 1996; Pharris et al. 1997; Coupe 2001). These include a history of receiving treatment for psychiatric problems, frequent church attendance, a high level of academic achievement, family attention and supportive networks, the degree of caring displayed by the family, good models in adults and tribal leaders, enjoyment of school, involvement in traditional activities, coping skills, high self-esteem, a sense of belonging through family and/or school connections, and cultural identity.

## Preventive programmes

In the US, Canada, Greenland, Australia and New Zealand, there are national and regional guidelines, goals and objectives to produce effective suicide-preventive programmes for the indigenous populations of these countries. Many are currently being implemented and have yet to be evaluated. Although there are many obstacles to implementing such interventions—language barriers, cultural differences and even mistrust on the part of the indigenous groups—some studies have implemented minor preventive programmes, with a degree of success (Capp et al. 2001; Echohawk 2006).

Coupe (2000), who drew attention to the fact that suicide is a major issue among the Maori, suggested that application of the present national suicide prevention strategy in New Zealand is somewhat restrictive to the Maori community. However, a culturally specific strategy reflecting suicide trends amongst the Maori now exists in New Zealand (Associate Minister of Health 2006).

Capp et al. (2001) stated that concern about the high suicide rate of Aboriginal people on the south coast of New South Wales had led to the development of a project aimed at preventing youth suicide in the Aboriginal communities of the Shoalhaven region. The main focus was a series of community gatekeeper training workshops, intended to increase the capacity of members of the Aboriginal community to identify and support people at risk of suicide and to facilitate their access to health and social care services (Cantor and Baume 1999). The present suicide-preventive strategy in Australia is adapted to indigenous people's needs.

## Conclusion

Overall, suicide interventions should take into consideration the difficulties in intervening in societies with heterogeneous ethnic and cultural backgrounds, languages and values. It is important to involve the tribal leaders in the communities, clergy and schools, and to sustain the indigenous heritage of the region. Involving local tribal leaders and councils, and fostering distinctive protective factors in these communities, as well as reducing risk factors, may enhance the prospects of a suicide intervention proving successful and bringing about a truly significant change.

## References

Advisory Group on Suicide Prevention (Canada) (2002). *Acting on What we Know: Preventing Youth Suicide in First Nations*. Health Canada, Ottawa.

Alaska Department of Health and Social Service (2003). *Children's Injury Disparities in Alaska. Alaska Injury Facts, No. 2*. Anchorage, Alaska.

Alaska Injury Prevention Center (2006). *Alaska Suicide Follow-back Study Final Report 2003–2006*. Retrieved 25 April 2007 at: http://www.alaska-ipc.org/intent.htm.

Alberta Centre for Injury Control and Research (2005). *Injury-related Health Services use by First Nations in Alberta. Hospital Admissions, 2000 and Emergency Department Visits, 2000*. Alberta Centre for Injury Control and Research, Edmonton.

American Indian Heritage Foundation (2005). *Indian Tribes*. Retrieved 26 April 2007 at: http://www.indians.org.

Andreeva E (2005). *Spatial Portrait of Mortality due to External Causes of Death in the Russian Federation*. Retrieved 26 April 2007 at: http://www.transitionhealth.org/andreeva.htm.

Associate Minister of Health 2006. *New Zealand Suicide Prevention Strategy 2006–2016*. Wellington, New Zealand.

Australian Institute of Health and Welfare (2005). *The Health and Welfare of Australia's Aboriginal and Torres Strait Islander Peoples*. Australian Institute of Health and Welfare, Cat. No. IHW14, Canberra.

Barnhardt C (2001). A history of schooling for Alaska native people. *Journal of American Indian Education*, **40**, 1–30.

Bartholomew D (2004). Indigenous education and the prospects for cultural survival. *Cultural Survival Quarterly*, **27**, 4.

Beautrais AL, Wells JE, McGee MA *et al.* (2006). Suicidal behaviour in the Te Rau Hinengaro: the New Zealand Mental Health Survey (NZMHS). *Australian and New Zealand Journal of Psychiatry*, **40**, 896–904.

Bjerregaard P and Curtis T (2002). The Greenland Population Study. Cultural change and mental health in Greenland: the association of childhood conditions, language and urbanization with vulnerability and suicidal thoughts among the Inuit of Greenland. *Social Science and Medicine*, **54**, 33–48.

Borowsky IW, Resnick MD, Ireland M *et al.* (1999). Suicide attempts among American Indian and Alaska Native youth: risk and protective factors. *Archives of Pediatric Adolescent Medicine*, **153**, 573–580.

Cantor CH and Baume PJ (1999). Suicide prevention: a public health approach. *Australian and New Zealand Journal of Mental Health Nursing*, **8**, 45–50.

Capp K, Deane FP, Lambert G (2001). Suicide prevention in Aboriginal communities: application of community gatekeeper training. *Australian and New Zealand Journal of Public Health*, **25**, 315–321.

Clelland N, Gould T, Parker E (2007). Searching for evidence: what works in indigenous mental health promotion? *Health Promotion Journal Australia*, **18**, 208–216.

Chandler M and Lalonde C (1998). Cultural continuity as a hedge against suicide in Canada's First Nations. *Transcultural Psychiatry*, **35**, 191–219.

Coloma C, Hoffman JS, Crosby A (2006). Suicide among Guarani Kaiowa and Nandeva youth in Mato Grosso do Sul, Brazil. *Archives of Suicide Research*, **10**, 191–207.

Coupe NM (2001). *The Epidemiology of Maori Suicide in Aotearoa/New Zealand*. Retrieved 26 April 2007 at: http://spjp.massey.ac.nz/books/bolitho/Chapter_4.pdf.

Day GE and Lanier AP (2003). Alaska Native mortality 1979–1998. *Public Health Reports*, **118**, 518–530.

Echohawk M (2006). Suicide prevention efforts in one area of Indian Health Service, USA. *Archives of Suicide Research*, **10**, 169–176.

Elliott-Farrelly T (2004). Australian Aboriginal suicide: the need for an Aboriginal suicidology? *Australia e-Journal for the Advancement of Mental Health*, **3**, 1–8.

Grove O and Lynge J (1979). Suicide and attempted suicide in Greenland. A controlled study in Nuuk (Godthaab). *Acta Psychiatrica Scandinavica*, **60**, 375–391.

Harrison J, Moller J, Bordeaux S (1997). Yééouth suicide and self-injury. The *Australian Injury Prevention Bulletin*, Supplement 15.

Henderson A (2003). *Report on the Workshop on Best Practices in Suicide Prevention and the Evaluation of Suicide Prevention Programs in the Arctic*. Iqaluit, Nunavut.

Helps YLM and Harrison JE (2006). *Hospitalised Injury of Australia's Aboriginal and Torres Strait Islander people: 2000–02*. Injury Technical Paper Series Number 8. AIHW, Cat. No. INJCAT 94, Adelaide.

Hunter E and Harvey D (2002). Indigenous suicide in Australia, New Zealand, Canada and the United States. *Emergency Medicine*, **14**, 14–23.

Indian Health Service (2004). *Regional Differences in Indian Health 1998–99*. Rockville, Maryland.

Kirmayer LJ, Malus M, Boothroyd LJ (1996). Suicide attempts among Inuit youth: a community survey of prevalence and risk factors. *Acta Psychiatr Scand*, **94**, 8–17.

Leenaars AA (2006). Suicide among indigenous peoples: introduction and call to action. *Arch Suicide Res*, **10**, 103–115.

Leineweber M (2000). *Modernization and Mental Health: Suicide among the Inuit in Greenland*. Nijmegen University Press, Nijmegen.

Leineweber M, Bjerregaard, P, Baerveldt C *et al.* (2001). Suicide in a society in transition. *International Journal of Circumpolar Health*, **60**, 280–287.

Lester D (2006). Suicide in Siberian aboriginal groups. *Archives of Suicide Research*, **10**, 221–224.

Measey ML, Li SQ, Parker R *et al.* (2006). Suicide in the Northern Territory, 1981–2002. *Medical Journal of Australia*, **185**, 315–319.

Metha A and Webb LD (1996). Suicide among American Indian youth: the role of the schools in prevention. *Journal of American Indian Education*, **36**, 22–32.

Ministry of Health (2006). *New Zealand Suicide Trends: Mortality 1921–2003, Hospitalisations for Intentional Self-harm 1978–2004*. Monitoring Report No. 10, Ministry of Health, Wellington.

National Adolescent Health Information Center (2006). *Fact Sheet on Suicide: Adolescents and Young Adults*. University of California Press, San Francisco.

Olson LM and Wahab S (2006). American Indians and suicide: a neglected area of research. *Trauma, Violence and Abuse*, **7**, 19–33.

Perkins R (2005). *Alaska Suicide Hospitalizations 2001–2002*. Alaska Injury Prevention Center, Anchorage.

Pharris M, Resnick M, Blum R (1997). Protecting against hopelessness and suicidality in sexually abused American Indian adolescents. *Journal of Adolescent Health*, **21**, 400–406.

Ray A (1996). *I Have Lived here Since the World Began*. Lester Publishing Ltd, Toronto.

Sims J and Kuhnlein H (2003). *Indigenous Peoples and Participatory Health Research: Planning and Management/Preparing Research Agreements*. World Health Organization, Geneva.

Skegg K, Cox B, Broughton J (1995). Suicide among New Zealand Maori: is history repeating itself? *Acta Psychiatrica Scandinavica*, **92**, 453–459.

Wen CP, Tsai SP, Shih YT *et al.* (2004). Bridging the gap in life expectancy of the aborigines in Taiwan. *International Journla of Epidemiology*, **33**, 320–327.

Wexler L and Goodwin B (2006). Youth and adult community member beliefs about Inupiat youth suicide and its prevention. *International Journal of Circumpolar Health*, **65**, 448–458.

WHO (2002). *World Report on Violence and Health*. World Health Organization, Geneva.

Yang MS and Yang MJ (2000). Correlated risk factors for suicidal ideation in Aboriginal southern Taiwanese women of childbearing age. *Public Health*, **114**, 191–294.

Youth Violence Prevention Center (2003). *Under the Microscope: Asian and Pacific Islander Youth in Oakland*. API Youth Violence Prevention Center: National Council on Crime and Delinquency. Oakland, California. Retrieved 25 April 2007 at: http://www.api-center.org/documents/microscope_full_report.pdf.

# CHAPTER 31

# Suicide during war and genocide

David Lester

## Abstract

Research indicates that suicide rates decline during wartime. The most likely explanation for this decline is the greater social cohesion of societies during wartime, but changes in the economy, such as reduced rates of unemployment, may also play a role. The impact of civil wars on suicide rates is unclear since the data in the different reports are inconsistent. Prisoners of war who are treated harshly have higher suicide rates after release. The suicide rate of Jews was high during all phases of the Holocaust in the 1930s and 1940s.

## Introduction

Modern research and theory about the impact of war on suicide date from the classic work by Durkheim (1897). Durkheim noted that suicide rates decline during wars, in both men and women, as they do during other types of crises, and he presented data from the Denmark–Saxony war of 1864, the Austria–Italy war of 1866 and the France–Germany war of 1870 to 1871 to support his conclusion. Many studies have explored this phenomenon since Durkheim drew attention it, and this chapter will review the research.

## Research from the United States

MacMahon, Johnson and Pugh (1963) examined the changing pattern of suicide rates over this century in the United States and noted that, while the suicide rate for females did not change dramatically during the Second World War, the suicide rate for men dropped substantially. MacMahon and his colleagues argued that, since this drop was evident for men of all age groups except those older than 75 years, the drop was not due to suicides being concealed by the Armed Forces. Those aged 65 to 75, for example, would not have been in the Armed Forces. They also noted that the drop in the suicide rate was apparent from 1939 onwards, that is, before America became involved in the war. In 1939, only 3 per cent of American men aged 20–24 were serving in the Armed Forces.

After the war, the suicide rates for men aged 15–34 declined, the suicide rates for those aged 35–44 remained steady, while the suicide rates for those aged 45–75 increased until the outbreak of the Korean War in 1951. Detailed examination of the suicide rates by month indicated that the rise in the suicide rates after the Second World War ended began in the second half of 1945.

Marshall (1981) also noted the drop in the American suicide rate during the Second World War (1942–1945) but found little change during the Korean War (1950–1953) or the Vietnam War (1965–1973). However, Marshall found that the unemployment rate was a stronger predictor of the suicide rate than was wartime and, once he controlled for the impact of unemployment, the effect of wartime was no longer apparent. Biro and Selakovic-Bursic (1996) made a similar point about the increase in the suicide rate in Serbia after the war began in 1991. They noted that the increased rate of suicide could be a result of the dramatic drop in income.

The decrease in suicide rates is found both in the general population and in the military. For example, Yessler (1968) noted that the suicide rate of both officers and enlisted men decreased dramatically during the Second World War and decreased a little during the Korean War.

It appears, therefore, that suicide rates decline during major wars, but the impact that wars have on society that causes this decline remain unclear.

## New research

Lester and Yang have conducted a series of studies looking at the association of various measures of military involvement and suicide rates. For example, the greater the proportion of the population in the military, the lower the suicide rate from 1933 to 1986 (Lester and Yang 1991a). This measure peaked during the Second World War in 1945 at 86.3 per 1,000 residents, with minor peaks during the Korean War in 1952 (23.1) and the Vietnam War in 1968 (17.7). However, controlling for the unemployment rate eliminated this association (Lester and Yang 1991b).

The military participation rate was also associated with lower birth and marriage rates, but not divorce rates (Lester 1993b), higher alcohol consumption (Lester 1993c), reduced unemployment and business failures but not interest rates or growth in the gross national product (Yang and Lester 1994), and lower homicide rates and fewer prisoners sentenced for crimes (Lester 1997).

The association between a lower suicide rate and a high military participation rate was found also for the suicides of military personnel (Lester 1993d). A similar negative association was found between the number of war-related movies produced each year from 1940 to 1986 and the suicide rate (Lester 1991). However, the threat of nuclear war as measured by the 'time clock' published by the *Bulletin of the Atomic Scientists*, which measures how close the world is to a nuclear war, was not associated with the suicide rate (Lester 1992).

Thus, periods of war are associated with lower suicide rates and, for the United States during the present century, a higher military participation rate has been associated with lower suicide rates.

## Studies in other nations

Research on the impact of war on suicide has been conducted in several nations.

### Australia

Hassan and Tan (1989) found no impact of war on suicide rates in Australia from 1901 to 1985 after they controlled for the impact of the changes in urbanization, the extent to which women participated in the labour force, and unemployment rates.

### England

In England and Wales from 1876 to 1975, Low and his colleagues (1981) found that the number of suicides was negatively associated with the male participation rate in the armed forces. The larger the armed forces, the lower the suicide rate of the general population. Lester (1994b) also found lower suicide rates in England and Wales during times of war for the period 1901–1965.

### France

Lester (1993a) found lower suicide rates in France during times of war for the period 1826–1913. Lunden (1946/1947) noted that the suicide rate in France dropped during the First World War and increased afterwards. Lunden had more detailed data for Paris, and he found that the decline in the Parisian suicide rate during the war was found for both men and women and for all of the common methods for suicide.

Lunden did not have data from France as a whole for the beginning of the Second World War, but the suicide rate in Paris again showed a decrease from 1939 to 1943. During the first part of the Second World War, the Parisian suicide rate dropped for all methods, but the decline occurred sooner for firearms than for gas or hanging. The decline in the Parisian suicide rate was noticeable for both individual suicides and suicide pacts and for attempted suicide.

### Israel

Landau and Rahav (1989) obtained monthly measures in Israel of stress from worry about the economy, security, terrorism, and political instability. A combined measure of stress was positively associated with the monthly completed suicide rate of men and negatively with the monthly completed suicide rate of women, but had no association with the monthly rate of attempted suicide in either men or women. The more stress, the higher the suicide rate for men and the lower the suicide rate for women.

### Studies across nations

Lester (1994a) examined the evidence in as many nations as possible for the decline in the suicide rates during wartime. Not all nations had available data, and there may, of course, be systematic bias the official suicide rates reported by nations. For the First World War, the average suicide rate for all nations with available rates was 11.83 per 100,000 per year for 1910–1913, 10.03 for 1915–1918 and 10.95 for 1919–1922. The decline during the war was found both in participating nations and in non-participating nations and for both men and women.

For the Second World War, the average suicide rate for all nations with available data was 12.15 for 1933–1938, 10.51 for 1940–1945 and 10.65 for 1946–1951. As before, the decline during the war was found for both participating and non-participating nations, for men in all nations but only for women in participating nations. The reason for the lack of response to war of female suicide rates in non-participating nations is not clear.

## Explanations

MacMahon and his colleagues speculated that war itself was not the cause of the decline in suicide rates. They suggested that war has an impact on the economy, for example by reducing unemployment, and that these economic changes produce the association between war and suicide rates. Thus, the decrease in the suicide rate may have been a result of the industrial mobilization rather than the military mobilization. The increase in suicide rates of older men after the war may have been a result of the increasing competition for jobs as the young soldiers returned from the war and were demobilized. Those over 75, of course, would not have been affected so much by these economic changes.

Durkheim (1897) argued that, at least for major wars, war increases the degree of social integration and thereby lowers the suicide rate. To understand this explanation, we need to examine Durkheim's theory of suicide in a little more detail. Durkheim argued that the societal suicide rate was determined by two broad social factors: (1) the level of social integration which may be defined as the extent to which the members of the society are bound together in social networks, and (2) the level of social regulation which may be defined as the extent to which the desires and behaviour of the members of the society are governed by social norms, values and customs. Durkheim argued that suicide could result from very low levels of social integration leading to *egoistic* suicide, very high levels of social integration leading to *altruistic* suicide, very low levels of social regulation leading to *anomic* suicide and very high levels of social integration leading to *fatalistic* suicide. War is thought to increase the level of social integration, but not excessively, so that egoistic suicide becomes less common. However, Durkheim did not consider the possible role of individual variables such as psychological traits, psychiatric disorders, and personal values.

In contrast, Henry and Short (1954) used psychoanalytic theory to argue that suicide and homicide were similar but alternative acts of aggression. When suicide rates are high, homicide rates will be low and vice versa. Since war is a time of externally directed aggression, war is associated with a relative drop in the suicide rate. Henry and Short also argued that, when there is a clear external source to blame for our misery, we tend to be angry and direct our anger outward, thereby becoming assaultive and, in the extreme, murderous. On the other hand, when there is no clear external source to blame for our misery and we have only ourselves to blame, then we tend to become depressed and, in the extreme, suicidal. In times of war, there is a clear external cause on which we can pin the blame for our misery, and so anger will be more common and depression less common. Therefore, suicide rates should decrease during times of war. However, it is not clear whether this hypothesis would apply to non-participating nations as well as participating nations.

Rojcewicz (1971) tested competing hypotheses for the effects of war on suicide rates. Since the decrease in suicide rates during wars is found in all age groups and in both those nations at war and those not at war, the reasons for the decrease could not be that potential suicides go off to war and get killed in battle or that war legitimates outward-directed aggression. Yessler (1968) produced some interesting data which argued against the theory that, in wartime, potentially suicidal people get killed in battle so that their suicides are not registered as such. He found that the recorded suicide rate of American Army men in Korea during the Korean War (17.2 per 100,000 per year) was higher than that of American Army men in foreign nations other than Korea (13.4) and higher than that of American Army men at home in the United States (12.2).

Rojcewicz noted that the drop in the suicide rate during the Second World War occurred in 1941 for Sweden (neutral), Norway (invaded and resistant), and France (invaded and compliant). Thus, actual participation in the war was not necessary for the decline in suicide rates to occur. This lead Rojcewicz to conclude that only Durkheim's theory of the effect of war on social integration was a feasible explanation for the decline in suicide rates during wartime.

## Other issues

### Soldiers

Surprisingly, there are few data on the suicide rate of soldiers during wartime as compared to years with no wars. Although there are newspaper accounts of suicides among soldiers during wars, such as reports of suicides among American soldiers in Iraq in 2002 and 2003, estimates of the suicide rate (for example, 13.5 for American soldiers in Iraq [Nelson 2004]) are lower than would be expected for adult males in America (whose suicide rates are about 25). The reasons for this are unclear, but it may be that the military recruitment process screens out those with obvious psychiatric disturbance.

### Prisoners of war

Nefzger (1970) found that the suicide rate of American soldiers who had been prisoners of war in the Second World War or the Korean War was similar to that of American males in general, but the sample sizes were quite small. Hall and Malone (1976) studied six prisoners of war from the Vietnam War and found no evidence of suicidal ideation. However, more recent extensive compilations of mortality data have revealed some interesting trends.

Keehan (1980) followed up American veterans of the Second World War and the Korean War up until 1975. He found a high suicide rate only in prisoners of war in the Second World War held by the Japanese as compared to men of similar age in America. This increased mortality rate from suicide (of some 75 per cent) was not found in prisoners of the Germans, in combat veterans in both arenas who were not captured, or in prisoners or combatants from the Korean War. It is noteworthy, of course, that the treatment of prisoners of war by the Japanese was much more brutal than the treatment of prisoners of war held by other nations. Thus, it may be reasonable to conclude that it was the incredible harsh prison conditions that may have increased the subsequent risk of suicide.

### Civil war

Sri Lanka has long had a very high suicide rate (as high as 45 per 100,000 per year), and Bolz (2002) claimed, without presenting any data, that the civil war in Sri Lanka which began in 1983 had not markedly changed this. Bolz attributed the high suicide rate in Sri Lanka to its high level of collectivism, poor techniques for conflict resolution, repressive education, the influence of foreign media alienating the youth from their families, high rates of substance abuse, and post-traumatic stress disorder due to the civil war. On the other hand, Somasundaram (2003) asserted, without presenting data, that the suicide rate had declined during the period of civil war in Sri Lanka. Civil wars are occasionally accompanied by suicide bombings (Leenaars and Wenckstern 2004), including Sri Lanka, but these do not have a major impact on official suicide rates.

Studies of suicide during the civil war in Croatia in 1991–1995, during the break-up of Yugoslavia, have also produced inconsistent results. Grubisic-Ilic et al. (2002) noted that the suicide rates in Croatia as a whole declined slightly, but significantly, during the war (1991–1995). Furthermore, the suicide rate was lower during the war in those areas of Croatia more affected by the war than in those less affected. The methods for suicide changed during the civil war, with firearms and explosives becoming more popular. Similar results were reported by Jakovljevic et al. (2004) and Bosnar et al. (2005).

On the other hand, Bosnar et al. (2004, 2005) documented that the number of suicides in one region of Croatia increased during the wartime period by 20.9 per cent, and dropped after the war by 26.2 per cent. Interestingly, Loncar et al. (2004) found a similar trend in suicide rates among psychiatric patients in Split, Croatia, suggesting that institutionalized people respond to the same social forces as those in the larger society. Thus, the data from Croatia are inconsistent.

### Refugees

Contrary to their expectation, Slodnjak et al. (2002) found that Bosnian adolescents who had fled to Slovenia at the beginning of the war in Bosnia had lower rates of depressive symptomatology than the Slovenian adolescents used as a control group, but they did not differ in suicidal ideation. They attributed this to differences in national character and values and to the possibly greater social cohesion among the refugees who were sharing a common fate.

### Genocide

In the past, many scholars studied what survivors of the concentration camps have reported (Roden 1982) and concluded that suicide was rare among Jews in the concentration camps during the Second World War. However, recent attempts to calculate suicide rates in the camps by Lester (2005) have suggested that the suicide rates were incredibly high.

Krysinska and Lester (2002) were able to calculate the suicide rate in the Jewish ghetto in Lodz (Poland) from 1941 to 1942 based on written newspaper records that were buried and survived the war, and calculated a completed suicide rate of 44 per 100,000 per year.

Suicide rates among Jews in Germany and Austria were also high in the 1930s in the years prior to the outbreak of war. Kwiet (1984) calculated rates as high as 70, while Lester (2005) compiled all the available data to estimate a suicide rate of close to 160.

It has been difficult to estimate accurate suicide rates for Jews during the Holocaust, despite the fact that this particular genocide has been more thoroughly studied than any other genocide. It has been even more difficult to conduct studies of suicide during other genocides. However, there are hints that suicide rates were high in other genocides. For example, Miller and Miller (1993) reported that suicide was common during the Armenia genocide conducted by the Turks in 1915 and later.

# Conclusions

This chapter has identified several clear associations between war and suicide. During wartime, suicide rates decline, and the most likely explanations of this are the accompanying increase in social integration in nations during times of war and changes in the economy such as reduced unemployment rates resulting from war.

Second, prisoners of war who are treated harshly do have a higher rate of suicide after release. Third, suicide rates among Jews were very high during all phases of the Holocaust during the twentieth century.

Some issues, however, have not been well-researched, such as the suicide rates of soldiers during wartime, or have produced inconsistent results so far such as suicide rates during civil wars.

## References

Biro M and Selakovic-Bursic S (1996). Suicide, aggression and war. *Archives of Suicide Research*, **2**, 75–79.

Bolz W (2002). Psychological analysis of the Sri Lankan conflict culture with special reference to the high suicide rate. *Crisis*, **23**, 167–170.

Bosnar A, Stemberga V, Coklo M *et al.* (2005). Suicide and the war in Croatia. *Forensic Science International*, **147**(Suppl), S13–S16.

Bosnar A, Stemberga V, Cuculic D *et al.* (2004). Suicide rate after the 1991–1995 war in southwestern Croatia. *Archives of Medical Research*, **35**, 344–347.

Durkheim E (1897). *Le suicide*. Felix Alcan, Paris.

Grubisic-Ilic M, Kozaric-Kovacic D, Grubisic F *et al.* (2002). Epidemiological study of suicide in the Republic of Croatia. *European Psychiatry*, **17**, 259–264.

Hall RCW and Malone PT (1976). Psychiatric effects of prolonged Asian captivity. *American Journal of Psychiatry*, **133**, 786–790.

Hassan R and Tan G (1989). Suicide trends in Australia, 1901–1985. *Suicide and Life-Threatening Behaviour*, **19**, 362–380.

Henry AF and Short JF (1954). *Suicide and homicide*. Free Press, Glencoe.

Jakovljevic M, Martinac M, Marcino D *et al.* (2004). Update of suicide trends in Croatia 1966–2002. *Psychiatria Danubina*, **16**, 299–308.

Keehan RJ (1980). Follow-up studies of World War II and Korean conflict prisoners. *American Journal of Epidemiology*, **111**, 194–211.

Krysinska K and Lester D (2002). Suicide in the Lodz ghetto 1941–1944. *Polish Psychological Bulletin*, **33**, 21–26.

Kwiet K (1984). The ultimate refuge. *Leo Baeck Institute Yearbook*, **29**, 135–167.

Landau SF and Rahav G (1989). Suicide and attempted suicide. *Genetic, Social and General Psychological Monographs*, **115**, 273–294.

Leenaars AA and Wenckstern S (eds) (2004). Altruistic suicide. *Archives of Suicide Research*, **8**, 1–136.

Lester D (1991). The association between involvement in war and rates of suicide and homicide. *Journal of Social Psychology*, **131**, 893–895.

Lester D (1992). The threat of nuclear war and rates of suicide and homicide. *Perceptual and Motor Skills*, **75**, 1186.

Lester D (1993a). The effect of war on suicide rates. *European Archives of Psychiatry*, **242**, 248–249.

Lester D (1993b). The effect of war on marriage, divorce and birth rates. *Journal of Divorce and Remarriage*, **19**, 229–231.

Lester D (1993c). War and alcohol use. *Psychological Reports*, **72**, 1282.

Lester D (1993d). Suicide in the military as a function of involvement in war. *Acta Psychiatrica Scandinavica*, **88**, 223.

Lester D (1994a). Suicide rates before, during and after world wars. *European Psychiatry*, **9**, 262–264.

Lester D (1994b). Involvement in war and suicide rates in Great Britain, 1901–1965. *Psychological Reports*, **75**, 1154.

Lester D (1997). Effect of war on crime. *Psychological Reports*, **81**, 194.

Lester D (2005). *Suicide and the Holocaust*. Nova Science, Hauppauge, New York.

Lester D and Yang B (1991a). Association between war and suicide and homicide. *Psychological Reports*, **68**, 1030.

Lester D and Yang B (1991b). The effect of war on personal aggression. *Medicine and War*, **7**, 215–217.

Loncar C, Definis-Gojanovic M, Dodig G *et al.* (2004). War, mental disorder and suicide. *Collegium Antropologium*, **28**, 377–384.

Low AA, Farmer RDT, Jones DR *et al.* (1981). Suicide in England and Wales. *Psychological Medicine*, **11**, 359–368.

Lunden WA (1946/1947). Suicides in France, 1910–1943. *American Journal of Sociology*, **52**, 321–334.

MacMahon B, Johnson S, Pugh TF (1963). Relation of suicide rates to social conditions. *Public Health Reports*, **78**, 285–293.

Marshall JR (1981). Political integration and the effect of war on suicide. *Social Forces*, **59**, 771–785.

Miller DE and Miller LT (1993). *Survivors*. University of California Press, Berkeley.

Nefzger MD (1970). Follow-up studies of Word War II and Korean War prisoners. *American Journal of Epidemiology*, **91**, 123–138.

Nelson R (2004). Suicide rates rise among soldiers in Iraq. *Lancet*, **363**, 300.

Roden RG (1982). Suicide and Holocaust survivors. *Israel Journal of Psychiatry*, **19**, 129–135.

Rojcewicz SJ (1971). War and suicide. *Suicide and Life-Threatening Behaviour*, **1**, 46–54.

Slodnjak V, Kos A, Yule W (2002). Depression and parasuicide in refugee and Slovenian adolescents. *Crisis*, **23**, 127–132.

Somasundaram D (2003). Collective trauma in Sri Lanka. *Intervention*, **1**, 4–13.

Yang B and Lester D (1994). The effect of war on the economy. *Atlantic Economic Journal*, **22**, 81.

Yessler PG (1968). Suicide in the military. In HLP Resnik, ed., *Suicidal Behaviours*, pp. 241–254. Little Brown, Boston.

# PART 5

# Social and Economic Determinants of Suicide

# CHAPTER 32

# Labour market, work environment and suicide

Ilkka Henrik Mäkinen and Danuta Wasserman

## Abstract

Work is an important sphere of human life. Besides economic subsistence, it also furnishes workers with social status and influences their life conditions in a profound manner. Social class at large seems to be connected with suicidality, but studies on the effects of specific occupations have produced few lasting results, perhaps due to the different societies investigated. In addition, lack of adequate data and problems with the methods chosen cause problems in the estimates of suicide mortality by class or occupation. However, it seems that the most vulnerable position is that of those who do not work at all. There is abundant empirical evidence of a surplus risk for suicide among the unemployed, but the causal nature of this relationship still needs clarification. Globally, the labour markets differ greatly, and so does their connection with suicide. Labour-market oriented suicide prevention issues concern unemployment policies, reduction of work-related access to means of suicide, and the use of the workplace as a base for suicide prevention.

## The labour market

Work, the activity on which human beings base their subsistence, is one of the central parts of human life. In a modern society, work is not performed for the needs of the workers and their immediate families only, but for a larger group of potentially interested persons, economically speaking, for a market. At the same time, work itself is a market commodity, bought and sold on the 'labour market'.

The market, and the positions existing on it, varies between societies and over time. Agricultural, industrial, and post-industrial societies all have their specific divisions of labour, with specific positions and labour markets. Seen from this perspective, the sheer number of potential positions to be occupied varies greatly, as does the degree of spatial and chronological separation between work and home.

The seller side of the labour market comprises actively working persons, employed by others or by themselves. Since complex tasks require experience and/or education for their correct performance, an individual's general position on the labour market tends to be stable, reflecting their human capital. Not everyone performs paid work, however, their not doing so is still often related to the labour market, as in the case of the unemployed (persons who would like to work but cannot find employment), the sick (persons judged incapable of working), students (persons presumably in preparation for a position on the labour market), and the retired (mostly persons who have worked). Thus, a majority of any population is in one way or another connected to a labour market and its order, in which the positions are often more or less hierarchically related to each other.

## The importance of labour market positions in individual lives

Individuals' positions on the labour market determine, in broad terms, what kind of physical environment they will spend the major part of their days in, and what kind of stresses their bodies will thereby be exposed to. The same applies to the mental environment, although the variation between specific places of work may be larger in that regard. Moreover, different work situations offer different possibilities to stress relief such as, for example, independent decision-making (Karasek and Theorell 1990). In addition to the mental stimuli provided by the work itself, one must take into account the social work environment consisting of persons close to oneself in terms of location, activities, and status. This is likely to be the second most salient social environment in a working individual's life beside family, and like family, its members are rarely chosen by the individual.

An individual's position on the labour market is a strong social marker, and it is often used as an indicator of one's overall standing in society. Besides that, it is also a major determinant of one's life chances in general through the economic, sociopsychological, and physical conditions it implies. Work is not only a source of material subsistence, but a gateway to many other things, and one of the main ties between the individual and the larger society. This in turn is one important rationale behind the concept of *social class*, a group of people defined by its similar position on the labour market, and who is often supposed to share other significant characteristics as well. Within each class, there is then a number of *occupations*, each with its own qualities and conditions.

The various positions on the labour market are intimately related to the health of the individuals occupying them (Marmot 2004).

Mental health is no exception. Since suicidal behaviour is partly socially conditioned, it would seem logical that different positions on the labour market would also imply different frequencies of suicide, and so they do, to a certain extent. The influences related to the organization of labour can be divided into (a) the effects of different class (and occupational) positions; (b) the effects of immediate work environments; and (c) the effects of a lack of position on the labour market.

Existing models of suicidal behaviours do not usually put directly work-related issues in central positions. However, both stress and object loss are important constitutive parts of many models (see Maris 1997; Wasserman 2001), and these can certainly be related to work.

## Inside the labour market: class, occupation, and work environment

### Class

As regards the hierarchical, more fixed, and partly inherited aspect of the organization of labour in society, the social classes, many studies have at least indirectly investigated the relationship between class and suicide. In contemporary industrialized countries, clear signs of a 'class ladder' in regard to suicide exist among men. Those with low income or education tend to have higher rates of suicide than those with higher income or education, and those in manual work higher than those in non-manual work; even lower-ranking office clerks often have higher suicide rates than those in the higher echelons (Stack 1982, 2000; Platt and Hawton 2000; Blakely et al. 2002; Qin et al. 2003; Kwan et al. 2005; Kalediene et al. 2006; Kim et al. 2006; Stark et al. 2006). The differences in suicide rates between the lowest and highest positions are typically two- or threefold. Mäki and Martikainen (2007) have calculated that the class difference in suicide mortality contributed 0.6 years (or 10 per cent) to the general difference in the life expectancy (at age 25) between manual workers and upper-echelon non-manual workers in Finland in 1991–2000.

However, the steepness, and sometimes even the existence, of the class ladder depends on the method used to determine the suicide risk, the specific groups studied, the time of the study, and other factors controlled for (Stack 2001; Lostao et al. 2006). Comparisons between groups are sometimes made using proportional mortality ratios (PMR), which relate the mortality from suicide to that from all causes. This tends to highlight suicides in groups with lower overall mortality (Kelly et al. 1995; Platt and Hawton 2000; Stack 2001), and the results must be interpreted accordingly. To take an example: in Japan, standardized all-cause mortality among miners in the ages of 20–64 was five times higher than that among managers in 1985 (Fujioka et al. 2002). Thus, five miners' suicides would be needed to produce the same proportional measure of 'suicide risk' than one managerial suicide. However, there is no obvious reason why suicide mortality and mortality from other causes should be related to each other.

Stack (2001) found in the USA that the higher risks for suicide among manual workers were no longer significantly higher when the demographic differences between occupational groups were controlled for. Class differences are often closely intertwined with those in other matters: lower-class men may, for example, have an elevated risk for divorce due to their low, work-based social

position and the disadvantages it entails. Should a suicide in this situation be attributed to the divorce or the social position? Moreover, many occupational groups have their characteristic demographics which partly shape the prevailing work atmosphere, perhaps influencing even mental health and suicidality. The meaning and implications of the controls used in analyses is sometimes uncertain (Agerbo et al. 2007a).

The empirical evidence concerning the impact of social class on women's suicide is more mixed. Some studies find relations more or less similar to those prevailing among men (Pensola and Martikainen 2003; Steenland et al. 2003; Kim et al. 2006), while others would seem to indicate a surplus risk for suicide among women in *higher* classes (Kelly et al. 1995), and still others find either inconsistent relations (Blakely et al. 2002; Lorant et al. 2005), or none at all (Kwan et al. 2005). This may reflect women's various—and changing—roles in relation to the labour market in different societies, but also the fact that their general socio-economic position is less often defined by their own occupation or income than men's, which makes individual-based class definitions more insecure.

However, seen in a larger perspective, social class seems to be connected with suicide not mainly through the economic and status positions it implies, but through its cultural aspect, the specific ways of thinking and acting which may be connected with certain classes. Rather than having any absolute effect on suicidal behaviour, class membership 'organizes' it much in the same way as it patterns other behaviours. Thus, the relation between class and suicide must be understood in its specific context.

To take an example, higher classes were over-represented among suicides in Czarist Russia a century ago, while the opposite is true today (Mäkinen 2002, 2006). The reason for this shift can hardly be economic or status-related, since those differences between the different classes in Russia remain similar today. However, the individualism and secularism which separated the educated higher classes from others in the past and 'enabled' them culturally to commit suicide, have now spread to the whole society, turning the class ladder upside down. In France, the lower rates of suicide in poor areas led Emile Durkheim in 1897 to his famous hypothesis of the suicide-protective effect of poverty. However, later developments have shown that it did not stand the test of time (Rehkopf and Buka 2006).

### Occupation

There are differences in suicidal behaviour between the members of different occupational groups. Although Stack (2001) concludes, on the basis of studies in the USA and in England, that 'most occupations tend neither to drive people to suicide nor to offer protection against suicide', there are exceptions. However, the question has been studied in different circumstances and using different methodologies, and the studies have often been limited by the small numbers of suicide cases or otherwise insufficient data.

Studies analysing many occupational groups at once are not very numerous. In Stack's analysis in 21 US states in 1990, 12 occupations out of the 32 studied showed a significantly higher risk (PMR) for suicidal death, among them dentists, physicians, artists, and carpenters (Stack 2001). On the other hand, elementary school teachers, postal workers, and clerks were at a significantly lower risk. In Agerbo et al.'s (2007a) study of Denmark in 1991–1997, high suicide rates were observed among medical doctors, nurses, plant and machine operators, and drivers and mobile-plant operators, among others. Architects, engineers, and technicians were found to be at lowest risk.

Kposowa (1999), studying industrial and occupational groups in the USA in 1979–1989, found that persons employed in the mining industry had the highest relative suicide risk (RR), 4.39 times greater than that of the comparison group of finance, insurance, and real estate employees. Persons employed in construction and in business and repair services were also at a very high risk. When the material was divided according to the occupational positions within industries, only laborers differed significantly (with a two-fold surplus risk) from the reference group. Burnley (1995) on the other hand, in a study performed in New South Wales in Australia in 1985–1991, found that farmers, transport and production workers and labourers had high suicide mortality, while miners and quarrymen showed significantly lower rates. Kagamimori *et al.* (2004) found similar results in their study of Japan between 1965–1995.

Why would there be a relationship between one's occupation and the propensity for suicide? Different explanations may apply in different cases. First, there may be a relatively direct relation between occupation-related stress and suicide in cases where very stressful situations are regularly encountered in one's work, or where a more permanent stressful situation, such as one's income being dependent on customers, is a part of the conditions. Labovitz and Hagedorn (1971), comparing client-dependent occupations with others in the USA, found a 60 per cent higher suicide rate among persons in such occupations.

There are also more temporary situations, where some occupational groups—for example, over-indebted Southern Indian cotton farmers (Stone 2002)—encounter grave crises and may then respond suicidally. Farmers are a group with a very specific, 'lifestyle' work whose suicide risks are often discussed when different crises afflict agriculture. However, it has also been found that the rationalization of agriculture has not influenced the suicide rates in Europe discernibly during the post-war period (Mäkinen and Stickley 2006), possibly because of the existence of sufficient alternatives.

Secondly, some occupations provide knowledge of the means of suicide, and sometimes also a privileged access to them. Doctors and care personnel (Wasserman 1992; Kelly *et al.* 1995; Hawton *et al.* 2000; Stack 2001, 2004; Hawton *et al.* 2004; Stark *et al.* 2006; Agerbo *et al.* 2007a) are probably those most studied in this regard. Stack (2004) estimates the suicide risk of US physicians to be 2.45 times higher than the average of the working-age population, after controlling for demographic factors, while the surplus risk for dentists (Stack 2001) was calculated to 5.43. Access to means of suicide is the most frequently quoted cause in the discussions of health care personnel suicide. However, other factors such as work-related stress and client dependency should not be dismissed.

Military personnel (Desjeux *et al.* 2004; Mahon *et al.* 2005), policemen (Schmidtke *et al.* 1999), and even the large agricultural populations of many developing countries (Nwosu and Odesanmi 2001; Khan 2002; CDC 2004; Recena *et al.* 2006) are also thus endangered, although research on military or police suicide does not always witness of higher rates among these groups (Stack and Kelley 1994; Loo 2003; Aasland *et al.* 2005; see also Chapter 36 in this book). Agricultural workers with access to highly toxic pesticides constitute the numerically largest identifiable group in the world at high risk for occupation-related suicide. However, there may also be cases of beneficial *non-*access to means of suicide. Schwartz (2006), for example, ascribes the low suicide rate of American college students to the fact that firearms have been banned from the campuses.

Thirdly, there is the selection of people into occupations—for example, character traits necessary or desirable for certain work may also be more prevalent among persons who are more prone to commit suicide. An example of such a connection is Wasserman's (1992) hypothesis that persons with depressive symptoms would more often be found among psychiatrists. Also, socially downwards-spiralling life careers often lead to certain kinds of work, of necessity rather than free will, which might then show high suicide rates. The high rates observed among unskilled workers may be partly due to such processes. To this category of causes could also in part be included what Stack (2001) calls 'demographics', i.e. the fact that different occupational groups are differently composed as regards sex, age, ethnicity, marital state, and other properties. Here, the class aspect of occupation is clearly visible. According to Agerbo *et al.* (2007a), class is the main factor behind the observed differences in suicidality between occupations.

Finally, more refined theories may attribute the high suicide rates in certain occupations to the fact that their members are exposed to some more general circumstances that are thought to generate suicide. People in commercial professions were, for example, especially exposed to anomie in Durkheim's classical theory, while those whose work did not comply with their other roles were supposed to suffer from status incompatibility ('role strain') according to Gibbs and Martin (1964). Such generalizations provide alternatives to the classification principles besides stress, access, and selection.

## Work environment

The everyday work environment, connected with but not determined by the previous aspects of one's labour market position, also seems to exercise influence on suicidal behaviour. Theoretically, that influence is of a different order—a work environment situation is in most cases changeable, while occupation may not be, and class is even more permanent (Erikson and Goldthorpe 1992). In addition, the working conditions themselves may change rapidly due to new technologies and organisational changes, the effects being different for different groups involved (Smith 1997; Wikman 2004). At the same time, the effects—including the health effects—of class are partly mediated through the quality of one's working environment (Borg and Kristensen 2000), and the same is probably true of occupations (Arnetz 2001).

Work environment is usually ascribed a more active role in the causation of suicide than class or occupation, and it also affects the individual's life in a more direct manner. Its main potential influences can be divided into the more permanent, related to the character of the work itself, the less permanent, pertaining to the actual workload, and those related to the social relations at the place of work.

In the Swedish Five County Study, Karasek and Theorell (1990) found that a work situation with few possibilities to learn new things was associated with a surplus risk for suicide or attempt of 2.44 among men, while hectic and monotonous work more than doubled the risk for women. Feskanich *et al.* (2002) found an association between both very high and very low occupational stress and suicide among US nurses, especially when combined with domestic stress. Even knowledge of dangerous substances present at the place of work could be counted into these more permanent stress factors—the Chernobyl nuclear accident clean-up workers are a salient example (Rahu *et al.* 2006).

In a study of Japanese work-related suicide cases, Amagasa *et al.* (2005) noted the heavy workloads and long working hours relevant in the context. Even positive processes such as company expansion can lead to negative outcomes (Westerlund *et al.* 2004). The very importance of work and the hierarchic nature of its organization can also make the workplace a potential source of deep conflict. The style of conflict resolution at the workplace has been linked to mental well-being in general (Hyde *et al.* 2006). In extreme cases the conflicts may result in bullying, which is undoubtedly psychologically detrimental but has so far been little researched in relation to adult workplaces (Leymann 1990).

A parent's work conditions may also affect the children: Aleck *et al.* (2006) report finding a relationship between fathers' adverse psychosocial work conditions and suicides (and suicide attempts) among their children in a cohort of Canadian sawmill workers.

# Outside the labour market

## Who is outside the labour market?

In line with the classic theory of Durkheim, work can be understood as one of those important ties that integrate individuals into the larger society and regulate their everyday life, providing them with realistic means to fulfil some of their basic needs. Accordingly, just having a position in the labour market would in itself seem to be very important.

Not everyone works in a modern society. Even in the most employment-friendly societies, such as Denmark, 'only' 75 per cent of the working-age population is likely to be gainfully employed. The growing complexity of modern societies produces different groups of adults who for different reasons are permanently or temporarily outside the labour market. In addition to the traditional housewives, the severely ill and handicapped, conscript soldiers, and prisoners, we also have students, retired persons, unemployed persons, those on a disability pension, welfare recipients, asylum applicants, and others—there is little that is common for all these groups, except their not performing paid labour at the moment. Global comparisons are also more difficult here than in the case of social classes or occupations—the categories are very differently present in different societies, and those based on legal definitions are also often differently defined.

Of all the 'outsider' groups mentioned above, persons retired due to old age and students are the largest ones in contemporary Western societies. Persons older than 65 years typically constitute up to a fifth of the adult population (15+ years) in economically developed countries, while students of working age constitute roughly one-tenth of it. Depending on the society, housewives or disability pensioners may also be numerous, as may the unemployed in hard times. In Europe, Poland and Slovakia have lately shown unemployment rates around 15 per cent, corresponding to approximately 10 per cent of the entire working-age population. Together all these groups may easily constitute half of the adult population of any industrialized society.

The unemployed are probably the most researched group from the point of view of suicide. However, members of the other groups outside the labour market may live in equally detrimental situations.

## Suicide risk in groups outside the labour market

### Unemployment

Persons who commit suicide are generally less often employed than others (Heikkinen *et al.* 1995b; Agerbo 2005). A two-to-fourfold surplus risk for suicide has often been observed among the unemployed in different parts of the world, mostly even after controlling for other variables, in individual-level studies based on cases from national mortality registers (Iversen *et al.* 1987; Platt *et al.* 1992; Andrian 1996;, Kposowa 2001; Blakely *et al.* 2002, 2003; Qin *et al.* 2003), and even using twin registers (Voss *et al.* 2004). The risk is often assessed by comparing with the fully employed, or with some other average value. This, along with the different properties controlled for, may account for differing results. Despite the individual surplus risk, Qin *et al.* (2003) calculated, on the basis of Danish register data, a population attributable risk (PAR) of only 2.8 per cent to unemployment. Others (Platt *et al.* 1992: 4.5–9.6 per cent) have presented somewhat higher figures in a situation with higher unemployment.

The risk for suicide when unemployed is generally thought to be less for women than for men (Platt 1984; Platt *et al.* 1992; Qin *et al.* 2003), but this finding is not consistent (see Blakely 2003). Kposowa (2001) in her follow-up study points out that the surplus risk among unemployed women lasts for a longer time and even increases with time. Other studies suggest that the time between the onset of unemployment and the suicidal act is generally relatively short (Blakely *et al.* 2003).

### Retirement

It could seem that the suicide rates of the elderly in general would be influenced by factors other than work or retirement, since the form of the age curve of suicide seems to depend on the society in question. However, Girard (1993) argues that especially the propensity of men's suicides in achievement-oriented societies to increase towards old age witnesses of the fact that the status risks of life in these grow towards old age. Retirement, especially for men, seems to constitute a risky life event (Qin *et al.* 2000; Harwood *et al.* 2006). In Qin *et al.*'s study (2003), the suicide PAR measure for being an age pensioner was 10.2 per cent. However, since being an old age pensioner is almost equal with having reached certain age, that risk also contains the risk of being old.

### Disability pension

Currently, more information is needed concerning disability pensioners, who seem to show very high rates of suicide in the places where they have been researched. Agerbo *et al.* (2007b) found in Denmark that their 'rest' group, consisting of persons neither employed nor unemployed, had a surplus suicide risk of 4–6 times among women, and 4–8 among men. In Qin *et al.*'s study (2003), the PAR measure for being on a disability pension was 3.2 per cent. It is possible, depending on the society in question, that this group contains many members whose reasons for being on a disability pension are connected to a high risk of suicide, such as severe mental illness or substance abuse (Karlsson *et al.* 2007).

### Groups at a lesser risk

There are also groups outside the regular labour market, such as students and homemakers, who do not generally show elevated rates of suicide (Niemi and Lönnqvist 1993; Schwartz 2006). Thus the risk for suicide due to being outside the labour market seems to depend on the position occupied by the individual. Compared with many other categories, students, housewives and also motivated conscript soldiers might be able to construct more positive life-roles out of their social positions, which also entail work, although usually unpaid.

### Unemployment: ecological-level evidence

In addition to individual-level studies, the covariation of a social environment with a higher or lower level of unemployment with suicide mortality has also been researched. The evidence on the question whether the level of unemployment in a social grouping (most often persons living in the same geographical area) is connected to that group's suicide rate has been generally negative in contemporary societies (Platt 1984; Zimmerman 1995; Mäkinen 1997; Platt and Hawton 2000), although there are exceptions (Martikainen et al. 2004), and some authors (Rehkopf and Buka 2006) suggest that the fault may lie in deficient study designs. The relationship between unemployment and suicide has also been researched with the help of time-series studies, where the rates of unemployment and suicide are related over time. Here the results are mixed: both significantly positive (Morrell et al. 1993; Gruenewald et al. 1995; Norström 1995; Gunnell et al. 1999) and non-significant relationships (Mäkelä 1996; Lucey et al. 2005) have been found.

Nevertheless, the exact effect of any social position on suicide is determined by the specific context of the society and time in question. While the effects of unemployment were hard to find in the unemployment crises of Scandinavia in the beginning of the 1990s (Hintikka et al. 1999; Hagquist et al. 2000), they seemed unquestionable in the same societies—and others—in the mass unemployment situations of the 1920s and 1930s (Norström 1995; Gunnell et al. 1999). The difference may lie in the far less dramatic social consequences of contemporary unemployment in welfare societies.

The 'paradoxal' theory, on the other hand, has stated that lower suicide rates *among the unemployed* should be expected in areas with high unemployment, since unemployment would be less of a social stigma in places and times where it is common. So far the evidence seems to speak against this theory (Martikainen et al. 2004; Ahs and Westerling 2006; Agerbo et al. 2007b).

### The nature of the relationship between unemployment and suicide

The mechanisms thought to be responsible for the relationship between unemployment and suicide correspond to those proposed for the relationships between other work-related positions and suicide. Unemployment, a state of seeking but not currently having an important social position in life, is stressful and stigmatizing as such; furthermore, the blessings of work are missing, making the individual psychologically more vulnerable to any other adversities, and increasing the possibility of isolation, substance abuse, and general mental ill-health. All this can contribute to provoking emotional states conducive to suicidal behaviour.

Recent studies (Blakely et al. 2003; Gerdtham and Johannesson 2003) suggest that the weaker economic position per se does not cause the relationship between unemployment and suicide. Blakely et al. (2003) found instead that the main mechanism connecting unemployment to suicide is the fact that unemployment is likely to lead to worse mental health. In a Finnish study, Heikkinen et al. (1995a) found that unemployment, a common event preceding especially young men's suicide, was also associated with alcohol misuse.

However, selection, the possibility that some persons may end up both unemployed and suicidal due to a third factor, such as mental illness, is also generally thought to be relevant when discussing the relationship. The question is difficult to solve because prospective longitudinal studies, which could determine the correct chronological order of events, are very difficult to organize due to the long time intervals and the small number of cases involved. The question of causality between unemployment and suicide is being actively researched and discussed (see, for example, the August 2003 issue of the *Journal of Epidemiology and Community Health*).

Finally, unemployment is not only an individual issue but a macro-economic state of affairs. Norström (1995), interpreting the difference in the attributable risk for suicide due to unemployment between individual- and aggregate-level studies (the risk estimate in the latter being far higher), points out that unemployment in society has also indirect effects, affecting more persons than only the unemployed.

# Different societies, different labour markets, different lives

So far, this chapter has mostly considered suicide in relation to labour markets such as they appear in the countries of Europe, North America, and East Asia, where an overwhelming majority of the studies have been conducted. This is due to both the availability of statistics of suicide, and the register systems that allow us to track individuals' labour market status after their death. Without these, little can be said about differences in suicidality between social and occupational groups. Lacking the tools for more advanced studies, the sampling of consecutive cases at a morgue, for example, is a good alternative, but it can seldom produce so many cases that they could reveal more than the most obvious relations. Suicide waves pertaining to certain places and groups are reported, but their value for systematic research is at present uncertain.

The labour markets of the world are very different due to different natural environments, different development of the division of labour, and also different political steering and control systems modifying the markets in different societies. Moreover, they may also differ greatly within single countries, especially large ones, but even elsewhere as a result of the globalization process. Thus, the traditional division described below must be read with some caution, keeping in mind that even modern societies retain parts of the earlier ways of organization.

In those societies where market-based transactions have not fully replaced the earlier, gender- and kinship-based forms of labour division, the labour market is restricted by these factors; unemployment or retirement in the modern sense of the word do not really exist either. Where labour is performed as a part of socially and culturally ascribed role obligation, it is a part of individuals' set life careers. This organization may increase the risk for suicide greatly in those cases where the expected life career is not a desirable one. The situation of new brides in societies with arranged (or determined) marriages is an example of a such precarious situation, where one's kinship, social status, and labour follow a traditional 'script'. Bleak prospects plague also people with a background in tribal societies (Bjerregaard and Lynge 2006; CDC 2007), whose traditional ways are often being threatened, rendering their customary work trivial or superfluous.

Industrial societies have replaced (and merged) the traditional forms of residence, labour, and thinking with modern urbanity, mobility, wage-labour, and secularization, all of which advance the role of an individual no more dependent from her kin and tradition. For the 'rootless' modern individual, ties to the greater society, such as work, become increasingly important, and losing one's work through unemployment or even retirement may be a difficult challenge. In western Europe, the change from agricultural to industrial society brought about a dramatic rise in suicide mortality during the nineteenth and early twentieth centuries (Cavan 1928); in other parts of the world similar processes have taken place later. It is, however, an open question whether this development is the fate of all societies or not.

In the most affluent, post-industrial societies, workers are typically more protected, and the detrimental effects of unemployment, for example, can to some extent be mitigated (cf. above). However, there are some visible trends on the labour market which affect everyone participating in the global economy, but which are thought to deteriorate the current work conditions, especially in these countries because they affect the attained job security. Globalization, the process of increasing communication over national borders, has since the 1990s reached a new phase due to the Internet and the flow of multinational information that it brings to those able to use it. Together with the worldwide movement towards 'open trade' it sharpens the competition on those markets where foreign goods and services can be brought in. Producers attempt to increase their own mobility in turn. In the process workplaces, still relatively immovable only half a century ago, are created, closed, and moved at an ever-increasing pace.

For the working population in economically advanced countries, the prospects are uncertain. They face increasing demands of 'flexibility', which increase their work-related stress and can in some cases make planned life outside work difficult. Their work may become a target for outsourcing, the move of specific tasks outside the mother company at home or abroad, and they may either become unemployed or have to accept new work conditions at a new employer. Another trend is the 'outsourcing' of even relatively regular work, thereby forcing employees to become small entrepreneurs, with the risks that this entails. All this insecurity has, of course, its psychological consequences (Benavides et al. 2000; Cheng et al. 2005), of which increasing suicidality can be one. However, research on these issues in relation to suicide is still largely absent.

Among those in the weakest positions on the labour market, insecurity is only a part of what is known as 'underemployment' of the working poor, including involuntary part-time work, poverty-level wages, and insecurity, which all erode the benefits of regular work, incomes, social status, and set daily routines (Dooley et al. 1996). Stark et al. (2006) speculate on the possibility that underemployment might be one cause for the over-representation of low-income persons among suicides.

It is difficult to say anything truly universal about the relationship between labour market positions and suicide, and very little globally oriented research has been undertaken. Unemployment, due to its generally negative nature and adverse financial consequences, may be considered a rather general risk factor for suicide, as the studies from many different countries (Koronfel 2002; Gururaj et al. 2004; Chen et al. 2006) show. Vijayakumar et al. (2005a) think that low socio-economic position might also be a universal risk factor.

However, the consequences of seemingly similar positions are not identical in different societies, and their effects on suicide are not similar either. The perceived importance of work in life varies between different societies, too. Kölves et al.'s (2006) finding that suicide after a job loss was more common in Tallinn (Estonia) than in Frankfurt am Main (Germany) might be an illustration of this. Also, studies of individual motives for suicide show that these vary greatly between different cultures (Bhatia et al. 1987). All this once again underlines the importance of careful, nuanced analyses of the relations between different social status positions and suicide worldwide.

## The suicide prevention point of view

The effectiveness of suicide-preventive measures is sometimes questioned, and the relative rarity of completed suicides is a constant obstacle for their scientific evaluation (Goldney 2005). In the national plans for suicide prevention so far in force, features related to working life can be divided into three categories: work and unemployment policies, reduction of work-related access to means of suicide, and improved access to help for substance abuse and other mental problems through place of work (Taylor, Kingdom and Jenkins 1997; Singh and Jenkins 2000; Wasserman et al. 2002, 2004).

It is uncertain to what extent policies aimed at reducing unemployment should be motivated by the reduced suicide risk (Mäkinen 1999; Goldney 2005). However, De Leo and Russel (2004) are of the opinion that measures pertaining to social and economic policy in times of crisis might be effective in preventing especially younger persons' suicides. Morrell et al. (2007) found in Australia a statistically significant relation between the National Youth Suicide Prevention Strategy and the decline in suicide, while there was no relation between the prevention strategy and unemployment. The authors suggest that this means that young male suicide and unemployment are no more correlated. According to Preti (2003), work is suicide-preventive for 'mentally suffering' persons. Yet Agerbo (2005), on the basis of his Danish study showing less suicidality among the unemployed who were admitted to psychiatric care, compared to the employed, does not think that this would be effective. In fact, work-related stress could worsen the existing mental problems.

Preventive measures targeting the access to suicide methods are both easier to implement and more effective than many other approaches (Gunnell and Frankel 1994). An obvious goal here is the reduction of the number of suicides committed with the help of pesticides in the rural areas of developing countries (Gunnell and Eddleston 2003; Vijayakumar et al. 2005b). The World Health Organization (WHO) announced a global public health initiative in 2005 to come to terms with this problem (Bertolote et al. 2006).

The workplace can also be used as a platform for suicide prevention, where a large number of persons can be reached. At the same time, it is difficult due to the relative rarity of suicide and the ensuing difficulties in motivating employers to preventive action (Lewis *et al.* 1997). This may be easier with very large employers such as the US Air Force, whose suicide-preventive program, seeking to facilitate recognition and treatment of psycho-social problems in 1997–2002, was accompanied by a 33 per cent reduction in the rate of suicide compared to the period before the intervention (Knox *et al.* 2003).

However, programs designed to identify and help persons dependent on alcohol or drugs are, due to their immediate usefulness, more likely to meet acceptance. Programs aiming at an early detection of depression are also of interest in this context (Wasserman 2006). Platt and Hawton (2000) suggest more general health promotion initiatives targeted at the occupations at risk, such as farmers and medical personnel, designed to promote help-seeking, reduce organisational stressors, and facilitate stress management. The retraining programs at closing industrial sites could also be used to that end.

# Conclusions

Suicide prevention in relation to the labour market can entail both prevention of the negative consequences connected with some occupations and working environments and the use of the workplace as a platform for general suicide-preventive measures. The current national programmes focus mostly on unemployment policies and restrictions to the means of suicide. The programmes in workplaces promoting early detection of mental problems, depression, and alcohol/drug abuse should be encouraged.

There are many needs left to be fulfilled in this area of research. The most acute of these is the lack of data on suicide, which still hampers research in most countries. More systematic, replicable research is needed on social classes and occupations, and especially on the relation between the working environment and suicide. While unemployment studies belong to the more developed parts of suicide research, more knowledge is needed concerning both the 'underemployed' and the many different groups outside the labour market. Indirectly, this should lead to better recognition of what factors are important in having work (or not) in different societies. Obviously, any work-related suicide prevention programmes would have to take into account the reasons why certain groups have elevated suicide rates in order to better target their actions.

# References

Aasland OG, Ekeberg I, Haldorsen T *et al.* (2005). Suicide rates according to education with a particular focus on physicians in Norway 1960–2000. *Psychological Medicine*, **35**, 873–880.

Agerbo E (2005). Effect of psychiatric illness and labour market status on suicide: a healthy worker effect? *Journal of Epidemiology and Community Health*, **59**, 598–602.

Agerbo E, Gunnell D, Bonde JP *et al.* (2007a). Suicide and occupation: the impact of socio-economic, demographic and psychiatric differences. *Psychological Medicine*, **37**, 1131–1140.

Agerbo E, Sterne JA, Gunnell DJ (2007b). Combining individual and ecological data to determine compositional and contextual socio-economic risk factors for suicide. *Social Science and Medicine*, **64**, 451–461.

Ahs AM and Westerling R (2006). Mortality in relation to employment status during different levels of unemployment. *Scandinavian Journal of Public Health*, **34**, 159–167.

Aleck O, Stefania M, James T *et al.* (2006). The impact of fathers' physical and psychosocial work conditions on attempted and completed suicide among their children. *BMC Public Health*, **6**, 77.

Amagasa T, Nakayama T, Takahashi Y (2005). Karojisatsu in Japan: characteristics of 22 cases of work-related suicide. *Journal of Occupational Health*, **47**, 157–164.

Andrian J (1996). Suicide in the prime of life [in French]. *Cahiers de sociologie et démographie médicales*, **36**, 171–200.

Arnetz BB (2001). Psychosocial challenges facing physicians of today. *Social Science and Medicine*, **52**, 203–213.

Benavides FG, Benach J, Diez-Roux AV *et al.* (2000). How do types of employment relate to health indicators? Findings from the Second European Survey on Working Conditions. *Journal of Epidemiology and Community Health*, **54**, 499–501.

Bertolote JM, Fleischmann A, Eddleston M *et al.* (2006). Deaths from pesticide poisoning: a global response. *British Journal of Psychiatry*, **189**, 201–203.

Bhatia SC, Khan MH, Mediratta RP *et al.* (1987). High risk suicide factors across cultures. *International Journal of Social Psychiatry*, **33**, 226–236.

Bjerregaard P and Lynge I (2006). Suicide—a challenge in modern Greenland. *Archives of Suicide Research*, **10**, 209–220.

Blakely T, Woodward A, Pearce N *et al.* (2002). Socio-economic factors and mortality among 25–64-year-olds followed from 1991 to 1994: the New Zealand Census Mortality Study. *New Zealand Medical Journal*, **115**, 93–97.

Blakely T, Collings SC, Atkinson J (2003) Unemployment and suicide. Evidence for a causal association? *Journal of Epidemiology and Community Health*, **57**, 594–600.

Borg V and Kristensen T (2000). Social class and self-rated health: can the gradient be explained by differences in life style or work environment? *Social Science and Medicine*, **51**, 1019–1030.

Burnley IH (1995). Socioeconomic and spatial differentials in mortality and means of committing suicide in New South Wales, Australia, 1985–91. *Social Science and Medicine*, **41**, 687–698.

Cavan, RS (1928). *Suicide*. Chicago University Press, Chicago.

CDC (Centers for Disease Control and Prevention) (2004). Suicide and attempted suicide—China, 1990–2002. *Morbidity and Mortality Weekly Report*, **53**, 481–484.

CDC (Centers for Disease Control and Prevention) (2007). Suicide trends and characteristics among persons in the Guaraní Kaiowá and Nandeva communities—Mato Grosso do Sul, Brazil, 2000–2005. *Morbidity and Mortality Weekly Report*, **56**, 7–9.

Chen EY, Chan WS, Wong PW *et al.* (2006). Suicide in Hong Kong: a case–control psychological autopsy study. *Psychological Medicine*, **36**, 815–825.

Cheng Y, Chen CW, Chen CJ *et al.* (2005). Job insecurity and its association with health among employees in the Taiwanese general population. *Social Science and Medicine*, **61**, 41–52.

De Leo D and Russel E (2004). *International Suicide Rates and Prevention Strategies*. Hogrefe and Huber, Göttingen.

Desjeux G, Labarère J, Galoisy-Guibal L *et al.* (2004). Suicide in the French armed forces. *European Journal of Epidemiology*, **19**, 823–829.

Dooley D, Fielding J, Levi L (1996). Health and unemployment. *Annual Review of Public Health*, **17**, 449–465.

Erikson R and Goldthorpe JH (1992). *The Constant Flux: A Study of Class Mobility in Industrial Societies*. Clarendon Press, Oxford.

Feskanich D, Hastrup JL, Marshall JR *et al.* (2002). Stress and suicide in the Nurses' Health Study. *Journal of Epidemiology and Community Health*, **56**, 95–98.

Fujioka M, Morii H, Yoshinaga K *et al.* (2002). Comparison of occupational mortality between the Nordic countries and Japan, with analysis by age group in Japan, using micro-data and the Statistical Pattern Analysis (SPA) method. *Bulletin of Labour Statistics*, ILO, 1/2002.

Gerdtham UG and Johannesson M (2003). A note on the effect of unemployment on mortality. *Journal of Health Economics*, **22**, 505–518.

Gibbs J and Martin W (1964). *Status Integration and Suicide*. University of Oregon Press, Eugene.

Girard C (1993). Age, gender, and suicide: a cross-national analysis. *American Sociological Review*, **58**, 553–574.

Goldney RD (2005). Suicide prevention. a pragmatic review of recent studies. *Crisis*, **26**, 128–140.

Gruenewald PJ, Ponicki WR, Mitchell PR (1995). Suicide rates and alcohol consumption in the United States, 1970–89. *Addiction*, **90**, 1063–1075.

Gunnell D and Eddleston M (2003). Suicide by intentional ingestion of pesticides: a continuing tragedy in developing countries. *International Journal of Epidemiology*, **32**, 902–909.

Gunnell D and Frankel S (1994). Prevention of suicide: aspirations and evidence. *British Medical Journal*, **308**, 1227–1233.

Gunnell D, Lopatatzidis A, Dorling D *et al.* (1999). Suicide and unemployment in young people. Analysis of trends in England and Wales, 1921–1995. *British Journal of Psychiatry*, **175**, 263–270.

Gururaj G, Isaac MK, Subbakrishna DK *et al.* (2004). Risk factors for completed suicides: a case–control study from Bangalore, India. *Injury Control and Safety Promotion*, **11**, 183–191.

Hagquist C, Silburn SR, Zubrick SR *et al.* (2000) Suicide and mental health problems among Swedish youth in the wake of the 1990s recession. *International Journal of Social Welfare*, **9**, 211–219.

Harwood DM, Hawton K, Hope T *et al.* (2006). Life problems and physical illness as risk factors for suicide in older people: a descriptive and case-control study. *Psychological Medicine*, **36**, 1265–1274.

Hawton K, Clemets A, Simkin S *et al.* (2000). Doctors who kill themselves: a study of the methods used for suicide. *QJM*, **93**, 351–357.

Hawton K, Malmberg A, Simkin S (2004). Suicide in doctors. A psychological autopsy study. *Journal of Psychosomatic Research*, **57**, 1–4.

Heikkinen ME, Isometsä ET, Aro HM *et al.* (1995a). Age-related variation in recent life events preceding suicide. *The Journal of Nervous and Mental Disease*, **183**, 325–331.

Heikkinen ME, Isometsä ET, Marttunen MJ *et al.* (1995b). Social factors in suicide. *British Journal of Psychiatry*, **167**, 747–753.

Hintikka J, Saarinen PI, Viinamäki H (1999). Suicide mortality in Finland during an economic cycle, 1985–1995. *Scandinavian Journal of Public Health*, **27**, 85–88.

Hyde M, Jäppinen P, Theorell T *et al.* (2006). Workplace conflict resolution and the health of employees in the Swedish and Finnish units of an industrial company. *Social Science and Medicine*, **63**, 2218–2227.

Iversen L, Andersen O, Andersen PK *et al.* (1987). Unemployment and mortality in Denmark, 1970–80. *British Medical Journal*, **295**, 879–884.

Kagamimori S, Kitagawa T, Nasermoaddeli A *et al.* (2004). Differences in mortality rates due to major specific causes between Japanese male occupational groups over a recent 30-year period. *Industrial Health*, **42**, 328–335.

Kalediene R, Starkuviene S, Petrauskiene J (2006). Social dimensions of mortality from external causes in Lithuania: do education and place of residence matter? *Sozial und Präventivmedizin*, **51**, 232–239.

Karasek R and Theorell T (1990). *Healthy Work. Stress, Productivity and the Reconstruction of Working Life*. Basic Books, New York.

Karlsson N, Carstensen J, Gjesdal S *et al.* (2007). Mortality in relation to disability pension: findings from a 12-year prospective population-based study in Sweden. *Scandinavian Journal of Public Health*, **35**, 341–347.

Kelly S, Charlton J, Jenkins R (1995). Suicide deaths in England and Wales 1982–92: the contribution of occupation and geography. *Population Trends*, **80**, 16–25.

Khan MM (2002). Suicide on the Indian subcontinent. *Crisis*, **23**, 104–107.

Kim MD, Hong SE, Lee SY *et al.* (2006). Suicide risk in relation to social class: a national register-based study of adult suicides in Korea, 1999–2001. *International Journal of Social Psychiatry*, **52**, 138–51.

Knox KL, Litts DA, Talcott GW *et al.* (2003). Risk of suicide and related adverse outcomes after exposure to a suicide prevention programme in the US Air Force: cohort study. *British Medical Journal*, **327**, 1376.

Kölves K, Värnik A, Schneider B *et al.* (2006). Recent life events and suicide: a case–control study in Tallinn and Frankfurt. *Social Science and Medicine*, **62**, 2887–2896.

Koronfel AA (2002). Suicide in Dubai, United Arab Emirates. *Journal of Clinical Forensic Medicine*, **9**, 5–11.

Kposowa AJ (1999). Suicide mortality in the United States: differentials by industrial and occupational groups. *American Journal of Industrial Medicine*, **36**, 645–652.

Kposowa AJ (2001). Unemployment and suicide: a cohort analysis of social factors predicting suicide in the US National Longitudinal Mortality Study. *Psychological Medicine*, **31**, 127–138.

Kwan YK, Ip WC, Kwan P (2005). Gender differences in suicide risk by socio-demographic factors in Hong Kong. *Death Studies*, **29**, 645–663

Labovitz S and Hagedorn R (1971). An analysis of suicide rates among occupational categories. *Sociological Inquiry*, **41**, 67–72.

Lewis G, Hawton K, Jones P (1997). Strategies for preventing suicide. *British Journal of Psychiatry*, **171**, 351–354.

Leymann H (1990). Mobbing and psychological terror at workplaces. *Violence and Victims*, **5**, 119–126.

Loo R (2003). A meta-analysis of police suicide rates: findings and issues. *Suicide and Life-Threatening Behaviour*, **33**, 313–325.

Lorant V, Kunst AE, Huisman M *et al.* (2005). Socio-economic inequalities in suicide: a European comparative study. *British Journal of Psychiatry*, **187**, 49–54.

Lostao L, Joiner TE, Lester D *et al.* (2006). Social inequalities in suicide mortality: Spain and France, 1980–1982 and 1988–1990. *Suicide and Life-Threatening Behaviour*, **36**, 113–119.

Lucey S, Corcoran P, Keeley HS *et al.* (2005). Socioeconomic change and suicide: a time-series study from the Republic of Ireland. *Crisis*, **26**, 90–94.

Mahon MJ, Tobin JP, Cusack DA *et al.* (2005). Suicide among regular-duty military personnel: a retrospective case–control study of occupation-specific risk factors for workplace suicide. *American Journal of Psychiatry*, **162**, 1688–1696.

Mäkelä P (1996). Alcohol consumption and suicide mortality by age among Finnish men, 1950–1991. *Addiction*, **91**, 101–112.

Mäki NE and Martikainen PT (2007). Socioeconomic differences in suicide mortality by sex in Finland in 1971–2000: a register-based study of trends, levels, and life-expectancy differences. *Scandinavian Journal of Public Health*, **35**, 387–395.

Mäkinen I (1997). Are there social correlates to suicide? *Social Science and Medicine*, **44**, 1919–1929.

Mäkinen IH (1999). Effect on suicide of having reduced unemployment is uncertain. *British Medical Journal*, **318**, 941–942. Letter.

Mäkinen IH (2002). Sorokin on suicide: an introduction to his essay 'Suicide as a social phenomenon'. In D Vågerö, ed., *The Unknown Sorokin: his Life in Russia and the Essay on Suicide*, pp. 32–61. Almqvist and Wiksell, Stockholm.

Mäkinen IH (2006). Suicide mortality of Eastern European regions before and after the Communist period. *Social Science and Medicine*, **63**, 307–319.

Mäkinen IH and Stickley AM (2006). Suicide mortality and agricultural rationalization in post-war Europe. *Social Psychiatry and Psychiatric Epidemiology*, **41**, 429–434.

Maris RW (1997). Social forces in suicide. A life review, 1965–1995. In RW Maris, MM Silverman and SS Canetto, eds, *Review of Suicidology*, pp. 42–60. Guilford Press, New York.

Marmot M (2004). *Status Syndrome: How your Social Standing Directly Affects your Health and Life Expectancy*. Bloomsbury, London.

Martikainen P, Mäki N, Blomgren J (2004). The effects of area and individual social characteristics on suicide risk. A multilevel study of relative contribution and effect modification. *European Journal of Population*, **20**, 323–350.

Morrell S, Taylor R, Quine S *et al.* (1993). Suicide and unemployment in Australia 1907–1990. *Social Science and Medicine*, **36**, 749–756.

Morrell S, Page AN, Taylor RJ (2007). The decline in Australian young male suicide. *Social Science and Medicine*, **64**, 747–754.

Niemi T and Lönnqvist J (1993). Suicides among university students in Finland. *Journal of American College Health*, **42**, 64–66.

Norström T (1995). The impact of alcohol, divorce, and unemployment on suicide. *Social Forces*, **74**, 293–314.

Nwosu SO and Odesanmi WO (2001). Pattern of suicides in Ile-Ife, Nigeria. *West African Journal of Medicine*, **20**, 259–262.

Pensola TH and Martikainen P (2003). Effect of living conditions in the parental home and youth paths on the social class differences in mortality among women. *Scandinavian Journal of Public Health*, **31**, 428–438.

Platt S (1984). Unemployment and suicidal behaviour: a review of the literature. *Social Science and Medicine*, **19**, 93–115.

Platt S and Hawton K (2000). Suicidal behaviour and the labour market. In K Hawton K and K van Heeringen, eds, *The International Handbook of Suicide and Attempted Suicide*, pp. 309–384. John Wiley and Sons, Chichester.

Platt S, Micciolo R, Tansella M (1992). Suicide and unemployment in Italy: description, analysis, and interpretation of recent trends. *Social Science and Medicine*, **34**, 1191–1201.

Preti A (2003). Unemployment and suicide. *Journal of Epidemiology and Community Health*, **57**, 557–558.

Qin P, Agerbo E, Westergård-Nielsen N *et al.* (2000). Gender differences in risk factors for suicide in Denmark. *British Journal of Psychiatry*, **177**, 546–550.

Qin P, Agerbo E, Mortensen PB (2003). Suicide risk in relation to socioeconomic, demographic, psychiatric, and familial factors: a national register-based study of all suicides in Denmark, 1981–1997. *American Journal of Psychiatry*, **160**, 765–772.

Rahu K, Rahu M, Tekkel M *et al.* (2006). Suicide risk among Chernobyl cleanup workers in Estonia still increased: an updated cohort study. *Annals of Epidemiology*, **16**, 917–919.

Recena MC, Pires DX, Caldas ED (2006). Acute poisoning with pesticides in the state of Mato Grosso do Sul, Brazil. *The Science of the Total Environment*, **357**, 88–95.

Rehkopf DH and Buka SL (2006). The association between suicide and the socio-economic characteristics of geographical areas: a systematic review. *Psychological Medicine*, **36**, 145–157.

Schmidtke A, Fricke S, Lester D (1999). Suicide among German federal and state police officers. *Psychological Reports*, **84**, 157–166.

Schwartz AJ (2006). Four eras of study of college student suicide in the United States: 1920–2004. *Journal of American College Health*, **54**, 353–366.

Singh B and Jenkins R (2000). Suicide prevention strategies—an international perspective. *International Review of Psychiatry*, **12**, 7–14.

Smith V (1997). New forms of work organisation. *Annual Review of Sociology*, **23**, 315–339.

Stack S (1982). Suicide: a decade review of the sociological literature. *Deviant Behaviour*, **4**, 41–66.

Stack S (2000). Suicide: a 15-year review of the sociological literature. Part I: cultural and economic factors. *Suicide and Life-Threatening Behaviour*, **30**, 145–162.

Stack S (2001). Occupation and suicide. *Social Science Quarterly*, **82**, 384–397.

Stack S (2004). Suicide risk among physicians: a multivariate analysis. *Archives of Suicide Research*, **8**, 287–292.

Stack S and Kelley T (1994). Police suicide: an analysis. *American Journal of Police*, **13**, 73–90.

Stark C, Belbin A, Hopkins P *et al.* (2006). Male suicide and occupation in Scotland. *Health Statistics Quarterly*, **29**, 26–29.

Steenland K, Halperin W, Hu S *et al.* (2003). Deaths due to injuries among employed adults: the effects of socioeconomic class. *Epidemiology*, **14**, 74–79.

Stone GD (2002). Biotechnology and suicide in India. *Anthropology News*, **43**, 5.

Taylor SJ, Kingdom D, Jenkins R (1997). How are nations trying to prevent suicide? An analysis of national suicide prevention strategies. *Acta Psychiatrica Scandinavica*, **95**, 457–463.

Vijayakumar L, John S, Pirkis J *et al.* (2005a). Suicide in developing countries (2): risk factors. *Crisis*, **26**, 112–119.

Vijayakumar L, John S, Pirkis J *et al.* (2005b). Suicide in developing countries (3): prevention efforts. *Crisis*, **26**, 120–124.

Voss M, Nylen L, Floderus B *et al.* (2004). Unemployment and early cause-specific mortality: a study based on the Swedish twin registry. *American Journal of Public Health*, **94**, 155–161.

Wasserman D (2001). *Suicide—An Unnecessary Death*. Martin Dunitz, London.

Wasserman D (2006). *Depression: The Facts*. Oxford University Press, Oxford.

Wasserman D, Mittendorfer-Rutz E, Rutz W *et al.* (2002). *Suicide Prevention in Europe—the WHO Monitoring Surveys of National Suicide Prevention Programmes and Strategies*. World Health Organization, Geneva.

Wasserman D, Mittendorfer-Rutz E, Rutz W *et al.* (2004). *Suicide Prevention in Europe—The WHO Monitoring Surveys of National Suicide Prevention Programmes and Strategies*. Swedish National Centre for Suicide Research and Prevention of Mental Ill-Health, Stockholm.

Wasserman I (1992). Economy, work, occupation and suicide. In R Maris, A Berman, J Maltsberger *et al.*, eds, *Assessment and Prediction of Suicide*, pp. 520–539. Guilford, New York.

Westerlund H, Ferrie J, Hagberg J *et al.* (2004). Workplace expansion, long-term sickness absence, and hospital admission. *Lancet*, **363**, 1193–1197.

Wikman A (2004). Indicators of changed working conditions. In RÅ Gustafsson and I Lundberg, eds, *Worklife and Health in Sweden*, pp. 39–77. National Institute for Working Life, Stockholm.

Zimmerman SL (1995). Psychache in context. States' spending for public welfare and their suicide rates. *Journal of Nervous and Mental Disease*, **183**, 425–434.

# CHAPTER 33

# Suicide study and suicide prevention in mainland China

Xiao Shuiyuan

## Abstract

Detailed descriptions of suicide can be found in Chinese historical writing, novels, and poetry, yet empirical suicide research has only developed in the past decade in China. Rigorous statistics on suicide have not been available until recently, and the systematic study of suicide is still at its preliminary stages. In this chapter, existing epidemiological data of suicide in mainland China is reviewed, ensued by a brief discussion about cultural views on suicide. Subsequently, there is an analysis of the possible influences of socio-economic and sociocultural changes leading to transitions in public health and suicidal behaviour. The available suicide statistics reveal certain dissimilarities to other statistics across the world: China is the only country with statistics showing an equal amount or more of female suicides. Furthermore, about one-third of the persons who commit suicide have no diagnosis of mental illness. In China, the suicide rate among rural residents is three to five times higher than that of urban residents. The high suicide rates among rural residents are strongly linked to the most frequent suicide method, which is the consumption of poisons, especially pesticides. The final section of the chapter is a discussion of the implications of available suicide studies on suicide prevention.

## Epidemiology of suicide

Before 1949, there were no official statistics about suicide in China. During this time, in the People's Republic of China, suicide statistics were not accessible for public information or academic research. For the first time in 1987, the Ministry of Health reported official mortality statistics that include deaths from suicide to the World Health Organization (WHO 1989). However, exact annual suicide rates are still not available at national and local levels for three major reasons. First, there is no systematic check for the cause of death in China. The cause of death is investigated in depth only when the death is suspected to be a crime, otherwise it is reported by physicians or family members. Second, China has not had a functioning registration system at national or provincial levels until today. The official mortality statistics provided to the WHO are based on data from about 10 per cent of the population (more than 100 million individuals). Finally, in almost all official reports on mortality, suicide

is categorized within 'injury and poisoning' (Ministry of Health 2007), a category that encompasses death by various injuries, traffic accidents, foodpoisoning, suicide, and homicide.

## Estimated suicide rates

Estimations of China's suicide rate have mainly been based on two data resources: the first data resource is the Death Registry in Certain Regions (DRCR), provided by the Ministry of Health. The DRCR data is provided by China's provinces and municipalities, who collect data in selected counties and cities with a relatively good reporting mechanism. The sample of DRCR covers about 100 million people but it is not a randomized one. The second data resource is the Disease Surveillance Point system (DSP) established by the Chinese Centre for Disease Control and Prevention (China CDC), formerly the Chinese Academy of Preventive Medicine. DSP used stratified technology to sample *xiang*/town (a *xiang* is an administrative unit between a *cun*—village—and county) or districts in cities and obtained a sample size of more than 10 million people (Ministry of Health Department of Disease Control and Chinese Academy of Preventive Medicine 1995). The DSP sample is more representative than the DRCR sample, but 15 per cent of the disease surveillance points are not included in the sample originally collected (Yang *et al.* 1992) and replaced by neighbourhood *xiang* instead. In addition, urban residents are over-represented in the sample (Phillips *et al.* 2002a). Based on these two data resources, a wide range of suicide rates have been estimated. For example, reported rates for 1990 range from 13.9 (He and Lester 1999) to 30.3 (Murry and Lopez 1996b). Among all studies of suicide rates performed in China, those mentioned below are influential.

### Official estimation by the Ministry of Health

At a WHO–Ministry of Health joint meeting held in Beijing in November 1999, the vice minister of the Ministry of Health officially reported a national suicide rate of 22.2 per 100,000 in 1993 (Yin 2000), and estimated that over 250,000 individuals died from suicide every year. A recently released official report (Disease Prevention and Control Bureau of MOH *et al.* 2007) estimated the number of suicide death was 193,000 in 2005.

## Suicide reported by WHO

The 1999 World Health Report (WHO 1999) estimated a suicide rate of 32.9/100,000 (413,000 suicides) in 1998 in China, much higher than the official figures. The 2001 *World Health Report* (WHO 2001b) dramatically down-tuned the suicide rate of China, reporting the average suicide rate for the years 1996 to 1998 to be 14.0/100,000, thus the average suicide rate decreased by 17 per cent from the period between 1988 to 1990.

## The estimation by Global Burden of Disease Study

The *Global Burden of Disease (GBD) study* (Murry and Lopez 1996a, b) applied several adjustments to the mortality data from DSP to estimate 343,000 suicides in 1990 (30.3 per 100,000).

## Estimation from DRCR

Based on the DRCR data from 1995 to 1999, adjusted according to unreported deaths and projected to the corresponding population, Phillips *et al.* (2002) reported an average annual suicide rate of 23 per 100,000 and a total of 287,000 suicide deaths per year.

# Features of suicide

## Gender difference

In most countries of the world, the sex ratio (male to female) of completed suicides is around 3:1, and at the same time, women attempt suicide approximately three times more often than men (Murry and Lopez 1996a; WHO 2002; Sudak 2005). Some studies have shown that in Asian countries the male to female ratio is much lower than that of Western countries (Murry and Lopez 1996a; He and Lester 1997). However, studies in China present a different picture. Our studies in local samples show that the male: female ratio of suicide is about 1:1 (Xu *et al.* 1999, 2000), while most other studies show that women committed suicide more often than males (Murry and Lopez 1996a, b; Yang *et al.* 1997; Philipps *et al.* 2002; Yip *et al.* 2005).

## Age difference

For all demographic groups, suicide is rare before puberty, though mass media reports that suicide among young people has increased in recent years. Generally, rates increase in nearly direct proportion to age, with the highest suicide rates in the elderly and a peak in the 19–34 age group. Studies in Western countries reveal that the suicide rate of adolescents and young adults has increased since 1950 (Bertolote 2001). Studies in China show that the age distribution of suicide follows the general picture of Western countries, but that the peak suicide rate in the 15–34 age group is much higher (Yang *et al.* 1997; Phillips *et al.* 1999; Xu *et al.* 1999; Phillips *et al.* 2002a). According to a widely cited study (Phillips *et al.* 2002a) suicide is the leading cause of death in individuals 15–34 years of age, accounting for 18.9 per cent of all deaths. The average suicide rate of this age group was 26.0/100,000 from 1995 to 1999, while at the same stage the average suicide rate of the group aged 60 to 84 was 68.0/100,000.

## Difference between rural and urban residents

According to French sociologist Emile Durkheim, strong social cohesion leads to lower suicide rates in rural areas, and individualism or egoism contributes to the high suicide rates in urban centres (Durkheim 1897, 1951). Based on an analysis of the suicide rate in Finland between 1800 and 1984, Stack linked suicide with urbanization (Stack 2000c). In China, however, almost all epidemiological studies reveal that the suicide rate of rural residents is three to five times higher than that of their urban counterparts (Phillips *et al.* 1999; Xu *et al.* 1999; Xu *et al.* 2000; Phillips *et al.* 2002a; Yip *et al.* 2005). Generally, the suicide rate of urban residents is around 10/100,000, lower than the world average of 15.7/100,000 (WHO 2001a), while the suicide rate is over 25/100,000 in Chinese rural areas, much higher than the world average (Murry and Lopez 1996a, b; Yang *et al.* 1997; Yip 2001; Xiao *et al.* 2003). A methodological question of this comparison is that suicide statistics only covered regular residents in cities. Currently, we don't know how the urban suicide rate will change if suicide of mobile workers from rural areas are counted.

## Suicide methods

Reduction of means, for example, limiting the availability of guns and poison, is widely believed to be an effective strategy of suicide prevention (see also Part 10C in this book). Epidemiological studies indicate that suicide methods employed are not only related to the availability of means (Kellermann *et al.* 1992), but also to socioeconomic and cultural variables (Lee *et al.* 2005). Overall, males use violent and lethal means while females use less violent and less lethal methods. In countries with large agricultural communities such as China, India and Sri Lanka, pesticides are widely used for suicide. In China, ingesting poisons, particularly pesticide, is the most frequently used method of suicide. Almost all epidemiological and psychological autopsy studies find that nearly two-thirds of all committed suicides were due to poisoning (Yang *et al.* 1997; Xu *et al.* 1999, 2000; Phillips *et al.* 2002b).

## Mental illness and suicide

It is reported that psychiatric disorders are present in at least 90 per cent of suicides (Rich and Runeson 1992; Appleby *et al.* 1999; Beautrais 2001; Mann *et al.* 2005; Sudak 2005). Depression is the most frequently cited illness linked with suicide, followed by schizophrenia, alcohol abuse disorder, other substance abuse disorders and personality disorder (Roy 2000). In China, retrospective studies utilizing the official death registry report that less than one-third of all suicides have a diagnosis of mental disorders (Xu *et al.* 1999, 2000; Zhang *et al.* 2000; Zhao and Ji 2000; Xiao *et al.* 2003). These studies underestimate the prevalence of mental disorders among those who commit suicide because disorders remain under-diagnosed and under-reported in the death registry. Recently, more rigorous psychological autopsy studies show that about two-thirds of all suicides have a diagnosis of mental disorder (Phillips *et al.* 2002b; Zhang *et al.* 2004). This figure is still much lower than those reported in Western countries.

## Explanations of the unique features of suicide in China

To summarize, the main feature of suicide in China is that rural females have a higher suicide rate than expected according to statistics from many areas across the world. Although there has been no systematic investigation of this unique pattern of suicide, several theories have been put forward to explain the phenomena. First, the availability of pesticides and other poison substances may convert a significant proportion of rural female suicide attempters into completed suicides. In Western countries, suicide attempts in females are more numerous than in males, and the usual method is poisoning by different types of medications. In China, the equivalent means for poisoning are pesticides, which are a lot more toxic and more often lead to suicide. Limiting access to poisons, thus has been suggested to be a priority in suicide prevention in China by many domestic and international researchers (Yang *et al.* 2005).

Second, the health care system in Chinese rural areas is often not qualified when a suicide attempter needs emergency rescue (Zhou *et al.* 2008). Clinics in *cun* (villages) are accessible to most suicide attempters, but there is barely any equipment or technology to rescue individuals with pesticide ingestion. Health care providers in village clinics generally receive less than two years of medical training. About half of the health stations and all county general hospitals can provide qualified emergency service to suicide attempters, but in many cases, suicide attempters have died before they are sent to such institutions for help, as there is no convenient transportation available and the distance to qualified institutions is often too far.

Third, mental health service is not available in most Chinese rural areas. Less than 50 per cent of counties (the population size of most counties vary from 300,000 to 1,500,000) have a mental hospital providing basic service to patients with psychotic disorders. Most rural health care providers only receive three years or less of medical education and have very limited knowledge and skills in mental health (Tang *et al.* 2005). As a result, it is estimated that only 5 per cent of patients with depression and 30 per cent of the patients with schizophrenia receive systematic treatment. There has been no crisis intervention and suicide prevention in Chinese rural areas until today.

Finally, socio-conomic and cultural variables such as stigmatization, pressure on delivering male babies, poverty due to low educational level and low socio-economic status may contribute to distress and to the high suicide rate of rural women.

## Attempted suicide

There is no community registry for attempted suicide in China, and consequently, it is very difficult to estimate the prevalence of attempted suicide in the country. Generally, the prevalence of attempted suicide is estimated to be 8–10 times that of completed suicides. If this estimation is applicable to China, then there are about 3 million individuals attempting suicide every year. Hence, attempted suicide is also an important social and public health concern (Beijing Huilongguan Hospital Center of Clinical Epidemiology 2000).

Small-scale community epidemiological studies reported a variety of attempted suicide rates in China. In the WHO multi-site intervention study on suicidal behaviours (SUPRE-MISS), China's chosen site, the Yuncheng County, reported lifetime suicide attempts of 2.4 per cent, while the range of all 10 participated sites varied from 0.4 per cent (Hanoi) to 4.2 per cent (Brisbane) (Bertolote *et al.* 2005). In a sample of junior high school students, the lifetime prevalence was reported to be 4.74 per cent (Zhou *et al.* 2005). Several studies using samples from emergency services indicate that the male to female ratio is around 2.5:1; that less than 50 per cent of the attempters have a diagnosis of mental disorders; and that more than 70 per cent tried to attempt suicide by self-poisoning (Zhang *et al.* 2000; Li *et al.* 2001, 2005; Pearson *et al.* 2002; Liu and Xiao 2002).

## Cultural reactions to suicide

Although there is scant empirical research, two different points of view have been advanced in the literature concerning cultural notions in relation to suicide and its prevention. Hsieh and Spence (1982) suggested, based on their historical study of suicide in pre-modern China, that suicide in Chinese culture was often positively evaluated and was actually encouraged by the state. In a cross-cultural study of suicide in Chinese and American societies, Chiles *et al.* (1989) suggested that, when compared to suicidal patients in the United States, Chinese suicidal patients are less likely to communicate suicidal intent and to experience concerned, supportive care. Using a quantitative questionnaire, Yang *et al.* (1999) found that health care providers in China hold a positive attitude toward suicide. In a recent qualitative study in northern China, Li *et al.* (2004) reported that most individuals interviewed expressed tolerant and sympathetic attitudes toward suicide.

Chinese perspectives on suicidal behaviour have been shaped throughout the long history of Chinese civilization. Thus, it is essential to begin our analysis with a brief examination of Chinese cultural and religious traditions.

Among all Chinese cultural influences, Confucianism, both as a philosophy and a religion, is the most important. Daoism and Buddhism are also important doctrines in Chinese history, but they have not been as influential as Confucianism (see Part 1, Chapter 3 in this book). Chinese attitudes toward death, including suicide, are influenced by such Confucian virtues as *zhong* (faithfulness), *xiao* (filial piety), *ren* (humanness) and *yi* (righteousness or justice). In feudal China, the Confucian Analects, the classic of Filial Piety and other Confucian classics were used as textbooks for primary education for almost all students, who were required to recite them fluently. In the period of the Republic of China (1911–1949), as China gradually opened the door to Western science and culture, particularly because of the influence of the 'new cultural movement', Confucian classics were no longer used in most public schools, but private schools continued to teach them. More importantly, the Confucian tradition was officially emphasized by the Kuomintang, which was the dominant political force in this period. Since 1949, the Confucian tradition has been criticised by both the Chinese government and some intellectuals influenced by Western cultural beliefs. During the Cultural Revolution (1966–1976), Confucianism was systematically condemned. Nonetheless, traditional Confucian beliefs still remain central to the lived experience of people in mainland China and have recently been re-emphasized by the mainstream culture.

## Filial piety and negative evaluations of suicide

Filial piety, which means showing respect and taking care of one's parents and ancestors, is among the most ancient and central values in Chinese culture. The *Xiao Jing*, the classic text on filial piety, which was written two thousand years ago, states:

> Filial piety is the basis of virtue and the source of culture. The body and the limbs, the hair and the skin, are given to one by one's parents, and to them no injury should come: this is where filial piety begins.
> (Zeng Zi pp. 326–327)

Because the body is held in trust to the parents and ancestors, the classic of filial piety ruled out neglect of the body, and most certainly suicide. Zeng Zi, one of the most famous disciples of Confucius, said he had been very careful to protect his body from injury and he was proud that he could take care of his own body until his death. Lun Yu, records the following story in the Analects of an unknown author, which is a collection of dialogues between Confucius and his disciples.

The philosopher Zeng Zi was sick and called to him the disciples of his school, to say to them:

> Uncover my feet, uncover my hands. It is said in the *Book of Poetry*, 'We should be apprehensive and cautious, as if standing on the brink of a deep gulf, as if treading on ice', and so have I been. Now and hereafter, I know my escape from all injury to my person, O! ye, my little children.

Anonymous (1992)

Although the Confucian virtue of filial piety is not explicitly taught in public education in the People's Republic of China, it is implicitly encouraged by the government and the mass media. For instance, all three editions of the Constitution of China published in 1952, 1980, and 1986 respectively, insist that every person should take care of their parents. Beliefs about filial piety and family cohesion are still highly valued across Chinese society.

The vignette below is an example of how filial beliefs have a strong hold in China today and can be related to suicidal behaviour and attitudes. In the following case, drawn from research conducted in China, a relative of a suicidal patient tries to convince her that suicide is not acceptable behaviour for a good daughter.

### Vignette

Ms Wu, a 19-year-old high school graduate, was sent to the emergency room at a large teaching hospital in south central China for loss of consciousness. According to her parents, Ms Wu was in a coma when they returned home from work. Ms Wu, their only child, 'had a good record of health history, cooked breakfast for the family and showed no sign of any disease when we left for work that morning'. After a careful examination, the emergency physician made a diagnosis of possible attempted suicide by taking an overdose of sleeping pills. Upon inquiring, Ms Wu's mother noted that Ms Wu failed to pass the university entrance examination three months earlier, while nearly half of her classmates passed it. Her father, a construction worker, wanted Ms Wu to continue to attend an extension course in the local high school to prepare for the next year's examination. However, Ms Wu, ashamed by her failure, was reluctant to return to school and considered instead becoming a worker. A few days before this interview, Ms Wu applied for a job in a textile manufacturing factory. Her father was very angry about this and, after he quarrelled with her, said he no longer wanted Ms Wu to be his daughter.

After having recovered from the coma, Ms Wu told the interviewer that her parents had been very good to her, but their expectations were too high. Before and after she failed this year's examination, her parents put great pressure on her to take the next examination, but she felt that she lacked the talent to pass this very competitive test and would rather quit school to be a worker. She did not want to face further failure and to continue to disappoint and anger her parents. Therefore, she attempted suicide.

Influenced by the idea of filial piety, Ms Wu could not rebel against her parents, and leave the family to start an independent life like many Western young adults might do in the same situation. The following dialogue, recorded by the author of this chapter, took place between Ms Wu and her aunt, a high school teacher in her late 30s, in the hospital ward four days after Ms Wu's attempted suicide. Informed consent to describe this dialogue was obtained orally:

Aunt: How are you doing, my child?

Wu: I am OK now. Thank you for coming to see me.

Aunt: Here are some apples for you. My child, how can you be so silly to take so many sleeping pills? They could have killed you!

Wu: Aunt … I know.

Aunt: My child, do you know you are the only child of your parents? They love you so much. In these two days they have eaten nothing. Your mother told me yesterday that if you do not recover, she cannot live any more.

Wu: I, I …

Aunt: You do not know how your parents take care of you. When you were ill, even with a light cold, they worried a lot about you. Your father has only a primary education and he wishes you to have the highest education they can afford. How could they live if you died? (She cries.) Nowadays children do not understand how to respect their parents.

Wu (crying): Aunt, I know I was wrong. I will not do this again.

Aunt: My good child!

According to Chinese cultural beliefs, one should take care of one's parents by respecting and obeying their ideas and attitudes, helping them to be happy when they are alive and giving them the best food and living conditions. When the parents die one should honour them and work to immortalize them. Many Chinese parents feel deep guilt if their offspring die when they remain alive because they believe parents should always die before their children. In this case, although Ms Wu's aunt did not mention the importance of being filial, the idea that suicide goes against ideas of respect for one's parents is quite clear. When Ms Wu's aunt says 'Do you know you are the only child of your parents?', this can be understood as 'how can you leave your parents alone?'. At the end of the conversation it seems that Ms Wu is convinced that her attempted suicide is unfilial to her parents, something she must have considered both before and after her suicide attempt.

In modern Chinese societies, suicide victims are sometimes openly accused of being irresponsible, selfish, individualistic, acting against filial values, and even being immoral. An example was the suicide of Shamao in the beginning of 1991. Shamao, a well known 39-year-old essay writer in Taiwan, was, in a newspaper, accused of being 'greatly unfilial' and 'irresponsible', because she committed suicide when her mother was suffering from late stage cancer and needed her love and care (Zhong 1991). Individuals who commit suicide are frequently accused for similar reasons. Wei Minlun, a famous writer in modern China, has recently criticised those fans who committed suicide following Zhang Guorong, an influential singer who committed suicide in 2005, as 'totally inconsiderate to their parents' and causing them extreme pain (Sichuan News Net 2005).

## Faithfulness and positive evaluations of suicide

Faithfulness is another traditional Chinese cultural belief that has great influence on the evaluation of suicidal actions. In the Confucian classics, being faithful is an important part of *ren* (humanness) and *yi* (*righteousness or justice*), the correct approach to human relations and a proper way for persons to deal with each other, leading to positive efforts for the good of others. In order to achieve the virtue of *ren* and *yi*, it is necessary to be faithful to both others and oneself. As discussed in the previous section, the Confucian school generally objects to deliberate destruction of one's own body. However, the virtues of *ren* and *yi* were considered more important than one's life by Confucius and his followers. For example, Confucius said in the Analects that 'The determined scholar and the men of virtue will not live at the expense of injuring their virtue. They will sacrifice their lives to preserve their virtue' (Anonymous 1992).

Mencius, the Confucian scholar next only to Confucius himself in importance, said:

> I like fish and I like bear's paws. If I cannot have the two together, I will let the fish go, and take the bears paws. So, I like life, and I also like righteousness. I like life indeed, but there is that which I like more than life, and therefore, I will not seek to possess it in any improper way. I dislike death indeed, but there is that which I dislike more than death, and therefore there are occasions when I will not avoid danger.
>
> Mencius (1992)

Although suicide is not directly mentioned here, the idea that one might have to give up one's own life for faithfulness to *ren* and *yi* has influenced the attitudes of Chinese toward suicide for nearly twenty-five centuries. Until today, the words *ren* and *yi* are still used in Chinese society in sayings such as 'to kill oneself to achieve the virtue of *ren*' or 'to achieve the goal or to die'.

In Chinese history, suicide committed because of faithfulness can be found in three categories:

1 Suicide due to loyalty to the government or the nation;

2 Suicide due to loyalty to one's ideals;

3 Suicide because of loyalty to a relationship with others.

### Suicide due to loyalty to the government or the nation

This type of suicide often takes place in order to keep national secrets or for national interests. Chinese culture openly admires this kind of behaviour. Many stories have been devoted to honouring those who killed themselves in wartime, when their sacrifices were important to national or group interests. Because many Chinese believe that to be killed or to be captured is a humiliation only for themselves and their country, they killed themselves when being killed or captured by an enemy seemed inevitable.

### Suicide due to loyalty to one's ideals

This has been expressed very clearly in the well-known saying 'If we have no freedom, we would rather die.' In China, as in some other East Asian countries such as Korea and Japan, committing suicide to express one's ideal is not uncommon. For example, almost everyone in China knows the death of Qu Yuan, a patriotic poet who is said to have drowned himself more than two thousand years ago when the emperor refused to heed his advice (Ning 1998). Chinese people believe that Qu Yuan's suicide was a protest to the emperor, and a sacrifice to society.

An often used method to express one's loyalty is hunger strike. Although the purpose of it or a similar self-destructive demonstration may not be to kill oneself, it is considered to be a kind of suicidal action for one's ideals, and is thus supposed to receive a sympathetic response from society.

### Suicide because of loyalty to a relationship with others

This was widely practised in feudal China and its traces can still be found in modern Chinese societies. One commonly practised form of suicide is that of the wife's out of loyalty to her husband. Hsieh and Spence (1982), in their historical study, described four circumstances for a wife's suicide:

1 When the husband dies;

2 When the wife's death is necessary for the transmission of her husband's propriety;

3 When the wife is put in the position of inevitably breaking the laws of propriety if she remains alive;

4 When an intolerable pressure is placed on the wife because of all her divided loyalty within a particular family situation.

Many stories, such as *A biography of women*, written by Liu Xiang of the Han dynasty and revised by others in feudal China (Liu 2003), have been devoted to recording this kind of suicide in Chinese history.

In Chinese society, it is not only having voluntary extra-marital affairs that are regarded as being unfaithful to one's husband: in some cases, even having been raped is considered unfaithful. The practice of a wife committing suicide because of loyalty to her husband has in some cases been extended to committing suicide for the culturally idealized state of keeping oneself clean and pure. For example, if an unmarried girl is raped or has a voluntary pre-marital affair she is still considered by some Chinese people to be 'unclean', or polluted because she can no longer present a 'pure' body to her future husband. Suicide for the sake of faithfulness is positively evaluated by Chinese society as heroic, romantic, aesthetic, and moral behaviour. There are even biographies specially designed to honour women who committed suicide out of loyalty to their husbands or to protect the purity of their bodies (Hsieh and Spence 1982).

## Suicide in the period of transition

Many biological, psychological, and biopsychosocial factors have been linked with suicidal behaviour at the level of the individual (Jacobs 1999; Sudak 2005). Explanation of suicide rates and its changes in large populations, however, should be focused on macro social, economic and cultural variables (Durkheim 1951; Phillips *et al.* 1999; Xiao *et al.* 2003; Yip *et al.* 2005). According to an estimation by Phillips *et al.* (1999), China accounts for 21 per cent of the world's population, but comprises 44 per cent of all suicides in the world. While not everyone agrees with this estimate, there is no doubt that suicide is a major public health and social problem in China. In addition to this, China has experienced huge socio-economic changes in the past three decades. Obviously, it is of great interest to suicidology how macro-demographic, socio-economic, cultural and health transitions have influenced the suicide rates in China.

## Recent changes of suicide rate in China

Studies on the trends of suicide rate in China are scarce, perhaps because of the unavailability of qualified data. According to the 2001 *World Health Report* released by the WHO, from the 1988–1990 period to the 1996–1998 period, the suicide rate of China decreased to 17.2 per cent (WHO 2001b). Using data from the *World Statistics Annual*, a study shows that the suicide rates had slightly decreased from 22.6 (22.5–22.7) in 1987 to 19.9 (19.8–20.0) per 100 000 (Qin and Mortensen 2001). Recently, Yip *et al.* (2005) studied the trends of suicide rates from 1991 to 2000 based on data from the Ministry of Health (i.e. DRCR). They found that national, urban, and rural suicide rates of both men and women decreased significantly for the period of 1991–2000; age-specific suicide rates, however, showed that there were different patterns of changes in suicide rates in rural and urban areas. Suicide rates among the elderly showed the most significant decrease in urban areas, and younger women showed the largest decrease in rural areas; the male to female ratio in suicide increased significantly in the urban areas, but no significant changes were found in rural areas (Yip *et al.* 2005). The recently released *Report on injury prevention in China* (Disease Prevention and Control Bureau of MOH *et al.* 2007) reported the number of suicide deaths to be 226,000, 224,000, 221,000, 193,000 and 193,000 in 1995, 1998, 2000, 2003 and 2005 respectively (Figure 33.1), but suicide rates and its specific distribution are not available from the report.

While the results of the above studies are encouraging, more evidence is needed in order to fully comprehend the change of suicide rates in China.

## Socio-economic and sociocultural transitions effects on suicide

China's economic reform, which started in 1978, has resulted in the most rapidly expanding economy in the world. Roughly, the per capita income in China has increased from less than

300 USD in 1978 to over 2000 USD in 2006: 43.9 per cent of the whole population lived in cities and towns in 2006 while more than 80 per cent of the population were rural residents at the beginning of the 1980s (National Bureau of Statistics of China 1978–2006). The formerly strict planning economy has become market-oriented.

Studies on the relationship between socio-economic changes and suicide in other countries have provided inconsistent results (Durkheim 1951; Kowalski *et al.* 1987; Simpson and Conklin 1989; Stack 1993, 2000a, b; Xiao *et al.* 2003; Otsu *et al.* 2004; Yip *et al.* 2005). Epidemiological studies consistently show that in China, the suicide rate of rural residents is three to five times higher than that of urban residents. This strongly suggests that urban life in China is not necessary linked to an increased suicide rate. Conversely, economic development may decrease China's suicide rate in the following ways:

1  Higher income and expectancy for better life conditions may meet the material demands of most people, so that less interpersonal conflict between family members will arise;

2  Better education can provide individuals with better knowledge about psychological distress and coping alternatives;

3  A more optimistic expectation of individual life may lead to more emphasis on the value of health and life;

4  Improvements of transportation and communications may facilitate individuals to obtain needed social links and social support from distant resources;

5  More opportunities for women in general and rural women in particular to improve their economic and social status;

6  Technical advances in agriculture, particularly the availability of good quality seeds, as well as effective and less lethal pesticides, may decrease the storage and use of highly lethal pesticides by rural residents;

7  Increased accessibility to qualified medical cares, particularly mental health care and emergency services, may improve the outcomes of individuals with mental disorders and prevent suicide attempters from death, especially in rural areas;

8  More investment from governments and private agencies in crisis intervention and suicide prevention may improve mental health and decrease suicide.

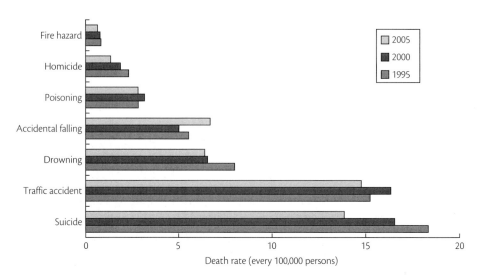

**Fig. 33.1** Suicide rates of selected urban and rural areas of China in 1995, 2000 and 2005, as compared with other injuries. Disease Prevention and Control Bureau of MOH *et al.* (2007).

Economic development, however, also brings social problems that may increase suicide rates in a society. Phillips *et al.* (1999) listed seven social changes that may result in the increase of suicide rates:

1  The increasing prevalence of major economic losses for individuals and families due to participation in risky ventures or pathological gambling;

2  Increasing rates of marital infidelity and divorce;

3  Increasing rates of alcohol and drug abuse;

4  Rapidly increasing costs of health care, which may make some older individuals prefer to end their lives rather than deplete family resources to receive treatment for chronic conditions;

5  Weakening of family ties, which results in less social support for individuals;

6  Large numbers of rural residents migrating to urban areas for temporary or seasonal work;

7  The increasing economic and social gap between the rich and poor, which may result in higher levels of dissatisfaction with one's social and economic situation.

One could add more to this list, for example, conflicts of values and lifestyles between old and younger generations, more complicated interpersonal relationships, and more stressful work and living demands, etc.

It is unclear today which of the above mentioned factors of a society in transition will prevail on suicide rates in the future China. It seems reasonable to assume that the distribution of suicide will change, and possibly, the suicide rate will decrease in rural areas, while in urban areas, it may remain stable or increasing in the near future.

## Health transitions and suicide

The term health transition is used to describe the changes over time in a society's health (Caldwell 1996). It encompasses three major components: the decrease of fertility and premature mortality, the increase of life expectancy, the transition of morbidity and death causes from infectious diseases to chronic non-infectious diseases and degenerative diseases. Health transition has been evidenced since the 1950s, with more complete transition in countries with a higher gross domestic product (GDP) and less complete in countries with lower GDP.

China is perhaps one of the countries that have experienced the most rapid health transitions in the world. The total mortality rate of China's population has dropped from 20/1000 in 1949 to 6.43/1000 in 2001. The infant mortality rate has dropped from 200/1000 in 1949 to 28.4/1000 in 2000. The maternal mortality rate has dropped from 150/10,000 in 1949 to 50.2/100,000 in 2001. The average life expectancy has increased from 35 years in 1949 to 71.4 years in 2000 (Lee 2004). The one child per parents policy imposed since the later 1970s has decreased the national fertility from 17.8 per 1000 in 1985 to 12.09 per 1000 in 2006 (Figure 33.2) (National Bureau of Statistics of China 1978–2006).

Although there are almost no systematic epidemiological studies that have investigated the links between health transitions and suicide, there are three major concerns that China's health transition will increase suicide rates nationwide. First, there is a rapid trend of ageing in China. The number of people aged 65 and over accounted for 7 per cent of the total population in 2000 (National Bureau of Statistics of China 2003). From 1982 to 1999 the proportion of people aged 60+ years increased from 7.64 per cent to 10.1 per cent (Lee 2004). It is predicted that this trend will be continue in the first half of the twenty-first century (Figure 33.3) (Wang and Mason 2005).

As the age structure of China keeps changing, the absolute number of elderly will increase rapidly, especially in rural areas where more and more young people are moving to cities and the elderly are left alone, with the traditional family support interrupted. Similar to other parts of the world, the elderly have the highest suicide rate in China and the increased proportion of the elderly may lead to increased suicide rates.

Second, non-infectious diseases have become the leading causes of death and morbidity with the continuing heavy burden of infectious diseases. Chronic course of disease, lowered quality of life and painful experiences can increase suicides (Kelly *et al.* 1999)

Finally, the one child per parent policy has resulted in serious gender imbalance, especially in rural areas. The male to female ratio at age 1 and age 10 reached 122.65 and 111.39 in 2000, respectively (National Bureau of Statistics of China 2003). Less females, who by tradition are responsible for the care of elderly parents, will impose great stress on both genders and may lead some to suicide.

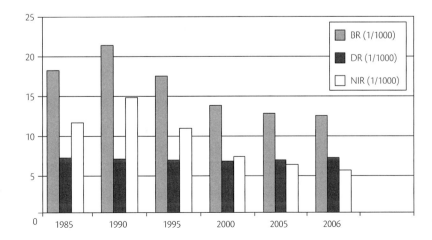

**Fig. 33.2** Changes of birth rate (BR), mortality rate (MR), and natural increase rate (NIR, the percentage growth of a population in a year, computed as the crude birth rate minus the crude death rate) in China (1980–2006). Data source: National Bureau of Statistics of China (1978–2006).

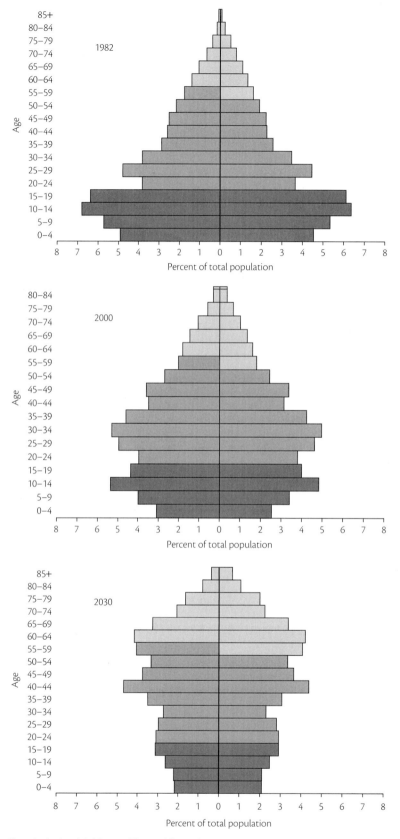

**Fig. 33.3** Population age structure, China (male, female). (a) 1982, (b) 2000, (c) 2030 (Wang & Mason 2005).

# Implications for suicide prevention in China

Suicide was a culturally and politically sensitive topic in China before the late 1980s. A recent analysis of media reports on suicide found that the *People's Daily*, the largest Chinese newspaper mainly publishing news about Mainland China, had totally ignored suicide during the period 1966–1976 (Liu and Xiao 2007). As China began to provide death statistics that include death by suicide to the WHO since 1987, suicide has been gradually recognized to be an important public health issue in China. A few centres and hotline services dedicated to crisis intervention and suicide prevention have recently been opened in large cities such as Nanjing, Beijing, Shanghai, Shenzhen, Dalian, Changsha, etc. The National Mental Health Schedule 2002–2010, released jointly by the Ministry of Health, Ministry of Public Security, Ministry of Civil Affaires, and China Disabled Person's Federation in 2002, also listed suicide prevention as one of the priorities in mental health development in the first decade of the twenty-first century.

Based on the unique features of suicide in China, the following suicide-prevention strategies have been suggested by both domestic and international experts in the field (Zhai 1997; WHO 2001a; Xiao *et al.* 2003; Phillips 2004):

1 Develop a national strategy for suicide prevention;

2 Develop national institutions, networks and programmes for promoting suicide prevention;

3 Monitor suicides and suicide attempts nationwide;

4 Stimulate ongoing public education programmes about suicide, reduce stigmatization imposed on individuals who have attempted suicide or who have suicidal ideation;

5 Control access to agricultural chemicals that are frequently employed in suicides; control access to dangerous medication;

6 Train individuals who come into contact with persons who are at high risk of suicide in the basic principles of suicide prevention;

7 Improve access and comprehensiveness of mental health services, particularly in rural areas;

8 Develop professional suicide-prevention services in urban areas;

9 Provide increased social support for at-risk groups, particularly rural women, the elderly and the mentally ill;

10 Mobilize all possible resources and a multidisciplinary approach to suicide prevention and suicide study; increase national and local investment in suicide study and suicide prevention.

## References

Anonymous (1992). Lun Yun (The Analects of Confucius) In James Legge (translator): *The Four Books* (revised and annotated by Liu Zhongde and Luo Ziye). Hunan Press, Changsa.

Appleby L, Cooper J, Amos T *et al.* (1999). Psychological autopsy study of suicides by people aged under 35. *British Journal of Psychiatry*, **175**, 168–174.

Beautrais AL (2001). Suicide and serious suicide attempters: two populations or one. *Psychological Medicine*, **31**, 837–845.

Beijing Huilongguan Hospital Center of Clinical Epidemiology (2000). Reports on the Ministry of Health/World Health Organization March 22–24 meeting on the prevention of suicide. *Chinese Mental Health Journal*, **14**, 295–298.

Bertolote JM (2001). Suicide in the world: an epidemiological overview 1959–2000. In D Wasserman, ed., *Suicide—An Unnecessary Death*, pp. 3–10. Martin Dunitz, London.

Bertolote JM, Fleischman A, Leo DD *et al.* (2005). Suicide attempts, plans, and ideation in culturally diverse sites: the WHO SUPRE-MISS community survey. *Psychological Medicine*, **35**, 1–9.

Caldwell JC (1996). Mortality, epidemiological, and health transition. In A Kuper and J Kuper, eds, *The Social Science Encyclopedia*, pp. 10071–10075. Routledge, London.

Chiles JA, Strosahl KD, ZhengYP *et al.* (1989). Depression, hopelessness and suicidal behaviour in Chinese and America psychiatric patients. *American Journal of Psychiatry*, **146**, 339–344.

Disease Prevention and Control Bureau of MOH, Statistical Information, MOH and Chinese Center for Disease Prevention and Control (2007). *Report on Injury Prevention in China*. People's Medical Publishing House, Beijing.

Durkheim E (1897). *Le suicide*. Felix Alcan, Paris.

Durkheim E (1951). *Suicide*. Free Press, New York.

He ZX and Lester D (1997). The gender difference in Chinese suicide rates. *Archives of Suicide Research*, **3**, 81–89.

He ZX and Lester D (1999). What is the Chinese suicide rate? Perceptual Motor Skills, **89**, 898.

Hsieh A and Spence J (1982). Suicide and family in pre-modern China. In A Kleinman and TY Lin, eds, *Normal and Abnormal Behavior in Chinese Culture*, pp. 29–48. D. Reidel, Dordrecht.

Jacobs DG (1999). *Guide to Suicide Assessment and Intervention*. Jossey-Bass, San Francisco.

Kellermann AL, Rivara FP, Somes GS *et al.* (1992). Suicide in the home in relation to gun ownership. *New England Journal of Medicine*, **327**, 467–472.

Kelly MJ, Mufson MJ, Rogers MP (1999). Medical settings and suicide. In DG Jacobs, ed., *The Harvard Medical School Guide to Suicide Assessment and Intervention*, pp. 491–519. Jossey-Bass, San Francisco.

Kowalski GS, Faupel CE, Starr PD (1987). Urbanism and suicide: a study of American counties. *Social Forces*, **66**, 85–101.

Lee DT, Chan KP, Yip PS (2005). Charcoal burning is also popular for suicide pacts made on the Internet. *British Medical Journal*, **330**, 7491.

Lee LM (2004). The current state of public health in China. *Annual Review of Public Health*, **25**, 327–339.

Li XY, Phillips MR, Ji HY *et al.* (2005). Characteristics of serious suicide attempts living in villages. *Chinese Journal Nervous and Mental Disease*, **31**, 272–277.

Li XY, Phillips MR, Wang AW, Liang H, Wang CL, Li C (2004). Current attitudes and knowledge about suicide in community members: a qualitative study. *Chinese Journal of Epidemiology*, **25**, 296–301.

Li XY, Yang YS, Zhang C *et al.* (2001) A case–control study on attempted suicide. *Chinese Journal of Epidemiology*, **22**, 281–283.

Liu LZ and Xiao SY (2002). A follow-up study on suicide attempters. *Chinese Mental Health Journal*, **16**, 253–256.

Liu X (2003). *A Biography of Women*. Jiangsu Ancient Books Press, Nanjing.

Liu YS and Xiao SY (2007). Social Representation of Suicide in the *People's Daily*. Unpublished manuscript, Central South University, Changsha.

Mann JJ, Apter A, Bertolote J *et al.* (2005). Suicide prevention strategies: a systematic review. *JAMA*, **294**, 2064–2074.

Mencius: Meng Zi (The Works of Mencius) (1992). In James Legge (translator): *The Four Books*, pp. 260–556 (revised and annotated by Liu zhongde and Luo Ziye). Hunan Press, Changsha.

Ministry of Health Department of Disease Control and Chinese Academy of Preventive Medicine (1995). *Annual Report on Chinese Diseases Surveillance*. People's Medical Publishing House, Beijing.

Ministry of Health (2007). *Chinese Health Statistics Digest*. Available at http://www.moh.gov.cn/open/2007tjts/P45.htm

Murry CJL and Lopez AD (1996a). *Global Health Statistics: A Compendium of Incidence, Prevalence, and Mortality Estimates for over 200 Conditions*. Harvard University Press, Cambridge.

Murry CJL and Lopez AD (1996b). *The Global Burden of Disease: A Comprehensive Assessment of Mortality and Disability from Diseases, Injuries, and Risk Factors in 1990 and Projected to 2020*. Harvard University Press, Cambridge.

National Bureau of Statistics of China (2003). *Bulletin of Fifth National Population Census*. Chinese Statistics Press, Beijing.

National Bureau of Statistics of China (1978–2006). *Annual National Statistics Communiqué*. http://www.stats.gov.cn/tjgb, accessed on 2 October 2007.

Ning (1998). *FX Qu Yuan*. Changjiang Culture and Art Press, Wuchang.

Otsu G, Araki S, Sakai R et al. (2004). Effects of urbanization, economic development, and migration of workers on suicide mortality in Japan. *Social Sciences and Medicine*, **58**, 1137–1146.

Pearson V, Phillips MR, He FS et al. (2002). Attempted suicide among young rural women in the People's Republic of China: possibilities for prevention. *Suicide and Life-Threatening Behavior*, **32**, 359–369.

Phillips MR (2004). Current status and future directions for suicide research and prevention in China. *Chinese Journal of Epidemiology*, **25**, 277–279.

Phillips MR, Li XY, Zhang YP (2002a). Suicide rate in China, 1995–99. *Lancet*, **359**, 835–840.

Phillips MR, Liu HQ, Zhang YP (1999). Suicide and social change in China. *Culture, Medicine and Psychiatry*, **23**, 25–50.

Phillips MR, Yang GH, Zhang YP et al. (2002b). Risk factors for suicide in China: a national case–control psychological autopsy study. *Lancet*, **360**, 1728–1736.

Qin P and Mortensen PB (2001). Specific characteristics of suicide in China. *Acta Psychiatrica Scandinavica*, **103**, 117–121.

Rich GL and Runeson BS (1992). Similarities in diagnostic comorbidity between suicide among young people in Sweden and the United States. *Acta Psychiatrica Scandinavica*, **86**, 335–339.

Roy A (2000). Suicide (monograph on CD-ROM). In BJ Sadock and VA Sadock, eds, *Comprehensive Textbook of Psychiatry*. Lippincott Williams and Wilkins, Philadelphia.

Sichuan News Net (2005). Wei Minglun condemned some fans angrily for not respecting their parents. Retrieved from http://www.newssc.org/gb/Newssc/scnews/sfxw/userobject1ai410098.html

Simpson M and Conklin G (1989). Socioeconomic development, suicide and religion: a test of Durkhiem's theory of religion and suicide. *Social Forces*, **67**, 945–964.

Stack S (1993). The effect of modernization on suicide in Finland: 1800–1984. *Sociological Perspectives*, **36**, 137–148.

Stack S (2000a). Suicide: a 15-year review of the sociological literature. Part I. Cultural and economic factors. *Suicide and Life-Threatening Behavior*, **30**, 145–162.

Stack S (2000b). Suicide: a 15-year review of the sociological literature. Part II. Modernization and social integration perspectives. Cultural and economic factors. *Suicide and Life-Threatening Behavior*, **30**, 163–176.

Stack S (2000c). The effect of modernization on suicide in Finland: 1800–1984. *Sociological Perspective*, **36**, 137–148.

Sudak HS (2005). Suicide. In BJ Sadock and VA Sadock, eds, *Kaplan and Sadock's Comprehensive Textbook of Psychiatry*, pp. 2443–2454. Lippincott Williams and Wilkins, Philadelphia.

Tang Y, Zhou L, Xiao SY et al. (2005). Awareness of suicide, emergency treatment for poisoning, and mental health among rural health care providers in Liuyang, Hunan Province. *Clinical Journal of Psychiatry*, **15**, 235–237.

Wang F and Mason A (2005). Demographic Dividend and Prospects for Economic development in China. United Nations Expert Group Meeting on Social and Economic Implications of Changing Population Age Structures, UN/POP/PD/2005/5

WHO (1989). *World Health Statistics Annual*. World Health Organization, Geneva.

WHO (2001a). *Report on a Workshop on Suicide Prevention in China*. World Health Organization, Geneva.

WHO (2002). *World Report on Violence and Health*. World Health Organization, Geneva.

WHO (1999). *World Health Report 1999: Making a Difference*. World Health Organization, Geneva.

WHO (2001b). *World Health Report 2001. Mental Health: New Understanding, New Hope*. World Health Organization, Geneva.

Xiao SY, Wang XP, Xu HL (2003). Several issues in suicide study and suicide prevention in China. *Chinese Journal of Psychiatry*, **36**, 129–131.

Xu HL, Xiao SY, Chen JP et al. (1999). Epdemiological study on suicide among urban and rural residents. *Clinical Journal of Psychiatry*, **9**, 196–198.

Xu HL, Xiao SY, Chen JP et al. (2000). Epdemiological study on suicide among elderly in selected urban and rural areas of Hunan Province. *Chinese Mental Health Journal*, **14**, 121–124.

Yang GH, Huang ZJ, Chen AP (1997). Accidental injuries and its changes of Chinese population. *Chinese Journal of Epidemiology*, **18**, 142–145.

Yang GH, Phillips MR, Zhou MG et al. (2005). Understanding the unique characteristics of suicide in China: national psychological autopsy study. *Biomedical and Environmental Sciences*, **18**, 379–389.

Yang GH, Zheng XW, Zeng G et al. (1992). The representiveness and districts of second stage of the Disease Surveillance Point System. *Chinese Journal of Epidemilogy*, **13**, 197–200.

Yang H, Xiao SY, Dong CH (1999). Attitude towards suicide among Buddhists and health care providers in China. *Chinese Mental Health Journal*, **10**, 116–117.

Yin DK (2000). Current status of mental health work in China: problems and recommendations. *Chinese Mental Health Journal*, **14**, 4–5.

Yip PS (2001). An epidemiological profile of suicide in Beijing, China. *Suicide and Life-Threatening Behavior*, **31**, 62–70.

Yip PS, Liu KY, Hu JP et al. (2005). Suicide rates in China during a decade of rapid social changes. *Social Psychiatry and Psychiatric Epidemiology*, **40**, 792–798.

Zhai ST (1997). *Crisis Intervention and Suicide Prevention*. People's Medical Publishing House, Beijing.

Zhang B, Yang YS, Zhang C et al. (2000). An Analysis on suicide in Fengshan County, Shanghai. *Shanghai Journal of Preventive Medicine*, **12**, 282–283.

Zhang C, He FS, Phillips MR et al. (2000). Case-control study on the general conditions of uncommitted suicides with oral pesticide. *Medicine and Society*, **13**, 13–15.

Zhang J, Yeates C, Zhou L et al. (2004). Culture, risk factors and suicide in rural China: a psychological autopsy case–control study. *Acta Psychiatrica Scandinavica*, **110**, 430–437.

Zhao M and Ji JL (2000). Current status of suicide research in China and abroad. *Shanghai Archives of Psychiatry*, **12**, 222–227.

Zhong P (1991). *The Mysterious World of Sanmao*. Guangxi People's Press, Nanning.

Zhou L, Xiao SY, Tang Y et al. (2005). Suicidal ideation and its psychological risk factors in junior high school students in rural areas of Liuyang. *Chinese Journal of Behavioral Medical Sciences*, **14**, 1108–1109.

Zhou L. Xioa SY, Liu ZH et al. (2008). Intoxication emergency services' ability and accessibility at town hospitals in two counties of Hunan province. *Chinese Journal of Social Medicine*, **25**, 114–116.

# CHAPTER 34

# Prevention of suicidal behaviour in females

## Opportunities and obstacles

Silvia Sara Canetto

## Abstract

Females have higher rates of suicidal ideation and behaviour, and lower rates of suicide mortality than males. This is a dominant, but not a universal pattern, both across and within countries. One of few national exceptions is China, a country where both non-fatal and fatal suicidal behaviours are most common in women. There is also cultural heterogeneity in meanings of, and attitudes about female suicidal behaviour. In some cultures, suicide is viewed more negatively in women, while in other cultures in men. This cultural diversity in gender patterns and meanings of suicidal behaviour challenges essentialist perspectives on female suicidal behaviour, and calls for culture and gender-grounded theory, research and prevention. The perception, dominant in industrialized countries, that suicide is a male behaviour is a challenge, but can also be an opportunity in prevention in that it may discourage female suicide. Evidence indicates that critical to the prevention of female suicidal behaviour is attention to social, economic and political factors, including structures of social inequality.

## Introduction

Suicidal behaviour is a significant problem for girls and women around the world. In countries where the epidemiology of suicidal behaviours is recorded, females have higher rates of suicidal ideation and behaviour than males. Suicide mortality tends to be lower in females than in males, though this pattern is not universal (Canetto 2005). The problem of female suicidality, however, is under-regarded and under-studied (Beautrais 2006).

In this chapter I focus on female suicidal behaviour around the world. First, I address the cultural variability in definitions and recording practices of suicidal behaviour. This is to note the limitations of comparing epidemiological patterns across cultures, and the difficulty of theorizing based on cross-cultural data. Next, I review epidemiological trends in female suicidal behaviour. I then present and discuss theories and research on female suicidal behaviour from around the world. Following that, I provide a summary of the international evidence on female suicidal behaviour, as well as highlights of a theory building on these global data. In the last section, I address the implications of our current global knowledge for the prevention of female suicidal behaviour, with attention to obstacles and opportunities.

## What is suicidal behaviour?

A fundamental issue when examining suicidal behaviour across cultures is how suicidal behaviour is defined. This is because what one culture considers critical for an act to be labelled suicidal may not coincide with what another culture considers essential.

In industrialized countries suicide is defined as deliberately self-inflicted death. In other countries, however, it is not necessary for a death to be self-induced to be considered a suicide. One example is the case of ritual killing of older widows by male kin among the Lusi in the Kaliai district of Papua New Guinea. The Lusi view the ritual killing of widows as suicides, since widows presumably demand to be killed to avoid becoming dependent on their children. By contrast, the German and Australian local authorities consider widow-killing a murder (Counts 1980, 1984). It is noteworthy that widow-killing by kin does not reflect a Lusi attitude about widowhood in general. It is an attitude about female widowhood. Among the Lusi, widowers are not subject to ritual killing by kin.

In industrialized countries suicide is generally assumed to involve individual choice. Suicide voluntariness may, however, be difficult to establish. Consider, for example, the case of sati, a mode of death that has been outlawed, but is not extinct in modern India. Sati involves a widow climbing on the funeral pyre of the deceased husband to be burned with him. Sati is presumably voluntary, which would make it a suicide, at least by industrialized countries' standards. The meanings and social consequences of widowhood and sati do, however, raise questions about choice in sati. According to Hindu tradition, if a husband dies before his wife, it is because of a wrong the wife committed. In traditional communities a Hindu widow is expected to submit to social and economic restrictions, ranging from exclusion from festive events to the prohibition to marry, to banishment without possessions to an ashram, a widows' house. By contrast, a Hindu widow who dies by sati is thought to bring great fortune to herself and her kinship. Thus, in Hindu tradition, a widow does not have 'good life' choices, only a 'good suicide' choice (Andriolo 1998; Cheng and Lee 2000).

The complexity in the determination of a behaviour as suicidal is further illustrated by cases of women's deaths by domestic burning. These deaths, which typically result from having caught fire while around a household open stove, have been reported in India, Sri Lanka, Iran, South Africa and Zimbabwe. What makes these suicides questionable is that they typically occur in the context of dowry or other disputes with in-laws. Even those deaths that appear and are recorded as suicides or accidents may be murders, either directly perpetrated or indirectly triggered through psychological pressure (Waters 1999; Mzezewa *et al.* 2000; Laloe and Ganesan 2002; Sukhai *et al.* 2002; Batra 2003; Groohi *et al.* 2003; Kumar 2003; Aaron *et al.* 2004; Laloe 2004; Maghsoudi *et al.* 2004; Mohanty *et al.* 2005; Lari *et al.* 2007; Rastegar *et al.* 2007).

In conclusion, the determination of a behaviour as suicidal is influenced by cultural and political factors. Under the influence of cultural and political factors, female homicides may be recorded as suicides, while female suicides may be registered as accidents or undetermined deaths. These cultural and political influences are a liability in that they introduce unaccounted variance in epidemiological data. They are also an oppotunity in that they challenge, and ultimately expand frameworks for understanding suicidal behaviour.

## The epidemiology of female suicidal behaviour

In countries where the epidemiology of suicidal behaviours is recorded, females tend to have higher rates of suicidal ideation and behaviour than males. This is a common, but not a universal pattern. One exception is Finland, where women and men have similar rates of nonfatal suicidal behaviour (Schmidtke *et al.* 1996). A caveat with regard to the data on suicidal ideation and non-fatal suicidal behaviour is that they come from selected sources and communities that is, mostly from hospital records, urban-areas and industrialized countries.

According to World Health Organization (WHO) records, suicide mortality is lower in females than in males, though this pattern is also not universal (2007). Specifically, suicide is most frequent in women in China, a country with 21 per cent of the world's population and 56 per cent of the world's female suicide (Murray and Lopez 1996). A strength of the suicide data is that they are collected on a national basis and reported to the WHO by approximately 130 of the world's 192 nations recognized by the United Nations (Bertolote 2001). A limitation is that the national suicide mortality reported to the WHO come from a selected group of countries, with industrialized countries being over-represented in the sample (Vijayakumar *et al.* 2005b).

The over-representation of females among the suicidal, and their under-representation among the dead by suicide is a paradox. One would expect the group with the highest number of life-threatening acts to also have the highest mortality from those acts (Canetto and Sakinofsky 1998). The gender paradox of suicidal behaviour is particularly common in industrialized countries, where it is often taken as a manifestation of essential and stable female–male differences. However, the gender paradox of suicidal behaviour is not consistently found even in industrialized countries. For example, in the US, there are exceptions to the gender paradox of suicidal behaviour when one examines female–male suicidality patterns by age, ethnicity or region. US exceptions are the similar rates of nonfatal suicidal behaviour recorded among female and male adolescents of Native Hawaiian descent (Yuen *et al.* 1996) as well as among female and male Pueblo Indian adolescents (Howard-Pitney

*et al.* 1991). Exceptions to the gender paradox of suicidal behaviour are also found in Central American, South American and Asian countries. For example, in Brazil, Cuba, the Dominican Republic, Ecuador, Hong Kong, Paraguay, the Philippines, Singapore, and Thailand, young females' suicide mortality exceeds that of young males (Canetto and Lester 1995a).

It is also noteworthy that the gender paradox of suicidal behaviour is not always a stable pattern. Historical analyses of suicide mortality trends show that in some of the countries where the gender paradox had been documented, gender patterns of suicide mortality have been shifting. For example, in Denmark the gender gap in suicide mortality has been narrowing (Canetto and Sakinofsky 1998).

In conclusion, the diversity in gender patterns of suicidal behaviours within and between countries as well as across time, combined with the selectivity of the data on suicidal behaviours, suggest that the gender paradox of suicidal behaviour does not represent a universal and fixed female–male difference in suicidal behaviour, as industrialized countries' suicidologists have often assumed (Canetto 2005). Rather, the gender paradox of suicidal behaviour is a culturally and historically specific phenomenon. When one takes a global and historical perspective, one finds that there is not a distinctly female (or a uniquely male) way 'to do suicide'. Rather, female and male patterns of suicidal behaviour are in some cases similar, and in other cases different, depending on cultural context and time period (Kushner 1995; Canetto and Lester 1998).

## Theories and research on female suicidal behaviour

Internationally influential theories and research on suicidal behaviour are generated mostly in industrialized countries. As a result, these theories and research tend to focus on industrialized countries' own dominant epidemiological gender pattern—that is, females' high suicidal morbidity and their low suicidal mortality. As noted earlier, this gender pattern is common, but neither universal nor stable, even within industrialized countries. This means that industrialized countries' dominant theories and findings are culture- and time-specific, though they often purport to be universally relevant (Canetto 2005). Given their global influence, these theories and research, however, deserve attention. This section opens with a review of dominant, industrialized countries-focused theories of female suicidal behaviour. These theories are critiqued in light of evidence from both industrialized, emerging and developing countries.

A most notable feature of industrialized countries' theories and research on suicidal behaviour is their under-regard for female suicidality. Simply put, dominant theories and research mostly ignore female suicidal behaviour (Beautrais 2006).

A factor contributing to the under-investment in female suicidal behaviour is females' lower rates of suicide mortality, relative to males. The paradox is that females have much higher rates of suicidal ideation and non-fatal suicidal behaviour than males. In fact, when morbidity and mortality from suicidal behaviour are considered together, females emerge as the most suicidal group (Beautrais 2006).

Another factor likely contributing to industrialized countries' limited attention to female suicidal behaviour is a long-standing tradition of conceptualizing suicide as a male behaviour (see Kushner 1993, 1995 for reviews). Many industrialized countries' authoritative theorists, including Durkheim (1897/1951), argued that suicide requires a degree of courage and intelligence they believed could be found only in men. Specifically, according to Durkheim, women are too timid, too weak, too conformist, and too dull to kill themselves. According to this theory, women are immune to suicide—at least as long as they act 'like women', that is as long as they stay subordinate to men and subsumed within 'traditional' institutions, such as 'traditional' marriage. Women who suicide, Dublin claimed, must have experienced a 'marked increase in ... schooling and employment. ... Greater economic and social independence ... played a role' (Dublin 1963). This perspective also assumes that when women act 'masculine', that is when they venture into such masculine domains and activities as education and employment, they risk becoming suicide casualties, like men.

A major theme in dominant industrialized countries' theories and research is that female suicidal behaviour is an expression of individual pathology. Females are thought to be naturally protected from suicide—since suicide is considered masculine behaviour. Therefore, suicidal women who kill themselves, are believed to be especially abnormal and unfeminine (Canetto 1997a; Deluty 1988–1989; Kushner 1995).

In industrialized countries there has been continuous interest in the role of female-specific biological factors in the risk for, and protection from suicidal behaviour—an interest that contrasts with the consistent lack of concern for male-specific biological factors (Canetto 1995b, 1997a). The evidence for female-specific biological factors in suicidal behaviour is, however, at best equivocal. For example, some studies from industrialized countries find pregnancy and motherhood to be protective against suicidality (Lindahl et al. 2005; Stallones et al. 2007). At the same time, pregnancy and motherhood are less protective when pregnancy is unwanted or the mother is younger than 20 (Appleby 1991; Gissler and Lonnqvist 1996; Vaiva et al. 1997). There is also evidence, from some developing countries (e.g., China, India, Kuwait), of an association between female suicidal behaviour and childlessness (Wolf 1975; Batra 2003; Fido and Zahid 2004). However, in these developing countries, mothers are also at risk for suicidal behaviour if they have girls, the culturally devalued children (Wolf 1975; Pearson 1995; Waters 1999; Ji et al. 2001; Meng 2002; Batra 2003). Together, these findings suggest that what may be protective about motherhood are not some universal biological processes, but rather, its social meanings, when positive.

In industrialized countries, much attention has been given to the role of mental disorders in female suicidality, particularly depression (Canetto 1997a). This emphasis on female psychopathology fits the dominant industrialized countries discourse on suicide. In industrialized countries, mental disorders are considered critical precursors of suicidal behaviour. By contrast, in developing countries, mental disorders are not viewed as significant in suicidal behaviour, with external stressors being believed to be most influential (Marecek 1998; Vijayakumar et al. 2005b,). Industrialized countries' psychopathology perspective is consistent with their mental disorders epidemiology trends. In these countries, girls and women are more likely to be diagnosed with the mental disorders (e.g., depression) considered precursors of suicidal behaviour (Canetto 1997b). Industrialized countries' psychopathology perspective on female suicidal behaviour has many limitations,

a key one being that it does not explain their own gender paradox of suicidal behaviour. If suicidal behaviour were simply a function of psychopathology, females, the group with the highest rates of precursor mental disorders and of non-fatal suicidal behaviour, should also have highest rates of suicide mortality, which is not typically the case.

Female suicidal behaviour is often explained as a response to interpersonal problems (Canetto1997a). This theory is prevalent in industrialized countries and in developing countries, with the difference being that in developing countries, interpersonal problems are often viewed as critical to male suicidal behaviour as well (Canetto and Lester 1998; Marecek 1998; Canetto 2005). In industrialized countries, suicidal women are believed to be psychologically impaired, and to break into suicidal behaviour in response to trivial, private interpersonal problems. By contrast, in these countries, male suicide is constructed as a decision in response to important impersonal adversities and losses, such as work problems or illnesses (Canetto 1992–1993; Canetto 1997a). Women's suicidal behaviour is also often assumed to be impulsive, 'not serious' and 'manipulative', as compared to men's suicidal behaviour, which is presumed to be planned, 'serious', and death-aiming (Canetto 1997a).

Research does not support these assumptions. First, while there is evidence that interpersonal factors play a role in female suicidal behaviour, it does not appear that suicidal behaviour is more interpersonally driven in women than in men. For women, as well as for men, both interpersonal and impersonal factors appear significant in suicidal behaviour (Canetto and Lester 1995b, 2002; Hjelmeland et al. 2002b). For example, interpersonal difficulties emerge as the dominant issues in women and men's suicide notes (Canetto and Lester 2002). Also, evidence shows that employment protects both women and men from suicidal behaviour (Kposowa 2001; Stallones et al. 2007).

Second, the kind of interpersonal problems associated with female suicidal behaviour are anything but trivial. Studies from both industrialized as well as developing countries find that rates of suicidal behaviour are higher in women who have experienced abuse. This abuse, which may be sexual, physical and/ or psychological, often takes place within family relationships (Counts 1980, 1984, 1987; Stark and Flitcraft 1995; Ji et al. 2001; Batra 2003; Fergusson et al. 2005; Verona et al. 2005; Roy and Janal 2006,).

Third, research findings challenge the idea that the interpersonal problems associated with female suicidal behaviour represent 'simply' private, domestic matters. Studies from developing countries are particularly enlightening in this regard. Some argue that for single young women, suicidality is associated with private turmoil, instability, and family conflict. However, for young single suicidal women from non-industrialized societies (e.g., in East Kwaio, Malaita, in the Solomon Islands, or among the Aguaruna of the Peruvian Amazon), family conflict typically revolves around culturally-based restrictions on women's self-determination and mobility, including a culturally-specific sexual impropriety, the choice of marriage partner, or interest in education (Akin 1985; Brown 1986). Under these circumstances, the young woman's suicide is viewed as culturally understandable, if not expected. Consider next how, in several developing countries, suicidality among married women is frequently associated with conflict with, and abuse from intimate partners and/or in-laws. For example, in rural China, conflict with, and abuse from in-laws often follows childlessness or the failure to produce a son, a situation revealing a cultural tradition of female devaluation and oppression (Wolf 1975; Ji *et al.* 2001). These married women's vulnerability to abuse by their husbands and in-laws is enabled by cultural traditions, including patrilocal marriages and patrilineal inheritance traditions. Having moved away from their natal village uneducated and with no personal assets, married women end up isolated and vulnerable. Female suicide in response to family conflict and abuse is culturally sanctioned behaviour in these societies. It is a way for women to obtain justice against their abusers, though only post-mortem. For example, in China, a married woman's suicide may oblige her in-laws to provide her kin with financial compensation (Wolf 1975; Pearson 1995; Pritchard 1996; Ji *et al.* 2001; Meng 2002; Pearson and Liu 2002). Finally, suicidality in older women is also often based in cultural practices of female devaluation and oppression, though not necessarily in family conflict. In communities where older women have high suicide rates, one frequently finds the belief that older women, particularly older widows, are a burden, with suicide being considered acceptable or even expected of widows. An example is Papua New Guinea's ritual killing of widows, a practice which the Lusi considered suicide (Counts 1980, 1984). What these examples illustrate is that the presumed private relationship problems associated with female suicidality, including abuse by family members, are often grounded in, and supported by cultural traditions. Another important point highlighted by these examples is how suicidal behaviour is culturally grounded. In each culture, there are circumstances when suicidal behaviour is socially understandable, and even expected (Healey 1979; Counts 1980; Heshusius 1980; Johnson 1981; Counts 1984; Canetto 1997a; Counts 1987; Ji *et al.* 2001; Canetto 2005). As noted by Kroeber, 'culture[s] not only define[s] certain situations that call for suicide but often indicate[s] the correct way to execute it' (1948, cited in Jeffreys 1952, p. 118). The fact that one can better see the influence of culture in foreign suicidal scenarios than in one's own is an indication of the difficulty of stepping out of one's own cultural habits and norms.

Finally, research does not support the assumption that female suicidal behaviour is more impulsive and less 'serious' than male suicidal behaviour. Industrialized countries studies of impulsivity, motives and intent indicate that suicidal females and males may be more similar than different in these domains, with the wish to die being the dominant intent reported by all (Hjelmeland *et al.* 2000; Hjelmeland *et al.* 2002a). What then may account for women's lower rates of suicide mortality? We know that the fatality of a suicidal act is a function of several factors beside intent, including the suicide method, the place of the suicide, the likelihood to be quickly found, and the likelihood of effective care. The more rapidly-lethal the method, and the less public the suicidal act, the lower the likelihood of survival. It has been speculated that women's generally lower suicide mortality is a function of their being less likely to use immediately-lethal suicide methods. In industrialized countries, suicide by firearms, a method more commonly used by men, carries higher fatality potential than poisoning, a method more commonly used by women, hence men's higher suicide mortality than women's, despite their possibly similar intent. By contrast, in developing countries, suicide by poisoning, even one that is carried out in a public area, carries a high fatality potential due to the toxicity of the poisons used (e.g. agrochemicals), and the

likelihood that effective medical care may not be available quickly enough to make a difference. At the same time, it is important to remember that the choice of suicide method as well as the outcome of the suicidal act are influenced by cultural norms, that is, by what cultures consider permissible method and outcome for particular persons, given their personal characteristic and situation. The fact that firearms are the dominant suicide method for males, and that most males die of suicide in the US, are likely influenced by the association of firearms, suicide and masculinity in US culture. Similarly, in the US, non-fatal female suicidality takes place in a cultural context in which 'attempted' suicide is considered more feminine and appropriate for women (Canetto 1997a; Canetto and Lester 1998; Canetto 2005).

## Female suicidal behaviour from a global perspective

In this chapter, I examined women's suicidal behaviour from a global perspective. This examination was constrained by the cultural diversity in definitions of suicidal behaviour. Naming and registering an act as suicidal is a cultural and political act.

Studies reveal suicidal behaviour to be a significant problem for girls and women around the world. When morbidity and mortality are considered together, girls and women bear the greatest burden of suicidality. Research also shows that a common risk factor for female suicidal behaviour is the experience of abuse.

Global evidence challenges widespread assumptions about women and suicidal behaviour. One such assumption, based on Durkheim's (1897/1951) theory, is that women are immune from suicide as long as they remain 'feminine', family-bound, and socially subordinate. In fact, studies show that membership in tightly structured social units, especially patriarchal families, is a risk factor for female suicidal behaviour in some cultures (Ji *et al.* 2001; Altindag *et al.* 2005; Kushner and Sterk 2005; Vijayakumar *et al.* 2005a; van Bergen *et al.* 2006). There is also evidence that, contrary to dominant theory, individualism and social equality protect women from suicide, especially among the young. A recent study of thirty-three developing and industrialized countries found that women's suicide rates were lower in countries with social structures emphasizing individualism and social equality (Rudmin *et al.* 2003).

Global evidence also highlights the heterogeneity in women's risk for, and typical forms of suicidal behaviour across and within cultures. For example, female suicide mortality is higher than male suicide mortality in China, but lower than male suicide mortality in the US. Also, among European Americans, female adolescents have high rates of non-fatal suicidal behaviour than males. However, among Native Hawaiians, female and male adolescents have similar rates of nonfatal suicidal behaviour. Furthermore, there is heterogeneity within and across cultures in the conditions, meanings and consequences of female suicidal behaviour. For example, in some cultures suicide is viewed more negatively in women, while in other cultures in men.

## Cultural scripts theory

This review has shown that dominant, industrialized-countries theories have disregarded female suicidality and also ignored the cultural variability in female suicidal behaviour. To explain women's suicidal behaviour across cultures, theory needs to start from a foundation on gender and culture. An example of such approach is cultural scripts theory (Canetto 1997a, 1997b, Canetto and Lester 1998, Canetto 2005). Cultural scripts can be thought of as norms of suicidal behaviour, that is, beliefs about, and practices of suicidal behaviour. A cultural script defines the meanings of suicidal behaviour, and the conditions under which suicidal behaviour is relatively acceptable, or even expected. A cultural script has also to do with the suicidal scenario, that is the events leading to the suicidal behaviour, the protagonists of the suicidal situation, the emotions and motives associated with the suicidal behaviour, and the suicide method. Furthermore, cultural scripts guide community responses to the suicidal behaviour, including those of experts and authorities.

Cultural script theory is grounded on the observation of a correspondence between scripts of suicidal behaviour and patterns of suicidal behaviour. Ideology and epidemiology likely reinforce each other. The fact that in some countries females are less likely to die of suicide likely contributes to the belief in the masculinity of suicide. This belief, in turn, can act as a social norm and a model, discouraging female suicide. The belief in the masculinity of suicide may also contribute to the under-recording of female deaths as suicide, especially when they are ambiguous, further perpetuating the norm and belief in the masculinity of suicide (Kushner 1993, 1995; Canetto and Sakinofsky 1998).

According to this theory, the risk for suicidal behaviour needs to be evaluated in light of local cultural scripts. This is based on the observation that those most at risk for suicidal behaviour are not necessarily the individuals who are most psychologically impaired, or the persons facing the greatest adversities. Rather the persons who engage in suicidal behaviour are those whose characteristics and circumstances also fit local scripts of suicidal behaviour. In other words, suicidal behaviour is most likely when it is socially expected. This does not mean that there is minimal individual agency in suicidal behaviour. It only means that individual agency is articulated in relation to cultural scripts (Canetto 2005). Individuals draw on local scripts in defining their suicidal action and in giving their suicidal behaviour public significance (Rubinstein 1992; Canetto 2005)

Cultural script theory overcomes the limitations of a purely individual perspective on female suicidal behaviour, including industrialized countries conceptualization of suicide as individual psychopathology. Cultural script theory also overcomes the limitations of pure ecological perspectives on suicidal behaviour, such as those dominant in developing countries. By focusing on meanings of gender and suicidality, cultural script theory integrates individual and ecological influences, and accounts for the apparent paradox that those who are most oppressed are not always the most suicidal. Consider, for example, that in the US, suicide rates are highest among older men of European-American descent, and lowest among older women of African-American descent. According to cultural script theory, this is because suicidal behaviour is most likely when it is the culturally-supported response (Canetto 2005).

## The prevention of female suicidal behaviour: obstacles and opportunities

What are the suicide prevention directions suggested by the global data on female suicidal behaviour? These data challenge essentialist perspectives on female suicidal behaviour. They also call attention to both environmental and individual factors in female suicidal behaviour. Finally, they highlight the importance of attending to culture and gender in prevention work. A culture- and gender-grounded suicide prevention approach means avoiding one size fits all programmes. This approach may take the form of a programme exploring, and educating about local scripts of suicidal behaviour. In a country like the US, where suicide 'attempts' are associated with femininity, educational programmes might challenge the notion that non-fatal suicidal behaviour is a feminine way to cope with problems. This notion is not only problematic for females in that it may inadvertently encourage female non-fatal suicidal behaviour. It is also dysfunctional for males in that it may push suicidal males toward killing themselves. As argued by Linehan, 'due to social pressures against attempted suicide, males ... [might] "skip" over the less drastic solution of attempting suicide and go directly to suicide' (Linehan 1973, pp. 31–32).

There are many obstacles to the prevention of female suicidal behaviour. A major one is the belief, dominant in industrialized countries, that suicide is a male problem. This belief contributes to under-evaluating the severity of the problem of female suicidality. It also obscures the variability in female suicide mortality between and across countries. Educating about females' significant involvement in suicidal behaviour may draw needed attention to it. Studies of female suicidal behaviour will not only provide critical information about female suicidal behaviour, but likely also promote greater understanding of male suicidal behaviour, as issues relevant to both that most readily emerge through the study of women may have been overlooked in studies of men (Canetto 1995a). Education on the seriousness of female suicidal behaviour problem may also improve the care of suicidal females. Studies indicate that care-providers are particularly unhelpful and hostile toward suicidal females out of the misguided view that their suicidality is not serious (see Canetto 1995b for a review).

The belief in females' immunity to suicide is an obstacle, but can also be a resource in the prevention of female suicidal behaviour. Women who believe in the masculinity of suicide may be more reluctant to kill themselves. When working with suicidal women, caregivers can reframe the false negative belief of the masculinity of suicide into an empowering positive belief. Reinforcing women's rejection of suicide as a solution to their problems as well as women's expectation of efficacy in coping with suicidal ideation may support actual effective coping.

Yet, another obstacle to effective suicide prevention in females is the over-emphasis on individual factors, and the under-appreciation of social, economic and cultural factors in female suicidal behaviour. Studies suggest that significant progress in the prevention of female suicidal behaviour will require a paradigmatic shift of focus, from individual to ecological factors (Douglas 1967; Counts 1987; Canetto and Lester 1995a; Corin 1996; Canetto 1997a, b; Canetto and Lester 1998; Waters 1999; Ji et al. 2001; Meng 2002; Pearson and Liu 2002; Laloe 2004; Canetto 2005; Rudmin et al. 2003; Mitra and Singh 2007). Critical in this regard is attention to the role of social equality in females' protection against suicidal behaviour.

## References

Aaron R, Joseph A, Abraham S et al. (2004). Suicides in young people in rural southern India. *The Lancet*, **363**, 1117–1118.

Akin D (1985). Suicide and women in East Kwaio, Malaita. In FX Hezel, DH Rubinstein, GM White, eds, *Culture, Youth and Suicide in the Pacific: Paper from an East-West Center Conference*, pp. 198–210. Pacific Island Studies Program, University of Hawaii, Honolulu.

Altindag A, Ozkan M, Oto R (2005). Suicide in Batman, Southeastern Turkey. *Suicide and Life-Threatening Behavior*, **35**, 478–482.

Andriolo KR (1998). Gender and the cultural construction of good and bad suicides. *Suicide and Life-Threatening Behavior*, **28**, 37–49.

Appleby L (1991). Suicide during pregnancy and in the first postnatal year. *British Medical Journal*, **302**, 137–140.

Batra AK (2003). Burn mortality: recent trends and sociocultural determinants in rural India. *Burns*, **29**, 270–275.

Beautrais AL (2006). Women and suicidal behavior. *Crisis*, **27**, 153–156.

Bertolote JM (2001). Suicide in the world: an epidemiological overview, 1959–2000. In D Wasserman, ed., *Suicide—An Unnecessary Death*, pp. 3–10. Martin Dunitz, London.

Brown MF (1986). Power, gender, and the social meaning of Aguaruna suicide. *Man*, **21**, 311–328.

Canetto SS (1992–1993). She died for love and he for glory: gender myths of suicidal behavior. *Omega—Journal of Death and Dying*, **26**, 1–17.

Canetto SS (1995a). Elderly women and suicidal behavior. In SS Canetto and D Lester, eds, *Women and Suicidal Behavior*, pp. 215–233. Springer, New York.

Canetto SS (1995b). Suicidal women: intervention and prevention strategies. In SS Canetto and Lester, eds, *Women and Suicidal Behavior*, pp. 237–255. Springer, New York.

Canetto SS (1997a). Gender and suicidal behavior: theories and evidence. In RW Maris, MM Silverman and SS Canetto, eds, *Review of Suicidology*, pp. 138–167. Guilford, New York.

Canetto SS (1997b). Meanings of gender and suicidal behavior among adolescents. *Suicide and Life-Threatening Behavior*, **27**, 339–351.

Canetto SS (2005). Patterns and scripts of women's and men's suicidal behavior across cultures. *Pogled—The View III /Acta Suicidologica Slovenica*, **1–2**, 21–35.

Canetto SS and Lester D (1995a). Gender and the primary prevention of suicide mortality. *Suicide and Life-Threatening Behavior*, **25**, 58–69.

Canetto SS and Lester D (1995b). The epidemiology of women's suicidal behavior. In SS Canetto and D Lester, eds, *Women and Suicidal Behavior*, pp. 35–57. Springer, New York.

Canetto SS and Lester D (1998). Gender, culture, and suicidal behavior. *Transcultural Psychiatry*, **35**, 163–191.

Canetto SS and Lester D (2002). Love and achievement motives in women's and men's suicide notes. *Journal of Psychology*, **136**, 573–576.

Canetto SS and Sakinofsky I (1998). The gender paradox in suicide. *Suicide and Life-Threatening Behavior*, **28**, 1–23.

Cheng ATA and Lee CS (2000). Suicide in Asia and the Far East. In K Hawton and K van Heeringen, eds, *The International Handbook of Suicide and Attempted Suicide*, pp. 29–48. Wiley, Chichester.

Corin E (1996). From a cultural stance: suicide and aging in a changing world. In JL Pearson and Y Conwell, eds, *Suicide and Aging: International Perspectives*, pp. 205–228. Springer, New York.

Counts DA (1980). Fighting back is not the way: suicide and the women of Kaliai. *American Ethnologist*, **7**, 332–351.

Counts DA (1984). Revenge suicide by Lusi women: an expression of power. In D O'Brien and WT Sharon, eds, *Rethinking Women's Roles: Perspectives from the Pacific*, pp. 71–93. University of California Press, Berkeley.

Counts DA (1987). Female suicide and wife abuse: a cross-cultural perspective. *Suicide and Life-Threatening Behavior*, **17**, 194–204.

Deluty RH (1988–1989). Factors affecting the acceptability of suicide. *Omega: Journal of Death and Dying*, **19**, 315–326.

Douglas JD (1967). *The Social Meanings of Suicide*. Princeton University Press, Princeton.

Dublin LI (1963). *Suicide: A Sociological and Statistical Study*. Ronald, New York.

Durkheim, E. (1897). *Suicide: A Study in Sociology*. JA Spaulding and G Simpson, trans. 1951. The Free Press, Glencoe.

Fergusson DM, Horwood LJ, Ridder E (2005). Partner violence and mental health outcomes in a New Zealand birth cohort. *Journal of Marriage and the Family*, **67**, 1103–1119.

Fido A and Zahid MA (2004). Coping with infertility among Kuwaiti women: cultural perspectives. *International Journal of Social Psychiatry*, **50**, 294–300.

Gissler HE and Lonnqvist J (1996). Suicides after pregnancy in Finland, 1987–1994: register linkage study. *British Medical Journal Clinical Research*, **313**, 1431–1434.

Groohi B, Alaghehbandan R, Lari AR (2003). Analysis of 1089 burn patients in the province of Kurdistan, Iran. *Burns*, **28**, 569–574.

Healey C (1979). Women and suicide in New Guinea. *Social Analysis*, **2**, 89–107.

Heshusius L (1980). Female self-injury and suicide attempts: culturally reinforced techniques in human relations. *Sex Roles*, **6**, 843–857.

Hjelmeland H, Hawton K, Nordvik H *et al.* (2002a). Why people engage in parasuicide: a cross-cultural study of intentions. *Suicide and Life-Threatening Behavior*, **32**, 380–393.

Hjelmeland H, Knizek LK, Nordvik H (2002b). The communicative aspect of nonfatal suicidal behavior—are there gender differences? *Crisis*, **23**, 144–155.

Hjelmeland H, Nordvik H, Bille-Brahe U *et al.* (2000). A cross-cultural study of suicide intent in parasuicide patients. *Suicide and Life-Threatening Behavior*, **30**, 295–303.

Howard-Pitney B, LaFramboise TD, Basil M *et al.* (1992). Psychological and social indicators of suicide ideation and suicide attempts in Zuni adolescents. *Journal of Consulting and Clinical Psychology*, **60**, 473–476.

Jeffreys MDW (1952). Samsonic suicides: or suicide of revenge among Africans. *African Studies*, **99**, 118–122.

Ji J, Kleinman A, Becker AE (2001). Suicide in contemporary China: a review of China's distinctive suicide demographics in their sociocultural context. *Harvard Review of Psychiatry*, **9**, 1–12.

Johnson PL (1981). When dying is better than living: female suicide among the Gainj of Papua New Guinea. *Ethnology*, **20**, 325–335.

Kposowa, AJ (2001). Unemployment and suicide: a cohort analysis of social factors predicting suicide in the US National Longitudinal Mortality Study. *Psychological Medicine*, **31**, 127–138.

Kumar V (2003). Burnt wives—a study of suicides. *Burns*, **29**, 31–35.

Kushner HI (1993). Gender and the irrelevance of medical innovation: the social construction of suicide as a male behavior in nineteenth century psychiatry. In I Lowy, ed., *L'innovation en Medicine: Etudes Historiques et Sociologiques*, pp. 421–445. Les Editions INSERM/Libby Eurotext, Paris.

Kushner HI (1995). Women and suicidal behavior: epidemiology, gender and lethality in historical perspective. In SS Canetto and D Lester, eds, *Women and Suicidal Behavior*, pp. 11–34. Springer, New York.

Kushner HI and Sterk CE (2005). The limits of social capital: Durkheim, suicide, and social cohesion. *American Journal of Public Health*, **95**, 1–5.

Laloe V (2004). Patterns of deliberate self-burning in various parts of the world. A review. *Burns*, **30**, 207–215.

Laloe V and Ganesan M (2002). Self-immolation: a common suicidal behavior in eastern Sri Lanka. *Burns*, **28**, 475–480.

Lari AR, Joghataei MT, Adli YR, ZadehYA, Alaghehbandan R (2007). Epidemiology of suicide by burns in the province of Isfaham, Iran. *Journal of Burn Care and Research*, **28**, 307–311.

Lindahl V, Pearson JL, Colpe L (2005). Prevalence of suicidality during pregnancy and the postpartum. *Archives of Women's Mental Health*, **8**, 77–87.

Linehan MM (1973). Suicide and attempted suicide: study of perceived sex differences. *Perceptual and Motor Skills*, **37**, 31–34.

Maghsoudi H, Garadagi A, Jafary GA *et al.* (2004). Women victims of self-inflicted burns in Tabriz, Iran. *Burns*, **30**, 217–220.

Marecek J (1998). Culture, gender, and suicidal behavior in Sri Lanka. *Suicide and Life-Threatening Behavior*, **28**, 69–81.

Meng L (2002). Rebellion and revenge: the meaning of suicide of women in rural China. *International Journal of Social Welfare*, **11**, 300–309.

Mitra A and Singh P (2007). Human capital attainment and gender empowerment: the Kerala paradox. *Social Science Quarterly*, **88**, 1227–1242.

Mohanty MK, Arun M, Monteiro FNP *et al.* (2005). Self-inflicted burn fatalities in Manipal, India. *Medicine, Science and the Law*, **45**, 27–30.

Murray CJL and Lopez AD eds (1996). *The Global Burden of Disease: A Comprehensive Assessment of Mortality and Disability from Diseases.* Harvard University Press, Cambridge.

Mzezewa S, Jonsson K, Aberg M *et al.* (2000). A prospective study of suicide burns admitted to the Harare burns unit. *Burns*, **26**, 460–464.

Pearson V (1995). Goods in which one loses: women and mental health in China. *Social Science and Medicine*, **41**, 1159–1173.

Pearson V and Liu M (2002). Ling's death: an ethnography of a Chinese woman's suicide. *Suicide and Life-Threatening Behavior*, **32**, 347–358.

Pritchard C (1996). Suicide in the People's Republic of China categorized by age and gender: evidence of the influence of culture on suicide. *Acta Psychiatrica Scandinavica*, **93**, 362–367.

Rastegar A., Joghataei MT, Adli YR *et al.* (2007). Epidemiology of suicide by burns in the province of Isfahan, Iran. *Journal of Burn Care and Research*, **28**, 307–311.

Roy A and Janal M (2006). Gender in suicide attempt rates and childhood sexual abuse rates: is there an interaction? *Suicide and Life-Threatening Behavior*, **36**, 329–335.

Rubinstein DH (1992). Suicide in Micronesia and Samoa: a critique of explanations. *Pacific Studies*, **15**, 51–75.

Rudmin FW, Ferrada-Noli M, Skolbekken JA (2003). Questions of culture, age and gender in the epidemiology of suicide. *Scandinavian Journal of Psychology*, **44**, 373–381.

Schmidtke A, Bille-Brahe U, De Leo D *et al.* (1996). Attempted suicide in Europe: rates, trends, and socio-demographic characteristics of suicide attempters during the period 1989–1992. *Acta Psychiatrica Scandinavica*, **93**, 327–338.

Stallones L, Leff M, Canetto SS *et al.* (2007). Suicidal ideation among low-income women on family assistance programs. *Women and Health*, **45**, 65–83.

Stark E and A Flitcraft (1995). Killing the beast within: woman battering and female suicidality. *International Journal of Health Services*, **25**, 43–64.

Sukhai A, Harris C, Moorad RGR *et al.* (2002). Suicide by self-immolation in Durban, South Africa. *American Journal of Forensic Medical Pathology*, **23**, 295–298.

Vaiva G, Tiessler E, Cottencin O *et al.* (1997). Letter to the editor: On suicide and attempted suicide in pregnancy. *Crisis*, **20**, 27.

van Bergen DD, Smit JH, Kerkhof A *et al.* (2006). Young Hindustani immigrant women in The Netherlands. *Crisis*, **27**, 181–188.

Verona E, Hicks BM, Patrick CJ (2005). Psychopathy and suicidality in female offenders: mediating influences of personality and abuse. *Journal of Consulting and Clinical Psychology*, **73**, 1065–1073.

Vijayakumar L, John S, Pirkis J *et al.* (2005a). Suicide in developing countries (2): risk factors. *Crisis*, **26**, 112–119.

Vijayakumar L, Nagaraj K, Pirkis J *et al.* (2005b). Suicide in developing countries (1): frequency, distribution, and association with socio-economic indicators. *Crisis*, **26**, 104–111.

Waters A (1999). Domestic dangers: approaches to women's suicide in contemporary Maharashtra, India. *Violence against Women*, **5**, 525–547.

Wolf M (1975). Women and suicide in China. In M Wolf and R Witke, eds, *Women in Chinese Society*, pp. 111–141. Stanford University Press, Stanford.

World Health Organization (2007). Suicide rates per 100,000 by country, year and sex (Table) Retrieved 2 December 2007 from http://www.who.int/mental_health/prevention/suicide_rates/en/index.html

Yuen N, Andrade N, Nahulu L *et al.* (1996). The rate and characteristics of suicide attempters in the Native Hawaiian adolescent population. *Suicide and Life-Threatening Behavior*, **26**, 27–36.

# CHAPTER 35

# Suicide in men

## Suicide prevention for the male person

Wolfgang Rutz and Zoltán Rihmer

## Abstract

Male life expectancy in Europe is between 5–15 years lower than that of women. This might, in part, be related to the fact that men in general approach and consume medical services only half as often as females. Between 70–90 per cent of all suicides are committed in a clinical condition of major depression and, paradoxically, men commit suicide 3–10 times more often than women in spite of being only half or less frequently diagnosed as depressive than women. Male depressive symptoms are different from those reported by females, mainly because of men's alexythymic difficulty in recognizing and reporting depressive symptoms. In addition, male depression can manifest itself as abusive, aggressive or antisocial behaviour. Moreover, in the case of suicidal behaviour, males more frequently use violent or lethal methods. Training of health care workers on earlier and better detection of male depression (including the use of the Gotland male Depression Scale) and increasing public awareness for depression are promising tools in the prevention of suicide in males.

## Morbidity and mortality in European societies—a question of male ill-being and suicide

Both genders define and influence each other's identity and societal situation. This means that men and women in a societal and individual crisis situation often become each other's problem, which can cause violence as well as suicide, abuse, risk-taking behaviour and stress-related somatic disorders. Thus, increasing the understanding and communicative ability, as well as social interaction between the two genders on a political level, in society as a whole, in families and between individuals seems to be one of the best health promotional activities. Such efforts should be made in parallel with improving early detection and possibilities for therapeutic intervention, especially concerning common but atypical conditions of 'male depression' as well as depression related to aggression and suicidality.

Danish men commit suicide seven times more often than women do during the first year after a divorce (Qin et al. 2000). Male life expectancy in the WHO European region is between five and fifteen years lower than that of women, and a widening gap between female and male life-expectancy seems to be a reliable indicator for an increasing stress load in a society (WHO 2005). In the European Union, mental ill-health is considered to be 'Europe's unseen killer'. The European Commissioner for Health declares that 'the societies we have created generate mental ill health', and the mental ill-health related and stress-related mortality in Europe is predominantly a male problem (European Commission 2005; WHO 2005).

In some Eastern European societies that are undergoing heavy and dramatic transitions, male life expectancy decreased during the 1990s within one decade by more than ten years, whereas female morbidity and mortality patterns remained unchanged. Increased numbers of suicide were one of the most important contributing factors to the decrease in male life expectancy (Wasserman et al. 1994; Notzon et al. 1998; Värnik et al. 1998; Rutz 2001).

The examples above may lead us to believe that males are more vulnerable than females in times of stressful transition and change. Looking at male suicide figures as the expression of mental ill-being, and comparing them to female suicides in Eastern Europe's countries of transition, we find that females seem to be more protected in times of change. Male suicidality seems to reflect almost unequivocally the stress load in a society, often related to challenged traditional role expectations and status losses in society, working places and as family providers (Taylor et al. 1998; Qin et al. 2000). It strongly correlates with mortality due to violence, risk-taking, accidents, injuries and cardio- and cerebrovascular disorders, a mortality that increased five to nine times compared to that of women.

## Determinants of mental health

There is consensus in the medical world today that the following conditions are crucial determinants for physical and mental health (Wilkinson and Marmot 1998): a sense of control, that is, the absence of helplessness; a feeling of social connectedness and significance, i.e. the absence of alienation, marginalization and social deprivation; a sense of cohesion, that is to say an absence of meaninglessness and existential emptiness; and finally, the feeling of dignity, status and integrity in life.

It is known from animal trials that males and females respond to stress differently (Jackson et al. 2005). The loss of social significance seems to be the most important risk factor in women, whereas males are especially sensitive to impairments in societal status and dignity (Taylor *et al.* 1998). Male individuals are most sensitive to hierarchical degradation, whereas females react more strongly to social deprivation and the loss of family cohesion. A recent Danish study on more than 800 suicide victims found that beside mental illness, which was the strongest risk factor for suicide for both genders, unemployment, retirement, being single and sickness absence were significant risk factors for men, and having a child at home was a significant protective factor for women (Qin *et al.* 2000). Related to this, there are indications that stressful societal and even individual transition in life due to unemployment and the loss of the capacity to be the family provider heavily afflicts males, whereas women even in times of crisis and transition often have the protective capacity to retain social networks, family responsibility and a feeling and ability to create control and meaning in life (Taylor *et al.* 1998; Qin *et al.* 2000).

## Gender related public health paradoxes

Two paradoxes of public health can be detected in Europe today. First, men in general approach and consume medical services, with the intention to ask for help only half as often as females, yet die, five (European Union) to fifteen (Russian Federation) years earlier than women (WHO 2005). The second one is attributed to the gender specificity of depression and suicide. We know today that between 70–90 per cent of all suicides are committed in a clinical condition of major depression and a consecutive depressive distortion of emotional and cognitive perception (Wasserman 2001; Rihmer *et al.* 2002). Paradoxically, men commit suicide three to ten times more often than women (Isometsa and Lönnqvist 1998; Wasserman 2001; Rihmer *et al.* 2002; Levi *et al.* 2003), despite being diagnosed as depressive only half as often, or less, as women (Picinelli and Wilkinson 2000; Szádóczky *et al.* 2002). Suicide attempts are much more frequent among females, yet males are markedly over-represented among suicide victims, and one of the explanations could be their use of more violent/lethal methods (Isometsa and Lönnqvist 1998; Wasserman 2001; Rihmer *et al.* 1995, 2002; Levi *et al.* 2003). The probable factor behind this is the failure of detection of male depressive conditions (Rutz 1999).

An exception from the European male preponderance of committed suicides can be found in central Asian and Asian countries, such as Kazakhstan, Kyrgyzstan, China and India. In these countries, young females are heavily exposed to the social consequences of gender role transition. In China, suicide-preventive subjection of females due to responsibilities for family and children has been weakened due to birth control and family restrictions (Yang *et al.* 2005). Furthermore, the easy access to heavily poisonous pesticides and insecticides is widespread.

Today, there is epidemiological evidence as well as clinical experience that the prevalence of diagnosed depression is inversely correlated to the frequency of suicide (Rihmer *et al.* 1993). Such evidence contrasts our knowledge about the specific and causal links between depression and suicide (Wasserman 2001; Rihmer *et al.* 2002) that would suggest an increase of suicides when depression more frequently occurs. This 'prima vista' paradox can only be explained by the postulate that adequately diagnosed and acknowledged depression leads to adequate treatment, thus preventing 'depressiogenic' suicides (Rihmer and Akiskal. 2006).

In accordance with this, Hungarian research shows that a statistically low prevalence of diagnosed depression in a population correlates with a high number of committed suicides, but also that a high number of recognized and consequently properly treated depression correlates with a lower suicide frequency (Rihmer *et al.* 1990, 1993; Rihmer 2004a; Berecz *et al.* 2005). These findings have been replicated in different studies. They show that improvements of the detection and monitoring of depression, e.g. through education of professionals in primary health or psychiatric care, but also by awareness raising activities in the society as a whole, often result in an increase of specific antidepressive prescriptions to an adequate population level and are correlated with lowered suicide rates (Rutz *et al.* 1990, 1997; Rihmer *et al.* 1995; Isacsson 2000; Oravecz *et al.* 2003; Rihmer 2004a; Grunebaum *et al.* 2004; Ludwig and Macrotte 2005; Rihmer and Akiskal 2006; Henriksson and Isacsson 2006). However, one must be conscious of methodological fallacies when analyses are performed on an aggregate level (Khan *et al.* 2003; Ferguson *et al.* 2005).

## Symptoms of male depression and suicidality—a question of gender specificity?

Male depression is often overlooked and not recognized, due to one or many of the following reasons: concomitant abusive and alcoholic behaviour, drug addiction, poor impulse control and an aggressive and violent acting out that misleads to an incomplete diagnosis of personality disorder, psychopathy or addiction (Rutz *et al.* 1995, 1997). Apparently, male depressive symptoms are different from those symptoms generally reported by females. Diagnostic criteria in conventionally used depression assessments are most often developed on the basis of reported symptoms of depression (Wasserman 2006). Such criteria could be inadequate or non-sufficient in male depression because of men's alexithymic incapacity to acknowledge depression and to report depressive symptoms (Rutz *et al.* 1997).

Two large-scale, community-based epidemiological studies showed that untreated depressive males reported depressed moods significantly less frequently than females, and that depressive males report fewer symptoms than females (Angst *et al.* 2002; Szádóczky *et al.* 2002). In addition, Angst *et al.* (2002) also found that there were marked gender differences in coping style: men coped by increasing their sports activities and consumption of alcohol and tobacco and women through emotional release, religion and reading. The high degree of abuse in males related to their helplessness and depression points to self-medication in the absence of specific help, where, for example, the alcohol consumption in a vicious circle reinforces the depressive underlying condition (Bech 2001; Angst *et al.* 2002).

## Lower prevalence of depression in males—an artefact?

In the American Amish population, aggressive and violent acting out as well as addiction and alcohol abuse are strictly stigmatized (Egeland *et al.* 1983). Similarly, in many American Jewish communities, as well as among Israeli orthodox Jews, alcohol abuse is taboo and considerably less frequent than in other ethnical and religious groups (Levav *et al.* 1993). Interestingly, the rate of depression in these populations is as high in males as in females, and suicide figures are equally low in both genders.

On the other hand, in those European countries where alcohol abuse frequently exists and has a relatively low stigma, the prevalence of female depression is considered to be two or three times higher than in males. Male completed suicides, however, are two to three times more frequent than in females (Picinelli and Wilkinson 2000; Wasserman 2001; Szádóczky *et al.* 2002; Angst *et al.* 2002; Rihmer *et al.* 2002; Levi *et al.* 2003.) Alcoholism that may camouflage depression is nine to ten times higher in Russian males than in females. Accordingly, the female to male ratio in completed suicide is 1:6 (Wasserman *et al.* 1994) and depression in certain Russian male populations are hardly ever diagnosed (Levi *et al.* 2003; Krasnov 2004). This, again, may exemplify the problematic under-diagnosis of depression in males resulting in high male suicide rates.

Thus, the following question can be asked: are European men today, as shown in Hungarian research (Rihmer et al 1990, 1993), under-treated and under-diagnosed in their depression and, therefore, 'over-suiciding' and exposed to the self-destructive consequences of risk-taking, self-neglecting and careless behaviour? Is the preponderance of female depression explained by insufficient diagnostic and therapeutic efforts in relation to depressed men, and as such an artefact? Can a solution be found through the improvement of the diagnosis and treatment compliance of depressive males?

## Problems of detecting male depression and suicidality

The WHO collaborative study 'Psychological problems in general health care', performed in 1991 on more than 25,000 primary care patients in 14 countries found that only 15 per cent of the patients with ICD-10 diagnosis of major depression were recognized as such by their general practitioners (Lecrubier 1998). However, more recent studies from the United States and Europe report a higher rate of recognition (Berardi *et al.* 2005). Considering the above, the recognition and treatment of the atypical male depression in medical and social services is still problematic. The biggest challenge, however, seems to be to identify depressive and suicidal males outside all supportive services, the ones who do not seek help, and who sometimes act out and often self-medicate their depression through addictions or addictive comportments such as gambling, fighting, excessive exercise, 'workaholism' or hypersexuality. This challenge is emphasized in a recent community study from Australia reporting that in both adolescents and adults the belief that one can deal with depression alone (i.e. without medical help) was significantly associated with the male gender. A less favourable view regarding mental health professionals could be detected, and a more favourable attitude toward substance use, such as alcohol, nicotine, marijuana, to cope with depression was widespread among men (Jorm *et al.* 2006). Another large-scale Australian survey also showed that compared to females, males more frequently contended with their suicidal crisis by an over-consumption of alcohol and or a misuse/overuse of drugs (De Leo *et al.* 2005).

## Males suicides—the case of Lithuania

According to WHO data, the highest suicide rates in the world can be found in the Baltic States, especially in Lithuania, predominantly in rural areas characterized by high male alcoholic consumption,

a low degree of male help-seeking and low prevalence of diagnosed and statistically registered depression in males.

Suicides in Lithuania are in 90 per cent of all cases committed by males, generally in the countryside. In order to tackle this issue, crisis intervention centres have been established in most communities, professionally staffed and working intensively around the clock. The problem is, however, that 80–90 per cent of their clients are female, and the suicide figures remain as high as before. However, the centres have existed for no longer than a few years, and results of intervention activities take time to evaluate correctly (O Davidoniene, personal communication 2005).

The lesson here is that male suicidality has to be met by innovative approaches. Availability and accessibility of services is not enough: they have to be acceptable and adapted to value systems favouring traditional and, worst, stagnant views on masculinity and the male self-imagination. However, to create services acceptable to male farmers and fisherman exposed to dramatic stress and work insecurity in a countryside in transition is not an easy task. Non-conventional platforms and arenas have to be used—the workplace, public spaces, religious congregations, sports clubs or trade union associations. Additionally, the willingness and engagement of relatives and friends to invest in socially difficult and life-threatening situations is essential.

## Suicide, aggression and violence

Male suicidality can be studied through the quite intricate context of depression, suicide, auto-aggressive self neglect and hetero-aggressive violence. Together with suicides, homicides in Russia have increased nine times during the 1990s, in parallel with an increase of alcohol intoxication related deaths, accidents and cardio- and cerebral vascular mortality (Rutz 2006). In the Balkan countries, especially in Islamic cultures, suicidality is relatively rare, even in times of societal stress and inner conflicts. Instead, premature mortality due to cardiovascular disorders, accidents, and homicides have increased dramatically since the conflict in former Yugoslavia, mainly related to different types of addiction as well as to aggressive behaviour and general misconduct (A Marusic, personal communication 2004). In Latin American countries, depression in males is also rarely diagnosed and the prevalence of female depression is up to ten times higher. However, aggression, violence, homicide and alcoholism, but not suicides, are to be found up to ten times more often among males (I Levav, personal communication 2004.)

The interrelationship between depression, suicide, abuse and violence is elaborated in the WHO's *World Health Report on Mental Health 2001* and the *World Health Report on Violence 2003*. Both reports point to the idea that an increase of male suicidality and a high prevalence of aggression, family violence, male carelessness and self-destruction could be related to male depression, and could be tackled by an improvement of detecting, treating and monitoring male depressive conditions (WHO 2001, 2003).

## What can be done? The Gotland experience

An educational approach on the prevention, treatment and monitoring of depression and suicide was directed to all general practitioners on the Swedish island of Gotland from 1984 to 1985 (Rutz *et al.* 1990, 1997). A drastic increase of suicidality during the 1970s and early 1980s led to a situation that primary health care doctors no longer felt able to deal with. On their demand, a comprehensive educational programme was started that resulted in a significant improvement of the GPs ability to detect and treat depressive conditions. The outcome was an obvious decrease of completed suicides and violent suicide attempts on the island, together with a decrease of depression-related morbidity, workplace absence and health care consumption. However, the positive results almost exclusively concerned the female depression-related suicides (Rihmer *et al.* 1995). Male suicidality was unchanged and remained very high (Rutz *et al.* 1995, 1997*)*.

The findings of the Gotland Study have been replicated in Jämtland county in Sweden, which also showed that the improvement in the treatment of depression and preventing suicide was more pronounced in women (Henriksson and Isacsson 2006).

To investigate the reasons for the unchanged male suicide rate, a psychological autopsy was performed on all male suicides committed on Gotland after the educational intervention. The study showed that the male suicide victims were unknown to the medical system, be it the psychiatric one or the primary care one. The men had not asked for help, but appeared to be quite disturbed on a personal level to themselves, their families and friends and the police, to taxation authorities and to the social welfare system, especially the units for alcohol and addiction. The men displayed misconduct through frequent verbal and physical manifestations of aggression, irritation, dissatisfaction, disturbed personality traits and a subjective feeling of uneasiness as well as bad impulse control together with abuse and a general negativism. They were generally not seeking help and had, in the few cases of seeking assistance, a non-compliant attitude to eventual treatment attempts (Rutz *et al.* 1995, 1997; Rutz 1999).

When a scientific evaluation of the original educational intervention was finalized in 1994 and showed the described positive results on female suicides (Rihmer *et al.* 1995), a programme, of continued education on depression was started in 1994 and offered to the general practitioners on Gotland. In this programme, information about the male depressive and suicidal syndrome was added and given to primary health care, but also to other caregivers and the general population, by dissemination via mass media and in complementary educational programmes. The public response was mostly from women asking for help for male relatives who they easily could recognize in the published descriptions of male depression and suicidality (Rutz *et al.* 1997; Rutz 1999). However, this was enough to motivate an increasing number of males to seek and keep therapeutic contact with the medical system and get their depressive and suicidal condition treated. As a result of this approach, the number of male suicides on Gotland significantly decreased for the first time in the mid and late 1990s (Rutz *et al.* 1997).

## Improving the recognition, early intervention and monitoring of male depression and suicidality

Males hardly ever report depression, depressive feelings or symptoms. Therefore, screening instruments in primary care and other medical settings should be used. An assessment instrument for male depression, the Gotland Male Depression Scale (see the Appendix to this chapter), can detect the phenomenology and depressive symptoms that have been found to be typical of depressed and suicidal males (Rutz 1999; Wälinder and Rutz 2001).

Such symptoms have been considered atypical, and thus have been overlooked in a medical world where therapeutic efforts depend on the gender bias in the diagnostic efforts. The subsequent lack of awareness and incorporation of gender data lead to blind spots, and a failure to see the differences as well as similarities between men and women in experience, conditions and symptoms. Today, the Gotland Male Depression Scale has been scientifically validated; it is translated into different languages and is met nationally and internationally with increasing interest. It is with good results used as a screening instrument in primary health care, but also by social welfare authorities in the treatment of masked depression in alcoholics and substance abusers, even among young men (Bech 2001; Zierau *et al.* 2002; Möller-Leimkühler *et al.* 2004). In addition to conventional depression diagnostic instruments in primary care, the Gotland Male Depression Scale is a helpful tool. Another useful screening method is the WHO 5 Well-Being Scale, which does not ask for depressive symptoms, but for a greater or lesser state of well-being in ways that those who is not used to verbalizing emotions appear able and willing to answer. This scale has been used in different large investigations, and it is one of most useful first screening steps to a diagnosis of male depression, even in non-medical arenas (Bech 2001, Möller-Leimkühler 2002). The engagement of families, friends and partners is also necessary (Wasserman 2006).

However, since the majority of the symptoms of male depression—irritability, anger attacks, aggressiveness, etc.—are also the leading features of mixed depression (three or more intra-depressive hypomanic symptoms in the frame of 'unipolar major depression'), it has been suggested that male depressive syndrome could be strongly related to the bipolar mood spectrum (Rihmer 2004b). However, the eventual gender specificity of the different types of bipolar mood disorders are still unclear and further investigations are needed. A link can be detected from the male depressive syndrome to the concept of a stress-provoked, cortisone-induced serotonin-related anxiety-driven depression, and studies suggest a male preponderance of such depression (van Praag 2004; Rihmer 2004b).

## Prevention measures in public spaces

To improve, alert and sensitize the health care system is not enough. Depressive, aggressive, violent and abusive males often generate immense problems for themselves and their close environment. Such men should actively be searched for in order to prevent suicides and domestic violence, as well as depressive, self-destructive and careless risk-taking and its consequences. Areas of such intervention should be public spaces such as workplaces, restaurants, social networks of friends and families, trade unions, sport associations, political organizations, but also institutions for abusers and criminals.

Activities should focus on sensitization, motivation, awareness, education and capacity building, by lecturing and networking in professional structures that are capable of intervention, treatment and monitoring follow-up.

## Specific services

Furthermore, society's unrealistic self-ideation of conventional masculinity, e.g. 'to always be strong', needs to be questioned. It is probable that men's ability to ask for help would be increased after cognitive programmes focusing on such issues. Such programmes could also play a curative role. However, it is especially important to create services where trained staff with a high degree of apprehension and the ability to see beyond stereotypes, recognizing and supporting male patients with broken or lost identities and/or rampant traditional masculinity.

## Design services

An additional problem here is that outpatient services in psychiatric and mental health care are often aimed at the female patients, as most of the outpatients in psychiatric services are females. Psychiatric and mental health care professionals may be unprepared to recognize and deal with the indications of male depressive pathology because of blind spots of gender-bias in medical practice. Also, the employment of female professionals is widespread in the mental health care arena, in part because it has traditionally been a female profession, one that is of low status and low pay. Perhaps these female professionals may be even less equipped to identify male depression because of their sex, although there are no studies or findings to confirm such statements.

Thus, in this vicious circle, a situation appears in which the frequency of help-seeking at psychiatric services does not reflect the real prevalence of mental ill-being, suffering and depression in males. An example: psychiatric and outpatient mental health services in many countries presuppose typical features of female help-seeking, such as motivation, compliance, insight and the willingness to change as inclusion criteria for offering help, thus excluding those patients who act out and behave abusively. These demands may be hard to fulfil by males (or females) in deep trouble who are desperately acting out suicidal depression.

One result of this gender-related imbalance is an artificial situation in many countries, where the huge majority of compulsive, custodial and forensic inpatient services are utilized by males, whereas 80 per cent of supportive psychiatric and mental health outpatient care facilities are consumed by females. Another is the poor treatment rate of depressed men, which is the consequence both of their less frequent treatment-seeking behaviour and lower recognition rate (du Fort *et al.* 1999; Angst *et al.* 2002; Möller-Leimkühler 2002). This again points to the importance of not only considering the accessibility, but also the acceptability of services when designing structures of service provision. The former is also true for suicidal persons. An extensive literature review (Luoma *et al.* 2002) shows that the rates of medical contact during the last year among suicide victims are much higher for primary care providers (77 per cent) relative to mental health services (32 per cent), and this rate is much higher for females than for males. Looking at the medical contacts in the last four weeks before suicide, the figures for females are 45 per cent and for males 19 per cent, respectively. It has also been demonstrated that the widespread use of antidepressants in the new 'SSRI-era' is particularly striking for women who, compared to men, seek more help for depression (Rihmer and Akiskal 2006).

It should be said that male depression can be treated and male suicides can be prevented. Antidepressive pharmacological interventions seem to be effective on male depression and suicidality, provided they are initiated and given by empathic and understanding services that create compliance and are embedded in a holistic approach.

## Some scientific challenges

The shortcomings in male help-seeking behaviour, and the health care professionals failing in identifying such behaviour when help is actually sought, as well as men's lack of compliance to treatment and preparedness to show weakness, leads to the delineation of gender-specific types of 'suicidal behaviour' in research. Such gender types are intrinsically linked to a wide range of sociocultural categories and specificities such as age, ethnicity, demography, sexuality, and such cultural phenomenon of identification, social images and belonging have to be considered. In the case of gender-specific types, one can detect two large groups: one completing suicides or committing aggressive, decisive suicide attempts that often are failed suicides, consisting predominantly of males, and another committing repetitive, multiple and less intentional acts of self-harm, consisting mainly of females (Isometsa and Lönnqvist 1998; Wasserman 2001; Rihmer *et al.* 2002). In the second group, many suicide attempts have the character of a 'cry for help' (Farberow & Schneidman 1961) and are often suicide-preventive as such (Rutz 2003). Consequently, it is scientifically questionable to put completed suicides and multiple suicide attempts together in a category of 'suicidal' or 'self-harming' behaviour for the purpose of creating a scientific context. This is, however, often done today, for example in investigations regarding outcomes of treatment studies, in order to gain statistical power in a research setting where completed suicides are rare. Such shortcuts in research methods lead to heterogeneity in the material, thus, complicating scientific and prognostic conclusions, more specifically regarding the risk for completed suicides later on. The stimulation of multi-centre studies could be a solution. Future research on self-harming behaviour should take into account gender specificity and other sociocultural differences as well as psychological and genetic factors in different types of self-harming behaviour, suicide attempts and completed suicides (Rutz 2004).

## Conclusion

A high rate of male suicide is the most evident proof for males' mental ill-being. When considering the links between men's individual depression and their suicidality a major challenge appears: the importance of improving the determinants and preconditions for men's well-being and health on a societal level. That is to say to identify and increase men's levels of autonomy, to counteract their helplessness, to facilitate a mutual and pluralistic gender tolerance, to support and resituate men's sense of social cohesion and existential meaning, and to provide a place for such traditional values of masculinity such as integrity, pride, status and dignity in modern societies of gender transition

In line with the World Psychiatric Association's new strategy of 'psychiatry for the person', improving the diagnoses and treatment of male depression is imperative. They should be directed to the male person taking into account the specific role expectations and weaknesses that are prevalent, such as sensitivity for change and status loss, and the often over-compensated inability to keep control and establish meaning and self-confidence in modern life. In order to do this, focus should be given to the overwhelming gender transitions across the world, that more or less stressfully affect both genders. Subsequently, one of the major suicide preventive and public health promoting strategies to perform in the near future is a positive interest for male-specific responses to stressful factors in societal change. Furthermore, an improvement of communication and a mutual interest of both genders with regard to the specificity of their respective circumstances is essential.

## References

Angst J, Gamma A, Gastpar M *et al.* (2002). Gender differences in depression. Epidemiological findings from the European DEPRES I and II studies. *European Archives of Psychiatry and Clinical Neurosciences*, **252**, 201–209.

Bech P (2001). Male depression: stress and aggression as pathways to major depression. In A Dawson and A Tylee, eds, *Depression—Social and Economic Timebomb*, pp. 63–66. British Medical Journals Books, London.

Berardi D, Menchetti M, Cevenini N *et al.* (2005). Increased recognition of depression in primary care. *Psychotherapy and Psychosomatics*, **74**, 225–230.

Berecz R, Cáceres M, Szlivka A *et al.* (2005). Reduced completed suicide in Hungary from 1990 to 2001: relation to suicide methods. *Journal of Affective Disorders*, **88**, 235–238.

De Leo D, Cerin E, Spathoris K *et al.* (2005). Lifetime risk of suicidal ideation and attempts in an Australian community: prevalence, suicidal process, and help-seeking behaviour. *Journal of Affective Disorders*, **86**, 215–224.

Du Fort GG, Newman SC, Boothroyd LC *et al.* (1999). Treatment-seeking for depression: role of depressive symptoms and comorbid psychiatric diagnoses. *Journal of Affective Disorders*, **52**, 31–40.

Egeland JA, Hostetter AM, Eshleman SK (1983) Amish Study III: the impact of cultural factors on diagnosis of bipolar illness. *American Journal of Psychiatry*, **140**, 67–71.

European Commission (2005). *The Green Paper*. The European Commission, Luxembourg.

Farberow N and Schneidman ES (1961) *The Cry for Help*. McGraw Hill, New York.

Ferguson D, Doucette S, Glass KC *et al.* (2005). Association between suicide attempts and selective serotonin reuptake inhibitors: systematic review of randomised controlled trials. *British Medical Journal*, **19**, 330–359.

Grunebaum MF, Ellis SP, Li S *et al.* (2004). Antidepressants and suicide risk in the United States, 1985–1999. *Journal of Clinical Psychiatry*, **65**, 1456–1462.

Henriksson S and Isacsson G (2006). Increased antidepressant use and fewer suicides in Jamtland county, Sweden, after a primary care educational programme on the treatment of depression. *Acta Psychiatrica Scandinavica*, **114**, 159–167.

Isacsson G (2000). Suicide prevention—a medical breakthrough? *Acta Psychiatrica Scandinavica*, **102**, 113–117.

Isometsa ET and Lönnqvist JK (1998). Suicide attempts preceding completed suicide. *British Journal of Psychiatry*, **173**, 531–535.

Jackson ED, Payne JD, Nadel L *et al.* (2005). Stress differentially modulates fear conditioning in healthy men and women. *Biological Psychiatry*, **59**, 516–522.

Jporm Af, Kelly CM, Wright A *et al.* (2006). Belief in dealing with depression alone: results from community surveys of adolescents and adults. *Journal of Affective Disorders*, **96**, 59–65. Epub 30 June.

Khan A, Khan S, Kolts RM *et al.* (2003) Suicide rates in clinical trials of SSRIs, other antidepressants, and placebo: analysis of FDA reports. *American Journal of Psychiatry*, **160**, 790–792.

Krasnov V (2004). Key note lecture at the WHO symposium on premature mortality in Eastern Europe, Moscow.

Lecrubier Y (1998). Is depression under-recognised and undertreated? *International Clinical Psychopharmacology* **13**, 3–6.

Levav I, Kohn R, Dohrenwend BP *et al.* (1993). An epidemiological study of mental disorders in a 10-year cohort of young adults in Israel. *Psychological Medicine*, **23**, 691–707.

Levi F, La Vecchia C, Lucchini F *et al.* (2003). Trends in mortality from suicide, 1965–99. *Acta Psychiatrica Scandinavica*, **108**, 341–349.

Ludwig J and Marcotte DE (2005). Anti-depressants, suicide, and drug regulation. *Journal of Policy Analysis and Management*, **24**, 249–272.

Luoma JB, Martin CE, Pearson JL (2002). Contact with mental health and primary care providers before suicide: a review of the evidence. *American Journal of Psychiatry*, **159**, 909–916.

Möller-Leimkühler A, Bottlender R, Strauss A *et al.* (2004). Is there evidence for male depressive syndrome in patients with major depression? *Journal of Affective Disorders*, **80**, 87–93.

Möller-Leimkühler AM (2002). Barriers to help-seeking by men: a review of cross-cultural and clinical literature with particular reference to depression. *Journal of Affective Disorders*, **71**, 1–9.

Notzon FC, Komarov YM, Ermakov SP *et al.* (1998). Causes of declining life expectancy in Russia. *JAMA*, **279**, 793–800.

Oravecz R, Czigler B, Leskosek L (2003). Correlation between suicide rate and antidepressant use in Slovenia. *Archives in Suicide Research*, **7**, 279–285.

Picinelli M and Wilkinson G (2000). Gender differences in depression. *British Journal Of Psychiatry*, **177**, 486–492.

Qin P, Agerbo E, Westergard-Nielsen N *et al.* (2000). Gender differences in risk factors for suicide. *British Journal Of Psychiatry*, **177**, 546–550.

Rihmer Z (2004a). Decreasing national suicide rates—fact or fiction ? *World Journal of Biological Psychiatry*, **5**, 55–56.

Rihmer Z (2004b). Is 'male depressive syndrome' bipolar rather than unipolar? *Journal of Bipolar Disorders*, **3**, 19.

Rihmer Z and Akiskal HS (2006). Do antidepressants t(h)reat(en) depressives? Toward a clinically judicious formulation of the antidepressant-suicidality FDA advisory in light of declining national suicide statistics from many countries. *Journal of Affective Disorders*, **94**, 3–13.

Rihmer Z, Barsi J, Vég K *et al.* (1990). Suicide rates in Hungary correlate negatively with reported rates of depression. *Journal of Affective Disorders*, **20**, 87–91.

Rihmer Z, Belső N, Kiss K (2002). Strategies for suicide prevention. *Current Opinion in Psychiatry*, **15**, 83–87.

Rihmer Z, Rurt W, Pihlgren H (1995). Depression and suicide on Gotland. An intensive study of all suicides before and after a depression-training programme for general practitioners. *Journal of Affective Disorders*, **35**, 147–152.

Rihmer Z, Rutz W, Barsi J (1993). Suicide rate, prevalence of diagnosed depression and prevalence of working physicians in Hungary. *Acta Psychiatrica Scandinavica*, **88**, 391–394.

Rutz W (1999). Improvement of care for people suffering from depression: the need for comprehensive education. *International Clinical Psychopharmacology*, **14**, 27–33.

Rutz W (2001). Mental health in Europe: problems, advancements, challenges. *Acta Psychiatrica Scandinavica Suppl*, **410**, 15–20.

Rutz W (2004). Suicidal behaviour: comments, advancements, challenges. A European perspective. *World Psychiatry*, **3**, 161–162.

Rutz W, von Knorring L, Pihlgren H *et al.* (1995). Prevention of male suicides: lessons from Gotland study (Letter). *Lancet*, **345**, 524.

Rutz W, von Knorring L, Wälinder J *et al.* (1990). Effect of an educational program for general practitioners on Gotland on the pattern of prescription of psychotropic drugs. *Acta Psychiatrica Scandinavica*, **82**, 399–403.

Rutz W, Wälinder J, von Knorring L *et al.* (1997). Prevention of depression and suicide by education and medication: impact on male suicidality. *International Journal of Psychiatry in Clinical Practice*, **1**, 39–46.

Szádóczky E, Rihmer Z, Papp Z *et al.* (2002). Gender differences in major depressive disorder in a Hungarian community survey. *International Journal of Psychiatry in Clinical Practice*, **6**, 31–37.

Taylor R, Morrell S, Slaytor E *et al.* (1998). Suicide in urban South-Wales, Australia 1985–1994: socioeconomic and migrant interactions. *Social Science and Medicine*, **47**, 1677–1686.

Van Praag H (2004). *Stress, Brain and Depression*. Cambridge University Press, Cambridge.

Varnik A, Wasserman D, Dankowicz M *et al.* (1998). Marked decrease in suicide among men and women in the former USSR during perestroika. *Acta Psychiatrica Scandinavica Suppl*, **394**, 13–19.

Wälinder J and Rutz W (2001). Male depression and suicide. *International Clinical Psychopharmacology*, **16**, S21–S24.

Wälinder J and Rutz W (2001). Male depression and suicide. *International Clinical Psychopharmacology*, **1**(Suppl 2), S 21–S24.

Wasserman D (2006). *Depression: The Facts*. Oxford University Press, New York.

Wasserman D (ed.) (2001). *Suicide. An Unnecessary Death*. Martin Dunitz, London.

Wasserman D, Varnik A, Eklund G (1994). Male suicides and alcohol consumption in the former USSR. *Acta Psychiatrica Scandinavica*, **89**, 306–313.

Wilkinson R and Marmot M (eds) (1998). *Social Determinants of Health—The Solid Facts*. WHO Regional Office for Europe, Copenhagen.

World Health Organization (2001). *The World Health Report 2001. Mental Health: New Understanding, New Hope*. World Health Organization, Geneva.

World Health Organization (2003). *World Health Report on Violence*. World Health Organization, Geneva.

World Health Organization (2005). *Regional Office for Europe*. Health for All (HFA) Database, Copenhagen.

Yang GH, Phillips MR, Zhou MG *et al.* (2005). Understanding the unique characteristics of suicide in China: national psychological autopsy study. *Biomedical and Environmental Sciences*, **18**, 379–389.

Zierau F, Bille A, Rutz W *et al.* (2002). The Gotland Male Depression Scale: a validity study in patients with alcohol use disorders. *Nordic Journal of Psychiatry*, **56**, 265–271.

# Appendix 1

## The Gotland Scale for assessing male depression (Rutz 1999)

During the past month, have you or others noticed that your behaviour is different than usual, and if so, in what way?

0 = not at all; 1 = to some extent; 2 = very true; 3 = extremely so

1 Lower stress threshold/more stressed than usual.

2 More aggressive, outward reacting, difficulty keeping self-control.

3 Feeling of being burned out and empty.

4 Constant, inexplicable tiredness.

5 More irritable, restless and frustrated.

6 Difficulty making ordinary everyday decisions.

7 Sleep problems: sleeping too much/too little/uneasily, difficulty falling asleep/waking up early in the morning especially, having a feeling of disquiet/anxiety/displeasure.

8 Over-consumption of alcohol and pills in order to achieve a calming and relaxing effect. Being hyperactive or blowing off steam by working hard and restlessly, jogging or practising some other form of sport, under- or overeating.

9 Do you feel your behaviour has altered in such a way that neither you yourself, nor others can recognize you, and you are difficult to deal with?

10 Have you felt, or have others perceived you as being gloomy, negative or characterized by a state of hopelessness in which everything looks bleak?

11 Have you or others noticed that you have a greater tendency for self pity, to be plaintive or to seem pathetic?

12 In your biological family, is there any tendency to abuse, depression/dejection, suicide attempts or proneness to some behaviour involving danger?

### Points

0–13 No signs of depression

14–26 Depression possible. Specific therapy, including psychopharmacological, possibly indicated

27–39 Clear signs of depression. Specific therapy, including psychopharmacological, clearly indicated

# CHAPTER 36

# Suicide in military settings
## Combatants and veterans

Vsevolod Rozanov, Lars Mehlum and Richard Stiliha

## Abstract

Suicide rates in military units are lower than in civilian populations and differ considerably from nation to nation. The processes that may influence suicide rates within the armed forces can be different from that of the civilian life, especially when armed forces are under reformation, downsizing and economic pressure.

Risk factors vary between groups and settings, such as active duty versus reservist/veteran or war versus peacekeeping mission. However, common risk factors are: easy access to firearms, exposure to traumatic stress, lack of social support, and the military life style with frequent relocations. Two subgroups are considered as equally important to target for suicide prevention: young conscripts and war veterans. In the first case, screening and crisis intervention are in focus, and in the second, treatments for post-traumatic stress syndrome, depression and substance abuse. Leadership interventions and changes in firearm regulations are other preventive measures.

## Introduction

Combatants have committed suicide throughout the history of armed conflicts. Soldiers sometimes killed themselves in order to avoid capture and slavery, commanders would do so rather than accept defeat. Officers have committed suicide to avoid revealing secrets under interrogation or torture. Today, armies are usually not involved in large battles, and the nature of conflicts has changed a lot, e.g. guerilla warfare. The military is often regarded as a profession, not only for males, since the number of females in service is growing, especially in the Western world. When suicide rates in the military are compared with those of other professional groups, it is found that they are generally lower in the military than in civilian populations of the same gender and age (Wasserman 1992). This is usually seen as a so called 'healthy worker' effect—a result of ruling out a variety of psychiatric conditions on the stage of admittance to the army, as well as ongoing control throughout the appointment. However, suicide rates in military units may differ considerably from nation to nation and in different types of military units. In this chapter, we will discuss results and experiences from recent studies addressing the problem of suicide in the military and provide some recommendations for future preventive strategies and policies.

## Suicide in the military: common risk factors

Recently, we have tried to outline some common features of suicide within the military environment (Rozanov *et al.* 2002). The following issues may be associated with an increased risk of suicide in the military context:

1. The loss of or lack of personal freedom experienced by people entering such a closed and authoritarian system;

2. The aggressive masculine culture in many military communities, which may leave little room for self-disclosure and peer support;

3. The risk for personal traumatic stress exposure and subsequent traumatic stress reactions;

4. The easy access to firearms;

5. The military lifestyle with frequent relocations and the break-up of supportive social structures;

6. Profound changes in social structures due to downsizing and reorganizing processes taking place in most countries armed forces; and

7. The danger of suicide contagion and clustering of suicides in military units.

In spite of the existence of some risk factors specific to the military environment that must be added to risk factors in the general population, suicide rates in military populations remain, in most cases, lower than the civilian population of men of the same age. This could possibly be attributed to the existence of protective factors that may balance the situation. We shall discuss these factors later, after a short review of epidemiological situation data on suicide from military populations in different parts of the world in diverse cultural and socio-economic contexts.

## Suicide in the army in war and peace: cross-national comparisons

When addressing military systems in different countries, it is necessary to take into consideration the military forces' level of involvement in various types of operations and actions, and the result of such actions. In view of this, the situation of the US Army is distinctive.

## North America

Regardless of involvement in military actions, for members of the US Army, suicide is the second leading cause of death after accidents, unintentional injuries or combat loss (Ritchie *et al.* 2003). This is distinctly different from the general population, where suicide is the second or third leading cause of death in the age group 15–34 years; and in older groups, it is the fifth–sixth leading cause of death (National Strategy for Suicide Prevention 2001). Suicide rates in the US Army declined from 14.8 per 100,000 in 1995 to 9.1 in 2001. With deployment to several missions in recent years (Iraq 1991, Afghanistan, Iraq 2003) large military contingents have been exposed to combat stress, as well as to complicated geographical, climatic and unfamiliar sociocultural situations. While the Iraq 1991 war and Afghanistan missions did not seem to cause any major change in suicide rates in the US Army, the painful Iraq 2003 war seems to have had a distinct impact on these rates. In a review of soldier suicides (2003), the Mental Health Advisory Team reports that the suicide rate for soldiers deployed to Operation Iraqi Freedom II (OIF-II, starting in mid-March 2003) from January to October 2003 was higher than recent Army historical rates (15.6 per 100,000 compared to the average annual rate of 11.9 for the period 1995–2002). Compared to historical army suicide rates, the OIF-II suicide rates were higher for active component male and female soldiers and lower compared to reserve component soldiers. Firearms were the predominant method of suicide. The majority of suicides were committed by young males (Annex D 2003).

In another extensive document, focusing on the mental health and well-being of soldiers experiencing numerous combat stressors, acute and post-traumatic stress is the top mental health concern (Walter Reed Army Institute of Research 2005). The extent of the problem may be seen from the following figures: a survey of 1700 soldiers and marines serving in Iraq since 2003 revealed that 94.5 per cent saw dead bodies or human remains, 92 per cent reported being attacked or ambushed, 86.2 per cent knew someone killed or seriously wounded, and 55.7 per cent caused the death of an enemy combatant (Walter Reed Army Institute of Research 2005). The percentage of study subjects whose responses met the screening criteria for major depression, generalised anxiety or post-traumatic stress disorder (PTSD) was significantly higher after duty in Iraq (15.6 to 17.1 percent) than after duty in Afghanistan (11.2 percent) or before deployment to Iraq (9.3 percent); the largest difference was in the rate of PTSD. For example, PTSD (strict definition) was found in approximately 12.5 per cent of the personnel in army and marine contingents (Hoge *et al.* 2004), while the estimated lifetime prevalence of PTSD among adult Americans is 7.8 per cent. Women (10.4 per cent) are twice as likely as men (5 per cent) to have PTSD at some point in their lives (Kessler *et al.* 1995). Knowing the link between PTSD, depression and suicide, there is no surprise that suicides are increasing (Mehlum 2005). On the other hand, those who are in the army still demonstrate high levels of adaptation, supported by the following data.

Despite the fact that personnel having served in the US Army in Iraq have higher suicide rates than the average US Army rates, both the Iraq contingent rate and the overall army rate remain below the civilian male population (13.5 per 100,000 troops

compared with 17.5 per 100.000 of population or approximately 25 per 100,000 for men aged 20–55) (National Strategy for Suicide Prevention 2001; Nelson 2004). Lower suicide rates in the army have been reported for decades (Rothberg *et al.* 1990; Senteil *et al.* 1997; Nelson 2004). Most recent reports confirm that military rates for the period 1990 to 2000 were approximately 20 per cent lower than the civilian rate (Eaton *et al.* 2006). On the other hand, those who had been in the army (veterans) have almost twice the suicide risk of non-veterans in the general population, as reported by Kaplan and colleagues (2007). In addition, some authors argue that some of the suicides in the army remain underestimated, the classification errors may account for about 21 per cent of additional suicides (Carr *et al.* 2004). In general, among the 1.4 million active duty US military service members, 6 per cent receive outpatient treatment for mental health disorders each year (Hoge *et al.* 2003).

In every army, there may be differences in suicide rates in different types of forces, which may depend on exposure to stress, traditions, policies and other factors. This is also the case in the US Army, and official sources provide extensive information regarding this subject. Regular suicide statistics from the US military testify that suicide rates in the Navy are the lowest, followed by the Air Force, Army and Marine Corps, which are at highest risk according to Department of Defence statistics (Allen *et al.* 2005). In the Air Force, suicide accounted for 23 per cent of all deaths and was the second leading cause of death (MMWR 1999). If speaking only about recruits, from 276 recruit deaths in the US military from 1997 through 2001, 28 per cent (77 deaths) were classified as traumatic (suicide, unintentional injury, homicide), and after age-adjustment, traumatic death rates were highest in the army (four times higher than in the Navy and Air Force, and 80 per cent higher than in the Marine Corps). The majority (60 per cent) of traumatic deaths was due to suicide, followed by unintentional injuries (35 per cent), and homicide (5 per cent) (Scoville *et al.* 2004).

## Western Europe

Sociocultural, economical and other societal peculiarities, as well as structural particularities, traditions and policies may influence such phenomenon as suicide in the military. Several reports were published recently in France (Desjeux *et al.* 2001, 2004). In a short review covering suicides and suicide attempts in the French armed forces during the course of the year 1998, the authors found a very typical pattern: from 145 records surveyed, 40 were suicides and 105 suicide attempts, suicide cases were exclusively males, average age 36, while attempts were distributed evenly between males and females, average age 30. In cases of completed suicide, main methods were firearms and hanging, while in attempted suicides—drug overdose and self-cuttings—previous suicide attempts were found in 21 per cent of attempters and 10 per cent of completers. The rate of completed suicides was reported, to be 14 per 100,000 of military troops (compared with the male French general population level, about 22 per 100,000) (Desjeux *et al.* 2001; European Health for all Database 2008). In a later report, the same authors have analysed the situation from the year 1997 to 2000 inclusive. During that period, 230 suicides occurred among 315,934 persons, making the overall annual suicide rate 18.2 per 100,000 of active duty personnel. In comparison to national rates for men of similar age categories, the rate in the army is lower. The main suicide methods used were firearms (51 per cent) and hanging (28 per cent). The incidence rate in the gendarmerie, a military body in charge of police duties among civilians, was twice as high as in the land forces. Men under 25 and aged 40–44 were at the highest risk (Desjeux *et al.* 2004). The overall conclusion of these reports is that despite global lower risk than general populations, gendarmerie personnel and younger people need specific surveillance measures.

Micklewright recently reported on deliberate self-harm in personnel of the Royal Navy (Micklewright 2005) and concluded that these acts should be viewed in the context of the environment that often imposes psychological, emotional and social pressures on servicemen. In the UK, detailed information on suicide in the regular Armed Forces are published by the Defence Analytical Services Agency (DASA). The report from 1984 to 2006 includes a comparison with the UK general population. For the 23-year period, suicide rates in the Army ranged from 12 to 20 per 100,000, suicide rates in the naval service ranged from 6 to 14, and from 3 to 15 per 100,000 in the Royal Air Force. Rates were rather high in the end of 1980s and first half of the 1990s, and from 1999, rates are decreasing in all of the armed forces (DASA 2007). Overall, suicide rates in the armed forces were lower than the general population (around 18 per 100,000 males of all ages) and changed over time in a very similar pattern, as the rates in the general population. However, there is an exception—young army members, aged 20 years and under showed periodically higher suicide rates than their civilian counterparts (DASA 2007).

In an Irish defence forces study (Mahon *et al.* 2005) of all regular duty personnel for the period from 1970 to 2002, the average annual suicide rate was found to be 15.3 per 100,000 (rates in the general population for men in this period in Ireland increased from 5 to 22 per 100,000) (European Health for all Database 2008). Firearm suicides accounted for 53 per cent of all cases. A history of previous episodes of deliberate self-harm, morning duty and a recent medical downgrading were identified as independent risk factors predicting suicide in the military (Mahon *et al.* 2005).

Several studies on risk factors for suicidal behaviour among military personnel have been conducted in Norway. Engelstad's (1968) and Hytten's (1985) epidemiological studies document a fourfold increase in suicide rates of young soldiers—reaching 13.6/100,000) during the period 1977–1984. This was, however, still considerably lower than in the general population of young males (28.1) in the corresponding time period. Clinical and descriptive studies from Norway (Mehlum 1990, 1992, 1994, 1998) revealed that suicidal behaviour in young soldiers was in many cases impulsive, and about one third of the suicide attempts were made under the influence of alcohol (Mehlum 1990). In cases of completed suicide, the self-destructive method was very often the use of firearms (Hytten 1985), whereas suicide attempters usually ingested drugs or poisons and/or cut their wrists (Mehlum 1990). Similar results were obtained in Finland, where suicide in the military is also lower than the general population. One of the major triggering factors for suicide among soldiers was situational stress, and alcohol was identified as a factor in many suicides (Marttunen *et al.* 1997).

Several reports have been published recently regarding suicide in the Italian military environment (Mancinelli *et al.* 2001, 2003). For the period 1986 to 1998, the authors have revealed 122 suicides and 136 suicide attempts, subjects age ranged from 17 to 60 years, and the most frequent ages both for suicides and suicide attempts were 19–22 years. The predominance of suicides in the Italian military was also found to be lower than in the general population. Authors attribute these figures to existing screening procedures of military personnel, excluding the mentally disturbed at an early age, and the development of a positive feeling of belonging to a group among young soldiers.

## Suicide in post-Soviet countries: experience from the Russian and Ukrainian military

The military cannot be separated from the rest of society, and many internal problems in the military may originate from current social problems in the surrounding larger society. With this in mind, it is interesting to look at the situation in the armies of the Russian Federation and the Ukraine. These two post-Soviet countries have high suicide rates, reflected also in the military setting. A report by Litvintsev *et al.* (2003) shows that suicide rates in the Russian Federation Army increased from 14.0 to 32.1/100,000 in the period 1993 to 1999. Suicide rates in the military, as in other countries, were well below the rates in the general population of males during the same period (increased from 59.3 to 74.3). On the other hand, changes in rates over time had their own peculiarities. It is well known that in most of the former USSR countries, since the perestroika in 1986, there was a sharp reduction in suicide rates until 1991, when a dramatic rise occurred (Värnik 1997; Wasserman *et al.* 1998) peaking in 1995–1996. After this, a slow and steady decrease was observed until the present (Rozanov 2007). These changes, especially shortly after the perestroika, were explained by the lowering of alcohol consumption due to a strong anti-alcohol campaign started by Gorbachev at that time (Värnik 1997; Wasserman *et al.* 1998). However, while general population suicide rates in the Russian Federation were reduced from 42.4 to 35.5 per 100,000 during the period 1994 to 1998, suicide rates in the army showed the exact opposite tendency, increasing from 14 to 32–30 during the period 1994 to 1997–1998, and substantially declining in 1999 (Litvintsev *et al.* 2003).

This tendency can be attributed to specific risk factors within the army, and especially to financial limitations, low salaries and poor social protection of those who were leaving the army, especially officers and warrants. Russian specialists consider socio-economic factors and the lowering of prestige of the military service to be the main explanatory factors for the relatively high suicide rates in the Russian Federation army as compared with armies of Western countries (Litvintsev *et al.* 2003). The authors state that 80 per cent of those who committed suicide had no diagnosis of severe psychiatric disorder, whereas 60 per cent seemed to have stress-related disturbances, and in most cases, unfavourable social and psychological factors were present: 65.8 per cent of the suicides were committed by soldiers and sergeants drafted on a conscription basis (two-thirds of suicides occurred during the first year of service). Altogether, 16.2 per cent of the suicides were committed by officers, 9.8 per cent by ensigns, and 8.2 per cent by other categories (Litvintsev *et al.* 2003).

A comparison of mental problems in a group of military officers who were engaged on a contract basis and completed suicide, with a sample of suicide completers from the general population, gave the following results: among 10 per cent of the officers, mental disorders were present, whereas 15–25 per cent were reported as having mental disorders in the general population; in 20–25 per cent of the officers, borderline neurotic disorders were found, compared to 35–40 per cent in the general population; and about 70 per cent of the officers were without any disorder compared to the drastically lower figure of 40–50 per cent in the general population (Litvintsev *et al.* 2002). In the army of the Russian Federation, suicides account for one-third to one-fifth of all deaths. Regarding different kinds of forces, the navy personnel were at biggest risk, followed by the air force, strategic missile forces and landing forces. The predominate methods of suicide were those with firearms as well as hanging, and in about 16 per cent of suicides, a farewell letter was found (Litvintsev *et al.* 2001a, b).

In the navy, the time course of suicides also differed distinctly from the general population: while in the whole USSR there was lowering of suicides in 1986 (see above for the suicide preventive effect of the perestroika), in the navy there was a rise in the percentage of suicides in general death structure during the period 1986 to 1995 (period of serious economical problems, fleet downsizing, lowering of the prestige of the marine professions). Only from 1998 to 2000 did the percentage of suicides start to diminish. In the navy, two-thirds of all suicides occur among conscripted personnel during their first year of service. In 65 per cent of the cases, the method of suicide was hanging, 20 per cent firearms, 5.5 per cent intoxications, 5.2 per cent self-cutting, 2.2 per cent jumping and finally, 1.8 per cent drowning (Sharaevskiy *et al.* 2002).

In the Russian Federation army, contingents in the Northern Caucasus region have been involved in the conflict in Chechnya, and the situation among these troops gives us an idea of how the involvement in action affects suicides and mental health in general. In an observation by Bogachenko *et al.* (2003) of 4953 soldiers in the Northern Caucasus military district, mental health instability was found in about 10.5 per cent of the cases. In 1999, 732 persons were relieved due to mental health problems, 457 of these had once attempted suicide, in 68.8 per cent of the cases, suicide attempts were provoked by interpersonal conflicts due to bullying and harassment. More than half of all suicide attempts occurred during the first year of service. These results are confirmed in another paper analysing soldiers with neurotic reactions that were admitted to the hospital. It was found that neurotic reactions in soldiers during two year periods of service had several distinct exacerbations in the third, sixth, twelfth and eighteenth months of service; suicidal behaviour showed the same temporal profile. The authors suggest an explanation for each peak of neurotic reactions, starting with poor adaptation to the military environment, with later shifts towards interpersonal conflicts, and a combination of poor adaptation, conflicts and family problems. It is important to note that suicidal behaviours have the same time profile: the general tendency is a lowering of risk with time, with the last 4–5 months of service remaining almost free of suicidal tendencies (Fadeev *et al.* 2001).

Many authors from the Russian Federation underline bullying as an important stressful or triggering event in the suicidal behaviour of the soldiers. An important factor is the process of pre-enrolment screening of the conscripts, which often fails to prevent the conscription of soldiers with existing suicidal tendencies.

The situation in the Ukrainian army is rather similar to that of the Russian Federation. Army suicide rates were once reported to be alarmingly high (340 per 100,000 in 1996), though it seems to be a result of unchecked information or short-term evaluations (Chuprikov *et al.* 1998). Later studies have revealed that military suicide rates, as in many other countries, are below the rates for

men in the general population (46.7 for men of all ages, 52.5 for men aged 20–55, average for 1991–1999) and in a given military unit (the air forces, unit comprising almost half of the air forces rank and file) constituted 32.6 per 100,000 (average for 1991–1999) (Rozanov *et al.* 2002). The most at-risk categories of military in this unit appeared to be soldiers by conscription and warrants (ensigns), whilst officers were at lowest risk. In a study evaluating 66 cases of completed suicides of the soldiers by conscription, it was registered that in 42.5 per cent of the cases, the method of suicide was hanging, and in 46.9 per cent of the cases, firearms were chosen (Gichun 2000). In Ukrainian resources, suicides in the militia is much more extensively studied than those in the regular army. This contingent (which resembles the military very much) also has lower suicide rates than the general population (20 per 100,000 as compared with 28–30 per 100,000 in 1995–1998). The period of the most alarming rise in suicides during the last two decades was from 1990 to 1998, after which a lowering of the number of suicides has been observed (Chorny 2001). The change in rates was highly similar to that observed in the general population. Alcohol consumption was associated with about half of the suicides: in 63 per cent of the cases, the method used was hanging, and in 25 per cent, firearms (Chorny 2002).

## Conscripts and young soldiers' suicidal tendencies: predictions and signs

Many authors pay special attention to the screening process of conscripts, especially on conscription occasions. In every country, screening instruments may vary, but are generally based on psychological testing (cognitive style, psychological performance) and clinical interviews. Of course, screening procedures for risk of suicidal behaviour need to be introduced with caution in such settings where there could be a real risk of suicide contagion. In these circumstances, it seems advisable to screen explicitly for depressive symptoms (including suicidal ideation and hopelessness), alcohol and drug misuse, and signs of reduced coping. In the search for further possible dimensions to utilize in screening procedures, several authors have studied the Sense of Coherence (SOC), a dimension developed by Antonovsky (Antonovsky 1993), which is potentially very important in military units and companies. In a study by Mehlum (Mehlum 1998), a low SOC score was found to be a strong predictor of suicidal behaviour in 663 male Norwegian conscripts. The same was found in Greece. A study based on interviewing 1098 young conscripts revealed that subgroups with suicidal ideation and behaviour showed a significantly lower sense of coherence compared with the whole sample (Giotakos 2003). Similar results obtained in a Finnish study determined that a sense of coherence was impaired among those conscripts who committed suicide as well as those with mental health problems, alcohol and drug abuse (Ristkani *et al.* 2005).

In Sweden, a study examining the relation between self-rated health, risk factors in youth and adolescence and mortality among 49,321 young men participating in a nationwide military conscription survey was performed. It was found that poor self-rated health at conscription was associated with increased mortality during a 27-year follow-up (Larsson *et al.* 2002). In another study from Sweden, utilizing the Swedish military service conscription register and examining possible correlation between intelligence tests results at the age of 18 and suicides, it was found that there was a distinct correlation. The risk of suicide was two to three times higher in those who had the lowest scores. The greatest risk was seen among poorly performing offspring of well-educated parents (Gunnel *et al.* 2005). A certain predictive potential can be derived from the data of Jiang, Rasmussen and Wasserman (1999) who have followed more than 150 thousand young people in Sweden born in 1973–1975 and found that short stature and poor psychological performance (logic test) were significantly inversely associated with the risk of attempted suicide. These results were confirmed later on in a larger contingent (more than 1 million males conscripted from 1968 to 1999) showing that the risk of suicide decreases by 15 per cent for every five points of the body mass index (Magnusson *et al.* 2006).

The problem of prediction of performance (in an inverse way, with regards to pre-enrolment suicidal tendencies) during military service was studied in Israel. The authors paid special attention to adolescents who had records of attempted suicide prior to being drafted into the army. These showed much poorer performance during the military service (but not much difference regarding cognitive/educational abilities) compared with those who had no history of suicide attempt (Farbstein *et al.* 2002). Turning to other Israeli resources, it is interesting to mention a study which deals with greater susceptibility of men to contextual and situational factors, which contributes to completed suicide in the armed forces. This is based on the finding that suicide in the armed forces frequently occurs on the first working day, especially among men (Israeli soldiers can spend weekends at home in peacetime) (Weinberg *et al.* 2002).

An important issue is the so-called 'psychological portrait' of the suicidal soldier, and other (contextual) factors that may predict suicide patterns in the military. Background factors such as the presence of a mental disorder, accumulation of negative life events, developing the state of hopelessness, and emotional pain are the same for suicide in the general population and in soldiers. As mentioned before, the vulnerability to negative life events may be higher in young soldiers due to impairment of social support (Mehlum and Schwebs 2001). In Greece, Botsis and co-authors (1999) have studied psychological correlates of suicidal ideation in conscripts. It was found that those who had suicidal thoughts (17 per cent of the sample of 528 persons) had significantly higher scores for depression and hostility. It was also revealed that they had suffered much more stressful life events prior to conscription. From a case report, authors have concluded that a psychological complex of basic inferiority, low educational levels together with family problems and poor integration into a military unit may be strong determinants of soldier suicide (Cabarcapa and Pania 2004). One of the more recent papers from Israel compared psychological characteristics (from army records) of combatant and non-combatant soldiers who committed suicide, with others who did not commit suicide. It was found that combatant soldiers who committed suicide showed proof of greater behavioural adjustment, motivation to serve and a higher sense of duty. Those who were involved in combat had fewer referrals for psychological evaluation and fewer unit changes. This may reflect the tendency of perfectionism in these soldiers. The authors come to the conclusion that excessive motivation, and the tendency to be autonomous and independent may account for suicide in combatant soldiers, while in non-combatant soldiers the main predisposition for suicidal behaviour may be personality weakness (Bodner *et al.* 2006).

# War veterans and the role of PTSD

Whereas suicide in the military has been known for centuries, the awareness of the problem increased substantially after the introduction of post-traumatic stress disorder (PTSD) as a new diagnosis in the DSM-III system (American Psychiatric Association 1980) in the wake of the Vietnam war. Studies of veterans from this war have shown that there is a direct causal link between traumatic stress exposure and subsequent PTSD (Davidson 2000). The Vietnam veterans have also been shown to have a significantly increased standard mortality ratio (the ratio of the number of deaths observed in the study population to the number that would be expected if the study population had the same rate as the standard population) for suicide; particularly, those who had a diagnosis of PTSD (Bullman and Kang 1994) or had been wounded (Bullman and Kang 1996). In other studies, Vietnam veterans have also been shown to have increased levels of suicidal ideation and history of suicide attempts, and again these phenomena seem to be highly correlated with a diagnosis of PTSD. With additional diagnoses, particularly depression, there is an even stronger association (Hendin and Haas 1991; Kramer *et al.* 1994). Recently, Lester has again drawn attention to Vietnam veterans' suicides, highlighting a possible undercounting of suicides in this contingent (Lester 2005). Kaplan and colleagues in a prospective population-based study, compared about 104,000 veterans of different ages from the First and Second World Wars, Korean, Vietnam and post-Vietnam conflicts with more than 200,000 non-veterans. The comparison showed that suicide risk among veterans is twice as high as in non-veterans (Kaplan *et al.* 2007).

The Vietnam experiences led to new research efforts into the long-term psychological consequences of war and traumatic stress in general. Very soon, it became obvious that problems of war veterans are very similar across cultures notwithstanding social and economical differences. Though rates are not often calculated and compared to general population, suicides were reported among Russian (Afghanistan and Chechnya) veterans, British Falkland conflict veterans and US 1991 Iraq mission veterans. The extent of the problem can also be seen from the 1982 British-Argentine Falkland conflict where 256 British soldiers were killed: since then, 264 veterans have committed suicide, thus, suicides have taken more lives than the conflict itself (Spooner 2002).

Today, war veterans' mental health problems and suicide, in particular, are under even more intense investigation. For instance, Vietnam veterans continue to experience higher mortality rates due to external causes of death in comparison to non-veterans (Tegan *et al.* 2004). In the longitudinal model study of male Vietnam veterans in the USA, with a history of drug abuse it was found that PTSD, drug-dependence, non-fatal attempted suicides and suicidal ideation showed strong continuity over time (Price *et al.* 2004). Suicide attempters among veterans had higher psychiatric comorbidity, and more severe substance abuse, characteristics. In men, these problems were more significant than in women (Benda 2003, 2005). It is emphasized that auto-aggressive behaviour in veterans more often occurs in cases where PTSD is present (Begic and Jokic-Begic 2001). Different addictions, including gambling, are associated with suicide attempts. About 40 per cent of the veterans that are pathological gamblers have had attempted suicide (Kausch 2003). PTSD veterans appeared to own four times as many firearms as other subjects (Freeman *et al.* 2003).

In general, there seems that starting with Second World War veterans to the Korean and Vietnam war veterans, suicide rates are growing (Lester 2005). Unfortunately, there is no data of veterans of other war conflicts. Conclusively, the problem of suicide in veterans is mainly a problem of the most socially unprotected contingent, or those with PTSD and different addictions.

## Peacekeeping duties

Recently, with the wide role of peacekeeping duties worldwide, several researchers have studied suicide in former peacekeepers (Hall 1996; Ponteva *et al.* 2000; Wong *et al.* 2001; Thoresen *et al.* 2003; Thoresen and Mehlum 2004). The peacekeeping soldier is not expected to be engaged in regular war activities, but rather to act as a buffer between hostile parties. As a result, he or she has a more complex role, and in some crucial respects, a task completely different from soldiers traditionally trained for combat (Mehlum and Weisaeth 2002). Though, not involved directly in war, these contingents suffer great tension and psycho-emotional problems in the regions of ethnical and other conflicts. Recently, Thoresen *et al.* (2003) have reported the significant increase of suicide by firearms by Norwegian peacekeepers.

Some reports cannot give distinct evaluation of relative suicide risk in peacekeepers and concentrate on the most risky periods of the duty. For instance, four cases of suicide were reported among 4,000 Danish soldiers who took part in the UN mandated forces, two of them committed suicide less then one month before deployment, and two within a year after discharge from a mission (Hansen-Schwartz *et al.* 2002). On the other hand, a Canadian study does not confirm the higher risk of suicides among UN peacekeepers (Wong *et al.* 2001). In a Swedish study, 39,768 former peacekeepers were compared to the general population, and again, a lower number of suicides was found in this contingent. The authors focus mostly on military lifestyles and interpersonal relationship strains as possible factors contributing to suicide among peacekeepers. This research area has unique characteristics possibly revealing specific situations in each cultural and social context of the country of origin and the country of mission.

## Protective factors

Since suicides in the military setting are lower than in the general population, there are obviously some protective features in the military that may play a role in prevention. These may be:

1   The military is a highly organized structure and if the problem is well understood by commanders, prevention programmes may be implemented in a prompt and effective way;

2   There is a preliminary and ongoing medical control of those who are dealing with weapons and certain psychiatric conditions may be recognized early on;

3   Special prevention units may be easily organized and special means of reporting may be implemented that provide quick identification of suicidal persons along with their referral to specialists;

4   The military can discharge those with suicidal ideations or actions when this is needed to reduce suicide risk;

5   Every case of completed or attempted suicide is often thoroughly investigated producing important information for further prevention models (Rozanov *et al.* 2002).

## Army suicide prevention programmes: implementation and evaluation

The majority of publications on military suicide discuss their results from the point of view of how findings can help to identify suicidal persons, and how the results may be implemented in organizing suicide prevention programmes and strategies. However, few studies have been published regarding suicide prevention in the armies and evaluations of such preventive measures. Strategic approaches to suicide prevention are well described from the United States and Norwegian armies. In Norway, the army suicide prevention programme has been a part of the National Strategy for Suicide Prevention launched in 1994 (Mehlum and Schwebs 2001). It has primary, secondary and tertiary preventive components and includes five main domains: leadership interventions, information/ education, medical interventions, welfare, and 24-hour crisis telephone service. Much attention is paid to the role of commanders in military units, which is why a lot is invested in such leaders' competence. Several training packets extending from two hours to two days have been developed and disseminated, from the level of the private soldier to commanders. In recent years, the Norwegian army has also emphasized restricting access to firearms in private homes of officers, members of the home guard, and the military reserve; this initiative has been accompanied by a strong reduction in the number of military firearm suicides.

The US Army suicide prevention strategy (The Army Suicide Prevention Program) is based on the same principles as the Norwegian. They both focus on a proactive suicide prevention programme, which is fundamental in averting the needless tragedy of suicide in the military. Suicide is preventable, and leaders must play an active and sensitive role in showing care and concern for their soldiers. Positive leadership, careful listening and deep concern for soldiers are crucial for suicide prevention in the military. It is important for leaders to know their soldiers and their concerns, and never hesitate to obtain professional help for a soldier in need. The key to preventing suicide in the unit is to respond quickly to any verbal, behavioural or situational clues. Soldiers need to be taught to take any suicidal statement by a fellow soldier seriously, and to inform the chain of command immediately. Prevention efforts must also focus on the personal responsibility of commanders and leaders to care for the soldiers under their charge.

Recently, the US Army introduced a new suicide prevention campaign plan focusing on standardized suicide prevention training (Army News Service 2001a). The US Army suicide prevention model focuses on four major areas: developing soldiers' life-coping skills, encouraging help-seeking behaviour, raising vigilance through suicide awareness, integrating and synchronizing unit and community programs (Army News Service 2001b). Special teams are assessing the situation and present it to authorities (Jontz 2004). Psychological autopsies are gathered and used for lessons learned after suicide; in addition, special policy and training courses are developed (Ritchie and Gelles 2002). Introducing anger management intervention (as far as anger appeared to be a predominating emotion) in Bagram, Afghanistan, secured the absence of suicide cases in the 7000 contingent during a half-year period in 2002 (Reyes and Hicklin 2005). Special prevention programs exist in specific branches of service, such as the air force and the navy (Patterson *et al.* 2001; Stander *et al.* 2004).

The programme of the air force was recently thoroughly evaluated by Knox *et al.* (2003). The investigation was designed as a cohort study with a quasi-experimental approach and analysis of cohorts before (1990–1996) and after (1997–2002) the intervention. The intervention was targeted at reducing risk and enhancing protective factors and consisted of measures aimed to encourage personnel to seek help for mental health, psychological or relationship problems, and enhancing general understandings of mental health issues as well as changing policies and social norms. One of the important aspects of the intervention was training (education) in suicide prevention. It was found that implementation of the programme was associated with a sustained decline in the rate of suicides and other adverse outcomes (homicide, family violence). A 33 per cent relative risk reduction was observed for suicide after the intervention, reduction for other outcomes ranged from 18–54 per cent (Knox *et al.* 2003).

In the Ukraine, suicide preventive intervention targeting air force units with about 10,000 personnel was performed (Rozanov *et al.* 2002). This intervention was based on the US model of gatekeepers' education and included education/information of the responsible personnel, military psychologists and medical staff. Distribution of educational material to the distant subunits and yearly educational seminars collecting all relevant commanders and staff proved to be a good model of prevention. By introducing suicide prevention education, the rate of suicides quickly decreased, giving rise to enthusiasm and satisfaction among commanders. Nevertheless, it was soon revealed that only constant education and consultations of specialists will ensure success, an important experience similar to the one made in the Gotland study (Rutz *et al.* 1995).

In many armed forces across the world, suicide preventive efforts have been developed in recent years and some of these have been made part of a national programmes for suicide prevention: in the US, UK, Norway, Sweden and Germany to mention a few. There are also reports about existing prevention programmes in the Hellenic navy (Polychronidis 1999), in the army of Serbia and Montenegro (Dedic *et al.* 2006; Gordana and Milivoje 2007), and in the Turkish air force (Gerede 2006). There are no reports regarding evaluations of these programmes, some of which have just been launched. To our knowledge, the evaluation performed by Knox *et al.* (2003) remains the only example.

Introduction of suicide prevention measures in the military environment sometimes is not an easy thing to do. Part of military self-esteem is the ability to stand straight while facing different threats. Therefore, training military staff to ask for help may not be easily accepted, in that such help-seeking behaviour, as well as referral to mental health facilities, can be seen as the end of a career. Even screening for psychological illness in the military is evaluated in a specific way (Rona *et al.* 2005).

In most countries, a lot more could be gained through more coordinated action between the military and civil sectors, and through more focused strategies within the armed forces. An obstacle to such a development has probably been the downsizing of military forces seen nearly everywhere, depleting the military of resources in terms of experts, manpower and money.

## Conclusion

Suicide in military settings has been a subject of research in many countries. The problem is most excessively covered in countries with big armies (USA, Russian Federation), and those involved in peacekeeping missions (Norway, Sweden). Almost all EU countries, most of them members of NATO, are implementing research and prevention regarding military suicides. There are reports also from Canada, Israel, Poland, Serbia and Montenegro and Ukraine. In the resources available, we could not find any information regarding the armies of China, Pakistan or countries of the Middle East. Prevention is an important topic in all studies. Nevertheless, stringent studies regarding prevention measures and their evaluation are not very numerous. Suicide in military settings is generally lower than in the general population of the same gender and age (some exceptions can be seen when specific age groups are evaluated). There are some specific risk factors for suicide in the army, such as exposure to traumatic stress (in war and peacekeeping duty), the military lifestyle with frequent relocations and break-up of protective social structures, and the easy access to firearms and other dangerous equipment. The risk factors may sometimes be balanced by protective factors such as social support, medical support and additional possibilities for prevention. Many authors state that during pre-enrolment and regular medical examination of the mental health of conscripts, suicidal tendencies are often not identified successfully, pointing to the need for better screening at an early stage. Educational initiatives directed at military leaders and medical personnel within the armed forces are other recommended measures.

## References

Allen JP, Cross G, Swanner J (2005). Suicide in the Army: a review of current information. *Military Medicine*, **170**, 580–584.

American Psychiatric Association (1980). *Diagnostic and Statistical Manual of Mental Disorders*, 3rd edn. American Psychiatric Association, Washington.

Annex D (2003). *Review of Soldier Suicides*. Available at: http://www.armymedicine.army.mil/news/mhat/Annex_D.pdf

Antonovsky A (1993) The structure and properties of the sense of coherence scale, *Social Science and Medicine*, **36**, 725–733.

Army News Service (2001a). *Army to Field New Suicide Prevention Plan*. Available at: http://hooah4health.com/mind/suicideprev/suicideprevention.htm

Army News Service (2001b). *Declaring War on Suicides*. Available at: http://www.military.com/Content/MoreContent?file=NL_suicide_ans

Begic D and Jokic-Begic N (2001). Aggressive behavior in combat-veterans with post-traumatic disorder. *Military Medicine*, **166**, 671–676.

Benda BB (2003). Discrimination of suicide thoughts and attempts among homeless veterans who abuse substances. *Suicide and Life-Threatening Behavior*, **33**, 430–442.

Benda BB (2005). Gender differences in predictors of suicidal thoughts and attempts among homeless veterans that abuse substances. *Suicide and Life-Threatening Behavior*, **35**, 106–116.

Bodner E, Ben-Artzi E, Kaplan Z (2006). Soldiers who kill themselves: the contribution of dispositional and situational factors. *Archives of Suicide Research*, **10**, 29–43.

Bogachenko SM, Kozachenko VF, Kovalyova GM (2003). Autoagressive suicidal behavior in the military who are the subject to early discharge. *Voenno-Meditsinskiy Jurnal*, **324**, 11, 68–69.

Botsis AJ, Soldatos CR, Kokkevi A *et al.* (1999). *Suicidal Ideation in the Military Conscripts*. 20th Congress of the IASP Abstract Book, Athens, IASP, pp. 124.

Bullman TA and Kang HK (1994). Posttraumatic stress disorder and the risk of traumatic deaths among Vietnam veterans. *Journal of Nervous and Mental Disease*, **182**, 604–610.

Bullman TA and Kang HK (1996). The risk of suicide among wounded Vietnam veterans. *American Journal of Public Health*, **86**, 662–667.

Cabarcapa M, Pania M (2004) Suicide in the military environment. *Vojnosanitetski Pregled*, **61**, 199–203.

Carr JR, Hoge CW, Gardner J *et al.* (2004). Suicide surveillance in the US military—reporting and classification biases in rate circulation. *Suicide and Life-Threatening Behavior*, **34**, 233–241.

Chorny MV (2001). Socio-epidemiological evaluation of suicides among personnel of internal affairs of Ukraine. *Archiv Psychiatrii*, **7**, 35–37.

Chorny MV (2002). Evaluation of suicides associated with alcohol consumption of the personnel of internal affairs. *Vrachebnoe Delo*, **1**, 147–150.

Chuprikov AP, Pilyagina GY, Nikiforuk RI (1998). The problem of suicide in Ukraine. *Mezhdunarodniy Meditsinskiy Zhurnal*, **4**, 52–57.

DASA (2007) Suicide and open verdict death in the UK regular Armed Forces 1984–2006. Available at: http://www.DASA.mod.uk

Davidson JR (2000). Trauma: the impact of post-traumatic stress disorder. *Journal of Psychopharmacology*, **14**, 5–12.

Dedic G, Lopicic Z, Panic M *et al.* (2006) Importance of psychotherapeutic intervention in the crisis following suicide in the Army of Serbia and Montenegro. *Psychiatria Danubina*, **18**, 98–98.

Desjeux G, Lebarere J, Galoisy-Guibal L *et al.* (2004). Suicide in the French armed forces. *European Journal of Epidemiology*, **19**, 823–9.

Desjeux G, Lemardeley P, Vallet D *et al.* (2001). Suicide and attempted suicide in the armed forces in 1998. *Encephale*, **27**, 320–324.

Eaton KM, Messer SC, Garvey Wilson AL *et al.* (2006). Srenthening the validity of population-based suicide rates comparisons: an illustration using US military and civilian data. *Suicide and Life-Threatening Behavior*, **36**, 182–191.

Engelstad JC (1968). Suicides and attempted suicides in the Norwegian Armed Forces during peace time. *Military Medicine*, **133**, 437–448.

Fadeev AS, Kulikov VV, Chernov OE (2001). Neurotic disorders in military service in the peacetime. *Voenno-Meditsinskiy Jurnal*, **322**, 39–43.

Farbstein I, Dycian D, Kinf RA *et al.* (2002). A follow-up study of adolescents attempted suicide in Israel. *Journal of the American Academy of Child and Adolescents Psychiatry*, **41**, 1342–1349.

Freeman TW, Roca V, Kimbrell T (2003). A survey of gun collection and use among three groups of veterans patients admitted to veterans' affairs hospital treatment program. *Southern Medical Journal*, **96**, 240–243.

Gerede A (2006). Turkish Air Force suicide prevention program. *Psychiatria Danubina*, **18**, 98–99.

Gichun VS (2000). Evaluating factors of psychological trauma leading to auto-aggressive behavior in soldiers by conscription. *Archiv Psychiatrii*, **6**, 17–18.

Giotakos O (2003). Suicidal ideation, substance use, and sense of coherence in Greek male conscripts. *Military Medicine*, **168**, 447–450.

Gordana DJ and Milivoje P (2007). Suicide prevention program in the Army of Serbia and Montenegro. *Military Medicine*, **172**, 551–555.

Gunnel D, Magnusson PK, Rasmussen F (2005). Low intelligence test scores in 18-year-old men and risk of suicide: a cohort study. *British Medical Journal*, **230**, 167.

Hall DP (1996). Stress, suicide, and military service during Operation Uphold Democracy, *Military Medicine*, **161**, 159–162.

Hansen-Schwartz J, Jessen G, Andersen K *et al.* (2002). Suicide after deployment in UN peacekeeping mission—a Danish pilot study. *Crisis*, **23**, 55–58.

Hendin H and Haas AP (1991). Suicide and guilt as manifestations of PTSD in Vietnam combat veterans. *American Journal of Psychiatry*, **148**, 586–591.

Hoge CW, Castro CA, Messer SC *et al.* (2004). Combat duty in Iraq and Afghanistan, mental health problems and barriers to care. *New England Journal of Medicine*, **352**, 13–22.

Hoge CW, Messer SC, Engel CC *et al.* (2003). Priorities for psychiatric research in the US military: an epidemiological approach. *Military Medicine*, **168**, 182–185.

Hytten K (1985). Suicide among Norwegian soldiers between 1977 and 1984. A retrospective study. *Tidsskr Nor Laegeforen*, **105**, 1770–1773.

Jiang G-X, Rasmussen F, Wasserman D (1999) Short stature and poor psychological performance: risk factors for attempted suicide among Swedish male conscripts. *Acta Psychiatrica Scandinavica*, **100**, 433–440.

Jontz S (2004). Suicide reports make Army improve. *Stars and Stripes*, **29** March.

Kaplan M, Huguet N, McFarland BH *et al.* (2007) Suicide among male veterans: a prospective population-based study. *Journal of Epidemiology and Community Health*, **61**, 619–624.

Kausch O (2003). Suicide attempts among veterans seeking treatment for pathological gambling. *Journal of Clinical Psychiatry*, **63**, 1031–1038.

Kessler RC, Sonnega A, Bromet E *et al.* (1995). Posttraumatic stress disorder in the National Comorbidity Survey. *Archives of General Psychiatry*, **52**, 1048–1060.

Knox KL, Litts DA, Talcott GW *et al.* (2003). Risk of suicide and related adverse outcomes after exposure to a suicide prevention programme in the US air force: cohort study. *British Medical Journal*, **327**, 1376–1380.

Kramer TL, Lindy JD, Green BL *et al.* (1994). The comorbidity of post-traumatic stress disorder and suicidality in Vietnam veterans. *Suicide and Life-Threatening Behavior*, **24**, 58–67.

Larsson D, Hemmingsson T, Allebeck P *et al.* (2002). Self-rated health and mortality among young men: what is the relation and how it may be explained. *Scandinavian Journal of Public Health*, **30**, 259–266.

Lester D (2005). Suicide in Vietnam veterans: the suicide wall. *Archives of Suicide Research*, **9**, 385–387.

Litvintsev SV, Shamrey VK, Fadeev AC *et al.* (2003). On the state of psychiatric aid in the Russian Federation Armed Forces. *Voenno-Meditsinskiy Jurnal*, **324**, 13–20.

Litvintsev SV, Shamrey VK, Nechiporenko VV *et al.* (2001a). Diagnostics and prevention of suicidal behavior in the military (Part 1). *Voenno-Meditsinskiy Jurnal*, **322**, 18–22.

Litvintsev SV, Shamrey VK, Nechiporenko VV *et al.* (2001b). Diagnostics and prevention of suicidal behavior in the military (Part 2). *Voenno-Meditsinskiy Jurnal*, **322**, 23–29.

Litvintsev SV, Shamrey VK, Rustanovich AV *et al.* (2002). Suicidal behavior in the military serving on the contract basis. *Voenno-Meditsinskiy Jurnal*, **323**, 29–30.

Magnusson PKE, Rasmussen F, Lawlor DA *et al.* (2006). Association of body mass index with suicide mortality: a prospective cohort study of more than one million men. *American Journal of Epidemiology*, **163**, 1–8.

Mahon MJ, Tobin JP, Cusack DA *et al.* (2005). Suicide among regular-duty military personnel: a retrospective study of occupation-specific risk factors for workplace suicide. *American Journal of Psychiatry*, **162**, 1688–1696.

Mancinelli I, Lazanio S, Comparelli A *et al.* (2003) Suicide in Italian military environment (1986–1998). *Military Medicine*, **168**, 146–152.

Mancinelli I, Tomaselli P, Comparelli A *et al.* (2001). Suicide in military circles in Italy (1986–1998). *European Psychiatry*, **16**, 432–433.

Marttunen M, Henriksson M, Pelkonen S *et al.* (1997). Suicides among military conscripts in Finland: a psychological autopsy study. *Military Medicine*, **162**, 14–18.

Mehlum L (1990). Attempted suicide in the armed forces: a retrospective study of Norwegian conscripts. *Military Medicine*, **155**, 596–600.

Mehlum L (1992). Prodromal signs and precipitating factors in attempted suicide. *Military Medicine*, **157**, 574–577.

Mehlum L (1994). Young male suicide attempters 20 years later: the suicide mortality rate. *Military Medicine*, **159**, 138–141.

Mehlum L (1998). Suicidal ideation and sense of coherence in male conscripts. *Acta Psychiatrica Scandinavica*, **98**, 487–492.

Mehlum L (2005). Traumatic stress and suicidal behaviour: an important target for treatment and prevention. In K Hawton, ed., *Suicidal Behaviour—From Science to Practice*, pp. 121–138. Oxford University Press, Oxford.

Mehlum L and Schwebs R (2001). Suicide prevention in the military. Recent experience from the Norwegian Armed Forces. *International Review of the Armed Forces Medical Services*, **74**, 71–74.

Mehlum L and Weisaeth L (2002). Predictors of posttraumatic stress reactions in Norwegian U.N. peacekeepers 7 years after service. *Journal of Trauma and Stress*, **15**, 17–26.

Micklewright S (2005). Deliberate self-harm in the Royal Navy. An audit of cases presenting to the Department of Community Mental Health. *Journal of the Royal Navy Medical Services*, **91**, 12–25.

MMWR (1999). *Morbidity and Mortality Weekly Report*, **48**, 1053–1057.

National Strategy for Suicide Prevention (2001). *National Strategy for Suicide Prevention, Goals and Objectives for Action*. US Department of Health and Human Services, Rockville.

Nelson R (2004). Suicide rates rise among soldiers in Iraq. *Lancet*, **363**, 300.

Patterson JC, Jones DR, Marsh W *et al.* (2001). Aeromedical management of US air force aviators who attempt suicide. *Aviation, Space, and Environmental Medicine*, **72**, 1081–1085.

Polychronidis I (1999). Epidemiological and clinical characteristics of suicides in the Hellenic Navy. In 20th Congress of the IASP, Athens, IASP, 125.

Ponteva M, Jormanainen V, Nurro S *et al.* (2000). Mortality after the UN service. Follow-up study of the Finnish peacekeeping contingents in the years 1969–96. *International Review of the Armed Forces Medical Service*, **73**, 235–239.

Price RK, Risk NK, Lewis CE *et al.* (2004). Post-traumatic stress disorder, drug dependence and suicidality among male Vietnam veterans with a history of heavy drug use. *Drug and Alcohol Dependence*, **76**(Suppl. 1), 31–43.

Reyes VA and Hicklin TA (2005). Anger in the combat zone. *Military Medicine*, **170**, 483–487.

Ristkani T, Sourander A, Helenius H *et al.* (2005). Sense of coherence among Finnish young men—a cross-sectional study at military call-up. *Nordic Journal of Psychiatry*, **59**, 473–480.

Ritchie EC and Gelles MG (2002). Psychological autopsies: the current Department of Defense effort to standardize training and quality assurance. *Journal of Forensic Sciences*, **47**, 1370–1372.

Ritchie EC, Keppler WC, Rothberg JM (2003). Suicide admission in the US military. *Military Medicine*, **168**, 177–181.

Rona RJ, Hyams KC, Wessely S (2005). Screening for psychological illness in military personnel. *Journal of American Medical Association*, **293**, 1257–60.

Rothberg JM, Bartone PT, Holloway HC *et al.* (1990). Life and death in the US army. *Journal of American Medical Association*, **264**, 2241–2244.

Rozanov VA (2007). Suicides in the countries of the former Soviet Union. *European Psychiatry*, **22**, 35–36.

Rozanov VA, Mokhovikov AN, Stiliha R (2002). Successful model of suicide prevention in the Ukraine military environment. *Crisis*, **23**, 171–177.

Rutz W, von Knorring L, Pihlgren H *et al.* (1995). Prevention of male suicides: lessons from the Gotland study. *Lancet*, **345**, 524.

Scoville SL, Gardner JW, Potter RN (2004). Traumatic deaths during US Armed Forces basic training, 1977–2001. *American Journal of Preventive Medicine*, **26**, 194–200.

Senteil JW and Lacroix M (1997). Predictive patterns of suicidal behavior; the United States Armed Services versus the civilian population. *Military Medicine*, **162**, 168–171.

Sharaevskiy GY, Kolkutin VV, Fetisov VA (2002). Medical-forensic evaluation of deaths from external causes in the Navy. *Voenno-Meditsinskiy Jurnal*, **323**, 7–10.

Spooner MH (2002). Suicide claiming more veterans than fighting did. *Canadian Medical Association Journal*, **166**, 1453.

Stander VA, Hilton SM, Kennedy KR *et al.* (2004). Surveillance of completed suicide in the Department of Navy. *Military Medicine*, **169**, 301–306.

Tegan K, Boehmer C, Flanders D *et al.* (2004). Post-service mortality in Vietnam veterans. *Archives of Internal Medicine*, **164**, 1908–1916.

The Army Suicide Prevention Program. Available at: http://www.medtrng.com/suicideprevention/

Thoresen S and Mehlum L (2004). Risk factors for fatal accidents and suicides in peacekeepers: is there an overlap? *Military Medicine*, **169**, 988–93.

Thoresen S, Mehlum L, Moller B (2003). Suicide in peacekeepers—a cohort study of mortality from suicide in 22,275 Norwegian veterans from international peacekeepers operations. *Social Psychiatry and Psychiatric Epidemiology*, **38**, 605–610.

Varnik A (1997). Suicide in the Baltic countries and in the former republics of the USSR, pp. 1–169. Karolinska Institute, Doctoral dissertation, Stockholm.

Walter Reed Army Institute of Research (2005). *Walter Reed Army Institute of Research (WRAIR) Report on the Mental Health and Well-being of Soldiers in Operation Iraqi Freedom (OIF-II)*. Available at: http://www.armymedicine.army.mil/news/mhat_ii/annex_a.pdf

Wasserman D, Varnik A, Dankowicz M (1998). Regional differences in the distribution of suicide in the former Soviet Union during perestroika, 1984–1990. *Acta Psychiatrica Scandinavica*, **394**, 5–12.

Wasserman IM (1992). Economy, work, occupation and suicide. In RW Maris, AL Berman, JT Maltsenberger *et al.*, eds, *Assessment and Prediction of Suicide*, pp. 520–540. The Guilford Press, New York.

Weinberg I, Lubin G, Shmushkevich M *et al.* (2002). Elevated suicide rate on the first working day: a replication in Israel. *Death Studies*, **26**, 681–688.

Wong A, Excobar M, Lessage A *et al.* (2001). Are UN peacekeepers at risk of suicide? *Suicide and Life-Threatening Behavior*, **31**, 103–112.

World Health Organization (2008). *Health for All Database (HFA-DB)*. World Health Organization Regional Office for Europe, Copenhagen. Available at http://www.euro.who.int./hfadb.

# CHAPTER 37

# Suicide in prisons and remand centres

## Screening and prevention

Ad Kerkhof and Eric Blaauw

## Abstract

Early identification of prisoners with suicide risk, and the prevention of suicide, are of great importance given the high suicide rates in correctional facilities. General suicide screening instruments are not very useful in prisons and remand centres. A new screening instrument has been developed and tested consisting of eight questions. The cut-off score, retrospectively, allowed the identification of 82 per cent of all Dutch prisoner suicides. By screening new inmates, this set of questions classified 18 per cent of all prisoners in a high-risk group. All of these inmates require immediate and further assessment by a medical or mental health care officer. However, even without screening, these prisoners will visit medical or mental health services sometime later during their incarceration, because of their level of psychopathology. Regular follow-up interviews are necessary to assess the suicide risk. Suicidal prisoners, most of whom have severe psychiatric disorders, should receive standard treatment in the same way as ordinary people would receive treatment beyond prison walls.

## Introduction

Suicide rates in correctional facilities are several times higher than in the larger community (Backett 1987; Hayes 1989; Dooley 1990; Kerkhof and Bernasco 1990; Liebling 1992; Davis and Muscat 1993; Blaauw and Kerkhof 1999; Shaw et al. 2004; Blaauw et al. 2005; Fazel et al. 2005). Many people are affected by prison suicides: prison officers, the psycho-medical staff, fellow prisoners, relatives and partners. Prison officers can develop feelings of guilt for not having interpreted warning signs correctly. A suicide confronts fellow prisoners with a model of applying a drastic change to their lives. For relatives and partners, coming to terms with a suicide is difficult in itself, but a suicide in a penal institution may be painful as it often leaves even more questions unanswered. A suicide can cause disturbance in the institution and be the cause of negative publicity, because it seems to indicate that the authorities failed in their responsibilities regarding the safety of their prisoners. In view of all this, both the early identification of prisoners having a high suicide risk and the prevention of suicide are of great importance.

## Screening for suicidal risk

General suicide screening instruments are unlikely to be very useful in a population that is characterized by suicide vulnerability, in a situation, in which even mentally strong individuals are being tested to the limits of their coping resources.

The high prevalence of suicidal behaviours in prisons is the result of a complex interaction between the highly demanding prison environment and the vulnerability of large numbers of prisoners (Liebling 1992; Blaauw et al. 2005). Many prisoners enter prison with alcohol or drug dependence (Walker 1983; Gibbs 1987), poor coping skills (Liebling 1992; Toch 1992), histories of suicidal behaviour (Anno 1985; Hatty and Walker 1986; Marcus and Alcabes 1993) and current mental disorders (for a meta-analysis see Fazel and Danesh 2002), such as schizophrenia (4–6 per cent) and major depression (10–12 per cent). In addition, many prisoners struggle with severe personality disorders. A meta-analysis on almost 23,000 prisoners revealed that of men, 65 per cent had a personality disorder, including 47 per cent with antisocial personality disorder (Fazel and Danesh 2002). Of women, 42 per cent had a personality disorder, including 21 per cent with antisocial personality disorder. Furthermore, there is no debate that imprisonment is stressful (Sykes 1966; Toch 1992). Prisoners are deprived of their liberty, decisional authority, contacts with their loved ones, work activities, etc. They are also forced to live in a situation in which they are more likely to be confronted with individuals with addiction problems, mental disorders and/or with increased needs than individuals in the community. Therefore, it is not surprising that the vast majority of prisoners suffer from negative mood states (Gibbs 1987; Ostfeld et al. 1987; Zamble and Porporino 1988) such as hostility, depression, hopelessness and anxiety. Suicidal gestures, therefore, occur at high rates in prisons and remand centres. Unfortunately, due to their long-term vulnerability, prisoners continue to have high suicide figures even after their release from prisons (156 per 100,000 person-years, Pratt et al. 2006), indicating that we are dealing with persons who have been, are, and will be suicidal: before, during and after their stay in prisons.

## Suicidal behaviour in prisons: specific correlates

Studies on differences between prison suicide victims and general prisoners have yielded equivocal findings with regard to over-representations of males, whites, unemployed, old, and single or unmarried inmates among suicide victims (Blaauw *et al.* 2005). There is an abundance of studies that found prior incarcerations and current charges of violent crimes to be more common among suicide victims than among general inmates. Furthermore, histories of suicide attempts, psychiatric illnesses, drug abuse and alcohol abuse may be useful for the assessment of vulnerability for suicide in penal institutions. These findings suggest that demographic characteristics may be less useful for screening on suicide risk than criminal characteristics, and that psychiatric characteristics are the most useful characteristics to assess suicide risk.

An Austrian study (Fruehwald *et al.* 2004) showed that the most important predictors of suicide among pre-trial prisoners were psychopharmacological treatment while incarcerated, known previous suicide attempt, single-cell accommodation and a high level of violence in the last offence. In a sample of sentenced prisoners, the most important predictors of suicide were suicide threat, psychiatric diagnosis, single-cell accommodation, a high level of violence in the last offence and psychopharmacological treatment while incarcerated. Thus, both psychiatric and criminal characteristics were found to be indicative of suicide risk.

A Dutch study (Blaauw *et al.* 2005) examined combinations of demographic, psychiatric and criminal characteristics for their capability of distinguishing suicide victims from general inmates in the Netherlands. With regard to demographic characteristics, this study found that the suicide victims and a comparison group had different distributions of age, marital status and living situation. Suicide victims were more often over 40 years, separated, divorced or widowed and of no fixed abode, and less often living in a home with other people. The two samples did not differ with regard to gender, country of birth, race and employment. With regard to criminal characteristics, suicide victims more often had a history of only one prior incarceration in a jail or prison, and they were more often charged with (or convicted for) violent offences and less often with alcohol or drug offences or other offences. With regard to psychiatric characteristics, suicide victims more often had histories of hard drug abuse, multiple substance abuse, psychiatric care and suicide attempts. The two samples did not have different histories of alcohol abuse or soft drug abuse. Of 70 suicide victims (25 missing cases), 73 per cent had received a psychiatric diagnosis (excluding alcohol or drug dependence) during their imprisonment, most often a psychotic disorder (44 per cent), personality disorder (43 per cent) or affective disorder (21 per cent). Among the respondents of the comparison group, 12 per cent had received a psychiatric diagnosis.

Regression analysis showed that a good prediction of suicide vulnerability was formed by a model that successively included history of psychiatric care, aged over 40 years, violent offence, homelessness, one prior incarceration and history of hard drug abuse. With each indicator assigned the beta weight and with a specificity of 82 per cent, the model correctly classified 82 per cent of the Dutch suicides. Thus, a combination of two demographic characteristics, two criminal characteristics and two indicators of psychiatric problems proved capable of identifying 82 per cent of the suicide victims in the Netherlands at a specificity of 0.82 in the general inmate population.

## Characteristics of the screening instrument

The Dutch screening instrument (see Figure 37.1) was constructed by making use of the results of the regression techniques. Each characteristic in the screening instrument was assigned the logistic regression beta weight, multiplied by 100. Hereby, the indicator 'violent offence' was replaced by the indicator 'a history of suicide attempts or self-destructive behaviours' because this latter indicator proved to be a more powerful indicator in subsamples of the Dutch dataset.

The resulting screening instrument consists of eight questions, each with its corresponding weight, and with six questions directly resulting from the regression analyses. Weighing 27 points, a history of (intramural or outpatient) mental health care has the highest predictive value for suicide risk. It concerns the question whether the prisoner ever received treatment for psychiatric problems (addictions excluded) at the psychiatric department of a general hospital, in a psychiatric hospital, any institute for outpatient mental health, or from an independent psychologist or psychiatrist. The lack of a fixed residence in the months prior to confinement (of which the week immediately preceding confinement is the most decisive), weighing 23 points, ranks as the next strongest indicator of increased suicide risk. Thirdly, belonging to the age group of 40 years and over is a strong indicator of increased suicide risk: this characteristic weighs 17 points. As the fourth characteristic, weighing 14 points, a past with one previous period of confinement distinguishes clearly between the suicides and the non-suicidal prisoners. A multiple addiction to hard drugs and a history of suicide attempts or self-destructive behaviours appear to be equally important in making a clear distinction; both characteristics weigh 13 points. Addiction, as a characteristic, applies when the prisoner used hard drugs (at least once a week) in combination with soft drugs, large amounts of alcohol or non-therapeutic quantities of medication. Examples of previous suicide attempts or self-destructive behaviours are: taking an overdose of drugs or medication, cutting one's wrists, trying to hang oneself, and trying to come to grief in other ways.

In regards to two important characteristics, no statistically determined weight could be assigned. It may be expected, certainly on the basis of the Dutch and Austrian studies, that psychiatric disorders, particularly psychotic disorders, are of a highly predictive value with regards to risk of suicide. Therefore, it was decided to give attention in the instrument to prisoners, who in the previous five years had contact with a psychologist or a psychiatrist who made such a diagnosis—this can be an Axis-1 diagnosis according to the *Diagnostic and Statistic Manual of Mental Disorders* (DSM) as well as a diagnosis according to the *International Classification of Diseases* (ICD). In addition, as mentioned before, recent suicidal expressions or self-destructive behaviours have predictive value. In this regard, attention was given to the prisoner who expressed himself in this manner or showed such behaviour during his stay at the police station, at the courthouse, or during his transportation to the prison.

A German study (Dahle *et al.* 2005) underlined the value of the instrument for the identification of suicide victims in German penal systems. The study consisted of all adult male pre-trial

| Name of prisoner: | | Date of birth: | | Cell number: | | |
| Interview date: | | | | Interview time: | | |
| Name of nurse: | | | | Institution: | | |

| | Characteristic | Description | | No | Yes |
|---|---|---|---|---|---|
| 1 | Aged 40+ | Prisoner is aged 40 years or older | | 0 | 17 |
| 2 | No fixed address or residence | In the time **shortly before confinement** the prisoner has not had a fixed address or residence | | 0 | 23 |
| 3 | One prior confinement | **In the past** the prisoner was held **once** previously in a detention centre or a prison. The current confinement is the second time. | | 0 | 14 |
| 4 | History of multiple hard drug abuse | **In the past** the prisoner has taken **hard drugs** (at least once a week) **in combination with**: (at least one of the following)<br>a. soft drugs (at least 3 times a week)<br>b. large quantities of alcohol (at least 3 times a week)<br>c. non-therapeutic amounts of medication (at least once a week) | | 0 | 13 |
| 5 | Treatment history for psychiatric symptoms | The prisoner has **at any time** been treated for **psychiatric symptoms** in a psychiatric (ward of a general) hospital, at an outpatient mental health centre or by an independent psychologist or psychiatrist. | | 0 | 27 |
| 6 | Psychotic disorder or other DSM-IV As-1 disorder * | **In the past five years** the prisoner has been diagnosed as schizophrenic (or another psychotic disorder), or suffering from anxiety, mood, somatoform or dissociative disorder. | | 0 | 24 |
| 7 | Previous suicide attempts or self-destructive behaviours | In the past the prisoner has **intentionally** cut, poisoned or wounded himself, or has tried to hang himself, drown or come to grief in other ways. | | 0 | 13 |
| 8 | Suicidal utterances or suicide attempts during current (court) procedure | During the admission interview the prisoner has made **remarks** that may point at suicidality or has done so during confinement at the police station, in the court house or during transport *or* has attempted suicide in one of these situations. | | 0 | 24 |
| | **Total score** | If 24 points or over, alert mental health staff member | **Total points** | | |

\* This question is to be answered in the affirmative only if a definitive diagnosis was made. A mental health care history is no sufficient indication for the existence of a diagnosable disorder.

If the prisoner gives the impression of being suicidal without it showing from the screening instrument, a mental health staff member must be informed of this suspicion.

**Referred to.......................(mental health staff member) on ...........................(date) at ....................hrs (time).**

**Fig. 37.1** A screening instrument for suicide risk (Blaauw and Kerkhof 1999).

detainees who committed suicide in Berlin between 1991 and 2000 (suicide group N = 30) and inmates who were booked with the following booking number into the same jail (comparison group N = 30). Based on the 24-point cut-off value, 25 of 30 suicidal inmates (83 per cent) would have been correctly classified as high-risk persons, at the expense of 7 false alarms in the comparison group (23 per cent). A cut-off score of 40 would have led to 7 per cent false positive classifications and 68 per cent proper identifications in the suicide group.

## Using the instrument

At a demarcation value of 24 points, around 18 per cent of all prisoners are placed in high risk of the suicide group. Although the majority of these prisoners will not commit suicide, most of them suffer from serious mental and emotional problems. When the separate predictors of suicide risk are considered, it becomes obvious that each of these characteristics points at special circumstances. During their confinement, prisoners with a history of mental health care will often suffer from the problems that required

earlier treatment. Prisoners with a psychotic or other psychiatric disorder require extra care, whereas those with no fixed address, in many cases, experience social or psychological problems. Relatively older prisoners in the institution may feel isolated compared to other, usually much younger, fellow prisoners. Prisoners who were imprisoned once before often do not feel comfortable during their confinement, and prisoners with a history of multiple hard drug abuse still tend to struggle with their addiction problems and withdrawal symptoms. Prisoners with a history of suicide attempts, and those who recently expressed themselves as such or showed self-destructive behaviours, are also a cause of concern. In short, the majority of those prisoners who meet one or more characteristics from the screening instrument probably belong to the group that should usually be referred for a further interview.

It is advisable to have the screening for suicide risk performed by a prison nurse, because the questions of the screening instrument are likely to have a major overlap with the questions that are usually asked during admission interviews in order to assess mental or addiction problems. In addition, it is recommended that the screening instrument be applied immediately on arrival, because many suicides occur during the first hours, nights and weeks of confinement (Crighton and Towl 1997; Frottier *et al.* 2002; Shaw *et al.* 2004).

## What to do after applying the screening instrument?

A prisoner scoring 24 points or more on this instrument, and as such belonging to the high-risk group, should be referred immediately to a psychologist, psychiatrist or in psychiatry trained nurse for a further diagnostic interview. Almost all prisoners in the high-risk group have mental problems, many have attempted suicide previously, but it is unknown which prisoners from this group will attempt suicide in the future. In order to prevent suicides, this entire group should immediately receive extra attention, to begin with a diagnostic interview to be carried out by trained staff. In the diagnostic interview, insight must be acquired into the prisoner's suicide risk. It is important to explore the thoughts, intentions and preparations in connection with possible previous suicide attempts and possible intended future suicide attempts. The degree of suicide ideation may differ in the course of time and can be influenced by certain events. For instance, some prisoners have a higher than normal chance of becoming the victim of bullying, which is related to heightened suicide risk in prisoners (Blaauw *et al.* 2001b; Ireland 2002; Blaauw *et al.* 2002). Therefore, regular follow-up interviews are necessary to assess the suicide risk at later moments in time. It is important to record all findings on a registration form. This form should be included in the prisoner's medical file. It is of the utmost importance that the findings of the suicide risk assessment are shared with the prison officers who are responsible for the daily care of these prisoners as these officers usually do not have access to the medical files of prisoners. Inclusion in the medical file promotes the transfer of information between the various members of the medical and mental health staff, and will contribute to the continuity of care in case of relocation to other penal institutions. However, after relocation it is necessary to screen prisoners again (Blaauw *et al.* 1997, 2001a).

## Conclusions about screening

Early identification of suicidal prisoners is an important first step to reduce the number of suicides in penal institutions. Therefore, it is promising that the Dutch research project resulted in a screening instrument that has proved to be easy and requires little time and effort. It is also an instrument that is unobtrusive as it makes use of a few historical characteristics that can be easily obtained, possibly even from files. As such, working with the screening instrument will most likely not conflict with other strategies to prevent suicide. It is even more promising that this instrument was found to be accurate in the prediction (actually post-diction) of suicides in prison systems in The Netherlands, England and Wales, the United States and Germany. Suicides in different countries share more similarities than differences (Blaauw *et al.* 2005).

## Further prevention of suicide in correctional facilities

### Mental health care

As said before, the prevention of suicide should start as soon as possible, immediately following the reception of inmates in the facility.

Attention should be paid immediately to the high vulnerability levels of many prisoners. Since many prisoners have psychiatric problems, the immediate routine provision of psychiatric care, including medication and, if necessary, psychotherapy should be self-evident. However, many European prison systems have only very limited mental health care provisions (Themeli *et al.* 1999). Anxiety, depression, psychosis, suicidal feelings—all these common mental disorders should receive standard treatment in the same way as ordinary people would receive outside the prison walls. When a prisoner breaks his leg, he will be immediately transferred to a hospital. Likewise, when a prisoner develops psychotic symptoms, he should be transferred to a psychiatric ward within or outside the prison. There is no excuse for withholding adequate mental health care. Since many addicted inmates enter the system, detoxification units and sustained medication (e.g. opiate-antagonists) should be available. After detoxification, psychological treatment should be available to help prisoners remain abstinent. The principles of Community Reinforcement Approach would be appropriate here, adapted to the prison system (Roozen 2005). Since many prisoners have problems in self-regulation or lack capacities for stress management, simple stress reduction techniques should become available. Prisoners have high levels of pathological worrying (Kerkhof and Van 't Veer 2004). Worrying may be one of the prodromes for suicidal behaviours. Simple exercises fighting excessive worrying are available and could be handed over upon reception in the form of leaflets. In such leaflets, worry regulation techniques can be proposed such as to postpone worry to specific worry episodes (30 minutes in the morning, 30 minutes in the evening), to spend time thinking about positive memories, about skills and characteristics one is proud of, to think about possible positive future prospects, and to challenge over-generalized negative self-statements.

Because suicidal vulnerability waxes and wanes over time, prison staff should assess suicidal ideation regularly. Prison staff, therefore, should be trained accordingly.

For the many prisoners with borderline personalities, who regularly engage in suicidal threats, gestures and acts, dialectical behaviour therapy (Linehan *et al.* 2006) is available and is already applied in some prison settings. Adequate treatment of psychiatric disorders during incarceration may as well prevent post-release suicides.

All of these recommendations are self-evident, and they are shared by all international experts in the field (Konrad *et al.* 2007; Daigle *et al.* 2007). However, there is not yet much empirical evidence that these recommendations are effective, because prevention programmes are extremely difficult to evaluate due to methodological difficulties. Only very few methodologically sound studies have been performed. The status, therefore, is a widely shared consensus that applying these recommendations would lower the suicide rates in correctional facilities. Directors of prison systems tend to point to this lack of empirical evidence and use this to justify doing nothing to prevent suicides.

### Training

Correctional officers and prison staff have to be educated and trained in suicide assessment and management. They have to know the motivation behind suicidal behaviour. In Australia, a specific suicide awareness training for all custodial staff has been implemented, including work supervision by professionals (Eyland *et al.* 1997). The State of New York developed a comprehensive training programme within its upstate local remand facilities, including a training manual, a videotape, an officer handbook, and pre- and post evaluations leading to certification (Cox *et al.* 1988, 1989; Cox and Morschauser 1997). Despite a nearly 100 per cent increase in the jail population, there has been more than a 150 per cent decrease in jail suicides since programme implementation. In the Netherlands, suicide prevention courses for correctional officers were set up by the training institute of the Dutch prison system, almost all psychologists working in Dutch remand centres and prisons receive postgraduate courses in suicide prevention. All experiences with suicide awareness programmes and risk-assessment course point to the excellent evaluations by the correctional officers and prison staff, who were happy to receive help in dealing with behaviour they often did not understand.

### Housing

Architectural design is important in suicide prevention. Safe cells provide safe conditions for the observation of inmates who require special supervision (no potential ligature points, no electrical outlets, no toxic materials, rounded corners for the walls, no exposed pipes, hooks, hinges, door knobs, etc.). However, suicide-proof cells may increase the feelings of loneliness and despair of suicidal inmates. It is also advisable to minimize the amount of time suicidal prisoners are in segregation units.

### Monitoring

Close and constant observation at different levels of supervision should be geared to the risk of individual prisoners. Closed-circuit television is not enough, since there are numerous examples of inmates committing suicide in full view of television equipment. Sometimes buddies are trained to observe suicide risk in peers and provide peer counselling in crisis. Monitoring, however, can only be successful in combination with face-to-face contact.

### Communication

The most powerful deterrent for suicide is personal contact. Communication between inmates and prison officers and mental health care workers may relieve feelings of isolation, hopelessness and crisis. Prison officers should be attentive to signs of excessive worrying, depression and despair, and should communicate with inmates about these signs. They should be able to provide emotional support. A common finding in prison suicides is a recent breakdown of communication between inmate and correctional officers. Prison officers can be attentive to the sense of hopelessness about the future, a characteristic that will only grow stronger in the absence of personal communication. Listeners scheme's including the availability of telephonic contact with Samaritans, or buddy schemes, trained by organizations such as the Samaritans, seem to help (selected) prisoners to survive their crises (Schlosar 1997). Confidential reporting of suicidal communications by fellow inmates should be encouraged.

Prison officers and psychologists and psychiatrists should have a routine communication of inmates' suicidal ideation. All prison officers in consecutive shifts should be aware of the pending danger. The oscillation of suicidal intent should be registered on a daily to weekly base.

### Contact with family and friends

Essential feature of suicide prevention is the involvement of family members and friends, if applicable. Suicidal inmates can be helped enormously by granting additional contact with next of kin. Several suicide prevention programmes do offer this extra contact for suicidal inmates. Relatives are the connection to the future. They embody future perspectives for the period upon release. As such, they are the first to help suicidal inmates re-orient themselves regarding the hopelessness of their future perspectives.

## Conclusion

Suicide prevention in remand centres and prisons and other correctional facilities should start as soon as possible when inmates enter the system. Thorough and systematic screening is the cornerstone, followed by immediate and adequate mental health care. Suicide prevention is only a small part of the more general mental health care remand centres and prisons offer. In this respect, the quality of suicide prevention is a performance indicator for the more general management of the emotional needs of prisoners. There is reason to believe that, in many countries, suicide prevention in detention could be improved considerably (Daigle *et al.* 2007; Konrad *et al.* 2007), and the WHO has issued a resource booklet called *Preventing suicide—a resource for prison officers* (WHO 2000).

## References

Anno BJ (1985). Patterns of suicide in the Texas Department of Corrections, 1980–1985. *Journal of Prisons and Jail Health*, **5**, 82–93.

Backett SA (1987). Suicide in Scottish prisons. *British Journal of Psychiatry*, **151**, 218–221.

Blaauw E and Kerkhof AJFM (1999). *Suïcides in Detentie* [suicides in prison]. Elsevier, The Hague.

Blaauw E, Arensman E, Kraaij V *et al.* (2002). Traumatic life-events and suicide risk among jail inmates: the influence of types of events, time period and ignificant others. *Journal of Traumatic Stress*, **15**, 9–16.

Blaauw E, Carrière R, Schilder F *et al.* (1997). Prevention of suicides in penal institutions in The Netherlands. *Crisis*, **18**, 170–177.

Blaauw E, Kerkhof AJFM, Hayes LM (2005). Identification of suicide vulnerability in inmates on the basis of demographic and criminal characteristics and indicators of psychiatric problems. *Suicide and Life-Threatening Behavior*, **35**, 63–75.

Blaauw E, Kerkhof AJFM, Winkel FW *et al.* (2001a). Identifying suicide risk in penal institutions in the Netherlands. *British Journal of Forensic Practice*, **3**, 22–28.

Blaauw E, Winkel FW, Kerkhof AJFM (2001b). Bullying and suicidal behavior in jails. *Criminal Justice and Behavior*, **28**, 279–299.

Cox JF and Morschauser PC (1997). A solution to the problem of jail suicide. *Crisis*, **18**, 178–184.

Cox JF, Landsberg G, Paravati MP (1989). The essential components of a crisis intervention program for local jails. *Psychiatric Quarterly*, **60**, 103–117.

Cox JF, Mc Carthy DW, Landsberg G *et al.* (1988). A model for crisis intervention services within local jails. *International Journal of Law and Psychiatry*, **11**, 391–407.

Crighton D and Towl G (1997). Self-inflicted deaths in prison in England and Wales: an analysis of the data for 1988–90 and 1994–95. *Issues in Criminological and Legal Psychology*, **28**, 12–20.

Dahle KP, Lohner JC, Konrad N (2005). Suicide prevention in penal institutions: validation and optimization of a screening tool for early identification of high-risk inmates in pretrial detention. *International Journal of Forensic Mental Health*, **4**, 53–62.

Daigle MS, Daniel AE, Dear GE *et al.* (2007). Preventing suicide in prisons: Part II: International comparisons of suicide prevention services in correctional settings. *Crisis*, **28**, 122–130.

Davis MS and Muscat JE (1993). An epidemiologic study of alcohol and suicide risk in Ohio jails and lockups, 1975–1984. *Journal of Criminal Justice*, **21**, 277–283.

De Leo D, Burgis S, Bertolotte JM *et al.* (2004). Definitions of suicidal behaviour. In D de Leo, U Bille Brahe, A Kerkhof *et al.*, eds, *Suicidal Behaviour: Theories and Research Findings*, pp. 17–39. Hogrefe and Huber, Gőttingen.

Dooley E (1990). Prison suicide in England and Wales, 1972–87. *British Journal of Psychiatry*, **156**, 40–45.

Eyland S, Corben S, Barton J (1997). Suicide prevention in New South Wales correctional centers. *Crisis*, **18**, 163–169.

Fazel S and Danesh J (2002). Serious mental disorder among 23000 prisoners: systematic review of 62 surveys. *Lancet*, **359**, 545–550.

Fazel S, Benning R, Danesh J (2005). Suicides in male prisoners in England and Wales, 1978–2003. *Lancet*, **366**, 1301–1302.

Frottier P, Fruehwald S, Ritter K et al. (2002). Jailhouse blues revisited. *Social Psychiatry and Psychiatric Epidemiology*, **37**, 68–73.

Fruehwald S, Frottier P, Matschnig T *et al.* (2004). Suicide in custody: a case–control study. *British Journal of Psychiatry*, **185**, 494–498.

Gibbs JJ (1987). Symptoms of psychopathology among jail prisoners: the effects of exposure to jail environment. *Criminal Justice and Behaviour*, **14**, 288–310.

Hatty SE and Walker JR (1986). *A National Study of Deaths in Australian Prisons*. Australian Institute of Criminology, Canberra.

Hayes LM (1989). National study of jail suicides: seven years later. *Psychiatric Quarterly*, **60**, 7–29.

Ireland JL (2002). Official records of bullying incidents among young offenders: what can they tell us and how useful are they? *Journal of Adolescence*, **25**, 669–679.

Kerkhof AJFM and Bernasco W (1990). Suicidal behavior in jails and prisons in The Netherlands. *Suicide and Life-Threatening Behavior*, **20**, 123–137.

Kerkhof AJFM and Van't Veer E (2004). Piekeren in Detentie (Worrying in detention). *Sancties*, **6**, 334–340.

Konrad N, Daigle MS, Daniel AE *et al.* (2007). Preventing suicide in prisons: Part I: Recommendations from the international association for suicide prevention task force on suicide in prisons. *Crisis*, **28**, 113–121.

Liebling A (1992). *Suicides in Prison*. Routledge, London.

Linehan MM, Comtois KA, Murray AM *et al.* (2006). Two-year randomized controlled trial and follow-up of dialectical therapy vs therapy by experts for suicidal behaviors and borderline personality disorder. *Archives of General Psychiatry*, **63**, 757–66.

Marcus PD and Alcabes PD (1993). Characteristics of suicides by inmates in an urban city jail. *Hospital and Community Psychiatry*, **44**, 256–261.

Ostfeld AM, Kasl SV, D'Atri DA *et al.* (1987). *Stress, Crowding, and Blood Pressure in Prison*. Lawrence Erlbaum, Hillsdale.

Pratt D, Piper M, Appleby L *et al.* (2006). Suicide in recently released prisoners: a population-based cohort study. *Lancet*, **368**, 119–123.

Roozen HG (2005). Community reinforcement approach and naltrexone in the treatment of addiction. Ph.D. dissertation, Vrije Universiteit, Amsterdam.

Schlosar H (1997). Befriendeing in prisons. *Crisis*, **18**, 148–151.

Shaw J, Baker D, Hunt IM *et al.* (2004). Suicide by prisoners: national clinical survey. *British Journal of Psychiatry*, **184**, 263–267.

Sykes G (1966). *The Society of Captives: A Study of a Maximum Security Prison*. Atheneum, New York.

Themeli O, Blaauw E, Kerkhof AJFM (1999). *Suicide Prevention in Penal Institutions*. Vrije Universiteit, Amsterdam.

Toch H (1992). *Living in Prison: The Ecology of Survival*. American Psychological Association, Washington.

Walker N (1983). Side-effects of incarceration. *British Journal of Criminology*, **23**, 61–71.

WHO (2000). *Preventing Suicide—A Resource for Prison Officers*. The World Health Organization, Geneva.

Zamble E and Porporino FJ (1988). *Coping, Behaviour, and Adaptation in Prison Inmates*. Springer-Verlag, New York.

# PART 6

# Psychiatric and Somatic Determinants of Suicide

# CHAPTER 38

# Major psychiatric disorders in suicide and suicide attempters

Jouko Lönnqvist

## Abstract

Suicidal behaviour is closely connected with mental disorders. Virtually all mental disorders carry an increased risk of suicidal ideation, suicide attempt, and suicide. Psychiatric disorder may be an almost necessary, yet insufficient, risk factor for suicide. About 90 per cent of individuals who attempt or commit suicide meet diagnostic criteria for a psychiatric disorder, most often mood disorder, substance use disorders, psychoses, and personality disorders. The risk of suicidal behaviour in anxiety disorders and eating disorders, both having strong comorbidity with depression, is often underestimated. Under-treatment, comorbidity, treatment non-compliance and poor adherence, as well as a high frequency of non-responders are common problems and challenges in the treatment of suicidal persons. On the other hand, there is growing evidence of lower risk of suicidal behaviour during closely monitored long-term treatment of suicidal patients, indicating that treatment adherence is an important factor in medical suicide prevention.

## Suicidal behaviour and mental disorder: two interacting processes and a chance of preventing suicide

Suicidality and, in a more narrow meaning, suicidal behaviour can be conceptualized as a continuum ranging from suicidal ideation and communications to suicide attempts and completed suicide. A complex developmental process, which leads to suicidal ideation, suicidal communication, self-destructive behaviour, in some cases even to suicide, and its consequences to the survivors is often referred to as a suicidal process (Table 38.1). A long-term suicide process is shaped by a number of interacting cultural, social, psychological, biological, and situational factors. Mental health and mental disorders of a person modulate the risk of suicidal behaviour among all risk and protective factors.

A suicidal act usually has no single cause, not even a mental disorder. However, suicidal behaviour is tightly connected with mental disorders. About 90 per cent of individuals who commit suicide meet diagnostic criteria for a psychiatric disorder, most often mood disorders, substance use disorders, psychoses, and personality disorders (Henriksson *et al.* 1993). Diagnostic distribution of those

**Table 38.1** The process model of suicidal behaviour

| Risk and protective factors |
| --- |
| **Cultural, societal, social and interpersonal factors** |
| Attitudes |
| Beliefs |
| Norms |
| Regulations |
| Integration–disintegration |
| Social networks and social support |
| Connections vs isolation |
| Services |
| **Individual factors** |
| Genetic and biological factors predisposing to or protecting from suicidal behaviour |
| Personality and specific personality traits (impulsivity, hopelessness, extraversion, hopefulness) |
| Symptoms (no symptoms, distress, anxiety and depressiveness) |
| Mental health and disorders |
| Physical health and illnesses |
| **Situational factors** |
| Stressful life events |
| Recent stressors |
| Availability of suicide methods and access to lethal means |
| Contact, help and services |
| **Suicidal ideation** |
| Severity of suicidal intention |
| Suicidal communication |
| External intervening factors |
| **Suicidal act: suicide attempt and suicide** |
| Personal reactions and behaviour |
| External reactions, help, and treatment |
| Outcome: survival or death |
| Aftermath |

attempting suicide is very similar (Suominen *et al.* 1996). Many suicidal persons have a family history of mental disorders and suicidal behaviour (Mann 2003; Brent and Mann 2005). Almost all suicidal persons have mental problems and symptoms, and they have often had contact with psychiatric services.

Virtually all mental disorders carry an increased risk of suicidal ideation, suicide attempt, and suicide. Suicidal ideation, and even suicide attempts, are common in mental disorders. However, it is only a minority of people who will eventually commit suicide. Psychiatric disorder may be an almost necessary, yet insufficient, risk factor for suicide. The greatest risk of suicide among all clinical states is in attempted suicide, which carries about forty times the expected value (Table 38.2). The suicide risk in mood disorders is high, about five- to twentyfold higher than expected. In schizophrenia, substance use disorders, and personality disorders, the suicide risk is at a lower level, but still about five to ten times higher than expected value in the total population. In various substance use disorders, the risk is dependent on the severity and type of disorder. In dementia and mental retardation, suicide risk is lower than in the general population (Harris and Barraclough 1997).

Mental disorder can be a risk factor for suicidal behaviour for several reasons. Mental disorders often cause difficulties in adaptation to society, and may even lead to negative stigmatization. The burden of mental disorder varies from society to society, and from time to time. Mental disorder can also be a predisposing factor for suicidal behaviour solely based on its signs and symptoms as an illness. It may cause loss of functional capacity and quality of life, and very often painful feelings like anxiety, anger, and depression. Mental disorder can also predispose in many ways to situational acute stress. Effective treatment can decrease the risk of suicidal behaviour. On the other hand, dissatisfaction with the course of illness can precipitate suicidal feelings. In the worst case, prescribed psychotropic drugs can offer an easy way to attempt suicide. The course of mental disorder and the outcome of suicidality are, in many ways, two tightly connected parallel developmental processes.

Both mental disorders and suicidal behaviour aggregate in families (Mann 2003; Brent and Mann 2005). Family studies indicate that first-degree relatives of suicide victims have a fivefold risk for suicide. Neuropsychological functions and some personality traits, such as emotional or cognitive styles, can be studied as intermediate phenotypes, which could explain association between psychopathology and suicidal behaviour. Some maladaptive personality traits, such as impulsivity, aggressiveness, hostility, neuroticism and introversion, correlate with psychopathology and suicidality. Several susceptibility genes associating both with psychopathology and suicidal behaviour have been identified: serotonin transporter, tryptophan hydroxylase, monoamine oxidase A, serotonin receptors (1A, 1B and 2A), cathecol-O-methyltransferase and dopamine receptors (2 and 4). It seems possible that genetic predisposition to impulsive and aggressive behaviour, and early negative life events and other stressors in the family, might lead to early psychopathology, and later in life, the tendency toward suicidal behaviour (Turecki 2005; Bondy *et al.* 2006).

Suicidal behaviour can be studied as part of the course and outcome of severe mental disorders using prospective studies. The most reliable picture of the role of suicidal behaviour can be drawn from the representative population studies on specific mental disorders and meta-analyses, using them as a source of information in long-term follow-up studies. Clinically, it is very important to follow unselected real-life patient cohorts to see the realistic outcome of specific mental disorders treated in health care. To some degree, we can get useful information on risk factors explaining suicidal behaviour by using a case–control setting to compare suicidal and non-suicidal patient groups.

In a nationwide population-based follow-up study from Finland, the cause-specific mortality of the adult population over 30 years of age was followed in the years 1978–1994 (Joukamaa *et al.* 2001). The age-adjusted risk of suicide in mental disorders among males was five times, and among females, twelve times higher than expected. The highest risk was among males in psychoses (12–15×), and among females in mood disorders (about 10×).

In a more recent population-based mortality study on individuals who have had psychiatric treatment in Nova Scotia in the years 1995–2000, the risk of suicide for those treated as inpatients was sixteenfold, and as outpatient two- to threefold, greater than among those treated in primary care. Suicide risk was highest among personality disorders, substance use disorders, and mood disorders (Kisely *et al.* 2005).

In a national clinical survey of a 4-year (1996–2000) sample of cases of suicide (N = 4859) in England and Wales (Hunt *et al.* 2006), where there had been a recent (less than one year) contact with mental health services, the principal primary diagnoses were in rank order as follows: depressive disorder (34 per cent), schizophrenia (20 per cent), personality disorder (9 per cent), alcohol dependence (9 per cent), bipolar disorder (8 per cent), drug dependence (5 per cent), anxiety disorder (4 per cent), adjustment disorder (3 per cent), dementia (0.5 per cent), eating disorder (0.4 per cent), and other specified disorders (3 per cent). Also, in this sample, the major diagnostic categories of suicide are mood disorders (42 per cent), schizophrenia (20 per cent) and substance use disorders (13 per cent), which together form three-quarters of all suicides of psychiatric patients (Hunt *et al.* 2006). More than half of the patients had a prior suicide attempt. In the same study, half of the people who committed suicide during 1996–1998 had been in contact with mental health services during the week before death, and one-fifth during the previous 24 hours. A quarter of all suicides occurred within three months of discharge from inpatient care (Appleby *et al.* 1999).

The association of suicide and mental disorders has been widely documented, suggesting a key role for the management of mental disorders in suicide prevention. If we apply treatment effectiveness

**Table 38.2** Rank order of suicide in mental disorders: studies from the years 1966–1993 (Harris and Barraclough 1997)

| Mental disorder | Standardized mortality ratio | 95% CI |
|---|---|---|
| Suicide attempt | 4737 | 3762–5887 |
| Major depression | 2035 | 1827–2259 |
| Bipolar disorder | 1505 | 1225–1844 |
| Dysthymia | 1212 | 1150–1277 |
| Schizophrenia | 845 | 798–895 |
| Substance use disorder | 574 | 541–609 |
| Personality disorder | 708 | 477–1010 |
| Anxiety disorder | 629 | 533–738 |
| Mental retardation | 88 | 18–258 |

of 50 per cent to major mental disorders, and suppose that an average of 50 per cent of people were correctly recognized, diagnosed and properly treated, we could expect a reduction of suicide rate of about 20 per cent (Bertolote *et al.* 2003). The official quantitative goal of the National Suicide Prevention Project in Finland in 1986 was to decrease the suicide rate by 20 per cent in 10 years (Lonnqvist 1988). We believed that it would be possible by using a comprehensive suicide prevention strategy, the core of which would be a proper treatment and better services for people with mental disorders, especially for those suffering from depression. Suicide mortality in Finland decreased from the beginning of the implementation phase of the national suicide prevention programme in 1990 by 40 per cent during the course of the following 15 years, from 30/100,000 in 1990 to 18/100,000 in 2005.

# Psychological autopsy studies on mental disorders in suicide

The ultimate goal of suicide research is to get useful information for the development of suicide prevention. For these purposes, we can study the role of mental disorders in various kinds of suicidal subpopulations, which are to some degree different, yet partially overlapping. We can use persons having suicidal ideation, patients treated for deliberate self-harm, or even severe suicide attempts, and finally, suicide victims after completed suicide by using a psychological autopsy method.

Psychological autopsy studies have been used to construct an overall view of suicide by collecting all available relevant information on the victim's life preceding his or her death by interviewing those closest to the deceased, and examining all relevant health care case notes, social work reports, and police and criminal records. Based on all available data, an assessment of the suicide victim's mental health and mental disorders is possible by using proper diagnostic criteria. The validity and reliability of the psychological autopsy method has been criticized, but its use has been increasing at the same time (Pouliot and De Leo 2006).

A systematic review of psychological autopsy studies on suicide identified 154 reports up to June 2000; 54 were case series and 22 were case–control studies (Cavanagh *et al.* 2003). The median proportion of cases with mental disorders was 91 per cent, and the confidence interval (CI) (95 per cent) was from 81–98 per cent. In the case-control series, the finding was very similar in the cases, 90 per cent had a mental disorder (95 per cent CI: 81–98 per cent). The lifetime prevalence of mental disorders among controls was 27 per cent (95per cent CI: 14–48 per cent), which is close to the findings usually received from general population studies, supporting the reliability of the diagnostic assessments conducted in autopsy studies. Population-attributable fraction for mental disorders was calculated from seven case-control studies. Between 47–74 per cent of the suicides were attributable to mental disorder, and 21–57 per cent to affective disorders, indicating that a major part of suicides could be avoided where it is possible to have effective treatment or prevention of mental disorders.

In a recent meta-analysis, from the period of 1986–2002, 27 psychological autopsy studies were selected from a total of 152 initial studies using appropriate diagnostic criteria for further analysis (Arsenault-Lapierre *et al.* 2004). There were 14 studies carried out in Europe (N = 1488), seven from North America (N = 794), three others from Australia (N = 258) and three from Asia (N = 735).

**Table 38.3** Diagnostic distribution of suicides (%) in psychological autopsy studies from Europe (EU), North America (NA), Australia (AU) and Asia (AS) in 1986–2002 (Arsenault-Lapierre *et al.* 2004)

| Diagnostic category | EU | NA | AU | AS |
|---|---|---|---|---|
| Mood disorders | 48 | 34 | 33 | 51 |
| Substance use disorders | 19 | 40 | 24 | 27 |
| Schizophrenia and other psychoses | 8 | 4 | 24 | 8 |
| Personality disorders | 17 | 13 | 18 | 18 |
| Any diagnosis | 89 | 90 | 79 | 83 |

Overall, 87.3 per cent of all included suicide cases had a history of psychiatric disorders. In all excluded studies, the mean percentage of suicides with a psychiatric diagnosis was 78.7 per cent. Diagnostic distribution across different regions of the world differed to some degree. On average, 43 per cent of suicide cases were diagnosed with mood disorder, 26 per cent with substance use disorder, 16 per cent with personality disorder, and 9 per cent with psychotic disorder. The highest risk was received for psychotic disorders, (0R = 15) (Table 38.3).

When the odds ratios (OR) and their confidence intervals (95 per cent CI) were calculated from all psychological autopsy studies having a control group, the probability of a mental disorder among suicide victims was, on average, about tenfold for any mental disorder, and about sixfold for depressive disorders and psychoses (Table 38.4).

Comorbidity has been a major finding in psychological autopsy studies, most commonly major depression with substance disorder (Henriksson *et al.* 1993). Comorbidity of mental disorders with substance abuse is very high among suicides, differing significantly from that among controls, 38 vs 6 per cent (Cavanagh *et al.* 2003). Several recent studies have also underlined the role of personality disorder as a comorbid risk factor for suicide (Schneider *et al.* 2006).

The diagnostic distribution of mental disorders in attempted suicides has been very similar to that in completed suicide. Substance use disorders and personality disorders are even more prevalent among attempters (Suominen *et al.* 1996).

Mental disorders, particularly depressive disorders, substance abuse, and antisocial behaviour, have an important role in adolescent suicides. The diagnostic distribution of mental disorders

**Table 38.4** Diagnostic distribution of suicides in psychological autopsy studies compared with the control groups (Arsenault-Lapierre *et al.* 2004)

| Diagnostic category | Odds ratio | 95% CI |
|---|---|---|
| Depressive disorders | 6.2 | 5.4–8.1 |
| Bipolar disorders | 3.0 | 1.5–9.9 |
| Substance problems | 3.5 | 3.1–4.5 |
| Psychoses | 6.6 | 3.9–11.9 |
| Personality disorders | 4.5 | 3.5–6.4 |
| Anxiety disorders | 2.4 | 1.7–3.6 |
| Adjustment disorders | 1.3 | 0.7–2.4 |
| Any mental disorder | 10.5 | 9.6–13.4 |

**Table 38.5** Mental disorders and comorbidity (%) in attempted suicides (Suominen *et al.* 1996)

| Mood disorders | 75 |
|---|---|
| Alcohol dependence and abuse | 53 |
| Other substance dependence/abuse | 12 |
| Personality disorders | 40 |
| Anxiety disorders | 18 |
| Psychotic disorders | 11 |
| Comorbid mental disorders | 82 |
| Any mental disorder | 98 |

among adolescents and young adults is surprisingly similar to that of older adults (Marttunen *et al.* 1991). However, the prevalence of adjustment disorders is higher, ranging between 5–34 per cent (Portzky *et al.* 2005). Suicidal patients with adjustment disorder more often had, compared with non-suicidal young patients, a psychiatric background; they also had lower levels of psychosocial functioning, and they were more dysphoric and restless (Pelkonen *et al.* 2005).

## Depressive disorders

Major depressive disorder has a point prevalence of about 5 per cent in a general population, and the lifetime risk is about 15 per cent. Milder depressive symptoms are much more common. The essential feature of depression is either depressed mood, or the loss of interest, or pleasure in all activities (major depression), and a chronically depressed mood (dysthymia). The risk of suicidal behaviour has always been connected with depression. More than half of clinically depressed persons have suicidal ideation, which is directly related to the severity of depression. One of the nine possible diagnostic criteria of a major depressive episode in DSM-IV-R contains 'recurrent thoughts of death, recurrent suicidal ideation without a specific plan, a suicide attempt or a specific plan for committing suicide' (Wasserman 2006).

The multifactorial aetiology of depression makes it a special challenge for prevention. Environmental and genetic factors, combined with the brain reactions, seem to determine together in a complex and dynamic way the final mood condition, and whether it is classified as normal or pathological. Response to environmental and stressful experiences leads to depression and suicidality, more often in some vulnerable people than in all others, depending on their genetic make-up (Caspi *et al.* 2003). Depression, at least short-term depressive symptoms, can and should be effectively prevented (Jane-Llopis *et al.* 2003). Major depressive disorders are, in principle, predictable and treatable, although the challenge is very demanding in practice.

A special challenge is to prevent the familial transmission of depression and associated early-onset suicidal behaviour in offspring. In a prospective high-risk study (Melhem *et al.* 2007) on offspring of parents with mood disorders, suicide attempts, or emergency referrals for suicidal ideation or behaviour, were compared with offspring without such events. Offspring of probands who had made suicide attempts had a much higher rate of suicide attempts (RR: 6.5), as well as overall suicidal events (RR: 4.4). Mood disorder and impulsive aggression in offspring, and a history

of sexual abuse and depression in parents predicted earlier time of suicidal event. These results suggest that efforts to prevent the familial transmission of early-onset suicidal behaviour could lead to successful suicide prevention among high-risk youths.

The most common predictive depressive symptom for suicidal ideation in depression is hopelessness. Feelings of guilt, loss of interest and low self-esteem is also associated with suicidal thoughts. Because depressiveness is very often comorbid in many mental disorders like anxiety disorders, substance use disorders, personality disorders, and even in schizophrenia, it may be a clinically significant reminder of the risk of suicidal behaviour. Comorbid depression is also of the utmost importance for suicide prevention in the treatment of somatic illnesses like cancer, cardiovascular diseases, neurological diseases, delirium, and any severe and chronic disease.

A systematic review, from the period 1966 to 1996, found 35 studies that reported rates of suicide as a percentage of deaths among the depressed with a mean of 11 per cent (Wulsin *et al.* 1999). Among the twenty-three psychiatric samples, including mainly former inpatients, suicide accounted for a mean of 16 per cent of all deaths. The best evidence came from three most qualified studies, which had a mean of 19 per cent. This figure is consistent with the often quoted rate of 15 per cent of completed suicide among psychiatric patients with severe depressive disorders, which comes from the results of the original twelve studies from the years 1937–1968, re-analysed and published by Guze and Robins in 1970. However, the real lifetime risk of suicide for major depression is lower than 15 per cent. The overestimation is due to sampling biases. A majority of studies have been conducted on severely depressed inpatients, which were followed-up during the years of the highest risk for suicide. In reality, the risk of suicide varies markedly across the subclasses of depressive disorders, and is related to the intensity of psychiatric treatment, indicating the selection of depressed patients to treatment settings, also according to the severity of their suicidal intent. The risk is lowest among the depressive primary care patients, clearly higher in psychiatric outpatients, and highest among former inpatients (Simon and Von Korff 1998).

In a meta-analysis of suicide risk in affective disorders conducted by Bostwick and Pankratz (2000), all available studies from 1937 to 1999 were identified. Fifty-eight studies were selected for further analysis, and case fatality prevalence (suicides divided by total subjects) was calculated. The results of the meta-analysis showed a clear hierarchy of lifetime suicide prevalence defined by history of treatment and suicidality: 8 per cent in people ever admitted for suicidality, 4 per cent in patients admitted with affective disorder, but not for suicidality, and 2 per cent in mixed inpatient and outpatient populations. Those recently hospitalized with a suicide attempt or suicidal ideation are clearly at highest risk. Suicide prevention efforts should be focused on recently or repeatedly hospitalized suicidal depressed patients.

The Lundby Study is a longitudinal cohort study from Sweden, which has followed-up 3563 subjects since 1947, and 344 subjects had their first onset of depression during the 50-year follow-up. Only 5 per cent (N = 17) of them have, to date, committed suicide. The proportion of suicides from all deaths has decreased as the follow-up time has increased. The suicides occurred early in the course of depression, and 12 of 17 suicides took place in connection with a registered episode of depression (Mattisson *et al.* 2007).

Depression of suicide victims differs qualitatively from that of living controls; it seems to be more severe and accompanied more often by insomnia, weight or appetite loss, feelings of worthlessness or inappropriate guilt, and thoughts of death or suicidal ideation (McGirr *et al.* 2007a, b). Suicide victims were significantly less likely to have felt fatigued, and to have difficulty in concentrating or making decisions. In addition, impulsive and aggressive behaviour, alcohol and drug abuse and dependence, and cluster B personality disorders increase the risk of suicide in individuals with major depression. Alcohol problems and cluster B personality disorder were found to be two independent predictors of suicide (Dumais *et al.* 2005).

Inadequate and inefficient antidepressant treatment of depressed suicide victims and suicide attempters has been a persistent finding in several studies (Isometsä *et al.* 1994a; Suominen *et al.* 1998; Oquendo *et al.* 2002). Less than half of suicide victims with major depression have been in contact with psychiatric care at the time of suicide. However, there is some evidence that good monitoring and maintenance treatment in high-risk groups of patients may be able to decrease their suicide rates.

Among consecutive suicide attempters visiting emergency rooms in Helsinki, Finland, 75 per cent of patients had a research diagnosis of depression. The prevalence of major depression was 38 per cent, 44 per cent for females, and 30 per cent for males. Half of all depressed patients had comorbid alcohol abuse or dependence. Depressed attempters without alcohol problems had higher suicide intent and lower impulsiveness than depressed attempters with alcohol problems (Suominen *et al.* 1996).

The prevalence of mood disorders among consecutive medically serious suicide attempts in Canterbury, New Zealand, was 77 per cent, and in comparison subjects from the general population, 7 per cent (OR: 33). The prevalence of major depression was 62 and 6 per cent, respectively (Beautrais *et al.* 1996). These findings mean, theoretically, that effective prevention and treatment of mood disorders might reduce the amount of severe suicide attempt by more than half.

Depression and attempted suicide are both risk factors for suicide. A recent suicide attempt by a person with depression means a higher risk of recurrent attempt and suicide after discharge from hospital, especially during the first week after the discharge. In a recent Finnish study, we showed that among all individuals hospitalized due to severe suicide attempt in Finland from 1997 to 2003 (N = 23,321) mood disorder (N = 5164) raised the risk of suicide by 72 per cent and suicide attempt by 59 per cent during the mean follow-up time of 3.6 years. The risk was very high just after discharge from hospital (Haukka *et al.* 2008).

Comorbidity in connection with attempted suicide means difficulties in the diagnostic and clinical assessment in the emergency situation, and is a real challenge to suicide prevention during the post-discharge period. Treating suicidal depressed patients actively and intensively might offer an effective way of preventing suicide. Few depressed suicide attempters receive adequate treatment for their depression, even after their attempts (Suominen *et al.* 1998; Oquendo *et al.* 2002).

Despite extensive research, it has not been possible to demonstrate that the use of any antidepressant medication directly decreases the risk of suicide. The use of antidepressants and the risk of suicidal behaviour have been under widespread public discussion. There has been controversy over whether selective serotonin reuptake inhibitors (SSRIs) might trigger suicidal ideation or behaviour. Treatment-emergent suicidal ideation and behaviour seem to be infrequent, about 4 per cent for antidepressants and 2 per cent for placebo. In our own high-risk study (Tiihonen *et al.* 2006a), we showed that the risk of suicide attempt among subjects who had previously attempted suicide, and then used antidepressants, increased by 39 per cent during all antidepressant treatments, when compared with no antidepressant use, but what is important is that at the same time the risk of completed suicide among them decreased by 32 per cent.

## Bipolar disorders

Bipolar disorder is characterized by the varying consequences of manic and depressive episodes over the course of life. The lifetime prevalence of bipolar I disorder is about 0.5 per cent or even higher, and for bipolar I and II disorders together up to 3.9 per cent. It has high heritability (80 per cent) and often familial background. The majority of episodes are characterized by depression. Numerous studies have documented an association between bipolar disorder and suicidal behaviour. Bipolar disorders and suicidal behaviours are often aggregated in the same families. Family history of completed suicide is a significant risk factor associated with suicide attempts in patients with bipolar disorder (Romero *et al.* 2007).

Suicidal ideation is highly prevalent in bipolar disorders, and it is commonly estimated that as much as half of people with bipolar disorder attempt suicide at least once. In a psychological autopsy study, a significant proportion of suicide victims were found to have died in their lifetime at first suicide attempt, after having had communicated about suicidal ideation (Isometsä *et al.* 1994b). During the current episode, more than half have suicidal ideation and about 20 per cent will attempt suicide. During their lifetime, most (80 per cent) of the bipolar persons have had suicidal ideation and half (51 per cent) have attempted suicide. Severity of depressive episode and hopelessness are independent risk factors for suicide ideation, whereas hopelessness, previous suicide attempt and comorbid personality disorder were risk factors for suicide attempts (Valtonen *et al.* 2005). Hopelessness predicts suicidal behaviour during the depressive phase, and the severity of depression predicts suicide attempts during mixed phases (Valtonen *et al.* 2007). During the 18-month follow-up, 20 per cent of bipolar I and II patients attempted suicide. Previous suicide attempts, depressive phase at index episode and younger mean age at intake (32 vs 39 years) were independent risk factors for suicide attempt during the follow-up (Valtonen *et al.* 2006). Clinically, it is important to manage the depressive phases quickly and effectively, as the time spent in depressive phases involves a high risk period of suicidal behaviour.

Suicide mortality rate of bipolar disorder has been assumed to be, based on several more or less selected samples, 15 times that of the general population (Harris and Barraclough 1997). In a population-based mortality study (Ösby *et al.* 2001) from Sweden, including all hospitalized bipolar patients (N = 15,386) from 1973 to 1995, standardized mortality ratio (SMR) was as high as 15.0 for males and 22.4 for females. The suicide rate was especially high during the first years after the first diagnosis. A recent study (Dutta *et al.* 2007) analysed suicide mortality in the cohort of 235 bipolar I patients from a defined area of south-east London over the years 1965–1999, compared suicide mortality with that of a general population, and found eight suicides, giving a surprisingly low SMR: 9.8 (95per cent CI: 4.2–19.2). Only alcohol abuse (hazard ratio 6.8) and deterioration in premorbid function (hazard ratio 5.2) remained in multivariate modelling as statistically significant and independent predictors of suicide.

It is generally known that the total Axis I lifetime comorbidity is high in all bipolar patients, about 60–80 per cent. The reported prevalences of substance use disorders among suicide victims diagnosed as bipolar cases are clearly higher in American studies (33–72 per cent) than in European studies (15–26 per cent). Substance use comorbidity in bipolar patients in Europe means almost exclusively the use of alcohol. In the USA, the suicide risk is raised by the use of many illegal drugs.

Isometsä and colleagues (1994b) made a careful diagnostic study of all bipolar suicides (N = 31) committed in Finland during a 1-year period. The mean age of the completed suicides was 43 for men and 55 for women. Most suicides (79 per cent) occurred during a depressive phase, or during a mixed state (11 per cent), and the rest were associated with psychotic mania. The final episode had been psychotic in 12 out of 31 suicide victims. Most were very complicated and comorbid cases of bipolar disorder. More than a half of male patients, but none of the women, were alcohol-dependent. Despite contact with psychiatric care, most subjects had not received adequate treatment or adhered to it. The use of lithium or antidepressants at optimal doses and serum levels was rare. On the contrary, on the basis of the existing observational and randomized evidence there have been continuous claims that lithium may substantially reduce the risk of suicide in bipolar disorder, and should be used as an antisuicidal drug for bipolar patients.

The meta-analysis of the risk factors for suicide and attempted suicide in bipolar disorder was published by Hawton and colleagues in 2005 (Hawton et al. 2005a). The search strategy started from 2142 articles, and the final analysis included 13 studies of suicide from the years 1976–2003, and 23 studies of attempted suicide from the period 1980–2003. The main findings concerning suicide were that suicide risk appeared to be elevated among males and where there was a history of attempted suicide and, probably, hopelessness. There were no statistically significant associations of suicide with any personal, social or family history characteristics. Other clinically relevant and important risk factors of suicidal behaviour, however not of suicide, were a family history of suicide, a history of abuse, early age at onset of bipolar disorder, extent of depressive symptoms and hopelessness, increasing severity of affective episodes, the presence of mixed affective states, rapid cycling, comorbid Axis I disorders like anxiety disorders, and abuse of alcohol and drugs. Hawton and his co-workers also found that attempted suicide was significantly more common among non-married bipolar persons.

Cipriani and colleagues (Cipriani et al. 2005) conducted a systematic review and meta-analysis of all 32 randomized trials available to investigate the effectiveness of long-term use of lithium in 1389 patients with mood disorders, compared to placebo and other active treatments in 2069 controls, on the risk of suicide. This meta-analysis indicated that lithium reduces the risk of suicide in patients with mood disorders (not only in bipolar patients!). Lithium patients were less likely to die by suicide (2 vs 11 suicides), odds ratio was 0.26 (95 per cent CI: 0.09–0.77), and odds ratio for suicide and attempted suicide combined was 0.21 (95 per cent CI: 0.08–0.50). The conclusion was that lithium should be a first-line therapy

for bipolar patients, including those at risk of suicidal behaviour. Similar positive findings were published by Kessing et al. (2005) from Denmark using a nationwide observational lithium cohort. The results indicated that continued lithium treatment was associated with a reduced suicide rate, being only about a half of that found in the comparison group not using lithium continuously. Also, other studies support growing evidence of lower risk of suicidal acts during closely monitored and highly adherent, long-term treatment with lithium, and indicate that treatment adherence is an important factor in suicide prevention in general. Baldessarini et al. (2006) published a meta-analysis on long-term lithium treatment of bipolar disorder patients including 31 studies since 2001 and involving over 85,000 person-years of risk-exposure. This meta-analysis showed that the overall risk of suicides and suicide attempts were five times less among lithium-treated subjects than among those bipolar patients not treated with lithium.

## Anxiety disorders

Anxiety disorders are the most common mental disorders and, at the same time, highly under-recognized and undertreated in the community. DSM-IV lists twelve anxiety disorders:

1 Panic disorder (PD) with agoraphobia;

2 PD without agoraphobia;

3 Agoraphobia without history of PD;

4 Specific phobia;

5 Social phobia;

6 Obsessive–compulsive disorder (OCD);

7 Post-traumatic stress disorder (PTSD);

8 Acute stress disorder;

9 Generalized anxiety disorder (GAD);

10 Anxiety due to a general medical condition;

11 Substance-induced anxiety disorder; and

12 Anxiety disorder not otherwise specified.

One-year prevalence of anxiety disorders has been estimated between 15–25 per cent with significant comorbidity, especially with mood and substance use disorders. Whether anxiety disorders are risk factors for suicidal behaviour has long been a controversial issue. However, it is likely that, due to high comorbidity, the significance of suicidality in anxiety disorders has, until now, been underestimated (Hawgood and de Leo 2008).

In the Netherlands Mental Health Survey and Incidence Study (NEMESIS), which is the first population-based, prospective and longitudinal examination of the impact of anxiety disorders on suicidal ideation and suicide attempts, Sareen and colleagues (2005) showed that pre-existing anxiety disorder is an independent risk factor for subsequent onset of suicidal ideation and attempts. In the cross-sectional analysis, the adjusted odds ratio was 2.3 for suicidal ideation and 2.4 for attempts. In the longitudinal analysis, OR was 2.3 for suicidal ideation and 3.6 for suicide attempts. The likelihood of suicide attempts was higher in anxiety disorders combined with mood disorder than in mood disorders alone. Examination of specific lifetime anxiety disorder was strongly associated with lifetime suicidal ideation and suicide attempts. Cross-sectionally odds ratios for suicide attempts were 10.0 in OCD, 7.6 in panic disorder, 5.9 in GAD, 5.5 in simple phobia, 5.0 in agoraphobia without panic, 4.9 in social phobia and 7.5 in any anxiety disorder OCD, social phobia, and GAD were strongly linked with suicidal ideation at baseline and follow-up.

In the Christchurch Health and Development Study (Boden *et al.* 2007), anxiety disorders were strongly associated with suicidal ideation and attempts in adolescence and young adulthood, and the estimates of the population-attributable risk suggested that they accounted for 7–10 per cent of the suicidality in the cohort. Any single anxiety disorder increased the odds of suicidal ideation by 8.0 times and increased the rate of suicide attempts by 5.8 times.

There are rather limited data on suicidal behaviour in obsessive–compulsive disorder. The British National Psychiatric Morbidity Survey of 2000 (Torres *et al.* 2006) identified 114 persons with OCD, with a prevalence of 1 per cent. Lifetime prevalence of suicide attempts was 26 per cent, 10 times higher than in the comparison group, showing that OCD had a higher risk for suicide attempts than expected. Most persons with OCD were not in contact with a mental health professional, and very few were receiving appropriate treatments. Kamath and colleagues (2007) published a study of one hundred consecutive OCD patients attending the specialty OCD clinic in Bangalore, India. The findings of this study revealed that OCD is associated with high rates of lifetime suicidal ideation (59 per cent) and attempts (27 per cent).

Diaconu and Turecki (2007) demonstrated that association between panic disorder and suicidal behaviour is mainly accounted for by comorbidity with depressive disorders. In clinical practice, suicidality should be taken into consideration when treating persons with panic disorder and comorbid depressive disorder.

Post-traumatic stress disorder, having lifetime prevalence of about 8 per cent, has strong association with suicidality predicting subsequent suicide attempt with an odds ratio of 6 (Kessler *et al.* 1999). In New Orleans, after Hurricane Katrina, suicidal ideation and suicide plans significantly increased in the population during the follow-up period (Kessler *et al.* 2008). In many PTSD studies, suicidality is associated with comorbid depression and substance use.

## Alcohol and other substance use disorders

The acute and chronic use of alcohol, cannabis, amphetamine, cocaine, opioids, nicotine products, and many other chemical substances have an effect on the brain and can lead to intoxication, abuse, dependence, withdrawal, delirium, psychosis, mood and anxiety disorders, and many other syndromes diagnosed as substance use disorders (SUD). The prevalence of SUD is high, the lifetime risk is about 15 per cent, and the 12-month prevalence about 4 per cent. Alcohol is still the most often used substance. All substance disorders increase the risk of suicidal behaviours. In most countries, the role of alcohol as the risk factor of suicidal behaviour is more important than any other substance. In the National Comorbidity Survey Replication (Kessler *et al.* 2005), lifetime prevalence estimates were as follows: alcohol abuse 13, alcohol dependence 5, drug abuse 8, drug dependence and any substance use disorder 15 per cent.

Alcohol, often combined with drugs, is a major risk and precipitating factor for suicidal behaviour, although the relationship between alcohol and suicidal behaviour is complex. Alcohol has short-term effects on mood, cognitive processes and impulsivity. As an intoxicating substance, alcohol impairs judgement and problem-solving skills, and may cause impulsivity and lower the threshold to suicidal behaviour. The state of alcohol intoxication represents a state of elevated suicide risk, especially the binge-drinking of young people. The long-term effects of alcohol misuse are probably mediated through interrelated effects on mood and social processes. Alcohol misuse and alcohol dependence predispose to impulsivity, aggression, depression, hopelessness, and negative effects increasing the risk for suicidal ideation, suicide attempts and completed suicide (Pirkola *et al.* 2004; Brady 2006).

In a large national after-care study (Ilgen *et al.* 2007) of substance use treatment, 4 per cent of patients reported a suicide attempt within the past 30 days before a 1-year post-treatment assessment. Suicide attempt associated with the following baseline predictors: suicidal and psychiatric symptoms, more recent problematic alcohol use and longer duration of cocaine use. A reduction in suicide risk correlated with contact with the criminal justice system and greater engagement in SUD treatment. Suicide prevention among SUD patients would benefit from a high-risk approach and longer treatment episodes.

Almost half of treatment-seeking persons with an alcohol use disorder report ever having attempted suicide. Over half of all suicide attempters had acted under the influence of alcohol (Suokas and Lonnqvist 1995). Attempters with alcohol dependence had lower suicidal intent and were more impulsive than those with depression alone, suggesting that impulsivity is an important factor in suicide attempts of alcohol dependent persons (Suominen *et al.* 1997). A prospective study of suicidal alcohol-dependent persons indicated a further suicide attempt was predicted by prior suicide attempts, younger age, being separated or divorced, drug dependence, other substance-induced mental disorders, and indicators of a more severe course of alcoholism (Preuss *et al.* 2003).

The lifetime risk of suicide has been estimated at 7 per cent for alcohol dependence, with only slight variation during lifetime, in a meta-analysis based on twenty-seven modern studies on alcohol dependence (Inskip *et al.* 1998). The suicide rates in heavy drinking are 3.5 times, and in alcohol use disorders, 10 times higher than that in the general population. In drug dependence and abuse, suicide rate was about 15 times higher than expected in the systematic review analysed by Harris and Barraclough (1997) from the years 1966–1993.

Wilcox and his colleagues (Wilcox *et al.* 2004) published a systematic review on the association of alcohol and other substance use disorders and completed suicide, based on the 81 cohort studies from the years 1966–2002. Suicide mortality risk (Table 38.6) was highest among drug users (thirteen- to sixteenfold greater risk than in a general population), and clearly lower, but still high among persons with alcohol use disorder (nine- to tenfold) and heavy drinking (three to fourfold). The overall standardized mortality ratio (SMR) for opioid use was 1351, 756 for males and 357 for females. Eight studies conducted in seven countries reported data on mixed intravenous (IV) drug use (opioid, cocaine, amphetamine, etc.) and SMR was 1373. General (mixed) drug use gave a SMR which was at the same level: 1685, 1000 for women and 329 for men. Data on amphetamine users was obtained from one Swedish study yielding SMR of 1136. SMR for heavy alcohol use was 351. Although alcohol use disorders are 2–3 times more common among males than females, alcohol use disorders mean

**Table 38.6** Suicide substance use disorders (Wilcox *et al.* 2004)

| Substance use | Standardized mortality ratio | 95% CI |
| --- | --- | --- |
| Mixed drug use | 1685 | 1473–1920 |
| Intravenous drug use | 1373 | 1029–1796 |
| Opioid use | 351 | 1047–1715 |
| Alcohol use disorders | 979 | 898–1065 |
| Heavy drinking | 351 | 251–478 |

a relatively higher risk of suicide among females (seventeenfold) than among males (fivefold).

In a case-control study opioid-dependent patients have, compared with non-opioid-dependent controls, significantly elevated levels of suicidal behaviour (suicidal thoughts in 66 versus 55 per cent, and suicide attempts 31 versus 20 per cent (Maloney *et al* 2007*)*. In a 20-year prospective cohort study (Bjornaas *et al.* 2008), 7 per cent of 185 opioid addicts committed suicide. The SMR was elevenfold for suicide. Opioid-dependent patients who had attempted suicide had experienced significantly more comorbidity with lifetime cocaine and alcohol dependence when compared with nonsuicidal opioid-dependent patients (Roy 2002).

Use of stimulants like amphetamine, methamphetamine, cocaine and ecstasy is associated with an elevated risk for suicidal behaviour which is, however, in most countries much lower than among opioid-dependent persons. Suicidal stimulant users often have comorbidity with alcohol and opioid dependence.

In a psychological autopsy study (Henriksson *et al.* 1993) in Finland, 44 per cent of suicide victims were found to be suffering from alcohol dependence or abuse, and most of them had comorbid mental disorders, usually personality disorder and depression. A post-mortem study (Ohberg *et al.* 1996) showed detectable blood alcohol in 36 per cent of all suicides, in significantly more males than females. Suicide victims who had a prior misuse of alcohol were more often younger, male, divorced or separated and were more often recently unemployed. They had experienced more often recent adverse life events possibly dependent on their own behaviour. They were also far more likely to be alcohol-intoxicated at the time of suicide (69 per cent vs 23 per cent), and tended to die from drug overdose more often than other suicide victims. Alcohol misuse is likely to have a deteriorating influence on the life course of those who eventually succumb to suicide, and its adverse consequences are common in misusers during the final month (Pirkola *et al.* 2000).

The role of alcohol and other substance use disorders, as a risk factor of suicidal behaviour, varies greatly by country, and is related to the consumption of alcohol and other substances in a general population. In psychological autopsy studies (Arsenault-Lapierre *et al.* 2004) conducted around the world, the percentage of substance use disorders varied from 19 per cent in Europe to 40 per cent in North America (Table 38.3). However, the substance use disorders everywhere were much more prevalent among male than female suicides (42 per cent vs 24 per cent). Globally, substance use disorders were present in at least a quarter (26 per cent) of suicide cases, more often among males (42 per cent) than females (24 per cent). Odds ratios across sexes were 3.6 in all substance problems and 2.2 in alcohol problems. In a recent psychological autopsy study from Estonia, a country which has a high suicide rate and high alcohol consumption, alcohol abuse and dependence was found in 61 per cent of suicide victims, 68 per cent among males and 29 per cent among females (Kolves *et al.* 2006). The corresponding figures for controls selected from general practioners' list were 7 and 14 per cent respectively.

National alcohol policy can have a marked positive or negative impact on suicide mortality (Wasserman *et al.* 1994). Easy availability and low prices of alcohol usually means increasing use and more harmful effects, especially more substance use disorders and increasing rates of suicidal behaviours. On the contrary, reducing levels of consumption can lead to reduced overall suicide rate. Public health measures that have been shown to be most effective in limiting alcohol use and misuse are taxing alcoholic beverages, restricting availability and consumption, and stricter drink-driving laws. Selective prohibition may, especially, protect young persons from becoming suicidal. On the other hand, lowering the minimum drinking age may increase the suicide rate among youth.

# Schizophrenia and other psychoses

Schizophrenia is a debilitating mental disorder with a mixture of characteristic signs and symptoms, both positive and negative, which may predispose secondarily to suicidal behaviour. The positive symptoms include: distortions in thought content (delusions), perception (hallucinations), language and thought process (disorganized speech), and self-monitoring of behaviour (grossly disorganized or catatonic behaviour). Negative symptoms are the core symptoms of schizophrenia including: restrictions in the range and intensity of emotional expression (affective flattening), in the fluency and productivity of thought and speech (alogia), and in the initiation of goal-directed behaviour (avolition). Lifetime prevalence of schizophrenia is between 0.5–1.0 per cent. Other psychoses are, together, more prevalent than schizophrenia, but the risk of suicide associated with them is not as well known as in schizophrenia (Perälä *et al.* 2007).

Deliberate self-harm or suicide attempt is common (25–45 per cent) in patients with schizophrenia and other psychotic disorders (Radomsky *et al.* 1999). About 15 per cent have made at least one suicide attempt by their first treatment contact, and another 15 per cent will occur within the next five years (Addington *et al.* 2004; Gonzales-Pinto *et al.* 2007). The systematic review of international literature (Haw *et al.* 2005) shows that the increased risk of deliberate self-harm of schizophrenia patients is associated with past and present suicidal ideation, previous suicidal behaviour, past depressive episode, drug abuse or dependence and higher mean number of psychiatric admissions. Suicidality in this patient group seems to be associated with more depressive, comorbid and severe forms of schizophrenia, needing intensive treatment and careful follow-up. Early detection programmes directed toward high-risk groups, by lowering the threshold for the first treatment contact and bringing patients into treatment earlier, can possibly reduce rates of serious suicidal behaviour (Melle *et al.* 2006).

In a nationwide Finnish high-risk study, 3373 schizophrenia patients were followed up 3.6 years on average after a severe suicide attempt, which had led to hospitalization (Haukka *et al.* 2008). During the follow-up, they had a significantly higher risk of suicide attempt (58 per cent) and suicide (78 per cent) compared with attempters without any psychiatric diagnosis before the attempt. Schizophrenic patients who have once attempted suicide are in a real risk for further attempts and suicide, especially shortly after the discharge from hospital treatment.

The suicide risk in schizophrenia is clearly higher than in the general population (Harris and Barraclough 1997), but not as high as it has often been presented. In a meta-analysis on the lifetime risk of suicide in schizophrenia, Palmer and his colleagues (Palmer *et al.* 2005) identified 632 articles on the topic and selected 29 studies, including 22,598 subjects at either illness onset or first admission. They showed that suicide in schizophrenia will occur in approximately 5.6 per cent (95 per cent confidence interval was 3.7–8.5 per cent) of subjects over their lifetimes. Suicides are concentrated in the early course of illness, meaning that intervention and prevention efforts have to be directed toward the early stages of the illness.

The systematic review of mortality in schizophrenia was conducted by Saha and colleagues (Saha *et al.* 2007). They found seven population-based studies on suicide showing that people with schizophrenia had twelve times the risk of dying of suicide compared with the general population. In addition, schizophrenia patients have a two- to threefold increased risk of dying due to other causes. Heritability of schizophrenia is about 80 per cent; the risk of schizophrenia among first-degree relatives is about 5–10 per cent, and the risk for all psychoses even higher. These facts raise the question of elevated suicide risk in offspring and need for suicide prevention in the families. Suvisaari *et al.* (2007) found that the prior suicide attempts of psychotic mothers, most having schizophrenia, were associated with eight times higher suicide mortality in offspring from late adolescence until middle age. Among mothers with psychotic disorder, a maternal suicide attempt is a strong predictor of offspring's suicide. Previous studies have already found substantially increased risk for suicide attempt in offspring of mothers who had attempted suicide (Lieb *et al.* 2005).

Hawton and his colleagues (Hawton *et al.* 2005b) selected twenty-nine case–control studies conducted before 2005 for the systematic review of suicide risk factors. They found robust evidence of increased risk of suicide on previous depressive disorders and recent depression, previous suicide attempts, drug misuse or dependence, agitation and motor restlessness, fear of mental disintegration, poor adherence to treatment and recent loss events. Suicide risk was not related to coming from a broken home or having lost a parent. The living circumstances of patients appeared to be important. Persons having schizophrenia and living alone or not living with their families were at greater risk of suicide. Suicide risk is related more to affective symptoms and less to the core psychotic symptoms in schizophrenia. Prevention of suicide would benefit from active treatment of affective symptoms, improving adherence to treatment, use of anti-suicidal medication and special vigilance in patients having several risk factors, especially when faced with significant loss events.

The great majority of schizophrenic patients commit suicide in the active phase of the disorder, after having suffered depressive symptoms. Suicide in schizophrenia is, thus, less of a surprise; it is typically preceded by a previous attempt, and suicidal intent has been communicated at least as often as in non-schizophrenic suicides (Heilä *et al.* 1977, 1999; Heilä and Lönnqvist 2002). In both groups, suicidal warnings typically are absent immediately preceding suicide. Hallucinations commanding suicide are occasionally present (about 10 per cent). Schizophrenic suicide victims differ from other schizophrenic patients by being male, having suicidal thoughts and previous suicide attempts, being more depressive and having more positive symptoms (Heilä *et al.* 1997; Kelly *et al.* 2004). Suicidal persons may deny or conceal their suicidal intent, or due to their psychotic thinking, they are not able to express their intention. For these, and many other reasons, the prediction of suicidal risk may be difficult. At the moment, we do not have any specific instrument to assess accurately the risk of suicide in schizophrenia. In estimating the degree of suicidality, we have to rely on case histories, interviews and clinical judgement (Sakinofsky *et al.* 2004). The prevention of post-discharge suicides is a real challenge in the treatment of schizophrenia patients. The first month after hospital treatment is a real high-risk period for suicide. In many countries, there have been claims that suicide mortality would increase among schizophrenia patients during a period of declining psychiatric beds. The major restructuring and downsizing of mental health services has not been associated with any increase in suicides. Instead, the risk of suicide among schizophrenia patients has decreased in many countries, like Finland, showing that the downsizing of psychiatric hospital can be successfully conducted (Heilä *et al.* 2005).

Effectiveness of antipsychotic treatments was studied in a nationwide cohort of 2230 consecutive adults hospitalized in Finland for the first time between 1995 and 2001, because of schizophrenia or schizoaffective disorder (Tiihonen *et al.* 2006b). Twenty-six suicides occurred in patients not taking antipsychotic drugs (3362 person years) compared with only one suicide in patients taking drugs (4664 person years). Adjusted relative risk was 37.4 (95 per cent CI 5.1–276). Patients who currently took any antipsychotic drug had decreased suicide mortality compared with the no-treatment group.

Some evidence suggests that clozapine might reduce suicide risk in chronically psychotic patients. Meta-analysis of six clozapine studies (Hennen and Baldessarini 2005) indicated a substantially lower overall risk of suicidal behaviours with clozapine compared with other treatments (RR: 3.3, 95 per cent CI: 1.7–6.3), for completed suicide RR was 2.9 (95 per cent CI: 1.5–5.7).

Under-treatment, comorbidity, treatment non-compliance and poor adherence, and a high frequency of non-responders are common problems among schizophrenic suicide victims. Adequacy of comprehensive care is crucial for suicide prevention in schizophrenia, especially among actively psychotic young patients with recent suicidal behaviour, affective symptoms and syndromes. We should improve adherence to treatment and give more emphasis on the continuation and maintenance of drug treatment and outreach programmes that actively contact patients or their family.

## Eating disorders

Anorexia nervosa and bulimia nervosa are both characterized by the individual's overemphasis on body image. Anorexia requires an abnormally low body weight, less than 85 per cent of that expected, and, in women, amenorrhea. Most individuals with bulimia have normal or above-normal weight, and all display a pattern of sequential binge eating and inappropriate compensatory and dangerous behaviours to avoid gaining weight. Anorexia is commonly associated with depression, social phobia and obsessive–compulsive features and an increased risk of premature death. Suicide is a common cause of death in anorexia nervosa, and suicide attempts occur often in both eating disorders.

In a prospective longitudinal study (Franko *et al.* 2004), 15 per cent of subjects reported a suicide attempt during an 8-year follow-up, 22 per cent in anorexia and 11 per cent in bulimia. Suicide attempt was predicted by the severity of depressive symptoms and the use of drugs in anorexia, and by a history of drug use and the use of laxatives in bulimia. Standardized mortality ratio for suicide in anorexia was high in an American study (Keel *et al.* 2003), SMR: 56.9 (95 per cent CI: 15.3–145.7), but not as high as has been previously presented by Harris and Barraclough (1997). In this study, one of the strongest predictors of fatal outcome was severity of alcohol use disorder during the follow-up. Lowering the threshold for hospitalization of anorexic patients may reduce the risk of suicide. In a meta-analysis, including nine anorexia studies comprising of 1536 patients and 36 suicides, Pompili and his colleagues (Pompili *et al.* 2003) showed that the suicide rate of anorexia patients was eight times higher than in the general population. A recent systematic review (Berkman *et al.* 2007) has analysed outcomes of eating disorders based on the studies published between 1980 and 2005. Mortality risk of anorexia nervosa was significantly higher than expected, and the risk of suicide was particularly pronounced. Although bulimia is associated with depression, its mortality was not significantly different from the rate expected in the population.

## References

Addington J, Williams J, Young J *et al.* (2004). Suicidal behaviour in early psychosis. *Acta Psychiatrica Scandinavica*, **109**, 116–120.

Appleby L, Shaw J, Amos T *et al.* (1999). Suicide within 12 months of contact with mental health: national clinical survey. *British Medical Journal*, **318**, 1235–1239.

Arsenault-Lapierre G, Kim C, Turecki G (2004). Psychiatric diagnoses in 3275 suicides: a meta-analysis. *BMC Psychiatry*, **4**, 37.

Baldessarini RJ, Tondo L, Davis P *et al.* (2006). Decreased risk of suicides and attempts during long-term lithium treatment: a meta-analytic review. *Bipolar disorder*, **8**, 625–639.

Beautrais AL, Joyce PR, Mulder RT *et al.* (1996). Prevalence and comorbidity of mental disorders in persons making serious suicide attempts: a case–control study. *American Journal of Psychiatry*, **153**, 1009–1014.

Berkman ND, Lohr KN, Bulik CM (2007). Outcomes of eating disorders: a systematic review of the literature. *International Journal of Eating Disorders*, **40**, 293–309.

Bertolote JM, Fleischmann A, De Leo D *et al.* (2003). Suicide and mental disorders: do we know enough? *British Journal of Psychiatry*, **183**, 382–383.

Bjornaas MA, Bekken AS, Ojlert A *et al.* (2008). A 20-year prospective study of mortality and causes of death among hospitalized opioid addicts in Oslo. *BMC Psychiatry*, **13**, 8.

Boden JB, Ferguson DM, Horwood LJ (2007). Anxiety disorders and suicidal behaviours in adolescence and young adulthood: findings from a longitudinal study. *Psychological Medicine*, **37**, 431–440.

Bondy B, Buettner A, Zill P (2006). Genetics of suicide. *Molecular Psychiatry*, **11**, 336–351.

Bostwick JM and Pankratz VS (2000). Affective disorders and suicide risk: a reexamination. *American Journal of Psychiatry*, **157**, 1925–1932.

Brady J (2006). The association between alcohol misuse and suicidal behaviour. *Alcohol and Alcoholism*, **41**, 473–478.

Brent DA and Mann JJ (2005). Family genetic studies, suicide, and suicidal behaviour. *American Journal of Medical Genetics (Seminars in Medical Genetics)*, **133**, 13–24.

Caspi A, Sugden K, Moffit TE *et al.* (2003). Influence of life stress on depression: moderation by a polyphormism in the 5-HTT gene. *Science*, **301**, 386–389.

Cavanagh JTO, Carson AJ, Sharpe M *et al.* (2003). Psychological autopsy studies of suicide: a systematic review. *Psychological Medicine*, **33**, 395–405.

Cipriani A, Pretty H, Hawton K *et al.* (2005). Lithium in the prevention of suicidal behaviour and all-cause mortality in patients with mood disorders: a systematic review of randomized trials. *American Journal of Psychiatry*, **162**, 1805–1819.

Diaconu G and Turecki G (2007). Panic disorder and suicidality: is comorbidity with depression the key? *Journal of Affective Disorders*, **104**, 203–209.

Dumais A, Lesage AD, Alda M *et al.* (2005). Risk factors for suicide completion in major depression: a case–control study of impulsive and aggressive behaviours in men. *American Journal of Psychiatry*, **162**, 2116–2124.

Dutta R, Boydell J, Kennedy N *et al.* (2007). Suicide and other causes of mortality in bipolar disorder: a longitudinal study. *Psychological Medicine*, **6**, 839–847.

Franko DL, Keel PK, Dorer DJ *et al.* (2004). What predicts suicide attempts in women with eating disorders? *Psychological Medicine*, **34**, 843–853.

Gonzales-Pinto A, Aldama A, Gonzales C *et al.* (2007). Predictors of suicide in first-episode affective and nonaffective psychotis in patients: five-year follow-up of patients from a catchment area in Vitoria, Spain. *Journal of Clinical Psychiatry*, **68**, 242–247.

Guze SB and Robins E (1970). Suicide and primary affective disorders. *British Journal of Psychiatry*, **170**, 437–478.

Harris EC and Barraclough B (1997). Suicide as an outcome for mental disorders. A meta-analysis. *British Journal of Psychiatry*, **170**, 205–228.

Haukka *et al.* (2008) has this been published?

Haukka J, Suominen K, Partonen T *et al.* (2008). Determinants and outcomes of serious attempted suicide: a nationwide study in Finland from 1996 to 2003. *American Journal of Epidemiology*, in press.

Haw C, Hawton K, Sutton L *et al.* (2005). Schizophrenia and deliberate self-harm: a systematic review of risk factors. *Suicide and Life-Threatening Behavior*, **35**, 50–62.

Hawgood J and de Leo D (2008). Anxiety disorders and suicidal behaviour: an update. *Current Opinion in Psychiatry*, **21**, 51–64.

Hawton K, Sutton L, Haw C *et al.* (2005b). Schizophrenia and suicide: systematic review of risk factors. *British Journal of Psychiatry*, **187**, 9–20.

Hawton K, Sutton L, Haw C *et al.* (2005a). Suicide and attempted suicide in bipolar disorder: a systematic review of risk factors. *Journal of Clinical Psychiatry*, **66**, 693–704.

Heilä H and Lönnqvist J (2002). The clinical epidemiology of suicide in schizophrenia. In R Murray, P Jones, E Susser *et al.*, eds, *The Epidemiology of Schizophrenia*, pp. 288–316. Cambridge University Press, Cambridge.

Heilä H, Haukka J, Suvisaari J *et al.* (2005). Mortality among patients with schizophrenia and reduced psychiatric hospital care. *Psychological Medicine*, **35**, 725–732.

Heilä H, Isometsä E, Henriksson MH *et al.* (1997). Suicide and schizophrenia: a nationwide psychological autopsy study on age- and sex-specific clinical characteristics of 92 suicide victims with schizophrenia. *American Journal of Psychiatry*, **154**, 1235–1242.

Heilä H, Isometsä E, Henriksson MH *et al.* (1999). Suicide victims with schizophrenia in different treatment phases and adequacy of antipsychotic medication. *Journal of Clinical Psychiatry*, **60**, 200–208.

Hennen J and Baldessarini RJ (2005). Suicidal risk during treatment with clozapine: a meta-analysis. *Schizophrenia Research*, **73**, 139–145.

Henriksson MH, Aro HA, Marttunen MJ *et al.* (1993). Mental disorders and comorbidity in suicide. *American Journal of Psychiatry*, **150**, 935–940.

Hunt IM, Kapur N, Robinson J *et al.* (2006). Suicide within 12 months of mental health service contact in different age and diagnostic groups. National clinical survey. *British Journal of Psychiatry*, **188**, 135–142.

Ilgen MA, Harris AHS, Moos RH *et al.* (2007). Predictors of a suicide attempt one year after entry into substance use disorder treatment. *Alcoholism: Clinical and Experimental Research*, **31**, 635–642.

Inskip HM, Harris EC, Barraclough B (1998). Lifetime risk of suicide for affective disorder, alcoholism and schizophrenia. *British Journal of Psychiatry*, **172**, 35–37.

Isometsä E, Henriksson MM, Aro HM *et al.* (1994b). Suicide in bipolar disorder in Finland. *American Journal of Psychiatry*, **151**, 1020–1024.

Isometsä ET, Henriksson MM, Aro HM *et al.* (1994a). Suicide in major depression. *American Journal of Psychiatry*, **151**, 530–536.

Jane-Llopis E, Hosman C, Jenkins R *et al.* (2003). Predictors of efficacy in depression prevention programmes. Meta-analysis. *British Journal of Psychiatry*, **183**, 384–397.

Joukamaa M, Heliövaara M, Knekt P *et al.* (2001). Mental disorders and cause-specific mortality. *British Journal of Psychiatry*, **179**, 498–502.

Kamath P, Reddy YCJ, Kandavel T (2007). Suicidal behaviour in obsessive–compulsive disorder. *Journal of Clinical Psychiatry*, **68**, 1741–1750.

Keel PK, Dorer DJ, Eddy KT *et al.* (2003). Predictors of mortality in eating disorders. *Archives of General Psychiatry*, **60**, 179–183.

Kelly DL, Shim J-C, Feldman SM *et al.* (2004). Lifetime psychiatric symptoms in persons with schizophrenia who died by suicide compared to other means of death. *Journal of Psychiatric Research*, **38**, 531–536.

Kessing LV, Sondergard L, Kvist K *et al.* (2005). Suicide risk in patients treated with lithium. *Archives of General Psychiatry*, **62**, 860–866.

Kessler RC, Berglund P, Demler O *et al.* (2005). Lifetime prevalence and age-of-onset distributions of DSM-IV disorders in the National Comorbidity Survey Replication. *Archives of General Psychiatry*, **62**, 593–602.

Kessler RC, Borges G, Walters EE (1999). Prevalence and risk factors for lifetime suicide attempts in the National Comorbidity Survey. *Archives of General Psychiatry*, **56**, 617–626.

Kessler RC, Galea S, Gruber MJ *et al.* (2008). Trends in mental illness and suicidality after Hurricane Katrina. *Molecular Psychiatry* **13**, 374–384.

Kisely S, Smith M, Lawrence D *et al.* (2005). Mortality in individuals who have had psychiatric treatment. Population-based study in Nova Scotia. *British Journal of Psychiatry*, **187**, 552–558.

Kõlves K, Värnik A, Tooding L-M *et al.* (2006). The role of alcohol in suicide: a case–control psychological autopsy study. *Psychological Medicine*, **36**, 923–930.

Lieb R, Bronisch T, Höfler M *et al.* (2005). Maternal suicidality and risk of suicidality in offspring: findings from a community study. *American Journal of Psychiatry*, **162**, 1665–1671.

Lonnqvist J (1988). National suicide prevention project in Finland: A research phase of the project. *Psychiatria Fennica*, **19**, 125–132.

Maloney E, Degenhardt L, Darke S *et al.* (2007). Suicidal behaviour and associated risk factors among opioid-dependent individuals: a case–control study. *Addiction*, **102**, 1933–1941.

Mann JJ (2003). Neurobiology of suicidal behaviour. *Nature Reviews Neuroscience*, **4**, 819–828.

Marttunen MJ, Aro HM, Henriksson MM *et al.* (1991). Mental disorders in adolescent suicide: DSM-III-R axes I and II diagnoses in suicides among 13- to 19-year-olds in Finland. *Archives of General Psychiatry*, **48**, 834–839.

Mattisson C, Bogren M, Horstmann V *et al.* (2007). The long-term course of depressive disorders in the Lundby Study. *Psychological Medicine*, **37**, 883–891.

McGirr A, Paris J, Lesage A *et al.* (2007a). Risk factors for suicide completion in borderline personality disorder: a case–control study of cluster B comorbidity and impulsive aggression. *Journal of Clinical Psychiatry*, **68**, 721–729.

McGirr A, Renaud J, Seguin M *et al.* (2007b). An examination of DSM-IV depressive symptoms and risk for suicide completion in major depressive disorder: a psychological autopsy study. *Journal of Affective Disorders*, **97**, 203–209.

Melhem NM, Brent DA, Ziegler M *et al.* (2007). Familial pathways to early-onset suicidal behaviour: familial and individual antecedents of suicidal behaviour. *American Journal of Psychiatry*, **164**, 1364–1370.

Melle I, Johannesen JO, Friis S *et al.* (2006). Early detection of the first episode of schizophrenia and suicidal behaviour. *American Journal of Psychiatry*. **163**, 800–804.

Ohberg A, Vuori E, Ojanpera I *et al.* (1996). Alcohol and drugs in suicides. *British Journal of Psychiatry*, **169**, 75–80.

Oquendo MA, Kamali M, Ellis SP *et al.* (2002). Adequacy of antidepressant treatment after discharge and the occurrence of suicidal acts in major depression: a prospective study. *American Journal of Psychiatry*, **159**, 1746–1751.

Ösby U, Brandt L, Correia N *et al.* (2001). Excess mortality in bipolar and unipolar disorder in Sweden. *Archives of General Psychiatry*, **58**, 844–850.

Palmer BA, Pankratz VS, Bostwick JM (2005). The lifetime risk of suicide in schizophrenia. *Archives of General Psychiatry*, **62**, 247–253.

Pelkonen M, Marttunen M, Henriksson M *et al.* (2005). Suicidality in adjustment disorder—clinical characteristics of adolescent outpatients. *European Child and Adolescent Psychiatry*, **14**, 174–180.

Perälä J, Suvisaari J, Saarni SI *et al.* (2007). Lifetime prevalence of psychotic and bipolar I disorders in a general population. *Archives of General Psychiatry*, **64**, 19–28.

Pirkola S, Suominen K, Isometsä E (2004). Suicide in alcohol-dependent individuals. Epidemiology and management. *CNS Drugs*, **18**, 423–36.

Pirkola SP, Isometsä ET, Heikkinen ME *et al.* (2000). Suicides of alcohol misusers and non-misusers in a nationwide population. *Alcohol and Alcoholism*, **35**, 70–75.

Pompili M, Mancinelli I, Girardi P *et al.* (2004). Suicide in anorexia nervosa. A meta-analysis. *International Journal of Eating Disorders*, **36**, 99–103.

Portzky G, Audenaert K, van Heering K (2005). Adjustment disorder and the course of the suicidal process in adolescents. *Journal of Affective Disorders*, **87**, 265–270.

Pouliot L and De Leo D (2006). Critical issues in psychological autopsy studies. *Suicide and Life- Threatening Behavior*, **36**, 491–510.

Preuss UW, Schuckit MA, Smith TL *et al.* (2003). Predictors and correlates of suicide attempts over 5 years in 1,237 alcohol-dependent men and women. *American Journal of Psychiatry*, **160**, 56–63.

Radomsky ED, Haas GL, Mann JJ *et al.* (1999). Suicidal behaviour in patients with schizophrenia and other psychotic disorders. *American Journal of Psychiatry*, **156**, 1590–1595.

Romero S, Colom F, Iosif A *et al.* (2007). Relevance of family history of suicide in the long-term outcome of bipolar disorders. *Journal of Clinical Psychiatry*, **68**, 1517–1521.

Roy A (2002). Characteristics of opiate dependent patients who attempt suicide. *Journal of Clinical Psychiatry*, **63**, 403–407.

Saha S, Chant D, McGrath J (2007). A systematic review of mortality in schizophrenia. Is the differential mortality gap worsening over time? *Archives of General Psychiatry*, **64**, 1123–1131.

Sakinofsky I, Heila H, Krishnan R (2004). Estimating suicidality as an outcome measure in clinical trials of suicide in schizophrenia. *Schizophrenia Bulletin*, **30**, 587–598.

Sareen J, Cox BJ, Afiti TO *et al.* (2005). Anxiety disorders and risk for suicidal ideation and suicide attempts: a population-based longitudinal study of adults. *Archives of General Psychiatry*, **62**, 1249–1257.

Schneider B, Wetterling T, Sargk D *et al.* (2006). Axis I disorders and personality disorders as risk factors for suicide. *European Archives of Psychiatry and Clinical Neuroscience*, **256**, 17–27.

Simon GE and VonKorff M (1998). Suicide mortality among patients treated for depression in an insured population. *American Journal of Epidemiology*, **147**, 155–160.

Suokas J and Lonnqvist J (1995). Suicide attempts in which alcohol is involved: a special group in general hospital emergency rooms. *Acta Psychiatrica Scandinavica*, **91**, 36–40.

Suominen K, Henriksson M, Suokas J *et al.* (1996). Mental disorders and comorbidity in attempted suicide. *Acta Psychiatrica Scandinavica*, **94**, 234–240.

Suominen K, Isometsä E, Henriksson M *et al.* (1997). Hopelessness, impulsiveness and intent among suicide attempters with major depression, alcohol dependence, or both, *Acta Psychiatrica Scandinavica*, **96**, 142–149.

Suominen K, Isometsä E, Henriksson M *et al.* (1998). Inadequate treatment for major depression both before and after attempted suicide. *American Journal of Psychiatry*, **155**, 1778–1780.

Suvisaari *et al.* (2007) – has this been published?

Suvisaari J, Häkkinen L, Haukka J *et al.* (2007). Mortality in offspring of mothers with psychotic disorder. *Psychological Medicine*, in press.

Tiihonen J, Lönnqvist J, Wahlbeck K *et al.* (2006a). Antidepressants and the risk of suicide, attempted suicide, and overall mortality in a nationwide cohort. *Archives of General Psychiatry*, **63**, 1358–1367.

Tiihonen J, Wahlbeck K, Lönnqvist J *et al.* (2006b). Effectiveness of antipsychotic treatments in a nationwide cohort of patients in community care after first hospitalisation due to schizophrenia and schizoaffective disorder: observational follow-up study. *British Medical Journal*, **333**, 224–227.

Torres AR, Prince MJ, Bebbington PE *et al.* (2006). Obsessive-compulsive disorder: prevalence comorbidity, impact, and help-seeking in the British National Psychiatric Morbidity Survey of 2000. *American Journal of Psychiatry*, **163**, 1978–1985.

Turecki G (2005). Dissecting the suicide phenotype: the role of impulsive-aggressive behaviours. *Journal of Psychiatry and Neuroscience*, **30**, 398–408.

Valtonen H, Suominen K, Mantere O *et al.* (2005). Suicidal ideation and attempts in bipolar I and II disorders. *Journal of Clinical Psychiatry*, **66**, 1456–1462.

Valtonen HM, Suominen K, Mantere O *et al.* (2007). Suicidal behaviour during different phases of bipolar disorder. *Journal of Affective Disorders*, **97**, 101–107.

Valtonen M, Suominen K, Mantere O *et al.* (2006). Prospective study of risk factors for attempted suicide among patients with bipolar disorder. *Bipolar Disorder*, **5**, 576–585.

Wasserman D (2006). *Depression: The Facts*. Oxford University Press, Oxford.

Wasserman D, Värnik A, Eklund G (1994). Male suicides and alcohol consumption in the former USSR. *Acta Psychiatrica Scandinavica*, **89**, 306–313.

Willcox HC, Conner KR, Caine ED (2004). Association of alcohol and drug use disorders and completed suicide: an empirical review of cohort studies. *Drug and Alcohol Dependence*, **76S**, S11–S19.

Wulsin LR, Vaillant GE, Wells VE (1999). A systematic review of the mortality of depression. *Psychosomatic Medicine*, **61**, 6–17.

# CHAPTER 39

# Risk for suicidal behaviour in personality disorders

Barbara Stanley and Jennifer Jones

## Abstract

While borderline personality disorder (BPD) and major depressive disorder (MDD) are the only two disorders in the *Diagnostic Statistical Manual for Mental Disorders IV* that list suicidal behaviour as a criterion, studies have shown that other personality disorders also increase one's risk for suicide. Among Axis II personality disorders, suicide has also been found to be associated with antisocial personality disorder and avoidant personality disorder, and there is a possibility that schizoid personality disorder increases the risk for suicide (Duberstein and Conwell 1997). Moreover, stressful life events, such as those involving interpersonal distress and loss, confer a significant risk for those with personality disorders, possibly due to poor coping strategies. Reliable instruments with good psychometric properties need to be established that are sensitive to detecting Axis II personality disorders. This chapter reviews the literature on suicidal behaviours in personality disorders.

## Introduction

According to several studies, approximately 90 per cent of the identified accomplished suicides are committed by people with *Diagnostic and Statistical Manual* (DSM) (APA 1994) Axis I psychiatric disorders, leaving Axis II diagnoses in arrears. (Beautrais *et al.* 1996; Cheng *et al.* 1997; Foster *et al.* 1997; Mann *et al.* 2005). Suicide has traditionally been most strongly associated with depression, substance dependence and schizophrenia, yet personality disorders have been shown to be related to suicidality and self-injurious behaviours in both the general population and among psychiatric populations, inpatient and outpatient equally (Duberstein and Conwell 1997; Bertolote *et al.* 2004; Mann *et al.* 2005). Thus, while it is well known that Axis I psychiatric illness is a major risk factor for suicide, Axis II personality disorder also confers a significant risk and has been under-studied.

The majority of studies examining suicide among those with personality disorders have focused on borderline personality disorder, referred to as emotionally unstable personality disorder according to ICD-10 (WHO 1992). Among the DSM-IV disorders, only borderline personality disorder and major depressive disorder list suicidal behaviour as a criterion. However, according to preceding studies, borderline personality disorder is not the only personality disorder that increases the risk for suicide. Suicide has been found to be associated with antisocial personality disorder and avoidant personality disorder, and there is a possibility that schizoid personality disorder increases the risk for suicide (Duberstein and Conwell 1997).

## Prevalence of personality disorders among suicides

In a study of comorbid Axis I and Axis II personality disorders, Hawton and colleagues (2003) found that 44 per cent of their sample of suicide attempters had a comorbid Axis I and Axis II disorder. Furthermore, studies have shown that 55–70 per cent of suicide attempters meet diagnostic criteria for a personality disorder (Cheng *et al.* 1997; Chioqueta and Stiles 2004; Schneider *et al.* 2006). In a psychological autopsy study in Finland, Marttunen and colleagues (1991) reported that 17 per cent of adolescents who had completed suicide met criteria for conduct disorder or antisocial personality disorder. Among those with non-fatal suicidal behaviours, 45 per cent of the males and 33 per cent of the females were characterized by antisocial behaviours.

## Typology of personality disorders

As defined in the DSM-IV, personality disorders are characterized by a chronic inflexible pattern of inner experience and behaviours that are pervasive across situations. These behaviours clearly depart from the expectations of the individual's culture and, similar to Axis I disorders, cause significant distress or impairment in social and occupational situations, as well as in other areas of functioning. The pattern of inflexibility is manifest in the individual's perception and interpretation of themselves and others; the way in which the individual experiences emotions, including the range, intensity, and appropriateness of the individual's emotional response; how the individual experiences interpersonal relationships; and in the experience of the individual's ability to control their impulses. The DSM-IV categorizes its ten personality disorders into three clusters based on similarities in symptom clusters. Below, is a discussion of each cluster, with a focus on its currently known association with suicidal behaviour: cluster A: paranoid, schizoid, and schizotypal personality disorders; cluster B: antisocial, borderline, histrionic, and narcissistic personality disorders; cluster C: avoidant, dependent, obsessive-compulsive, and passive-aggressive personality disorders.

## Cluster A personality disorders

Individuals with prominent cluster A characteristics such as paranoid, schizoid, and schizotypal ones tend to be distrustful, guarded, emotionally restricted, interpersonally disconnected, and exhibit odd or eccentric behaviours, ideas, and appearance. To date, cluster A personality disorders have not been implicated as a risk factor in studies of suicide; however, there is some evidence, albeit minor, that schizoid personality disorder may be associated with suicide (Duberstein and Conwell 1997). This disorder is characterized by an inability and lack of desire to form close relationships with others, poor or inappropriate response to social cues, restriction of affect, and odd and eccentric behaviour. Schizoid personality disorder is a rare phenomenon overall in the general and clinical population, and there is little data on it. For this reason, it is difficult to estimate true prevalence rates among those with suicidal behaviours adequately.

## Cluster B personality disorders

Individuals with cluster B personality disorders include antisocial personality disorder, borderline personality disorder (BPD), histrionic personality disorder, and narcissistic personality disorder. Cluster B personality disorders are marked by dramatic, emotional, and erratic behaviour. Among cluster B personality disorders, BPD has been shown in studies to be a significant risk factor for suicide, and is the only personality disorder that lists recurrent suicidal and self-harm behaviours as a criterion (Isometsa et al. 1996; Linehan et al. 2000; Black et al. 2004). Studies have reported that up to three-quarters of patients with BPD attempt suicide, and approximately 10 per cent eventually complete suicide (Black et al. 2004). In a psychological autopsy study of completed suicides among adolescents, Brent and colleagues (1994) found cluster B personality disorders to be significantly associated with victims, even after controlling for Axis I disorders. Studies have shown that among subjects with BPD, suicide risk is particularly high when comorbid with affective disorders or substance use disorders (Isometsa et al. 1996; Yen et al. 2003). Individuals with BPD tend to exhibit poor impulse control, affective instability, unstable identity and self-image, and they are likely to experience real or imagined abandonment. Regardless of psychiatric diagnoses, researchers and clinicians alike have implicated poor impulse control and affective instability as risk factors in suicidal behaviours. Indeed, among those with cluster B personality disorders, an inability to plan for and think about the future in positive terms, a focus on the present, as well as problems in interpersonal relationships, are central features of the disorders. These characteristics may make it less likely that a person with cluster B personality disorder could effectively solve problems or use positive past satisfying experiences in relationships, to mitigate and protect against current interpersonal loss or conflict that may trigger suicidal behaviours.

Another cluster B personality disorder that has been found to increase the risk for suicide is antisocial personality disorder (Linehan et al. 2000). Antisocial personality disorder often leads to criminal behaviour and includes the disregard for or the violation of the rights of others. Like BPD, antisocial personality disorder includes problems with planning for the future alongside impulsivity and aggressiveness, but the DSM-IV's description of this disorder does not list suicide attempts as a criterion. Because deceit and manipulation of others is considered to be a core feature of this disorder, rates of suicide attempts may be inaccurate since individuals with this disorder may feign an attempt in order to avoid incarceration and gain hospital admission. One study found prevalence rates of suicide attempts to have been reported in 72 per cent of individuals with antisocial personality disorder (Garvey and Spoden 1980); while other studies have found that 23 per cent of outpatients who met criteria for antisocial personality disorder had made a previous suicide attempt (Woodruff et al. 1971). Robins (1966) found that 11 per cent of those with sociopathic behaviour (a common element in cluster B personality disorders) had attempted suicide. Garvey and Spoden (1980) reported that most suicide attempts among this group had low lethality. The authors suggest that the motivation among this group may be to manipulate others or act out their frustration, rather than a serious intent to die.

Few data exist among individuals with narcissistic personality disorder and histrionic personality disorder regarding suicidal behaviour. Although studies have reported an association between cluster B personality disorders and suicide, none that we are aware of have specifically identified narcissistic or histrionic personality disorders as a risk factor for suicide (Chioqueta and Stiles 2004).

## Cluster C personality disorders

Cluster C personality disorders include avoidant, dependent, and obsessive–compulsive disorders. There has been some evidence linking avoidant personality disorder with suicidal behaviour (Duberstein and Conwell 1997). Among those with avoidant personality disorder, prevalence rates of suicide have been estimated to be 5.2 per cent (as reported in Chioqueta and Stiles 2004). In a study by Brent and colleagues (1994) among adolescent suicide completers, they found that, after controlling for the presence of Axis I disorders, cluster C personality disorders were not strongly associated with suicide. Chioqeta and Stiles (2004) examined suicide risk among psychiatric outpatients with cluster C personality disorders and found that at 35 per cent, the dependent group had the highest percentage of suicide attempts, compared to 18 per cent in the avoidant group and 14 per cent in the obsessive–compulsive group. Dependent personality disorder was the only cluster C personality disorder that was found to be significantly associated with suicide attempt; however, this association was no longer significant after controlling for the presence of concurrent and lifetime depressive disorder. The authors did find that the cluster A and B personality disorders remained significantly associated with suicide attempt, independent of co-occurring lifetime and concurrent depressive disorder and severity of depression. The authors postulate that the lack of findings among the cluster C group may be due to the characteristics associated with this disorder including avoidance of risk-taking behaviours, and, among dependent personality disorder, a reluctance to engage in self-destructive behaviour due to their submissive and passive tendencies.

## Post-mortem diagnosis of personality disorders

Studies that have examined completed suicide often use the psychological autopsy to identify psychiatric diagnoses retrospectively. The psychological autopsy involves interviews with suicide victim's family, friends, and relatives in order to determine a comprehensive understanding of the victim, including psychiatric diagnoses and psychological functioning. Relying on friends and family to report on the psychological functioning of the suicide victim prior to their suicide may result in unreliable rates. Prevalence rates of personality disorders vary in psychological autopsy studies. This has led researchers to suggest that this method of ascertaining diagnosis may be effective for Axis I disorders, but less sensitive in identifying Axis II disorders (Ernst *et al.* 2003), resulting in unreliable estimates regarding personality disorders among suicide completers. Rates may not be reliable because most psychological autopsy studies have focused on Axis I disorders and have not used structured interviews. Previous studies have shown that reliability rates for personality disorder are typically low without structured interviews (Schneider *et al.* 2004). Researchers have suggested that the decreased sensitivity in detecting Axis II disorders is due to inherent limitations of the proxy-based interview method such as recall bias, the way bereavement can affect a relative's perception and distort the information they provide, and the way some suicide victim's social withdrawal prior to the suicide can affect information an informant can provide (Ernst *et al.* 2003). Lower rates of personality disorders among victims with comorbid axis I and II disorders have also been reported when axis II disorders were not in the forefront of the psychiatric constellation (Schneider *et al.* 2006).

Although previous studies reported poor reliability for detecting personality disorders due to unstructured instruments and small sample sizes, Schneider and colleagues (2004) recently published good psychometric properties of the Structured Clinical Interview for DSM-IV Disorders Axis II personality disorders (SCID-II) in post-suicide population. Unlike previous studies that have employed non-standardized interview methods in the psychological autopsy, the SCID-II is a semi-structured interview administered to an informant, including third parties, and is consistent with DSM-IV diagnostic criteria for personality disorders. Schneider and colleagues reported that all interviewers were trained by senior clinicians to administer a modified version of the SCID-II, including viewing multiple interviews by expert raters and conducting patient interviews. Inter-rater reliability for personality disorders was reported to be excellent for all subtypes of personality disorders (Schneider *et al.* 2004). Future studies utilizing this instrument may show an increase in the rates of personality disorders among suicide completers.

## Risk factors for suicidal behaviour in personality disorders

Studies have identified important factors that place individuals with axis I and axis II personality disorders at increased risk for suicide attempts and completed suicide. Specifically, hopelessness, suicidal ideation, history of suicide attempts and non-suicidal self-injury and severity of depression are all significant risk factors in psychiatric populations (Mann *et al.* 1999; Stanley *et al.* 2001; Keilp *et al.* 2006). Brown and colleagues (2000), in a prospective study of psychiatric outpatients between 1975 and 1995, found that current suicidal ideation, diagnosis of major depression, bipolar disorder, personality disorder, and unemployment status all contributed to the individual estimates of risk for eventual suicide. They also found that previous suicide attempts, previous psychiatric hospitalization, and increasing age all contributed individually to suicide risk. In this study, after controlling for the risk associated

with mood disorders, personality disorder did not add a unique contribution to the prediction of suicide.

Patients with depressive disorder, who have a comorbid axis II personality disorder, exhibit more suicidal ideation and attempts than those without a comorbid personality disorder (Charney *et al.* 1981; Kelly *et al.* 2000; Black *et al.* 2004). Among those with BPD, psychiatric comorbidity has been identified as a strong risk factor in suicide attempts and completions (Black *et al.* 2004). Childhood sexual abuse has been shown in studies to be a significant risk factor for suicide attempts among individuals with BPD (Brodsky *et al.* 1997; Black *et al.* 2004; Yen *et al.* 2004). Others have found that among those with a history of childhood abuse, post-traumatic stress disorder comorbid with BPD increases the risk for suicidal behaviours (Heffernan and Cloitre 2000; Oquendo *et al.* 2005).

Studies implicating life events in increasing risk for suicidal behaviour indicate the perceived negative life events, particularly those involving interpersonal distress and loss, are more likely to be precipitants to suicidal behaviour for individuals with personality disorder compared to suicidal individuals who do not have PD (Heikkinen *et al.* 1997; Horesh *et al.* 2003; Yen *et al.* 2005; Brodsky *et al.* 2006). Some studies have also shown that stressful love events, particularly ones related to love/marriage and legal problems, may increase imminent risk for suicidal behaviour among those with schizoid, avoidant, borderline and obsessive–compulsive personality disorders (Heikkinen *et al.* 1997; Yen *et al.* 2005). Paykel and colleagues (1975) compared suicide attempters to non-suicidal depressed patients and to controls from the general population. They found that suicide attempters had higher scores on life events in the previous six months compared with both groups. Also, suicide attempters reported an increase in the number of life events in the month preceding the suicide attempt. In a more recent study, Kelly and colleagues (2000) examined social adjustment, recent life events and suicidal behaviours among a sample of psychiatric inpatients with current major depressive episode (MDE), compared to patients with BPD, and a group with co-morbid BPD and MDE. The authors found that patients with BPD and BPD comorbid with MDE were significantly more likely to have attempted suicide than those with MDE alone. Furthermore, social adjustment—especially regarding relationships with immediate family—was also a significant predictor for the suicide attempter status for BPD and comorbid BPD/MDE patients. The reason why stressful life events may be particularly problematic for those with personality disorders is possibly a consequence of poor coping strategies that individuals with personality disorders exhibit. Particularly, among those with cluster B personality disorders, characteristics such as reactivity, impulsivity, dramatic and erratic behaviour—core symptoms of these disorders—are commonly associated with suicide and self-destructive behaviours (Corbitt *et al.* 1996). A study of suicide attempters by MacLeod and colleagues (2004) found that deficits in thinking about the future, which the authors posit to be related to hopelessness and impulsivity, were significantly associated with the diagnosis of cluster B disorders, particularly borderline and antisocial personality disorder. Because hopelessness has been found to be a significant risk factor for suicide, deficits in one's ability to positively think about one's future is key and has significant implications for treatment. Other studies have found high levels of aggression and suicidal ideation among first-degree relatives of suicide completers with cluster B personality disorders (Kim *et al.* 2005); and among borderline personality disorder with self-harm behaviours. Deficits were found in time perception and orbitofrontal cortex dysfunction was evident (Berlin and Rolls 2003). In a study by Stanley and colleagues (2001) that compared cluster B suicide attempters who engage in non-suicidal self injury with those who did not engage in non-suicidal self-injury, the authors found that while both groups had attempts that were equal in degree of lethality, the self-injurers group perceived their suicide attempts as less lethal, and with less certainty of death. Thus, the authors noted that the underestimation of lethality in the context of lethal attempts makes this group of self-injurers at particularly high risk.

Keilp and colleagues (2006) examined the significance of impulsivity, aggressive behaviour and hostility among depressed suicide attempters and non-attempters, controlling for the effects of comorbid BPD. The authors found that comorbid BPD subjects were significantly more impulsive, hostile and aggressive than non-BPD subjects. However, after controlling for the effect of BPD status, the authors did not find impulsiveness or hostility to be significantly related to past suicide attempts, only aggressiveness remained significant. Soloff and colleagues (2000) examined suicide attempts in patients with BPD, MDE and comorbid BPD with MDE. The authors found that the comorbid group had significantly more suicide attempts, greater level of self-reported depression and hopelessness. Impulsivity and hopelessness independently predicted lifetime number of suicide attempts in this study. Like the previous study, Brodsky et al. (2006) also found that suicide attempters with comorbid BPD plus MDD had a higher number of lifetime suicide attempts, higher lifetime aggression, hostility and impulsivity than suicide attempters with MDD only. These authors also found that the comorbid group were younger at the first suicide attempt and reported interpersonal triggers for their first and subsequent attempts.

## Co-occurring axis I and axis II disorders and suicide risk

Co-occurrence of axis I with axis II personality disorders has been increasingly recognized as a major factor in suicide. In studies examining suicidal behaviours, comorbidity with depressive disorders has been found to be highly prevalent among individuals with BPD (Corbitt et al. 1996; Yen et al. 2003; Pompili et al. 2004; Zanarini et al. 2004); comorbidity of substance use and BPD (Links et al. 1995); and comorbidity of psychiatric and personality disorders in general (Hawton et al. 2003; Zanarini et al. 2004; Schneider et al. 2005; Skodol et al. 2005). Other studies have identified impulsivity (Brodsky et al. 1997; Soloff et al. 2000; Yen et al. 2004) and affective instability as the key ingredient in the risk for suicide independent of lifetime depression and substance use (Yen et al. 2004). The reasons why comorbid personality disorders and axis I psychiatric disorders increase the risk for suicide has received relatively little attention in the research literature (Hawton et al. 2003). The studies that have been conducted have suggested that difficulties with problem-solving, aggressive behaviour, and impulsivity are thought to increase the risk for suicide, traits typically found among those with axis II disorders (Brodsky et al. 1997; Mann et al. 1999; Soloff et al. 2000; Hawton et al. 2003; Keilp et al. 2006). Mann and colleagues (1999), in a study that examined 347 psychiatric patients with axis I or II disorders, reported that suicide attempters had significantly higher scores for lifetime aggression,

impulsivity, and had higher rates of comorbid cluster B personality disorders.

A stress–diathesis model has been proposed by Mann and colleagues (1999) to explain the factors that underlie one's propensity for suicidal behaviours. The stressors involved in the prediction of suicide are the onset or worsening of a psychiatric disorder and a psychosocial crisis or life event that leads to feelings of hopelessness and depression, suicidal ideation, impulsivity and aggressivity. This, in combination with vulnerability factors, including negative childhood experiences, poor psychosocial support, access to high lethal suicide methods, familial and genetic factors, and substance use, can contribute to suicide risk.

Hawton et al. (2003) found that suicide attempters with co-occurring axis I and axis II disorders showed marked differences from those without comorbidity. Individuals with comorbid disorders were more likely to have made previous suicide attempts, with 37 per cent having made multiple attempts. Not being able to make friends and having an addiction significantly differentiated those with comorbid disorders compared to those without comorbid disorders. Suicide attempts in the comorbid group were also associated with wanting to make others feel guilty, finding their situation unbearable, and wanting to get help. In the follow-up interview, the comorbid group reported higher suicidal ideation and had made more suicide attempts than those without a comorbid disorder. In terms of psychological characteristics, those with comorbid disorders were more depressed, hopeless, aggressive and impulsive. They also had poorer problem-solving skills and lower self-esteem.

## Treatment implications

One of the most promising treatments, with the most empirical support to date for individuals with borderline personality disorder and self-harm behaviours, was manualized and published by Linehan in 1994 (Linehan et al. 1994, 1997, 2006) and is described by Brodsky and Stanley in Chapter 57 of this book.

Bateman and Fonagy (1999, 2001) published results of an 18-month follow-up randomized controlled trial showing superior gains for a psychoanalytically oriented partial hospitalization over standard psychiatric treatment (Bateman and Fonagy 2001). The treatment consisted of up to eighteen months of individual and group psychotherapy designed to focus on the relational characteristic of BPD. The partial hospitalization consisted of four parts:

1 Once-weekly individual psychoanalytic psychotherapy;

2 Three-times-a-week group analytic psychotherapy;

3 Once-weekly expressive therapy using psychodrama techniques; and

4 A weekly community meeting.

## Conclusion

Historically, suicide has been associated with axis I disorders; however, this chapter highlights empirical evidence that demonstrates the prevalence of axis II disorders among those with suicidal behaviours, particularly when comorbid with an axis I disorder. Although the literature to date implicates suicidality in borderline personality disorder in particular, antisocial, avoidant, and schizoid personality disorders need further study. Some studies have grouped together separate categories of personality disorders often due to low base rates of suicidal behaviours; however, future studies need to examine individual personality disorders in order to gain an understanding about their associated risk in suicide. Finally, better tools to assess both suicidal behaviour in personality disorders more reliably and accurately, both prospectively and in post-mortem studies, are needed. Research efforts in this direction need to be further developed (Stanley *et al.* 1986; Nimeus *et al.* 2000; Posner *et al.* 2007).

## References

APA (American Psychiatric Association) (1994). *Diagnostic and Statistical Manual for Mental Disorders*, 4th edn. American Psychiatric Association, Washington.

Bateman A and Fonagy P (1999). Effectiveness of partial hospitalization in the treatment of borderline personality disorder: a randomized controlled trial. *American Journal of Psychiatry*, **156**, 1563–1569.

Bateman A and Fonagy P (2001). Treatment of borderline personality disorder with psychoanalytically oriented partial hospitalization: an 18-month follow-up. *American Journal of Psychiatry*, **158**, 36–42.

Beautrais AL, Joyce PR, Mulder RT *et al.* (1996). Prevalence and comorbidity of mental disorders in persons making serious suicide attempts: a case–control study. *American Journal of Psychiatry*, **153**, 1009–1014.

Berlin HA and Rolls ET (2004). Time perception, impulsivity, emotionality and personality in self-harming borderline personality disorder patients. *Journal of Personality Disorders*, **18**, 358–378.

Bertolote JM, Fleischmann A, DeLeo D *et al.* (2004). Psychiatric diagnosis and suicide: revisiting the evidence. *Crisis*, **25**, 147–155.

Black DW, Blum N, Pfohl B *et al.* (2004). Suicidal behaviour in borderline personality disorder: prevalence, risk factors, prediction and prevention. *Journal of Personality Disorders*, **18**, 226–239.

Brent D, Johnson BA, Perper J *et al.* (1994). Personality disorder, personality traits, impulsive violence, and completed suicide in adolescents. *Journal of American Child and Adolescent Psychiatry*, **33**, 1080–1086.

Brodsky BS, Groves SA, Oquendo MA *et al.* (2006). Interpersonal precipitants and suicide attempts in borderline personality disorder. *Suicide and Life-Threatening Behaviour*, **36**, 313–322.

Brodsky BS, Malone KM, Ellis SP *et al.* (1997). Characteristics of borderline personality disorder associated with suicidal behaviour. *American Journal of Psychiatry*, **154**, 1715–1719.

Brown GK, Beck AT, Steer RA *et al.* (2000). Risk factors for suicide in psychiatric outpatients: a 20-year prospective study. *Journal of Consulting and Clinical Psychology*, **68**, 371–377.

Charney DS, Nelson JC, Quinlan DM (1981). Personality traits and disorder in depression. *American Journal of Psychiatry*, **138**, 1601–1604.

Cheng AT, Mann AH, Chan KA (1997). Personality disorder and suicide. A case–control study. *The British Journal of Psychiatry* **170**, 441–446.

Chioqueta AP and Stiles TC (2004). Assessing suicide risk in cluster C personality disorders. *Crisis*, **25**, 128–133.

Corbitt MC, Malone KM, Hass GL *et al.* (1996). Suicidal behaviour in patients with major depression and comorbid personality disorders. *Journal of Affective Disorders*, **39**, 61–72.

Duberstein PR and Conwell Y (1997). Personality disorders and completed suicide: a methodological and conceptual review. *Clinical Psychology: Science and Practice*, **4**, 359–376.

Ernst C, Lalovic A, Lesage A *et al.* (2003). Suicide and no axis I psychopathology. *BMC Psychiatry*, **4**, 359–364.

Foster T, Gillespie K, McClelland R (1997). Mental disorders and suicide in Northern Ireland. *The British Journal of Psychiatry*, **170**, 447–452.

Garvey MJ and Spoden F (1980). Suicide attempts in antisocial personality disorder. *Comprehensive Psychiatry*, **21**, 146–149.

Hawton K, Houston K, Haw C *et al.* (2003). Comorbidity of axis I and axis II disorders in patients who attempted suicide. *American Journal of Psychiatry*, **160**, 1494–1500.

Heffernan K and Cloitre M (2000). A comparison of posttraumatic stress disorder with and without borderline personality disorder among women with a history of childhood sexual abuse: etiological and clinical characteristics. *Journal of Nervous and Mental Disease*, **188**, 589–595.

Heikkinen ME, Henriksson MM, Isometsa ET *et al.* (1997). Recent life events and suicide in personality disorders. *The Journal of Nervous and Mental Disease*, **185**, 373–381.

Horesh N, Sever J, Apter A (2003). A comparison of life events between suicidal adolescents with major depression and borderline personality disorder. *Comprehensive Psychiatry*, **44**, 277–283.

Isometsa ET, Henriksson MM, Heikkinen ME *et al.* (1996). Suicide among subjects with personality disorders. *American Journal of Psychiatry*, **153**, 667–673.

Keilp JG, Gorlyn M, Oquendo M *et al.* (2006). Aggressiveness, not impulsiveness or hostility distinguishes suicide attempters with major depression. *Psychological Medicine*, **12**, 1–10.

Kelly TM, Soloff PH, Lynch KG *et al.* (2000). Recent life events, social adjustment, and suicide attempts in patients with major depression and borderline personality disorder. *Journal of Personality Disorders*, **14**, 316–326.

Kim CD, Seguin M, Therrein N *et al.* (2005). Familial aggregation of suicidal behaviour: a family study of male suicide completers from the general population. *American Journal of Psychiatry*, **162**, 1017–1019.

Linehan MM, Armstrong HE, Suarez A *et al.* (1997). Cognitive-behavioural treatment of chronically parasuicidal borderline patients. *Archives of General Psychiatry*, **48**, 1060–1064.

Linehan MM, Comtosis KA, Murray AM *et al.* (2006). Two-year randomized controlled trial and follow-up of dialectical behaviour therapy vs. therapy by experts for suicidal behaviours and borderline personality disorder. *Archives of General Psychiatry*, **63**, 757–766.

Linehan MM, Rizvi SL, Welsh SS *et al.* (2000). Psychiatric aspects of suicidal behaviours: personality disorders. In K Hawton and K van Heeringen, eds, *The International Handbook of Suicide and Attempted Suicide*, pp. 148–178. John Wiley & Sons.

Linehan MM, Tutek DA, Heard HL *et al.* (1994). Interpersonal outcome of cognitive behavioural treatment for chronically suicidal borderline patients. *American Journal of Psychiatry*, **151**, 1771–1776.

Links PS, Heselgrave RJ, Mitton JE *et al.* (1995). Borderline personality disorder and substance abuse: consequences of comorbidity. *Canadian Journal of Psychiatry*, **40**, 9–14.

MacLeod AK, Tata P, Tyrer P *et al.* (2004). Personality disorders and future-directed thinking in parasuicide. *Journal of Personality Disorders*, **18**, 459–466.

Mann JJ, Apter A, Bertolote J *et al.* (2005). Suicide prevention strategies: a systematic review. *Journal of the American Medical Association*, **294**, 2064–2074.

Mann JJ, Waternaux C, Hass GL *et al.* (1999). Toward a clinical model of suicidal behaviour in psychiatric patients. *American Journal of Psychiatry*, **156**, 181–189.

Marttunen MJ, Aro HM, Henrikson MM *et al.* (1991). Mental disorders in adolescent suicide. DSM-III-R axes I and II diagnosis in suicides among 19-year-olds in Finland. *Archives of General Psychiatry*, **48**, 834–839.

Nimeus A, Alsen M, Traskman-Bendz L (2000). The suicide assessment scale: an instrument assessing suicide risk of suicide attempters. *European Psychiatry*, **15**, 416–423.

Oquendo M, Brent DA, Birmaher B *et al.* (2005). Postraumatic stress disorder comorbid with major depression: factors mediating the association with suicidal behaviour. *American Journal of Psychiatry*, **162**, 560–566.

Paykel ES, Prusoff BA, Myers JK (1975). Suicide attempts and recent life events. A controlled comparison. *Archives of General Psychiatry*, **32**, 327–333.

Pompili M, Ruberto A, Girardi P *et al.* (2004). Suicidality in DSM IV cluster B personality disorders. An overview. *Ann Ist Super Sanità*, **40**, 475–483.

Posner K, Oquendo MA, Stanley B, Davies M, Gould M (2007). Columbia Classification Algorithm of Suicide Assessment (C-CASA): Classification of Suicidal Events in the FDA's Pediatric Suicidal Risk Analysis of Antidepressants. *American Journal of Psychiatry*, **164**(7), 1035–1043.

Robins L (1966). *Deviant Children Grown Up: A Sociological and Psychiatric Study of Sociopathic Personality*. Williams & Wilkins, Baltimore.

Schneider B, Maurer K, Sargk D *et al.* (2004). Concordance of DSM-IV Axis I and II diagnoses by personal and informant's interview. *Psychiatry Research*, **127**, 121–136.

Schneider B, Wetterling T, Sargk D *et al.* (2006). Axis I disorders and personality disorders as risk factors for suicide. *European Archives of Psychiatry and Clinical Neoroscience*, **256**, 17–27.

Skodol AE, Gunderson JG, Shea MT *et al.* (2005). The collaborative longitudinal personality disorders study: overview and implications. *Journal of Personality Disorders*, **19**, 487–504.

Soloff PH, Lynch KG, Kelly TM *et al.* (2000). Characteristics of suicide attempts of patients with major depresive episode and borderline personality disorder: a comparative study. *American Journal of Psychiatry*, **157**, 601–608.

Stanley B, Gameroff MJ, Michalsen BA *et al.* (2001). Are suicide attempters who self-mutilate a unique population? *American Journal of Psychiatry* **158**, 427–432.

Stanley B, Traskman-Bendz L, Stanley M (1986). The suicide assessment scale: a scale evaluating change in suicidal behaviour. *Psychopharmacologyl Bulletin*, **22**, 200–205.

WHO (World Health Organization) (1992). *International Statistical Classification of Diseases and Related Health Problems*, 10th revision. World Health Organization, Geneva.

Woodruff RA, Guze SB, Clayton PJ (1971). The medical and psychiatric implications of antisocial personality (sociopathy). *Diseases of the Nervous system*, **32**, 712–714.

Yen S, Pagano ME, Shea MT *et al.* (2005). Recent life events preceding suicide attempts in a personality disorder sample: findings from the collaborative longitudinal personality disorders study. *Journal of Consulting and Clinical psychology*, **73**, 99–105.

Yen S, Shea MT, Pagano M *et al.* (2003). Axis I and axis II disorders are predictors of prospective suicide attempts: findings from the collaborative longitudinal personality disorders study. *Journal of Abnormal Psychology*, **112**, 375–381.

Yen S, Shea MT, Sanislow CA *et al.* (2004). Borderline personality disorder criteria associated with prospectively observed suicidal behaviour. *American Journal of Psychiatry*, **161**, 1296–1298.

Zanarini MC, Frankburg FR, Hennen J *et al.* (2004). Axis I comorbidity in patients with borderline personality disorder: 6-year follow-up and prediction of time remission. *American Journal of Psychiatry*, **161**, 2108–2114.

# CHAPTER 40

# Somatic diseases and suicidal behaviour

Elsebeth Stenager and Egon Stenager

## Abstract

The association between chronic somatic disorders and the risk of suicide has been examined in many studies. Common features in the studies are a large variation in quality and choice of study method. The studies performed, in more recent decades, have substantially improved knowledge not only on the extent of risk, but also on factors influencing the risk. Most of the studies on completed suicides have been made in European countries, the United States of America and Australia, one single study is from Japan (Whitlock 1985; Allgulander and Fisher 1990; Stenager and Stenager 1992; Harris and Barraclough 1994; Stenager and Stenager 1997; Ruzicka *et al.* 2005).

The majority of studies on the association between chronic somatic disorders and suicidal behaviour, including suicidal thoughts and suicide attempts, studies have demonstrated a correlation. The studies have been performed in Europe (DeLeo *et al.* 1999; Pajonk *et al.* 2002), the US (Druss and Pincuss 2000) and Australia (Lawrence *et al.* 2000).

This chapter is a review on present knowledge on suicide and suicidal behaviour in selected somatic disorders and pain syndromes, with focus on studies from different parts of the world, and whether or not this reflects variation in the estimated risk of suicidal behaviour.

## Suicide attempts and somatic disorders

Studies on the association between somatic disorders and suicide are qualitatively better than those investigating the association between somatic disorders and suicide attempts. Three types of studys have been performed: first, frequency and diagnosis of somatic disorders in patients who have made suicide attempts (Kontaxakis *et al.* 1988; Nielsen *et al.* 1990; Dietzfelbinger *et al.* 1991; Öjehagen *et al.* 1991; Wedler 1991; Stenager *et al.* 1992). Next, follow-up studies on patients with suicide attempts and somatic disorders, where the risk of repetition of suicidal behaviour has been estimated (Nielsen *et al.* 1990; DeLeo *et al.* 1999). Thirdly, studies on the risk of suicide attempts in defined populations and studies in defined populations in comparison to a control group (Hawton *et al.* 1980). The above mentioned studies have shown a frequency of 27–50 per cent of somatic disorders differing between in- and outpatients and depending on the definition of the somatic disorder.

Painful disorders and disorders involved with an increased risk of depression are most common in suicide attempters. Furthermore, somatic disorders in older people are of significant importance.

## Psychosocial consequences of somatic disorders

Suicidal behaviour in a human being can be considered, as a consequence of life, being unbearable. Reasons for this are manifold and may be of physical, psychological and social character. The threshold for suicidal behaviour in individuals varies, and a single cause may only be a precipitating factor. The hard task is to predict when a given person reaches the threshold and, before that occurs, provide relevant help. In this context, knowledge about which disorders might entail increased risks of suicide may be helpful.

Somatic disorder involves troubles of physical, psychological, and social character. The somatic disorder may imply pains, handicaps, as well as distress about whether or not it is life-threatening. Complicating, simultaneously present, psychic disorders give limitations in social performance, loss of the capability to work and need for public social services. The risk of suicide may change during the course of a disorder. There may be periods during the course where the risk may be increased, for instance, before or after the diagnosis is made, or when the patient has had the disease for a long period. Age may also be a parameter of importance (Juurlink *et al.* 2004). Other factors influencing the risk of suicide could be depression, cognitive deficits, anxiety, and medically induced abuse of medication due to pains, psychosis and organic mental disorders, e.g. vascular or Alzheimer's dementia. Attention should be given to psychosomatic disorders that have been increasingly recognized during the last decade.

## Pain and suicide

Studies concerned with the association between pain and suicide come across considerable methodological problems, such as the definition of pain and the selection of a study group. A controlled study in England of 6569 persons with pains found a fivefold increased risk of suicide, accidents and violence. The study involved persons with extensive pain, among which many were cancer patients (Macfarlane *et al.* 2001). A review of eighteen studies on chronic pain and suicidal behaviour concluded that suicidal behaviour is frequent in patients with pain. It was recommended to be aware of this aspect in a psychiatric setting (Fishbain 1999). A British study of 1665 suicide attempters showed that in 4 per cent of the cases, pain was of importance (Theodoulou *et al.* 2005). The patients differed from other studies in that they were older, had a higher suicidal intention score and were rarely seen in a psychiatric setting.

As many patients with cancer have pain, an increased risk of suicide can be expected in these patients.

## Methodological demands in studies on somatic disorders and risk of suicide

A number of conditions need to be considered when designing studies of this sort. The most important is the presence of, and access to, adequate information about the health care given to the studied population. This puts a limitation on the number of communities where such studies can be performed. Furthermore, this implies that the disorder should be well characterized with accepted diagnostic criteria. The course of the disorder should be well described in order to be able to ascertain during which periods the risk of suicide increases. It is of great interest to know whether it is a genetic disorder, and if it is possible to screen for the disorder.

### Parameters of importance

When studies are evaluated regarding the quality of design, the following three parameters should be taken into consideration. In the choice of study population, one should consider whether the selected population is at a high or low risk of suicide. Regarding the registration of suicide, one should bear in mind how the suicide data is validated. Finally, it is important to reflect upon how the control group is selected. When studying the risk of suicide in somatic disorder, there are quite a few prerequisites. A disorder with an adequate diagnostic criterion is of prime importance as well as large and representative groups to study. Furthermore, the control group should include a complete background population. Usually the normal population in the study area are used, i.e the Danish population. Only validated registry of death causes should be used and statistical analyses with calculation of standard mortality ratio (SMR) controlling for at least sex and age and preferably with survival curves. SMR is a statistical measure for the relative risk adjusted for age and sex. An SMR of 2 means a doubled suicide risk.

A number of early studies were based on autopsy studies. Such studies are not useful if the purpose is to estimate the risk of suicide, but are valuable when studying characteristics of patients and risk factors in patients who have committed suicide.

Follow-up studies in well-defined groups of patients have frequently been performed. The studies follow the patients with a defined disorder for a certain period and, by comparing with controls, estimate the number of suicides. The studies are often part of studies on mortality of the disorder. Such studies can be biased by a number of factors: first, a lack of defined diagnostic criteria; also, in the selection process of the patients, if, for example, only inpatients are included. Further, there may be great variation of follow-up periods, not well-defined controls and far from optimal statistic sources. From a methodological point of view, studies based on regional or nationwide registries on disorders with well-defined diagnostic criteria, compared to the background population using the sex- and age-standardized mortality ratio (SMR), are advantageous. The benefits of such studies are many: they deal with well-defined patients

on a regional/national basis found in registries of causes of death during a defined period. Moreover, they compare risks of suicide in patients and the background population and calculate a standardized SMR for sex and age. Generally speaking, the quality of the studies has increased in recent years, concurrently with the improvement of registries on specific disorders and causes of death and improved statistics in many parts of the world. Many studies are now based on validated registries and large populations in contrast to earlier studies, which were based on case stories or small populations.

## Cancer

The diagnosis of cancer can be associated with troublesome treatments, pains, bad prognosis, economical troubles and, as a possible consequence, of depression and crisis reaction. Many cancers are ultimately lethal. Thus, it is not surprising that a diagnosis of cancer is associated with an increased risk of suicide. Numerous studies have dealt with the association of cancer and risk of suicide. They include autopsy studies and register-based studies in large populations, particularly from Scandinavia and the US (Louhivouri and Hakama 1979; Fox *et al.* 1982; Allebeck *et al.* 1989; Levi *et al.* 1991; Storm *et al.* 1992). Studies from Japan also demonstrate an increased risk of suicide in cancer patients compared to the background population (Tanaka *et al.* 1999; Akechi *et al.* 2002). These methodologically well-performed studies estimate the SMR in males between 1.9 and 2.8, while there is disagreement whether or not women have an increased risk. There is no significant difference cross-nationally in the results. Few studies found an elevated risk of suicide in certain types of cancer. In patients with cancer in the oesophagus, an increased suicide risk of 35× was found (Innos *et al.* 2003). The risk was especially increased in the period after the diagnosis was made. A Swedish study found an increase of suicide by 16× in all males with cancer in the first year after diagnosis (Allebeck *et al.* 1989). However, Norwegian and Danish studies could not confirm this elevated risk during the first year after the diagnosis (Storm *et al.* 1992; Hem *et al.* 2004; Yousaf *et al.* 2005).

## Neurological disorders

Next to cancer, neurological disorders are the most thoroughly investigated disorders. This is obvious considering that many neurological disorders have an increased risk of psychic disorders such as depression. Some of the neurological disorders do not always have well-defined diagnostic criteria, or have not been studied in populations with good registries. As a consequence, not all disorders have been subjected to well-designed studies. Most of the studies have been conducted in Europe, Australia, the US and Japan. Despite the different geographic areas investigated, the results are fairly consistent. A study from Japan (Kishi *et al.* 2001) examined the extent of suicidal thoughts in patients with stroke, traumatic brain injury, myocardial infarction and spinal cord injury. A total of 7.3 per cent had suicidal thoughts, and among patients with depression, the figure was 25 per cent. The study stressed the importance of being aware of, and carefully treating, depression in these patients as a preventive measure.

## Multiple sclerosis

The largest study on the frequency of suicide in patients with multiple sclerosis (MS) is from the Danish MS Registry and based on approximately 5000 patients (Stenager *et al.* 1992). The SMR for males diagnosed before the age of 40 years was 3.12, and the SMR for females diagnosed before the age of 40 years was 2.12. There was no increased risk of suicide for patients diagnosed after the age of 40 years. The risk was largest in the first five years after diagnosis. The cumulated lifetime risk of suicide was approximately twice that of background population. There was a follow-up study from the MS Registry (Brønnum-Hansen et al. 2005) comprising 10,174 patients with MS diagnosed in the period 1953 to 1996 and a follow-up the 1 January 1999. This study confirmed a doubled risk of suicide in MS patients, as well as new findings that an increased risk of suicide was also found 20 years after the diagnosis was made. A study from Sweden (Frederikson et al. 2003), based on 122,834 persons followed from 1969 to 1996, confirmed the Danish results with a SMR of 2.3 in MS patients, and an increased risk within the first 5 years after the diagnosis was made. However, a Canadian study (Sadovnick et al. 1985) found a substantially increased risk of suicide by a factor of 7.5 compared to the Scandinavian results, yet this study did not calculate the SMR or standardize for sex and age, which is a bias as the sex distribution is skewed in MS patients. Yet, another study from the US (Feinstein et al. 2002) examined suicidal intention in 140 MS patients and found that it was associated with depression, abuse of alcohol and social isolation.

## Huntington's chorea

Most studies demonstrate an increased risk of suicide in patients with Huntington's chorea, but all studies have methodological problems and, subsequently, the conclusions on the size of the risk should be taken with caution (Schoenfeld et al. 1984; Farrer 1986). A study from The Huntington study Group Database from the US (Paulsen et al. 2005) examined the suicidal thoughts of 4171 patients, who were in different stages of the disease, from healthy carriers to severely disabled. Among the healthy carriers, i.e. with normal neurological signs, 9.1 per cent had suicidal thoughts. In the group with slight neurological signs, 19.8 per cent had suicidal thoughts, and in the group with signs of a possible disease, the figure was 23.5 per cent. In the group where the disease was active with certainty, patients in the early stages had a high risk, while the risk decreased with the progression of the disease. The study showed that the risk of suicidal thoughts was the largest immediately before the diagnosis was made, and when the disorder resulted in loss of capability of taking care of oneself. Similar results were found in a study from Hungary (Baliko et al. 2004), which found more suicides in the early stages of the disease compared to the later stages.

Huntington's chorea is an autosomal dominant disorder that can be diagnosed in healthy family members. A Canadian study (Almquist et al. 1999) examined 4527 persons who had been genetically tested with the purpose of estimating whether or not the test results made a difference in the number of persons who committed suicide, made suicide attempts or were admitted to a psychiatric ward. The study concluded that the behaviour of the tested persons was not dependent on whether or not they tested positive on the diagnosis. Instead, suicidal behaviour was dependent on whether the tested persons had previous psychiatric disorders or were unemployed.

## Spinal cord lesions

Spinal cord lesions are most frequently the result of accidents in young males, and may result in life-long dependence on a wheelchair. Many studies have been performed on the risk of suicide in patients with spinal cord lesions. Most studies have methodological problems, but a well conducted North American study found a 4.9 increased risk of suicide (DeVivo et al. 1991).

## Epilepsy

Epilepsy is one of the somatic disorders, in which the association of risk of suicide has been examined most thoroughly. A review (Barraclough 1987) of the existing literature on suicidal risk in different groups of epilepsies found that patients with epileptic seizures generated in the temporal lobes had a five times increased risk of suicide, and patients with difficult treatable epilepsy, an increased risk of 25 per cent.

A methodologically adequate British study (White et al. 1979) followed 2000 patients admitted between 1931 and 1971 and on anticonvulsant treatment to 1977. In estimating the mortality, consideration of sex, age and period of risk was made. The study found an increased risk of suicide of 5.4. A mortality study from Sweden (Nilsson et al. 1997), based on 9061 patients diagnosed with epilepsy, found an SMR of 3.6. When including death due to injuries and poisoning, conceivably hidden suicides, the SMR was 5.6. A follow-up study (Nilsson et al. 2002) examined risk factors for suicide and suicide attempts in 6880 patients with epilepsy. The risk of suicide was increased 9× times in patients with a psychiatric disorder. The risk was increased 10× if the patients were also on an anti-psychotic treatment. In patients with onset of epilepsy before the age of 18, the risk was increased 16× compared to patients with onset after the age of 18 years.

A Russian study (Kalinin and Polianski 2003) on risk factors for suicidal behaviour in patients with epilepsy confirmed that patients with organic affective disorders, personality changes and cognitive deterioration had substantially increased risk of suicide.

An British study examined the frequency of epilepsy in patients admitted due to a suicide attempt during a two-year period. Compared to the prevalence of epilepsy in the background population, the number of suicide attempts in patients with epilepsy increased 5×. Patients with epilepsy had more frequently been in psychiatric treatment and had more suicide attempts compared to the background population. A US study (Mendez et al. 1989) comparing suicide attempts in matched groups, with and without epilepsy, concluded that patients with epilepsy more frequently had borderline personality, psychotic disorders and previous suicide attempts.

## Migraine

A US study (Breslau et al. 1991) compared diagnosed migraine patients, with and without aura, and found an increased risk of suicide attempts with an odds ratio of 3.0 in patients with migraine with aura.

## Brain injuries

All studies on suicidal risk in patients with brain injuries are based on studies on wounded soldiers from the Second World War. These studies do not fulfil the present methodological demands on studies in suicidology. However, they report an increased risk of suicide.

Oquendo et al. (2004) have found that traumatic brain injury is associated with psychiatric illness, suicidal ideation, suicide attempts and completed suicide. The study was retrospective and has to be confirmed in a prospective design.

An Australian study (Simpson and Tate 2005) has examined the importance of demographic, clinical and other parameters in suicidal behaviour in 172 patients with traumatic brain injury. They found that patients with a previous psychiatric disorder and history of abuse had a 21× increased risk of suicidal behaviour compared to patients with no previous psychic disorders or abuse.

## Parkinson's disease

Few studies on suicidal risk in Parkinson's disease (PD) have been performed. In a Danish study (Stenager *et al.* 1994) on 485 patients followed in an outpatient clinic for a little less than 20 years, a reduced risk of suicide was found in males with PD, while the risk in females was the same as in the background population. The low risk was explained as the result of late age at onset and good possibilities for treatment. Only a small number of patients participated, so the results have to be treated with caution. In the study from USA of 144,364 patients with PD were found to be at a 10× reduced risk of suicide, that was reduced 10× compared to the background population (Myslobodsky *et al.* 2001). This study, thus, confirms the results previously found.

## Stroke

In a Danish study (Stenager *et al.* 1998) of 37,869 patients with stroke admitted to hospital and followed up to 17 years, the risk of suicide in females below 60 years of age was increased 13× and in males 6×. Patients older than 60 years had an increased risk of 1.5–2×. Part of the increased risk could be explained by an increased risk of depression in females after a stroke. A recent Danish study (Teasdale and Engberg 2001) confirms the doubled risk of suicide in stroke patients. In patients below 50 years of age, the SMR was 2.85, i.e. lower than in the first study. The risk was the largest in the first five years after diagnosis and in patients discharged after a short admittance.

## Motor neuron disease

A single study (Bak *et al.* 1994) did not find any increased risk of suicide in motor neuron disease. Only 116 patients participated.

## Mental retardation

In recent years, studies on mental retardation have been published. A Swedish study (Gunnell *et al.* 2005) on 987,308 males examined for military service showed that males with low intelligence scores in the psychological tests had 2–3× increased risk of suicide compared to males with high intelligence scores.

On the other hand, a Finnish study (Patja *et al.* 2001) in a population of persons with mental retardation found that females had a risk comparable to the total Finnish population, while males had a lower risk than the background population. Persons who committed suicide had only mild retardation and a psychic disorder. The mental retardation being of different magnitude in these two studies may explain the difference in results.

## Heart and lung disorders

Recent studies on the risk of suicide in patients with cardiac diseases have dealt with whether or not cholesterol-reducing medication increases the risk of suicide and other types of violent deaths in these patients. A US study (Neaton *et al.* 1992) of 350,000 males followed for 12 years found a 1.6× increased risk of suicide in males with low cholesterol count.

In Jacobs' *et al.* (1992) meta-analysis, a similar conclusion was reached. People with low cholesterol level had an increased risk of dying from reasons other than heart disorders, including suicide. Other studies (La Rosa *et al.* 1995) did not find any association between low cholesterol level and mortality from other disorders apart from heart diseases. More studies are needed to reach a reliable conclusion.

Two US studies have estimated the risk of suicide in asthma patients. One study examined suicidal thoughts in 1285 young American patients in the age interval of 9–17 years of age. Patients with asthma had an increased risk of 3× for suicidal thoughts. Controlling for the comorbidity of a psychiatric disorder did not change the result. A study (Goodwin and Eaton 2005) on the association of suicidal thoughts and suicide attempts in patients with asthma, controlling for psychiatric disorders, confirmed the result. Hence, the studies indicate that asthma may increase the risk for suicidal behaviour.

## Bowel disorders

Disorders like Crohn's disease and ulcerative colitis often affect young people and are associated with pains, operations, and discomfort. Crohn's disease is also associated with the risk of depression. An Italian study (Palli *et al.* 1998) showed a non-significant tendency to increased mortality due to suicide in patients with Crohn's disease and ulcerative colitis. A Danish study (Winther *et al.* 2003) found an increased risk of suicide in females with ulcerative colitis. Previous studies found an increased risk of suicide in females with Crohn's disease in the UK (Prior *et al.* 1981). Another English study (Cooke *et al.* 1980) demonstrated an increased risk in both males and females. In conclusion, patients with bowel disorders seem to have an increased risk of suicide.

## Liver transplantations

Liver transplantation implies much strain on the patients, it is also expensive and the number of available organs is small. Candidates for treatment usually display symptoms of depression, anxiety, cognitive disorders and fear of the future. The reported number of suicides has been rare in candidates for liver transplantation. On the other hand, case reports (Riether and Mahler 1994) have indicated an increasing number of patients attempting or committing suicide. Thus, it is important to be aware of the risk for suicide in candidates for liver transplantation. However, the small number of transplantations, and an even smaller number of suicides makes difficult to draw any conclusion as to whether or not patients with liver transplantations have an increased risk of suicide.

## Kidney disorders

The risk of suicide in patients with kidney disorders, and especially in patients with renal failure and kidney transplants, has been studied. Patients with renal failure have an increased risk of suicide (Haenel *et al.* 1980). Methodological difficulties in the studies do not allow an exact estimation of the size of the risk. The studies have not found any difference in the risk in transplanted patients compared to non transplanted patients. Part of the explanation may be that transplanted patients need lifelong medication and they have a risk of renal failure in the transplant.

## Diabetes mellitus

A number of studies have examined the risk of suicide in diabetes mellitus, but only one (Kyvik *et al.* 1994) has dealt satisfactorily with the methodological demands previously described. This is a Danish study of 1682 male patients with diabetes mellitus treated with insulin. Twelve had committed suicide, and the study found that males in the age interval of 20–24 years of age had an increased risk with a SMR of 2.98. The study concluded that the number of suicides may have been underestimated as a large number of patients died from unknown reasons. This problem was later discussed in a German study on mortality in diabetes mellitus (Mulhauser *et al.* 2002).

A number of studies on mortality in diabetes have been performed, primarily European ones (Sartor and Dahlquist 1995; Swerdlow and Jones 1996; Warner *et al.* 1998; Podar *et al.* 2000). The SMR for suicide has not been calculated, but an increased mortality, especially in young diabetics with bad control of the disease, could indicate that some of these deaths are due to suicide.

### Suicide attempts in diabetes mellitus

The frequency of suicide attempts in diabetes mellitus has been discussed frequently. In this disorder, abuse of insulin through self-destructive behaviour can result in an insulin chock. A review of the literature on the abuse of insulin (Kaminer and Robbins 1989) revealed 17 cases of suicide and 80 cases of attempted suicide. The sex ratio was 1:1, the age distribution among the attempters was even, and about 50 per cent of the attempters were repeaters. A study of overdoses of insulin (Gale 1980) found that 4 of 204 episodes were suicide attempts, and holds that suicidal overdoses of insulin are not uncommon. A British study (Jefferys and Volans 1983) of self-poisoning in diabetic patients referred to the National Poisons Service in London in the period 1978 to 1979 found that 64 among 386 diabetic patients used hypoglycaemic drugs. The rest had used other drugs. Among those taking hypoglycaemic drugs, ten died from brain damage. The authors concluded that self-poisoning was common in diabetic patients and suggested toxicological screening in patients with prolonged keto-acidotic coma. A study from the United States has concluded that suicide attempts and suicide with insulin in diabetics are not uncommon (Arem and Zoghbi 1985). However, one must bear in mind that, in certain cases, an overdose of insulin might be a mistake.

## Diseases of locomotory system

The studies have concentrated on arthritis and amputated patients. Studies on the last mentioned group are old and mainly on soldiers from the Second World War. A study by Dorpat and Ripley (1960) from the US based on forensic material found that patients with arthritis had an increased risk of suicide in the order of 2–3 times compared to the background population. Another forensic study (Whitlock 1985) did not find any association between suicide and arthritis. The study was based on 1000 suicides in England and Wales. The frequency of suicides in patients with arthritis was compared with the number of patients with arthritis in the UK. The method is questionable. On the other hand, a Finnish study (Timonen *et al.* 2003) found an association between depression, suicide attempts and suicide in patients with rheumatoid arthritis, and thus confirms the result of the forensic study. A British study of 300 patients with lupus erythematosis disseminatus has indicated that this group of patients may have an increased risk of suicide, especially in patients with neuro-psychiatric symptoms. The SMR was not calculated (Karassa *et al.* 2003).

## Tinnitus

Tinnitus involves an increased risk of depression. An American study has found a life-time prevalence of depression of 62 per cent compared to 21 per cent in a control group (Harrop-Griffiths *et al.* 1987). A study from the UK (Lewis *et al.* 1994) on 28 patients with tinnitus who committed suicide demonstrated that they were predominantly males, elderly and socially isolated. Most had psychiatric disorders (97 per cent), mainly depression (70 per cent). Forty per cent of the suicides were committed within one year after the onset of tinnitus and 50 per cent within two years, indicating that tinnitus was an important risk factor. It was estimated that the risk of suicide was increased compared to the background population. However, SMR was not calculated.

## AIDS

Almost from the start of the AIDS epidemic, it has been discussed whether or not this disorder resulted in an increased risk of suicide. A US study (Marzuk *et al.* 1988) found a 36× increased risk of suicide in males with AIDS compared to controls. The possibilities of treatment have improved considerably since then. Moreover, the social stigmatisation has decreased in the United States. This could be part of the explanation of the reduced risk of suicide reflected in another study from US (Coté *et al.* 1992), which found an increased risk of suicide of 7.4 compared to controls. Another study performed in the US (Marzuk *et al.* 1997) on suicide risk in the HIV positive in the period 1991–93 demonstrated that HIV infection is associated with other risk factors for suicide, such as abuse of narcotics and other social factors.

A review of literature (Komiti *et al.* 2001) from studies in the United States of America, Europe and Australia on suicidal risk in patients with HIV/AIDS concluded that the risk of suicide is the same order as in other chronic somatic disorders. In AIDS, there is an additional problem of psychiatric disorders, abuse and social consequences that are difficult to control for. A US study (Perry *et al.* 1990) on suicide risk in patients tested for HIV showed that both zero-positive and zero-negative patients had suicidal thoughts in the period of waiting for the result of the test, and that the thoughts were resolved in the following two months.

# Conclusion

In this chapter, we have shown that a number of somatic disorders are associated with increased risk of suicidal behaviour. Suicidal behaviour can be considered as the final indicator of a life with insurmountable physical, psychological and social problems. There are fairly robust studies on increased risk of suicide in a number of neurological disorders and cancer, while the studies in cardiac, lung, rheumatologic disorders and other somatic disorders are fewer and far less thorough. A usually well accepted perception of disease as being a biological, psychological, and social process could be expected to be reflected in studies on suicidal behaviour. However, this is not the case. Suicidal behaviour is often considered solely as a psychiatric problem, which is a far too simplistic view (Fredriksen *et al.* 2005). In line with this, studies controlling for psychiatric disorders still show increased risk of suicide in somatic disorders. Signs of depression, anxiety, hopelessness, crisis reaction, pain, previous suicide attempts, suicidal thoughts, complicated social conditions (family situation, work, finance, leisure time) and the waiting time for somatic diagnosis can be signals of increased risk in somatic patients. Prophylactic measures are obviously of importance in somatic disorders. Depression and pain should be treated adequately. Measures to ease the social–medicinal consequences of disease in the patient, involvement of social workers, psychologists and others should take place.

A final point to be made is that despite the fact that the studies have been made on different continents and populations, they do not show significant differences. However, the majority of studies have been conducted in Western Europe, the USA and Australia, which are countries and continents where many similarities as far as social systems, cultural history and religion exist. When more studies emerge from the remaining continents, further differences may be revealed. Today, there is great need for studies from other parts of the world.

## References

Allebeck P, Bolund C, Ringbäck G (1989). Increased suicide rate in cancer patients. *Journal of Clinical Epidemiology*, **42**, 611–616.

Allgulander C and Fisher LD (1990). Clinical predictors of completed suicide and repeated self-poisoning in 8,895 self-poisoning patients. *European Archives of Psychiatrical and Neurological Science*, **239**, 270–276.

Akechi T, Nakano T, Akizuki N et al. (2002). Clinical factors associated with suicidality in cancer patients. *Japan Journal of Clinical Oncology*, **32**, 506–511.

Almquist EW, Bloch M, Brinkman R et al. (1999). A worldwide assessment of the frequency of suicide, suicide attempts, or psychiatric hospitalization after predictive testing for Huntington's disease. *American Journal of Human Genetics*, **64**, 1293–1304.

Arem R and Zogbi W (1985). Insulin overdose in eight patients: insulin pharmacokinetics and review of the literature. *Medicine*, **64**, 323–332.

Bak S, Stenager EN, Stenager E et al. (1994). Suicide in patients with motor neuron disease. *Behavioural Neurology*, **7**, 3–4.

Baliko L, Csala B, Chopf J (2004). Suicide in Hungarian Huntington's disease patients. *Neuroepidemiology*, **23**, 258–260.

Barraclough BM (1987). The suicide rate of epilepsy. *Acta Psychiatrica Scandinavica*, **76**, 339–345.

Breslau N, Davis GC, Andreski P (1991). Migraine, psychiatric disorders and suicide attempts: an epidemiological study of young adults. *Psychiatry Research*, **37**, 11–23.

Brønnum-Hansen H, Stenager E, Stenager EN et al. (2005). Suicide among Danes with multiple sclerosis. *Journal of Neurology. Neurosurgery and Psychiatry*, **76**, 1457–1459.

Cooke WT, Mallas E, Prior P et al. (1980). Chrohn's disease: course, treatment and long-term prognosis. *Quarterly Journal of Medicine*, **49**, 363–384.

Coté TR, Biggar RJ, Dannenberg AL (1992). Risk of suicide among persons with AIDS. A national assessment. *JAMA*, **268**, 2066–2068.

DeLeo D, Scocco P, Marietta P et al. (1999). Physical illness and parasuicide: evidence from the European Parasuicide Interview Schedule (EPSIS) WHO/Euro. *International Journal of Psychiatry Medicin*, **29**, 149–163.

DeVivo Mj, Blask KS, Scott Richards J et al. (1991). Suicide following spinal cord injury. *Paraplegia*, **29**, 620–627.

Dietzfelbinger T, Kurz A, Torhorst A et al. (1991). Körperliche ind seelishe Krankheit als Hintergrund parsuizidalens Verhaltens. In H Wedler and HJ Möller, eds, *Körperliche Krankheit und Suizid*, pp. 101–115. Roderer Verlag, Regensburg.

Dorpat TL and Ripley HS (1960). A study of suicide in the Seattle area. *Comprehensive Psychiatry*, **1**, 349–359.

Druss B and Pincus H (2000). Suicidal ideation and suicide attempts in general medical illnesses. *Archives of Internal Medicine*, **160**, 1522–1526.

Farrer LA (1986). Suicide and attempted suicide in Huntington disease. Implications for preclinical testing of persons at risk. *American Journal of Medical Genetics*, **24**, 305–311.

Feinstein A (2002). An examination of suicidal intent in patients with multiple sclerosis. *Neurology*, **59**, 674–678.

Fishbain DA (1999). The association of chronic pain and suicide. *Seminnars of Clinical Neuropsychiatry*, **4**, 221–227.

Fox BH, Stanek EJ, Boyd SC et al. (1982). Suicide rates among cancer patients in Connecticut. *Journal of Chronic Diseases*, **35**, 89–100.

Frederiksen A, Pedersen LB, Præstekjær SC et al. (2005). *Årsager til Selvmordsforsøg i et Socialpsykologisk og Sociologisk Perspektiv*. Aalborg University, Aalborg.

Fredrikson S, Cheng Q, Jiang GX et al. (2003). Elevated suicide risk among patients with multiple sclerosis in Sweden. *Neuroepidemiology*, **22**, 46–52.

Gale E (1980). Hypoglycaemia. *Clinics in Endocrinology and Metabolism*, **9**, 461–475.

Goodwin RD and Eaton WW (2005). Asthma, suicidal ideation, and suicide attempt: findings from the Baltimore epidemiologic cathment area follow-up. *American Journal of Public Health*, **95**, 717–722.

Goodwinn RD and Marusic A (2004). Asthma and suicidal ideation among youth in the community. *Crisis*, **25**, 99–102.

Gunnell D, Magnusson PK, Rasmussen F (2005). Low intelligence test scores in 18-year-old men and risk of suicide: cohort study. *British Medical Journal*, **22**, 167.

Haenel T, Brunner F, Battegay R (1980). Renal dialysis and suicide. Occurrence in Switzerland and Europe. *Comprehensive Psychiatry*, **21**, 140–154.

Harris EC and Barraclough BM (1994). Suicide as an outcome for medicial disorders. *Medicine*, **73**, 281–296.

Harrop-Griffiths J, Katon W, Bobie R et al. (1987). Chronic tinnitus: association with psychiatric diagnosis. *Journal of Psychosomatic Research*, **31**, 613–621.

Hawton K, Harriss L, Zahl D (2006). Deaths from all causes in a long-term follow-up study of 11583 deliberate self-harm patients. *Psychological Medicine*, **10**, 1–9.

Hawton K and Fagg J (1988). Suicide and other causes of death following attempted suicide. *British Journal of Psychiatry*, **152**, 259–266.

Hawton K, Fagg J, Marsack P (1980). Association between epilepsy and attempted suicide. *Journal of Neurology Neurosurgery and Psychiatry*, **43**, 168–170.

Hem E, Loge JH, Haldorsen T et al. (2004). Suicide risk in cancer patients from 1960–1999. *Journal of Clinical Oncology*, **22**, 4209–4216.

Innos K, Rahu K, Rahu M et al. (2003). Suicides among cancer patients in Estonia: a population-based study. *European Journal of Cancer*, **39**, 2223–2238.

Jacobs D, Blackburn H, Higgins M et al. (1992). Report of the conference on low blood cholesterol mortality associations. *Circulation*, **86**, 1046–1060.

Jefferys DB and Volans GN (1983). Self-poisoning in diabetic patients. *Human Toxicology*, **2**, 345–483.

Juurlink DN, Herrmann N, Szalai JP et al. (2004). Medical illnes and the risk of suicide in the elderly. *Archives of Internal Medicine*, **164**, 1179–1184.

Kalinin VV and Polianskii DA (2003). Suicide risk factors in epileptic patients. *ZH Nevrol Psykhiatr Im SS Korsakova*, **103**, 18–21.

Kaminer Y and Robbins DR (1989). Insulin misuse: a review of an overlooked psychiatric problem. *Psychosomatics*, **30**, 19–24.

Karassa FB, Magliano M, Isenberg DA (2003). Suicide attempts in patients with systemic lupus erythematosus. *Annals of Rheumatological Disieases*, **62**, 58–60.

Kishi Y, Robinson RG, Kosier JT (2001). Suicidal ideation among patients with acute life-threatening physical illness: patients with stroke, traumatic brain injury, myocardial infarction, and spinal cord injury. *Psychosomatics*, **42**, 382–390.

Komiti A, Judd F, Grech P et al. (2001). Suicidal behaviour in people with HIV/AIDS: a review. *Australian and New Zealand Journal of Psychiatry*, **35**, 747–757.

Kontaxakis VP, Christodolou GN, Mavreas VG et al. (1988). Attempted suicide in psychiatric outpatients with concurrent physical illness. *Psychotherapy and Psychosomatics*, **50**, 201–206.

Kyvik K, Stenager EN, Green A et al. (1994). Suicides in men with IDDM. *Diabetes Care*, **17**, 210–212.

LaRosa JC (1995) Cholesterol lowering morbidity and mortality. *Current Opinion in Lipidology*, **6**, 62–65.

Lawrence D, Almeida OP, Hulse GK et al. (2000). Suicide and attempted suicide among older adults in Western Australia. *Psychological Medicine*, **30**, 813–821.

Levi F, Builliard JL, La Vecchia C (1991). Suicide risk among incident cases of cancer in the Swiss Canton Vaud. *Oncology*, **48**, 44–47.

Lewis JE, Stephens SDG, McKenna L (1994). Tinnitus and suicide. *Clinical Otolaryngology*, **19**, 50–54.

Louhivouri KA and Hakama M (1979). Risk of suicide among cancer patients. *American Journal of Epidemiology*, **109**, 59–64.

Macfarlane GJ, McBeth J, Silman AJ (2001). Widespread body pain and mortality: prospective population-based study. *British Medical Journal*, **323**, 662–665.

Marzuk PM, Tardiff K, Leon AC et al. (1997). HIV seroprevalence among suicide victims in New York City, 1991–1993. *American Journal of Psychiatry*, **154**, 1720–1725.

Marzuk PM, Tierney H, Tardiff K et al. (1988). Increased suicide risk of suicide in persons with AIDS. *JAMA*, **259**, 1333–1337.

Mendez MF, Lanska DJ, Manon-Espaillat R et al. (1989). Causative factors for suicide attempts by overdose in epileptics. *Archives of Neurology*, **46**, 1065–1068.

Muhlhauser I, Sawicki PT, Blank M et al. (2002). Reliability of causes of death in persons with Type I diabetes. *Diabetologia*, **45**, 1490–1497.

Myslobodsky M, Lalonde FM, Hicks L (2001). Are patients with Parkinson´s disease suicidal? *Journal of Geriatry, Psychiatry and Neurology*, **143**, 120–124.

Neaton JD, Blackburn H, Jacobs D et al. (1992). Serum cholesterol level and mortality findings for men screened in the Multiple Risk Factor Intervention Trial. *Archives of International Medicine*, **152**, 1490–1500.

Nielsen B, Wang AG, Bille-Brahe U (1990). Attempted suicide in Denmark IV: a five-year follow up. *Acta Psychiatrica Scandinavica*, **81**, 250–254.

Nilsson L, Ahlbom A, Farahmand BY et al. (2002). Risk factors for suicide in epilepsy: a case–control study. *Epilepsia*, **43**, 644–651.

Nilsson L, Tomson T, Farahmand BY et al. (1997). Cause-specific mortality in epilepsy: a cohort study of more than 9,000 patients once hospitalized for epilepsy. *Epilepsia*, **38**, 1062–1068.

Öjehagen A, Regnell G, Träskman-Bendz L (1991). Deliberate self-poisoning: repeaters and non-repeaters admitted to an intensive care unit. *Acta Psychiatrica Scandinavica*, **84**, 266–271.

Oquendo MA, Frieman JH, Grunebaum MF et al. (2004). Suicidal behaviour in mild traumatic brain injury in major depression. *Journal of Nervous and Mental Disease*, 1992, 430–4.

Pajonk FG, Gruenberg KA, Moecke H et al. (2002). Suicides and suicide attempt in emergency medicine. *Crisis*, **23**, 68–73.

Palli D, Trallori G, Saieva C et al. (1998). General and cancer specific mortality of a population based cohort of patients with inflammatory bowel disease: the Florence Study. *Gut*, **42**, 175–179.

Patja K, Iivanainen M, Raitasuo S et al. (2001). Suicide mortality in mental retardation: a 35-year follow-up study. *Acta Psychiatrica Scandinavia*, **103**, 307–311.

Paulsen JS, Hoth KF, Nehl C et al. (2005). Critical periods of suicide risk in Huntington´s disease. *American Journal of Psychiatry*, **162**, 725–731.

Perry S, Jacobsberg L, Fishman B (1990). Suicidal ideation and HIV testing. *JAMA*, **263**, 679–682.

Podar T, Solntsev A, Reunanen A et al. (2000). Mortality in patients with childhood-onset type 1 diabetes in Finland, Estonia, and Lithuania: follow-up of nationwide cohorts. *Diabetes Care*, **23**, 290–294.

Prior P, Gyde S, Cooke WT et al. (1981). Mortality in Chrohn´s disease. *Gastroenterology*, **80**, 307–312.

Riether AM and Mahler E (1994). Suicide in liver transplant patients. *Psychosomatics*, **35**, 574–577.

Ruzicka LT, Choi CY, Sadkowsky K (2005). Medical disorders of suicides in Australia: analysis using a multiple-cause-of-death approach. *Journal of Social Science in Medicine*, **61**, 333–541.

Sadovnick AB, Ebers GC, Paty DW et al. (1985). Causes of death in multiple sclerosis. Canadian *Journal of Neurological Science*, **12**, 189.

Sartor G and Dahlquist G (1995). Short-term mortality in childhood onset insulin-dependent diabetes mellitus: a high frequency of unexpected deaths in bed. *Diabetes Medicine*, **12**, 607–611.

Schoenfeld M, Myers RH, Cupples LA et al. (1984). Increased rate of suicide among patients with Huntington's disease. *Journal of Neurology, Neurosurgery and Psychiatry*, **47**, 1283–1287.

Simpson G and Tate R (2005). Clinical features of suicide attempts after traumatic brain injury. *Journal of Nervous and Mental Disease*, **193**, 680–685.

Stenager EN (1996). *Attempted Suicide. Treatment and Outcome*. Odense University Press, Odense.

Stenager EN, Madsen C, Stenager E et al. (1998). Suicide in stroke patients. An epidemiological study. *British Medical Journal*, **316**, 1206.

Stenager EN and Stenager E (1992). Suicide in patients with neurological diseases. Methodological problems. Literature review. *Archives of Neurology*, **49**, 1296–1303.

Stenager EN and Stenager E (1997). *Disease, Pain and Suicidal Behaviour*. The Haworth Press, New York.

Stenager EN, Stenager E, Koch-Henriksen N et al. (1992). Multiple sclerosis and suicide. An epidemiological study. *Journal of Neurology, Neurosurgery and Psychiatry*, **55**, 542–545.

Stenager EN, Wermuth L, Stenager E et al. (1994). Suicide in patients with Parkinson's disease. *Acta Psychiatrica Scandinavica*, **90**, 70–72.

Storm HH, Christensen N, Jessen OM (1992). Suicides among Danish patients with cancer: 1971 to 1986. *Cancer*, **69**, 1507–1512.

Swerdlow AJ and Jones ME (1996). Mortality during 25 years of follow-up of a cohort with diabetes. *International Journal of Epidemiology*, **25**, 1250–1261.

Tanaka H, Tsukuma H, Masaoka T et al. (1999). Suicide risk among cancer patients: experience at one medical center in Japan 1978–1994. *Japan Journal of Cancer Results*, **90**, 812–817.

Teasdale TW and Engberg AW (2001). Suicide after a stroke: a population study. *Journal of Epidemiological and Community Health*, **55**, 863–866.

Theodoulou M, Harriss L, Hawton K et al. (2005). Pain and deliberate self-harm: an important association. *Journal of Psychosomatic Results*, **58**, 317–320.

Timonen M, Viilo K, Sarkioja T et al. (2003). Suicides in persons suffering from rheumatoid arthritis. *Rheumatology*, **42**, 1571–1572.

Wärn M, Rubenowitz E, Runeson B et al. (2002). Illness burden in elderly suicides. A controlled study. *British Medical Journal*, **324**, 1355–1358.

Warner DP, MCKinney PA, Law GR et al. (1998). Mortality and diabetes from a population-based register in Yorkshire 1978–93. *Archives of Child Disease*, **78**, 435–438.

Wedler H (1991). Körperliche Krankheiten bei Suizidpatienten einer internistischen Abteilung. In H Wedler and HJ Möller, eds, *Körperliche Krankheit und Suizid*, pp. 87–101. Roderer Verlag, Regensburg.

White SJ, McLean AEM, Howland C (1979). Anticonvulsant drugs and cancer, *Lancet*, **2**, 458–461.

Whitlock FA (1985). Suicide and physical illness. In A Roy, ed., *Suicide*, pp. 151–170. Williams & Wilkins, Baltimore.

Winther KV, Jess T, Langholz E et al. (2003). Survival and cause-specific mortality in ulcerative colitis: follow-up of a population-based cohort in Copenhagen County. *Gastroenterology*, **125**, 1576–1582.

Yousaf U, Christensen ML, Engholm G et al. (2005). Suicides among Danish cancer patients 1971–1999. *British Journal of Cancer*, **92**, 995–1000.

# PART 7

# Suicide Risk Assessment

# PART 7A

# Suicide Risk Assessment: Psychometric Measures

# CHAPTER 41

# Measurement of suicidal behaviour with psychometric scales

Per Bech and Suichi Awata

## Abstract

Among the many psychometric scales for assessing suicidal risk and behaviour, only short scales with high clinical validity have been selected. According to clinical focus, the scales have been classified into those including 'fixed' items outside the suicidal process (predictive factors) and 'flexible' items measuring the severity of the current suicidal state.

The SAD PERSONS scale supplemented by the NO HOPE scale are among the valid predictive scales, and the item of suicide severity in the Hamilton Depression Scale or the Paykel Suicidal Ladder are among the valid measurements of current suicidal severity.

The subjective dimension of suicidal thoughts has been especially contrasted against the dimensions of positive psychological well-being as measured by WHO-5. Such short questionnaires have been found important in modern Internet communication, especially with young people. The individual, idiographic approach has also been discussed by selecting individual items from the Reasons for Living Inventory.

## Introduction

The use of psychometric scales for the measurement of suicidal behaviour has, like the use of depression scales, still not become an appropriate routine aspect of patient care among front line mental health clinicians. This situation has been explained by Lam *et al.* (2005) with reference to the two prototypes of clinicians: Dr Gestalt (using a global clinical impression scale) and Dr Scales (who has incorporated the use of rating scales as a routine in the daily clinic). Apparently, the number of Gestalt clinicians is still larger than the number of Scales clinicians. In the assessment of suicidal behaviour it is, however, important to make inquiries about the suicidal process itself by using brief, relevant items to give the patient the impression that the doctor is able to handle positive answers. Capstick (1960) showed that approximately 80 per cent of suicides were actually under the care of their family doctors at the time of the act. Furthermore, online Internet communication has increased the need for brief self-report scales.

There are many scales for the measurement of suicidal behaviour. In this chapter, these scales will be evaluated by functional analyses

as proposed by Emmelkamp (2004). According to this proposal, we can speak about macroanalysis and microanalysis of rating scales. Macroanalysis focuses on the external factors of a scale relevant for the prediction of suicidal risk, while microanalysis focuses on the suicidal behaviour as a process in itself.

In these functional analyses of scales for the measurement of suicidal behaviour, we have tried to select simple and brief scales to be used in the setting of the daily clinic or on the Internet. Many of the scales for the measurement of suicidal behaviour have been developed with too many items to fulfil the classical psychometric criteria of internal consistency, which Feinstein (1987) has referred to as the 'psychosocial' investigator error. Such investigators lack sufficient clinical experience when they select scale items and they are, therefore, fascinated by the coefficient of consistency, which depends on the number of items in a rating scale: more items, higher coefficients (Feinstein 1987). In this chapter, the brief scales selected by the functional analyses should obviously have a high degree of clinical validity, i.e. they should cover the relevant domains of the dimension under investigation (e.g. suicide risk). Validity, thus, essentially refers to clinical validity. However, when measuring clinical states such as depression or suicidal behaviour, the epistemological process of validation, i.e. to what degree the total score of the items is a sufficient measure (Borsboom 2005), is scientifically also very important. To validate, in other words, is to evaluate psychometrically that, for instance, a higher total score signifies a higher risk of suicide.

The reliability of psychometric scales depends on their administration. Interview or clinician-rated scales should be tested for inter-rater reliability while self-reported questionnaires can be tested for intra-individual reliability by a test–retest coefficient. Finally, an approach to measure individual quality of life (the idiographic approach) will be included.

## Macro-analysis: suicide risk scales

When reviewing the psychometric scales originally developed for the measurement of the prediction of suicidal behaviour, Bürk *et al.* (1985) identified only two short scales: the Risk of Repetition Scale, which relatively heavily relies on the evidence of mental disorder

(Buglasz and Horton 1974), and the Post-attempt Risk Assessment Scale ('Short Risk Scale'), which places the greatest weight on previous suicide attempts (Pallis *et al.* 1982, 1984). This scale has a lower sensitivity and specificy than the SAD PERSON Scale.

Table 41.1 shows the SAD PERSONS scale (Patterson *et al.* 1983). Its modified version was validated by Hocksberger and Rothberg (1988), who showed a sensitivity of 93 per cent and a specificity of 74 per cent when it was used as a screening instrument for the need of hospitalization due to suicidal risk. The standardization (Table 41.1) is from Goldberg and Murray (2006).

It is very difficult to locate comparable psychometric characteristics for making an adequate conclusion as to these suicide prediction scales (Rothberg and Geer-Willimas 1992). In the daily clinical work, the SAD PERSONS, however, seems to cover the highest clinical validity within the limits of a brief scale, i.e. with around 10 items. The items are checklist items, i.e. scored as present or non-present. A proper psychometric validation of this scale is still lacking.

## Micro-analysis: the measurement of the suicidal process

According to Emmelkamp (2004), the micro-analysis of psychometric scales is an attempt to evaluate whether the total scale score is a sufficient measure of severity, e.g. of the suicidal state, which is considered to range from some doubtful, presuicidal signs or symptoms to the completed suicide seen as the end point of the process. This type of analysis, as discussed by Faravelli (2004), is based on certain assumptions:

1  The current state is the sum of its symptoms;

2  The symptoms are represented by numbers associated with specific thoughts and feelings;

3  Operations conducted statistically on these numbers reflect actual changes in the clinical reality;

4  The relationship among the numbers is represented by a simple additive effect, regardless of reciprocal interactions.

**Table 41.1** The SAD PERSONS Scale for assessing the risk of suicide (Patterson *et al.* 1983; Goldberg and Murray 2006)

| Acronym and domain (if present score 1) | | Score |
|---|---|---|
| **S**ex: Male | (0–1) | |
| **A**ge: Younger than 20 or older than 45 years | (0–1) | |
| **D**epression | (0–1) | |
| **P**revious attempts | (0–1) | |
| **E**thanol abuse | (0–1) | |
| **R**ational thinking loss, e.g. organic brain syndrome, affective disorders, schizophrenia | (0–1) | |
| **S**ocial support lacking | (0–1) | |
| **O**rganized plan for suicide | (0–1) | |
| **N**o spouse or not living with relation | (0–1) | |
| **S**ickness, poor physical health | (0–1) | |
| Total score | (0–10) | |

Standardization: total score 0–2, low risk; 3–4, moderate risk (close monitoring as outpatient, consider admission); 5–6, high risk (admission is advised); 7–10, very high risk of suicide (admission required).

**Table 41.2** The Suicidal Ladder (Paykel *et al.* 1974). Start with the step number 1, then step 2, etc. It is pertinent to specify the timeframe, e.g. 2 weeks, 2 months, 6 months, 12 months or lifetime

| 5 | Have you ever made an attempt to take your life? |
|---|---|
| 4 | Have you ever reached the point where you seriously considered taking your life, or perhaps make plans how you would go about doing it? |
| 3 | Have you ever thought of taking your life, even if you would not really do it? |
| 2 | Have you ever wished you were dead?—for instance, that you could go to sleep and not wake up? |
| 1 | Have you ever felt that life was not worth living? |

Source: Paykel ES, Myers JK, Lindenthal JJ, *et al.* (1974). Suidical feelings in the general population: a prevalence study. *British Journal of Psychiatry*, **124**, 460–469.

### Dr Gestalt and Dr Scales

One of the few examples identified by Borsboom (2005) linking variation in clinical states to variation in observed measurement outcome, i.e. fulfilling the assumption by Faravelli, is the domain of mood. Thus, the dimension of depression as well as the suicidal state refer to the same items within an individual patient at different periods as well as between different patients. These assumptions are the very focus of the dialogue between Dr Gestalt and Dr Scales, as outlined by Lam *et al.* (2005). However, in Faravelli's discussion, Dr Gestalt is a very experienced psychiatrist, in contrast to Dr Scales, while in Lam's discussion Dr Scales is as experienced as Dr Gestalt. The balanced approach of Lam *et al.* (2005) is used in the following.

It is a serious pitfall to believe that the use of a suicide rating scale is an attempt to replace the experienced clinician by a young and inexperienced clinician. In this context, it is important to be aware of the instructions for the Clinical Global Impression Scale (CGI) by Guy (1976). When using the CGI, the interviewer has to make his or her assessment on the basis of previous experiences with the category of patients under examination, e.g. the suicidal person. Thus, with reference to acquaintance, the clinician should make the comparison with other persons with suicidal risk he or she has previously treated.

As discussed by Ottosson, the suicidal process 'can be established with a reasonable degree of accuracy provided a good doctor-patient relationship is established and the right questions put to the patient' (Ottosson 1979, p. 264). Ottosson recommends the use of the 'Suicidal Ladder', as published by Paykel *et al.* (1974), which is shown in Table 41.2. Moreover, Ottosson emphasizes that whereas suicidal risk often is taken into account in depressed patients, it is not considered with the same regularity in other cases, e.g. the mixed bipolar state (Fagiolini *et al.* 2004; Hawton *et al.* 2005).

### The 'Suicidal Ladder'

The 'Suicidal Ladder' as shown in Table 41.2 is a five-item hierarchy of questions (Paykel *et al.* 1974). By validation of the interrelationships of the data collected in a general population sample it was shown that subjects who reported being on a higher step of the ladder also reported having been on the steps below (Paykel *et al.* 1974). In other words, the scale follows the performance of mounting a ladder. Thus, 3.5 per cent of the subjects felt that life was not worth living; 2.8 per cent wished themselves dead; 1.0 per cent had thought of taking their lives; and 0.6 per cent had made a suicide attempt over the past year. Thereby, Paykel *et al.* (1974) had confirmed that the five items in Table 41.2 are additive in Faravelli's sense (Faravelli 2004), i.e. the individual items can be rank-ordered consistently according to their relation to the severity of the suicidal process. This implies that scoring of lower prevalence items (higher number on the ladder in Table 41.2) presupposes scorings on higher prevalence items (lower number on the ladder in Table 41.2). Thus, a score on number 4 (thoughts of ending life) has to be preceded by scores on numbers 3, 2 and 1.

## The Hamilton Depression Scale, suicide item

The most adequate statistical analysis based on this criterion of additivity is the item response theory model (Licht *et al.* 2005). This psychometric analysis has been the most frequently analysis used to evaluate the Hamilton Depression Scale (HAM-D). The results, when reviewing all studies from 1980 to 2003 with this scale have shown that the item of suicide in the HAM-D should be analysed separately, as it has no clear additive interaction with the core items of depression (Bagby *et al.* 2004), even though it has no reciprocal interaction (Licht *et al.* 2005) as have anxiety items such as agitation, hypochondriasis and somatic anxiety (Grunebaum *et al.* 2005).

Table 41.3 shows the HAM-D suicide item in the version accepted by Hamilton (Bech *et al.* 1986). When used separately, the inter-rater reliability of the HAM-D item of suicide (which follows the Suicide Ladder in Table 41.2 very closely) has obtained a coefficient of 0.92 (Reynolds 1991). The predictive validity of the HAM-D suicide item has been investigated in a prospective study of risk factors in psychiatric outpatients, and the results showed that patients with a score of 2 or higher were 4.9 times (95 per cent confidence interval 2.7–9.0) were more likely to commit suicide than patients who score less than 2 (Brown 2004).

According to Carlat's practical interviewing form (Carlat 2005), it is essential to make not only the HAM-D suicide item assessment covering the past week or past 3 days, as conventionally recommended (Bech *et al.* 1986), but to elicit information concerning the past two months to explore what has kept the person from killing himself. Many desperate patients remain opposed to suicide for specific reasons, often because they have dependent children or religious considerations as discussed by Carlat (2005).

In the American version of the HAM-D, as published by Guy (1976), the spontaneous mentioning of a symptom is regarded as indicating greater severity of depression than if it had been elicited by questioning. This approach was criticised by Max Hamilton himself (Bech 2002): 'There are many reasons why patients may not mention a symptom at an interview. For example, they may not think it is relevant, they may be embarrassed or they may be too polite.' As recommended by Carlat (2005) 'By inquiring specifically about common suicidal behaviour, you are giving patients permission to be truthful and communicating, that you're familiar with this difficult topic and won't be put off by a positive answer.' There exists now a patient-related questionnaire of the HAM-D (Bent-Hansen *et al.* 1995) and the 'Suicide Ladder' has been used in a self-reported version (Meneese and Yutrzenko 1990).

## The additivity of the items and prediction of suicide

The additivity of the items in the clinician version of the Suicidal Ladder has been confirmed in a population sample of 85-year-olds (Skoog *et al.* 1990). The Suicidal Ladder is an individual item of Paykel's Clinical Interview for Depression (CID) (Paykel 1985). In the CID, the item of suicidal tendencies goes from 1 = absent to 7 = suicidal attempt. In the SADS (Schedule for Affective Disorders and Schizophrenia), item 246 is similar to the CID item of suicidal tendencies (Spitzer and Endicott 1997). In a study of clinical predictors of suicide in primary major depression it has recently been shown that this SADS item by far was the most robust predictor of eventual suicide (Coryell and Young 2005). In a recent prospective study of risk factors for attempted suicide among patients with DSM-IV major depression, it was shown that total time spent in major depression episodes was the most robust predictor, and the authors therefore concluded that reducing time spent depressed is a credible preventive measure (Sokero *et al.* 2005). The authors have used the total Hamilton Depression Scale (i.e. the summed score of all 17 items, HAM-D$_{17}$) for the measurement of depressive states. However, as this scale includes an item of suicidal ideation (Table 41.3) and as the difference between the patient groups 'no suicide attempt' and 'suicide attempt' was 18.6 versus 23.8 (mean scores) on the HAM-D$_{17}$, it might well be that the authors have been arguing in a circle. This study illustrates the importance of measuring severity of depression with a unidimensional scale such as the HAM-D$_6$ in which the item of suicide has been excluded. This approach has been used by Fountoulakis *et al.* (2004), who showed that depressed patients without thoughts of death scored 7.9 on HAM-D$_6$, while those with death thoughts, but without suicidal ideation, scored 10.7, and those with specific thoughts of suicide scored 13.1. Thereby, the HAM-D$_6$ discriminated significantly (p <0.05) between these three groups of patients, and a score of 9 or more indicates treatable major depression, while a score of 12 or more indicates severe major depression requiring more intensive care.

## The scale for suicide ideation

While the Suicidal Ladder (Table 41.2) is a five-item scale, the item of suicidal tendencies in CID, SADS or HAM-D is constructed as one global item. The most frequently used interview-based scale with more than five items is the Scale for Suicide Ideation (SSI) developed by Beck *et al.* (1979). It contains 19 items, each of which can be scored from 0 to 2, and the theoretical total score therefore ranges from 0 to 38. The higher the scores, the more suicidal thoughts. The original version covers current suicidal ideation (SSI-C).

The inter-rater reliability of the SSI-C is adequate, and the internal consistency is apparently high (Cronbach's coefficient alpha 0.89). However, as shown by Feinstein (1987), this coefficient depends on the number of items and is not an expression of additivity in

**Table 41.3** HAM-D suicide item (Bech *et al.* 1986)

| | |
|---|---|
| 0 | No suicidal thoughts |
| 1 | The patient feels that life is not worthwhile, but he expresses no wish to die |
| 2 | The patient wishes to die, but has no plans for taking his own life |
| 3 | It is problable that the patient contemplates committing suicide |
| 4 | If during the days prior to the interview the patient has tried to commit suicide or if the patient is under special observation due to suicide risk |

the sense of Faravelli (2004). This implies that many items are redundant. In a psychiatric outpatient setting (Beck *et al.* 1997) found that the SSI-C represents two dimensions of which 'preparation' includes 9 items and 'motivation' 8 items.

In 1999, Beck *et al.* (1999) published the Scale for Suicide Ideation including a measure of suicidal thoughts at the worst point in the patient's life (SSI-W). In this prospective study (Beck *et al.* 1999), it was found that psychiatric patients who scored in the high risk category (i.e. an SSI-W total score higher than 14) were over 10 times more likely to commit suicide than patients scoring in the lower risk category. The SSI-W has also been found significantly associated with the suicidal item of the HAM-D (Brown 2004). The SSI-W is an attempt to make a chronological assessment of suicide as recommended by (Carlat 2005), by eliciting information about any suicidal event across time.

### The Beck Hopelessness scale

Beck's work with the cognitive aspects of suicide and depression (e.g. the negative triad of viewing past, present and future as very dark) has suggested that hopelessness may be an even better indicator of suicidal behaviour than the severity of depressive mood (Brown 2004). With this background the Beck Hopelessness Scale (BHS) was developed (Beck *et al.* 1974), and this is one of the most frequently used self-reported questionnaires for the measurement of the suicidal process. The scale consists of 20 items, each of which is rated true of false. Thus, the total score has a theoretical range from 0 to 20, and people with a score of 10 or more have a high risk of suicide. However, the false positive rate is extremely high, even when using a score of 17 or more.

The internal consistency in terms of Cronbach's coefficient alpha is extremely high, indicating that many items are redundant. This was shown by Aish and Wasserman (2001) by using confirmative factor analysis. They found that one single item explained most of the variance: 'My future seems dark to me.' This item is directly derived from the negative triad of depression according to the cognitive therapy of depression and should rather be considered as a measure of depressed mood. Thus, hopelessness is included in the HAM-D item of depressed mood (Bech *et al.* 1986; Bech 2006).

### The No Hope scale

When exploring clinical factors in the suicidal process, Shea (1988) found the SAD PERSONS Scale (Table 41.1) very useful, but has made a supplemental scale for the more thorough evaluation of suicide potential with reference to hopelessness by the acronym NO HOPE, as shown in Table 41.4.

In the acute patient care, a higher score on the NO HOPE Scale is an indicator for considering hospitalization, similar to the SAD PERSONS Scale (Table 41.1). As discussed by Shea (1988), patients seem to kill themselves for one major reason, namely to escape what to them appears an inescapable pain. Feelings of hopelessness are obviously to be found in the items at the top of the NO HOPE Scale as listed in Table 41.4. This feeling overlaps the emotions covered by Frank's concept of demoralization as found in distressed persons who are 'unable to cope with some pressing problems. They feel powerless to change the situation themselves. Their life space is constricted' (Frank and Frank 1993, p. 35).

The excuses for dying are an important item to explore during the interview, asking the person about what has kept them from

**Table 41.4** The NO HOPE Scale modified after Shea (1988)

| Acronym and domain (if present score 1) | Score |
|---|---|
| **N**o framework for meaning | (0–1) |
| **O**vert change in clinical condition | (0–1) |
| **H**ostile interpersonal environment | (0–1) |
| **O**ut of hospital recently | (0–1) |
| **P**redisposing personal factors | (0–1) |
| **E**xcuses for dying are present and strongly believed | (0–1) |
| Total score | (0–6) |

killing themselves when the suicidal ideation was present some weeks ago. Analogously to the Bradburn Affect Balance Scale (Bradburn 1969), which measures both positive and negative well-being, attempts, have been made to measure both positive and negative suicide ideation (Osman and Gutierez 1988).

## Positive and negative well-being. The quality of life or the reason for living

From a rating scale point of view, psychological well-being is considered a core dimension of health-related quality of life. This is a subjective experience to such an extent that only self-report scales seem applicable (Bech 1998a). The most frequently used scale based on the Affect Balance Scale (Bradburn 1969) is the Psychological General Well-Being Scale, from which the WHO-Five Well-Being Index (WHO-5) has been developed (Bech *et al.* 2003).

Thus, the dialogue between Dr Gestalt and Dr Scales, when measuring well-being or reason for living, has by the subjective quality of life dimension to be expanded to a third person, 'Dr Self-Ratings', i.e. the patient themself. Quality of life has been defined as being what the patient says it is (Joyce 1987), i.e the patient is considered the expert. The impact of quality of life on the doctor–patient relationship is hopefully able to open a dialogue between them.

### The WHO-Five Well-Being Index

Table 41.5 shows the WHO-Five Well-Being Index together with the five suicide items identified by Paykel *et al.* (1974), including the suggestions made by Meehan *et al.* (1992). These two questionnaires are considered opposite poles of the bipolar well-being factor. The five suicide items were shown to be additive, and item response theory models have shown that the WHO-Five Well-Being Index is an unidimensional scale, i.e. the total score is a sufficient statistic (Bech 2006). In a recent study, with the Japanese version of WHO-5, it was shown that the WHO-5-J has a sensitivity of 75 per cent, and a specificity of 76 per cent in predicting suicide ideation (Awata et al. 2007). Compared to self-rating depression questionnaires, the WHO-5-J was found superior (Awata *et al.* 2007) in predicting suicide behaviour.

In a German study in the primary care setting, when screening patients with major depression, the WHO-5 was found superior to the General Health Questionnaire and a specific depression questionnaire (Henkel *et al.* 2003). Although, it is the more severely depressed persons who make contact with their family doctors (Angst 1998), and therefore have a higher risk of suicide (Sokero *et al.* 2005) than those who have no contact during the depressive

**Table 41.5** The WHO-Five and the Suicide-Five indices WHO-Five Well-Being Index

| Over the last two weeks | All of the time | Most of the time | More than half of the time | Less than half of the time | Some of the time | At no time |
|---|---|---|---|---|---|---|
| 1 I have felt cheerful and in good spirits | 5 | 4 | 3 | 2 | 1 | 0 |
| 2 I have felt calm and relaxed | 5 | 4 | 3 | 2 | 1 | 0 |
| 3 I have felt active and vigorous | 5 | 4 | 3 | 2 | 1 | 0 |
| 4 I woke up feeling fresh and rested | 5 | 4 | 3 | 2 | 1 | 0 |
| 5 My daily life has been filled with things that interest me | 5 | 4 | 3 | 2 | 1 | 0 |

**The suicide-five index**

| Over the last two weeks | All of the time | Most of the time | More than half of the time | Less than half of the time | Some of the time | At no time |
|---|---|---|---|---|---|---|
| 1 I have felt that life is not worth living | 5 | 4 | 3 | 2 | 1 | 0 |
| 2 I have felt I would be better off dead | 5 | 4 | 3 | 2 | 1 | 0 |
| 3 I have been occupied by thoughts of ending my life | 5 | 4 | 3 | 2 | 1 | 0 |
| 4 I have had thoughts of specific ways to take my life | 5 | 4 | 3 | 2 | 1 | 0 |
| 5 I have been at the edge of trying to hurt myself for ending my life | 5 | 4 | 3 | 2 | 1 | 0 |

episode with their family doctors, it is important to realize that lack of social contact (introversion) is, in itself, a symptom of depression. The online Internet use of self-report well-being scales has increased the proportion of depressed persons (especially in the younger generation) seeking help through their family doctors. Thus, the Internet has shown the potential of providing self-help interventions to people who do not seek for help against depression (Christensen and Griffiths 2002). In a study delivering interventions for depression by using the Internet, the Center for Epidemiologic Studies Depression Questionnaire (CES-D) was the scale for measurement of depression (Christensen *et al.* 2004). However, the CES-D includes no item for suicidal ideation. In community studies, the Beck Depression Inventory (BDI) has been found much less user-friendly than CES-D, not because of the item of suicidal thoughts, but because of its item content and layout in general (Naughton and Wiklund 1993).

## The Reasons for Living Inventory

Table 41.6 shows a brief version of the Reasons for Living Inventory. This questionnaire was developed by Linehan *et al.* (1983) with reference to the cognitive–behavioural view of suicidal behaviour, focusing on the factors that differentiate suicidal from non-suicidal persons. It might also be considered intra-individually as discussed by Carlat (2005) and Shea (1988) when comparing suicidal thoughts of two months ago with the current state. The original version of the Reasons for Living Inventory includes 48 items and factor analysis identified 6 factors: survival and coping beliefs, responsibility to family, child-related concerns, fear of suicide, fear of social disapproval, and moral objection. The selection of items shown in Table 41.6 includes only items from the factor of survival and coping beliefs, because these items refer directly to the positive pole of the bipolar well-being dimension, while suicidal ideation is the negative one.

The selected items of the Reasons for Living Inventory (Table 41.6) are an illustration of the eudaimonic approach to psychological well-being, while WHO-5 represents the hedonic approach. According to Ryan and Deci (2001), the eudaimonic approach to psychological well-being refers to the degree to which a person masters life, while the hedonic approach refers to the current degree of happiness the person is feeling.

In a recent review by one of the co-authors of the Reasons for Living Inventory (Chiles and Strosahl 2005), selection of several of the items in the inventory, during an interview with the suicidal patient, is recommended. The philosophy behind the scale has

**Table 41.6** Reasons for Living Inventory selected items from the survival and coping beliefs subscale. The original item number is shown in () brackets and the version by Chiles JA, and Strosahl KD (2005) in [] brackets

| (2) | I believe I can learn to adjust or cope with my problems [15] | [tick box] |
|---|---|---|
| (3) | I believe I have control over my life and destiny [23] | [tick box] |
| (12) | Life is all we have and it is better than nothing [22] | [tick box] |
| (13) | I have plans I am looking forward to carrying out [19] | [tick box] |
| (35) | I still have many things left to do [3] | [tick box] |
| (37) | I am happy and content with my life [12] | [tick box] |
| (40) | I have hope that things will improve and the future will be happier [4] | [tick box] |
| (44) | I believe that I can find a purpose in life, a reason to live [8] | [tick box] |
| | Total | 000 |

At each item, put a number to indicate the importance to you of each for not killing yourself. A score of less than 4 should be considered for suicidal risk.

1 = Not at all important

2 = Quite unimportant

3 = Somewhat unimportant

4 = Somewhat important

5 = Quite important

6 = Extremely important

been that suicide is one way of solving problems, but that there are usually better ways: 'As a clinician, always try to understand the totality of the patient's views of suicide and then reinforce the positive side of suicidal ambivalence.' The items selected in Table 41.6 are an attempt to reinforce the positively worded items of the full scale, while still taking into account that quality of life assessments are to reflect the total situation.

As shown in Table 41.6, a score of less than 4 on the individual items is an indication of suicidal risk (Schutte and Malouff 1995).

## Quality of life—a subjective measure

Because quality of life is a subjective measure, the use of standard questionnaires with fixed item categories may be unable to capture the unique problem for the individual patient in terms of reasons for living or quality of life (Bech 1998b). The best way to describe this idiographic approach has been illustrated by Eysenck, not when he developed his personality questionnaires, but when he published his autobiography, in which he says:

> In writing one's autobiography, one inevitably has to take the idiographic path of trying to see regularities in one's own life, look for behaviour patterns that repeat themselves, and try to discover variables that are important for oneself, even though they might not be of general interest.
>
> Eysenck (1990, p. 3)

The repertory grid model has been used to measure idiographic or individual quality of life. In suicide research, the religious dimension has been identified as an important area in the prevention of suicide behaviour (Kehoe and Gutheil 1994). This was confirmed in a review which systematically evaluated the negative association between religion and suicide (Neeleman *et al.* 1997). The idiographic approach is by self-rating to elicit what is of importance to the individual patient, although it might not be of importance to other patients, even though they all have suicidal ideation in common.

## Conclusion

The psychometric approach to measuring suicidal behaviour has been focusing on short scales with high clinical validity.

According to clinical focus, the scales were classified into those including a predicitve factor of suicidal behaviour outside the suicide process (through macro-analysis) and those measuring the suicidal process itself (through micro-analysis).

The scale selected by macroanalysis was the SAD PERSONS scale, which in the diagnostic process provides the predictors most relevant for the acute care of the suicidal patient.

Among the scales measuring the severity of the suicidal process itself, micro-analysis has identified the Paykel scale, i.e. the Suicidal Ladder, as being the most valid one, but the individual suicidal items on the HAM-D or the SADS have also been considered. As clinical depression in itself is a robust predictor of suicide risk, a brief depression scale such as the HAM-D$_6$ is of great relevance. Because hopelessness is a core feature of depression, the NO HOPE scale also has been recommended in this context.

As the subjective dimension is most important when measuring well-being or reason for living, brief self-rating scales have also been recommended. As modern equivalents to the Bradburn Affect Balance Scale, the WHO-Five Well-being Index and the Suicide-Five Index, based on Paykel's Ladder, are recommended. This approach is important when trying to capture those persons who in their depressive state can only use the Internet for communication.

As a consequence of the subjective approach to measuring the suicidal process, idiographic self-ratings have been discussed, i.e. the individual measurement of what is of importance and constitutes a reason for living to one patient, but possibly not to others, even though all of them have suicidal ideation in common.

## References

Aish A-M, Wasserman D (2001). Does Beck's Hopelessness Scale really measure several components? *Psychological Medicine*, **31**, 367–372.

Angst J (1998). Treated contra untreated major depressive episodes. *Psychopathology*, **31**, 37–44.

Awata S, Bech P, Koizumi Y *et al.* (2007). Validity of the Japanese version of the WHO-Five Well-Being Index in the context of detecting suicide risk in elderly community residents. *International Psychogeriatrics*, **19**, 77–88.

Bagby RM, Ryder AG, Schuller DR *et al.* (2004). The Hamilton Depression Rating Scale: has the gold standard become a lead weight? *American Journal of Psychiatry*, **161**, 2163–2177.

Bech P (1998a). *Quality of Life in the Psychiatric Patient*. Mosby-Wolfe, London.

Bech P (1998b). Quality of life measurements in chronic disorders. In GA Fava and H Freyberger, eds, *Handbook of Psychosomatic Medicine*, pp. 205–222. International University Press, Madison.

Bech P (2002). The Bech–Rafaelsen Melancholia Scale (MES) in clinical trials of therapies in depressive disorders: a 20-year review of its use as outcome measure. *Acta Psychiatrica Scandinavica*, **106**, 252–264.

Bech P (2004). Modern psychometrics in clinimetrics: impact on clinical trials of antidepressants. *Psychotherapy and Psychosomatics*, **73**, 134–138.

Bech P (2006). Rating scales in depression: limitations and pitfalls. *Dialogues in Clinical Neuroscience*, **8**, 207–215.

Bech P, Andersen MB, Bech-Andersen G (2005). Work-related stressors, depression and quality of life in Danish managers. *European Psychiatry*, **20**(Suppl 3), 318–324.

Bech P, Kastrup M, Rafaelsen OJ (1986). Mini-compendium of rating scales for states of anxiety, depression, mania, schizophrenia with corresponding DSM-III syndromes. *Acta Psychiatrica Scandinavica*, **326**, 7–37.

Bech P, Olsen RL, Kjoller M *et al.* (2003). Measuring well-being rather than the absence of distress symptoms: a comparison of the SF-36 Mental Health subscale and the WHO-Five Well-Being Scale. *International Journal of Methods in Psychiatric Research*, **12**, 85–91.

Beck AT (1979). Assessment of suicidal intention: the Scale for Suicide Ideation. *Journal of Consulting and Clinical Psychology*, **47**, 343–352.

Beck AT, Brown GK, Steer RA (1997). Psychometric characteristics of the Scale for Suicide Ideation with psychiatric outpatients. *Behaviour Research and Therapy*, **35**, 1039–1046.

Beck AT, Brown GK, Steer RA (1999). Suicide ideation at its worst point: a predictor of eventual suicide in psychiatric outpatients. *Suicide and Life-Threatening Behaviour*, **29**, 1–9.

Beck AT, Weissman A, Lester D *et al.* (1974). The measurement of pessimism: the hopelessness scale. *Journal of Consulting and Clinical Psychology*, **42**, 861–865.

Bent-Hansen J, Lauritzen L, Clemmensen L *et al.* (1995). A definite and semi-definite questionnaire version of the Hamilton/ Melancholia Scale. *Journal of Affective Disorders*, **33**, 143–150.

Borsboom D (2005). *Measuring the Mind. Conceptual Issues in Contemporary Psychometrics*. Cambridge University Press, Cambridge.

Bradburn NM (1969). *The Structure of Well-being*. Aldine, Chicago.

Brown GK (2004). *A Review of Suicide Assessment Measures for Intervention Research with Adults and Older Adults*. Bethesda, NIMH. (http://www.nimh.nih.gov/suicideresearch/adultsuicide.pdf)

Buglasz D and Horton J (1974). A scale for predicting subsequent suicidal behaviour. *British Journal of Psychiatry*, **124**, 573–578.

Bürk F, Kurz A, Möller HJ (1985). Suicide risk scales: do they help to predict suicidal behaviour? *European Archives of Psychiatry and Clinical Neuroscience*, **235**, 153–157.

Capstick A (1960). The recognition of emotional disturbances and the prevention of suicide. *British Medical Journal*, 1179–1181.

Carlat DJ (2005). *The Psychiatric Interview*. Lippincott, Philadelphia.

Chiles JA and Strosahl KD (2005). *Clinical Manual for Assessment and Treatment of Suicidal Patients*. American Psychiatric Publishing, Washington.

Christensen H and Griffiths KM (2002). The prevention of depression using the internet. *Medical Journal of Australia*, **177**, 122–125.

Christensen H, Griffiths KM, Jorm AF (2004). Delivering interventions for depression by using the internet: randomised conrolled trial. *British Medical Journal*, **328**, 265–276.

Coryell W and Young EA (2005). Clinical predictors of suicide in primary major depressive disorder. *Journal of Clinical Psychiatry*, **66**, 412–417.

Emmelkamp PMG (2004). The additional value of clinimetrics needs to be established rather than assumed. *Psychotherapy and Psychosomatics*, **73**, 142–144.

Eysenck HJ (1990). *Rebel with a Cause: An Autobiography*. WH Allen, London.

Fagiolini A, Kupfer DJ, Rucci P *et al.* (2004). Suicide attempts and ideation in patients with bipolar I disorder. *Journal of Clinical Psychiatry*, **65**, 509–514.

Faravelli C (2004). Assessment of psychopathology. *Psychotherapy and Psychosomatics*, **73**, 139–141.

Feinstein AR (1987). *Clinimetrics*. Yale University Press, New Haven.

Fountoulakis KN, Iacovides A, Fotiou F *et al.* (2004). Neurobiological and psychological correlates of suicide attempts and thoughts of death in patients with major depression. *Neuropsychobiology*, **49**, 42–52.

Frank JD and Frank JB (1993). *Persuasion and Healing. A Comparative Study of Psychotherapy*. Johns Hopkins University Press, Baltimore.

Goldberg D and Murray R (2006). *The Maudsley Handbook of Practical Psychiatry*. Oxford University Press, Oxford.

Grunebaum MF, Keilp J, Li S *et al.* (2005). Symptom components of standard depression scales and past suicidal behaviour. *Journal of Affective Disorders*, **87**, 73–82.

Guy W (1976). *Early Clinical Drug Evaluation (ECDEU) Assessment Manual for Psychopharmacology*. National Institute of Mental Health, Rockville.

Henkel V, Mergl R, Kohnen R *et al.* (2003). Identifying depression in primary care: a comparison of different methods in a prospective cohort study. *British Medical Journal*, **326**, 200–201.

Hawton K, Sutton L, Haw C *et al.* (2005). Suicide and attempted suicide in bipolar disorder: a systematic review of risk factors. *Journal of Clinical Psychiatry*, **66**, 693–704.

Hocksberger JM and Rothstein RJ (1988). Assessment of suicide potential by nonpsychiatrists using the SAD PERSONS score. *Journal of Emergency Medicine*, **6**, 99–107.

Joyce CRB (1987). Quality of life. The state of the art in clinical assessment. In SR Walker and RM Rosser, eds, *Quality of Life: Assessment and Application*, pp. 169–179. MTP Press, Lancaster.

Kehoe NC and Gutheil TG (1994). Neglect of religious issues in scale-based assessment of suicidal patients. *Hospital Community Psychiatry*, **45**, 366–369.

Lam RW, Michalak EE, Swinson RP (2005). *Assessment Scales in Depression, Mania and Anxiety*. Taylor and Francis, London.

Licht RW, Qvitzau S, Allerup P *et al.* (2005). Validation of the Bech-Rafaelsen Melancholia Scale and the Hamilton Depression Scale in patients with major depression: is the total score a valid measure of illness severity? *Acta Psychiatrica Scandinavica*, **111**, 144–149.

Linehan MM, Goodstein JL, Nielsen SL *et al.* (1983). Reasons for staying alive when you are thinking of killing yourself: the reasons for living inventory. *Journal of Consulting and Clinical Psychology*, **51**, 276–286.

Meehan PJ, Lamb JA, Saltzman LE *et al.* (1992). Attempted suicide among young adults: progress toward a meaningful estimate of prevalence. *American Journal of Psychiatry*, **149**, 41–44.

Meneese WB and Yutrzenko BA (1990). Correlates of suicidal ideation among rural adolescents. *Suicide and Life-Threatening Behaviour*, **20**, 206–212.

Naughton MJ and Wiklund I (1993). A critical review of dimension-specific measures of health-related quality of life in cross-cultural research. *Quality of Life Research*, **2**, 397–432.

Neeleman J, Halpern D, Leon D *et al.* (1997). Tolerance of suicide, religion and suicide rates: an ecological and individual study in 19 Western countries. *Psychological Medicine*, **27**, 1165–1171.

Osman O and Gutierrez PM (1998). The positive and negative suicidal ideation inventory: development and validation. *Psychological Reports*, **82**, 783–793.

Ottosson J-O (1979). Prevention of suicide. In Schou M and Strömgren E, eds, *Origin, Prevention and Treatment of Affective Disorders*, pp. 257–268. Academic Press, London.

Pallis DJ, Barraclough BM, Levey AB *et al.* (1982). Estimating suicide risk among attempted suicides. I. The development of new clinical scales. *British Journal of Psychiatry*, **141**, 37–44.

Pallis DJ, Gibbons JS, Pierce DW (1984). Estimating suicide risk among attempted suicides. II. Efficiency of predictive scales after the attempt. *British Journal of Psychiatry*, **144**, 139–148.

Patterson WM, Dohn HH, Bird J *et al.* (1983). Evaluation of suicidal patients: the SAD PERSONS scale. *Psychosomatics*, **24**, 343–352.

Paykel ES (1985). The clinical interview for depression. Development, reliability and validity. *Journal of Affective Disorders*, **9**, 85–96.

Paykel ES, Myers JK, Lindenthal JJ *et al.* (1974). Suicidal feelings in the general population: a prevalence study. *British Journal of Psychiatry*, **124**, 460–469.

Reynolds WM (1991). Psychometric characteristics of the Adult Suicidal Ideation Questionnaire in college students. *Journal of Personal Assessment*, **56**, 289–307.

Rothberg JM and Geer-Willimas C (1992). A comparison and review of suicide prediction scales. In RW Maris, AL Berman, JT Maltsberger *et al.*, eds, *Assessment and Prediction of Suicide*, pp. 202–217. Guilford Press, New York.

Ryan RM and Deci EL (2001). On happiness and human potentials: a review of research on hedonic and eudaimonic well-being. *Annual Review of Psychology*, **52**, 141–166.

Schutte NS and Malouff JM (1995). *Sourcebook of Adult Assessment. Applied Clinical Psychology*. Plenum Press, New York.

Shea SC (1988). *Psychiatric Interviewing. The Art of Understanding*. Saunders, Philadelphia.

Skoog I, Aevarsson O, Beskow J *et al.* (1996). Suicidal feelings in a population sample of non-demented 85-year-olds. *American Journal of Psychiatry*, **153**, 1015–1020.

Sokero TP, Melartin TK, Rytsala HJ *et al.* (2005). Prospective study of risk factors for attempted suicide among patients with DSM-IV major depressive disorder. *British Journal of Psychiatry*, **186**, 314–318.

Spitzer RL and Endicott J (1997). *Schedule for Affective Disorders and Schizophrenia* (SADS). Biometric Research, State Psychiatric Institute, New York.

# CHAPTER 42

# Instruments used in SUPRE-MISS

## The WHO Multisite Intervention Study on Suicidal Behaviours

Alexandra Fleischmann, José M Bertolote,
Diego De Leo and Danuta Wasserman

## Abstract

The WHO Multisite Intervention Study on Suicidal Behaviours (SUPRE-MISS) was launched on the five continents to increase knowledge about suicidal behaviours and effective interventions for suicide attempters in culturally diverse places around the globe, with the ultimate goal of reducing mortality and morbidity associated with suicidal behaviours.

The three components of SUPRE-MISS are a community description to grasp basic sociocultural characteristics, a community survey to identify suicidal behaviours, and a randomized controlled trial to evaluate treatment strategies for suicide attempters treated in emergency care settings of the same catchment area. Three specific instruments were used for the three components of the study and commonly applied in all participating sites. These assessment instruments were designed for SUPRE-MISS in particular, partly based on existing instruments and measurements and compiling them. They succeeded in fulfilling the requirements of being applicable across different cultures, manageable in low- and middle-income countries, assessing suicidal behaviours, and comprising well-established and widely recognized predictors of suicidal behaviours.

## Background

In 2000, the World Health Organization (WHO) launched the Multisite Intervention Study on Suicidal Behaviours (SUPRE-MISS) to address the emerging public health problem of attempted suicide. SUPRE-MISS is part of SUPRE, the WHO worldwide initiative for the prevention of suicide, which was launched in 1999, and shares its overall common goal to reduce mortality and morbidity associated with suicidal behaviours.

As attempted suicide is one of the strongest predictors of subsequent completed suicide, it is important to understand it properly, to identify effective interventions for suicide attempters,

and to provide adequate clinical care, in order to ultimately reduce suicide mortality and morbidity (Platt et al., 1992; World Health Organization 2001; Schmidtke et al. 2004). The amount of suffering cannot be underestimated, bearing in mind that every suicide also affects at least five other persons on average (Diekstra et al. 1995).

The rationale of SUPRE-MISS was to increase knowledge of suicidal behaviours, including effective interventions for suicide attempters in culturally diverse places around the globe. The participating sites of SUPRE-MISS represented all six WHO regions, including Campinas (Brazil), Chennai (India), Colombo (Sri Lanka), Durban (South Africa), Hanoi (Viet Nam), Karaj (the Islamic Republic of Iran), Tallinn (Estonia), and Yuncheng (People's Republic of China).

SUPRE-MISS had three components:

1 A randomized controlled trial to evaluate treatment strategies for suicide attempters treated in emergency care settings in defined catchment areas (Fleischmann et al. 2005, 2008);

2 A community survey to identify suicidal ideation and behaviour characteristics in the same catchment areas (Bertolote et al. 2005); and

3 A qualitative community description of the basic sociocultural characteristics of the target communities (Bertolote et al. 2005).

## Sociocultural instrument

Despite a strong interest in sociocultural studies of suicidal behaviour, the research in this area is not well advanced (Desjarlais et al. 1995). While much has been written about international variations of the rates and patterns of suicidal behaviours, little systematic research has been carried out on the specific contribution of sociocultural factors to suicidal behaviours. The absence of a systematic measurement instrument for assessing sociocultural variables across international and cultural settings has been a major obstacle in this effort. However, an international, multisite, collaborative study like SUPRE-MISS provided the opportunity for insights into the complex determinants of suicidal behaviours across different cultures.

Specifically for the purposes of SUPRE-MISS, a sociocultural instrument was developed to grasp the basic sociocultural characteristics of the target communities in participating sites. This instrument was an attempt to assess the sociocultural and community determinants of suicidal behaviour by profiling the culture and community in which the target population lived. It comprised a pool of indices and questions that could be helpful in contextualizing suicidal behaviours and understanding its nature and meaning.

Taking the physical and social environment into consideration, as well as economic, political, religious, communications, social deviancy, and health aspects, both objective (e.g. population density, divorce rates, unemployment rates) and subjective (e.g. perceived level of optimism, gender status and roles, rapid social change) indices were used to contextualize suicidal behaviours culturally (Marsella 1998; Marsella and Yamada 2000; Marsella et al. 2002). The final instrument, which can be accessed at the WHO website (WHO 2002), consists of a large number of sociocultural indices, the assessment of attitudes towards attempted and completed suicide towards those who are left behind after a suicide, and the description of the procedures for the ascertainment of suicide. It was to be completed by an experienced person in the field, e.g. a cultural psychologist, anthropologist, or sociologist. The joint role of these contextual variables and of individual risk factors may explain differences in suicidal behaviours noted between sites; results of multilevel (hierarchical) regression modelling are awaited.

## Community survey and intervention study instruments

Both the community survey and the intervention study of SUPRE-MISS were carried out in the same catchment area of each site. The community survey aimed at identifying suicidal thinking, plans to commit suicide, and suicide attempts in the community, including those people who, for various reasons, did not present themselves at emergency care departments with this specific complaint. All suicide attempters seen at the emergency care departments of the same catchment area were offered an opportunity to participate in the intervention study, which aimed at evaluating different treatment strategies for suicide attempters. The enrolled subjects were randomly assigned to either treatment as usual, according to the norms of the respective emergency care department, or brief intervention and contact, including a one-hour information session and follow-up contacts according to a specific time line up to 18 months after discharge.

The instruments of the SUPRE-MISS community survey and intervention study were largely based on the European Parasuicide Study Interview Schedule (EPSIS) (Kerkhof et al. 1999), which had been applied in the WHO/EURO Multicentre Study on Suicidal Behaviour (Schmidtke et al. 2004). In a WHO meeting of experts, the SUPRE-MISS instruments were discussed and refined. The final instruments (WHO 2002), which were commonly applied across all sites, were translated into the local languages of the sites, and modified to take into account cultural specificities, and then pilot tested.

In order to receive comparable data from the community survey and the intervention study, which were carried out in the same catchment area, the community survey used the same questions as the intervention study questionnaire, regarding sociodemographic information, physical health, contact with health services, mental health, alcohol- and drug-related questions, and family data (i.e. completed or attempted suicide by members of the family related by birth). In addition, the community survey asked questions about community stress and problems. To assess suicidal behaviours, the following questions were asked in the community:

1  'Have you ever seriously thought about committing suicide?'

2  'Have you ever made a plan for committing suicide?'

3  'Have you ever attempted suicide?'

If the answer was 'yes' to any of these questions, further questions were asked, such as 'How old were you the first time this happened?', 'Did this happen to you at all in the last twelve months?', 'How old were you the last time this happened to you?', and the first and last suicide attempt were assessed in more detail.

Community surveys of the general population, asking similar questions about suicidal thoughts, suicide plans and attempts, to pilot and compare with SUPRE-MISS were conducted in Queensland, Australia (De Leo et al. 2005) and Stockholm, Sweden (Ramberg and Wasserman 2000).

The questionnaire of the intervention study was much more extensive. It covered a detailed intake part using hospital data-collection procedures (e.g. routine medical records) already in place, comprising the method of the present suicide attempt (according to ICD-10 codes), physical consequences of the attempt, the type of care received and referral to other services as determined by the medical staff, as well as the most basic sociodemographic information.

The questions that were asked about sociodemographic information, physical health, contact with health services, mental health, alcohol- and drug-related questions, and family data overlapped with the community survey questionnaire. Additional parts of the intervention study questionnaire covered traumatic experiences, psychosocial difficulties, life satisfaction, the opportunity to talk about problems, antisocial behaviour, and the legal or offending history of the patient.

The current suicide attempt was further investigated using the Suicide Intent Scale (Beck et al. 1974a). The assessment of previous suicide attempts included the question 'when the last one occurred' as well as items about the number and methods of previous attempts.

Also, several scales (in full or in part) and measurements were used in the questionnaire of the intervention study, as follows: The WHO (Five) Well Being Index, 1998 version (Bech et al. 2003), the Beck Depression Inventory, revised copyright version 1978 (Beck et al. 1988; Groth-Marnat 1990) of the original (Beck et al. 1961), one item of the Hopelessness Scale, i.e. 'My future seems dark to me' (Beck et al. 1974b; Aish and Wasserman 2001), the Trait Anger Scale (Spielberger 1980), an instrument to measure Social Support (Bille-Brahe et al. 1999; Bille-Brahe and Jensen 2004), and the Social Role Performance instrument, section 2 of the WHO Psychiatric Disability Assessment Schedule (WHO 1988).

Finally, an attempt was made to establish, if applicable, a psychiatric diagnosis for the patients, preferably, according to

ICD-10 or DSM-IV criteria. However, as psychiatric assessment was not routine in the participating sites, not all of the sites could comply with this request. At any rate, a psychological exam was carried out in all sites to provide a minimum of information. The items used for this purpose derived from the second part (Manifest abnormalities) of the Clinical Interview Schedule (CIS), which is a standardized interview, developed in the late 1960s for use in general practice and community settings (Goldberg *et al.* 1970).

The follow-up questions, at the different time points, asked whether the patient was still alive, if not, what the cause of death would have been, if yes, whether any further suicide attempts had been committed, how the patient felt, and whether the patient needed any support. However, at the final follow-up point at 18 months, further questions covered thoughts and plans of suicide, the hopelessness item, and the WHO (Five) Well-Being Index.

When refining and finalizing the SUPRE-MISS instruments, it was of major concern to only keep those instruments that had previously been translated into different languages and validated. Also, the relevance of the measures and items in different cultures was carefully scrutinized. This procedure resulted, for instance, in discarding the Impulsiveness scale (Eysenck and Eysenck 1978) and allowing it as an optional measurement only in those sites where its validity had been demonstrated.

Different legal and logistic reasons made it impossible to keep a biological component as part of the general study, as originally intended. This component was meant to identify biological factors in suicidal behaviours by assessing several biochemical and genetic markers. However, most of the countries participating in the study were not in a position to perform all the biological analyses, particularly those more relevant to the genetic markers. This meant that blood samples would have had to be sent abroad to centres accepting the task of conducting these analyses; but in some countries, the law did not authorize the shipment abroad of biological samples for some analyses (e.g. DNA). Also, given previous contamination of blood samples (particularly with HIV), biological samples from some of the countries could not be accepted by the centres to perform the analyses. Therefore, the biological component was dropped (as originally conceived) and left as an option, both in terms of its inclusion at all and its extent, for those sites in a position to conduct it.

## Conclusion

The SUPRE-MISS instruments (i.e. for the sociocultural description, the community survey, and the intervention study) successfully compiled the most powerful predictors of suicidal behaviours.

For the first time, an instrument to grasp basic sociocultural characteristics of communities around the world was applied. Whereas this instrument would certainly need revision after wider application, it provided the necessary information for using contextual variables to explain differences in suicidal behaviours between sites.

The community survey and intervention study instruments were comprehensive, but not over-inclusive. They represented the best possible compromise of including essential measurements to capture well-established predictors of suicidal behaviours in different places of the world; though not overly time-consuming in their completion, it was manageable even with scarce resources, both financial and personnel (as it was the case in the participating sites of low- and middle-income countries), and at the same time of being relevant to different cultures across the globe.

## References

Aish A and Wasserman D (2001). Does Beck's Hopelessness Scale really measure several components? *Psychological Medicine*, **31**, 367–372.

Bech P, Olsen RL, Kjoller M *et al.* (2003). Measuring well-being rather than the absence of distress symptoms: a comparison of the SF-36 Mental Health subscale and the WHO-Five Well-Being Scale. *International Journal of Methods in Psychiatric Research*, **12**, 85–91.

Beck AT, Schuyler D, Herman I (1974a). Development of suicidal intent scales. In AT Beck, HLP Resnik and DJ Lettieri, eds, *The Prediction of Suicide*, pp. 45–56. Charles Press, Bowie.

Beck AT, Steer RA, Garbin MG (1988). Psychometric properties of the Beck Depression Inventory: twenty-five years of evaluation. *Clinical Psychology Review*, **8**, 77–100.

Beck AT, Ward CH, Mendelson M *et al.* (1961). An inventory for measuring depression. *Archives of General Psychiatry*, **4**, 561–571.

Beck AT, Weissman A, Lester D *et al.* (1974b). The measurement of pessimism: the hopelessness scale. *Journal of Consulting and Clinical Psychology*, **42**, 861–865.

Bertolote JM, Fleischmann A, De Leo D *et al.* (2005). Suicide attempts, plans, and ideation in culturally diverse sites: the WHO SUPRE-MISS community survey. *Psychological Medicine*, **35**, 1457–1465.

Bille-Brahe U, Hegebo H, Crepet P *et al.* (1999). Social support among European suicide attempters. *Archives of Suicide Research*, **5**, 215–231.

Bille-Brahe U and Jensen B (2004). The importance of social support. In D De Leo, U Bille-Brahe, AJFM Kerkhof *et al.*, eds, *Suicidal Behaviour: Theories and Research Findings*, pp. 197–208. Hogrefe and Huber, Göttingen.

De Leo D, Cerin E, Spathonis K *et al.* (2005). Lifetime risk of suicide ideation and attempts in an Australian community: prevalence, suicidal process, and help-seeking behaviour. *Journal of Affective Disorders*, **86**, 215–224.

Desjarlais D, Eisenberg L, Good B *et al.* (1995). *World Mental Health: Problems and Priorities in Low-income Countries*. Oxford University Press, London.

Diekstra RFW, Gulbinat W, Kienhorst I *et al.* (1995). *Preventive Strategies on Suicide*. Brill, Leiden.

Eysenck SBG and Eysenck HJ (1978). Impulsiveness and venturesomeness: their position in a dimensional system of personality description. *Psychological Reports*, **43**, 1247–1255.

Fleischmann A, Bertolote JM, De Leo D *et al.* (2005). Characteristics of attempted suicides seen in emergency care settings of general hospitals in eight low- and middle-income countries. *Psychological Medicine*, **35**, 1467–1474.

Fleischmann A, Bertolote JM, Wasserman D *et al.* (2008). Eeffectiveness of brief intervention and contact for suicide attempters: a randomized controlled trial in five countries. *Bulletin of the World Health Organization*, **86**, 703–709.

Goldberg DP, Cooper B, Eastwood MR *et al.* (1970). A standardised psychiatric interview for use in community surveys. *British Journal of Preventive and Social Medicine*, **24**, 18–23.

Groth-Marnat G (1990). *The Handbook of Psychological Assessment*, 2nd edn. Wiley, New York.

Kerkhof AJFM, Bernasco W, Bille-Brahe U *et al.* (1999). European Parasuicide Study Interview Schedule (EPSIS). In U Bille-Brahe, ed., *Facts and Figures: WHO/EURO*, pp. 1–4. WHO Regional Office for Europe, (WHO/EUR/ICP/PSF), Copenhagen.

Marsella AJ (1998). Urbanization, mental health, and social deviancy: a review of issues and research. *American Psychologist*, **53**, 624–634.

Marsella AJ and Yamada A (2000). Culture and mental health: an introduction and overview of foundations, concepts, and issues. In I Cuellar and F Paniagua, eds, *The Handbook of Multicultural Mental Health: Assessment and Treatment of Diverse Populations*, pp. 3–24. Academic Press, New York.

Marsella AJ, Kaplan A, Suarez E (2002). Cultural considerations for understanding, assessing, and treating depressive experience and disorder. In M Reinecke and M Davison, eds, *Comparative Treatments of Depression*, pp. 47–78. Springer, New York.

Platt S, Bille-Brahe U, Kerkhof A *et al.* (1992). Parasuicide in Europe: the WHO/EURO multicentre study on parasuicide. I. Introduction and preliminary analysis for 1989. *Acta Psychiatrica Scandinavica*, **85**, 97–104.

Ramberg IL and Wasserman D (2000). Prevalence of reported suicidal behaviour in the general population and mental health-care staff. *Psychological Medicine*, **30**, 1189–1196.

Schmidtke A, Bille-Brahe U, De Leo D *et al.* (2004). *Suicidal Behaviour in Europe: Results of the WHO/EURO Multicentre Study on Suicidal Behaviour*. Hogrefe and Huber, Göttingen.

Spielberger CD (1980). Preliminary manual for the State-Trait Anger Scale (STAS). Unpublished manuscript, University of South Florida, Tampa, USA.

World Health Organization (1988). *WHO Psychiatric Disability Assessment Schedule (WHO/DAS)*. World Health Organization, Geneva.

World Health Organization (2001). *The World Health Report 2001: Mental Health: New Understanding, New Hope*. World Health Organization, Geneva.

World Health Organization (2002). *Multisite Intervention Study on Suicidal Behaviours SUPRE-MISS: Protocol of SUPRE-MISS*. World Health Organization, Geneva. Retrieved 3 April 2008 at: http://www.who.int/mental_health/resources/suicide/en/index.html.

# Suicide Risk Assessment: Clinical Measures

# CHAPTER 43

# The clinical interview as a method in suicide risk assessment

Mark Schechter and John T Maltsberger

## Abstract

In this chapter we describe the role of the clinical interview in the assessment of suicide risk. In the course of the interview the clinician must endeavour to understand the patient's crisis from both the 'objective/descriptive' and the 'experiential' perspectives, each of which we describe in detail. A focus on both of these perspectives is critical in the clinician's coming to the best possible understanding of the patient. In addition to the role of the clinical interview in *assessing* risk, this critical clinical interaction is also the beginning of the treatment relationship and crisis intervention; thus it has a role in *reducing* risk as well. Finally, we comment briefly on the clinician's conscious as well as unconscious responses to the patient, or 'countertransference', that can arise in the interview of potentially suicidal patients and influence the clinical assessment.

## Introduction

The clinical interview remains the fundamental instrument in the assessment of suicide risk. In considering this aspect of clinical assessment we discuss the interview as a single encounter, though it may in fact encompass a series of interviews and clinical interactions depending on the clinical situation and venue. We conceptually divide the functions of the interview into what we call the 'objective/descriptive' and the 'experiential' perspectives. The objective/descriptive perspective, commonly given greatest emphasis, is that from which the clinician performs a medically oriented psychiatric evaluation. Equally important, however, is that the clinician also hold the experiential perspective; that is, in addition to observation and gathering objective data, the clinician must endeavor to understand the subjective inner experience of the patient. Thus, the clinician who is attempting to come to the best possible understanding of the patient's risk for suicide has the challenging task of holding and moving back and forth between these perspectives in the course of the clinical evaluation.

## The objective/descriptive perspective

This perspective encompasses the use of the clinical interview to gather objective data about the patient that can aid in assessing the degree of suicide risk. In addition to taking a clinical psychiatric history, this includes recognizing the overt manifestations of a suicidal crisis, identifying risk factors for suicide, and assessing high-risk clinical symptoms. We will discuss each of these in turn.

## Recognizing manifestations of a suicidal crisis

It is of paramount importance that the clinician recognize those observable signs that signal that the patient is in a crisis that could lead to suicide. Most obvious, of course, is the patient's direct expression of suicidal thoughts. The clinician's task is to recognize the intensity of these thoughts and whether the patient has associated intent, or suicidal urges even in the absence of conscious intent. Other questions include whether the patient has had a specific plan for suicide, the potential lethality of the plan, and whether the patient has access to lethal means. Also important is whether the patient has been rehearsing for suicide—either overtly or cognitively—and whether they have been behaving in such a way that appears to reflect preparation for suicide.

Of note, a patient's denial of suicidal thoughts is not necessarily reassuring in the context of other signs pointing to a suicidal crisis. While patients often give some indication of suicidal thoughts or intent, this communication is not always direct, and is often to others in his life but not to the clinician (Robins 1981; Wolk-Wasserman 1987b; Fawcett *et al.* 1990, 1993; Pallaskorpi *et al.* 2005). In a chart review of 76 inpatient suicides, 78 per cent had documented denial of suicidal thoughts just prior to the event (Busch *et al.* 2003). Thus, the clinician must not only attend to the patient's words, but also ask: is there anything about the patient's clinical situation and mental status that makes me question whether he might still be at risk? In this context collateral information from family, friends, and other clinicians—regarding both the patient's recent statements as well as behaviour—can be critical to the assessment. For example, has the patient who currently appears calm and denies suicidal thoughts been making what appear to be preparations for suicide, such as giving away possessions, getting affairs in order, or planning a funeral?

Why might a suicidal patient deny suicidal thoughts when interviewed by the clinician? One possibility is that the patient is lying about, or at least minimizing, the extent of his suicidal thoughts and intent. The patient may, for example, have an explicit suicide plan and want to avoid discovery. Another possibility, however, is that the patient might believe that the prospect of suicide is anxiety-provoking to the clinician and might put the relationship at risk; thus, concealment might be in the service of preserving the relationship. Still another possibility is that the patient is not lying or consciously minimizing at all. Perhaps he has experienced transient relief in the context of being in the therapist's office or emergency department, and genuinely does not recognize the degree to which they are likely to feel overwhelmed and suicidal shortly after leaving (Wolk-Wasserman 1987a). Perhaps the patient is so disconnected from his inner experience (as sometimes occurs in psychotic illnesses) that the denial of suicidal thoughts is genuine, even as the patient might the next moment be seized by an overwhelming suicidal urge.

## Identification of risk factors

A full review of suicide risk factors is beyond the scope of this chapter, and precipitating events to suicide are discussed by Hendin in the next chapter. One area of potential confusion, however, is to what degree the identification of risk factors can aid the clinician in the clinical assessment. Risk factors are helpful in identifying patients who fall into high-risk groups, which can help to heighten the vigilance of the clinician in the assessment of these patients. Unfortunately, however, the number of risk factors does not inform the clinician about the risk of suicide in an individual patient (Pokorny 1983; Goldstein et al. 1991; Powell et al. 2000). Conversely, the absence of identified risk factors is not at all protective in the face of other clinical variables. For example, a history of previous suicide attempts is well known as a strong risk factor for completed suicide (Owens et al. 2002). In the context of other reasons for concern, however, the absence of such a history is not reassuring in that approximately two-thirds of completed suicides occur on the first attempt (Mann et al. 1999).

There is another way in which the significance of a history of previous self-harm as a risk factor is at times misunderstood by clinicians. Patients with repetitive low-lethality, low-intent self-harm are often seen as having interpersonal manipulative motives; the fact that they have not made higher lethality attempts is taken as an indication that they are at low risk of ever actually completing suicide, as implied by the commonly used term 'suicide gesture'. This can be a dangerous over-simplification. First, it is important for the clinician to be aware of a variety of possible motivations for self-harm, including the possibility that it may serve to relieve intolerable tension. Secondly, the assessment of suicide risk in these patients is often not a simple matter. While it is true that patients who make high lethality attempts are statistically at greatest risk (Rosen 1976; Douglas et al. 2004), low-lethality self-harm—even in the absence of suicidal intent—still increases the risk of eventual suicide (Gunderson and Ridolfi 2001; Oldham 2006). In particular, the clinician should be vigilant to changes in affective state or psychosocial situation that might put the patient at increased risk, and not be lulled into a false sense of security.

## High-risk clinical symptoms

It is widely known that patients with affective disorders are at highest risk for eventual suicide, and that psychotic features and concomitant substance abuse (particularly alcohol) increase the risk (Robins 1981; Roose et al. 1983; Fawcett et al. 1990; Chirpitel

et al. 2004; Pallaskorpi et al. 2005). We will focus here on three other high-risk clinical symptoms that are less widely known to clinicians: hopelessness, anxiety, and sleep disturbance.

### Hopelessness

Prospective studies of psychiatric patients after hospital discharge have found that the extent of a patient's hopelessness is more highly correlated with suicidal thoughts, intensity of suicidal intent, and eventual suicide than is depression (Bedrozian and Beck 1979; Wetzel et al. 1980; Beck et al. 1985, 1993). Outpatients with severe hopelessness are have also been found to be at significantly increased risk of eventual suicide (Brown et al. 2000). The association between hopelessness and suicide makes clinical sense, in that the hopeless patient is less likely to see alternatives to suicide in times of crisis.

Hopelessness is a subjective experience, often without outward manifestations, and thus can easily be missed if the interviewer does not understand the need for specific assessment. It is particularly easy to underestimate the degree to which a patient may continue to feel hopeless even after apparent clinical improvement and the remission of other affective symptoms. Attunement to this continued 'trait' hopelessness is important in the assessment of suicide risk, as it has been associated with an increased risk of suicide attempts (Young et al. 1996).

The clinician should try to answer a number of questions in the interview. To what extent if any was the patient able to generate alternatives at the moment of crisis? What about now? Does the patient continue to feel hopeless at the time of evaluation? Is there any experience of relief and hope for help? In the ambivalent internal struggle around suicide, the extent to which a patient experiences a continued wish to die—as opposed to a competing increase in hopefulness and wish to live—increases the risk of eventual suicide (Brown et al. 2005; Henriques et al. 2005).

The clinical assessment of the patient who is persistently hopeless can be very challenging. The patient's life situation is often so difficult, and his hopelessness about the possibility of any change so genuine and persuasive, that the clinician can easily begin to feel that the patient is right: nothing will ever actually help. It is important that the clinician recognize such an internal response, particularly since the patient is likely extremely sensitive to even subtle signs of hopelessness in the clinician. A recent study on a trial of cognitive therapy is helpful in this regard, in that patients who had attempted suicide showed improvement in both hopelessness and depression—and a 50 per cent lower risk of repeat attempts—at 18 months (Brown et al. 2005).

### Anxiety

Also often under-appreciated is that the assessment of the patient's level of anxiety is a critical aspect of the clinical evaluation of suicide risk. In prospective studies of patients with affective disorders both panic attacks and 'psychic' anxiety were strongly associated with increased *short-term* risk of suicide, within weeks to one year (Fawcett et al. 1990; Maser et al. 2002). It may often be anxiety that makes the experience of depression and hopelessness intolerable, adding a potentially lethal urgency to act (Fawcett et al. 1993). It is essential that the clinician explicitly assess the extent of the patient's anxiety, particularly since it may readily be treatable both pharmacologically (i.e., benzodiazepines, atypical antipsychotics) and psychotherapeutically (i.e., cognitive skills, coping strategies).

The extent of a patient's anxiety can easily be missed in the clinical interview, particularly if it is a quiet form of anxiety. A good example was a 46-year-old female inpatient who had been admitted for suicidal ideation and was seen by one of the authors (M.S.) several days after admission. The patient had spent most of the first few days of her hospitalization sitting in her room, appearing quietly depressed. She did not seem outwardly anxious, and had not received any doses of the benzodiazapine that had been ordered on an 'as needed' basis by the admitting physician. When the author interviewed her he explicitly asked about anxiety, despite the lack of outward manifestations. The patient described feeling severely anxious, as though she 'could not take it any more', she felt she would 'do anything' to put a stop to the experience. She was treated with a standing order for a benzodiazepine, the clinical focus shifted to specifically helping with her anxiety, and she subsequently experienced rapid improvement.

### Sleep disturbance

Sleep disturbance is another potentially treatable clinical symptom that may be associated with increased risk of suicidality in depression. Like anxiety, global insomnia has been identified as one of the factors associated with increased *short-term* risk of suicide, within weeks to one year (Fawcett *et al*. 1990). Depressed patients who report suicidal ideation have been found to have greater subjective sleep disturbance that those who do not (Ağargün *et al*. 1997), and both insomnia and frequent nightmares have been associated with increased suicidal ideation in depressed patients (Bernert *et al*. 2005). In a prospective study of elderly patients a correlation was found between subjective sleep disturbance and a higher risk of eventual completed suicide (Turvey *et al*. 2002). Like anxiety, sleep disturbance is a symptom that may be readily treatable but is not always spontaneously reported by the patient. Thus, it is essential that the clinician specifically assess sleep in the evaluation of depressed and potentially suicidal patients.

## The experiential perspective

As Birtchnell (1983) has pointed out, the 'medicalization' of the clinical interview—by which he means a focus on medically oriented symptoms without sufficient emphasis on understanding the patient's subjective experience—carries the risk of unintentionally curtailing the exchange for both clinician and patient:

> The therapist conveys to the patient that the suicidal urge is a manifestation of the illness, that it has nothing to do with the patient himself. If the patient can allow the doctor to eliminate the illness he will find that his suicidal urge has gone away... The psychiatrist asks the patient whether he feels that life is worth living; whether he feels like putting an end to it all. Once the patient has answered yes, the symptom has been elicited, and the psychiatrist wishes to know no more.
>
> Birtchnell (1983, p. 27)

Thus it is essential that the clinician also try to understand the patient's subjective inner experience of the suicidal crisis. What was/is the patient actually *feeling*, beyond a delineation of clinical symptoms? In what way(s) are the patient's suicidal thoughts or actions understandable given that experience? (Linehan 1993, 1997). The clinician who focuses exclusively on the elicitation of symptoms runs the risk of not meeting the patient's basic need to be seen, understood, and accepted; this can paradoxically can leave the patient feeling more alone, even in the context of seeking help.

As we will discuss, the clinician's effort to understand the patient's subjective experience includes eliciting the patient's personal narrative, understanding his affective experience, assessing sustaining resources, and identifying underlying beliefs, motivations, and fantasies. We will also discuss the clinician's capacity for empathy as an important tool in this aspect of the clinical interview.

### The patient's personal narrative

In eliciting the patient's personal narrative the clinician's goal is to understand what led to the suicidal crisis from the patient's perspective. The hope is to engage the patient—to the extent possible—in arriving at a shared understanding of his distress, and how it was that he came to see suicide as the solution. While this may sound obvious, it is a goal that is frequently far from attained in clinical practice. In fact, there is often discontinuity between a patient's understanding of the reasons for his suicidal behaviour and those attributed by the clinician. Patients most often describe a wish for relief from unbearable mental anguish as the reason for a suicide attempt; clinicians commonly identify interpersonal communication and manipulation as primary motives (Bancroft *et al*. 1979; Michel *et al*. 1994). It is therefore essential that the clinician be alert to any preconceived notions, biases, feelings, and past experiences that may lead to premature inferences and conclusions about the patient's experience.

Our emphasis on understanding suicidality from the patient's perspective can readily be misunderstood. It does not mean that the clinician must take the patient's perspective on his suicidal crisis at face value, eschewing critical thinking, clinical inference, and independent judgement. It is in fact essential that the clinician understand that patients often have many levels of motivation for their behaviour, some less readily identified and disclosed than others, and some truly outside of awareness. However, if the patient's own experience is not the *starting* place for exploration a major opportunity is lost, and the chances of arriving at the best possible understanding damaged. The patient is likely not to feel heard and understood, and is subsequently less likely to feel able and willing to be open and forthcoming.

### The patient's affective experience

Shneidman describes suicide as 'a combined movement toward cessation and away from intolerable, unendurable, unacceptable anguish' (1992, p. 6). There is widespread agreement that this effort to escape psychological pain and an intolerable affective state is a primary driver of suicidal behaviour (Buie and Maltsberger 1983; Maltsberger 1988; Shneidman 1992; Linehan 1993; Hendin *et al*. 2004). Hendin *et al*. (2004) found that therapists reported a higher number of intense affective states in their patients who completed suicide in the course of treatment than in a non-suicidal comparison group with severe depression. The most frequently cited affect was desperation, defined as a state of anguish accompanied by an urgent need for relief. Under the pressure of such unbearable affective intensity cognition narrows, the experience can feel interminable, and the capacity for such functions as self-soothing and problem-solving can transiently be lost. Patients often report breakdowns in self-control; they will say that they are losing their grip, and of this they are often very ashamed. They may know better than to do or to say certain things, but unable to restrain themselves under the pressure of intense feeling, they act or speak out anyway. The dread accompanying the self's breaking up, sometimes called annihilation anxiety, is a profound experience of helpless horror. When the patient sees no alternative, no end point or escape from unbearable suffering, the risk of suicidal behaviour is increased.

It is essential to be aware that under certain circumstances, such as in the holding environment of a hospital or a therapist's office, even overwhelming affect and unbearable psychological pain can transiently be relieved. The clinician must therefore be attuned not only to the patient's affective experience at the time of the interview, but also to their experience in the moment of crisis. The challenge is to understand to what degree the relief experienced by the patient is transient and unstable, and to help the patient to understand this as well. Ideally clinician and patient can use the opportunity of temporary calm to problem-solve, work on coping strategies, and develop a crisis plan so that the patient will be better prepared to deal with the next affective storm.

Clinicians often undervalue the role of intolerable affect, and mistakenly see suicidal thoughts and behaviour as arising only as symptoms of clinical depression. Thus, a patient who describes feeling suicidal in the absence of current clinical signs and symptoms of depression is likely to be seen as motivated by secondary gain, and perhaps to be malingering. While this is at times undoubtedly true, the clinician should be aware of other possibilities as well. For example, a patient who is calm and apparently euthymic after admission to the hospital may inaccurately be using the term 'depression' to describe an intolerable experience of anguish and desperation that has now transiently been relieved by hospitalization. The danger here is that the clinician will mistake this either for manipulation or for improvement in the patient's 'depression'. In either case, both physician and patient may misunderstand the patient's current euthymia to mean a decrease in suicide risk, when in fact he is just as vulnerable to being overwhelmed by intolerable affect when once again outside the office or hospital.

## The patient's sustaining resources

All of us rely on outside resources such as spouses, friends, school, or job to support our sense of self; for some, however, this is a critical need, the loss of which leads to an experience of aloneness, overwhelming affect, and unbearable psychological pain. The experience of aloneness is an unbearable psychological state; it differs from loneliness in that it leaves the individual unable to feel the presence of comforting and sustaining supports, even if they are genuinely available. From a psychoanalytic perspective (Adler and Buie 1979; Buie and Maltsberger 1983; Maltsberger 1988) this vulnerability is seen as a developmental deficit: the patient has not had the opportunity to internalize and thus later to be able to evoke soothing introjects (i.e., images of others, inner voices), which leads to an over reliance on others (i.e., self-objects) to modulate negative affect and sustain the sense of self. In this context the loss—*real or perceived*—of a critical sustaining resource such as a relationship or a job can lead to a suicidal crisis.

This inability to make use of available sustaining resources can also be a 'state' experience in the absence of clear developmental deficit. The severely depressed and/or psychotic patient can transiently lose the capacity to evoke soothing introjects, and thus be unable to feel even the genuine presence and support of others; this can evoke an overwhelming experience of aloneness and increase the risk of suicidal behaviour.

In assessing suicide risk, then, the clinician should keep the following questions in mind. Who/what does the patient have to live for? Who/what does the patient rely on to sustain his sense of self? Has there been a change, particularly a real or perceived loss of any of these critical supports? Is patient able to make use of available sustaining resources given his current mental status? What about once the patient is outside the interview room or hospital, at a moment of crisis?

## Beliefs, motivations, and fantasies

A frequently neglected aspect of the suicide risk assessment is the importance of the patient's beliefs about suicide. The clinician's goal here is to find out what the patient actually thinks will happen if he attempts suicide; to assess the strength and rigidity of these beliefs; and to see if the patient can entertain other alternatives. For example, does the patient believe that he will complete the attempt and end up dead? What consequences does the patient believe this would have on others, such as spouse, children, family, friends? To what degree has the patient been able and willing to genuinely explore these consequences, and can he do so now? If the patient views suicide as an effective solution, the risk of future suicide attempts is increased (Chiles *et al.* 1985).

Also important are the patient's overall beliefs and attitudes about suicide. In general, patients who endorse 'reasons for living'—such as positive beliefs about capacity to cope, concerns for family/children, fear of social disapproval and moral/religious objections to suicide—have been found to have less suicidal ideation, to make fewer suicide attempts, and to have less suicidal intent than those who do not (Linehan *et al.* 1983; Strosahl *et al.* 1992; Malone *et al.* 2000). In addition, strong moral/religious objections to suicide have been correlated with lower lethality suicide attempts (Malone *et al.* 2000). The caveat here is that the clinician must be careful not to allow generalizations based on clinical research to preclude a genuine inquiry into the meaning of an individual patient's beliefs and attitudes. For example, the clinician might assume that a mother's concern for the well-being of her children is a mitigating factor against suicide. But what if her concerns have turned to a belief that she has been an utter failure as a parent, and that her children would ultimately be better off without her? In this case, what might have been seen as a 'protective' factor may be such a source of shame that it actually worsens the patient's despair and increases her risk of suicide.

The clinician should also be aware that the idea of suicide can have very different meanings and be motivated by different sets of fantasies. Some fantasies and motivations are fully or partially conscious, and some may be outside of awareness. For example, the patient may feel he deserves punishment, may long for a fantasized reunion with a lost other, may wish for retaliation (and paradoxically have a fantasy that they will experience the pleasure of retaliation even in the context of suicide), or wish to destroy a hated aspect of self such as an identification with an abuser (Maltsberger and Buie 1980; Maltsberger 2004).

Essential to this aspect of the clinical assessment is the clinician's willingness not only to ask about but also to offer respectful alternatives to the patient's stated beliefs. Is the mother who believes that her child would be better off without her able/willing to consider that she may be misreading the situation because of her depression, and that her child would likely be irrevocably damaged by her suicide? Is the man who has felt utterly alone since his father's death, and longs for a reunion through suicide, able/willing to consider the possibility that suicide might *not* mean blissful reunion?

Is the woman who has strong religious objections to suicide but has decided that God sure would forgive her about this, or is she open to the possibility that she might be wrong? The clinician's willingness to enter into this kind of dialogue with the patient allows for an assessment of the strength and rigidity of beliefs that may predispose the patient to suicidal behaviour. It also helps in starting to build a treatment alliance, demonstrating the clinician's interest in a genuine and full understanding of the patient's experience. Finally, this level of inquiry is the beginning of crisis intervention and treatment, offering a challenge to the cognitive constriction—the no alternative/no option thinking—that characterizes the patient's suicidal crisis.

### The role of empathy

The clinician's capacity for empathy— that is, to understand and to feel intuitively the perspective and experience of another—is critical to the clinical interview. In addition to listening to the patient's words, the clinician picks up something else from patient—a non-verbal affective communication—that stimulates an empathic resonance, a sense of understanding what the other is feeling. As part of this process clinicians makes reference to their own past experiences that inform this intuitive sense of affective understanding. The process of empathy is often preconscious or even completely out of the clinician's awareness, yet it is a critical source of clinical data (Wolk-Wasserman 1987a).

Often the clinician's empathic experience is consonant with the patient's conscious and stated declaration of his emotional state, adding a resonance and a deepening of connection. At times, however, there may be a discordance between what the patient says and what the clinician picks up empathically, a time when the 'words and the music' don't seem to match. A patient may, for example, deny suicidal thoughts while the clinician is picking up empathic cues of distress that raise a question about safety. Alternatively, a patient may express suicidal thoughts while the clinician's empathic experience is that the patient is overstating the degree of distress, raising a question about the possibility of secondary gain. In either case the clinician's empathic experience is an important tool, but the clinician must be aware that as a sole source of data it is prone to error. Thus, the clinician must ask: 'Why doesn't this fit? Where is my concern coming from?' This leads the clinician to integrate his empathic experience with the other sources of clinical data about the patient.

## The interview as crisis intervention

In addition to its essential role in suicide risk assessment, the clinical interview is also the starting point of the treatment relationship and crisis intervention. This beginning is often complicated by the feelings that the patient brings to the encounter, such as shame, self-blame, hopelessness, aloneness, anger, distrust (Leenaars 1994). At this moment the patient is quite likely to believe that help is not possible, and that full engagement is not even worthwhile. Thus, an additional major goal of the interview is to enhance motivation, to join with the patient in initial problem-solving, and to increase the likelihood that the patient will follow through with recommended treatment.

Perhaps the most important tool available to the clinician in this regard is an attitude of non-judgmental acceptance and validation of the patient's experience (Linehan 1993, 1997; Schechter 2007).

It is essential that the patient feel heard by the clinician to the extent possible, and that the clinician demonstrate an understanding of the way or ways in which suicidal thoughts and/or behaviour are at least understandable given his situation and internal experience. This serves a number of functions: it helps to relieve to some degree acute distress and aloneness, minimizes the patient's propensity for self-blame, models a hopeful attitude about problem-solving and treatment, and offers at least the possibility that the patient can be understood and ultimately helped. Ideally, this increases the likelihood that the patient can become a full and active participant in the evaluation and treatment planning process, and enhances motivation for treatment adherence

## Countertransference issues in the clinical interview

A full review of the countertransference issues involved in the evaluation of suicidal patients is beyond the scope of this chapter, and will be covered elsewhere. There are, however, a few issues that we will highlight in the context of our discussion of the clinical interview.

Hendin *et al.* (2006) aptly describe the universal difficulty involved in assessing and treating potentially suicidal patients:

> The added gravity common problems assume when suicide is a risk … invariably involves unique anxieties related to the possibility that despite the therapist's best efforts, the patient may kill himself and the therapist may be blamed. Therapists' fear that a patient may commit suicide frequently impedes their ability to deal effectively with the danger.
>
> (2006, p. 70)

While the goal of the clinical interview is an objective assessment of suicide risk, the assessment cannot help but be affected by the feelings, biases, and pre-existing inclinations that the clinician brings to a clinical encounter in which the stakes truly are life and death. Each of us bears anxiety, ambiguity, and risk in characteristic ways. Some, for example, are more likely to take control and thus to minimize uncertainty; others have a greater tolerance for anxiety and are willing to bear greater risk in the hope of promoting to the extent possible a patient's autonomy. What is essential is that clinicians have as much self-knowledge as possible about where they fall on this continuum, and that real-time consultation is sought as needed.

One clinical scenario that has major potential for countertransference difficulties is that in which the clinician encounters an angry, hostile, and/or devaluing patient. This presents an inherently problematic situation: no matter how disrespectfully the patient behaves, the clinician still must come away from the interview with an objective assessment of suicide risk. It is not uncommon for the clinician to experience anger toward such a patient. This emotional response may conflict with the clinician's ideals, which increases the likelihood that it will defensively be kept from his full awareness. In addition, the clinician may unconsciously accept the patient's devaluing projections, leading to feelings of incompetence, guilt, and increased anxiety. The clinician's capacity to be aware of the feelings engendered is of utmost importance, so that the countertransference pressures experienced do not lead to a distortion of the risk assessment. Of greatest concern are unrecognized feelings of aversion toward the patient (Maltsberger and Buie 1974; Wolk-Wasserman 1987a, c), which can lead to unconscious withdrawal and increase the possibility that the clinician will not fully appreciate the extent of the patient's suicidal crisis and immediate needs.

## Conclusion

In this chapter we have reviewed the functions of the clinical interview, which depending on setting and clinical need may in fact encompass a series of interviews and clinical interactions over time. We have divided these functions conceptually into the 'objective/descriptive' and the 'experiential' perspectives. The clinician must be able to move comfortably between these perspectives in order to come to the best possible understanding of the patient's suicide risk. In addition to its role in risk assessment, the clinical interview is also the beginning of the treatment relationship and crisis intervention. Finally, it is important that the clinician be aware of countertransference issues that commonly arise in the evaluation of suicidal patients, which if unrecognized can have an inadvertent influence on the clinical assessment.

## References

Adler G and Buie DH (1979). Aloneness and borderline psychotherapy: the possible relevance of child developmental issues. *Journal of Psychoanalysis*, **60**, 83–96.

Ağargün MY, Kara H, Somaz M (1997). Subjective sleep quality and suicidality in patients with major depression. *Journal of Psychiatric Research*, **31**, 377–381.

Bancroft J, Hawton K, Simkin S *et al.* (1979). The reasons people give for taking overdoses: a further inquiry. *British Journal of Medical Psychology*, **52**, 553–565.

Beck AT, Steer RA, Kovacs M *et al.* (1985). Hopelessness and eventual suicide: a longer prospective study of patients hospitalized with suicidal ideation. *American Journal of Psychiatry*, **142**, 559–563.

Beck AT, Steer RA, Beck JS *et al.* (1993). Hopelessness, depression, suicidal ideation, and clinical diagnosis of depression. *Suicide and Life-Threatening Behavior*, **123**, 139–145.

Bedrozian RC and Beck AT (1979). Cognitive aspects of suicidal behavior. *Suicide and Life-Threatening Behavior*, **9**, 87–96.

Bernert RA, Joiner TE, Cukrowicz KC *et al.* (2005). Suicidality and sleep disturbances. *Sleep*, **28**, 1039–1040.

Birtchnell J (1983). Psychotherapeutic considerations in the management of the suicidal patient. *American Journal of Psychotherapy*, **1**, 24–36.

Brown, GK, Beck AT, Steer RA *et al.* (2000). Risk factors for suicide in psychiatric outpatients: a 20-year prospective study. *Journal of Consulting and Clinical Psychology*, **68**, 371–377.

Brown GK, Steer RA, Henriques GR *et al.* (2005). The internal struggle between the wish to die and the wish to live: a risk factor for suicide. *American Journal of Psychiatry*, **162**, 1977–1979.

Brown GK, Ten Have T, Henriques GR *et al.* (2005). Cognitive therapy for the prevention of suicide attempts: a randomized controlled trial. *JAMA*, **294**, 563–570.

Buie DH and Maltsberger JT (1983). *The Practical Formulation of Suicide Risk*. Firefly Press, Cambridge.

Busch KA, Fawcett J, Jacobs DG (2003). Clinical correlates of inpatient suicide. *Journal of Clinical Psychiatry*, **64**, 14–19.

Chiles JA, Strosahl KD, McMurtray L *et al.* (1985). Modeling effects of suicidal behavior. *Journal of Nervous and Mental Disease*, **173**, 477–481.

Chirpitel CJ, Guilherme LG, Wilcox HC (2004). Acute alcohol use and suicidal behavior: a review of the literature. *Alcoholism, Clinical and Experimental Research*, **28**, 18–28.

Douglas J, Cooper J, Amos T, Webb R, Guthrie E, Appleby L (2004). 'Near fatal' deliberate self-harm: characteristics, prevention, and implications for prevention of suicide. *Journal of Affective Disorders*, **79**, 263–268.

Fawcett J, Clark DC, Busch KA (1993). Assessing and treating the patient at risk for suicide. *Psychiatric Annals*, **23**, 244–255.

Fawcett J, Scheftner WA, Fogg L *et al.* (1990). Time related predictors of suicide in major affective disorders. *American Journal of Psychiatry*, **147**, 1189–1194.

Goldstein RB, Black DW, Nasrallah A *et al.* (1991). The prediction of suicide. *Archives of General Psychiatry*, **48**, 418–422.

Gunderson JC and Ridolfi ME (2001). Borderline personality disorder. Suicidality and self-mutilation. *Annals of the New York Academy of Science*, **932**, 61–72.

Hendin H, Haas AP, Maltsberger JT *et al.* (2006). Problems in psychotherapy with suicidal patients. *American Journal of Psychiatry*, **163**, 67–72.

Hendin H, Maltzberger JT, Haas AP *et al.* (2004). Desperation and other affective states in suicidal patients. *Suicide and Life-Threatening Behavior*, **34**, 386–394.

Henriques G, Wenzel A, Brown GK *et al.* (2005). Suicide attempters' reaction to survival as a risk factor for eventual suicide. *American Journal of Psychiatry*, **162**, 2180–2182.

Leenaars A (1994). Crisis intervention with highly lethal suicidal people. In A Leenaars, JT Maltsberger and R Neimeyer, eds, *Treatment of Suicidal People*, pp. 45–59. Taylor and Francis, London.

Linehan MM (1993). *Cognitive–Behavioral Treatment of Borderline Personality Disorder*. The Guilford Press, New York.

Linehan MM (1997). Validation and psychotherapy. In A Bohart and L Greenberg, eds, *Empathy Reconsidered: New Directions in Psychotherapy*, pp. 353–392. APA, Washington.

Linehan MM, Goodstein JL, Nielson SL *et al.* (1983). Reasons for staying alive when you are thinking about killing yourself. The Reasons for Living Inventory. *Journal of Consulting and Clinical Psychology*, **51**, 276–286.

Malone KM, Oquendo MA, Haas GL *et al.* (2000). Protective factors against suicidal acts in major depression: reasons for living. *American Journal of Psychiatry*, **157**, 1084–1088.

Maltsberger, JT (1988). Suicide danger: clinical estimation and decision. *Suicide and Life-Threatening Behavior*, **18**, 47–54.

Maltsberger JT (2004). The descent into suicide. *International Journal of Psychoanalysis*, **85**, 653–668.

Maltsberger JT and Buie DH (1974). Countertransference hate in the treatment of suicidal patients. *Archives of General Psychiatry*, **30**, 625–633.

Maltsberger JT and Buie DH (1980). The devices of suicide. Revenge, riddance, and rebirth. *International Review of Psycho-analysis*, **7**, 61–72.

Mann JJ, Waternaux C, Haas G *et al.* (1999). Toward a clinical model of suicidal behavior in psychiatric patients. *American Journal of Psychiatry*, **156**, 181–189.

Maser JD, Akiskal HS, Schettler P *et al.* (2002). Can temperament identify affectively all patients who engage in lethal or near-lethal suicidal behavior? A 14-year prospective study. *Suicide and Life-Threatening Behavior*, **32**, 10–32.

Michel K, Valach L, Waeber V (1994). Understanding deliberate self-harm: the patient's views. *Crisis*, **15**, 172–178.

Oldham JM (2006). Borderline personality disorder and suicidality. *American Journal of Psychiatry*, **163**, 20–26.

Owens D, Horrocks J, House A (2002). Fatal and non-fatal repetition of self-harm. *British Journal of Psychiatry*, **181**, 193–199.

Pallaskorpi SK, Isometsa ET, Henriksson MM *et al.* (2005). Completed suicide among subjects receiving psychotherapy. *Psychotherapy and Psychosomatics*, **74**, 388–391.

Pokorny AD (1983). Prediction of suicide in psychiatric patients. *Archives of General Psychiatry*, **40**, 249–257.

Powell J, Geddes J, Deeks J *et al.* (2000). Suicide in psychiatric hospital inpatients. *British Journal of Psychiatry*, **176**, 266–272.

Robins E (1981). *The Final Months*. Oxford University Press, New York.

Roose SP, Glassman AH, Walsh T *et al.* (1983). Depression, delusions, and suicide. *American Journal of Psychiatry*, **140**, 1159–1162.

Rosen DH (1976). The serious suicide attempt: five-year follow-up study of 886 patients. *JAMA*, **235**, 2105–2109.

Schechter M (2007). The patient's experience of validation in psychoanalysis. *JAPA*, **55**, 105–130.

Shneidman E (1992). What do suicides have in common? Summary of the psychological approach. In B Bongar, ed., *Suicide: Guidelines for Assessment, Management, and Treatment*, pp. 3–15. Oxford University Press, New York.

Strosahl K, Chiles JA, Linehan MM (1992). Prediction of suicide intent in hospitalized parasuicides: reasons for living, hopelessness, and depression. *Comprehensive Psychiatry*, **6**, 366–373.

Turvey CL, Conwell Y, Jones MP *et al.* (2002). Risk factors for late-life suicide: a prospective, community-based study. *American Journal of Geriatric Psychiatry*, **10**, 398–406.

Wetzel RD, Margulies T, Davis R *et al.* (1980). Hopelessness, depression and suicide intent. *Journal of Clinical Psychiatry*, **41**(5), 159–160.

Wolk-Wasserman D (1987a). Contacts of suicidal alcohol and drug abuse patients and their significant others with public care institutions before the suicide attempt. *Acta Psychiatrica Scandinavica*, **76**, 394–405.

Wolk-Wasserman D (1987b). Contacts of suicidal neurotic and prepsychotic/psychotic patients and their significant others with public care institutions before the suicide attempt. *Acta Psychiatrica Scandinavica*, **75**, 358–372.

Wolk-Wasserman D (1987c). Some problems connected with the treatment of suicide attempt patients: transference and countertransference aspects. *Crisis*, **1**, 69–82.

Young MA, Fogg LF, Scheftner W *et al.* (1996). Stable trait components of hopelessness: baseline and sensitivity to depression. *Journal of Abnormal Clinical Psychology*, **105**, 155–165.

# CHAPTER 44

# Recognizing a suicide crisis in psychiatric patients

Herbert Hendin

## Abstract

Data from therapists who were treating patients when they committed suicide were examined. Comparable information was obtained on depressed, non-suicidal patients treated by the same therapists. Three factors were identified as markers of a suicide crisis: precipitating events, changes in behaviour, and intense affective states. Of these, intense affective states appeared to be the most significant. The suicide patients had a significantly greater number of intense affects than did the comparison patients. The affect that most distinguished the two groups was desperation, which was intense in 30 of 36 (83 per cent) of the suicide patients but in none of the comparison patients. The study permitted us to develop a scaled Affective States Questionnaire (ASQ) which is being tested prospectively.

## Introduction

Suicide risk is a broad term that weighs factors such as age, gender, diagnosis, past suicide attempts, and such traits and behaviours as impulsivity (Åsberg et al. 1987; Apter et al. 1993) and substance abuse (Murphy 1986; Flavin et al. 1990) known to be correlated with suicide. Most work in the last century dealing with risk factors for suicide did not distinguish a suicide crisis—an immediate or acute danger of suicide—from longer-term risk.

The work of Fawcett and colleagues was a notable exception. Based on data from a prospective study of suicide in patients with major affective disorders, they differentiated acute risk—defined by them as occurring within a year—from chronic risk, with the suicide occurring after a year (Fawcett et al. 1990). The symptoms associated with acute risk were anhedonia, anxiety, insomnia, a diminished ability to concentrate, and moderate alcohol abuse. Associated with longer-term risk were hopelessness, suicidal ideation, and previous suicide attempts. Recent work has stressed the need for a shorter timeframe than a year for defining a more imminent danger of suicide (Rudd et al. 2006).

## Difficulties in identifying a suicide crisis

- Patients often withhold their suicide intentions and plans from their treatment providers.
- They deny suicide intent when asked.
- They do so particularly when they fear frank response may lead to involuntary hospitalization, delayed discharge if they are already hospitalized, or interfere with a suicide plan.
- Standard measures of suicide intent or ideation have significant limitations as measures of acute suicide risk.

My colleagues and I have been accumulating and analysing information from therapists who were treating patients with open-ended psychotherapy and medication when suicide occurred (Hendin et al. 2001, 2004, 2007). Participating therapists completed semi-structured questionnaires on thirty-six patients dealing with their patient's background, clinical history, medication history, affective states, and psychodynanmic factors related to the suicide. Therapists also prepared case narratives in which a section focused on the treatment process (Hendin et al. 2006).

We examined three factors identified as markers of acute risk for suicide: a precipitating event; behavioural changes; and intense affective states. Although information from all three markers made some contribution to identifying a suicide crisis, the markers were of varying degrees of value in independently signalling the crisis.

## Precipitating events

An event was defined as precipitating if it was experienced within a few months of the suicide, and there was evidence that it played a role in triggering the suicide.

Therapists identifying such an event were asked to describe the event and to note the specific evidence that linked it to the patient's suicide. Past studies have identified 'negative life events' in 80 per cent of cases (Heikkinen et al. 1997) which is consistent with what we found. Among the cases we examined, however, where there was a precipitating event, therapists identified the event, and had evidence for doing so, 75 per cent of the time. In the other 25 per cent, however, there was a tendency to identify a potentially upsetting event as having precipitated the suicide, even though the therapist had no evidence that this was so.

Precipitating events could be distinguished by whether they had been instigated by the patient or were essentially beyond the patient's control. In a small number of cases the circumstances were not clear enough to make this determination. Those beyond the patient's control ranged from the death or probable death of a loved one or rejection in a relationship to financial difficulties or to events related to treatment. In cases where no precipitating event could be linked to the suicide, deterioration in the patient's emotional condition appeared to be more significant than any particular event. What follows are some case examples (Maltsberger et al. (2003).

---

**Box 44.1** Case studies of suicides

Among the patients whose behaviour precipitated the event that was seen as the trigger for their suicide was a Vietnam veteran with post-traumatic stress disorder who drank heavily and when drinking was abusive to his wife. He attributed his suicidal feelings to his wife's leaving him, but his behaviour was responsible for her doing so. In other patients, erratic behaviour related to their bipolar disorder destroyed their careers. Humiliation and desperation related to their career failures were a dominant feature in their therapy and identified as triggering their suicides.

Several such patients structured the precipitating events that led to their suicide. A 44-year-old artist announced to his psychiatrist at the onset of treatment that he would kill himself unless he was able to open an art gallery within the next six months. There was virtually no possibility of his doing so but when after six months he could not, he hanged himself.

Among the patients who reacted with suicide to events that were beyond their control was a 34-year-old non-commissioned officer who developed a major depressive disorder after his infant son was diagnosed with leukaemia. He treated the illness as a personal failure in his role as protector of the family. His immediate reaction had been to suggest to his wife that they kill themselves and their two children by immolation in the family car. Continuing symptoms of irritability and euphoria interfered with his work and led to serious conflicts with his supervisor. Faced with the imminent loss of his son and his military career, he saw his life as falling apart. He ended it by shooting himself in the family car.

A therapist's misidentification of a precipitating event involved a young woman with schizoaffective disorder who had increasingly frequent hallucinations aggravated by substance abuse, worsening of her depression, and akathisia resulting from her medication. In her last session which was on the day of her suicide, she complained of these symptoms, but also reported a minor accident. Her car had been parked with the engine running. She had not kept her foot firmly on the brake, so the car slid into the rear of the car in front of her. Although no damage was done, the therapist listed the accident as the precipitating event to the suicide, although recognizing its relevance as uncertain. The event was not likely to have been precipitating, but her mentioning the incident was probably a way of expressing that she felt her life was slipping out of control and, if explored, might have made clearer the extent of her distress.

---

Reviewing the kinds of evidence that were used to link patients to a precipitating event led us to develop the following schema of evidence:

- Patient's statements, writings or recordings linking thoughts or plans of suicide to an event, or making living contingent on an event occurring or not occurring.

- Patient's dreams containing images of death linked to an event.

- Worsening of patient's affective state, symptoms and/or behaviour following an event (usually accompanied by preoccupation with the event).

- Prior suicide attempt following a similar event.

- Information obtained from persons knowledgeable about an event related to a patient's suicidal feelings or behaviour.

Disturbing events, if linked by a depressed patient to suicidal thoughts, should certainly alert a treating clinician to the danger of suicide. The events by themselves, however, are of limited help in signaling a suicide crisis.

## Behavioural changes

Almost 80 per cent of the suicides showed at least one of three behavioural signs that warned of the suicide crisis: speech or actions indicated they were contemplating suicide; deterioration in social or occupational functioning; or increased alcohol abuse.

Seventeen patients showed by speech or actions that they were contemplating suicide. The patient with PTSD and alcohol abuse began shooting at trees while intoxicated. When the police were called, he challenged them to shoot him. Seven patients made suicide attempts while in their current therapy and within three months of their suicide.

Over half of the patients showed a marked deterioration in social and/or occupational functioning immediately before their suicide. At times this was signalled by increasing loss of control and rage.

A nurse's aide, for example, who worked with retarded children, hit one shortly before killing herself. She was terrified by her loss of control.

Socially, the patients' deterioration was expressed in frequent arguments, break ups in relationships, or social withdrawal. Several gave up long-standing professional careers; one quit a long-held job. Others were in danger of losing their jobs because of growing absenteeism or were experiencing difficulties with employers or supervisors. Two patients used the last session before their suicide to announce that they were stopping therapy.

Over half of the patients had a history of substance abuse. Over a third were currently abusing and an increase in alcohol abuse, used to deal with increasing anxiety, characterized this group.

Although these behavioural symptoms are a better warning sign than disturbing events, apart from speech or actions indicating that patients were contemplating suicide, they are seen too frequently in patients who are not suicidal to be by themselves a predictor of short-term risk for suicide.

## Intense affective states

Past studies have suggested the importance of looking at certain affective states found to distinguish depressed patients who die by suicide from depressed patients who are not suicidal, to see if they could help signal a suicide crisis and perhaps help identify a crisis independent of a patients' acknowledging suicidal intentions. Among the affects that have been linked to suicide are hopelessness (Beck et al. 1985, 1993); rage (Weissman et al. 1973; Plutchik et al. 1989); guilt (Hendin and Haas 1991); feelings of abandonment (Van der Kolk et al. 1994; Blaauw et al. 2002) and severe anxiety (Fawcett et al. 1990, 1993). Other affective states that have been suggested to contribute to suicidality include persistent feelings of loneliness (Heikkinen et al. 1997; Koivumaa-Honkanen et al. 2001; Stravynski and Boyer 2001); humiliation (Shneidman 1999), and self-hatred (Shneidman 1999; Orbach 2001).

Our own early work with suicide crises with fatal outcomes also strongly suggested that intense affects are the most potent indicators of acute risk for suicide. A recent analysis of an expanded sample of patients who died by suicide, with a comparison group of patients who had been seriously depressed but not suicidal, provided new insights into the role that intense affects can play in helping clinicians recognize a suicide crisis (Hendin *et al.* 2007).

Therapists had been asked to rate their patients' depression during the period just before the suicide (mild, moderate, severe). They also rated nine affective states (no evidence, present, intense): rage, abandonment, guilt, desperation, hopelessness, loneliness, anxiety, humiliation, self-hatred. Participating therapists were asked to identify recent patients who were depressed but had no persistent suicide ideation and no history of suicide attempts. They completed the same affective states questionnaire for the comparison patients as for the suicide patients, focusing on the period when the patient's depressive symptoms were at their worst. Structured case narratives were also provided for these patients. Twenty-six comparison cases were selected that best matched the suicide patients on age and sex.

## Diagnosis

The patients who died by suicide and those who were depressed were similar with regard to the distribution of their axis I diagnoses, with about two-thirds of each group having a primary diagnosis of major depressive disorder, and a tenth of each group having a diagnosis of bipolar disorder. All the patients showed at least a minimal degree of depression. The patients who died by suicide, however, were more likely to have a severe depression and were also more likely to have a comorbid axis I disorder, primarily either substance abuse or anxiety disorder. In addition, the suicide patients more frequently had axis II diagnoses, most frequently borderline personality disorder, occurring in about 20 per cent of this group, but in none of the patients who were depressed but not suicidal.

## Intense affective states

Just before their deaths, the suicide patients evidenced an average of (4.8) of the nine intense affects explored, a significantly higher number than the average of (1.4) (p < 0.001) of the comparison patients when their symptoms were at the worst. The factors that distinguished the suicidal patients from the patients who were depressed but were not suicidal, i.e. the severity of their depression, the greater frequency of comorbidity among them, and their greater frequency of borderline personality disorders, were potentially explanatory variables for the affective state differences in the two groups. When these factors were controlled for, however, the strikingly significant differences in affective states remained.

The severely depressed suicidal patients had an average of 5.4 intense affects, compared with an average of 2.0 among the severely depressed comparison patients (p < 0.001). Similarly, the suicide patients with comorbid axis 1 diagnoses had an average of 4.8 intense affects compared with an average of 1.6 among the comparable patients in the nonsuicide group (p < 0.001). Finally, when the analysis omitted the suicide patients with a diagnosis of borderline personality disorder, in whom increased affective lability may have been expected, the remaining suicidal patients continued to show a significantly higher number of intense affects (4.8) than the comparison patients (1.4) (p < 0.001). No difference was found in the number of intense affects evidenced among the suicidal patients treated primarily as hospital inpatients and those treated as outpatients.

## Desperation and interrelated affects

The most striking difference between the two groups was seen in regard to desperation (defined as an 'urgent need for relief from pain or distress that has become intolerable') which was rated as intense in 30 of the 36 (80 per cent) of the patients who died by suicide, but in none of the comparison patients. Hopelessness, rage, abandonment, loneliness, self-hatred, and anxiety were also significantly more frequent in the suicide patients than in the comparison patients.

Rather than having a singular impact among these thirty suicide patients, however, intense desperation was found to coexist with an average of 4.2 among the other intense affects.

Intense hopelessness was seen in 70 per cent of the suicide cases who were intensely desperate and, in most of them, hopelessness about the future appeared to have been more long-standing than the feeling of desperation. Many of these patients appeared to have long abandoned the hope they could ever feel better, but they did not become acutely suicidal until their present anguish became intolerable and they were overwhelmed by a need for immediate relief. For most patients, desperation thus appeared to be a better marker than hopelessness of an acute suicide crisis.

In addition to hopelessness, desperation frequently arose in unrelieved experiences of intense rage, anxiety, and abandonment. Intense rage frequently contributed to the sense of disintegration and loss of control that led to desperation. Anguish and the urgent need for relief, the essence of desperation, often grew out of intense anxiety or from panic over intense feelings of abandonment. For such patients, choosing to be the one who leaves through death appeared to provide an illusion of control over their affective turmoil, and over the person they felt was abandoning them. For a smaller proportion of the suicidal patients, the roots of desperation lay in long-standing feelings of loneliness, guilt, or humiliation.

Surprisingly, guilt and humiliation were not significantly more frequent among the patients who died by suicide than among the depressed comparison patients. Among the comparison patients, however, guilt and humiliation were most related to their diminished sense of functional capacity secondary to their depression. In the suicide patients both guilt and humiliation seemed more frequently related to concrete experiences or events and were associated with other affects such as enraged, abusive behaviour that led to the break up of a family and were associated with feelings of abandonment and desperation. Although guilt and humiliation in themselves did not appear to be indicators of acute suicide risk, in the presence of other intense affects they provided important information about the patient's suicidality.

Desperation appeared to be the final common pathway for patients with intense affects who went on to suicide. The other intense affects that were present, however, pointed to what these patients were desperate about.

### Case example

Ms A, an executive in a large corporation and a divorced mother of two teenage children, entered therapy because of problems she was having with her 16-year-old daughter and anxiety that she related to financial problems resulting from her first husband's refusal to pay adequate child support. Her former husband was an older company executive who had helped support her career. Four years earlier she had left him because of physically abusive behaviour, and was now engaged to be remarried. She described her fiancé as caring and supportive of her and her children, but she criticised and seemed to devalue him because he lacked her first husband's accomplishments and prestige.

She appeared depressed as well as anxious, and admitted to heavy use of alcohol. Although her history indicated that she was chronically dysthymic and preoccupied with dreams and thoughts of death since adolescence, she had not been diagnosed as depressed previously and had no history of suicide attempts.

In treatment she focused on her increasingly acrimonious relationship with her former husband, and the escalating battles with both her children. She also provoked fights with her fiancé, whom she married several months after beginning treatment. Although her former husband continued to be emotionally and physically abusive, she clung to the unrealistic hope that they could be friends and was unable to express anger towards him. She spoke of her inability to feel close to anyone and of having no close friends.

In the months before her suicide, Ms A's situation deteriorated. Her daughter became depressed and was hospitalized after taking an overdose of aspirin. She blamed Ms A for not spending time with her or listening to her problems. Her 14-year-old son grew increasingly rude and obstinate, spending almost all his time with his father and the father's girlfriend. When Ms A's new husband reproached her son for his disrespectful behaviour, she became angry, saying that only she had the right to hate her kids as she was their mother. She dreamed of her children being roasted to death over a fire while no one noticed. The dream seemed to reflected her rage toward them, and perhaps also toward their father. Increasingly she felt trapped in an intolerable situation she could not control and from which she could not escape. She dreamed of a car crashing and finding her own dead body, signalling her sense of loss of control and hinting at suicide. The night of her suicide she drank heavily, fought with her husband, kicked him in front of a friend who was visiting, then announced she would sleep in the car. She asphyxiated herself by running the car in the locked garage (Hendin *et al.* 2007).

Her sense of being alone and abandoned, even though she had a family and a psychiatrist, as well as her rage contributed to her desperation (Hendin *et al.* 2007).

At the core of the intense affective turmoil experienced by most of the patients who died by suicide was an acute sense that their lives were collapsing or falling apart. Their distress had become intolerable, and they saw death as the only way to attain both relief and control. In other words, these patients were intensely desperate.

## Next steps

The role of desperation in the period immediately preceding suicide is striking. So is the significant difference in the average number of intense affects seen among the patients who died by suicide, compared to those who were depressed but not suicidal. Taken together these facts suggested that an instrument measuring the full range of intense affects would be both a useful clinical tool, and a sensitive indicator of the emotional dyscontrol related to suicide.

The Affective States Questionnaire we have developed permits a prospective study which is the best way to validate the findings of a retrospective study. Promising results in preliminary testing encouraged testing it on a larger scale at a major medical centre. A scale effective in identifying a suicide crisis would make a contribution to the challenging task of helping clinicians identify patients at acute risk for suicidal behaviour and suicide.

## References

Apter A, Plutchik R, Van Praag HM (1993). Anxiety, impulsivity and depressed mood in relation to suicidal and violent behaviour. *Acta Psychiatrica Scandinavica*, **87**, 1–5.

Åsberg M, Schalling D, Traskman L *et al.* (1987). Psychology of suicide, impulsivity and related phenomena. In HY Meltzer, ed., *Psychopharmacology: The Third Generation of Progress*, pp. 655–668. Raven Press, New York.

Beck AT, Steer RA, Beck JS *et al.* (1993). Hopelessness, depression, suicidal ideation, and clinical diagnosis of depression. *Suicide and Life-Threatening Behaviour*, **23**, 139–145.

Beck AT, Steer RA, Kovacs M *et al.* (1985). Hopelessness and eventual suicide: a 10-year prospective study of patients hospitalized with suicidal ideation. *The American Journal of Psychiatry*, **142**, 559–563.

Blaauw E, Arensman E, Kraaji V *et al.* (2002). Traumatic life events and suicide risk among jail inmates: the influence of types of events, time period and significant others. *Journal of Traumatic Stress*, **15**, 9–16.

Fawcett J, Sheftner W, Fogg L *et al.* (1990). Time-related predictors of suicide in major affective disorders. *The American Journal of Psychiatry*, **147**, 1189–1194.

Fawcett J, Clark DC, Busch KA (1993). Assessing and treating the patient at risk for suicide. *Psychiatric Annals*, **23**, 244–255.

Flavin DK, Franklin JE, Frances RJ (1990). Substance abuse and suicidal behaviour. In S Blumenthal and D Kupfer, eds, *Suicide over the Lifecycle*, pp. 177–204. American Psychiatric Press, Washington.

Heikkinen M, Isometsa ET, Henrikson MM *et al.* (1997). Psychosocial factors and completed suicide in personality disorders. *Acta Psychiatrica Scandinavica*, **95**, 49–57.

Hendin H and Haas AP (1991). Suicide and guilt as manifestations of PTSD in Vietnam combat veterans. *The American Journal of Psychiatry*, **148**, 586–591.

Hendin H, Haas AP, Maltsberger J *et al.* (2006). Problems in psychotherapy with suicidal patients. *American Journal of Psychiatry*, **163**, 67–72.

Hendin H, Maltsberger J, Lipschitz A *et al.* (2001). Recognizing and responding to a suicide crisis. *Suicide and Life-Threatening Behaviour*, **31**, 115–128.

Hendin H, Maltsberger JT, Haas AP *et al.* (2004). Desperation and other affective states in suicidal patients. *Suicide and Life-Threatening Behaviour*, **34**, 386–394.

Hendin H, Maltsberger JT, Szanto K (2007). The role of intense affective states in signaling a suicide crisis. *Journal of Nervous and Mental Disease*, **195**, 363–368.

Koivumaa-Honkanen H, Honkanen R, Viinamaki H *et al.* (2001). Life satisfaction and suicide: a 20-year follow-up study. *American Journal of Psychiatry*, **158**, 433–439.

Maltsberger JT, Hendin H, Haas AP *et al.* (2003) Determination of precipitating events in the suicide of psychiatric patients. *Suicide and Life-Threatening Behaviour*, **33**, 111–119.

Murphy, GE (1986). Suicide in alcoholism. In A Roy, ed., *Suicide*, pp. 89–96. Williams & Williams, Baltimore.

Orbach I (2001). Therapeutic empathy with the suicidal wish: principles of psychotherapy with suicidal individuals. *American Journal of Psychotherapy*, **55**, 166–184.

Plutchik R, Van Praag HM, Conte HR (1989). Correlates of suicide and violence risk: III. A two-stage model of countervailing forces. *Psychiatry Research*, **28**, 215–225.

Rudd MD, Berman AL, Joiner T *et al.* (2006). Warning signs for suicide: theory, research, and clinical applications. *Suicide and Life-Threatening Behaviour*, **36**, 255–262.

Shneidman ES (1999). The psychological pain assessment scale. *Suicide and Life-Threatening Behaviour*, **29**, 287–294.

Stravynski A and Boyer R (2001). Loneliness in relation to suicide ideation and parasuicide: a population-wide study. *Suicide and Life-Threatening Behaviour*, **31**, 32–40.

Van der Kolk BA, Hostetler A, Herron N *et al.* (1994). Trauma and the development of borderline personality disorder. *Psychiatric Clinics of North America*, **17**, 715–730.

Weissman M, Fox K, Klerman GL (1973). Hostility and depression associated with suicide attempts. *The American Journal of Psychiatry*, **130**, 450–455.

**PART 7C**

# Suicide Risk Assessment: Biological Measures

# CHAPTER 45

# Biological predictors of suicidal behaviour in mood disorders

J John Mann and Dianne Currier

## Abstract

Predicting suicide is difficult due to the low base rate, even in high-risk groups, and the multi-causal nature of suicidal behaviour. Retrospective and cross-sectional studies have identified a number of biologic abnormalities associated with suicide and suicide attempt. Prospective studies provide estimates of the predictive utility of biologic measures. Here, we review prospective studies of suicidal behaviour and serotonergic, noradrenergic, dopaminergic systems and the hypothalamic–pituitary–adrenocortical (HPA) axis function in mood disorders. The most promising biologic predictors are low CSF (cerebrospinal fluid) 5-hydroxyindoleacetic acid ( 5-HIAA) and HPA axis dysfunction as demonstrated by dexamethasone non-suppression that are each associated with about 4.5-fold greater risk of suicide.

## Introduction

Identifying individuals at imminent risk for suicidal behaviour is a major challenge for clinicians. However, prediction of suicidal behaviour is difficult due to the relative rarity of the event as well as the multidetermined causes of such behaviour.

This chapter reviews prospective studies of the serotonergic, dopaminergic and noradrenergic systems and hypothalamic–pituitary–adrenal axis, and systems in relation to suicidal behaviour in mood disorders, to assess the potential of biologic measures for improving the prediction of suicidal behaviour.

## Serotonergic system

Prospective studies of suicide completion and the serotonergic system consistently report that, in mood disorder individuals, low baseline cerebrospinal fluid levels of 5-HIAA (the serotonin metabolite) levels and a history of attempting suicide predict those who go on to complete suicide (Åsberg et al. 1976a, 1976b; Roy et al. 1989; Träskman-Bendz et al. 1992a; Samuelsson et al. 2006). The association between CSF 5-HIAA and suicide attempts is less clear (see Mann et al. 1996 for a review). Cross-sectional and retrospective studies find little evidence for a relationship between violent suicide attempt method and CSF 5-HIAA levels. Rather, it seems that the choice of a violent method is more dependent on what methods are available or commonly used in a society. However, greater planning and medical lethality of suicide attempt correlate with lower CSF 5-HIAA (Mann and Malone 1997; Placidi et al. 2001; Oquendo et al. 2003b). Insofar as the time between sampling CSF 5-HIAA and suicide attempt did not affect this relationship to lethality (Mann and Malone 1997) it appears that CSF 5-HIAA is a stable biochemical trait that may prospectively predict suicide and the lethality of non-fatal suicidal behaviour.

Suicidal acts are associated with aggressive and impulsive traits that, in turn, are also associated with serotonergic dysfunction (Oquendo and Mann 2000; Baca-Garcia et al. 2001; Placidi et al. 2001; Oquendo et al. 2003b). In prospective studies of alcoholic fire setters and violent offenders, lower levels of CSF 5-HIAA predict future aggression against property or homicide (Virkkunen et al. 1989, 1996). A 15-year follow-up study of army veterans (Faustman et al. 1993), supports the association between suicide, aggression and lower CSF 5-HIAA insofar as it found that those under 40 years of age who died by suicide, accident, or homicide, had significantly lower CSF 5-HIAA and homovanillic acid (HVA) compared with living controls.

Lower CSF 5-HIAA has also been associated with severity of lifetime aggressivity and a history of higher lethality suicide attempt (Träskman-Bendz et al. 1992a; Mann et al. 1996; Placidi et al. 2001). It is likely that definitions of impulsiveness and aggressive traits need to be refined. Perhaps greater suicide intent correlates with greater aggression, but inversely with impulsiveness, in which case serotonin system deficiency would more likely be related to intent rather than impulsiveness. Alternatively, different parts of the serotonin system may modulate intent and impulsiveness, as we have reported in depressed suicide attempters using positron emission tomography (PET) scanning (Oquendo et al. 2003b). The causal relationship between lower serotonin function and aggressive and/or impulsive behaviours has been demonstrated by the increase in aggressiveness and impulsiveness following lowering serotonin function transiently by acute tryptophan depletion in healthy male volunteers (Salomon et al. 1994; Cleare and Bond 1995; Moeller et al. 1996). Clearly the same kind of study would be unethical in those at risk for suicidal behaviour.

Clinical prospective studies have suggested that risk for suicidal acts might be associated with phase of depressive episode or subtype of depressive disorder (Berglund and Nilsson 1987; Leon et al. 1999; Brinkman-Sull et al. 2000; Coryell et al. 2002). Serotonergic abnormality has been observed in euthymic patients with a history of major depression, via a depressive response to tryptophan depletion (Price *et al.* 1991; Heninger *et al.* 1992; Delgado *et al.* 1994; Moreno *et al.* 1999; Smith *et al.* 1999) and a blunted prolactin response to serotonin release by fenfluramine during remission (Flory *et al.* 1998; Smith *et al.* 1999), suggesting that an abnormality in serotonergic function may underlie a predisposition to recurrent episodes of major depression. A prospective study of CSF 5-HIAA across the course of depressive illness found that, while CSF 5-HIAA increased on recovery, levels remained lower in individuals who had the lowest levels during a depressive episode compared to those with higher levels during a depressive episode and who achieved recovery (Träskman-Bendz *et al.* 1984). It is crucial to note that the abnormalities in serotonergic function associated with suicidal behaviour can be distinguished from those of a major depressive episode/disorder by their anatomical distribution in the brain (Mann *et al.* 2000). Thus, individuals that have mood disorders have a widespread abnormality in serotonin function affecting most of the prefrontal cortex and many other cortical and subcortical areas (Milak *et al.* 2005). In contrast, in post-mortem brain tissue from suicides, or in depressed suicide attempters identified by PET, is the abnormality is localized to parts of the prefrontal cortex, perhaps reflecting those brain regions involved in suicide intent, decision-making, and impulse regulation (Mann *et al.* 2000; Oquendo *et al.* 2003b). The generalizability of this localized serotonin system deficit and suicidal behaviour is supported by findings of low CSF 5-HIAA in suicide attempters with schizophrenia or personality disorders compared to psychiatric controls (Brown *et al.* 1982; Ninan *et al.* 1984; Gardner *et al.* 1990; Cooper *et al.* 1992).

Genetic studies may shed light on the origins of serotonergic system dysfunction in suicidal behaviour. In a longitudinal genetic study, Caspi *et al.* (2003) found a functional polymorphism in the promoter region of the serotonin transporter (5-HTTLPR) was associated with the likelihood of developing major depression and suicidality in relation to stressful life events in adulthood.

## Dopaminergic system

Abnormality in the dopaminergic system has been documented in major depression (for reviews see Mann and Kapur 1995; Dailly *et al.* 2004), however, with regard to suicidal behaviour, post-mortem and retrospective studies of dopaminergic function are few and inconclusive (see Mann 2003). Prospective studies of dopaminergic system function and suicidal behaviour have also produced divergent findings. (Roy *et al.* 1986; Roy 1992).

## CSF HVA:5 -HIAA ratio

The ratio between monoamine metabolites has shown a stronger association with suicidal behaviour, although the predictive value of these ratios is unclear. Such ratios factor out common variance due to characteristics such as the shared CSF transport system and effects on monoamine metabolites levels related to CSF gradient due to variation in length of the spinal canal.

Engstrom *et al.* (1999) found lower HVA/5-HIAA and HVA/MHPG (3-methoxy-4-hydroxyphenylglycol) ratios in individuals with a history of suicide attempt compared with surgical controls at baseline, although there was no difference during follow-up between past attempters and those who completed suicide. Roy *et al.* (1986) reported a lower baseline CSF HVA/ 5-HIAA ratio in depressed subjects compared to controls. Moreover,

among depressed subjects who had a history of suicide attempts, dexamethasone suppression test (DST) non-suppressors had a significantly lower mean CSF HVA/ 5-HIAA ratio than suppressors. This may indicate that depressed individuals who attempt suicide have a more marked imbalance between the turnover of dopamine and serotonin in terms of relatively lower dopaminergic activity or turnover.

## Noradrenergic system

There is evidence that abnormal functioning in the noradrenergic system is associated with both major depression and suicidal behaviour. In post-mortem studies fewer noradrenergic neurons in the locus coeruleus in the brainstem have been observed in depressed suicide victims (Arango *et al.* 1996), along with indications of cortical noradrenergic overactivity such as decreased alpha and high affinity beta$_1$-adrenergic receptor binding (Arango *et al.* 1993). While data are limited on the role of the noradrenergic system in suicidal attempt and suicide (see Mann 2003), severe anxiety and/or agitation increase suicide risk and are associated with noradrenergic overactivity (Fawcett *et al.* 1997).

Additional support for a role for increased noradrenergic activity as a predictor of suicidal behaviour is provided by a treatment study of a norepinephrine reuptake inhibitor (NRI), maprotiline, that found that individuals maintained on the NRI after remission of depressive episode have higher rates of suicidal behaviour than those on placebo despite a lower likelihood of depression relapse (Rouillon *et al.* 1989).

## Hypothalamic–pituitary–adrenal axis

HPA axis abnormalities, most commonly dexamethasone resistance, have been observed in suicidal patients in diagnostically heterogeneous populations (Bunney *et al.* 1969; Meltzer *et al.* 1984; Nemeroff *et al.* 1988; Roy 1992; Träskman-Bendz *et al.* 1992b; Inder *et al.* 1997; van Heeringen *et al.* 2000; Brunner *et al.* 2001; Coryell and Schlesser 2001). Prospective biological studies of suicidal behaviour have investigated HPA function using both urinary measures of cortisol and the dexamethasone suppression test (DST).

## Dexamethasone suppression test

In prospective studies of mood disorder samples that include both individuals with and without prior suicide attempts, seven of nine studies reported that the majority of subjects who completed suicide over the course follow-up were DST non-suppressors (Boza *et al.* 1988; Carroll *et al.* 1981b; Coryell 1990; Coryell and Schlesser 1981; Norman *et al.* 1990; Roy *et al.* 1986; Yerevanian *et al.* 1983) while two studies found no relation (Black *et al.* 2002; Träskman-Bendz *et al.* 1992a). Coryell and Schlesser (2001) estimated that, over a 15-year follow-up period, DST non-suppressors had a fourteenfold higher risk of suicide compared to suppressors. In that study, the next most powerful predictor, a prior serious suicide attempt, indicated only a threefold increase in risk.

For suicide attempt, three of seven studies found an association between DST non-suppression and seriousness of suicide attempts at baseline (Targum *et al.* 1983; Norman *et al.* 1990), and over the follow-up period (Coryell 1990). Serious suicide attempts, including attempts prior to baseline resulting in high medical damage (Norman *et al.* 1990) and necessitating hospitalization

(Targum *et al.* 1983) were associated with DST non-suppression. In the third study, DST non-suppressors were more likely to make a psychologically, rather than medically, serious attempt in follow-up (Coryell 1990). Three further studies (Carroll *et al.* 1981b; Roy 1992; Träskman-Bendz *et al.* 1992a) reported baseline associations between violent method of suicide attempt and abnormal HPA axis function, however, only one study achieved statistical significance. In that study Roy (1992) found that at baseline individuals who had a previous violent attempt had significantly higher maximum post-DST plasma cortisol levels than those who had a previous non-violent attempt, however, no significant differences were observed between attempters, violent or not, and non-attempters during a 5-year follow-up.

Non-suppression on the DST may be associated with suicide because it predicts non-response to antidepressant treatment or a tendency for early relapse. Prospective studies provide evidence for both possibilities. Two studies (Yerevanian *et al.* 1983; Targum 1984) noted that DST non-suppressors, particularly those who fail to normalize over the course of inpatient treatment, had worse outcomes in terms of depression remission and relapse, circumstances which clinical follow-up studies have suggested increase risk for future suicidal acts (Oquendo *et al.* 2002). Targum *et al.* (1983) found that MDD subjects who normalized during treatment had the same relapse rate as non-suppressor psychiatric controls, while those who did not normalize had a higher incidence of relapse and poorer treatment response compared to normalizers.

## Conclusions

### Biological markers and the prediction of future suicidal behaviour

Developing sensitive prediction models for suicide and suicide attempt is crucial for prevention but is difficult due to the multiplicity of contributory risk factors and the low base rate of suicidal behaviour. Anomalies in several biological systems have been associated with suicidal behaviour in mood disorders and prospective biological studies, while not yet conclusive, suggest some potential for prediction based on biological measures. Meta-analysis of prospective studies of completed suicide show that CSF 5- HIAA levels and dexamethasone non-suppression yielded odds ratios for prediction of suicide of 4.48 and 4.65 respectively (Mann *et al.* 2006). Given the multi-determined nature of suicidal behaviour no one biological index will be adequate to predict suicidal behaviour, however including multiple biological markers in a model, for example CSF 5-HIAA and dexamethasone response, in order to assess both trait and state related risks (Mann *et al.* 2006) may increase predictive power. Including more than one tests results in some trade-off of sensitivity (requiring a positive result on any single test) versus specificity (requiring a positive result on more than one test). Therefore, also integrating other biological tests reviewed elsewhere, into multivariate predictive models alongside clinical and genetic risk factors to develop still more sensitive and specific predictive models, is a major challenge for this field of research (Mann and Currier 2007).

## References

Arango V, Ernsberger P, Sved AF *et al.* (1993). Quantitative autoradiography of α1- and α2-adrenergic receptors in the cerebral cortex of controis and suicide victims. *Brain Research*, **630**, 271–282.

Arango V, Underwood MD, Mann JJ (1996). Fewer pigmented locus coeruleus neurons in suicide victims: preliminary results. *Biological Psychiatry*, **39**, 112–120.

Åsberg M, Thoren P, Träskman L *et al.* (1976a). 'Serotonin depression'— A biochemical subgroup within the affective disorders? *Science*, **191**, 478–480.

Åsberg M, Träskman L, Thoren P (1976b). 5-HIAA in the cerebrospinal fluid. A biochemical suicide predictor? *Archives of General Psychiatry*, **33**, 1193–1197.

Baca-Garcia E, Diaz-Sastre C, Basurte E *et al.* (2001). A prospective study of the paradoxical relationships between impulsivity and lethality of suicide attempts. *Journal of Clinical Psychiatry*, **62**, 560–564.

Berglund M and Nilsson K (1987). Mortality in severe depression. A prospective study including 103 suicides. *Acta Psychiatrica Scandinavica*, **76**, 372–380.

Black DW, Monahan PO, Winokur G (2002). The relationship between DST results and suicidal behavior. *Annals of Clinical Psychiatry*, **14**, 83–88.

Boza RA, Milanes FJ, Uorente M *et al.* (1988). The DST and suicide among depressed alcoholic patients. *American Journal of Psychiatry*, **145**, 266–267.

Brinkman-Sull DC, Overholser JC, Silverman E. (2000). Risk of future suicide attempts in adolescent psychiatric inpatients at 18-month follow-up. *Suicide and Life-Threatening Behavior*, **30**, 327–340.

Brown GL, Ebert MH, Goyer PF *et al.* (1982). Aggression, suicide, and serotonin: relationships to CSF amine metabolites. *American Journal of Psychiatry*, **139**, 741–746.

Brunner J, Stalla GK, Stalla J *et al.* (2001). Decreased corticotropin-releasing hormone (CRH) concentrations in the cerebrospinal fluid of eucortisolemic suicide attempters. *Journal of Psychiatric Research*, **35**, 1–9.

Bunney WE Jr, Fawcett JA, Davis JM (1969). Further evaluation of urinary 17-hydroxycorticosteroids in suicidal patients. *Archives of General Psychiatry*, **21**, 138–150.

Carroll BJ, Feinberg M, Greden JF *et al.* (1981a). A specific laboratory test for the diagnosis of melancholia. Standardization, validation, and clinical urility. *Archives of General Psychiatry*, **38**, 15–22.

Carroll BJ, Greden JF, Feinberg M (1981b). Suicide, neuroendocrine dysfunction and CSF 5H1AA concentrations in depression. In B Angris, ed., *Recent Advances in Neuropsychopharmacology: Selected Papers from the 12th Congress of the Collegium Internationale Neuro-Psychophannacologicum, Goteborg, Sweden, 22–26 June 1980*, pp. 307–313. Pergamon Press, Oxford, New York.

Caspi A, Sugden K, Moffitt TE *et al.* (2003). Influence of life stress on depression: moderation by a polymorphism in the 5-HTT gene. *Science*, **301**, 386–389.

Cleare AJ and Bond AJ (1995). The effect of tryptophan depletion and enhancement on subjective and behavioural aggression in normal male subjects. *Psychopharmacology*, **118**, 72–81.

Cooper SJ, Kelly CB, King DJ (1992). 5-Hydroxyindoleacetic acid in cerebrospinal fluid and prediction of suicidal behaviour in schizophrenia. *Lancet*, **340**, 940–941.

Coryell W (1990). DST abnormality as a predictor of course in major depression. *Journal of Affective Disorders*, **19**, 163–169.

Coryell W, Haley J, Endicott J *et al.* (2002). The prospectively observed course of illness among depressed patients who commit suicide. *Acta Psychiatrica Scandinavica*, **105**, 218–223.

Coryell W and Schlesser MA (1981). Suicide and the dexamethasone supression test in unipolar depression. *American Journal of Psychiatry*, **138**, 1120–1121.

Coryell W and Schlesser MA (2001). The dexamethasone suppression test and suicide prediction. *American Journal of Psychiatry*, **158**, 748–753.

Dailly E, Chenu F, Renard CE *et al.* (2004). Dopamine, depression and antidepressants. *Fundamentals of Clinical Pharmacology*, **18**, 601–607.

Delgado PL, Price LH, Miller HL *et al.* (1994). Serotonin and the neurobiology of depression: Effects of tryptophan depletion in drug-free depressed patients. *Archives of General Psychiatry*, 51, 865–874.

Engstrom G, Alling C, Blennow K *et al.* (1999). Reduced cerebrospinal HVA concentrations and HVA/5-HIAA ratios in suicide attempters. Monoamine metabolites in 120 suicide attempters and 47 controls. *European Neuropsychopharmacology, 9*, 399–405.

Faustman WO, Ringo DL, Faull KF (1993). An association between low levels of 5-HIAA and HVA in cerebrospinal fluid and early mortality in a diagnostically mixed psychiatric sample. *British Journal of Psychiatry*, 163, 519–521.

Fawcett J, Busch KA, Jacobs D *et al.* (1997). Suicide: a four-pathway clinical–biochemical model. *Annals of the New York Academy of Sciences*, **836**, 288–301.

Flory JD, Mann JJ, Manuck SB *et al.* (1998). Recovery from major depression is not associated with normalization of serotonergic function. *Biological Psychiatry*, 43, 320–326.

Gardner DL, Lucas PB, Cowdry RW (1990). CSF metabolites in borderline personality disorder compared with normal controls. *Biological Psychiatry*, 28, 247–254.

Goldstein RB, Black DW, Nasrallah A *et al.* (1991). The prediction of suicide: sensitivity, specificity, and predictive value of a multivariate model applied to suicide among 1906 patients with affective disorders. *Archives of General Psychiatry*, 48, 418–422.

Heninger GR, Delgado PL, Charney DS *et al.* (1992). Tryptophan-deficient diet and amino acid drink deplete plasma tryptophan and induce a relapse of depression in susceptible patients. *Journal of Chemical Neuroanatomy*, 5, 347–348.

Inder WJ, Donald RA, Prickett TC *et al.* (1997). Arginine vasopressin is associated with hypercortisolemia and suicide attempts in depression. *Biological Psychiatry*, 42, 744–747.

Leon AC, Keller MB, Warshaw MG *et al.* (1999). A prospective study of fluoxetine treatment and suicidal behavior in affectively ill subjects. *American Journal of Psychiatry*, 156, 195–201.

Mann JJ (2003). Neurobiology of suicidal behaviour. *Nature Reviews Neuroscience*, 4, 819–828.

Mann JJ and Currier D (2007). A review of prospective studies of biologic predictors of suicidal behavior in mood disorders. *Archives of Suicide Research*, 11, 3–16.

Mann JJ, Currier D, Stanley B *et al.* (2006). Can biological tests assist prediction of suicide in mood disorders? *International Journla of Neuropsychopharmacology*, 9, 465–474.

Mann JJ, Huang YY, Underwood MD *et al.* (2000). A serotonin transporter gene promoter polymorphism (5-HTTLPR) and prefrontal cortical binding in major depression and suicide. *Archives of General Psychiatry*, 57, 729–738.

Mann JJ and Kapur S (1995). A dopaminergic hypothesis of major depression. *Clinical Neuropharmacology*, 18, 557–565.

Mann JJ and Malone KM (1997). Cerebrospinal fluid amines and higher-lethality suicide attempts in depressed inpatients. *Biological Psychiatry*, 41, 162–171.

Mann JJ, Malone KM, Sweeney JA *et al.* (1996). Attempted suicide characteristics and cerebrospinal fluid amine metabolites in depressed inpatients. *Neuropsychopharmacology*, 15, 576–586.

Meltzer HY, Perline R, Tricou BJ *et al.* (1984). Effect of 5-hydroxytryptophan on serum cortisol levels in major affective disorders. II. Relation to suicide, psychosis and depressive symptoms. *Archives of General Psychiatry*, 41, 379–387.

Milak MS, Parsey RV, Keilp J *et al.* (2005). Neuroanatomic correlates of psychopathologic components of major depressive disorder. *Archives of General Psychiatry*, 62, 397–408.

Moeller FG, Dougherty DM, Swann AC *et al.* (1996). Tryptophan depletion and aggressive responding in healthy males. *Psychopharmacology (Berl)*, 126, 97–103.

Moreno FA, Gelenberg AJ, Heninger GR *et al.* (1999). Tryptophan depletion and depressive vulnerability. *Biological Psychiatry*, 46, 498–505.

Nemeroff CB, Owens MJ, Bissette G *et al.* (1988). Reduced corticotropin-releasing factor binding sites in the frontal cortex of suicide victims. *Archives of General Psychiatry*, **45**, 577–579.

Ninan PT, van Kammen DP, Scheinin M *et al.* (1984). CSF 5-hydroxyindoleacetic acid levels in suicidal schizophrenic patients. *American Journal of Psychiatry*, 141, 566–569.

Norman WH, Brown WA, Miller LW *et al.* (1990). The dexamethasone suppression test and completed suicide. *Acta Psychiatrica Scandinavica*, **81**, 120–125.

Oquendo MA, Echavarria G, Galfalvy HC *et al.* (2003b). Lower cortisol levels in depressed patients with comorbid post-traumatic stress disorder. *Neuropsychopharmacology*, 28, 591–598

Oquendo MA, Kamali M, Ellis SP *et al.* (2002). Adequacy of antidepressant treatment after discharge and the occurrence of suicidal acts in major depressive episode in patients with depressive disorder or bipolar disorder. *American Journal of Psychiatry*, 161, 1433–1441.

Oquendo MA and Mann JJ (2000). The biology of impulsivity and suicidality. *Psychiatric Clinics of North America*, 23, 11–25.

Oquendo MA, Placidi GP, Malone KM *et al.* (2003b). Positron emission tomography of regional brain metabolic responses to a serotonergic challenge and lethality of suicide attempts in major depression. *Archives of General Psychiatry*, 60, 14–22.

Placidi GP, Oquendo MA, Malone KM *et al.* (2001). Aggressivity, suicide attempts, and depression: Relationship to cerebrospinal fluid monoamine metabolite levels. *Biological Psychiatry*, **50**, 783–791.

Price LH, Charney DS, Delgado PL *et al.* (1991). Serotonin function and depression: neuroendocrine and mood responses to intravenous L-tryptophan in depressed patients and healthy comparison subjects. *American Journal of Psychiatry*, 148, 1518–1525.

Rouillon F, Phillips R, Serrurier D *et al.* (1989). Rechutes de depression unipolaire et efficacite de la maprotiline. *L'Encephale*, **XV**, 527–534.

Roy A (1992). Hypothalamic–pituitary–adrenal axis function and suicidal behavior in depression. *Biological Psychiatry*, 32, 812–816.

Roy A, Ågren H, Pickar D *et al.* (1986). Reduced CSF concentrations of homovanillic acid and homovanillic acid to 5-hydroxyindoleacetic acid ratios in depressed patients: relationship to suicidal behavior and dexamethasone non-suppression. *American Journal of Psychiatry*, 143, 1539–1545.

Roy A, De Jong J, Linnoila M (1989). Cerebrospinal fluid monoamine metabolites and suicidal behaviour in depressed patients. A 5-year follow-up study. *Archives of General Psychiatry*, 46, 609–612.

Salomon RM, Mazure CM, Delgado PL *et al.* (1994). Serotonin function in aggression: The effect of acute plasma tryptophan depletion in aggressive patients. *Biological Psychiatry*, **35**, 570–572.

Samuelsson M, Jokinen J, Nordstrom AL *et al.* (2006). CSF 5-HIAA, suicide intent and hopelessness in the prediction of early suicide in male highrisk suicide attempters. *Acta Psychiatrica Scandinavica*, **113**, 44–47.

Smith KA, Morris JS, Friston KJ *et al.* (1999). Brain mechanisms associated with depressive relapse and associated cognitive impairment following acute tryptophan depletion. *British Journal of Psychiatry*, **174**, 525–529.

Targum SD (1984). Persistent neuroendocrine dysregulation in major depressive disorder: a marker for early relapse. *Biological Psychiatry*, 19, 305–318.

Targum SD, Rosen L, Capodanno AE (1983). The dexamethasone supression test in suicidal patients with unipolar depression. *American Journal of Psychiatry*, **140**, 877–879.

Träskman L, Åsberg M, Bertilsson L *et al.* (1981). Monoamine metabolites in CSF and suicidal behavior. *Archives of General Psychiatry*, **38**, 631–636.

Träskman-Bendz L, Alling C, Oreland L *et al.* (1992a). Prediction of suicidal behavior from biologic tests. *Journal of Clinical Psychopharmacology*, 12, 215–226.

Träskman-Bendz L, Åsberg M, Bertilsson L *et al.* (1984). CSF monoamine metabolites of depressed patients during illness and after recovery. *Acta Psychiatrica Scandinavica*, **69**, 333–342.

Träskman-Bendz L, Ekman R, Regnell G *et al.* (1992b). HPA-related CSF neuropeptides in suicide attempters. *European Neuropsychopharmacology*, **2**, 99–106.

van Heeringen K, Audenaert K, Van de WL *et al.* (2000). Cortisol in violent suicidal behaviour: association with personality and monoaminergic activity. *Journal of Affective Disorders*, **60**, 181–189.

Virkkunen M, De Jong J, Bartko J *et al.* (1989). Relationship of psychobiological variables to recidivi in violent offenders and impulsive fire setters. A follow-up study. *Archives of General Psychiatry*, **46**, 600–603.

Virkkunen M, Eggert M, Rawlings R *et al.* (1996). A prospective follow-up study of alcoholic violent offenders and fire setters. *Archives of General Psychiatry*, **53**, 523–529.

Westrin Å, Ekman R, Ragnell G *et al.* (2001). A follow up study of suicide attempters: Increase of CSF-somatostatin but no change in CSF-CRH. *European Neuropsychopharmacology*, **11**, 135–143.

Yerevanian BI, Olafsdottir H, Milanese E *et al.* (1983). Normalization of the dexamethasone suppression test at discharge from hospital. Its prognostic value. *Journal of Affective Disorders*, **5**, 191–197.

# CHAPTER 46

# Neuroimaging of suicidal behaviour

## Where does the field stand?

Maria A Oquendo, Tresha Gibbs and Ramin Parsey

## Abstract

Consistent evidence implicates serotonin system dysfunction in the neurobiology of suicidal behaviour. Neuroimaging studies link brain structure and function *in vivo* and contribute to our understanding of neural pathways. Areas of the prefrontal cortex and limbic structures are targeted in neuroimaging studies of suicidal behaviour, which have focused on structural, haemodynamic, metabolic, and neuroreceptor changes in the brains of suicide attempters. Neuroimaging studies have revealed that signal hyperintensities, perfusion and metabolic abnormalities, processing of affect and serotonin receptor and transporter changes, may each play a role. Knowledge regarding the neurobiology of suicidal behaviour must rely on study designs utilizing robust methodologies, including improved patient and control group selection, improved neuroimaging techniques, and adequate statistical analysis to enhance the validity, consistency, and conclusiveness of the data. Ongoing development of new radioligands and imaging methodologies promise to enhance our ability to delineate the neurobiology of suicidal acts.

## Introduction

There is consistent evidence implicating serotonin system dysfunction in the neurobiology of suicidal behaviour. In early studies by Åsberg and colleagues (1976), depressed suicide attempters were found to have lower cerebrospinal fluid (CSF) serotonin metabolite, 5-hydroxyindoleacetic acid (5-HIAA), than depressed non-attempters. High-lethality suicide attempters had lower CSF 5-HIAA levels when compared to those who used a low-lethality method (Mann and Malone 1997; Placidi *et al.* 2001). Through post-mortem studies of suicide victims, the dorsal raphe nucleus and the ventral prefrontal cortex (PFC) have been identified to have serotonin abnormalities such as decreased serotonin transporter (SERT) binding and increased serotonin (5HT)-1A receptor binding (for a review see Mann *et al.* 1999).

Neuroimaging studies provide the opportunity to link brain structure and function *in vivo* and can contribute to our understanding of neural pathways in suicidal behaviour. Based on post-mortem findings and current understanding of serotonin pathways in the brain, areas of the PFC and structures of the limbic system are targeted in many neuroimaging studies of suicide (Oquendo and Mann 2001). Using available imaging modalities, these studies have focused on structural, haemodynamic, metabolic, and neuroreceptor changes in the brains of suicide attempters.

## Method

In order to identify relevant neuroimaging studies of suicidal behaviour for this review, we conducted a search in PubMed using the following key words: suicide (or suicide attempt or suicidal behaviour) and MRI (magnetic resonance imaging)—or fMRI (functional magnetic resonance imaging) or diffusion tensor imaging (DTI) or PET (positron emission spectography) or single photon emission computerized tomography (SPECT). All articles identified were reviewed, and those with original data regarding suicidal behaviour were included. Those articles that did not specifically address the topic of suicidal behaviour were excluded from this review. In addition, bibliographies were scanned to identify additional relevant publications not found with our search strategy.

## Results

We identified thirteen studies using this strategy, with significant variations in study design and methodology. Data from each study is presented in Table 46.1 to highlight design, number of study participants, imaging modality used, major findings reported by the authors, and major limitations.

The thirteen neuroimaging studies highlighted in Table 46.1 suggest that underlying brain abnormalities reflected by signal hyperintensities, perfusion or metabolic abnormalities, functional differences in processing of affect, and serotonin receptor and transporter changes may play a role in suicidal behaviour. Although these results are intriguing, due to differences in study design, most of them cannot be directly compared. It is also difficult to draw firm conclusions.

**Table 46.1** Neuroimaging studies of suicide attempters

| Author/study design | Study participants | Imaging modality/tracer, ligand | Major findings (as stated in paper) | Limitations |
|---|---|---|---|---|
| **Structural MRI studies** | | | | |
| Ahearn 2001 Case–control, retrospective | 20 outpatients with MDD with SA history. 20 MDD without SA | T1- and T2-weighted images | Higher number of subcortical grey matter hyperintensities in those with history of SA. | No control for history of drug, alcohol use or method of SA. Comorbid diagnoses not specified. |
| Ehrlich 2005 Cross-sectional, retrospective | 102 inpatients with MDD, 62/102 with SA history. | T2 weighted | Higher prevalence of PVH but not DWMH in patients with history of SA when compared to those without SA history. Severity of PVH a significant predictor of past SA. | No information on methods of SA. Three different scanners used. Group level differences in white matter hyperintensities (DWMH+PVH) between SA and non-attempters not significant. |
| Monkul 2007 Case–control, Brain volume | 7 female MDD with history of SA 10 female MDD without history of SA 17 HC | T1 or T2? ROI: OFC, cingulate, amygdala, hippocampus | SA with decreased bilateral OFC grey matter volumes, and increased right amygdala volumes. | No information on methods or lethality of SA, or time from last attempt. 2 different image analysis programs were used. |
| **Blood flow studies** | | | | |
| Audenaert 2002 Activation Study: Verbal fluency test | 20 MDD patients with recent SA (less than 7 days prior) 20 HC | SPECT/b, 99mTc-ECD ROI: none specified | During CFT, SA had blunted perfusion of left inferior PFC, R inferior parietal gyrus, L and R ACC. During LFT, SA had blunted perfusion in L and R med temporal gyrus, R ACC, and R hypothalamus. | No psychiatric control group. Patients on psychotropic drugs not excluded. Lower IQ in SA group. P values for regions of activation non-significant. Pixel by pixel analysis showed difference but not cluster level differences. |
| Fountoulakis 2004 Cross-sectional, retrospective | 50 MDD patients Subgroups: 18 SA vs. 32 Non-SA; 17 No current thoughts of death 23 No specific thoughts of death 10 With suicidal thoughts | SPECT/a, 99mTc HMPAO ROI: cerebellum, thalamus, caudate nucleus, GP, FL, PL, TL, OL. | After Bonferroni correction, no difference in rCBF between SA versus non-SA. No difference between three subgroups based on thoughts of death. | Included patients with GAD and panic disorder, disorders which may involve the serotonin system. Did not study inferior frontal lobe. |
| **Functional MRI studies** | | | | |
| Jollant 2008 | All euthymic male subjects 13 SA with MDD 14 MDD 16 HC | Event-related fMRI on 1.5 T magnet | Compared to MDD alone, SA with MDD showed increased activity in R lateral orbitofrontal cortex (BA 47) in response to angry faces Decreased activity in R superior frontal gyrus (BA 6) in response to angry faces Greater activity in R cerebellum in response to mild angry expressions. No differences in response to neutral or happy faces Greater activity in the R anterior cingulate gyrus (BA 32), extending to the medial frontal gyrus (BA 10) in response to mild happy versus mild happy versus neutral faces. | No description of comorbidities such as anxiety or cluster B personality disorders, common in SA and which may impact affect processing Time since most recent SA not given |

**Serotonin studies**

| Study | Sample | Method | Results | Comments |
|---|---|---|---|---|
| Audenaert 2001 Case–control 5HT2a receptor study | 9 SA (<8 days prior) Axis I diagnoses: 4 MDD 4 adjustment disorder 1 brief psychotic disorder 13 HC | SPECT, resting/ d[123I]5-I-R91150 ROI: bilateral frontal cortex, OFC, dorsolateral PFC | After Bonferroni correction, frontal 5HT 2a BP lower in SA versus HC; 0.39 vs. 0.68. | No psychiatric control. No intent measure in SA. Multiple psychiatric diagnoses represented. Small groups, 3 patients in deliberate self-injury group. Use of SEM instead of SD in analysis. SA by overdose in 5/9 patients. Regions of PFC not specified. Multiple post-hoc comparisons with small sample sizes. |
| Van Heeringen 2003 Case–control | See Audenaert 2001 | See Audenaert 2001 | Lower 5HT 2a receptor antagonist binding in PFC in SA (140.7) vs non- SA (168). | See above. |
| Oquendo 2003 Cross-sectional. Activation study, fenfluramine challenge | 25 MDD with SA (mean 4 years prior) 16 high-lethality SA 9 low-lethality SA | PET/FFDG ROI: anterior cingulate and medial frontal gyri; anterior cingulate and right superior frontal gyrus. | Lower rCMRglu in ventral, medial, lateral PFC in high-lethality vs low-lethality SA. Lower VM PFC activity associated with lower impulsivity, intent, and lethality. Pre-fenfluramine: Lower rCMRglu in bilateral superior frontal, ACC, and inferior frontal gyri in high-lethality group. Post-fenfluramine: Lower rCMRglu in same areas above and superior frontal gyri. | No psychiatric control group. No HC group. Comorbid diagnoses not discussed. Methods of suicide attempt not discussed. |
| Lindstrom 2004 Case–control 5HT transporter | 12 SA with high intent Axis I diagnoses: 6 mood disorder 1 social phobia 3 adjustment disorder 12 HC | SPECT/cocaine analogue, [123I]-β CIT ROI: cerebellum and whole brain | No significant differences in whole brain BP of 5HTT. No significant differences in BP for violent SA vs. nonviolent SA vs controls. | Heterogeneous diagnoses. SPECT automatic scaling- increases error in ROI. No regional anatomic structures specified. β-CIT also binds the dopamine transporter. |
| Leyton 2006 Case–control Tryptophan uptake | 10 high lethality SA (mean 14.7days) Methods: 8 by overdose, 1 by hanging, 1 by jumping Axis I diagnoses: 2 Mood disorder 6 Substance abuse 16 HC | PET/ α[11C]Methyl-L-tryptophan ROI: medial OFG, left OFG, medial PFG | SA with decreased normalized tryptophan trapping in OFC and VM PFC. Increased tryptophan trapping seen in L thalamus, R paracentral lobule, L middle occipital cortex, L hippocampal gyrus. Suicide intent negatively correlated with tryptophan trapping in OFG and R medial PFG. | No psychiatric controls. Unclear which toxins used in SA. Multiple comorbid diagnoses, including substance abuse. Utility of labelled tryptophan as a marker of serotonin synthesis has been questioned. In planned comparisons of trapping rate constants in VOI, main effect of group not significant. |

**Table 46.1** (Continued) Neuroimaging studies of suicide attempters

| Author/study design | Study participants | Imaging modality/tracer, ligand | Major findings (as stated in paper) | Limitations |
|---|---|---|---|---|
| Cannon 2006 Case–control 5HT transporter | 18 BD, current MDE (8 SA history) 37 HC | PET/ g[11C] DASB ROI: thalamus, striatum, insula, midbrain, sgACC, pgACC, DCC, PCC | In SA, increased pgACC binding and decreased midbrain binding compared to 10 without SA. Compared to controls, increased binding in thalamus, insula, DCC, and increased in midbrain. | Use of SEM distorts the small effect size. SPM reported with uncorrected p-values. No arterial sampling documented. Comorbid diagnoses include OCD, panic attacks. No account for cerebellum uptake (in bipolar disorder). |
| Oquendo 2007 Case–control 5HT transporter | 18 BD, current MDE (9 SA history) 41 HC | PET/h[11C] McNeil 5652 ROI: midbrain, amygdala, hippocampus, thalamus, putamen, ACC | No difference in BP between SA and non-SA. Bipolar patients had lower 5HTT BP in midbrain, amygdala, hippocampus, thalamus, putamen and ACC No correlation between depression severity and BP. | 11% of patients with remission of symptoms during washout is concerning for change in synapses. Multiple comorbid diagnoses (OCD, PTSD, GAD, binge eating, simple phobia), some of which involve the serotonin system. |

AD = antidepressant.

BD, bipolar disorder; BP, binding potential; CFT, category fluency test; CBF, cerebral blood flow; CV, cardiovascular risk factors; DR, dorsal raphe; DWMH, deep white matter hyperintensity; FL, frontal lobe; GAD, generalized anxiety disorder; GP, globus pallidus; HC, healthy controls; L, left; LFT, letter fluency test; MDD, major depressive disorder; MDE, major depressive episode; MPFC, medial prefrontal cortex; MRI,magnetic resonance imaging; OCD, obsessive–compulsive disorder; OFG, orbitofrontal gyrus; OL, occipital lobe; OPFC, orbital prefrontal cortex; PET, positron emission tomography; PFG, prefrontal gyrus; pgACC, pregenual anterior cingulate cortex; PL, parietal lobe; PTSD, post-traumatic stress disorder; PVH, periventricular hyperintensity; R, right; rCBF, regional cerebral blood flow; rCMRglu, regional cerebral glucose utilization; ROI, regions of interest; SA, suicide attempters; SCH, subcortical grey matter hyperintensity; SEM, standard error of the mean; sgACC, subgenual anterior cingulate cortex; SPECT, single photon emission computed tomography; SPM, statistical parametric mapping; TL, temporal lobe; VM, ventromedial; VOI- voxel of interest; WM, white matter.

Tracers/ligands: a[99mTc]-HMPAO, 99mTc hexamethylpropyleneamine oxime;b[99mTc]-ECD, 99mTc-Ethyl Cystine Dimer; cFDG, 18F- flourodeoxyglucose; d[123I]5-I-R91150, 4-amino-N-[1-[3-(4-fluorophenoxy) propyl]-4-methyl-4-piperidinyl]-5-iodo-2-methoxybenzamide; f[123I]-(β-CIT), 123I-β-carbomethoxy-3-beta (4-iodophenyl)-tropane; g[11C] DASB, [11C]-3-amino-4-(2-dimethylaminomethylphenyl-sulfanyl)-benzonitrile; h[11C] McNeil 5652, 11C(+) trans 1;2;4;5;6; 10-β-hexahydro-6-[4-(methylthio)phenyl]-pyrrolo[2;1-a]isoquinoline.

# Discussion

Several methodological recommendations may improve the likelihood of determining the neurobiological basis of suicidal acts. These include improved sample selection, imaging technique, and statistical analysis. Below, we detail strategies that may improve our fund of knowledge regarding the biological basis for suicide attempts.

## Sample selection

From a sampling point of view, future studies would benefit from utilizing a standardized definition of suicidal behaviour, well-matched controls, as well as sufficient subjects to ensure the statistical power to detect clinically relevant abnormalities.

### Uniformity in definitions of suicidal behaviour

To date, imaging studies have used a variety of definitions regarding suicidal behaviour, as researchers differ on the definition of a suicide attempt. One widely accepted definition of a suicide attempt is the 'potentially self-injurious behaviour with non-fatal outcome for which there is evidence that that the person intended at some level, to kill himself' (O'Carroll *et al.* 1996). This definition involves three components: self-injury, non-fatal outcome, and intent to die as a consequence of the behaviour. However, some studies have included patients with a history of deliberate self-harm, irrespective of the intent of the act. In other studies, descriptions are not detailed enough to permit a clear definition of suicide attempt for comparison to other studies. Such inclusion criteria discrepancies can create potential confounders when interpreting results. The definition of suicide attempt is important, not only because we seek to elucidate the underlying biological basis of as uniform a phenotype as possible, but also because there is evidence that the degree of suicidal intent and lethality of suicide attempt correlate with neurobiological markers such as tryptophan uptake and cerebral perfusion in the PFC (Oquendo *et al.* 2003; Leyton *et al.* 2006).

The use of appropriate controls groups is another key sampling issue. Although many of the studies have used healthy volunteers as controls, this type of matching does not permit full characterization of the abnormalities that are specific to suicidal behaviour. The inclusion of psychiatric control groups may help clarify the role of underlying psychopathology in observed abnormalities. Thus, well-matched, well characterized, control groups that take into account drug abuse history and comorbid psychiatric conditions, may clarify the confounding effect of these factors in the development of abnormalities observed in neuroimaging studies. Similarly, the method of suicide attempt used by the subject may have key effects on observed neuroimaging abnormalities.

Patient inclusion criteria based on time from suicide attempt varies in the studies reviewed, and points to an underlying question of whether propensity for suicidal behaviour and associated biological findings are enduring traits. Indeed, some studies image patients within an average of 1 or 2 weeks post suicide attempt (Audenaert *et al.* 2001, 2002; van Heeringen *et al.* 2003; Leyton *et al.* 2006), while others imaged patients with a lifetime history of suicide attempt, even if the attempt was over 4 years in the past or time from suicide attempt was not reported (Ahearn *et al.* 2001; Oquendo *et al.* 2003; Monkul *et al.* 2007; Jollant *et al.* 2008). Suicidal behaviour may be a state in which brain changes involved are only detectable at the time of the suicide attempt and given the plasticity

of the brain, there are advantages to studying suicide attempters close to the time of the attempt. However, serious methodological issues must be grappled with. For example, acute and long-term effects of drug overdose on brain chemistry, use of alcohol during the attempt, and relative hypoxia experienced during certain types of suicide attempts can affect the central nervous system. Of course, damage from suicide attempts can be long lasting and, thus, even those studies of attempters with a lifetime history of suicidal behaviour may be affected by the consequences of the suicidal acts themselves. For these reasons, these issues require consideration during the design phase of the study.

## Technical study design

There are several factors that may improve the validity of the data acquired in neuroimaging studies and neuroreceptor studies in particular (Audenaert *et al.* 2001; Parsey *et al.* 2002; Oquendo *et al.* 2003; Lindstrom *et al.* 2004; Leyton *et al.* 2006; Cannon *et al.* 2006; Oquendo *et al.* 2007). First, initial studies should be conducted with full quantification of binding potential through the use of metabolite corrected input functions. The use of arterial input functions or arterialized venous input functions should be standard practice until reference regions are determined to be measures of free and non-specific binding and are found to be invariant between suicide attempters and non-attempters. Once it is determined in a sample of sufficient size that the reference region is adequate, future studies can be carried out with reference tissue modelling approaches.

Second, choice of PET as the imaging modality would lead to improved data collection, since PET imaging offers much higher resolution than current commercially available SPECT imaging systems. Given the small volume of some structures of interest, the higher resolution of PET offers a distinct advantage.

Third, each year we see the development of new and improved radioligands for use in human studies. State of the art radioligands ideally have good blood–brain barrier permeability, stable tracer kinetics, absence of radioactively labelled metabolites that have affinity for the target, and measurable free fraction. Key considerations also include ease of production and a favourable safety profile in humans. For example, [$^{11}$C]DASB is an excellent alternative to the previous serotonin transporter radioligand [$^{11}$C]McNeil 5652. Namely, it has a measurable free fraction (Ogden *et al.* 2007), kinetics that are more amenable to accurate modelling, and it generates a higher signal to noise ratio. Utilization of superior radioligands will improve the accuracy and reliability of the data collected.

Our literature search revealed few blood flow studies and only one metabolism study and one functional imaging study (Audenaert *et al.* 2002; Oquendo *et al.* 2003; Fountoulakis *et al.* 2004; Jollant *et al.* 2008). In order to assess functional differences and establish the presence or absence of a functional neurocircuitry of suicidal behaviour, these studies are essential. Again, initial studies should be conducted with metabolite input functions as there may be global changes in flow or metabolism that are not detectable using qualitative scans.

## Statistical analysis

To analyse neuroimaging data, statistical parametric mapping (SPM) software is commonly used, but it requires care in interpretation. This is due to the issue of multiple comparisons.

While the program has the capability to perform analyses to test the difference in regions of interest (ROI) that are defined a priori, most commonly, the statistical approach used is not hypothesis-driven. In this type of exploratory analysis, the statistical program makes inferences about differences in signal across the brain. Specifically, it morphs individual brains to fit a standardized brain space and creates a three dimensional matrix or 'map', also referred to as a 'glass brain'. The program assigns a value to individual volumes in the space referred to as voxels. By literally calculating millions of t-tests, voxel by voxel across the entire brain volume, it makes estimates about group differences. It generates two different types of output. First, it identifies points in the brain where the signal from the imaging methodology is significantly different from other regions. These brain locations are identified by the p value calculated for that specific point in the 'glass brain' but the p value, referred to as an 'uncorrected p value' in the output, is not corrected for multiple comparisons. Then, utilizing sophisticated statistical theory, SPM generates two additional types of output. One type of output is an estimate of the probability that a given cluster of adjacent or colocalized voxels, that together exceed a threshold in terms of a predetermined size of the cluster, is a region of significant difference between groups. This cluster is assigned a p value. SPM also generates 'corrected p values' for points within the significantly different cluster that are significantly different in the groups being compared. The threshold for significance can be set by the user. Although this powerful, data-mining methodology can be useful for hypothesis generation, it requires that the output be interpreted within its limitations. For example, not every p value that is 'significant' is meaningful (uncorrected p values) because the problem of multiple testing confounds the results. However, as mentioned, the program does generate p values that are 'corrected'. These are the p values that are most reliable. Uncorrected p values or analyses conducted in which the threshold for generating images that demonstrate regions of 'significant difference' is too low, and cannot be interpreted meaningfully.

## Interpretation of results

In general, there are several key challenges in the interpretation of neuroimaging studies of suicidal behaviour. For example, some structural studies have focused on presence of signal hyperintensities (Ahearn et al. 2001; Erlich et al. 2005). However, the presence or location of signal hyperintensities is not specific to suicidality. Signal hyperintensities are regions of decreased regional cerebral blood flow (Wen et al. 2004) reflecting areas of vascular, neuronal, or other brain parenchymal damage. They are associated with ageing, geriatric depression, dementia, cardiovascular disease, methamphetamine, cocaine and opiate abuse (Greenwald et al. 1998; Barber et al. 1999; Breeze et al. 2003; Lyoo et al. 2004; Bae et al. 2006). Nonetheless, the studies of signal hyperintensities are instructive since key brain pathways involved in mood regulation and behavioural inhibition may be affected. Signal hyperintensities may disrupt neural communication between PFC, limbic and other pivotal regions. They may result in impaired impulse regulation and other functions central to decision-making, which may impact on the emergence of suicidal acts.

Similarly, interpretation of studies using C-α-methyl-L-tryptophan is hampered by studies that question the use of labelled tryptophan in CNS as a marker of serotonin synthesis (Leyton et al. 2006). Indeed, in anesthetized rhesus monkeys, labelled tryptophan appeared to be a marker of tryptophan uptake, rather than serotonin synthesis (Shoaf et al. 2000). In light of such disagreement, caution must be used in interpretation of results using this radioligand.

## Future directions

Among the newer modalities for neuroimaging, diffusion tensor imaging (DTI), may help elucidate neural substrates for suicidal behaviour. While it is a new technology in schizophrenia research (Hoptman et al. 2002; Kanaan et al. 2005), DTI may provide a measure of white matter integrity and, therefore, an assessment of the degree of connectivity among brain regions involved in mood regulation and executive functioning. DTI uses MRI scanners and has two common outcome measures, fractional anisotropy and probabilistic tractography, or trace. Fractional anisotropy reflects the direction of diffusion of water between nerve tissue, with lower values reflecting axonal disorganization. Trace is the diffusion coefficient across all directions, with higher values reflecting increased extracellular space, suggesting an abnormality (Hoptman et al. 2002). Potentially, this technology could more specifically identify regions of neural disconnection which may contribute to manifestation of suicidal behaviour.

# Conclusion

There is much to learn from *in vivo* neuroimaging studies of suicidal behaviour. Neuroimaging studies have revealed that factors such as signal hyperintensities, perfusion and metabolic abnormalities, and serotonin receptor and transporter changes, may each play a role in suicidal behaviour. As discussed, the advancement of knowledge regarding the neurobiology of suicidal behaviour relies on the design of studies utilizing robust methodologies, including improved patient and control group selection, improved neuroimaging techniques, and adequate statistical analysis to further enhance the validity, consistency, and conclusiveness of the data. The ongoing development of new radioligands and imaging methodologies are likely to enhance our ability to uncover the underlying neurobiology of suicidal acts.

## References

Ahearn EP, Jamison KR, Steffens DC et al. (2001). MRI correlates of suicide attempt history in unipolar depression. *Biological Psychiatry*, **50**, 266–270.

Åsberg M, Träskman L, Thorén P (1976). 5-HIAA in the cerebrospinal fluid. A biochemical suicide predictor? *Archives of General Psychiatry*, **33**, 1193–1197.

Audenaert K, Goethals I, Van Laere K et al. (2002). SPECT neuropsychological activation procedure with the Verbal Fluency Test in attempted suicide patients. *Nuclear Medicine Communications*, **23**, 907–916.

Audenaert K, Van Laere K, Dumont F et al. (2001). Decreased frontal serotonin 5HT 2a receptor binding index in deliberate self-harm patients. *European Journal of Nuclear Medicine*, **28**, 175–182.

Bae SC, Lyoo IK, Sung YH et al. (2006). Increased white matter hyperintensities in male methamphetamine abusers. *Drug and Alcohol Dependence*, **81**, 83–88.

Barber R, Scheltens P, Gholkar A et al. (1999). White matter lesions on magnetic resonance imaging in dementia with Lewy bodies, Alzheimer's dementia, vascular dementia, and normal aging. *Journal of Neurology, Neurosurgery, and Psychiatry*, **67**, 66–72.

Breeze JL, Hesdorffer DC, Hong X *et al.* (2003). Clinical significance of brain white matter hyperintensities in young adults with psychiatric illness. *Harvard Review of Psychiatry*, **11**, 269–283.

Cannon DM, Ichise M, Fromm SJ *et al.* (2006). Serotonin transporter binding in bipolar disorder assessed using [11C] DASB and positron emission tomography. *Biological Psychiatry*, **60**, 207–217.

Ehrlich, S, Breeze JL, Hesdorffer DC *et al.* (2005). White matter hyperintensities and their association with suicidality in depressed young adults. *Journal of Affective Disorders*, **86**, 281–287.

Fountoulakis KN, Iacovides A, Fotiou F *et al.* (2004). Neurobiological and psychological correlates of suicide attempts and thoughts of death in patients with major depression. *Neuropsyschobiology*, **49**, 42–52.

Greenwald BS, Kramer-Ginsberg E, Krishnan K *et al.* (1998). Neuroanatomic localization of magnetic resonance imaging signal hyperintensities in geriatric depression. *Stroke*, **29**, 613–617.

Hoptman MJ, Volavka J, Johnson G *et al.* (2002). Frontal white matter microstructure, aggression, and impulsivity in men with schizophrenia: a preliminary study. *Biological Society*, **52**, 9–14.

Jollant F, Lawrence NS, Giampietro V *et al.* (2008). Orbitofrontal cortex response to angry faces in men with histories of suicide attempts. *American Journal of Psychiatry*, **165**, 740–748.

Kanaan RAA, Kim Jin-Suh, Kaufmann WE *et al.* (2005). Diffusion tensor imaging in schizophrenia. *Biological Psychiatry*, **58**, 921–929.

Leyton M, Paquette V, Gravel P *et al.* (2006). α-[11C] Methyl-L-tryptophan trapping in the orbital and ventral medial prefrontal cortex of suicide attempters. *European Neuropsychopharmacology*, **16**, 220–223.

Lindström MB, Ryding E, Bosson P *et al.* (2004). Impulsivity related to brain serotonin transporter binding capacity in suicide attempters. *European Neuropsychopharmacology*, **14**, 295–300.

Lyoo IK, Streeter CC, Ahn KH *et al.* (2004). White matter hyperintensities in subjects with cocaine and opiate dependence and healthy comparison subjects. *Psychiatry Research*, **131**, 135–145.

Mann JJ and Malone KM (1997). Cerebrospinal fluid amines and higher lethality suicide attempts in depressed inpatients. *Biological Psychiatry*, **41**, 162–171.

Mann JJ, Oquendo MA, Underwood MD *et al.* (1999). The neurobiology of suicide risk: a review for the clinician. *The Journal of Clinical Psychiatry*, **60**, 7–11.

Monkul ES, Hatch JP, Nicoletti MA *et al.* (2007). Fronto-limbic brain structures in suicidal and non-suicidal female patients with major depressive disorder. *Molecular Psychiatry*, **12**, 360–366.

O'Carroll PW, Berman Al, Maris RW *et al.* (1996). Beyond the tower of Babel: a nomenclature for suicidology. *Suicide and Life-Threatening Behaviour*, **26**, 237–252.

Ogden RT, Ojha A, Erlandsson K *et al.* (2007). *In vivo* quantification of serotonin transporters using [11C]DASB and positron emission tomography in humans: modeling considerations. *Journal of Cerebral Blood Flow & Metabolism*, **27**, 205–217.

Oquendo MA, Hastings RS, Huang YY *et al.* (2007). Brain serotonin transporter binding in depressed patients with bipolar disorder using positron emission tomography. *Archives of General Psychiatry*, **64**, 201–208.

Oquendo MA and Mann JJ (2001). Neuroimaging findings in major depression, suicidal behaviour and aggression. *Clinical Neuroscience Research*, **1**, 377–380.

Oquendo MA, Placidi GP, Malone KM *et al.* (2003). Positron emission tomography of regional brain metabolic responses to a serotonergic challenge and lethality of suicide attempts in major depression. *Archives of General Psychiatry*, **60**, 14–22.

Parsey RV, Oquendo MA, Simpson NR *et al.* (2002). Effects of sex, age, and aggressive traits in man on brain serotonin 5-HT1A receptor binding potential measured by PET using [C-11]WAY-100635. *Brain Research*, **954**, 173–182.

Placidi GPA, Oquendo MA, Malone KM *et al.* (2001). Aggressivity, suicide attempts and depression: Relationship to cerebrospinal fluid monoamine metabolite levels. *Biological Psychiatry*, **50**, 783–791.

Shoaf SE, Carson RE, Hommer D *et al.* (2000). The suitability of [11C]-alpha-methyl-L-tryptophan as a tracer for serotonin synthesis: studies with dual administration of [11C] and [14C] labeled tracer. *Journal of Cerebral Blood Flow and Metabolism*, **20**, 244–252.

Van Heeringen C, Audenaert K, Van Laere K *et al.* (2003). Prefrontal 5HT 2a receptor binding index, hopelessness, and personality characteristics in attempted suicide. *Journal of Affective Disorders*, **74**, 149–158.

Wen W, Sachdev P, Shnier R *et al.* (2004). Effect of white matter hyperintensities on cortical cerebral blood volume using perfusion MRI. *NeuroImage*, **21**, 1350–1356.

# CHAPTER 47

# Electrodermal hyporeactivity and suicide risk

Lars-Håkan Thorell

## Abstract

Electrodermal hyporeactivity is related to the incidence of suicide and violent attempted suicide in depressed patients. The electrodermal reactivity test is a non-invasive examination of habituation to a standardized tone stimulus. Further testing of electrodermal hyporeactivity in clinical conditions is needed.

## Introduction

The electrodermal response, i.e. momentary light sweating in palms and soles, is conceived as part of the neutral response to unexpected non-noxious events. The response to a repeated neutral stimulus successively diminishes until it disappears—an expression of habituation (Sokolov 1963).

A typical investigation, as described by Edman *et al.* (1986), proceeds as follows: After standardized verbal preparatory information has been given, electrodes are applied to the subject's fingertips for continuous measurement of electrodermal activity during a habituation examination. Following an initial period of silence, a series of repeated identical, brief and moderately strong tone stimuli are administered at intervals, varying from approximately 20–60 seconds and sometimes more.

## Electrodermal hyporeactivity and suicidal propensity

Swedish studies (Edman *et al.* 1986; Thorell 1987) reported that electrodermal hyporeactivity, i.e. none or very few initial responses (rapid habituation), was related to the incidence of suicide or attempted suicide, particularly in depressed patients.

These studies were followed by a series of German publications (Keller *et al.* 1991; Diepers 1994; Wolfersdorf and Straub 1994; Wolfersdorf *et al.* 1993, 1995, 1996, 1999). However, the reported statistical significance of the relationship between electrodermal hyporeactivity and suicide and attempted suicide, particularly if the suicidal act was violent, has varied from non-significant (Wolfersdorf *et al.* 1993, 1996; Diepers 1994) to significant (Keller *et al.* 1991; Wolfersdorf and Straub 1994; Wolfersdorf *et al.* 1995) and highly significant (Thorell 1987; Wolfersdorf *et al.* 1999). These widely varying results are probably due to the heterogeneity of the groups investigated.

Peripheral cholinergic dysfunction (dry mouth, urine retention, etc.), which may be seen in patients who are in a depressive state or in conjunction with antidepressant pharmacological treatment, might possibly influence habituation of the cholinergically mediated electrodermal response, but does not appear to do so according to several reviews (Williams *et al.* 1985; Thorell *et al.* 1987; Bernstein *et al.* 1988; Wolfersdorf *et al.* 1999).

## Time extension of electrodermal hyporeactivity

In an unpublished meta-analysis performed by the author, electrodermal hyporeactivity was found to be statistically significantly related to the incidence of attempted suicide up to 20 years before, and to suicide or attempted suicide up to 20 years after, the test date (Thorell *et al.* 2008). A series of observations have shown that electrodermal hyporeactivity is influenced very little by successful antidepressive treatment (Noble and Lader 1971; Dawson *et al.* 1977; Toone *et al.* 1981; Storrie *et al.* 1981; Janes and Strock 1982), and does not fully normalize in remission within one year (Iacono *et al.* 1984), although a significant change towards normal, but still significantly lower levels than in healthy controls after two years was found (Thorell and d'Elia 1988).

Time-extended electrodermal hyporeactivity may possibly be seen as an indicator of long-term suicide risk, and may be used as a supplementary means of acute suicide risk assessment.

## Electrodermal hyporeactivity, serotonergic dysfunction and preattentive neglect

Electrodermal hyporeactivity in depressed patients was found to be unrelated to the concentration of 5-HIAA in cerebrospinal fluid (Edman *et al.* 1986). It, therefore, appears not to be directly influenced by serotonin activity. An interpretation derived from information-processing theories of the orienting reaction and its habituation (Sokolov *et al.* 2002) is that the hyporeactivity (rapid habituation) may represent a condition of a premature preattentive neglect of the event (Thorell 2008). However, the principle of premature preattentive neglect does not necessarily contradict the principles of dysfunctional impulse control and serotonergic dysfunction as discussed by others (Edman *et al.* 1986; Wolfersdorf and Straub 1994; Wolfersdorf *et al.* 1996 1999). Their possible functional interrelation and synergism in severe suicidal behaviour are an important target for future research.

## Electrodermal hyporeactivity and dexamethasone suppression

Some observations indicate that electrodermal hyporeactivity in depressed patients is related to nocturnal and morning hypercortisolism (Thorell *et al.* 1988), and non-suppression of cortisol production upon dexamethasone administration (Reus *et al.* 1985). However, some studies have found that no association with pathological dexamethasone suppression response can be demonstrated (Ward *et al.* 1983; Williams *et al.* 1985; Thorell *et al.* 1988).

## Conclusion

The results prompt further testing of electrodermal hyporeactivity in persons with depressive disorder, under clinical conditions, to detect a long-term risk of suicide.

## References

Bernstein AS, Riedel JA, Graae F *et al.* (1988). Schizophrenia is associated with altered orienting activity; depression with electrodermal (cholinergic?) deficit and normal orienting response. *Journal of Abnormal Psychology*, **97**, 3–12.

Dawson ME, Schell AM, Catania JJ (1977). Autonomic correlates of depression and clinical improvement following electroconvulsive shock therapy. *Psychophysiology*, **14**, 569–577.

Diepers M (1994). Zur Suizidalität in der Depression: Persönlichkeitsmerkmale und psychophysiologische Reaktionsmunster [On suicidality in depression: personality and psychophysiological pattern of reactions]. Dissertation. Universität Ulm, Ulm.

Edman G, Åsberg M, Levander S *et al.* (1986). Skin conductance habituation and cerebrospinal fluid 5-hydroxyindoleatic acid in suicidal patients. *Archives of General Psychiatry*, **43**, 586–592.

Iacono WG, Lykken DT, Haroian KP *et al.* (1984). Electrodermal activity in euthymic patients with affective disorders: one-year retest stability and the effects of stimulus intensity and significance. *Journal of Abnormal Psychology*, **93**, 304–311.

Janes CL and Strock BD (1982). Skin conductance responding following major depressive episode remission. *Psychophysiology*, **19**, 566.

Keller F, Wolfersdorf M, Straub R *et al.* (1991). Suicidal behaviour and electrodermal activity in depressive inpatients. *Acta Psychiatrica Scandinavica*, **83**, 324–328.

Noble P and Lader M (1971). The symptomatic correlates of the skin conductance changes in depression. *Journal of Psychiatric Research*, **9**, 61–69.

Reus VI, Peeke HVS, Miner C (1985). Habituation and cortisol dysregulation in depression. *Biological Psychiatry*, **20**, 980–989.

Sokolov EN (1963). *Perception and the Conditioned Reflex*. Pergamon Press, Oxford.

Sokolov EN, Spinks JA, Näätänen R *et al.* (2002). *The Orienting Response in Information Processing*. Lawrence Erlbaum Associates, Mahwah.

Storrie MC, Doerr HO, Johnson MH (1981). Skin conductance characteristics of depressed subjects before and after therapeutic intervention. *Journal of Nervous and Mental Disease*, **69**, 176–179.

Thorell LH (1987). Electrodermal activity in suicidal and nonsuicidal depressive patients and in matched healthy subjects. *Acta Psychiatrica Scandinavica*, **76**, 420–430.

Thorell LH (2008). Valid electrodermal hyporeactivity for depressive suicidal propensity offers links to cognitive theory. *Acta Psychiatrica Scandinavica*, accepted for publication.

Thorell LH and d'Elia G (1988). Electrodermal activity in depressive patients in remission and in matched healthy subjects. *Acta Psychiatrica Scandinavica*, **78**, 247–253.

Thorell LH, Kjellman BF, d'Elia G (1987). Electrodermal activity in antidepressant medicated and unmedicated depressive patients and in matched healthy subjects. *Acta Psychiatrica Scandinavica*, **76**, 684–692.

Thorell LH, Kjellman BF, d'Elia G *et al.* (1988). Electrodermal activity in relation to cortisol dysregulation in depressive patients. *Acta Psychiatrica Scandinavica*, **78**, 743–753.

Thorell LH, Alkhori L, Carlsson K *et al.* (2008). Electrodermal hyporeactivity in relation to suicidal acts 20 years before and 20 years after the depressive index episode. Unpublished manuscript.

Toone BK, Cooke E, Lader MH (1981). Electrodermal activity in the affective disorders and schizophrenia. *Psychological Medicine*, **11**, 497–508.

Ward NG, Doerr HO, Storrie MC (1983). Skin conductance: a potentially sensitive test for depression. *Psychiatry Research*, **10**, 295–302.

Williams KM, Iacono WG, Remick RA (1985). Electrodermal activity among subtypes of depression. *Biological Psychiatry*, **20**, 158–162.

Wolfersdorf M, Straub R, Hole G (1993). Electrodermal activity in depressive men and women with violent or non-violent suicide attempts. *Schweiz Arch Neurol Psychiatr*, **144**, 173–184.

Wolfersdorf M and Straub R (1994). Electrodermal reactivity in male and female depressive patients who later died by suicide. *Acta Psychiatrica Scandinavica*, **89**, 279–284.

Wolfersdorf M, Straub R, Keller F *et al.* (1995). Elektrodermale reaktivität bei suizidversuch und suizid depressiver. In M Wolfersdorf and WP Kaschka, eds, *Suizid—Die Biologische Dimension* [Suicide—The Biological Dimension], pp. 99–110. Heidelberg, Berlin.

Wolfersdorf M, Straub R, Barg T, Keller F (1996). Depression und EDA—kennwerte in einem habituations experiment [Depression and electrodermal response measures in a habituation experiment. Results from over 400 depressed inpatients]. *Fortschritte der Neurologie-Psychiatrie*, **64**, 105–109.

Wolfersdorf M, Straub R, Barg T *et al.* (1999). Depressed inpatients, electrodermal reactivity, and suicide—a study about psychophysiology of suicide behaviour. *Archives of Suicide Research*, **5**, 1–10.

# CHAPTER 48

# Post-mortem studies of serotonin in suicide

Hélène Bach-Mizrachi, Mark D Underwood, J John Mann and Victoria Arango

## Abstract

Abnormalities of the serotonergic system have been implicated in suicide. Post-mortem brain studies of suicides have begun to elucidate the underlying molecular changes in the brain serotonergic system that may provide an understanding of the biology of suicide. There is evidence for alterations in the presynaptic serotonin transporter and serotonergic receptors in both the serotonin-synthesizing neurons in the brainstem and their targets in the prefrontal cortex. Some of these changes may represent primary pathophysiology, while other changes may reflect homeostatic regulatory responses to low serotonin or even maladaptive non-specific stress responses. We review the post-mortem studies of suicides and discuss a model of homeostatic plasticity in the human brain in a serotonin-deficient environment.

## Introduction

Studies of post-mortem brain tissue from people who committed suicide is an important biological resource that can be used in direct study of the molecular underpinnings of underlying psychiatric disorders and suicide. To date, post-mortem studies indicate that multiple monoaminergic systems contribute to the complex etiology of major depressive disorder (MDD) and suicide (Arango et al. 1993; Mann and Arango 2001, 2003; Ordway et al. 2003; Stockmeier 2003).

A large body of post-mortem research has focused on the serotonergic system in suicides. Interest in the serotonergic system stemmed from the efficacy of serotonin (5-HT) specific reuptake inhibitors (SSRIs) in treating MDD and findings of low cerebrospinal fluid (CSF) 5-hydroxyindoleacetic acid, the 5-HT metabolite, in depressed suicide attempters and in brainstem of suicides (Åsberg et al. 1976; Carlsson et al. 1980; Träskman et al. 1981; Banki et al. 1984; Roy et al. 1986; Mann and Malone 1997; Placidi et al. 2001). In suicide attempters, 5-HT activity, measured by the release of prolactin in response to administration of the 5-HT releasing drug, fenfluramine, was found to be blunted (Mann et al. 1995; Malone et al. 1996; Pandey 1997; Weiss and Coccaro 1997; Corrêa et al. 2000; Dulchin et al. 2001). These findings suggest deficient 5-HT transmission in MDD and suicide and directed investigators to examine 5-HT-synthesizing brainstem nuclei (dorsal [DRN] and median raphe [MRN]) and brain areas, targeted by 5-HT neurons, that mediate complex behaviour.

This chapter focuses on post-mortem studies of suicide, examining data on the brain 5-HT system and its role in the pathophysiology of MDD and suicide. We discuss a model of MDD and suicide in which the brain attempts to compensate for deficient serotonergic neurotransmission by making homeostatic changes in expression levels and functioning of several of its molecular components.

## Serotonin and suicide

Serotonin modulates many human behaviours including mood, sleep–wake cycle, memory, impulsivity and aggressivity. Neurons synthesizing 5-HT and projecting to the forebrain are located in the DRN and MRN in the rostral brainstem (Baker et al. 1990; Törk 1990) and project, among many regions, to the prefrontal cortex (PFC, (Pierce et al. 1976; Wilson and Molliver 1991a, b). Serotonergic neurotransmission between the DRN/MRN and PFC is regulated by the presynaptic 5-HT transporter (SERT) and by pre- and post-synaptic serotonergic receptors. SERT acts to re-uptake 5-HT, terminating synaptic transmission following serotonin release by an action potential. The serotonergic receptors are encoded by fifteen known genes (see Barnes and Sharp 1999 for review) and are expressed both pre-synaptically on raphe serotonergic cell bodies and post-synaptically in neurons in multiple brain regions including the PFC (Azmitia and Whitaker-Azmitia 1991). Of the pre-synaptic receptors, $5\text{-HT}_{1A}$ and $5\text{-HT}_{1B}$ receptors act as autoreceptors, inhibiting the firing of 5-HT neurons and decreasing 5-HT release in the PFC (Aghajanian et al. 1987). Through the interactions of the SERT re-uptake mechanisms, the pre-synaptic regulation of 5-HT neurons and the post-synaptic transduction mechanisms through 5-HT receptors in the PFC, brain 5-HT levels are tightly regulated.

Current models of depression and suicide include a critical interaction between stressful life events and biochemical traits as a basis for the diathesis of recurrent MDD or suicidal behaviour. The most reproducible biochemical trait associated with suicidal behaviour is serotonergic hypofunction. Stressful life events may interact with hyperresponsive stress response systems such as the noradrenergic system and the hypothalamic–pituitary–adrenal

(HPA) axis and thereby contribute to the primary pathogenesis of depression and suicide. However, post-mortem studies reveal molecular changes in the 5-HT system which point to both deficient and to compensatory mechanisms (Mann and Currier 2006). Post-mortem studies have consistently, though not uniformly, uncovered changes in SERT, serotonergic receptors, signal transduction pathways and biosynthetic enzymes that, taken together, begin to draw a molecular picture of a plastic human brain in a 5-HT deficient environment.

## Post-mortem studies of serotonergic receptors and transporter

Early studies (Stanley et al. 1982; Stanley and Mann 1983; Mann et al. 1986) found fewer SERT binding sites and more 5-HT$_{2A}$ receptors in the frontal cortex. We and others have refined these studies to map receptor binding changes in many regions using quantitative autoradiography. For the 5-HT$_{1A}$ receptor and SERT, we use [$^3$H]-8-OH-DPAT and [$^3$H]-cyanoimipramine, respectively (Arango et al. 2001). For the 5-HT$_{2A}$ receptor, both agonists ($^{125}$I-LSD) and antagonists ($^3$H-Ketanserin) have been used (Arango et al. 1990; Turecki et al. 1999; Pandey et al. 2002; Oquendo et al. 2006). Using this technology, presynaptic serotonergic alterations in the brainstem (Stockmeier et al. 1998; Arango et al. 2001) and pre- and post-synaptic alterations in the PFC (Arango et al. 1990; Hrdina et al. 1993; Arango et al. 1995; Mann et al. 2000; Pandey et al. 2001; 2002) have been detected.

## Prefrontal cortex

Evidence suggests that a focal point for the pathology lies in the PFC. We found lower SERT binding in the ventromedial PFC (Arango et al. 2002) and more 5-HT$_{1A}$ receptor binding in the lateral PFC in suicides vs normal controls (Arango et al. 1995) and throughout the PFC the binding was inversely correlated. While our 5-HT$_{1A}$ finding was not replicated by some laboratories (Stockmeier et al. 1997), our SERT finding was replicated, as a deficit in the length and density of SERT immunoreactive axons in lateral PFC of depressed suicides (Austin et al. 2002). We also found lower SERT binding throughout the PFC in MDD and found that this finding extended to other brain regions in vivo, using PET (Parsey et al. 2006). Less SERT binding may represent accelerated transporter internalization as a homeostatic response to low 5-HT or lower gene expression among other explanations. Conversely, the postsynaptic 5-HT$_{1A}$ receptor may be upregulated in an attempt to increase serotonergic transmission (Arango et al. 1995). In addition, binding to the postsynaptic 5-HT$_{2A}$ receptor was found to be higher in the PFC of suicides, as were protein levels and mRNA expression (Stanley and Mann 1983; Mann et al. 1986; Arango et al. 1990; Hrdina et al. 1993; Turecki et al. 1999; Pandey et al. 2002). Paradoxically, we and others have found deficits in signal transduction for these two receptor types, raising questions about the state of target neurons in the cortex.

Further findings from post-mortem studies have begun to tease out differences in the molecular profiles of MDD and suicide. Less SERT binding in the ventromedial PFC of suicides was related to suicide independently of psychiatric diagnosis, while a deficiency in SERT binding across most of the PFC was found in MDD (Mann et al. 2000; Arango et al. 2002). The ventral PFC is involved in

behavioural inhibition (Shallice and Burgess 1996), thus low 5-HT input to this area may contribute to impaired inhibition and the propensity to act on suicidal thoughts.

The other 5-HT receptor that has been studied in suicides is the 5-HT$_{2C}$ receptor. This is the only known G-protein coupled receptor whose mRNA undergoes post-transcriptional editing resulting in the formation of 5-HT$_{2C}$ receptor isoforms, each having a different function (Burns et al. 1997). Suicides have more pre-mRNA editing of the 5-HT$_{2C}$ receptor in the dorsal PFC than controls, which may result in less efficient coupling and lower signal transduction (Gurevich et al. 2002). Furthermore, a study by Pandey and colleagues (2006) has revealed increased protein levels in the PFC of suicides, with no change in mRNA, further limiting the pathophysiology to post-translational modifications and an increased proportion of less functionally active edited isoforms.

## Dorsal raphe nucleus

The brainstem holds the 5-HT synthesizing neurons that project to the entire forebrain. These neurons reside in the DRN and MRN. We found fewer SERT-expressing DRN neurons and less 5-HT$_{1A}$ autoreceptor binding (Arango et al. 2001), indicative of homeostatic changes in serotonergic neurons consistent with upregulatory responses that would serve to enhance serotonergic neuron firing and slow reuptake in terminal fields to amplify the 5-HT signal. 5-HT$_{1A}$ binding was shown to be higher in the rostral 5mm of the DRN of depressed suicides by other investigators (Stockmeier et al. 1998). The discrepant findings may have been reconciled by our work (Boldrini et al. 2004) which shows higher 5-HT$_{1A}$ binding in the rostral 5mm of the DRN in suicides and lower binding in the remaining caudal 15mm. Females have higher 5-HT$_{1A}$ binding than males both post mortem (Arango et al. 2001), and in vivo demonstrated by PET (Parsey et al. 2002), highlighting the importance of matching controls and patient samples for sex and other demographic traits.

Tryptophan hydroxylase (TPH) is the rate-limiting enzyme in the biosynthesis of 5-HT, converting tryptophan to 5-hydroxytryptophan (5-HTP) on route to decarboxylation into 5-hydroxytryptamine (see Mockus and Vrana 1998 for review). Alterations in TPH expression or catalytic activity can potentially cause changes in the levels of 5-HT in the brain. At the transcript level, brain 5-HT in rodents is regulated by a neuron-specific isoform of TPH, known as TPH2 (Patel et al. 2004; Zhang et al. 2004). Prior to the discovery of TPH2 (Walther et al. 2003), quantitative studies of TPH gene expression in brain had been unknowingly measuring the almost undetectable level of peripheral TPH (TPH1), the non-neuronal isoform of the enzyme (Clark and Russo 1997; Austin and O'Donnell 1999).

Neuron-specific TPH is the product of the *TPH2* gene located on chromosome 12q15 (Walther et al. 2003; Zhang et al. 2004) and is specifically and robustly expressed in the DRN and MRN of humans (Bach-Mizrachi et al. 2006) and rats (Patel et al. 2004). We found elevated TPH2 protein expression in MDD suicides as shown by immunocytochemistry (Underwood et al. 1999), a finding we replicated in a second cohort using immunoautoradiography (Boldrini et al. 2005). Another group reported no change in TPH protein expression in depressed suicides (Bonkale et al. 2004), but found greater expression in the dorsal subnucleus of the DRN of depressed suicides who were also alcohol-dependent (Bonkale et al. 2006).

The inconsistency in immunoautoradiography findings may be explained by differences in methodologies. Bonkale and colleagues (2006) sampled five representative rostral sections while our group sampled the entire DRN at 1mm intervals, thereby increasing the resolution in which changes in expression can be found. TPH2 transcript expression was also found to be elevated in the DRN and MRN of depressed suicides (Boldrini *et al.* 2005; Bach-Mizrachi *et al.* 2006) and a modest positive correlation exists between protein and transcript levels, indicating that more protein may at least partly result from greater gene expression.

Immunocytochemistry studies have also revealed higher density and number of TPH immunoreactive (IR) neurons in the DRN of depressed suicides (Underwood *et al.* 1999). More TPH-IR neurons, when taken together with more TPH protein (Underwood *et al.* 1999; Boldrini *et al.* 2005), and more TPH2 mRNA (Bach-Mizrachi *et al.* 2006) would favour higher 5-HT levels and yet most studies report lower 5-HT levels in suicides. Higher TPH2 expression does not necessarily indicate increased catalytic capacity and certainly does not mean that there is greater release of 5-HT and higher intra-synaptic levels. Lower brainstem 5-HT levels in depressed suicides and lower CSF 5-HIAA suggest a compensatory mechanism in which the enzyme level may be increased but catalytic activity or release of 5-HT is impaired. However, the mechanism by which TPH2 gauges brain 5-HT levels remains unknown and furthermore, it is not clear whether this upregulation in the brainstem is a function of aberrant transcriptional or translational control or a naturally occurring normal response. In either case, it is possible that the TPH2 enzyme produced in affected individuals is of lower catalytic activity, perhaps due to a gene polymorphism in the TPH2 catalytic site since 5-HT production is ultimately compromised.

Post-mortem studies have found low levels of TPH2 transcript in the terminal fields of 5-HT neurons including the cortex, hippocampus and amygdala (De Luca *et al.* 2005; Zill *et al.* 2007) using quantitative RT-PCR. Interestingly, abundant levels of TPH protein were found in the PFC by Western blots (Ono *et al.* 2002). The presence of TPH2 in serotonergic terminals suggests a potential mechanism for the regulation of 5-HT synthesis locally, at synapses in terminal regions distant from the raphe nuclei. Therefore, it is possible that despite an upregulation in the brainstem, inefficient axoplasmic flow of TPH2 to cortical terminal fields can lead to deficits in TPH2 protein at terminals despite higher levels at cell bodies. This notion is proposed in one post-mortem study of Alzheimer's patients in which TPH activity and 5-HIAA were increased in the DRN and decreased in terminal fields in the amygdala. These authors propose that high levels of toxic serotonergic metabolites in the raphe contribute to degeneration of 5-HT neurons seen in Alzheimer's disease (Burke *et al.* 1990). However, more probable is a defect in catalytic activity because there are low 5-HT and 5-HIAA levels reported even in the brainstem.

Since its discovery, researchers have sought genetic variants in the *TPH2* gene in populations with MDD as a possible mechanism for a change in the enzyme that would affect its catalytic activity or alter its expression level, and ultimately lead to low levels of 5-HT (Bondy *et al.* 2006; Mann and Currier 2006). Recent studies report associations of the *TPH2* gene with MDD and suicide, involving the same single nucleotide polymorphism (SNP) for both, but it is not clear which is the primary association (Zhang *et al.* 2004, 2005; Zill *et al.* 2004a, b).

## Conclusions and future directions

If all findings in post-mortem studies of MDD suicides were to be considered pathogenic, it would be difficult to reconcile the seemingly paradoxical conclusions. However, an alternative interpretation of the data leads us to propose a model wherein some of the changes are part of the brain's normal adaptive response to low 5-HT levels, while others are associated with primary pathogenic effects. Pathogenic effects may include inefficient catalytic activity of TPH, impaired signal transduction, decreased activation of serotonergic receptors in the cortex due to RNA editing effects or enhanced expression of the autoreceptor and lower firing rates of 5-HT neurons. Compensatory changes would include a general upregulation of the functioning of the brainstem raphe nuclei, a downregulation of inhibitory regulators of 5-HT release and 5-HT reuptake.

Finally, gene–environment relationships have to be considered when analysing causality. Cross-fostering studies in mice (Francis *et al.* 2003) show that naturally occurring mouse strains exhibiting anxiety and depressive behaviours show marked improvement when fostered with mothers from non-anxious strains. These anxious inbred mouse strains have been shown to have specific genetic variants in the *TPH2* gene that are associated with low 5-HT levels (Zhang *et al.* 2004). Clearly, epigenetic studies in mice do not encompass the complex aetiology of human MDD and suicide. However, these findings make the point that environmental improvements can interact with genetic make-up and contribute to the functional state of the serotonergic system.

## References

Aghajanian GK, Sprouse JS, Rasmussen K (1987). Physiology of the midbrain serotonin system. In HY Meltzer, ed., *Psychopharmacology. The Third Generation of Progress*, pp. 141–149. Raven Press, New York.

Arango V, Ernsberger P, Marzuk PM *et al.* (1990). Autoradiographic demonstration of increased serotonin 5-HT2 and beta-adrenergic receptor binding sites in the brain of suicide victims. *Archives of General Psychiatry*, **47**, 1038–1047.

Arango V, Ernsberger P, Sved AF *et al.* (1993). Quantitative autoradiography of alpha 1- and alpha 2-adrenergic receptors in the cerebral cortex of controls and suicide victims. *Brain Research*, **630**, 271–282.

Arango V, Underwood MD, Boldrini M *et al.* (2001). Serotonin 1A receptors, serotonin transporter binding and serotonin transporter mRNA expression in the brainstem of depressed suicide victims. *Neuropsychopharmacology*, **25**, 892–903.

Arango V, Underwood MD, Gubbi AV *et al.* (1995). Localized alterations in pre- and postsynaptic serotonin binding sites in the ventrolateral prefrontal cortex of suicide victims. *Brain Research*, **688**, 121–133.

Arango V, Underwood MD, Mann JJ (2002). Serotonin brain circuits involved in major depression and suicide. *Progress in Brain Research*, **136**, 443–453.

Åsberg M, Träskman L, Thorén P (1976). 5-HIAA in the cerebrospinal fluid. A biochemical suicide predictor? *Archives of General Psychiatry*, **33**, 1193–1197.

Austin MC and O'Donnell SM (1999). Regional distribution and cellular expression of tryptophan hydroxylase messenger RNA in postmortem human brainstem and pineal gland. *Journal of Neurochemistry*, **72**, 2065–2073.

Austin MC, Whitehead RE, Edgar CL *et al.* (2002). Localized decrease in serotonin transporter-immunoreactive axons in the prefrontal cortex of depressed subjects committing suicide. *Neuroscience*, **114**, 807–815.

Azmitia EC and Whitaker-Azmitia PM (1991). Awakening the sleeping giant: anatomy and plasticity of the brain serotonergic system. *Journal of Clinical Psychiatry*, **52**, 4–16.

Bach-Mizrachi H, Underwood MD, Kassir SA *et al.* (2006). Neuronal tryptophan hydroxylase mRNA expression in the human dorsal and median raphe nuclei: major depression and suicide. *Neuropsychopharmacology*, **31**, 814–824.

Baker KG, Halliday GM, Tork I (1990). Cytoarchitecture of the human dorsal raphe nucleus. *Journal of Comparative Neurology*, **301**, 147–161.

Banki CM, Arato M, Papp Z *et al.* (1984). Biochemical markers in suicidal patients. Investigations with cerebrospinal fluid amine metabolites and neuroendocrine tests. *Journal of Affective Disorders*, **6**, 341–350.

Barnes NM and Sharp T (1999). A review of central 5-HT receptors and their function. *Neuropharmacology*, **38**, 1083–1152.

Boldrini M, Underwood MD, Mann JJ *et al.* (2005). More tryptophan hydroxylase in the brainstem dorsal raphe nucleus in depressed suicides. *Brain Research*, **1041**, 19–28.

Boldrini M, Underwood MD, Martini A *et al.* (2004). Distribution of serotonin-1A autoreceptors in the dorsal raphe nucleus of depressed suicide victims. ACNP 43rd Annual Meeting, San Juan, Puerto Rico

Bondy B, Buettner A, Zill P (2006). Genetics of suicide. *Molecular Psychiatry*, **11**, 336–351.

Bonkale WL, Murdock S, Janosky JE *et al.* (2004). Normal levels of tryptophan hydroxylase immunoreactivity in the dorsal raphe of depressed suicide victims. *Journal of Neurochemistry*, **88**, 958–964.

Bonkale WL, Turecki G, Austin MC (2006). Increased tryptophan hydroxylase immunoreactivity in the dorsal raphe nucleus of alcohol-dependent, depressed suicide subjects is restricted to the dorsal subnucleus. *Synapse*, **60**, 81–85.

Burke WJ, Park DH, Chung HD *et al.* (1990). Evidence for decreased transport of tryptophan hydroxylase in Alzheimer's disease. *Brain Research*, **537**, 83–87.

Burns CM, Chu H, Rueter SM *et al.* (1997). Regulation of serotonin-2C receptor G-protein coupling by RNA editing. *Nature*, **387**, 303–308.

Carlsson A, Svennerholm L, Winblad B (1980). Seasonal and circadian monoamine variations in human brains examined post mortem. *Acta Psychiatrica Scandinavica*, **280**, 75–85.

Clark MS and Russo AF (1997). Tissue-specific glucocorticoid regulation of tryptophan hydroxylase mRNA levels. *Brain Research Molecular Brain Research*, **48**, 346–354.

Corrêa H, Duval F, Mokrani M-C *et al.* (2000). Prolactin response to D-fenfluramine and suicidal behavior in depressed patients. *Psychiatry Research*, **93**, 189–199.

De Luca V, Likhodi O, Van Tol HH *et al.* (2005). Tryptophan hydroxylase 2 gene expression and promoter polymorphisms in bipolar disorder and schizophrenia. *Psychopharmacology, (Berl)*, 1–5.

Dulchin MC, Oquendo MA, Malone KM *et al.* (2001). Prolactin response to dl-fenfluramine challenge before and after treatment with paroxetine. *Neuropsychopharmacology*, **25**, 395–401.

Francis DD, Szegda K, Campbell G *et al.* (2003). Epigenetic sources of behavioral differences in mice. *Nature Neuroscience*, **6**, 445–446.

Gurevich I, Englander MT, Adlersberg M *et al.* (2002). Modulation of serotonin 2C receptor editing by sustained changes in serotonergic neurotransmission. *Journal of Neuroscience*, **22**, 10529–10532.

Hrdina PD, Demeter E, Vu TB *et al.* (1993). 5-HT uptake sites and 5-HT$_2$ receptors in brain of antidepressant- free suicide victims/depressives: increase in 5- HT$_2$ sites in cortex and amygdala. *Brain Research*, **614**, 37–44.

Malone KM, Corbitt EM, Li S *et al.* (1996). Prolactin response to fenfluramine and suicide attempt lethality in major depression. *British Journal of Psychiatry*, **168**, 324–329.

Mann JJ and Arango V (2001). Neurobiology of suicide and attempted suicide. In D Wasserman, ed., *Suicide: An Unnecessary Death*, pp. 29–34. Martin Dunitz Ltd, London.

Mann JJ and Arango V (2003). Abnormalities of brain structure and function in mood disorder. In DS Charney and EJ Nestler, eds, *Neurobiology of Mental Illness*, 2nd edn, pp.. Oxford University Press, San Francisco.

Mann JJ and Currier D (2006). Effects of genes and stress on the neurobiology of depression. *International Review of Neurobiology*, **73**, 153–189.

Mann JJ, Huang YY, Underwood MD *et al.* (2000). A serotonin transporter gene promoter polymorphism (5-HTTLPR) and prefrontal cortical binding in major depression and suicide. *Archives of General Psychiatry*, **57**, 729–738.

Mann JJ and Malone KM (1997). Cerebrospinal fluid amines and higher-lethality suicide attempts in depressed inpatients. *Biological Psychiatry*, **41**, 162–171.

Mann JJ, McBride PA, Malone KM *et al.* (1995). Blunted serotonergic responsivity in depressed patients. *Neuropsychopharmacology*, **13**, 53–64.

Mann JJ, Stanley M, McBride PA *et al.* (1986). Increased serotonin2 and beta-adrenergic receptor binding in the frontal cortices of suicide victims. *Archives of General Psychiatry*, **43**, 954–959.

Mockus SM and Vrana KE (1998). Advances in the molecular characterization of tryptophan hydroxylase [Review]. *Journal of Molecular Neuroscience*, **10**, 163–179.

Ono H, Shirakawa O, Kitamura N *et al.* (2002). Tryptophan hydroxylase immunoreactivity is altered by the genetic variation in postmortem brain samples of both suicide victims and controls. *Molecular Psychiatry*, **7**, 1127–1132.

Oquendo MA, Russo SA, Underwood MD *et al.* (2006), Higher postmortem prefrontal 5-HT2A receptor binding correlates with lifetime aggression in suicide. *Biological Psychiatry*, **59**, 235–243.

Ordway GA, Schenk J, Stockmeier CA *et al.* (2003). Elevated agonist binding to alpha(2)-adrenoceptors in the locus coeruleus in major depression. *Biological Psychiatry*, **53**, 315–323.

Pandey GN (1997). Altered serotonin function in suicide. Evidence from platelet and neuroendocrine studies. *Annals of the New York Academy of Sciences*, **836**, 182–200.

Pandey GN, Dwivedi Y, Ren X *et al.* (2006). Regional distribution and relative abundance of serotonin(2c) receptors in human brain: effect of suicide. *Neurochemical Research*, **31**, 167–176.

Pandey GN, Dwivedi Y, Ren X *et al.* (2001). Increased 5HT2A receptors and impaired phosphoinositide siginaling in the postmortem brain of suicide victims. In K Miyoshi *et al.*, eds, *Contemporary Neuropsychiatry*, pp. 314–321. Springer-Verlag, Tokyo.

Pandey GN, Dwivedi Y, Rizavi HS *et al.* (2002). Higher expression of serotonin 5-HT(2A) receptors in the postmortem brains of teenage suicide victims. *American Journal of Psychiatry*, **159**, 419–429.

Parsey RV, Oquendo MA, Ogden RT *et al.* (2006). Altered serotonin 1A binding in major depression: a [carbonyl-C-11]WAY100635 positron emission tomography study. *Biological Psychiatry*, **59**, 106–113.

Parsey RV, Oquendo MA, Simpson NR *et al.* (2002). Effects of sex, age, and aggressive traits in man on brain serotonin 5- HT(1A) receptor binding potential measured by PET using [C-11]WAY- 100635. *Brain Research*, **954**, 173–182.

Patel PD, Pontrello C, Burke S (2004). Robust and tissue-specific expression of TPH2 versus TPH1 in rat raphe and pineal gland. *Biological Psychiatry*, **55**, 428–433.

Pierce ET, Foote WE, Hobson JA (1976). The efferent connection of the nucleus raphe dorsalis. *Brain Research*, **107**, 137–144.

Placidi GP, Oquendo MA, Malone KM *et al.* (2001). Aggressivity, suicide attempts, and depression: relationship to cerebrospinal fluid monoamine metabolite levels. *Biological Psychiatry*, **50**, 783–791.

Roy A, Ågren H, Pickar D *et al.* (1986). Reduced CSF concentrations of homovanillic acid and homovanillic acid to 5-hydroxyindoleacetic acid ratios in depressed patients: relationship to suicidal behavior and dexamethasone nonsuppression. *American Journal of Psychiatry*, **143**, 1539–1545.

Shallice T and Burgess P (1996). The domain of supervisory processes and temporal organization of behaviour. *Philosophical Transactions of the Royal Society of London*, **351**, 1405–1412.

Stanley M and Mann JJ (1983). Increased serotonin-2 binding sites in frontal cortex of suicide victims. *Lancet*, **1**, 214–216.

Stanley M, Virgilio J, Gershon S (1982). Tritiated imipramine binding sites are decreased in the frontal cortex of suicides. *Science*, **216**, 1337–1339.

Stockmeier CA (2003). Involvement of serotonin in depression: evidence from postmortem and imaging studies of serotonin receptors and the serotonin transporter. *Journal of Psychiatric Research*, **37**, 357–373.

Stockmeier CA, Dilley GE, Shapiro LA *et al.* (1997). Serotonin receptors in suicide victims with major depression. *Neuropsychopharmacology*, **16**, 162–173.

Stockmeier CA, Shapiro LA, Dilley GE *et al.* (1998). Increase in serotonin-1A autoreceptors in the midbrain of suicide victims with major depression—postmortem evidence for decreased serotonin activity. *Journal of Neuroscience*, **18**, 7394–7401.

Törk I (1990). Anatomy of the serotonergic system. *Annals of the New York Academy of Sciences*, **600**, 9–35.

Träskman L, Åsberg M, Bertilsson L *et al.* (1981). Monoamine metabolites in CSF and suicidal behavior. *Archives of General Psychiatry*, **38**, 631–636.

Turecki G, Briere R, Dewar K *et al.* (1999). Prediction of level of serotonin 2A receptor binding by serotonin receptor 2A genetic variation in postmortem brain samples from subjects who did or did not commit suicide. *American Journal of Psychiatry*, **156**, 1456–1458.

Underwood MD, Khaibulina AA, Ellis SP *et al.* (1999). Morphometry of the dorsal raphe nucleus serotonergic neurons in suicide victims. *Biological Psychiatry*, **46**, 473–483.

Walther DJ, Peter JU, Bashammakh S *et al.* (2003). Synthesis of serotonin by a second tryptophan hydroxylase isoform. *Science*, **299**, 76.

Weiss D and Coccaro EF (1997). Neuroendocrine challenge studies of suicidal behavior. *Psychiatric Clinics of North America*, **20**, 563–579.

Wilson MA and Molliver ME (1991a). The organization of serotonergic projections to cerebral cortex in primates: regional distribution of axon terminals. *Neuroscience*, **44**, 537–553.

Wilson MA and Molliver ME (1991b). The organization of serotonergic projections to cerebral cortex in primates: retrograde transport studies. *Neuroscience*, **44**, 555–570.

Zhang X, Beaulieu JM, Sotnikova TD *et al.* (2004). Tryptophan hydroxylase-2 controls brain serotonin synthesis. *Science*, **305**, 217.

Zhang X, Gainetdinov RR, Beaulieu JM *et al.* (2005). Loss-of-function mutation in tryptophan hydroxylase-2 identified in unipolar major depression. *Neuron*, **45**, 11–16.

Zill P, Baghai TC, Zwanzger P *et al.* (2004a). SNP and haplotype analysis of a novel tryptophan hydroxylase isoform (TPH2) gene provide evidence for association with major depression. *Molecular Psychiatry*, **9**, 1030–1036.

Zill P, Buttner A, Eisenmenger W *et al.* (2007). Analysis of tryptophan hydroxylase I and II mRNA expression in the human brain: a post-mortem study. *Journal of Psychiatric Research*, **41**, 168–173.

Zill P, Buttner A, Eisenmenger W *et al.* (2004b). Single nucleotide polymorphism and haplotype analysis of a novel tryptophan hydroxylase isoform (TPH2) gene in suicide victims. *Biological Psychiatry*, **56**, 581–586.

# PART 8

# Cost of Suicide and Prevention Strategies

# CHAPTER 49

# An economic perspective on suicide across the five continents

David McDaid and Brendan Kennelly

## Abstract

In considering suicide prevention measures it is important to consider potential economic risk factors, as well as the costs and consequences of suicide. We provide a brief overview of some areas where economics has played a role in the analysis of suicide and suicide prevention strategies. Evidence on the wide-ranging socio-economic costs and consequences of suicide is provided, as well as a reflection on the development of economic theories on individual motivations for suicide. The evidence from econometric models at both cross-country and single country levels on the links between suicide and socio-economic risk factors such as poverty and unemployment are reviewed. Cost-effectiveness is increasingly used as part of decision-making processes in health and other sectors. In respect of suicide prevention, such evidence remains limited. The present review, nonetheless, suggests that suicide prevention measures may be highly cost-effective. Incorporating economic analyses into future effectiveness studies is likely to help strengthen the case for investment in suicide prevention. There is also scope to look at the economic implications of interventions already shown to be effective.

## Introduction

The impact of suicide is profound. In addition to the emotional suffering, caused by suicide and attempted suicide, the cost to the nation and/or region in the case of suicide or attempted suicide is increasingly recognized as a significant burden. While the avoidance of just one such tragedy provides a powerful motivation for action, the economic perspective may well be one additional incentive that hopefully will act as catalyst for noteworthy preventive measures. Policy-makers in health and other sectors are continually faced with many competing claims for resources, and economics is concerned with the optimal use of scarce resources. Investing in measures to reduce suicide is unlikely to be a cost-free exercise. A better understanding of the socio-economic risk factors and costs of suicide may provide valuable information to policy-makers considering whether or not to increase investment in suicide prevention strategies and programmes. Of course this is of little use

unless effective strategies are available, but assuming that they are, then it is also helpful to look at their cost-effectiveness.

This chapter provides a brief overview of some of the different areas where economic evidence and approaches can play a role. We begin by looking at the economic impact of suicide and by identifying its many costs and consequences. To provide effective suicide prevention interventions, it is also critical to have a better understanding of what the individual motivations for suicide might be. We look at what economic theory can contribute to this discussion. We also review the econometric work that has been undertaken to identify whether socio-economic factors such as poverty and unemployment are linked to suicide. Finally, we reflect on what is known about the cost-effectiveness of different measures to counter suicide, and how such information may be used to inform policy and practice across the five continents.

## The costs of suicide

As part of any process, considering whether or not to invest in suicide prevention, it is important to have information on the costs of *not* taking action; i.e. the costs of suicide. These are substantial impacts on many sectors of society and are long lasting. Most obviously, such costs include what economists call *direct costs*, including the demands placed on the emergency services, as well as use of potential life-saving interventions, police investigations and funerals. For those individuals who survive lengthy physical and psychological rehabilitation may follow (Meneghel *et al.* 1996; O'Sullivan *et al.* 1999).

There are also two kinds of *indirect costs*. Lost output costs refer to the fact that as a result of premature death, individuals lose the opportunity to contribute to the economy, whether this is through paid work, voluntary activities, or family responsibilities such as looking after one's children or parents. The most fundamental impact of suicide, of course, is the loss of the opportunity to experience all that life holds. The pain and grief caused to family and friends, as well as ensuing health consequences, can also be immense and take many years to subside. Suicide can be stigmatizing for families, particularly in cultures where suicide may be regarded as sinful or where it is illegal. Conversely, some individuals who complete suicide may believe this to be of benefit (or negative cost) to others; for instance it may be seen as a way of avoiding shame for failure or becoming a burden to family. All of these very personal, and often culturally driven impacts, are collectively known by economists as '*intangible costs*' because they are often hidden and difficult to evaluate. Increasingly, however, studies try and place a value on some of these complex costs.

Surprisingly, there are few cost estimates for suicide compared with those for other causes of premature death, such as illness or unintentional injury. Moreover, those available do not always include all costs, and values can vary considerably, but all indicate that preventing suicide would avert enormous costs to society. One of the earliest estimates from the Canadian province of New Brunswick, despite not including intangible costs, still estimated the cost of each suicide to be CAN$1,019,210 (Clayton and Barceló 2000). In the United States, the total costs of suicides for those aged 20 or less in 1996 were estimated to be more than US$15.5 billion, 75 per cent of which were intangible costs and 18 per cent indirect costs, due to the loss of opportunity to contribute to the economy (Cox and Miller 1999). The costs of the lost opportunity alone to earn a paid wage, as a result of all suicides in the US in 2002, have also been estimated at US$13 billion (Knox and Caine 2005).

One Australian study estimated the total costs of suicide or self-harm events in the state of Victoria at A$428 million in 1994, 25 per cent of these costs were for direct health sector and other sector costs (Watson and Ozanne-Smith 1997). There are also cost-of-illness studies for different mental disorders that include suicide. In England, the costs of depression in 2000 (excluding the value of intangible costs) included £562 million for premature mortality, much of which was due to suicide (Thomas and Morris 2003).

Several studies, using similar methods, include all three types of cost (see Table 49.1). In New Zealand, costs were estimated at £1,158,768 (NZ$3,094,243) per suicide (O'Dea and Tucker 2005) while in Ireland, the corresponding figure was some £1,402,438 (€1,982,667) (Kennelly *et al.* 2005). In Scotland, the average cost was £1.29 million per completed suicide (Platt *et al.* 2006).

From Table 49.1, it is clear that the direct costs of suicide account for just a tiny fraction of total cost. The lifetime lost opportunity to contribute to the economic output of a nation, as well as the additional value placed by society on the loss of life, are the main contributors. Given these high costs, the potential economic benefit, if the number of suicides can be reduced, may be substantial. In the Scottish case, for instance, a 1 per cent reduction in the number of suicides on average might avoid costs of up to £10.7 million over the lifetimes of these individuals. This is dependent on the availability and cost-effectiveness of interventions.

## Economic theories on suicide

Having illustrated the socio-economic costs of suicide, how and what can economics contribute to our understanding of individual

**Table 49.1** Mean cost per completed suicide (UK £s 2005 prices)

| Cost category | Ireland | New Zealand | Scotland |
|---|---|---|---|
| Direct | 2,682 | 4,033 | 8,509 |
| Indirect | 400,263 | 173,136 | 357,667 |
| Intangible | 999,494 | 981,599 | 926,760 |
| **Total** | **1,402,438** | **1,158,768** | **1,292,936** |

motivations to contemplate suicide? A better understanding of these motivations may help us to invest in interventions and strategies that address the underlying factors influencing motivation.

Durkheim, in his classic work, looked at the links between the structures and roles that individuals play in society and their risk of suicide, including some discussion of the role of income and changes in economic circumstances (Durkheim 1897). For instance, he suggested that a lifetime of poverty might be a protective factor against suicide, as the poor would have time to learn to live without material resources. In contrast, those individuals who experienced a downturn in their fortunes as a result of unemployment would be at higher risk of suicide. Similarly, he argued that suicides might increase in times of economic prosperity, when the demand for consumer goods might become insatiable, leading to anomie or social fragmentation, where social norms do not correspond with an individual's perception of the meaning of life.

This theory has been refined and/or challenged ever since. Ginsberg, for instance, writing in 1966, suggested that suicide would only increase in times of economic prosperity. During recessions, economic aspirations would decrease at a greater rate than economic growth, thus, individuals would expect less than what they would actually receive (Ginsberg 1980). Henry and Short, in contrast, suggested that suicides would only rise in times of recession, due to aggression and frustration being released when individuals realize that they cannot meet all their goals (Henry and Short 1954).

Despite this long-standing interest in the links between broad socio-economic factors and suicide by sociologists and others, it was not until the early 1970s that economists began to turn their attention to trying to explain the individual rationale behind suicide. While the number of economic papers on suicide is probably still too few to talk about any standard or basic model, the closest that any has come to attaining such status is the Lifetime Utility Model (Hamermesh and Soss 1974). This begins by noting Schopenhauer's famous statement that 'as soon as the terrors of life reach the point at which they outweigh the terrors of death, a man will put an end to his life' (Schopenhauer 1974, p. 310). Lifetime utility is determined by age and income and by a 'taste for living or distaste for suicide'. The basic assumption is that an individual kills himself when the total value of remaining lifetime reaches zero (or below some threshold required to continue to live).

This mainstream economic or 'rational choice' approach sees an individual's stock of health as a form of human capital, with skills and potential to be productive. The individual inherits an initial stock and invests over a lifetime to produce a stock of health which depreciates with age. The decision to invest in health is affected by income, the cost of health inputs, the return to investment in human capital and the time horizon over which this investment may be recouped. The theory suggests that suicide rates would increase with age as the costs of maintaining health increase with age.

This lifetime utility model has been criticised on several grounds. First, given that many suicidal individuals have mental disorders, it would be wrong to assume individuals to act rationally. Indeed, Hamermesh and Soss, themselves, acknowledged that the 'individual agony resulting in suicide does not stem solely from an economic calculation' (1974, p. 97). They, nonetheless, argued that their model illustrated the apparent links between macroeconomic conditions and the risk of some suicides. Others might argue that the economic model does not take rationality far enough—some individuals will have different views of the act of suicide and place a greater value on life after death depending on religious and cultural values.

A rational individual should also take into account the possibility that human life might improve. Given that suicide is an irreversible act, this 'option value' of staying alive could be extremely large (Dixit and Pindyck 1994). Indeed, those individuals who have enjoyed better fortunes in life might be more likely to survive into old age and, thus, may be less likely to contemplate suicide. Individuals might also wait to see if their circumstances improve before contemplating suicide. This would be consistent with evidence indicating that suicide actions are higher among the long-term unemployed (Platt 1986).

It is important to note that economic theories and models can be modified. One model, incorporating this option value on the potential of future life, no longer predicted any direct relationship between suicide and age (Cutler *et al.* 2001), in consistency with the increased rates of suicide in young people seen across the world (Wasserman *et al.* 2005). Economic models can potentially take account of a myriad of potential risk factors and socioeconomic contexts. For instance, relative income rather than absolute income may potentially have more effect on one's likelihood to commit suicide (Daly and Wilson 2006). The prior model is part of a rapidly growing body of literature in economics that suggests that interdependent preferences matter. It also harks back to some of the theories put forward by Durkheim and others about placing individual income into an appropriate context.

Game theory has also been applied by economists to estimate the trade-offs individuals may consider between the benefits of obtaining help for suicidal behaviour and the potential negative consequence of perhaps being involuntarily detained. In this model, health service professionals also have to weigh up the pros and cons of detaining individuals against providing community-based support, with a possibly higher risk of suicide. The likelihood that an individual will seek help will be dependent on the probability that support will remove suicidal tendencies with certainty (Yaniv 2001). From a policy perspective, this would suggest not only developing ever-more effective support and treatment, but engaging in campaigns to improve public awareness of the availability of such options.

Models can also be adapted to specific phenomena, such as Koo and Cox's model (2006), accounting for the rise in suicide among middle-aged men in Japan. Their model hypothesizes that any individual's human capital declines as a result of unemployment (because of the loss of on-the-job training etc.). During periods of sustained economic transition driven by technological shocks, the human capital of the middle-aged unemployed depreciates faster than that of younger workers, because they tend to be slower in adapting to new labour market conditions. This in turn (along with other factors such as a greater chance of divorce) drives down the expected relative lifetime utility of unemployed individuals, and thus increases the risk of suicide. From a policy perspective, if the model is validated, it might suggest that appropriate labour market interventions may include schemes to help re-skill older workers.

One feature of the economic approach that has not received as much attention is the way in which decreased utility or distress is produced. Lillard and Firestine's (2006) model focus on how a person chooses to manage such distress using what economists call 'a production function' approach. According to this model, the output, such as the emotional well-being that an individual enjoys, is dependent on certain inputs chosen or provided. These inputs might either be health-related goods (such as drugs, counselling) or non-market activities (relationships with friends or family). When an exogenous event, such as the onset of depression, substantially reduces the individual's emotional well-being, the mix of inputs in the production of emotional well-being needs to change. Their model predicts that a reduction in the availability of antidepressants (for instance as a result of an increase in price) should cause individuals to spend more time cultivating relationships with friends and family to bolster mental well-being.

In a similar fashion, another economic model considers child well-being as an output of a production function where the inputs are parental time and market goods (Mathur and Freeman 2002). Parental decisions to devote more time to work (or spend less time with children as a result of divorce) have a negative effect on child well-being, although this may be outweighed by the additional income earned. It might also imply that greater contact with relatives, e.g. grandparents or others through child care and/or after-school activities, might be needed to help counter some of the negative effects that may increase the risk of suicide.

Although not the focus of our chapter, it is worth noting that in addition to theories on motivations for completed suicide, economists have also sought to use game theory to explain motivations for attempted suicides, some of which may be perceived to be a 'cry for help'. One recent economic model assumes that such actions may be a rational attempt to elicit attention and care from family and friends. In the case where an individual assesses the potential additional care and long-term improved utility gained to outweigh the risk of death as well as the potential negative consequences of non-fatal but life-threatening self-harm events, the likelihood of such actions may increase (Marcotte 2003).

## What does the evidence actually show?

To what extent does empirical evidence support theories on the role of macro-economic factors and suicide?

Challenges remain in obtaining comprehensive individual-level data. Most empirical work to date is ecological in nature, making it impossible to definitively infer any individual behaviour from the aggregate data. The studies cited below at the cross-national, national and individual levels mainly report results that have reached conventional levels of significance in multivariable regression analysis. Many of the papers use fixed effects estimation techniques to control for differences in cross-country suicide cultures that are time invariant within countries. They also use time dummies that account for changes in suicide rates over time common to all countries.

### Income, economic growth and employment

A number of cross-country studies have looked at income levels as a risk factor for suicide in both developed and developing countries. The findings have been mixed: some report that there is a negative relationship between per capita income and male suicide rates (Neumayer 2003b; Helliwell 2004; Lin 2006). Another study states that per capita income has a non linear effect on male suicide rates, initially positive, but then negative for incomes above a threshold ($30,700) (Neumayer 2003a). The impacts of low income are particularly marked in transition countries in Eastern Europe, where the decline in gross domestic product (GDP) per capita and the employment/population ratio, accounted for nearly one third of the increase in male suicides in the 1990s (Brainerd 2001). On the other hand, an analysis of suicide rates in fifteen western European nations found that economic growth had a significant negative effect on both male and female suicide rates (Rodriguez-Andres 2005). Several studies did not find any significant association between suicide rates and income inequality (Helliwell 2004; Rodriguez-Andres 2005, 2006; Leigh and Jencks 2007).

Many studies report a positive relationship between unemployment and male suicide rates (Brainerd 2001; Neumayer 2003a). The rate of female participation in the labour force has also been shown to have a positive effect on male and female suicide rates (Neumayer 2003a; Rodriguez-Andres 2006). The evidence is again mixed with some studies not finding any association between unemployment and suicide rates (Helliwell 2004; Gerdtham and Ruhm 2006). A study of countries in western Europe found a positive effect for unemployment on suicide rates only for 45–64-year-old men, indicating the importance to policy-makers of looking at suicide by age group when considering potential suicide prevention measures (Rodriguez-Andres 2005).

Turning to single country analyses, again there is a mixed pattern of evidence on the links between macroeconomic factors and suicide. Some US studies suggest that state-level income is insignificant (Markowitz *et al.* 2003; Ludwig and Marcotte 2005; Cuellar and Markowitz 2007). Hamermesh and Soss, in contrast, reported a negative relationship between discounted permanent income and state suicide rates for men in the US (Hamermesh and Soss 1974). Another US study reported that county level median income also had a negative effect on youth suicide rates, although this result was sensitive to gun ownership (Cutler *et al.* 2001).

Not only income, but relative income, as some economic models contend, can be important, and this can differ by income group. In one recent US study, increased inequality between the average and the upper tail of the income distribution was linked to increased suicide rates, while increases in inequality between the average and the lower tail of the income distribution reduced suicide rates. This has been interpreted as meaning that individuals in the middle of the income distribution experience higher utility if they manage to keep up with those on higher incomes, while moving further ahead of those on lower incomes also increases their utility. If an analysis simply looked at the population as a whole, however, no relationship between income inequality and suicide would be observed (Daly and Wilson 2006).

A prior US study illustrates the importance not only of an individual's income, but also that of other family members. Increased parental income was found to be associated with declines in state suicide rates of 15–19-year-olds (Mathur and Freeman 2002). This outweighed the negative impact of reduced contact between parents and their children. The results are not confined to the US—two studies in Taiwan have reported a negative association between per capita income and regional suicide rates (Chuang and Huang 1997; Lin 2006).

A number of studies report that the male suicide rate increases with unemployment, e.g. Hamermesh and Soss (1974), in some instances this relationship is stronger for older age groups (Ruhm 2000). Unemployment has also been positively associated with the suicide rate for 15–19 year olds in two US studies

examined (Mathur and Freeman 2002; Cuellar and Markowitz 2007). Increased rates of female labour force participation have been linked to increased rates of suicides in young people at state level in the US (Cutler *et al.* 2001) and also in Japan (Koo and Cox 2006). The risk of suicide has also been shown to decrease in US counties when the proportion of the population with a university education increases (Markowitz *et al.* 2003; Daly and Wilson 2006).

Another US study used data from the 3 (NLMS) to follow a cohort of five national samples over a 10-year period from 1979 to 1989. Again the results suggest that an unemployed person is at greater risk of suicide, and that the effect may diminish over time, but be more enduring in women (Kposowa 2001). This dataset was also used to analyse differences in risk of suicide by occupation, after controlling for socio-economic factors. This suggested that risks are significantly higher for some occupations such as mining, retail and construction, but great care is needed in interpreting such findings (Kposowa 1999).

The positive relationship between unemployment and suicide can also be seen elsewhere around the world, for instance in Denmark, Sweden, Taiwan and Japan (Qin *et al.* 2003; Dahlberg and Lundin 2005; Lin 2006; Koo and Cox 2006). Agerbo and colleagues, making use of the rich data from Denmark's health, social and economic registers, were able to analyse individual level data and also area level-based factors. Again this study found that suicide risk was associated with a lack of employment and low income, combined with living alone or being divorced. It is also suggested that the characteristics of geographical areas do not have much impact on suicide, and thus policy-makers should target their efforts on the characteristics of individuals, which will include socio-economic and cultural factors, rather than their area of residence alone (Agerbo *et al.* 2007a, b). These socio-economic and culture factors might include ethnicity and sexuality, although evidence from economic models linking them to suicide remains limited.

As with cross-country studies, at country level not all evidence points in the same direction; no significant relationships between unemployment and suicide were found in some US studies (Markowitz *et al.* 2003; Ludwig and Marcotte 2005), while in Germany, for example, the economic downturn was associated with decreasing rates of suicide (Neumayer 2004). Again this illustrates the need for careful consideration of local contexts—for instance, the extent to which the social welfare safety net may cushion the economic impacts of recession.

## Social and behavioural factors

Many economic analyses have also considered social and behavioural factors as illustrated in one recent review (Rehkopf and Buka 2006). Consistent with results reported by others, divorce rates have been shown to have a positive effect on suicide rates in both developed and economic transition countries (Brainerd 2001; Neumayer 2003a, b; Helliwell 2004), while birth and marriage rates have a negative effect (Neumayer 2003a, b). Alcohol has also been associated with poor mental health and increased risk of suicide; evidence from econometric studies in the developed world indicates a positive effect of alcohol consumption on both male (Wasserman *et al.* 1994; Neumayer 2003a; Rodriguez-Andres 2005; Värnik *et al.* 2007) and female suicides (Wasserman *et al.* 1998; Brainerd 2001; Rodriguez-Andres 2006). Social networks and community well-being appear to be protective against suicide. One study found that two indicators of social capital—membership per capita in non-religious organizations and trust—were significantly associated with lower rates of suicide for both men and women. Belief in God was also found to be protective (Helliwell 2004). A later study using the same data also identified a positive relationship with poor subjective perceptions of health (Helliwell 2006). The links between suicide and the utilization of health care services, in particular antidepressants, have also been examined. While the impact on the use of selective serotonin re-uptake inhibitors (SSRIs) and suicide are complex and subject to debate (Simon *et al.* 2006), some studies indicate that the use of SSRIs may have a strong negative effect on suicide, with rates falling fastest in those countries that experienced the most rapid rate of growth in SSRI sales (Ludwig and Marcotte 2005).

At a country level, the US studies also indicate that divorce has a significant positive impact on suicide rates (Cutler *et al.* 2001; Mathur and Freeman 2002; Daly and Wilson 2006). In Japan, this relationship was only significant for male suicide, although there was weak support for a negative relationship between fertility and suicide rates, with a greater effect on women than on men (Koo and Cox 2006). In contrast, divorce had a significant negative effect on female suicide rates in a Swedish study (Dahlberg and Lundin 2005).

Most studies that looked at alcohol consumption at country level indicated that this was a risk factor, as for instance in Sweden (Dahlberg and Lundin 2005). Alcohol was shown to be a risk factor for 15–19-year-olds in one US study (Mathur and Freeman 2002), although this finding was contradicted by a more recent analysis, which indicated that beer consumption had a negative impact on suicide rates in this age group (Cuellar and Markowitz 2007). In another study of US states, a higher tax on beer was associated with lower male suicide rates—a 5.5 cent increase in the beer tax was estimated to save on average one male in the 15–19 and 20–24 age groups per state per year. The evidence on drink driving laws was mixed: in one study having only a limited effect on male suicides, while few regulatory measures had any impact on female suicide rates (Markowitz *et al.* 2003). Another US study did, however, find that the adoption of very tough underage drink driving laws were associated with reductions in the suicide deaths of 15–20-year-olds (Carpenter 2004). In the US, the consumption of SSRIs appeared to have a significant negative relationship with the state level suicide count 15–19-year-olds (Cuellar and Markowitz 2007), but

in Sweden, no relationship could be found between the use of anti-depressants and county suicide rates (Dahlberg and Lundin 2005).

## The contribution of economic evaluation to suicide prevention

We have briefly highlighted the importance of looking at the costs and consequences of suicide, and examined how economic models can help potentially identify areas where policy-makers may wish to focus suicide preventive efforts. At the start of this chapter, we emphasized the importance of taking action based on evidence not only of effectiveness, but also the undertaking of economic evaluation to assess cost-effectiveness, which is increasingly used as part of the process of evidence-based health policy making (Oliver and McDaid 2002). Below, a brief look at some different approaches and then a review of the extent to which economic evaluation has been used to date is given.

### Economic evaluation methods

Economic evaluation, in essence, compares both the costs and effectiveness of two or more alternative uses of resources. Figure 49.1 illustrates the range of possible cost-effectiveness results, and the way in which they can help inform policy-making.

Possible combinations of outcomes and costs when comparing two measures to prevent suicide are shown in Figure 49.1. Point B indicates that the new measure is both more effective in preventing suicide and less costly than the existing measure. In these circumstances, the task for the decision-maker is quite straightforward: recommend wider use of the new suicide prevention measure. It may be the case that a new measure is in fact at point A: producing better outcomes but at a higher cost. The decision now is more complex because a trade-off is needed: are the better outcomes worth the higher costs? There is no right or wrong answer to this question—decision-makers must decide how much they are willing to invest for improved health outcomes. In the UK, for instance, interventions that cost no more than £30,000 per life year gained are usually funded without great debate. Economic evaluation is just one source of information; many other factors will rightly influence decisions, not the least of which will be equity considerations.

There are different methods of economic evaluation; all estimate costs in the same way but differ in how they treat outcomes (Drummond *et al.* 1997; Byford *et al.* 2003b; Hale *et al.* 2005).

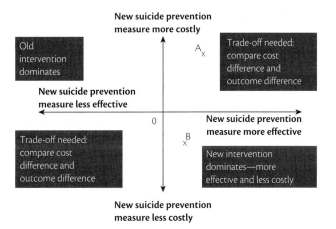

**Fig. 49.1** The cost-effectiveness plane

Cost-effectiveness analysis (CEA) measures outcomes using a natural measure, e.g. the number of suicides averted. Cost-utility analysis (CUA) uses a common health outcome measure, such as the Quality-adjusted life year (QALY) or the Disability-adjusted life year (DALY) (Murray and Lopez 1996). Both these measures can use values from the public or specific target groups for different health or disability states respectively. This has the advantage of allowing policy-makers to compare investments in suicide prevention with alternative health-promoting interventions. However, it can be difficult to make use of values for health states from individuals experiencing suicidal thoughts, who may rationally place (at least temporarily) a greater value on death compared to life (Chisholm et al. 2006).

Cost–benefit analysis (CBA) places a monetary value on all outcomes. With two or more alternatives, the intervention with the greatest net benefit would be deemed the most efficient. This is useful given that the costs and consequences of suicide go well beyond the health care system. CBA needs to obtain monetary values from individuals on the intangible value of life, which again can be problematic when considering suicide (Healey and Chisholm 1999), but the technique is widely used for assessing the value of comparable interventions such as transport-related injury prevention programmes (Department of Transport 2004). Nonetheless, because all outcomes (health and non-health) can be considered and valued, CBA can facilitate the comparison between suicide prevention measures and alternative investment in any sector such as housing, education or defence, for decision-makers to more easily compare.

## What is actually known about the cost-effectiveness of suicide prevention strategies?

The idea of assessing the costs of suicide prevention programmes, as well as the economic value of suicides averted, is not new (Diggory 1969; Lum 1973). Despite this, and the attention currently given to suicide prevention in national mental health policies worldwide, there are few economic evaluations of population-based measures to tackle suicide (US Preventive Services Task Force 2004). This is unsurprising, given that there is still relatively little evidence on the effectiveness of such complex community-based interventions (Beautrais 2005; Mann et al. 2005).

One rare example of the evaluation of an area-based prevention strategy, albeit with many limitations, one of them being that it is highly context-specific, is a retrospective analysis of a suicide prevention programme targeted at members of a reservation-based Native American group in New Mexico (Zaloshnja et al. 2003). The intervention focused primarily on young people aged 15–19, with the whole community as a secondary target group. It included peer training of young people, postvention outreach, community education programmes, and suicide-risk screening within local health and social care programmes. The rate of suicidal acts and suicides in the eight years prior to the programme was compared with suicides over the subsequent eight years. Direct and indirect costs were estimated. Overall the programme was deemed to have cost savings of $1.7 million due to the marked decrease in the rate of suicide from 59 per 1000 in the 15–19 age group, to a much lower rate varying between 10 and 17 per 1000 in subsequent years. Benefits gained were 43 times greater than costs incurred, while the cost per QALY saved was just $419, a value in most jurisdictions that is considered to be highly cost-effective. These findings must,

however, be treated cautiously, not least because of the lack of a comparator group and observed natural cyclical changes in suicide rates within this population group. Nonetheless, the study illustrates how economic analysis might be incorporated into the evaluation, and also how this may be done retrospectively making use of existing knowledge on the effectiveness of interventions.

Other powerful tools that economists can make use of include decision-analytical models. In the absence of long-term empirical data, these can be used to synthesise evidence on short-term costs and consequences of interventions and make long-term projections (Buxton et al. 1997). While rare for suicide prevention, modelling has been used in the US to estimate the potential cost-effectiveness of both a general suicide education and peer support group programme targeted at university students in Florida (de Castro et al. 2004). The model indicated that, because of the substantial lifetime costs avoided, both programmes would be highly cost-saving, with the peer support programme and the general education programme generating benefits 5.35 and 2.92 times, respectively, greater than costs. Another example is that of a regression model being used to assess the potential costs and consequences of suicide prevention centres in the US in the 1980s (Medoff 1986). These centres provided a 24-hour telephone service which would initiate crisis intervention services if appropriate. The model suggested that the value of human lives saved would be at least five times greater than the costs of running the centres.

Training to improve the recognition by primary care physicians of individuals at risk of suicide has also been highlighted as effective (Mann et al. 2005), but little economic analysis has been undertaken. One evaluation, set on the Swedish island of Gotland, looked at an educational programme for general practitioners to improve their ability to recognisze and treat the symptoms of depression (Rutz et al. 1992). Although there were methodological limitations in the assessment and attribution of the effectiveness of the data, the study suggests that the programme was cost-saving, in part because of the avoidance of costs associated with suicides averted. More recently, the costs of a training intervention in England that focused on the risk assessment and management of suicide was assessed alongside information on implementation and acquisition of skills and knowledge by front line health professionals. This study indicated that if a 2.5 per cent decrease in the suicide rate could be achieved, the cost per life year gained would be just £3391, a value considered to be highly cost effective in high income countries (Appleby et al. 2000).

There has also been some limited economic analysis of specific interventions to reduce the risk of suicide, including various safety measures (such as safety nets and barriers for bridges) and restriction of access to means such as firearms and poisons. Much more information is available, however, on a wide range of interventions intended to prevent unintentional injury which are also relevant to suicide, such as the installation of airbags in cars (Thompson et al. 2002). Thus, it is also important to look at the potential cost-effectiveness, in respect of suicide, of many measures to counter risky behaviours that may have many adverse health impacts. Alcohol control measures have been widely evaluated, although again these typically do not focus specifically on suicide. One recent study indicates that cost-effective measures are available right across the globe: in Europe the most cost-effective approach to reduce hazardous alcohol consumption is through taxation, whereas in parts of the world where heavy alcohol use is rare, e.g. in South East Asia, targeted interventions such as brief physician interventions or advertising bans appear to be more cost-effective (Chisholm *et al.* 2004).

For those already identified as being at high risk of suicide, there is some emerging evidence on the cost-effectiveness of different interventions. In England, a home-based social work intervention targeted at children, who had previously deliberately poisoned themselves, reported no statistically significant differences in overall health and social care costs between this treatment and routine care. However, it did record lower rates of suicidal ideation at 6-month follow-up in the subgroup of children without major depression, who received the social work intervention compared with those receiving routine care alone (Byford *et al.* 1999). Another study looked at the use of cognitive behavioural therapy (CBT) for people with a history of deliberate self harm in centres in both England and Scotland. It suggested that manual CBT was likely to be cost-effective in reducing the number of deliberate self-harm events, although it did not explicitly look at suicides averted (Byford *et al.* 2003a).

Some studies have also indicated that substantial costs can be avoided by providing treatment and support to people with depression (Wolfersdorf and Martinez 1998). While we do not propose here to enter into the debate about the relative merits of antidepressants as an effective suicide prevention intervention, it should be noted that such medications have been subject to much assessment of cost-effectiveness. Some of these evaluations include the economic impact of suicides averted (Barrett *et al.* 2005). Ludwig *et al.* (2007) estimate that an increase in SSRI sales of one pill per capita would reduce suicide mortality rates by around 5 per cent. Based on this the cost per statistical life saved from increasing SSRI used is around $20,000.

While economic evaluation has an important role to play, common sense needs to be applied to its use, as resources to undertake such evaluations are often scarce. Some interventions may be shown to be of sufficient effectiveness and have such low implementation costs that a comprehensive economic evaluation would add little to the case for investment. They are already clearly cost saving. This, for instance, might include simple, but effective, measures such as the erection of signs for support services in some areas known to be suicide black spots (King and Frost 2005).

## Conclusion

Economic evidence can play an important role in helping to understand how different risk factors influence individual motivations for suicide. Econometric techniques, both across and within countries, linked to economy theories, can add knowledge to ecological and epidemiological work already undertaken. Providing information on the profound socio-economic costs of suicide, in particular, emphasizing that these impacts go way beyond immediate costs to health care and emergency services, can help to strengthen the case for taking action to reduce suicide. Ultimately, such a case may stand or fall on evidence not only on the availability of effective interventions, but also on cost-effective interventions. Such information is increasingly part of evidence-based policy-making, but its use in suicide prevention remains limited, and is focused on high income countries. Incorporating economic analyses into new evaluations is one step that might be taken, but much can also be done through retrospectively considering what the crude economic costs would be of implementing effective prevention strategies in different contexts, and what the potential economic benefits of predicted suicides averted as a result might be. The limited evidence available to date would suggest that investment in effective interventions is likely to be highly cost-effective compared with other uses of public resources. The challenge is to expand on, strengthen and communicate findings from this emerging evidence base.

## References

Agerbo E, Gunnell D, Bonde JP *et al.* (2007b). Suicide and occupation: the impact of socio-economic, demographic and psychiatric differences. *Psychological Medicine*, **37**, 1131–1140.

Agerbo E, Sterne JA, Gunnell DJ (2007a). Combining individual and ecological data to determine compositional and contextual socio-economic risk factors for suicide. *Social Science and Medicine*, **64**, 451–461.

Appleby L, Morriss R, Gask L *et al.* (2000). An educational intervention for front-line health professionals in the assessment and management of suicidal patients (The STORM Project). *Psychological Medicine*, **30**, 805–812.

Barrett B, Byford S, Knapp M (2005). Evidence of cost-effective treatments for depression: a systematic review. *Journal of Affective Disorders*, **84**, 1–13.

Beautrais A (2005). National strategies for the reduction and prevention of suicide. *Crisis* **26**, 1–3.

Brainerd E (2001). Economic reform and mortality in the former Soviet Union: a study of the suicide epidemic in the 1990s. *European Economic Review*, **45**, 1007–1019.

Buxton MJ, Drummond MF, Van Hout BA *et al.* (1997). Modelling in economic evaluation: an unavoidable fact of life. *Health Economics*, **6**, 217–227.

Byford S, Harrington R, Torgerson D *et al.* (1999). Cost-effectiveness analysis of a home-based social work intervention for children and adolescents who have deliberately poisoned themselves. Results of a randomised controlled trial. *British Journal of Psychiatry*, **174**, 56–62.

Byford S, Knapp M, Greenshields J *et al.* (2003a). Cost-effectiveness of brief cognitive behaviour therapy versus treatment as usual in recurrent deliberate self-harm: a decision-making approach. *Psychological Medicine*, **33**, 977–986.

Byford S, McDaid D, Sefton T (2003b). *Because it's Worth It. A Practical Guide to Conducting Economic Evaluations in the Social Welfare Field*. York Publications, York.

Carpenter C (2004). Heavy alcohol use and youth suicide: evidence from tough drunk driving laws. *Journal of Policy Analysis and Management*, **23**, 831–842.

Chisholm D, Rehm J, Van Ommeren M *et al.* (2004). Reducing the global burden of hazardous alcohol use: a comparative cost-effectiveness analysis. *Journal of Studies on Alcohol*, **65**, 782–793.

Chisholm D, Salvador-Carulla L, Ayuso-Mateos JL (2006). Quality of life measurement in the economic analysis of mental health care. In H Katschnig, H Freeman and N Sartorius, eds, *Quality of Life in Mental Disorders*, 2nd edn, pp. 299–308. John Wiley & Sons Ltd, Chichester.

Chuang WL and Huang WC (1997). Economic and social correlates of regional suicide rates. A pooled cross-section and time-series analysis. *Journal of Socio-Economics*, **26**, 277–289.

Clayton D and Barceló A (2000). The cost of suicide mortality in New Brunswick, 1996. *Chronic Diseases in Canada*, **20**, 89–95.

Cox K and Miller TR (1999). *The Costs of Youth Suicide and Medically-treated Attempts by State*. Children's Safety Network, Landover.

Cuellar A and Markowitz S (2007). Medicaid policy changes in mental health care and their effect on mental health outcomes. *Health Economics, Policy and Law*, **2**, 23–49.

Cutler DM, Glaeser EL, Norberg KE (2001). *Explaining the Rise in Youth Suicide*. Harvard Institute of Economic Research, Cambridge.

Dahlberg M and Lundin D (2005). *Antidepressants and the Suicide Rate: Is There Really a Connection?* University of Uppsala, Uppsala.

Daly M and Wilson D (2006). *Well-being and Inequality: Evidence From Suicide Data*. Federal Reserve Bank of San Francisco, San Francisco.

de Castro S, Newman F, Mills G *et al.* (2004). Economic evaluation of suicide prevention programs for young adults in Florida. *Business Review Cambridge*, December, 14–20.

Department of Transport (2004). *Highways Economic Note No 1*. Department of Transport, London.

Diggory JC (1969). Calculation of some costs of suicide prevention using certain predicors of suicidal behaviour. *Psychological Bulletin*, **71**, 373–386.

Dixit A and Pindyck R (1994). *Investment Under Uncertainty*. Princeton University, Princeton.

Drummond M, O'Brien B, Stoddart G *et al.* (1997). *Methods for the Economic Evaluation of Health Care Programmes*. Oxford Medical Publications, Oxford.

Durkheim E (1897). *Le suicide. Etude de sociologie*. Felix Alcan, Paris.

Gerdtham U-G and Ruhm CJ (2006). Deaths rise in good times: evidence from the OECD. *Economics and Human Biology*, **4**, 298–316.

Ginsberg RB (1980). Anomie and aspirations: a reinterpretation of Durkheim's theory. Doctoral Thesis Columbia University 1966. Arno Press, New York.

Hale J, Cohen D, Ludbrook A *et al.* (2005). *Moving from Evaluation into Economic Evaluation: A Health Economics Manual for Programmes to Improve Health and Well-being*. National Assembly for Wales: Cardiff.

Hamermesh D and Soss N (1974). An economic theory of suicide. *Journal of Political Economy*, **82**, 83–98.

Healey A and Chisholm D (1999). Willingness to pay as a measure of the benefits of mental health care. *Journal of Mental Health Policy and Economics*, **2**, 55–58.

Helliwell JF (2004). *Well-Being and Social Capital: Does Suicide Pose a Puzzle?* National Bureau of Economic Research, Cambridge.

Helliwell JF (2006). Well-being, social capital and public policy. What's new? *The Economic Journal*, **116**, C34–C45.

Henry AF and Short JF (1954). *Suicide and Homicide*. Free Press, Glencoe.

Kennelly B, Ennis J, O'Shea E (2005). Economic cost of suicide and deliberate self harm. In *Reach Out. National Strategy for Action on Suicide Prevention 2005–2014*. Department of Health and Children, Dublin.

King E and Frost N (2005). The New Forest Suicide Prevention Initiative (NFSPI). *Crisis*, **26**, 25–33.

Knox KL and Caine ED (2005). Establishing priorities for reducing suicide and its antecedents in the United States. *American Journal of Public Health*, **95**, 1898–1903.

Koo J and Cox WM (2006). *An Economic Interpretation of Suicide Cycles in Japan*. Federal Reserve Bank of Dallas, Dallas.

Kposowa AJ (1999). Suicide mortality in the United States: differentials by industrial and occupational groups. *American Journal of Industrial Medicine*, **36**, 645–652.

Kposowa AJ (2001). Unemployment and suicide: a cohort analysis of social factors predicting suicide in the US National Longitudinal Mortality Study. *Psychological Medicine*, **31**, 127–138.

Leigh A and Jencks C (2007). Inequality and mortality: long run evidence from a panel of countries. *Journal of Health Economics*, **26**, 1–24.

Lillard D and Firestine T (2006). *Managing Despair: An Economic Model of Rational Suicide*. Department of Policy Analysis and Management, Cornell University, mimeo.

Lin S-J (2006). Unemployment and suicide: panel data analyses. *Social Science Journal*, **43**, 727–732.

Ludwig J and Marcotte D (2005). Anti-depressants, suicide and drug regulation. *Journal of Policy Analysis and Management*, **24**, 249–272.

Ludwig J, Marcotte D, Norberg K (2007). Anti-depressants and suicide. *National Bureau of Economic Research, Working Paper*, 12906.

Lum D (1973). How much is it worth to prevent suicides? Economic and public health issues in suicide prevention. *Hawaii Medical Journal*, **32**, 391–394.

Mann JJ, Apter A, Bertolote J *et al.* (2005). Suicide prevention strategies. A systematic review. *Journal of the American Medical Association*, **294**, 2064–2074.

Marcotte DE (2003). The economics of suicide, revisited. *Southern Economic Journal*, **69**, 628–643.

Markowitz S, Chatterji P, Kaestner R (2003). Estimating the impact of alcohol policies on youth suicides. *Journal of Mental Health Policy & Economics*, **6**, 37–46.

Mathur VK and Freeman DG (2002). A theoretical model of adolescent suicide and some evidence from US data. *Health Economics*, **11**, 695–708.

Medoff MH (1986). An evaluation of the effectiveness of suicide prevention centers. *Journal of Behavioural Economics*, **15**, 43–55.

Meneghel G, Scocco P, Dente A *et al.* (1996). Qualità della cura e costi del trattamento dei pazienti parasuicidari. *Giornale Italiano di Suicidologia*, **6**, 31–37.

Murray CJL and Lopez AD (eds) (1996). *The Global Burden of Disease: A Comprehensive Assessment of Mortality and Disability from Diseases, Injuries, and Risk Factors in 1990 and Projected to 2020*. Harvard University Press, Cambridge.

Neumayer E (2003a). Are socio-economic factors valid determinants of suicide? Controlling for national cultures of suicide with fixed-effects estimation. *Cross-Cultural Research*, **37**, 307–329.

Neumayer E (2003b). Socioeconomic factors and suicide rates at large-unit aggregate levels. *Urban Studies*, **40**, 2769–2776.

Neumayer E (2004). Recessions lower (some) mortality rates: evidence from Germany. *Social Science and Medicine*, **58**, 1037–1047.

O'Dea D and Tucker S (2005). *The Cost of Suicide to Society*. New Zealand Ministry of Health, Wellington.

O'Sullivan M, Lawlor M, Corcoran P *et al.* (1999). The cost of hospital care in the year before and after parasuicide. *Crisis*, **20**, 178–83.

Oliver A and McDaid D (2002). Evidence-based health care: benefits and barriers. *Social Policy and Society*, **1**, 183–190.

Platt S (1986). Clinical and social characteristics of male parasuicides: variation by employment status and duration of unemployment. *Acta Psychiatrica Scandinavica*, **74**, 24–31.

Platt S, Halliday E, Maxwell M *et al.* (2006). *Evaluation of the First Phase of Choose Life. Final Report*. Scottish Executive, Edinburgh.

Qin P, Agerbo E, Mortensen PB (2003). Suicide risk in relation to socioeconomic, demographic, psychiatric, and familial factors: a national register-based study of all suicides in Denmark, 1981–1997. *American Journal of Psychiatry*, **160**, 765–772.

Rehkopf D and Buka SL (2006). The association between suicide and the socio-economic characteristics of geographical areas: a systematic review. *Psychological Medicine*, **36**, 145–158.

Rodriguez-Andres A (2005). Income inequality, unemployment and suicide: a panel data analysis of 15 European countries. *Applied Economics*, **37**, 439–451.

Rodriguez-Andres A (2006). *Inequality and Suicide Mortality: A Cross-country Study*. Institute for Advanced Development Studies, La Paz.

Ruhm CJ (2000). Are recessions good for your health? *Quarterly Journal of Economics*, **115**, 617–650.

Rutz W, Carlsson P, von Knorring L *et al.* (1992). Cost–benefit analysis of an educational program for general practitioners by the Swedish Committee for the Prevention and Treatment of Depression. *Acta Psychiatrica Scandinavica*, **85**, 457–464.

Schopenhauer A (1974). *Parerga and Paralipomena: Short Philosophical Essays*. Clarendon Press, Oxford.

Simon GE, Savarino J, Operskalski B *et al.* (2006). Suicide risk during antidepressant treatment. *American Journal of Psychiatry*, **163**, 41–47.

Thomas C and Morris S (2003). Cost of depression among adults in England in 2000. *British Journal of Psychiatry*, **183**, 514–519.

Thompson KM, Segui-Gomez M, Graham JD (2002). Validating benefit and cost estimates: the case of airbag regulation. *Risk Analysis*, **22**, 803–811.

US Preventive Services Task Force (2004). *Screening for Suicide Risk*. Agency for Healthcare Research and Quality, Rockville.

Värnik A, Kölves K, Väli M *et al.* (2007). Do alcohol restrictions reduce suicide mortality? *Addiction*, **102**, 251–2546.

Wasserman D, Cheng Q, Jiang GX (2005). Global suicide rates among young people aged 15–19. *World Psychiatry*, **4**, 114–120.

Wasserman D, Värnik A, Eklund G (1994). Male suicides and alcohol consumption in the former USSR. *Acta Psychiatrica Scandinavica*, **89**, 306–313.

Wasserman D, Värnik A, Eklund G (1998). Female suicides and alcohol consumption during *perestroika* in the former USSR. *Acta Psychiatrica Scandinavica*, **98**, 26–33.

Watson WL and Ozanne-Smith J (1997). *The Cost of Injury to Victoria*. Monash University, Victoria.

Wolfersdorf M and Martinez C (1998). Suizid bei depression, verlorene lebensjahre und bruttosozialprodukt: wasbringt suizidpravention? [Suicide in depression, lost years of life and Gross National Product. Why prevent suicide?] *Psychiatrische Praxis*, **25**, 139–141.

Yaniv G (2001). Suicide intention and suicide prevention: an economic perspective. *Journal of Socio-Economics*, **30**, 453–468.

Zaloshnja E, Miller TR, Galbraith MS *et al.* (2003). Reducing injuries among Native Americans: five cost-outcome analyses. *Accident Analysis and Prevention*, **35**, 631–639.

# CHAPTER 50

# World Health Organization and European Union policy actions, responsibilities and solutions in preventing suicide

Danuta Wasserman, Elizabeth Mårtensson and Camilla Wasserman

## Abstract

Mental health policies in Europe have been driven, in recent years, by two key documents: *The Mental Health Declaration* (WHO 2005) and the European Commission Green Paper (2005). As such, these important papers have paved the way towards the development of a European Mental Health Pact (European Commission 2008) in which policy-makers and stakeholders are urged to act upon European, national and local policies and implement key measures to enable the prevention of suicide and depression, improvement of mental health in youth, older people and in working places.

## World Health Organization initiatives to prevent mental ill-health and suicide

The prevention of suicide and mental ill-health involves not only the individuals affected or at risk, but also families, peers, schools, workplaces, and communities. Any place where people live or work are key areas for targeting prevention initiatives (WHO 2002).

At the WHO Ministerial Conference on Mental Health, held in Helsinki 12–15 January 2005, the *Mental health declaration for Europe: facing the challenges, building solutions* was agreed upon and signed by the Ministers of Health of the 52 member states of WHO's European Region (WHO 2005).

Central to this document were several premises, in particular, that:

> There is no health without mental health. Mental health is central to the human, social and economic capital of nations and should therefore be considered as an integral and essential part of other public policy areas such as human rights, social care, education and employment.
>
> WHO (2005, p. 3)

This statement was strengthened by the call for more actions to support the implementation of evidence-based mental health policies, and to build sustainable means and structures to enable delivery of such supportive policies. It was clearly identified that within Europe there was a need to 'develop and implement measures to reduce the preventable causes of mental health problems, comorbidity and suicide' (WHO 2005, p. 3).

Responsibilities of the fifty-two participating member states in the WHO European Region included the committal to support several measures promoting mental health and prevent mental ill-health and suicide, namely:

◆ Work to deconstruct myths and reduce stigma and discrimination by increasing awareness in the general public in order to empower and increase the inclusion of people with mental ill-health or those at risk;

◆ Increase collaboration between different agencies, departments, non-governmental organizations etc., both within and outside of the health care arena, to promote positive mental health in different settings, including places of education and employment, and in communities.

◆ Acknowledge the importance of primary health care in detecting and supporting people who are at risk and support the development of capacity to take on responsibility for mental health;

◆ Focus on the prevention of suicide and causes of stress, depression and anxiety, and substance use disorders, including alcohol;

◆ Ensure all health care professionals have mental health education in the training curricula, and continuous professional education in the field of mental health;

◆ Identify areas where knowledge is missing and commission research where necessary;

◆ Disseminate findings and good practice points.

Agreement to implement identified measures by member states was achieved in relation to each of the separate countries national constitutional processes and policies, available resources, and identified needs.

The WHO Mental Health Programme EURO (Regional Advisor Dr Matt Muijen) coordinates the implementation, monitoring and evaluation of the activities in the Mental Health Declaration together with several WHO lead collaborating centres. NASP (National Prevention of Suicide and Mental Ill-Health at Karolinska Institute, Stockholm, Sweden) is responsible for coordination and promotion of activities concerning prevention of mental health problems and suicide across the WHO European region.

## European Commission's actions to promote mental health and prevent suicide

The European Commissions' response to the WHO invitation to continue working with member states on the implementation of the Mental Health Declaration's action framework, was the European Commission green paper: 'Improving the mental health of the population: Towards a strategy on mental health for the European Union' (European Commission 2005). The aim of the paper was in essence to create an European Commission strategy to enable more effective communication and cooperation between member states, and thus support political action both in the health care and public health policies. It also created a platform for experts and decision-makers to be involved in developing and driving forward effective solutions.

In the EU's green paper, the primary focus rests on the facts that one in four people have been, or are affected by mental ill-health, which can lead to suicide, and that improvements in the mental health of the European Commission population are attainable.

In 2006, 59,000 people in the 27 European Commission Member States (EU27) committed suicide, of which 45,000 were men and 14,000 were women (Eurostat 2008). In comparison, traffic accidents caused 50,000 deaths (Eurostat 2008). Every 9 minutes, 1 person dies due to suicide in the EU. Among the countries with the highest suicide rate for women, seven are European member states (WHO 2008). Non-fatal self-harm greatly increases the risk for suicide. The incidence of non-fatal self-harm is estimated to be 10–40 times more common than that of actual suicide (1:9 for males, 1:42 for females).

There is a strong need to adapt political policies into evidence based actions in the field of mental health. This has been successfully achieved in other areas, for example the European Commission public health programmes, which indicate that actions can be effective, generate knowledge and information and also be cost-effective (European Commission 2005).

Suicide prevention interventions, policies and strategies have been developed nationally throughout the EU (European Commission 2005; Mittendorfer and Wasserman 2004). There are increasing amounts of evidence to support various actions which can reduce the numbers of suicide (Wasserman 2001), in particular restricting access to the means of suicide (WHO 2006), training of healthcare providers (Ramberg and Wasserman 2003), training of general practitioners and follow-up services for suicide attempts (Mann *et al.* 2005), as well as stimulating collaboration between health care services and non-governmental agencies.

In 2008, the European Commission followed the green paper by creating an action-oriented approach in order to support mental health activities in the EU. On 12 June 2008, the EU initiated a high-level conference in Brussels; 'Together for Mental Health and Well-being' lead by the European Commissioner for Health, Androulla Vassiliou. A European pact on mental health and well-being was established, to encourage the governments of member states and various stakeholders to focus on mental health as a common goal and responsibility. The aim is to ensure long-term collaboration and sustained input into this important area concerning prevention of depression and suicide.

The pact acknowledges the importance of further actions within the field of mental health and agrees that there is a need for action within the following five priority areas:

1 Prevention of depression and suicide;

2 Mental health in youth and education;

3 Mental health in workplace settings;

4 Mental health of older people;

5 Combating stigma and social exclusion.

Concerning prevention of depression and suicide the pact encourages the following actions:

◆ Improve the training of health professionals and key actors within the social sector on mental health;

◆ Restrict access to potential means for suicide;

◆ Take measures to raise mental health awareness in the general public, among health professionals and other relevant sectors;

◆ Take measures to reduce risk factors for suicide such as excessive drinking, drug abuse and social exclusion, depression and stress;

◆ Provide support mechanisms after suicide attempts and for those bereaved by suicide.

The pact underlines the necessity of monitoring trends and activities in member states and among stakeholders. Supporting documents, which have drawn together key researchers and practitioners in the prevention of depression and suicide, highlight existing knowledge, key areas for development, examples of effective projects and programmes.

The European Commission, member states, the relevant international organizations and stakeholders have been invited to contribute to the implementation of the pact which calls for:

◆ The establishment of a mechanism for the exchange of information;

◆ To work together to identify good practices and success factors in policy and stakeholder action;

◆ To communicate the results of such work through a series of conferences on the pact's priority themes over the coming years;

◆ The European Commission to issue a proposal for a Council recommendation on mental health and well-being during 2009;

◆ The presidency to inform the Council of Ministers of the proceedings and outcomes of this conference.

A conference is expected to follow up this work in 2009–2010.

## Conclusion

European mental health policies have been highly influential factors in the stimulation of suicide preventive activities in many European countries. Significant benefits can be attained through effective international collaboration in research and dissemination. This was recognized, and strategies were identified to achieve this in the WHO Mental Health Declaration in 2005, signed by all Ministers of Health in fifty-two countries of the WHO European region and in the Mental Health Pact (European Commission 2008) that was agreed by the twenty-seven EU member states in June 2008. Both documents call for increased collaboration, exchanges of information, the identification and dissemination of good and successful practices in both direct and policy actions.

## References

European Commission (2005). *Green paper. Improving the mental health of the population: towards a strategy on mental health for the European Union*. European Commission, Brussels, 14.10.2005 COM (2005) 484.

European Commission (2008). *European Pact for Mental Health and Well-being*. EU High-Level Conference 'Together for Mental Health and Well-being'. Brussels, 12–13 June 2008. European Commission, Brussels.

Eurostat (2008). *Europe in Figures: Eurostat Year Book 2006–2007*. http:// www.ec.europa.eu/eurostat (latest review 22 June 2008).

Mann JJ, Apter A, Bertolote J *et al.* (2005). Suicide prevention strategies: a systematic review. *JAMA*, **16**, 2064–2074.

Mittendorfer Rutz E and Wasserman D (2004). The WHO European monitoring surveys on suicide preventive programmes and strategies. *Suicidologi*, **9(1)**, 23–25.

Ramberg I-L and Wasserman D (2003). Benefits of implementing a training-of-trainers model to promote knowledge and clarity in work with psychiatric suicidal patients. *Archives of Suicide Research*, **8**, 331–343.

Wasserman D (ed.) (2001). *Suicide: An Unnecessary Death*. Martin Dunitz, London.

WHO (2002). *Suicide Prevention in Europe: The WHO European monitoring survey on national suicide prevention programmes and strategies*. WHO Regional Office for Europe, Copenhagen.

WHO (2005). *Mental Health Declaration for Europe: Facing the Challenges, Building Solutions*. Finland 12–15 January 2005.

WHO (2006). *Safer Access to Pesticides: Community Interventions*. World Health Organization, Geneva.

WHO (2008). http://www.who.int/mental_health/prevention/auicide_rates/en/.

# CHAPTER 51

# The role of the state and legislation in suicide prevention

## The five continents perspective

Martin Anderson and Rachel Jenkins

## Abstract

This chapter explores the way in which current states intervene in suicide prevention. The broader context for the development of national policy will be discussed including guidance from the WHO and the United Nations. At the centre of this is the recognition of suicide as a global phenomenon and the need to ensure that countries do all they can to reduce suicide rates and help those bereaved by suicide. We examine how nations have been asked to consider suicide prevention in national public health policy and look at the common areas for state intervention. The chapter draws upon information from the five continents perspective and emphasizes the similarities, differences and areas in which state work is needed.

## Introduction

The emergence of suicide as one of the major causes of death across the world has led to clear recommendations from the World Health Organization (WHO) that governments worldwide should develop national suicide prevention programmes (WHO 1990; Jenkins and Singh 2000a). Indeed, as early as 1984, the WHO European member states drafted a health policy document that included, as one of its main targets, the reduction of suicide:

> By the year 2000 there should be a sustained and continuing reduction in the prevalence of mental disorders and improvement in the quality of life of all people with such disorders and a reversal of the rising trends in suicide and attempted suicide.
>
> WHO (1985, p. 50)

The World Health Organization has worked to ensure that suicide is fully recognized as a key health and social issue within the public health arena (Taylor *et al.* 1997). The following recommendations have been publicized to the WHO member states in order to facilitate and coordinate comprehensive national and international strategies:

1 To recognize the problems as a priority in public health;

2 To develop national suicide preventive programmes, where possible interlinked to other public health polices; and

3 Establish national coordinating management groups (WHO 1990).

The United Nations suggested five main components for the content of national suicide prevention strategies. The recommendations consists of an explicit government policy on suicide prevention, a coherent model for prevention of suicidal behaviour including general aims and goals, measurable objectives, and ongoing monitoring and evaluation (United Nations 1996; Singh and Jenkins 2000). At the WHO Ministerial Conference on Mental Health in Helsinki 2005, a mental health declaration was agreed upon and signed by the Ministers of Health of fifty-two member states of the WHOs European region. The declaration stated that mental health is central to the human, social and economic capital of actions and it should be part of other public policy such as human rights, social care, education and employment. This vision is echoed in the European Union's green paper on mental health, which also highlights the need to integrate mental health into other policies. Furthermore an increased visibility of mental health in health policies and other policies was emphasized, as well as the establishment of comprehensive mental health strategies and the reduction of suicide as an overall target (European Commission 2005). The six WHO lead collaborating centres (named below) took on specific roles in the spreading of policies such as tackling stigma discrimination and social exclusion, mental health promotion, dissemination of information about mental health, mental health services development and mental health problems and suicide (NASP 2006). The WHO lead collaborating centres are:

1 The WHO Lead Collaborating Centre for Tackling Stigma, Discrimination and Social exclusion. The Scottish Executive's National Programme for Improving Mental Health and well-being and NHS Health Scotland, UK.

2 The WHO Lead Collaborating Centre for Mental Health Promotion. The National Finnish Research and Development Centre of Welfare and Health (STAKES), associated with the Finnish Institute of Occupation Health (FIOH), Finland.

3 The WHO Lead Collaborating Centre on Mental Problems and Suicide. 6. The Swedish National Prevention of Suicide and Prevention of Mental Ill-Health (NASP), Karolinska Institute (KI), Sweden.

4 The WHO Lead Collaborating Centre for Dissemination of Information about Mental Health. The Trimbos Institute, The Netherlands.

5 The WHO Lead Collaborating Centre for Mental Health Services Development in Europe Trieste, Italy.

6 The WHO Lead Collaborating Centre for Research. Institute of Psychiatry Centre, London, UK.

This new organizational leadership, and the key targets and guidance provided, put in place the way forward for governmental leaders of countries.

While there has been guidance from the WHO and the UN has led to recognition of the need for national policies, public and societal views of suicide prevention remain an important influence. Such views may range from the norm that all suicides should be prevented to a clear acceptance of an individual's right to take their own life. The world currently faces a whole spectrum of suicide related issues: from the use of suicide bombers, to the question of an individual's right to end their life in the face of a degenerative disease, to physician assisted euthanasia. This chapter focuses on examining key issues faced by governments in establishing a national strategy embedded in public health policy, including examples of the impact of legislation in relation to suicide prevention.

## Developing a national suicide prevention strategy

Governments' health polices generally strive to promote health, prevent illness, reduce morbidity, disability and mortality. States tend to place particular emphasis on reducing mortality and many governments in the developed world have developed significant inter-ministry concerted action on such mortalities as deaths from road traffic accidents, from heart disease and from cancers. There is also significant and overriding emphasis on deaths from infectious diseases such as malaria and HIV in countries where the virus is widespread (Jenkins and Singh 2000a). A focus on suicide prevention has not been widely prioritized although premature death from suicide is a significant cause of mortality around the globe: official suicides alone are equivalent in magnitude to deaths from road traffic accidents and some tropical diseases. Suicide in all countries is heavily stigmatized and not all actual suicides are recorded as such (Jenkins and Singh 2000b).

Research has contributed a great deal to our understanding of suicide and related diseases and has underpinned investigations on the prevalence of suicide and the efficacy of preventative strategies. Epidemiological and psychological autopsy studies in a number of countries indicate that the rate of unofficial suicides is considerable and thus the rate of actual suicides may often be double that of official suicides. Premature death from suicide leaves a range of adverse consequences. Of greatest significance is the immediate loss of life, but there are also the direct consequences for the family of the loss of a breadwinner and parent. There is the long-lasting psychological trauma of children, friends and relatives,

and the loss of economic productivity for the country. These facts and the knowledge gleaned from research are essential to those charged with the responsibility in governmental office. For policy-makers and those responsible for implementing national and local strategies an appropriate model of prevention is essential.

## A model for prevention

A traditional model of prevention is described by Gerald Caplan and involves primary, secondary and tertiary prevention (Caplan 1964; Diekstra 1992). A contemporary explanation of the three concepts is offered in the context of a public health model (Jenkins and Singh 2000a). Initially, primary, secondary and tertiary prevention was developed for diseases with clear onsets followed by early and later phases.

*Primary prevention* focuses on populations, not individuals. When applied to an uncommon condition or behaviour (with a fatal outcome), it must have reduced potential to harm and be economically viable. It also has to be appropriate and acceptable to the population. Awareness programmes on suicide as examples of primary prevention strategies implemented in schools are discussed in Part 10B, Chapter 73, in this book, and teaching of coping and relationship skills have been found to be more effective and less harmful than raising awareness of suicide in young people. Primary prevention may also be focused on modification of environmental factors, for example diminishing the access to means of suicide (see Part 10C, in this book), on enhancing social support (Cantor and Baume 1999), and may focus on particular settings, e.g. prison environments (see Part 5, Chapter 37, in this book).

*Secondary prevention* includes the early treatment of all individuals at risk of harming themselves and people with an identified mental health problem (Diekstra 1992; Jenkins and Singh 2000b) . Secondary prevention involves the identification of and intervention with a wide range of individuals—many of whom may never commit suicide. This requires the training of front line professionals in general practice, mental health and emergency health care professionals. Those charged with the duty of commissioning and budgeting of services may consider such interventional strategies not to be an economic priority. However, it is argued that early treatment offers financial as well as health benefits (Cantor and Baume 1999).

*Tertiary prevention* encompasses people who present obvious concerns relating to suicidal behaviour. This population constitutes people who have already attempted suicide and those people affected by the death of others, including family, friends and survivors (Jenkins and Singh 2000b; Anderson and Jenkins 2003).

## General population strategies

While an accepted model is important to governments developing such policy, specific evidence relating to risk factors should be recognized and integrated into policy. There are a number of factors that appear to have immediate relevance to national suicide prevention strategies (Singh and Jenkins 2000). General population strategies in their evolution have come to focus on the treatment of depression. Further to this, there has been growing recognition of the role of alcohol and other substance misuse in the progression toward suicide (see Chapter 81, in this book). This is backed up by established and convincing evidence that suicides rarely occur without the presence of depression or some other form of breakdown in mental health well-being (Brainerd 2001). Yet the move from a classical infective disease model of health/illness to a broader concept of public health, integrating behaviours such as injury and suicide, has facilitated the development of programmes to deal with such issues.

Government activity in forming policy on suicide reduction has to focus on establishing, facilitating and monitoring the most relevant mechanisms and approaches. Thus, strategies for suicide prevention are seen in the divisions of the health care service and the public health approach (Wasserman 2001; WHO 2002). Effective suicide prevention campaigns will combine both approaches for optimal impact. Health care approaches focus on improving health care services and diagnostic procedures and ultimately treatment interventions. This will involve work to improve and maintain effective follow-up for people with mental health problems, those who have engaged in suicidal behaviour and hose with suicidal thoughts. There should also be efforts to increase awareness among health care staff of their own attitudes and taboos towards suicide prevention and mental illness (WHO 2002).

Public health perspectives are centred not only on restricting access to means of suicide and a responsible media policy, but also with changing condemnatory attitudes in society towards suicide prevention and mental illness (Jenkins and Singh 2000a; WHO 2002; Anderson and Jenkins 2005). One strategy that governments can adopt is to increase knowledge through public education (as mentioned above) about mental illness and its recognition at an early stage. Governments can disseminate information on the role of acute and chronic psychosocial stress and the importance of protective factors against psychological stress and suicidal behaviour. Factors that protect against mental ill health include psychosocial factors, such as good supportive networks and adequate coping abilities, as well as physical and environmental factors such as good sleep, a balanced diet, physical exercise and drug-free environment (Wasserman 2001; WHO 2002).

Governments in various countries share common themes within their national suicide prevention strategies, and experience from one country has often influenced policy in another country. Such themes for suicide prevention are detailed in Table 51.1 (Taylor et al. 1997). The WHO has carried out a survey on suicide prevention activities in Europe as of October 2003. Questionnaires were sent to 48 of the 52 Member States in 2001 in order to survey the level of activities in countries of the WHO European Region. Key persons were members of WHO European Multicentre Study, WHO national counterparts for mental health, or national representatives of the International Association for Suicide Prevention. Countries were split into two groups relating to the presence of a national suicide prevention initiative. Those with initiatives have country-wide integrated activities carried out by government bodies. Those without national initiatives carry out isolated activities in different parts of the country. The survey revealed that while most countries had official documents issued by governments or ministries, some did not. Approval of initiatives by parliaments varied. The coordination and comprehensiveness of suicide prevention activities also varied considerably between countries as described below (Wasserman et al. 2004).

**Table 51.1** Themes used in comprehensive National Prevention Strategies

| |
|---|
| Public education |
| Responsible media reporting |
| School-based programmes |
| Detection and treatment of depression and other mental disorders |
| Attention to those abusing alcohol and drugs |
| Attention to individuals suffering from somatic illness |
| Enhanced access to mental health services |
| Improvement in assessment of attempted suicide |
| Post-vention |
| Crisis intervention |
| Work and unemployment policy |
| Training of health professionals |
| Reduced access to lethal methods |

## Examples of state-led interventions in suicide prevention

### Europe

Across Europe national suicide prevention strategies have been developed by relevant governments and health departments, for example Finland, Sweden, Norway, Slovenia, Hungary, and Poland. The Finnish strategy was one of the first comprehensive approaches and provided an excellent model which undoubtedly assisted the development and implementation of subsequent national strategies (National Research and Development Centre for Welfare and Health 1993; Upanne et al. 1999). The WHO European monitoring survey on national suicide prevention programmes and strategies detected some common themes identified in the initiatives cross-nationally, such as a focus on improving access to health care services. Many also included the education of health care staff; however, not all countries had public suicide prevention activities with a focus on media portrayal and regulations to control access to means. Public education to increase awareness on suicide prevention featured in all initiatives (WHO 2002).

### England

England has used the approach of setting specific targets to be achieved in regard to suicide rates, first as part of the Health of the Nation policy, in 1992, to reduce suicides by 15 per cent over 10 years and then as part of the Our Healthier Nation policy [1999] to reduce suicide to 7.4 per 100,000 of the population (Department of Health 2004). Evidence up to this point suggests that such an approach has been successful as judged by falling rates following implementation of basic strategies, but more importantly by the attention that it puts on suicide as a preventable outcome which warrants a national approach. The strategy does, of course, receive criticism in that basing such a strategy on 'targets' to be achieved can paradoxically create a blame culture (Jenkins and Singh 2000b). Yet progress so far highlights that striking progress is being made with available data (for 3 years 2001/02/03) showing a rate of 8.6 per 100, 000 population—a reduction of 6 per cent from 1995/6/7) (Department of Health 2004).

### Scotland

An interesting example of state intervention is the Scottish National Strategy *Choose Life* which was launched in 2002. This formed part of a broader national programme to improve mental health and well-being and linked into other national policies on health and welfare (Scottish Executive 2002). The strategy has its own budget, which funds the local implementation of activities. A national implementation team supports local networks, develops and disseminates materials, best practices and information. As in other initiatives worldwide, focus has been on specific population 'priority groups' such as young people and people recently bereaved.

### Ireland

The framework described above is similar to the Northern Ireland Suicide Prevention Strategy Protect Life in which government guidance suggests links with other strategies such as those related to general health, mental health promotion, alcohol and drugs, and neighbourhood renewal. Yet again there is a focus on 'joined up' working, anti-stigma and identifying best practice (DHSSPS 2006).

### Australia and New Zealand

In Australia the Government Department of Health and Ageing produced a key document: *Living is for everyone: a framework for the prevention of suicide and self-harm in Australia* (LIFE Framework) (DHA 2000). This details the overall comprehensive state intervention for suicide prevention in Australia. The focus of this plan is to engender strategic partnerships and to embed suicide prevention action across all sectors. The National Advisory Council on Youth Suicide Prevention developed the programme initially. This was organized through consultation with key groups and recognition that suicide prevention requires a multifaceted approach involving collaboration between all levels of government and the community.

The LIFE Framework promotes six action areas for suicide prevention activity:

1 Promoting well-being, resilience and community capacity across Australia;

2 Enhancing protective factors and reducing risk factors for suicide and self-harm across the Australian Community;

3 Services and support within the community for groups at increased risk;

4 Services for individuals at high risk;

5 Partnerships with Aboriginal and Torres Strait Islander peoples;

6 Improving the evidence base for suicide prevention and good practice.

The New Zealand Suicide Prevention Strategy was launched in June 2006 and aimed to offer an all-ages approach to suicide prevention (Ministry of Health 2006). The strategy built on the work implemented by the New Zealand Youth Suicide Prevention Strategy (Ministry of Youth Affairs 1998). In a similar way to the Australian strategy a key element of the intervention is to build a multi-sectorial approach to reducing the rate of suicidal behaviour and its effects on the lives of New Zealanders.

Most important to both strategies is the involvement and targeting of the wider community groups. As in the case of the Australian government, state interventions have focused on ensuring that suicide prevention and life promotion respect the fundamental principle of self-determination and the empowerment of indigenous communities, their men and their elders, and supporting and respecting the role of the traditional healers. Principles central to aboriginal people and Torres Strait islanders were taken into consideration and working groups were established to ensure this approach. There is a need for the state to continue to be responsive to issues of social and emotional well-being, to political action including that of reconciliation, to community development and to culturally appropriate, effective and accessible mainstream services. Furthermore the adaptation of mainstream approaches (such as narrative therapy) that has proven potential with Aboriginal communities alongside traditional Aboriginal and Torres Strait Islander therapies should be encouraged (DHA 2000). Equally so, in New Zealand, recognition and responsiveness to Maori has been an important part of the overall intervention. Most important is the need to focus on issues relating to factors such as age (older people), gender (males) and the relative cultural/belief system of the Maori (Ministry of Health 2006).

### North America

In North America, there has been considerable academic and NGO focus on suicide prevention. In the US, the National Strategy for Suicide prevention was published by the US Department of Health and Human Services in 2001. Its goals were to promote awareness relating to suicide as a public health problem that is preventable. Further objectives were to develop broad support for suicide prevention, develop and implement strategies to reduce stigma associated with being a consumer of mental health, substance abuse and suicide prevention services. Suicide prevention programmes were to be developed and implemented, efforts to reduce access to lethal means and methods of self-harm were promoted and training was implemented for the recognition of at-risk behaviour and delivery of effective services, alongside the development and promotion of effective clinical and professional practices. Another important aspect was the improved access to mental health and substance abuse services, as well as community linkages with such services. Improved reporting and portrayals of suicide behaviour, mental illness and substance abuse on the entertainment and news media was emphasized and the promotion and support of research on suicide and suicide prevention. Lastly, improved and expanded surveillance systems were underlined.

### South and Central America

In South and Central America awareness about suicide is increasing and national suicide prevention programmes are in preparation.

### Asia

In Asia, only Sri Lanka has formulated a national suicide prevention plan. A Presidential Committee on Prevention of Suicide was appointed in 1997 in Sri Lanka. The recommendations were to recognize and address the mental health needs of youth and elderly, to provide mechanisms to intervene and help families and individuals with problems and to create a culture which discourages suicide. Moreover suicidal behaviour was decriminalized in 1998 and the government reduced the sale of certain toxic pesticides as stated in the prevention plan. A life skills programme was introduced into schools. The suicide rate declined, but unfortunately the committee ceased to function at the end of 2000 (Lakshmi *et al.* 2004).

In the West Pacific region, the government of China has sponsored the Beijing Suicide Research and Prevention Centre in 2002. A hotline was started and a workshop on a proposed national suicide prevention plan was hosted in 2003. The workshop brought about a consensus that the state and local governments in China should establish suicide prevention committees with the responsibility and resources to develop, implement and monitor national, regional and local suicide prevention plans.

Japan has a range of preventive efforts across the country, and the development of a national strategy has just begun. Some prefecture and regions have undertaken unique suicide prevention measures (Kimiko and Yoshiyuki 2003; Shiho *et al.* 2005).

### Iran

In the Middle East, Iran has introduced a national mental health programme, initially covering rural areas but now extended to urban areas. The front line health workers are trained in priority topics including depression, severe mental illness and suicide prevention, and are backed up by district level mental health services.

## The impact of a government setting targets

The impact of government setting targets occurs at different levels. In the first instance it influences priorities within the governmental health department or ministry in relation to time, resources and focus. There is also an impact across other government departments. However, the internal effect on governments is only one part of the process. Priorities, funding and management emphasis within the health service are affected. As a result, training, further education and clinical management amongst professionals are influenced. Finally, the attention provided by governments influences the shaping of priorities and role of voluntary bodies, charity organizations and commercial organizations in the formation of their health policies. Overall, it openly sets a framework in which the responsibility for achieving the targets does not sit with the individual alone but with all sectors of the nation (Jenkins and Singh 2000b).

## The impact of legislation

### Death certificates

Legislation has a key role within the public health agenda on suicide prevention. Of particular significance in England is the role played by the coroner. In England, 22,000 deaths each year are subject to public inquest (Tarling 1998). Suicide is one form of death that is dealt with by an inquest in a coroner's court. Some argue that unlike other inquests which may directly result in legislative change or preventative public health measures, it is more difficult to arrive at a modern day purpose for suicide inquests (Biddle 2003). Indeed, the legislative system relating to suicide and the use of the coroner is to some extent unique to England. The coroner has to conduct an independent inquiry for the Crown, which involves time-consuming procedures to gather information from psychiatrists, physicians, the police and other sources. This process impacts most notably on the family of the deceased, but it is the difficulty in reaching a verdict on cases that has implications for all parties (Biddle 2003).

In cases where the individual has written a note, the certification may be straight forward. If there is no note, and if stigma surrounding suicide and the distress to relatives is high, the coroner or other official responsible for recording deaths may not register the deaths as suicide but as 'undetermined' death/open verdict. Psychological autopsy studies have demonstrated that a large amount of such verdicts are in fact actual suicides (Jenkins and Kovess 2002). Therefore, it makes sense to use combined figures of official and undetermined deaths rather than official suicides figures alone which omit a significant proportion of actual suicides. International suicide data only reflects official suicides and therefore is a significant underestimate of actual suicides. Moreover, the extent to which the official suicide rate is an underestimate will vary between countries, and within (Jenkins and Kovess 2002).

### Medication package size

Another important example within England of the influence of legislation on suicidal behaviour is the more recent change in laws relating to pack sizes of paracetomol for 'over the counter' sale. Legislation to limit the size of packs of analgesics (paracetomol, salicylates and their compounds) sold in shops and pharmacist shops was introduced in the United Kingdom in 1998 to attempt to reduce the mortality and morbidity associated with deliberate overdoses, in particular with paracetomol (Hawton *et al.* 2004). The legislation reduced the uncontrolled sale of such medication to 32 tablets for pharmacies and 16 tablets (down from 24) in other shops/outlets (Committee on Safety of Medicines Control Agency 1997). The purpose of the legislation was to minimize the household keeping of analgesics and the associated danger of overdoses from such stocks (Hawton *et al.* 1995). A recent study has now demonstrated that suicide deaths from paracetomol and salicylates were reduced by 22 per cent in the year after the change in legislation and the fall continued in the subsequent two years (Hawton *et al.* 2004). Other countries have adopted the use of legislation to reduce medication pack size, for example this is a key part of the Australian strategy Life is for Everyone (DHA 2000). Thus, growing evidence exists to suggest that such public health interventions via the legislative system can impact on the incidence of suicidal behaviour. Sri Lanka successfully imposed restrictions on the sale of the more toxic pesticides.

### Other legislation

Further interventions may include promoting compliance with guns and firearms laws and control regulations. The New Zealand strategy has specifically referred to this requirement and this is also a key part of the Australian strategy (DHA 2000; Ministry of Health 2006).

## Researching the effectiveness of national strategy

Despite the fact that many suicide preventive interventions have been developed and implemented for quite some time, only a small amount have been formally evaluated for their effectiveness. Ultimately, governments need to include a clear evaluation programme when planning effective strategies (WHO 2004). In 1999 the Centres for Disease control in the USA established a framework for programme evaluation in public health. This framework is a synthesis of existing evaluation practices and a standard for further improvement. The WHO European Multicentre Study continues to carry out extensive monitoring research (WHO 2002).

However, the evaluation of suicide prevention has been difficult for methodological reasons as well as for lack of funding for suicidological research (Jenkins and Kovess 2002). Researchers face problems in experimental design and the issue of establishing an adequate sample size to demonstrate a reduction in the suicide rate (Jenkins and Kovess 2002). In the light of the need of more randomized controlled trails demonstrating the effectiveness of treatments, there are good arguments for taking a pragmatic view of evidence-based methods of suicide prevention (Goldney 2005).

# Conclusion

In an effort to increase life expectancies and to improve public health, governments have since long attempted to influence the way people live. These attempts involve changing people's living conditions as well as the way people choose to behave (Vallgarda 2001). This may well be an overarching aim of any public health strategy created by a government. The role of the state in a public health policy approach to suicide prevention is to respond to suicide as multifaceted phenomena with a multifaceted approach. This should preferably be built on disseminating policy through national, regional and local structures. Every government's policy on suicide should take forward both a health and public health/education approach.

It is striking that most national suicide prevention strategies are to be found in countries with higher GDP, when suicide rates are at least as high and often much higher in countries with lower GDP. This is related to the situation of mental health issues in general, where the burden is high in low and middle income countries, but has not achieved priority status for governments or donors. Frequently, other causes of mortality have achieved priority status, such as those from infectious diseases, e.g. HIV or malaria. Such priority status is not always related to mortality rates, and sometimes the respective mortalities of infectious diseases may be less than those from suicide or road traffic accidents, which have similar mortality to suicide. There is a need to support countries to develop national suicide prevention strategies as an integrated part of their health, social and economic sector reforms. Awareness raising needs to be targeted toward donors and those engaged in such national reforms if states are to be persuaded to take action.

It is worth noting that national strategies need to be sustained for long periods of time. The experience from countries with national strategies suggests that, while each individual component has an effect, the overall effect of visible national commitment from the state is of itself helpful and encouraging to those who implement the strategy. Where countries have discontinued their focus on suicide prevention, gains are quickly lost.

Even without the presence of a clear national strategy, much can still be done such as raising government awareness; financial support; technical support in development of suicide prevention strategies, establishing/promoting recommendations arising from clinical and scientific evidence; national assessments; professional training; expert exchange and consultations and management/network. All of these activities can be supported by the WHO (Wasserman *et al.* 2004).

# References

Anderson M and Jenkins R (2003). Mental health promotion and prevention. *Dynamic Psychiatry*, **36**, 231–246.

Anderson M and Jenkins R (2005). The challenge of suicide prevention: an overview of national strategies. *Disease Management and Health Outcomes*, **13**, 245–253.

Biddle L (2003). Public hazards or private tragedies? An exploratory study of the effect of coroners' procedures on those bereaved by suicide. *Social Science and Medicine*, **56**, 1033–1045.

Brainerd E (2001). Economic reform and mortality in the former Soviet Union: a study of the suicide epidemic in the 1990s. *European Economic Review*, **45**, 1007–1019.

Cantor CH and Baume PJM (1999). Suicide prevention: a public health approach. *Australian and New Zealand Journal of Mental Health Nursing*, **8**, 45–50.

Caplan G (1964). *Principles of Preventative Psychiatry*. Basic Books, New York.

Committee on Safety of Medicines Control Agency (1997). Paracetemol and aspirin. *Current Problems in Pharmacovigilance*, **23**, 9.

Department of Health (2002). *National Suicide Prevention Strategy for England*. HMSO, London.

Department of Health (2004). *National Suicide Prevention Strategy for England*. Annual Report on Progress. Department of Health, London.

DHA (2000). *Living is for Everyone: a Framework for the Prevention of Suicide and Self Harm in Australia (LIFE Framework)*. Department for Health and Ageing, Australia.

DHSSPS (2006). *Protect Life: A Shared Vision. The Northern Ireland Suicide Prevention Strategy and Action Plan 2006–2011*. Department of Health, Social Services and Public Safety, Ireland.

Diekstra RFW (1992). The prevention of suicidal behaviour: evidence for the efficacy of clinical and community based programs. *International Journal of Mental Health*, **21**, 69–87.

European Commission (2005). Green paper. Improving the mental health of the population. Towards a strategy on mental health for the European Union. European Commission, Brussels.

Goldney R (2005). Suicide prevention: a pragmatic review of recent studies. *Crisis*, **26**, 128–140.

Hawton K, Simkin S, Deeks J *et al.* (2004). UK legislation on analgesic packs: before and after study of long-term effect on poisonings. *British Medical Journal Online*. BMJ, **329**, 1076.

Hawton K, Ware C, Mistry H *et al.* (1995). Why patients choose paracetemol for self-poisoning and their knowledge of its dangers. *British Medical Journal*, **310**, 164.

Jenkins R and Kovess V (2002). Evaluation of suicide prevention: a European approach. *International Review of Psychiatry*, **14**, 34–41.

Jenkins R and Singh B (2000a). Policy and practice in suicide prevention. *British Journal of Forensic Practice*, **1**, 3–11.

Jenkins R and Singh B (2000b). General population strategies of suicide prevention. In K Hawton and K van Heeringen, eds, *The International Book of Suicide and Attempted Suicide*, pp. 597–615. John Wiley and Sons Ltd, Surrey.

Kimiko U and Yoshiyuki M (2003). National strategy for suicide prevention in Japan. *Lancet*, **361**, 882.

Lakshmi V, Nagaraj K, Sujit J (2004). *Suicide and Suicide Prevention in Developing Countries, Disease Control Prevention Project, Working paper no 27 June*. World Health Organization, Geneva.

Ministry of Health (2006) *The New Zealand Suicide Prevention Strategy 2006–2016*. Ministry of Health, Wellington.

Ministry of Youth Affairs (1998) The *New Zealand Youth Suicide Prevention Strategy*. Ministry of Youth Affairs, Wellington.

NASP (The Swedish National and Stockholm County Council's Centre for Suicide Research and Prevention of Mental Ill-Health at the Karolinska Institute) (2006). *Information Booklet*. NASP, Stockholm.

National Research and Development Centre for Welfare and Health, Finland (1993). *Suicide Can be prevented: Fundamentals of Target and Action Strategy*. NRDCWH, Helsinki, Finland.

Scottish Executive (2002). *Choose Life: A National Action Plan to Prevention Suicide in Scotland*. Scottish Executive, Scotland.

Shiho Y, Tohru T, Shuji A *et al.* (2005). Suicide in Japan: present conditions and prevention measures *Crisis*, **26**, 12 -19.

Singh B and Jenkins R (2000). Suicide prevention strategies—an international perspective. *International Review of Psychiatry* **12**, 7–14.

Tarling R (1998). *Coroner service survey*. The Research and Statistics Directorate, Home Office Research Studies, London.

Taylor SJ, Kingdon D, Jenkins R (1997). How are nations trying to prevent suicide? An analysis of national suicide prevention strategies. *Acta Psychiatrica Scandinavica*, **95**, 457–463.

United Nations (1996). *Prevention of Suicide—Guidelines for the Formation and Implementation of National Strategies*. United Nations, New York.

Upanne M, Hakanen J, Rautava M (1999). *Can Suicide be Prevented? The Suicide Prevention Project in Finland 1992–1996: Goals, Implementation and Evaluation*. National Research and Development Centre for Welfare and Health, Finland.

Vallgarda S (2001). Governing people's lives. Strategies for improving the health of the nations in England, Denmark, Norway and Sweden. *European Journal of Public Health*, **11**, 386–392.

Wasserman D (2001). *Suicide—An Unnecessary Death*. Martin Dunitz, London.

Wasserman D, Mittendorfer-Rutz E, Rutz W *et al.* (2004). *Suicide Prevention in Europe: The WHO European Monitoring Survey on National Suicide Prevention Programmes and Strategies*. NASP, Stockholm.

WHO (1990). *Consultation on Strategies for Reducing Suicidal Behaviours in the European Region. Summary Report*. World Health Organization, Geneva.

WHO (2002). *Suicide Prevention in Europe. The World European Monitoring Survey on National Suicide Prevention Programmes and Strategies*. World Health Organization, Copenhagen.

WHO Regional Office for Europe (1985). *Targets for All. Targets in Support of the European Regional Strategy for Health for All*. European Health for All Series, No. 1, World Health Organization, Copenhagen.

WHO Regional Office for Europe's Health Evidence Network (2004). *For Which Strategies of Suicide Prevention is there Evidence of Effectiveness?* World Health Organization, Denmark.

# CHAPTER 52

# Strategies in suicide prevention

Danuta Wasserman and Tony Durkee

## Abstract

Strategies in suicide prevention have developed throughout the years, and progressed into conceptual models that are defined by a set of restrictive definitions. In this chapter, classifications of two suicide preventive strategic models, namely the Primary/Secondary/Tertiary (PST) and Universal/Selective/Indicated (USI) are described, as well as a pragmatic suggestion for health care and public health-oriented strategies in suicide prevention. Health care-oriented strategies use the individual-centred approach with the focus on the treatment of patients. Public health strategies in prevention of suicide are directed toward groups and whole populations.

## Introduction

Preventive strategies age back decades and continue to develop and expand across a wide spectrum of disease and illness. Mental disorders, with suicide in particular, have increasingly gained special interest among the scientific community, essentially for the fact that aspects behind suicide entail many mental disorders, and prevention of those mental disorders would lead, in itself, to the prevention of suicide (Bertolote 2004).

Strategic preventive models are designed to target short- and long-term initiatives on either individual or population levels. The traditional preventive continuum often consists of targeting the early onset of a particular disease or disorder, treating those who currently endure the disease or disorder, and following up with those who have received intervention or treatment. Suicide preventive strategies too work along this prevention continuum by addressing the onset, treatment and follow-up aspects of suicide risks.

There are several conceptual models for suicide prevention as referenced in Silverman's commentary: 'Gordon's Universal/Selective/Indicated; Haddon's Injury Control Model (Pre-injury, Injury, Post-Injury); the classical triad of Primary/Secondary/Tertiary; and the alternative of Prevention/Intervention/Postvention' (Silverman 2004, p. 153).

## The primary/secondary/tertiary prevention model

Traditionally, in suicide preventive strategies, the primary/secondary/tertiary (PST) prevention model is, and has been, often employed as fundamental principles in the development of suicide preventive strategies. The primary/secondary/tertiary classification scheme has been noted to be attractive and simple in its design to effectively target risk factors associated with suicide in the short- and long-term goals. The strategic initiatives for this model are as follows.

### Primary prevention

Along the prevention continuum, the primary prevention addresses prophylaxis of the onset of the disease (Dwight et al. 2005).

Reducing the incidence of suicidal behaviours, by eliminating or reducing risk factors and strengthening the protective factors, is the goal of primary prevention, which falls outside the health care sector, involving for example, media, legislators, etc. However, mental health professionals should be actively involved in this type of prevention, as their profound knowledge of suicidal persons' mind and their social networks functioning is, at the moment, underestimated in this kind of preventive activity, which would gain a lot in effectiveness and precision. Good examples of the involvement of mental health professionals are: European Alliance Against Depression (EAAD) activities, as described by Hegerl and colleagues in Chapter 66 of this book, and Suicide awareness and mental health among youth in the community; Exposing dark secrets: what must be told by Hoven et al. in Chapter 67 of this book.

The primary prevention sets the foundation by increasing awareness of suicide and suicide risks before suicidal behaviour occurs. De Leo and Meneghel (2001) describe the primary prevention as approaching subjects (in this case the elderly) who currently do *not* feel suicidal, and decrease such risks that would later inflict suicidal feelings and ideations among this group. Of course, in order to decrease latter suicidal risks, one would have to identify target populations. Examples of interventions utilized in the primary prevention model for suicide are:

◆ *Suicide awareness* interventions are directed towards the whole population, or specific arenas (e.g. schools, workplaces, etc.) or group education, in order to diminish stigma and taboo surrounding suicide and mental disorders. Suicide awareness interventions are usually found in school-based programmes. Educating teens about mental health promotion is as a fundamental intervention strategy. The goal is of course to teach young people the signs of suicide behaviour, identifying peers at risk and how to take action (Beautrais 2006).

- *Skills training* with specific focus on improving problem-solving skills, coping skills, increased self-esteem and self-efficacy all of which can be established in school-based programmes.

- *Restriction of lethal methods:* limiting access to methods and means of suicide can be implemented in a universal or primary prevention scheme (Beautrais 2006). The strategy involves limiting or restricting access to methods that increase suicide, e.g. guns, pesticides, etc.

Other examples of primary prevention strategies are to involve media in responsible reporting of suicides, and supporting occupational groups with a high risk for suicide, such as doctors, farmers, pharmacists, and policemen.

## Secondary prevention

The next stage along the prevention continuum is referred to as secondary prevention. The ultimate goal of secondary prevention is reducing the prevalence of already existing mental disorders by treatment and early detection of unknown cases and their appropriate treatment (Dwight *et al.* 2005). The secondary preventive strategy addresses individuals at risk for self-harm, and those identified with a mental disorder, by providing early treatment that can be broadly accessible (Andersson and Jenkins 2006).

This type of prevention focuses also on reducing or eliminating suicidal risks factors by intervening and treatment (De Leo and Meneghel 2001). In other words, the secondary preventive strategy is intended to implement treatment to persons who are actively considering or even attempted suicide. Examples of interventions for this strategy are as follows:

- *Screening techniques* are vital strategies in identifying 'at-risk' individuals for suicidal behaviour in general populations; although at present, most research is conducted among adolescents. Screening for vulnerable adolescents by disseminating a questionnaire, which focuses on depression, suicidal ideation and previous suicide attempts is useful in identifying risk severity for suicidal behaviour (Gould *et al.* 2005).

- *Gatekeeper training* is an intervention strategy that may focus on schools, the community or be health care-related. The purpose is to train school staff and health care professionals in recognizing people at risk and referring them to appropriate professional treatment (Beautrais 2006).

## Tertiary prevention

The final strategy on the prevention continuum is tertiary prevention. The goal of tertiary prevention is to reduce the incidence of relapses through rehabilitation, after having experienced suffering from a disease or disorder, to prevent supplementary deterioration (Dwight *et al.* 2005).

In the ideal of suicide prevention, the tertiary approach attempts to reduce the consequences of individuals that surpassed at-risk status, after having previously been suffering from suicide ideation and attempts (Andersson and Jenkins 2006). De Leo and Meneghel (2001) describe this tactic as also a way to manage those who have already been inflicted and suffered a loss by a relative or loved one who committed suicide.

Tertiary suicide prevention requires multidisciplinary services according to the principles of the modern psychiatry with easy access, continuity of care and rehabilitation and inclusion of the family in the process. Reintegration into society, supply of housing, educational possibilities, prevocational and vocational training and work are the most important components. In some countries, legislation allows tailoring of comprehensive rehabilitation programmes.

## The Universal/Selective/Indicated prevention model

The primary/secondary/tertiary prevention strategy has proven effective in outlining and the formation of suicide preventive strategies. Below, a prevention model used in public health called universal/selective/indicated is presented.

The universal/selective/indicated classification scheme in forming suicide preventive strategies was proposed in a 1994 report (Mrazek and Haggerty 1994) by the Institute of Medicine (IOM) in Washington D.C. The definitions are based upon a classification proposed by Gordon (1983) a decade earlier, and are related to health behaviour and health risks in target populations. According to this conceptual model, all three strategies are aimed at target populations.

Universal prevention is aimed at general populations, selective prevention is aimed at populations who have an above average risk to develop diseases, and indicated prevention is directed at persons who have already experienced symptoms.

The strategic initiatives for this model are as follows.

## Universal strategies

The universal strategy method is beneficial for everyone in a population (Yip 2005). In a report by Kimokeo (2006), the author describes universal prevention as being directed towards entire populations (not individuals), and is principally aimed at decreasing risk factors for suicidal behaviour and increasing protective factors for suicidal behaviour (Greenberg *et al.* 2001). Activities target entire communities and programmes reach asymptomatic individuals at low risk.

Bertolote (2004) explains that an example of universal strategies for prevention of suicide could entail the limitation of access to toxic substances, which are used as means of suicide. This strategy also entails measures like different welfare, social, educational and working policies and improved health care availability, for example, different community-based programmes giving social support, or educational programmes teaching substance use dangers (Yip 2005).

## Selected strategies

The selected strategy is targeted at subgroups with increased risk of suicide, which could be based on age, gender, occupation or family history. Kimokeo (2006) states that the selected prevention scheme is targeted particularly at subgroups with signs of elevated biological or social risk factors for suicide or suicidal behaviour, although currently they may be clinically asymptomatic (Burns and Patton 2000). The group-level characteristics place them considerably higher than the average risk for suicide (Dwight *et al.* 2005), e.g. isolation, antisocial behaviour, negative life events, etc. (Burns and Patton 2000; Bertolote 2004).

Examples of an intervention for the selected scheme could be treatment of people with mental disorders and substance use disorders, psychological support to persons in crisis situations or with physical disabilities (Bertolote 2004). Intervention programmes for children with clinically depressed parents, or victims of physical or sexual abuse (Yip 2005) or an event-centred intervention focused on adverse life events (Burns and Patton 2000), or interventions focused on groups who are victims of war, violence and the bereaved are other examples.

### Indicated strategies

Indicated strategies are aimed at persons who display significant signs of a disorder or condition, which is known as a high risk for future development of an illness (Burns and Patton 2000; Katschnig and Schrank 2003; Yip 2005; Dwight *et al.* 2005; Kimokeo 2006). For instance, an intervention in the indicated scheme is treatment and close follow-up of people with depression, bipolar disorders, recurrent psychotic episodes and intensive psychosocial follow-up of suicide attempters (Bertolote 2004; Yip 2005).

Other examples are programmes for parents of children with high levels of aggression and behavioural disturbances.

## Similarities between Primary/Secondary/Tertiary (PST) and Universal/Selective/Indicated (USI) prevention models

There are substantial similarities and dissimilarities between the two conceptual models of PST and USI prevention.

Katschnig and Schrank (2003) suggests that the PST scheme has a temporal perspective, i.e. there are specific stages before and during the progression of the disease, whereas a USI scheme has both a temporal perspective and target populations perspective, in which the universal and selective strategies aim at those who are not ill yet (first in the general population, and second in subgroups with risk factors and exposure to risk situations); and indicated prevention intended for persons who currently display symptoms of a disorder, e.g. depression, substance abuse, etc. (Burns and Patton 2000; Katschnig and Schrank 2003; Dwight *et al.* 2005; Yip 2005; Kimokeo 2006).

In a closer analysis of PST, the primary prevention is compared to a prevention in the traditional sense, whereas secondary and tertiary prevention is equated with treatment and rehabilitation, accordingly (Katschnig and Schrank 2003). In the USI model, the universal prevention addresses prevention in the general population, similar to primary prevention in the PST model. Selective prevention addresses groups at risk, which is similar to secondary prevention and, to some extent, to primary prevention; the indicated prevention aims at those who individually have been identified as having a disorder, comparable to secondary prevention in the PST scheme (Katschnig and Schrank 2003).

The primary prevention can be universal or in cases when occupational groups with high risk for suicide are targeted, selective. The secondary prevention corresponds to both selective and indicated prevention (in which case the latter aims at persons known for having symptoms of mental disorders or suicidal behaviours). Tertiary prevention strives to avoid relapses, which are often seen among mentally ill and suicidal persons, and has no distinct place in the USI model (Katschnig and Schrank 2003). The tertiary suicide preventive strategies are essential when suicide prevention is concerned, as studies show that rehabilitation of suicide attempters diminishes relapses of suicidal behaviour, i.e., repetition of attempted suicide or completed suicide (Hawton *et al.* 1998; Fleishmann *et al.* 2008).

Both conceptual models are used in practical and preventive work. An American study was conducted to evaluate the effectiveness of a public health approach suicide prevention among American Indian tribal nations over a 15-year span. The universal/selected/indicated conceptual model was utilized. The results concluded that during the 15-year period, suicide gestures and attempts dropped dramatically (May *et al.* 2005).

In a systematic meta-analysis on suicide prevention by Mann *et al.* (2005), it was found that the primary and secondary suicide preventive measures according to the PST model, including treatment intervention strategies such as medication, education for physicians and restricting access to lethal means, were successful in lowering suicide rates.

## Practical suggestions for strategies in suicide prevention

The previous sections described classifications of two conceptual models used in suicide prevention. This section will focus on the assorted types of interventions that are implemented within those conceptual models.

Preventive intervention strategies can be applied according to (i) the health care approach, and (ii) the public health approach (Wasserman 2001).

1 The health care approach aims to improve;

   ◆ health care services;

   ◆ early diagnosis of psychiatric disorders like depression, psychoses, substance abuse;

   ◆ identification of psychosocial stress factors and suicidal behaviours;

   ◆ attitudes among health care staff towards persons with mental disorders, suicide behaviours;

   ◆ treatment;

   ◆ follow-up and rehabilitation for suicide attempters and persons with mental disorders.

   Target groups include patients, relatives, health care professionals as well as different health care settings and arenas.

2 The public health approach promotes legislation and policies concerning:

   ◆ social welfare;

   ◆ mental health;

   ◆ education;

   ◆ substance use;

   ◆ violence and child abuse, etc.

   The target group is the population in general or in specific arenas as schools, workplaces, military, housing, etc.

The objectives are to promote strong environmental protective factors, increase awareness through public education, improve societal attitudes and diminish stigma towards suicide and mental illness, diminish access to means of suicide and influence media policy to promote responsible reporting, which decreases the probability of contagion or cluster suicides.

For the sake of simplicity, evidence-based suicide preventive measures presented in the following chapters of this book are classified as having a health care or public health perspective.

# Conclusion

Strategies for suicide prevention are crucial in the struggle to reduce suicidal behaviours. As discussed in this chapter, conceptual models and intervention strategies have come a long way since their development, however, further research, evaluation and creativity is still needed in the arena of suicide prevention. As stated by Bertolote (2004), if a universal prevention programme existed, it would already have been adopted by everyone. Moreover, research of effective suicide prevention, a seemingly obvious task, has been until now heavily neglected and under-resourced area around the world, which calls for attention.

## References

Andersson M and Jenkins R (2006). The national suicide prevention strategy for England: the reality of a national strategy for the nursing profession. *Journal of Psychiatric and Mental Health Nursing*, **13**, 641–650.

Beautrais A (2006). Suicide prevention strategies 2006. Editorial. *Australian e-Journal for the Advancement of Mental Health*, **5**, http://www.auseinet.com/journal/vol5iss1/beautraiseditorial.pdf.

Bertolote JM (2004). Suicide prevention: at what level does it work? *World Psychiatry*, **3**, 147–151.

Burns JM and Patton GC (2000). Preventive interventions for youth suicide: a risk factor-based approach. *Australian and New Zealand Journal of Psychiatry*, **34**, 388–407. Cited in D Kimokeo (2006). *Research-Based Guidelines and practices for school based suicide*. Teachers College, Columbia University.

De Leo D and Meneghel G (2001). The elderly and suicide. In D Wasserman, ed., *Suicide—An Unnecessary Death*, pp. 195–207. Martin Dunitz, London.

Dwight EL, Foa EB, Gur RE *et al.* (eds) (2005). Prevention of Shcizophrenia. In Dwight EL, Foa EB, Gur RE, eds, *Treating and Preventing Adolescent*

*Mental Health Disorders. What We Know and What We Don't Know. A Research Agenda for Improving the Mental Health of our Youth*, pp. 130–134. Oxford University Press, USA.

Fleischmann A, Bertolote JM, Wasserman D *et al.* (2008). Effectiveness of brief intervention and contact for suicide attempters: a randomized controlled trial in five countries. *Bulletin of the World Health Organization*, **9**, 703–709. Accessed at: http://www.who.int/bulletin/volumes/86/07–046995.pdf

Gordon R (1983). An operational classification of disease prevention. *Public Health Reports*, **98**, 107–109.

Gould MS, Marrocco FA, Kleinman M *et al.* (2005). Evaluating iatrogenic risk of youth suicide screening programs: a randomized controlled trial. *JAMA*, **293**, 1635–1643.

Greenberg MT, Domitrovich C, Bumbarger B (2001). The prevention of mental disorders in school-aged children: Current state of the field. *Prevention &Treatment*, **4**(1). Cited in D Kimokeo (2006). *Research-Based Guidelines and practices for school based suicide*. Teachers College, Columbia University, New York.

Hawton K, Arensman E, Townsend E *et al.* (1998). Deliberate self harm: systematic review of efficacy of psychosocial and pharmacological treatments in preventing repetition. *BMJ*, **317**, 441–447.

Katschnig H and Schrank B (2003). Theme 3: needed supportive infrastructure for mental health promotion and prevention of common mental disorders. University of Vienna, Austria. In I Azueta, U Katila-Nurkka, Ville Lehtinen, eds, *Mental Health in Europe. New Challenges, New Opportunities*, pp. 83–110. Report from a European Conference 9–11 October. Bilbao, Spain.

Kimokeo D (2006). *Research-Based Guidelines and Practices for School-based Suicide*. Teachers College, Columbia University, New York.

Mann JJ, Apter A, Bertolote J *et al.* (2005). Suicide prevention strategies: a systematic review. *Journal of the American Medical Association*, **294**, 2064–2074.

May PA, Serna P, Hurt L *et al.* (2005). Outcome evaluation of a public health approach to suicide prevention in an American Indian tribal nation: 1988–2002. *American Journal of Public Health*, **95**, 1238–1244.

Mrazek PJ and Haggerty RJ (1994). *Reducing Risks from Mental Disorders: Frontiers for Preventive Intervention Research*. National Academy Press, Washington.

Silverman MM (2004). Preventing suicide: a call to action. Commentary. *World Psychiatry*, **3**, 152.

Wasserman D (2001). Strategy in suicide prevention. In D Wasserman, ed., *Suicide—An Unnecessary Death*, pp. 211–224. Martin Dunitz, London.

Yip PSF (2005). A public health approach to suicide prevention. *Hong Kong Journal of Psychiatry*, **15**, 29–31.

# Health Care Strategies

# PART 9A

# Health Care Strategies: Treatment of Suicidal Adults

# CHAPTER 53

# Countertransference in the treatment of suicidal patients

Mark J Goldblatt and John T Maltsberger

## Abstract

Countertransference is an inescapable component of all psychotherapy. Intense countertransference reactions often occur during the treatment of suicidal patients. Lack of awareness of countertransference reactions of malice and aversion may be suicide-inviting. On the other hand, awareness of these reactions may enhance the treatment by alerting therapists that the suicidal patient is fomenting issues he is unable or unwilling to articulate. Problems that arise in the course of psychotherapy of suicidal patients may be understood in relation to the therapist's countertransference reactions. In this chapter, we review case examples of countertransference manifestations and their effects on the treatment of the suicidal patient.

## Introduction

### 'What is countertransference?'

As originally conceived by Freud (1910), countertransference was an impediment to the analyst's optimal functioning, a difficulty arising from the patient's influence on the therapist's unconscious feelings. Paula Heimann elaborated the term, making it embrace 'all the thoughts and feelings that an analyst experiences towards his patient' (1950, p. 81). More modern usage of the term (Slakter 1987, p. 3) includes 'all those reactions of the analyst to the patient that may help or hinder treatment'. We now understand countertransference to be an inescapable component of all psychotherapy that can provide valuable information about patients (Gabbard 1995). Furthermore, countertransference enactments are increasingly recognized for the information they reveal about the therapist–patient dyad (Gabbard 2001). Although there is a small but significant literature dealing with the difficulties associated with countertransference problems, very little has been published about the use of the countertransference to facilitate treatment of the suicidal patient. Countertransference reactions arising in the treatment of suicidal patients are likely to be extremely intense. Lack of awareness of countertransference reactions of malice and aversion may provoke suicides in vulnerable individuals (Maltsberger and Buie 1973). On the other hand, countertransference reactions may enhance therapy by alerting therapists that the suicidal patient is fomenting issues he is unable or unwilling to

articulate. In this chapter, we review case examples of countertransference manifestations and their effects on the treatment of the suicidal patient, and discuss the ways countertransference can impede as well as help the treatment of suicidal patients.

A recent study of the psychotherapy of patients who had died by suicide while in treatment identified six recurrent problem areas. These were:

1 Poor communication with others in the treatment team;

2 Allowing patients or their relatives to control the treatment;

3 Avoidance of issues related to sexuality;

4 Ineffective or coercive actions resulting from the therapist's anxiety;

5 Not recognizing the meaning of the patient's communication; and

6 Inadequately treating symptoms (Hendin *et al.* 2006).

Although these problem areas are complex and probably determined by multiple factors, they may all be understood in relation to the therapist's countertransference reactions.

## Shame contributing to impaired clinical communication and consultation avoidance

### Clinical example 1

Susan began therapy with an experienced clinician in order to get help leaving an abusive boyfriend. She was 28 years old when she began treatment and revealed that she had struggled with depressive symptoms throughout most of her life. At that time, she denied significant suicidal ideation or self-harming behaviour. Dr A referred Susan to Dr B, a skilled psychopharmacologist whom she had known and respected for a long time. With the help of this treatment team providing psychotherapy and medication, Susan was able to regain a euthymic state. She left the destructive relationship and returned to her parents' home. However, after some initial relief, she sank into a state of self-loathing depression. Several years into the treatment Susan revealed to Dr A that she had begun cutting and burning herself in an increasing cycle of self-destructiveness. Dr A recommended that Susan reveal to Dr B the extent of her self-harming behaviour. There was no formal acknowledgement between the two clinicians of the importance of this information, however, nor of the secrecy in which Susan was cloaking her symptoms.

Both Dr A and Dr B were disturbed to see Susan become more regressed and dysfunctional. Medications and psychotherapy were only marginally helpful in stemming the tide of this downward spiral. Over time, Susan's depression worsened and her suicidal thoughts increased. Dr A and Dr B each separately questioned their own approaches and suspected that the other colleague was secretly critical. They refrained from discussing the case in depth, other than to check in with each other about vacation absences, and note Susan's difficulty with separation. Susan was eventually hospitalized during a severe episode of suicidal distress associated with Dr A's summer vacation. This prompted a re-evaluation of the treatment plan. Dr A was able to seek consultation with a therapists' suicide support group. As she prepared to present her case to her colleagues, she consulted with Dr B, who was then able to reveal his own misgivings about the patient's regression. It became clear to both that each had felt responsible for not recognizing the emergent diagnosis of borderline personality disorder. (The initial working diagnoses had been post-traumatic stress disorder and major depression.) Both clinicians feared exposure and blame for inadequately diagnosing the problem. They respected each other and feared the embarrassment of revealing their own incompetence: this had led to mutual avoidance of sufficient discussions about this case, as well as avoidance of outside consultation.

A treatment consultation at the time of the crisis led to the recommendation that the therapy with Dr A should be interrupted, and that Susan should be referred for dialectical behaviour therapy. However, both Dr A and Dr B felt that the rift in their communication had been sufficiently repaired for them to continue together, more open than before. The mutual shame about 'missing' the patient's true diagnosis of borderline personality disorder was articulated and discussed, as was the tendency to hide from their unbearable feelings. This mirrored Susan's style of dealing with her trauma at the hands of the abusive boyfriend. As a result of this communication, each clinician felt they could continue in their treatment roles, despite the consultation recommendations to the contrary. The patient was firmly allied with both members of the treatment team and would certainly have perceived a termination with Dr A as a serious abandonment, perhaps an intolerable one. Four years later, Susan remains in treatment with Drs A and B. She is no longer suicidal, and her self-destructive attacks have diminished, only appearing at times of severe interpersonal stress. The communication between the clinicians has remained open with regular telephone calls and email communication.

---

The therapist's inability to control the thoughts and actions of suicidal patients often reactivates his own primitive abandonment anxiety, stirring up countertransference reactions of rage and shame. Automatic self-preserving ego defence responses for repressing these powerful emotions often lead to therapists' isolation, withdrawal and denial. This passive countertransference reaction is linked to and mirrors the patient's transference experience of helplessness, shame and rage. An anti-therapeutic cycle of unconscious rage and shame leading to increasing passivity and silence in the therapist may then emerge. The suicidal patient experiences this as an abandonment and responds with increasing levels of panic. The patient then escalates his self-destructive behaviour

in order to mobilize a desperately needed sustaining object. The result, however, is increased countertransference feelings of anxiety, which further fuel the regressive cycle of helplessness, rage and hostility.

Problems in communication arise from various sources. In busy hospital and outpatient practices, overworked clinicians are often taxed to find time for clinical discussion with colleagues. Despite good intentions, sometimes even the most problematic cases may receive only minimal attention by the treatment team. Fears of criticism and exposure contribute to conscious and unconscious feelings of shame and lead to withdrawal and avoidance. Reactivation of primitive abandonment anxieties compounds this isolation. As a result, problems in communication are more likely to result from countertransference defence mechanisms than logistical challenges.

## Surrendering control of the therapy

### Clinical example 2

Jonathan, a 20-year-old college student, was seen at the student infirmary three times over the course of two weeks. His roommates had brought him in when they noticed he was perched on the windowsill outside their eighth floor apartment. On each occasion, Jonathan was assessed as being depressed with suicidal ideation, but each time he denied that he had meant to kill himself. The emergency room doctor had sent him home with a prescription for antidepressant medication. Because he was a handsome and intelligent young man and seemingly successful at the university, the consulting psychiatrist was reluctant to force a psychiatric admission that Jonathan was sure he did not need. Projecting onto Jonathan his own fears of having been depressed and confused when he himself had been a student, the psychiatrist wrongly decided Jonathan was not in great distress (which the young man claimed), in spite of the history of repeated dangerous recent behaviour. Allowed to leave the clinic, Jonathan immediately attempted to get up into a high tower with a plan to jump.

Finally, Jonathan's father came in from out of town and brought Jonathan to another psychiatrist for evaluation. This consultant, Dr C, diagnosed a major depressive episode with intense suicidal urges and advised inpatient admission. Jonathan once again refused, saying that he was only having occasional thoughts of death and he was not in danger at this point. Dr C also identified with Jonathan's distress, but reacted to his assessment of imminent danger. He insisted that Jonathan's father drive him immediately to hospital for an admission, which he hurriedly arranged. Dr C's action arose partly from his identification with the young patient and his memory of his own need to be taken care of as an adolescent in distress. He was unambivalent about the need for hospitalization, and acted in the patient's best interest, despite Jonathan's protestations to the contrary. After a short admission, which stabilized the depression, Jonathan was discharged to begin outpatient psychotherapy with Dr C. He continued in a productive long-term treatment that succeeded in resolving his needs to reject help and blame himself for all problems.

---

Suicidal patients often seek to dictate the terms of their treatment. When countertransference feelings of rage at excessive demands are unconsciously repressed through reaction formation, therapists can become excessively passive and unassertive. Reaction formation implies inhibited action; typically what gets warded off is some impulse to attack or punish the uncooperative patient. In the process of unconsciously turning the impulse to punitive action into passive (sometimes masochistic) surrender, many therapists will unwittingly inhibit therapeutically important activities such as limit setting. Limit setting is not intrinsically sadistic or punitive, but it may seem to be. The therapist who is unaware that the patient's efforts to take over control of the treatment make him angry may have difficulty in setting appropriate limits and acting in the best interests of the patient and the therapy. Such a therapist may find himself in the untenable position of going along with patients' demands for extraordinary concessions. To him, it may appear that the concessions are needed, because frustrating the patient would stir up narcissistic rage and invite suicide. Little does he appreciate that unconsciously the narcissistic rage is his own (coming from having the treatment hijacked), and that the fear of suicide really disguises his own wishes to get rid of a troublesome patient. Unaware that he fears his impulses to punish a dangerous patient, the therapist indulges the patient's increasingly regressive demands. Such coercion usually escalates into what has been termed 'therapeutic bondage' in which the therapist feels responsible for keeping the patient alive (Hendin 1981).

Such transference–countertransference interactions invariably lead to unworkable therapeutic entanglements, fraught with tricky potential for a lethal outcome. Appropriate assertion by the therapist is not sadistic, and is often an essential piece in the prudent management of suicidal patients.

## Avoidance of sexual issues

### Clinical example 3
Lee, a 19-year-old male, had been fantasizing about being a woman for most of his life. He consulted a psychiatrist, Dr D, in high school and was treated for depression with medication and psychotherapy. Dr D suggested that treatment focus of on overcoming depression and then becoming integrated into the community. In therapy, Lee discussed his homosexual longings, but avoided questions about gender identity. After two years of treatment Lee went to college in a town several hours away and had to terminate with Dr D. Soon after the start of classes, Lee's depression worsened into a suicidal crisis. Lee felt abandoned without Dr D and returned home, where he was found to be psychotic and in need of hospitalization.

With the resumption of therapy with Dr D, Lee confided that since he was a young boy he had fantasized about having a vagina instead of a penis. The issue of Lee's gender identity confusion was, thereby, brought directly into the treatment. Dr D realized after just a few sessions that his own castration fears had been aroused by Lee's unspoken wish for transsexual surgery. These countertransference fears had led Dr D to take up treatment of the depressive aspects in Lee's life, with a focus on integration into the community. Although this would have been a useful goal in the treatment of most adolescent depressions, in this case, it avoided Lee's central concern—gender identity—and was contributing to his suicidality.

Issues relating to patients' sexual lives are often problematic for therapists. Recognizing erotic transferences and homosexual longings may be difficult for therapists who are anxious about such concerns. In therapies with non-suicidal patients, the neglect of such topics may prove frustrating and lead to an impasse. With the suicidal patient, such avoidances may lead to lethal actions. Patients are inclined to understand the therapist's silence on sexual matters as tacit condemnation and ridicule. Patients struggling with feelings of shame and confusion related to their own sexual identity need to have such matters clarified. When the countertransference reaction to the erotic transference is to shut down in fear of arousing unmanageable closeness, patients can be left abandoned and hurt. In the case of suicidal patients, this abandonment may prove lethal.

## Coercive actions driven by the therapist's anxiety

### Clinical example 4
Margaret was a 28-year-old woman who began therapy with a new clinician after several years in treatment with other therapists. Work with a cognitive behavioural therapist and then later with a psychodynamic therapist had done little to ameliorate her suicidal depression. When she began with a new psychiatrist, Dr E, Margaret disclosed she was chronically suicidal. She told Dr E that what she feared most was not death, but that the therapist would try to take control of her life by forcing hospitalization. Dr E knew a control struggle with this treatment-refractory patient would be highly problematic, but she also feared the medico-legal consequences that might ensue if she failed to hospitalize a suicidal patient. In response, Dr E acknowledged Margaret's need for autonomy, but added that if she thought Margaret needed to be hospitalized, she might insist on it, despite the patient's expressed desire to the contrary. On hearing this, Margaret felt enraged and abandoned. She realized that she could not trust Dr E, and swore to herself that she would hide her innermost thoughts from Dr E. She regretted ever having raised the hope within herself of getting help for her chronic distress. As her feelings of loneliness increased in the therapy, Margaret's symptoms worsened, marked by escalating rage at family, friends, and pets. The therapy became a control struggle in which Margaret denied her hopelessness and concealed her suicidal plans. Eventually she hanged herself, leaving a note that attested to her rage and the betrayal she experienced at Dr E's threat to force hospitalization upon her, even though at the time, such a possibility seemed extremely remote.

Treating suicidal patients elicits almost unbearable anxiety in many therapists. Feeling responsible for someone else's life, with no real ability to control the patient, leaves many a novice clinician scared and tentative. When faced with the almost unbearable anxiety of the suicidal patient, the inexperienced clinician may feel prompted to try and take control of the patient's life. This is often seen in the escalating prescription of sedating medications, reframing mindsets, no-suicide contracts, and statements such as Dr E's, which could be construed as an effort on her part to assure herself that Margaret could not, in the long run, make her helpless.

Learning how to manage this unbearable reaction is the task of the trainee therapist, and takes many years for most clinicians. For that reason, good training programmes should provide supervision for novice therapists, so that they may learn how to interpret their own reactions, and how to appropriately assess the real level of suicidal danger that they are confronted with (See Chapter 68 by David Titelman). Unfortunately, many training programmes neglect this aspect of training, and new therapists may find themselves inadequately supported as they deal with life-threatening interactions. For more experienced clinicians, supervision and peer support groups may help in dealing with reactions to the suicidal patient.

## Not recognizing the meaning of patients' communications

When the therapist is preoccupied with his own fears of the patient's aggressiveness, he may well miss the usual signs that one picks up in the course of the therapeutic session. Frightened therapists unconsciously wish to minimize the implications of patients' communications, and tend to deny ominous signals, in the service of warding off countertransference helplessness (Maltsberger and Buie 1973; Wolk-Wasserman 1987).

Countertransference hate leads to aversive withdrawal that leaves the therapist without his usual sense of empathic attunement. Without that sense of relatedness, patients often feel a sense of abandonment, which may be suicide-inviting.

Psychotic patients endow special meaning to their communications that they expect the therapist and others to easily understand. Confusion and related anger in the countertransference may worsen the connection between therapist and patient, and strain the helpful connection that can sustain suicidal patients over long periods of time.

## Boundary crossings

Establishing a therapeutic alliance allows the therapist and patient to work together to increase the patient's safety and overcome depressive or conflictual issues that may be suicide-inviting. However, it is often very difficult to establish and maintain a therapeutic alliance with a patient who is in the throes of a suicidal crisis. Negative transference assumptions may hinder cooperation and promote distancing and suspicion. When the therapist is able to convey to the patient that he really is a safe, caring person, the treatment is more likely to proceed successfully and be suicide-preventing. Most of this therapeutic work is achieved through interventions such as clarification and interpretation, which help the patient become aware of his conscious and unconscious experience. However, suicidal patients more often need additional supportive measures. Sometimes these additional measures include actions on the part of the therapist: actions that are necessary therapeutic interventions in order to maintain the alliance and facilitate the treatment.

There is often a need for special accommodations in the treatment of suicidal patients. For example, they may need to be seen at inconvenient times, or they may need between-session phone calls or reduced fees. To ignore these communications, or refuse such accommodations, communicates to the sensitive and easily hurt suicidal patient a message of hostility and abandonment. Similarly, an interpretation of the patient's underlying aggression is likely to be experienced as an unwarranted assault. Such rejections may play a crucial role in precipitating a suicidal crisis. On the other hand, by making these essential accommodations, the therapist is extending himself, often without compensation. The issue of accommodating to the suicidal patient is further complicated by the defence mechanisms such as reaction formation, which may induce the therapist to provide more and more to the regressively functioning patient. Burdened with guilt at his rage at the suicidal patient, the therapist tries harder to provide more for the suicidal patient out of fear that the patient will kill himself. As in the case of coercive bondage, such treatment is untenable.

Actions involving the therapist and the patient have received increasing attention in the psychoanalytic literature concerning countertransference enactment. Although it originally implied something pathological, enactment has come to describe a normal range of interpersonal occurrences (Frank 1999). Goldberg (2002) narrowed the definition to those interactions 'that may be conceptualized as transference and countertransference issues' (2002, p. 882), usually operating outside of the therapist's awareness. Transference pressures that elicit countertransference reactions commonly complicate the treatment of the suicidal patient. Enactments may involve special accommodations on account of the patient's needs and (temporary) incapacity to care for himself. Some of these actions are clearly conscious and thought through by the therapist. In other cases, there may be less awareness of the unconscious psychological defence mechanisms involved. The therapist who is aware of his actions and understands their impact on the patient can best ensure that his countertransference enactments will be helpful.

Such accommodations to the treatment of the suicidal patient may be termed boundary crossings. Boundary violations that take advantage of the patient and aim primarily at narcissistic gratification of the therapist are, on the other hand, destructive. Awareness of the legitimate needs of the regressed suicidal patient can inform the therapist about the use of countertransference actions. Separating the need for supportive measures from coercive bondage is fundamental to successful treatment, and relies on countertransference awareness of intense primitive feelings in the therapist, doctor, or any caregiver that are activated in these treatments.

## Conclusion

Countertransference reactions are ubiquitous in the therapeutic and any treatment situation. In the treatment of suicidal patients, the problems that arise in the therapy appear most often related to countertransference enactments, which may produce therapeutic inaction, or inappropriate over-action. Awareness of the treater's own feelings of hatred, inadequacy, confusion and withdrawal are key to containing the enactments that stem from unconscious reactions. In the treatment of suicidal individuals, it is even more crucial that such awareness be made conscious so as to prevent the patient from interpreting the caregiver's communications as hostile, rejecting and suicide-inviting.

Therefore, ongoing education and supervision should be available to all personnel involved in the treatment of suicidal patients, independent of the treatment modality. All clinicians who treat suicidal patients, whether by pharmacological, behavioural or psychodynamic therapies, would greatly benefit from the insight developed through sharing clinical material with trusted peers or supervisors.

## References

Frank K (1999). *Psychoanalytic Participation, Action, Interaction and Integration*. Analytic Press, Hillsdale.

Freud S (1910). *The Future Prospects of Psycho-analytic Therapy*. Standard Edition 11.Hogarth Press, London.

Gabbard GO (1995). Countertransference: the emerging common ground. *International Journal of Psychoanalysis*, **76**, 475–485.

Gabbard GO (2001). A contemporary psychoanalytic model of countertransference. *Journal of Clinical Psychology*, **57**, 983–991.

Goldberg A (2002). Enactment as understanding and misunderstanding. *Journal of the American Psychoanalytic Association*, **50**, 869–883.

Heimann P (1950). On counter-transference. *International Journal of Psychoanalysis*, **31**, 81–84.

Hendin H (1981). Psychotherapy and suicide. *American Journal of Psychotherapy*, **35**, 469–480.

Hendin H, Haas AP, Maltsberger JT, Koestner B, Szanto K (2006). Problems in psychotherapy with a suicidal patient. *Am J Psychiatry*, **163**, 67–72.

Maltsberger JT and Buie DH (1973). Countertransference hate in the treatment of suicidal patients. *Archives of General Psychiatry*, **30**, 625–633.

Slakter E (ed.) (1987). *Countertransference*. Aronson, Northvale.

Wolk-Wasserman D (1987). Some problems connected with the treatment of suicide attempt patients: transference and countertransference aspects. *Crisis*, **1**, 69–82.

# CHAPTER 54

# Pharmacological and other biological treatments of suicidal individuals

Hans-Jurgen Möller

## Abstract

Due to the role of depressive disorders, as the most frequent cause of suicidal behaviour, antidepressants have the most prominent place in psychopharmacological prevention of suicidal behaviour. Based on clinical experience, antidepressants reduce suicidality in association with the reduction of depressive symptoms, and it is assumed that suicidal behaviour is also reduced as a consequence. However, based on the results of empirical studies, the evidence is not as clear as clinicians like to believe, which might, in part, be due to methodological problems. Other pharmacological and biological treatment methods with lithium, neuroleptics, benzodiazepines, anti-epileptics and ECT are described as well.

## Introduction

Besides counselling and other psychotherapeutic approaches, psychopharmacological treatment and other biological treatment procedures (e.g. electroconvulsive therapy) are indicated for many suicidal patients. In people at risk of committing suicide, these interventions are usually aimed at actual prevention of suicide, mostly through sedative–anxiolytic or sleep-inducing approaches, or specific treatment of psychiatric disorders that are the underlying cause of suicidality. It is of great importance for patients in a critical life situation to be able to get rid of anxieties, depression, agitation, sleeplessness and other disturbing symptoms, even if these are not part of a full syndrome of a psychiatric disorder, but only subsyndromal. In this chapter, the psychopharmacological treatment of patients suffering from suicidality in defined psychiatric disorders is described.

The first part of this chapter describes pharmacological treatments of suicidality in the context of psychiatric disorders, and psychopharmacological approaches as used in clinical settings. The evidence for beneficial, as well as potentially harmful, effects of antidepressants on suicidality in depressive patients is also reviewed.

## Treatment of suicidality in the context of psychiatric disorders

### Unipolar and bipolar depression

Depression is seen as the most frequent cause of suicidality and suicide. Although, the suicide lifetime risk in depressed patients is not much higher than, for example, in schizophrenic patients; depression is the most frequent reason for suicidality and suicide due to the high prevalence rate of depression. As to the differentiation between unipolar and bipolar depression, the suicide risk rate is more or less the same, i.e. about 10–15 per cent lifetime risk. Suicidal thoughts occur almost regularly in depression, especially in moderate or severe cases. Furthermore, a large number of patients think about suicidal acts, perform a suicide attempt or even die from suicide.

### Antidepressants

Antidepressants are the treatment of choice to reduce depressive symptoms of the depressive episode (Bauer et al. 2002, 2007), and also suicidal thoughts occurring in this context (Möller 2006a).

When selecting an antidepressant for severely suicidal depressive patients, traditionally, compounds with a sedative profile were favoured (e.g. amitriptyline or doxepin as representatives for the classic tricyclics, or mitrazepine as an example for a modern antidepressant [Möller and Volz 1996; Baghai et al. 2006]), although this view is not accepted by all experts. Drugs that increase drive, such as MAO inhibitors or desipramine, may increase the risk of suicide and should, therefore, be avoided (Möller 1992). Another aspect of drug selection is that the antidepressant should be safe in overdose, which is proven for most modern antidepressants, especially the selective serotonin reuptake inhibitors (SSRIs) (Wasserman 2006). If a tricyclic antidepressant (TCA) is chosen, the smallest package should be prescribed to avoid the risk of lethal intoxication in case of suicidal overdose. Most TCAs have a high risk of fatal outcome if dosages of 1000mg or more are taken. SSRIs are, nowadays, seen as the first-line treatment of depression, particularly under outpatient conditions, and especially with respect to tolerability and compliance (Möller 1992; Möller and Volz 1996). It should be remembered that SSRIs, as well as the selective serotonin–noradrenalin reuptake inhibitor venlafaxine (Baghai *et al.* 2006), have no sedative potential and, in some cases, even cause agitation.

The degree of sedation achieved by a sedative antidepressant in highly excited suicidal depressive patients is sometimes insufficient, so that it may be necessary to prescribe a benzodiazepine or a sedative neuroleptic (Möller 1999). The dose depends on the patient's condition and individual reaction. It should be chosen in a way that the inner restlessness and agitation wear off completely, or as far as possible, and significant sedation and promotion of nocturnal sleep are achieved. In the case of delusional depressions, highly potent neuroleptics (e.g. 5–10mg haloperidol orally or parenteral) are indicated in addition to antidepressant treatment. In cases of severe depression with extreme suicidality, electroconvulsive therapy (Fink 2005) should be considered, because of the rapid onset of action in comparison with antidepressants. Electroconvulsive therapy (ECT) is also an important option in patients who are refractory to antidepressant treatment (Möller 1994a).

### ECT

However, we lack systematic knowledge on potential suicide preventive effects of this type of treatment, since hardly any adequately controlled treatment studies have been conducted on ECT with suicidal behaviour as their focus. A large Finnish national psychological autopsy study found that a remarkably low number of suicide cases had received ECT during the final months before suicide, thus suggesting that ECT may indeed have a suicide-preventive effect, (Isometsa *et al.* 1996). In a Swedish retrospective case–control study, there seemed to be a reduced risk of suicide in those patients who had received follow-up treatment with antidepressant medication after ECT (Brådvik and Berglund 2000).

Attention should be paid to two additional problem points when antidepressants are given to suicidal depressive patients. First, immediate antidepressant therapy is contraindicated in cases of intoxication with psychotropic substances (e.g. in an attempted suicide). In case of need, the fading period of intoxication should be bridged with sedating neuroleptics. Secondly, an increase in drive or normalization of reduced drive often occurs during antidepressant treatment prior to brightening of mood (so-called drive–mood dissociation). This may require temporary prescription or dose increase of a concomitant sedative medication until mood starts to brighten, in order to counteract the increased risk of acting on suicide impulses. This is of special importance with certain drugs, like the SSRIs, which are not sedative and, sometimes, even induce agitation or akathisia (Möller 1992; Möller 2006b). As a general rule, it should be considered that depressive patients treated with antidepressants should be observed carefully in the first days/weeks after treatment indication to assess and counteract as soon as possible negative changes in their degree of suicidality.

Unipolar and bipolar depressions are usually recurrent. Thus, in patients who have had two or more recurrent episodes, treatment is required to prevent relapse subsequent to acute and maintenance treatment. Antidepressants or lithium are candidates for preventing relapse in unipolar depression (Bauer *et al.* 2002, 2007). In bipolar depression (Grunze *et al.* 2002), lithium is generally the first choice; carbamazepine and valproate are the alternatives in special indications, such as resistance to lithium treatment or lithium intolerance. Recently, atypical antipsychotics have demonstrated relapse/recurrence preventive properties, but hitherto only in patients recovering from a manic episode. Of great interest is the increasingly confirmed result that prophylactic treatment with lithium reduces the well-known excess mortality of patients with unipolar or bipolar depression to within the normal range. This effect is apparently not only due to the reduction of depressive relapses and related suicidal behaviour, but also seems to be the consequence of a direct effect on suicidal behaviour itself (Thies-Flechtner *et al.* 1996; Müller-Oerlinghausen and Berghofer 1999; Goodwin *et al.* 2003; Fleischhacker *et al.* 2005).

Cipriani and co-workers' review and meta-analysis (2005) of 32 randomized trials of lithium versus other compounds (active or placebo) showed that lithium reduced the suicide mortality with approximately 60 per cent and the risk of suicide and deliberate self-harm combined by about 70 per cent. Lithium prophylaxis should, therefore, clearly be considered for patients with bipolar disorder who have displayed suicidal behaviour.

Until now, no differentiation was made with respect to the drug treatment of depressive episodes occurring during unipolar or bipolar affective disorder. In the last decade, great emphasis was placed on the fact that the treatment of bipolar depression should consider some special issues, especially the risk that antidepressants may induce a switch into mania. Therefore, some guidelines recommended avoiding antidepressants, and favour a monotherapy with lithium or anticonvulsants used as mood stabilizers. However, it has not been proven that these compounds have antidepressive efficacy comparable to that of the antidepressants (Möller and Grunze 2000). For this reason, antidepressants should still be regarded as the treatment of choice in bipolar depression (Grunze *et al.* 2002; Goodwin 2003; Möller *et al.* 2006a). SSRIs should be preferred due to their almost complete lack of risk for switching to mania. If the prescription of TCAs, which induce switching to mania in about 10 per cent of patients, is deemed clinically necessary, co-medication with a mood stabilizer is recommended to reduce the risk of switching to mania.

In mixed states, i.e. the coexistence of depression and manic symptoms (Balazs *et al.* 2006), as well as in patients with rapid cycling, antidepressants should be completely avoided; in such cases, treatment has to rely on lithium or other mood stabilizers only. Based on recently published data on olanzapine and quetiapine (Calabrese *et al.* 2005; Perlis *et al.* 2006; Perlis 2007), it appears that these, and possibly other atypical neuroleptics, will become an option for the treatment of patients suffering from a depressive episode in the frame of a bipolar affective disorder.

### Schizophrenia

Schizophrenia has a virtually similar lifetime risk for suicide as unipolar or bipolar depression. The symptoms of schizophrenia can be easily treated with antipsychotics (Falkai *et al.* 2005). Second generation antipsychotics are increasingly in use in recent years, because of their lower liability to extra-pyramidal side effects, and a broader spectrum of efficacy (Möller 2000, 2002). Suicidality associated with a schizophrenic psychosis often requires medication in addition to the standard neuroleptic treatment of the schizophrenic symptoms, especially in cases of severe anxiety or excitation. Sedating neuroleptics or benzodiazepines are indicated in these conditions. If high doses of sedating neuroleptics are initially required to achieve adequate sedation, special attention must be paid to the risk of orthostatic hypotension.

A different approach is required for suicidality in schizophrenic patients who have depressive or negative symptoms. If depressive–apathetic symptoms with suicidality exist as part of a post-psychotic depression, or a deficit syndrome, pharmacotherapy should generally follow the guidelines for the treatment of these conditions. This means that treatment with antidepressants in the case of post-psychotic depression, and treatment with atypical neuroleptics, or SSRIs (or both) in the deficit syndrome, is necessary (Möller 2005b; Möller et al. 2006; Möller 2006a). If the suicidal symptoms are a side-effect of treatment with classical neuroleptics (pharmacogenic or akinetic depression), the neuroleptic dose should be reduced, if possible, or the patient should be switched to an atypical neuroleptic. An anti-parkinsonism drug, such as biperidon, is often advisable for some days to reduce the parkinsonian side-effects as soon as possible.

Atypical antipsychotics are the treatment of choice for long-term relapse prevention in schizophrenia, which is usually required subsequent to the acute episode, because they have no or a lower risk of inducing depression compared to the first generation antipsychotics, and may even have antidepressant effects (Möller 2005a, b). Atypical neuroleptics, thus, possibly reduce not only depression, but also related suicidality. Of special interest is that clozapine seems to have a special antisuicidal efficacy in the long-term treatment of schizophrenic patients (Meltzer and Okayli 1995; Meltzer et al. 2003). The study of Spivak et al. (2003) suggests that the reduction in suicidality following long-term clozapine treatment may be related to a reduction in impulsiveness and aggression.

### Anxiety disorders and obsessive–compulsive disorders

Anxiety disorders and anxiety are often associated with the risk of suicidality. In addition to psychotherapeutic procedures, nearly all anxiety disorders and obsessive–compulsive disorders (OCD) are an indication for psychopharmacological treatment. Serotonergic antidepressants, especially SSRIs, are the treatment of choice, but also the dual selective reuptake inhibitor venlafaxine has demonstrated efficacy in some of these conditions (Bandelow et al. 2002). Administration of a benzodiazepine is often necessary for the acute control of panic situations. Antidepressants are also very often indicated in so-called neurotic disorders, depending on the type and severity of the symptoms. Examples include dysthymia (for which TCAs of the amitriptyline type, monoamine oxidase [MAO] inhibitors or SSRIs are used, for example), anxiety disorders (for which imipramine and SSRIs are used, for example) and OCD (for which clomipramine and SSRIs are used, for example). If suicidality occurs during such disorders, monotherapy with an antidepressant is often not sufficient to overcome the critical situation as quickly as possible. Short-term administration of benzodiazepines or sedative neuroleptics, along with the antidepressant, may be necessary. However, the application of a benzodiazepine should be restricted to a short period of days or a few weeks to avoid the risk of a low-dose dependency.

### Personality disorders

Personality disorders are frequently associated with chronic, repetitive suicidality. At special risk are histrionic and borderline patients. In general, the efficacy of psychopharmacological treatment of personality disorders is not well established (Kapfhammer and Hippius 1998; Cardish 2007; Herpertz et al. 2007). In borderline cases, the occasional risk of paradoxical reactions to benzodiazepines or TCAs, and possibly also to modern antidepressants like the SSRIs, should be taken into consideration (Möller 1994b). In most cases, only pharmacological treatment of the acute critical condition seems indicated. Benzodiazepines, antidepressants with a sedative–anxiolytic profile or low potency neuroleptics in small dosages, can be administered in this indication as a short-term intervention. It should be taken into account that these suggestions are mostly based on clinical experience, but not on clinical trials. Long-term treatment with benzodiazepines should be avoided due to the risk of abuse.

Over the last years, atypical neuroleptics have gained more widespread use for patients with BPD and seems to have promising effects on impulsivity and suicidal behaviour (Zanarini and Frankenburg 2001; Hilger et al. 2003), especially when they are used in combination with psychotherapeutic measures (Soler et al. 2005). Low-dose neuroleptics or atypical neuroleptics may also be necessary to use in the treatment of patients with BPD, in order to strengthen reality control or to reduce dissociative symptoms.

There are very few studies that have investigated whether a medium-term psychopharmacological approach might be useful in the prevention of further suicide attempts in patients with a history of repeated suicide attempts. The studies that have been performed have mostly involved patients suffering from comorbidity with personality disorders of the impulsive, histrionic and borderline type (Montgomery et al. 1992).

### Adjustment disorders and post-traumatic stress disorders

When suicidality results from abnormal reactions to psychosocial stress, psychopharmacological interventions are mainly aimed at sedation, anxiolysis, sleep induction, or suppression of disturbing vegetative symptoms.

Anxiolytic benzodiazepines, or in cases of predominant sleep disturbances, sleep-inducing benzodiazepines, or the modern non-benzodiazepine hypnotics, are generally the treatment of first choice in adjustment disorders. The selection of the specific compound and of the dose varies according to the individual case. The aim should be to induce not only sedation, but also affective–emotional distancing. Some doctors tend to be very restrictive in prescribing benzodiazepines, even under these conditions, because they are afraid of the risk of dependency. They prefer to use sedating antidepressants, such as doxepin, or low doses of sedating neuroleptics as surrogates. However, given the extraordinary good tolerability of benzodiazepines and the high compliance of patients with these drugs, the risk–benefit assessment should favour the benzodiazepines under these special conditions, especially given the fact that, in general, only short-term medication is needed. An inadequate psychopharmacological regime could induce a high risk of continuation of suicidality, and for this reason, under-treatment with benzodiazepines, which seems to become a general problem in patients with a need for benzodiazepine treatment (Möller 1999), should be avoided. In cases of longer-lasting depressive reactions, antidepressants should be considered. Modern antidepressants with better tolerability than the TCAs should preferably be chosen.

The psychopharmacological treatment of post-traumatic stress disorder is not yet well defined. Most experts recommend SSRIs, while benzodiazepines are not seen to be a treatment of choice (Asnis *et al.* 2004; Davidson 2004; Ursano *et al.* 2004).

## Evidence base for beneficial effects of antidepressants on suicidality in depressive patients

Due to the role of depressive disorders, as the most frequent cause of suicidal behaviour, antidepressants have the most prominent place in psychopharmacological prevention of suicidal behaviour. Clinicians assume that antidepressants not only reduce depressive symptoms, but also the associated suicidality. This clinical experience is confirmed at least in terms of suicidal ideation by the results of controlled antidepressant studies, which show that if the depression subsides during treatment with antidepressants, the suicidal thoughts usually also diminish or disappear (Möller 2006a).

However, in the early publications on antidepressants, there are hardly any special studies on this topic. Much more interest in exploring this matter was shown later in the context of the question whether certain antidepressants reduce suicidal thoughts more quickly or effectively, particularly after the advent of the SSRIs.

A pooled analysis of all data from control group studies of the SSRI fluoxetine, involving a total of 1765 patients treated with fluoxetine, 569 with placebo and 731 with TCAs, found that suicidal ideation improved significantly more with fluoxetine than with placebo (72.0 per cent vs 54.8 per cent, p < 0.001), and was similar to the improvement with TCAs (72.5 per cent vs 69.8 per cent, p = 0.294) (Beasley *et al.* 1991). It is important to underline that, in terms of suicidal behaviour (suicide attempts and suicide), there is no relevant difference: the pooled incidence of suicidal acts was 0.3 per cent for fluoxetine, 0.2 per cent for placebo and 0.4 per cent for tricyclics. The slight numerical differences were not statistically significant. If only placebo-controlled fluoxetine studies were included in the pooled analysis, the rate in the fluoxetine and placebo groups was the same: 0.2 per cent (Beasley *et al.* 1991).

Similar results were also obtained in the pooled analysis of the results of a paroxetine study (Figure 54.1) (Lopez-Ibor 1993). The change in the Hamilton Depression Scale (HAM-D) suicidality item score over time showed that paroxetine and the active control were significantly superior to placebo in reducing suicidal thoughts from week 1 onward. In terms of frequency of attempted suicide and suicide, documented as adverse events, there were no statistically significant differences between the groups. The frequencies for suicides were as follows: 0.17 per cent for paroxetine, 0.26 per cent for active control and 0.36 per cent for placebo; the frequencies for attempted suicides were 1.3 per cent for paroxetine, 1.0 per cent for active control and 1.1 per cent for placebo.

Altogether, these findings provide some evidence that antidepressants are able to reduce suicidal thoughts in depressive patients. This effect is associated with the global antidepressive effect (Möller 2006a).

From a clinical perspective, one might hypothesize that the beneficial effect on suicidal ideation has consequences for the prevention of suicide attempts or even completed suicide. However, empirical data from randomized controlled studies, and even the pooled analyses of fluoxetine or paroxetine comparator trials, give no support to this hypothesis. Methodological limitations may not allow this question to be addressed adequately. The extremely low basal rate of suicide attempts, and especially completed suicide, is a limiting factor in short-term studies of antidepressants. Even meta-analytical approaches on huge datasets involving not only one experimental antidepressant but several, are apparently not able to overcome the respective statistical power problem of individual studies. Khan and colleagues (Khan *et al.* 2000, 2001, 2003) analysed several FDA databases on randomized, placebo- and/or active comparator-controlled trials on new antidepressants, mostly SSRIs. The analysis of this huge database did not find any significant differences between placebo, active comparator or investigational antidepressants in the rates of attempted or completed suicide. In a similar meta-analysis (Storosum *et al.* 2001), all randomized and placebo-controlled, double-blind, short- and long-term studies of an antidepressant that were part of a registration dossier submitted to the Dutch regulatory authority between 1983 and 1997 were reviewed for attempted suicide. In addition, all long-term, placebo-controlled antidepressant studies that were conducted in the

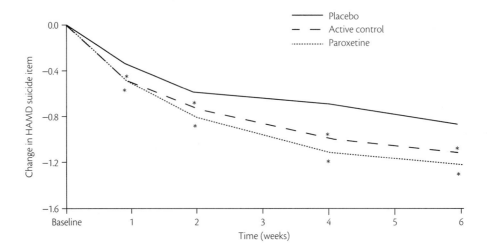

**Fig. 54.1** Change in HAMD suicide item score over time (Lopez-Ibor 1993).
* p < 0.05; paroxetine/active control vs placebo.

last decade in patients with major depression were identified by a Medline search and assessed for attempted suicide. The analysis of this huge database was unable to demonstrate a significant difference in the risk of suicide attempts between active compounds and placebo. When interpreting the results of the long-term studies, it should be considered that even under these long-term conditions (the duration of most of the studies was one year), the base rate of suicide attempts was low, i.e. up to 0.2 per cent.

In contrast, two other huge meta-analyses (Fergusson *et al.* 2005; Gunnell *et al.* 2005) found an increased risk of suicide attempts for antidepressants, where in the latter study, the risk was only small and did not reach statistical significance. Thus, the overall findings from pooled analyses/meta-analyses of results of randomized, controlled, short- and long-term trials (mostly up to one year) do not support the hypothesis that antidepressants reduce attempted or completed suicide (Möller 2006a). This astonishing result, which appears to contradict general clinical experience, together with the findings from randomized controlled trials that antidepressants reduce suicidal thoughts, might be due to methodological pitfalls, such as a low base rate of the outcome criteria suicide attempts or suicide, and recruitment of a low-risk population. The result of the meta-analysis by Fergusson and colleagues (Fergusson *et al.* 2005) shows that, in contrast to the general expectations, there might be an increased risk of suicidal behaviour as a consequence of treatment with antidepressants, which requires further discussion (Möller 2006b).

Interesting data demonstrating the capacity of antidepressants to reduce suicidal behaviour was obtained in recent years from epidemiological studies (Möller 2006a). In view of the fact that it appears to be extremely difficult to prove the anti-suicidal effect of antidepressants in randomized, control group studies, such a naturalistic approach, seems to be one of the best ways to obtain at least some evidence. These studies are backed up by data from awareness and follow-up trials. However, naturalistic studies, on an ecological level, are always difficult to interpret due to several potential confounding factors, which require careful consideration.

The prescription rate of antidepressants has increased in several countries in the past decades, partly associated with the fact that modern antidepressants are better tolerated and, therefore, easier to handle in the everyday routine care situation, especially in primary care. This increased prescription of antidepressants offers the possibility of a quasi-experiment, in which the suicide rates at the time of a lower and higher prescription rate can be compared.

For example, Isacsson analysed such data in a study on suicide rates in Sweden and other Scandinavian countries (Figure 54.2) (Isacsson 2000). He took into account relevant confounding factors, which might explain the change in suicide rates, like unemployment rates and alcohol consumption. However, this was not performed using complex statistical procedures, but only by looking at the development of each of these variables over time. The suicide rate in Sweden decreased by 19 per cent in parallel with the increased use of antidepressants, from 23.3 suicides per 100,000 inhabitants in 1991 to 18.8 in 1996 (rho = −0.90, p < 0.05). Considering subgroups in Sweden during 1990–1996, there were no demographic groups with regard to age, gender or county in which the suicide rate decreased in the absence of an increased use of antidepressants. In women under 30 and over 75 years of age, however, and in four of the 23 counties, suicide rates remained unchanged despite an increased use of antidepressants. Inverse correlations between the use of antidepressants and suicide rates were also seen in the three other Scandinavian countries, Denmark (rho = −0.94, p < 0.01), Norway (rho = −0.87, p < 0.05) and Finland (rho = −1.00, p < 0.01), during 1990–1996. There was no consistent correlation in Sweden (1978–1996), between suicide rates and alcohol consumption, or between suicide rates and unemployment rates (Isacsson 2000). In this epidemiological study, it appears that the increased use of antidepressants was one of the contributing factors to the decrease in the suicide rate.

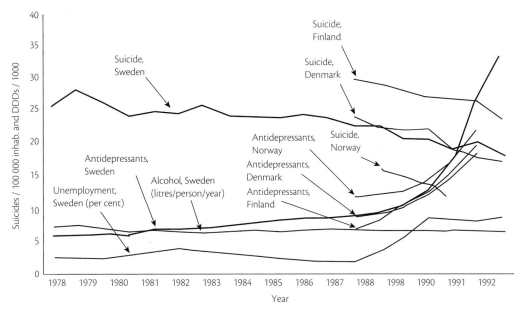

**Fig. 54.2** Correlations with Swedish suicide rates in the retrospective analysis of 1978–1991. Two-tailed tests: antidepressants: rho = −0.85, p < 0.01; unemployment: rho = +0.25, NS; alcohol: rho = +0.30, NS. Correlations with suicide rates in the prospective analysis of 1992–1996. One-tailed tests: antidepressants: rho = − 0.90, p < 0.05; unemployment: rho = − 0.25, NS; alcohol: rho = +0.70, NS (Isacsson 2000).

Grunebaum and colleagues (Grunebaum *et al.* 2004) presented the results of a methodologically sound analysis of the US-American data for the years 1985 to 1999 that took into account unemployment and alcohol consumption as confounding factors in a multivariate approach. The relationships between the suicide, antidepressant prescription, unemployment and alcoholic beverage consumption rates were studied using generalized linear models. Suicide rates by antidepressant overdose were compared in SSRIs and TCAs. From 1985 to 1999, the suicide rate fell 13.5 per cent, with a greater decline among women, and antidepressant prescription rates increased over fourfold, with the increase mostly due to SSRIs. Prescription rates for SSRIs, and other second-generation antidepressants, were both inversely associated with suicide rates ($p = 0.03$ and $p = 0.02$, respectively). In a multivariable analysis adjusting for unemployment and alcoholic beverage consumption rates, SSRI antidepressant prescription rates remained inversely associated with the national suicide rate ($p = 0.03$). The authors came to the conclusion that the decline in the national suicide rate (1985–1999) appears to be associated with greater use of non-tricyclic antidepressants. A similar study on suicide data from the USA performed by Gibbons and colleagues (Gibbons *et al.* 2005) obtained similar, but somewhat more differentiated results.

Other epidemiological studies confirmed the positive results (Rihmer 2001; Hall *et al.* 2003; Kelly *et al.* 2003; Rihmer 2004). In order to give a balanced overview, it should be mentioned that two studies were unable to support the findings of an association between an increased prescription rate of antidepressants and a decreased suicide rate (Barbui *et al.* 1999; Helgason *et al.* 2004).

These studies results on an epidemiological level show that it is evident that an increased utilization of antidepressants, especially SSRIs, was accompanied by a relevant decline of national suicide rates in several countries (Möller 2006a), particularly in those where the suicide rates were previously very high. The results of complex and sophisticated statistical analyses show that this relationship cannot only be explained by potential confounding variables. It can be considered to be a very robust epidemiological finding, due to the fact that it could be replicated in several countries under different psychosocial and care conditions (Möller 2006a). Apparently, in terms of suicide rates, certain subgroups of the population are influenced to different degrees by the prescription of antidepressants. The US Food and Drug Administration (FDA) analyses show a pattern of increasing benefits and decreasing risk of suicidal behaviour in treatment with antidepressant in all age groups, with the exception of those under the age of 18 and young adults aged 18–24 years (see Chapter 91 by David Brent).

The most common psychiatric illness seen to be associated with suicide is a depressive disorder (Möller 2003). Isacsson and colleagues (Isacsson *et al.* 1996), for example, found that the risk for suicide among depressed patients who were treated with antidepressants in Sweden was 141 per 100,000 person years and, among the untreated, 259 per 100,000 person years (i.e. 1.8 times higher among the untreated).

Although, a lot of patients seek professional help in the month before committing suicide (Isacsson *et al.* 1992), post-mortem studies show that most patients are untreated at the time of death (Isometsa *et al.* 1994; Isacsson *et al.* 1997; Oquendo *et al.* 1999). The huge proportion of under-diagnosed and undertreated depressive patients is also known from several studies on the care

of depressive patients, e.g. the DEPRES study (Lepine *et al.* 1997; Tylee *et al.* 1999a, b; Angst *et al.* 2002). Thus, it seems reasonable to suggest that the important strategy for lowering suicide rates should be to identify all individuals with depressive disorders and to intervene effectively.

Awareness and education campaigns seem to be an appropriate approach in achieving this goal (Mann *et al.* 2005). A milestone in this respect is the so-called Gotland study. In 1983–1984, the Swedish Committee for the Prevention and Treatment of Depression offered an educational programme on the diagnosis and treatment of depressive disorders to all general practitioners on the island of Gotland. The programme was carefully evaluated: 1982 was used as the baseline, and the main evaluation was carried out in 1985 (Rutz *et al.* 1992). After the educational programmes, the frequency of sick leave for depressive disorders decreased, and the frequency of inpatient care for depressive disorders decreased to 30 per cent of that at the baseline, the prescription of antidepressants increased, but prescription of major tranquillizers, sedatives and hypnotics decreased. The frequency of suicide on the island among females decreased significantly.

A programme called the Defeat Depression Campaign was carried out in Great Britain for five years from 1992 to 1996. It was aimed at enhancing public awareness of, and attitudes toward, depressive disorders by providing professional education for general practitioners and reducing the suicide rate (Paykel *et al.* 1997). The campaign was evaluated through three representative surveys of public attitudes (1991, 1995, 1997) (Paykel 2001). The surveys showed a progressive increase in the general population's knowledge about the biological causes of depressive disorders. However, the campaign did not result in a sustained improvement of patient care (Rix *et al.* 1999), or in a change of entrenched public attitudes, for example, the negative opinion about treatment with antidepressants (Paykel *et al.* 1998). The prescription rate of TCAs and SSRIs increased over the course of the campaign (Paykel 2001). A basic problem of the study is that there was no control region, so it cannot be elucidated whether the measured effects were related to the campaign or possible changes in the health care system.

The Nuremberg Alliance against Depression programme, which was carried out in the German city of Nuremberg, is another, even more complex, study that combined an educational programme addressed at general practitioners with a public awareness campaign for depression (Hegerl *et al.* 2003; Henkel *et al.* 2003; Althaus *et al.* 2005; Hegerl *et al.* 2008). It confirmed the principal results of the Gotland study, while using a more sophisticated evaluation methodology, for example, involvement of a control region in the evaluation.

As is always the case in such quasi-experimental, but complex intervention programmes, it is difficult to decide which factors are responsible for the achieved effects. Besides the improved diagnosis and treatment of depression, changes in the prescription rate of antidepressants are probably also relevant (Pfeiffer-Gerschel 2007).

Altogether, there seems to be reasonable evidence from different research approaches that antidepressants are able to reduce suicidal ideation, and also suicide in depressive patients. While the evidence for the beneficial effect on suicidal ideation comes from randomized, control group studies, some of which used a placebo arm, the evidence for the prophylactic effect on suicide was primarily obtained from well-designed epidemiological studies.

# Negative effects of antidepressants on suicidality in depressive patients

Finally, the question whether antidepressants can induce or aggravate suicidal ideation, or even stimulate suicidal behaviour, should be briefly addressed in this paper, because it has attracted so much attention in recent years, especially in the field of child and adolescent psychiatry. A review of the evidence concerning children and young people is given in this book (see Chapter 91).

A comprehensive review (Möller 2006b; Tandon *et al.* 2008) came to the following conclusions in this regard:

◆ Negative effects of antidepressants on suicidality are difficult to investigate in empirical studies due to several methodological limitations. A broad scientific approach, therefore, has to use complementary methods to obtain the most comprehensive evidence. As mentioned before, the empirical data seem to demonstrate a suicidality-decreasing effect of antidepressants (Möller 2006a).

◆ Case reports on suicidality-inducing effects of antidepressants should be interpreted very cautiously and different kinds of bias and misperceptions inherent in case reports should be considered carefully. Case reports should, therefore, be seen only as a source of hypotheses, but not as confirmation of hypotheses. If only single case data are available, the extreme uncertainty of the evidence should be addressed, and the drawing of relevant conclusions should be avoided.

◆ Randomized, controlled studies do not supply much evidence to support the hypothesis that antidepressants, in general or individual antidepressants, have suicidality-inducing effects. Several meta-analyses comparing datasets of individual antidepressants, mostly SSRIs, demonstrated a greater average reduction of the suicidal thoughts score under SSRIs, as well as comparator drugs like TCAs compared to placebo. In addition, the categories 'worsening of pre-existing suicidal thoughts' or 'new emergence of suicidal thoughts' were less frequent in the SSRI or TCA groups than in the placebo groups. Meta-analyses on datasets of novel antidepressants from national drug authorities, which took either the suicide attempt rate or suicide rate as the outcome criterion, often failed to demonstrate a suicidality-increasing effect of antidepressants (Gunnell *et al.* 2005). However, there are signals for suicidality-inducing effects, coming from meta-analyses of the most comprehensive datasets. The meta-analysis by Fergusson and colleagues (Fergusson *et al.* 2005) found an increased risk of suicide attempts for SSRIs compared to placebo, but not different from TCAs. The meta-analysis by Gunnell (Gunnell *et al.* 2005) supported this, but with a weaker level of evidence. A meta-analysis by the FDA of the antidepressant studies in children or adolescents found an increase of suicidal thoughts and behaviour, but not suicide (FDA Public Health Advisory 2004; Hammad 2004; Hammad *et al.* 2006a, b), which does not appear to be specific to the SSRIs.

◆ A comprehensive and methodologically differentiated meta-analysis was recently performed on this topic for a special FDA task force, reviewing the relationship between antidepressant drugs and suicidality in adults (Stone and Jones 2006). This meta-analysis included the most comprehensive database of placebo-controlled trials for various indications in this research field.

The estimated odds ratio for suicide-related behaviour (preparatory acts, attempts and completed suicide) associated with assignment to antidepressant drug treatment compared to placebo was 1.12 (95 per cent Cl, 0.79–1.58) for the whole dataset, indicating a non-significant risk with antidepressant drug treatment compared to placebo. However, for persons older than 18, the estimates of suicidality risk (ideation, preparatory acts, attempts and completed suicide) associated with assignment to antidepressant drug treatment compared to placebo showed a lower, but not statistically significant risk for suicidality for the group treated with antidepressant drugs. For persons over 64 years, the significantly protective effect of antidepressants was shown. Apparently, age effects play an important modulating role. Since suicidal behaviour is probably more meaningfully related to suicide risk in older age groups, these findings are moderately reassuring. Only younger adults, below the age of 24 (and children), appear to have a certain increased risk for suicide-related behaviour.

◆ Pharmaco–epidemiological studies, which search for associations between prescription rates of antidepressants and the risk of suicide attempts (not suicide!) in clinical cohorts on an individual level, are not fully conclusive.

◆ Related to this problem is the issue of differences in the fatal toxicity of antidepressants. There is clear evidence that most modern antidepressants like the SSRIs have a lower fatal toxicity risk than the TCAs.

◆ Even though statistical analyses of control group studies or epidemiological data about available psychopharmaceutical agents may not deliver strong indications for a suicidality-inducing effect of SSRIs or antidepressants in general, but possibly only in subgroups, the principle possibility of such an adverse effect in single cases should always be considered carefully; especially, in children, *adolescents and younger adults* with a frequently very complex clinical situation that is characterized by non-response, co-medication, comorbidity, personality factors and situational stress, among others.

◆ It should be considered that different mechanisms can lead to suicidality-enhancing effects. These might, for example, be related to the pharmacological mode of action related to different transmitter systems, or to special pharmacodynamic properties like activating/drive-enhancing effects. However, the data are generally not consistent enough to allow solid conclusions to be drawn. It might only be plausible, from the line of clinical thinking, to assume that activation or even agitation induced by an antidepressant can induce or enhance suicidality. Beside these mechanisms, idiosyncratic paradoxical effects also have to be taken into account; these are well known, not only from antidepressants, but also from other psychoactive drugs, such as the benzodiazepines. Special pre-dispositions of patients, including personality factors, such as borderline personality disorder, seem especially to contribute in the sense of a multifactorial aetiopathogenesis (Teicher *et al.* 1993).

◆ In the context of possible mechanisms for a potentially higher suicide rate, it deserves consideration that, as far as antidepressants are concerned, determination of the suicide risk of an individual patient, or the general suicide rate, is very complex and involves the integration of different factors. For example, the potential induction of suicidal thoughts or even suicidal ideation, of which the SSRIs are accused when compared to TCAs, may be compensated for by a much lower risk of a fatal outcome of a suicide attempt with an SSRI compared to a TCA. In the discussion about the potential suicide-enhancing risks of the SSRIs, it seems highly problematic not to equally consider the much higher fatal toxicity indices of the equally TCAs.

In everyday clinical practice, the discussion about the possible risks of the SSRIs or antidepressants, in general, should not result in clinicians forgetting the benefits of these drugs. The symptoms of depression require an effective drug treatment accompanied by the chance to reduce suicidal thoughts. Of course, particularly at the start of treatment, patients are often very labile; and in single cases, antidepressants, depending on their specific pharmacological and pharmacodynamic characteristics and in interaction with special characteristics of the patient, such as personality traits, comorbidity etc., can potentially induce or enhance suicidal thoughts, or even reduce the threshold potential for suicide attempts. It is a matter of good clinical practice to monitor the patient carefully, especially at the start of drug treatment, and try to avoid any kind of risk. If agitation, sleep disturbances or other drug side effects that may potentially induce or enhance suicidality occur, a sedating or sleep-inducing co-medication should be administered. It is also of greatest importance to offer the patient a substantial supportive psychotherapy. Finally, it should not be forgotten that depressive symptoms and suicidal thoughts can fluctuate during the day or over longer time periods. It is often difficult to follow this carefully enough on an outpatient basis, so that inpatient treatment might be a better option for patients at risk (Möller 2006b).

## Evidence base for beneficial effects of lithium on suicidality

Going beyond the antidepressants, the important role of another drug, lithium, in the field of suicide prevention should be mentioned. Several analyses of lithium prevention studies show that the excess mortality, usually shown by depressive patients in comparison to the general population, can be reduced to the normal level by lithium relapse prophylaxis. This effect of lithium could not only be explained by its relapse-prophylactic effect, but was interpreted as being a specific influence on suicidality, potentially by the serotonergic effects of lithium (Müller-Oerlinghausen 1989; Coppen *et al.* 1991; Tondo *et al.* 2001; Goodwin *et al.* 2003; Cipriani *et al.* 2005). The finding that a raised lithium concentration in drinking water correlates with a lower suicide rate is also of interest (Schrauzer and Shrestha 1990). Lithium relapse prevention in unipolar or bipolar patients seems therefore meaningful whenever there is an indication for lithium long-term treatment.

## Conclusions

Psychiatric disorders can cause suicidality. Given the high prevalence and lifetime risk of depressive disorders, depression is one of the major causes of suicidal behaviour. Adequate psychopharmacological treatment of depression and other psychiatric disorders associated with suicidality is recommended as a meaningful strategy to reduce suicidal thoughts and suicidal behaviour. Depending on the individual disorder and the specific conditions, this includes the administration of antidepressants, antipsychotics,

benzodiazepines and hypnotics. The psychopharmacological intervention should aim to have a positive effect on suicidality as soon as possible. In critical situations, co-medication is often clinically indicated, e.g. the combination of an antidepressant with a benzodiazepine.

The findings of randomized, control group studies in acute depressive patients supply good evidence that antidepressants are able to reduce suicidal thoughts in depressive patients. However, data from randomized, control group studies in acute depressive patients give no support to the hypothesis that antidepressants can reduce suicide attempts or suicide. The extremely low base rate of suicidal behaviour in these studies is, apparently, a principal methodological problem, which makes it almost impossible to demonstrate, under such conditions, a beneficial effect of antidepressants on suicidal behaviour. Even meta-analyses of huge datasets from randomized, controlled trials seem unable to overcome this problem. Thus, complementary methodological approaches have to be applied.

Over the past year, there have been intensive discussions about possible negative effects of antidepressants on suicidality. Although there is only weak evidence for such effects when treating individual patients with antidepressants, the potential, but rare risk, of inducing suicidality should be considered carefully. Optimal clinical management can avoid possible harmful consequences of treatment with antidepressants.

## References

Althaus D, Niklewski G, Pfeiffer-Gerschel T *et al.* (2005). Vom 'Nürnberger Bündnis gegen Depression' zur 'European Alliance against Depression'. Modelle zur Optimierung der Versorgung depressiver Patienten [From the 'Nuremberg League against Depression' to the European Alliance Against Depression'. Models for optimizing care of depressive patients]. *Nervenheilkunde*, **24**, 402–407.

Angst J, Gamma A, Gastpar M *et al.* (2002). Gender differences in depression. Epidemiological findings from the European DEPRES I and II studies. *European Archives of Psychiatry and Clinical Neuroscience*, **252**, 201–209.

Asnis GM, Kohn SR, Henderson M *et al.* (2004). SSRIs versus non-SSRIs in post-traumatic stress disorder: an update with recommendations. *Drugs*, **64**, 383–404.

Baghai TC, Volz HP, Moller HJ (2006). Drug treatment of depression in the 2000s: an overview of achievements in the last 10 years and future possibilities. *World Journal of Biological Psychiatry*, **7**, 198–222.

Balazs J, Benazzi F, Rihmer Z *et al.* (2006). The close link between suicide attempts and mixed (bipolar) depression: implications for suicide prevention. *Journal of Affective Disorders*, **91**, 133–138.

Bandelow B, Zohar J, Hollander E *et al.* (2002). World Federation of Societies of Biological Psychiatry (WFSBP) guidelines for the pharmacological treatment of anxiety, obsessive–compulsive and posttraumatic stress disorders. *World Journal of Biological Psychiatry*, **3**, 171–199.

Barbui C, Campomori A, D'Avanzo B *et al.* (1999). Antidepressant drug use in Italy since the introduction of SSRIs: national trends, regional differences and impact on suicide rates. *Social Psychiatry and Psychiatric Epidemiology*, **34**, 152–156.

Bauer M, Bschor T, Pfennig A *et al.* (2007). World Federation of Societies of Biological Psychiatry (WFSBP) Guidelines for Biological Treatment of Unipolar Depressive Disorders in Primary Care. *World Journal of Biological Psychiatry*, **8**, 67–104.

Bauer M, Whybrow PC, Angst J *et al.* (2002). World Federation of Societies of Biological Psychiatry (WFSBP) Guidelines for Biological Treatment of Unipolar Depressive Disorders, Part 1: Acute and continuation treatment of major depressive disorder. *World Journal of Biological Psychiatry*, **3**, 5–43.

Beasley CM Jr, Dornseif BE, Bosomworth JC *et al.* (1991). Fluoxetine and suicide: a meta-analysis of controlled trials of treatment for depression. *British Medical Journal*, **303**, 685–692.

Brådvik L and Berglund M (2000). Treatment and suicide in severe depression: a case–control study of antidepressant therapy at last contact before suicide. *Journal of ECT*, **16**, 399–408.

Calabrese JR, Elhaj O, Gajwani P *et al.* (2005). Clinical highlights in bipolar depression: focus on atypical antipsychotics. *Journal of Clinical Psychiatry*, **66**, 26–33.

Cardish RJ (2007). Psychopharmacologic management of suicidality in personality disorders. *Canadian Journal of Psychiatry*, **52**, 115S–127S.

Cipriani A, Pretty H, Hawton K *et al.* (2005). Lithium in the prevention of suicidal behavior and all-cause mortality in patients with mood disorders: a systematic review of randomized trials. *American Journal of Psychiatry*, **162**, 1805–1819.

Coppen A, Standish-Barry H, Bailey J *et al.* (1991). Does lithium reduce the mortality of recurrent mood disorders? *Journal of Affective Disorders*, **23**, 1–7.

Davidson JR (2004). Use of benzodiazepines in social anxiety disorder, generalized anxiety disorder, and posttraumatic stress disorder. *Journal of Clinical Psychiatry*, **65**, 29–33.

Falkai P, Wobrock T, Lieberman J *et al.* (2005). World Federation of Societies of Biological Psychiatry (WFSBP) Guidelines for Biological Treatment of Schizophrenia, Part 1: acute treatment of schizophrenia. *World Journal of Biological Psychiatry*, **6**, 132–191.

FDA Public Health Advisory (2004). *Suicidality in Children and Adolescents being Treated with Antidepressant Medications*. Available at http://www.fda.gov/cder/drug/antidepressants/SSRIPHA200410.htm, accessed 15 October 2004.

Fergusson D, Doucette S, Glass KC *et al.* (2005). Association between suicide attempts and selective serotonin reuptake inhibitors: systematic review of randomised controlled trials. *British Medical Journal*, **330**, 396.

Fink M (2005). Is the practice of ECT ethical? *World Journal of Biological Psychiatry*, **6**, 38–43.

Fleischhacker WW, Rabinowitz J, Kemmler G *et al.* (2005). Perceived functioning, well-being and psychiatric symptoms in patients with stable schizophrenia treated with long-acting risperidone for 1 year. *British Journal of Psychiatry*, **187**, 131–136.

Gibbons RD, Hur K, Bhaumik DK *et al.* (2005). The relationship between antidepressant medication use and rate of suicide. *Archives of General Psychiatry*, **62**, 165–172.

Goodwin FK, Fireman B, Simon GE *et al.* (2003). Suicide risk in bipolar disorder during treatment with lithium and divalproex. *Journal of the American Medical Association*, **290**, 1467–1473.

Goodwin GM (2003). Evidence-based guidelines for treating bipolar disorder: recommendations from the British Association for Psychopharmacology. *Journal of Psychopharmacology*, **17**, 149–173.

Grunebaum MF, Ellis SP, Li S *et al.* (2004). Antidepressants and suicide risk in the United States, 1985–1999. *Journal of Clinical Psychiatry*, **65**, 1456–1462.

Grunze H, Kasper S, Goodwin G *et al.* (2002). World Federation of Societies of Biological Psychiary (WFSBP) guidelines for biological treatment of bipolar disorders, Part I: Treatment of bipolar depression. *World Journal of Biological Psychiatry*, **3**, 115–124.

Gunnell D, Saperia J, Ashby D (2005). Selective serotonin reuptake inhibitors (SSRIs) and suicide in adults: meta-analysis of drug company data from placebo controlled, randomised controlled trials submitted to the MHRA's safety review. *British Medical Journal*, **330**, 385.

Hall WD, Mant A, Mitchell PB *et al.* (2003). Association between antidepressant prescribing and suicide in Australia, 1991–2000: trend analysis. *British Medical Journal*, **326**, 1008.

Hammad T (2004). *Review and Evaluation of Clinical Data: Relationship Between Psychotropic Drugs and Pediatric Suicidality*. Available at http://www.fda.gov/OHRMS/DOCKETS/AC/04/briefing/2004-4065b1-10-TAB08-Hammads-Review.pdf.

Hammad TA, Laughren T, Racoosin J (2006a). Suicidality in pediatric patients treated with antidepressant drugs. *Archives of General Psychiatry*, **63**, 332–39.

Hammad TA, Laughren TP, Racoosin JA (2006b). Suicide rates in short-term randomized controlled trials of newer antidepressants. *Journal of Clinical Psychopharmacology*, **26**, 203–207.

Hegerl U, Althaus D, Stefanek J (2003). Public attitudes towards treatment of depression: effects of an information campaign. *Pharmacopsychiatry*, **36**, 288–291.

Hegerl U, Bottner AC, Holtschmidt-Taschner B *et al.* (2008). Onset of depressive episodes is faster in patients with bipolar versus unipolar depressive disorder: evidence from a retrospective comparative study. *Journal of Clinical Psychiatry*, e1–e6.

Helgason T, Tomasson H, Zoega T (2004). Antidepressants and public health in Iceland. Time series analysis of national data. *British Journal of Psychiatry*, **184**, 157–162.

Henkel V, Mergl R, Kohnen R *et al.* (2003). Identifying depression in primary care: a comparison of different methods in a prospective cohort study. *British Medical Journal*, **326**, 200–201.

Herpertz SC, Zanarini M, Schulz CS *et al.* (2007). World Federation of Societies of Biological Psychiatry (WFSBP) guidelines for biological treatment of personality disorders. *World Journal of Biological Psychiatry*, **8**, 212–844.

Hilger E, Barnas C, Kasper S (2003). Quetiapine in the treatment of borderline personality disorder. *World Journal of Biological Psychiatry*, **4**, 42–44.

Isacsson G (2000). Suicide prevention—a medical breakthrough? *Acta Psychiatrica Scandinavica*, **102**, 113–117.

Isacsson G, Bergman U, Rich CL (1996). Epidemiological data suggest antidepressants reduce suicide risk among depressives. *Journal of Affective Disorders*, **41**, 1–8.

Isacsson G, Boethius G, Bergman U (1992). Low level of antidepressant prescription for people who later commit suicide: 15 years of experience from a population-based drug database in Sweden. *Acta Psychiatrica Scandinavica*, **85**, 444–448.

Isacsson G, Holmgren P, Druid H *et al.* (1997). The utilization of antidepressants—a key issue in the prevention of suicide: an analysis of 5281 suicides in Sweden during the period 1992–1994. *Acta Psychiatrica Scandinavica*, **96**, 94–100.

Isometsa E, Henriksson M, Heikkinen M *et al.* (1994). Suicide and the use of antidepressants. Drug treatment of depression is inadequate. *British Medical Journal*, **308**, 915.

Isometsa ET, Henriksson MM, Heikkinen ME, Lonnqvist JK (1996). Completed suicide and recent electroconvulsive therapy in Finland. *Convulsive Therapy*, **12**, 152–155.

Kapfhammer HP and Hippius H (1998). Special feature: pharmacotherapy in personality disorders. *Journal of Personality Disorders*, **12**, 277–288.

Kelly CB, Ansari T, Rafferty T *et al.* (2003). Antidepressant prescribing and suicide rate in Northern Ireland. *European Psychiatry*, **18**, 325–328.

Khan A, Khan S, Kolts R *et al.* (2003). Suicide rates in clinical trials of SSRIs, other antidepressants, and placebo: analysis of FDA reports. *American Journal of Psychiatry*, **160**, 790–792.

Khan A, Khan SR, Leventhal RM *et al.* (2001). Symptom reduction and suicide risk in patients treated with placebo in antidepressant clinical trials: a replication analysis of the Food and Drug Administration Database. *International Journal of Neuropsychopharmacology*, **4**, 113–118.

Khan A, Warner HA, Brown WA (2000). Symptom reduction and suicide risk in patients treated with placebo in antidepressant clinical trials: an analysis of the Food and Drug Administration database. *Archives of General Psychiatry*, **57**, 311–317.

Lepine JP, Gastpar M, Mendlewicz J *et al.* (1997). Depression in the community: the first pan-European study DEPRES (Depression Research in European Society). *International Clinical Psychopharmacology*, **12**, 19–29.

Lopez-Ibor JJ (1993). Reduced suicidality with paroxetine. *European Psychiatry*, **8**, 17s–19s.

Mann JJ, Apter A, Bertolote J et al. (2005). Suicide prevention strategies: a systematic review. Journal of the American Medical Association, **294**, 2064–2074.

Meltzer HY and Okayli G (1995). Reduction of suicidality during clozapine treatment of neuroleptic-resistant schizophrenia: impact on risk–benefit assessment. American Journal of Psychiatry, **152**, 183–190.

Meltzer HY, Alphs L, Green AI et al. (2003). Clozapine treatment for suicidality in schizophrenia: International Suicide Prevention Trial (InterSePT). Archives of General Psychiatry, **60**, 82–91.

Möller HJ (1992). Antidepressants—do they decrease or increase suicidality? Pharmacopsychiatry, **25**, 249–253.

Möller HJ (1994a). Non-response to antidepressants: risk factors and therapeutic possibilities. International Clinical Psychopharmacology, **9**, 17–23.

Möller HJ (1994b). Provocation of aggressive and autoaggressive behavior by psychoactive drugs. European Neuropsychopharmacology, **4**, 232–234.

Möller H-J (1999). Effectiveness and safety of benzodiazepines. Journal of Clinical Psychopharmacology, **19**, 2S–11S.

Möller HJ (2000). Definition, psychopharmacological basis and clinical evaluation of novel/atypical neuroleptics: methodological issues and clinical consequences. World Journal of Biological Psychiatry, **1**, 75–91.

Möller HJ (2002). Appearance of the first WFSBP treatment guidelines. World Journal of Biological Psychiatry, **3**, 2–3.

Möller HJ (2003). Suicide, suicidality and suicide prevention in affective disorders. Acta Psychiatrica Scandinavica Supplementum, **108**, 73–80.

Möller HJ (2005a). Antidepressive effects of traditional and second generation antipsychotics: a review of the clinical data. European Archives of Psychiatry and Clinical Neuroscience, **255**, 83–93.

Möller HJ (2005b). Antipsychotic and antidepressive effects of second generation antipsychotics. Two different pharmacological mechanisms? European Archives of Psychiatry and Clinical Neuroscience, **255**, 190–201.

Möller HJ (2006a). Evidence for beneficial effects of antidepressants on suicidality in depressive patients: a systematic review. European Archives of Psychiatry and Clinical Neuroscience, **256**, 329–343.

Möller HJ (2006b). Is there evidence for negative effects of antidepressants on suicidality in depressive patients? European Archives of Psychiatry and Clinical Neuroscience, **256**, 476–496.

Möller HJ and Grunze H (2000). Have some guidelines for the treatment of acute bipolar depression gone too far in the restriction of antidepressants? European Archives of Psychiatry and Clinical Neuroscience, **250**, 57–68.

Möller HJ and Volz HP (1996). Drug treatment of depression in the 1990s. An overview of achievements and future possibilities. Drugs, **52**, 625–638.

Möller HJ, Grunze H, Broich K (2006). Do recent efficacy data on the drug treatment of acute bipolar depression support the position that drugs other than antidepressants are the treatment of choice? A conceptual review. European Archives of Psychiatry and Clinical Neuroscience, **256**, 1–16.

Montgomery SA, Montgomery DB, Green M et al. (1992). Pharmacotherapy in the prevention of suicidal behavior. Journal of Clinical Psychopharmacology, **12**, 27S–31S.

Müller-Oerlinghausen B (1989). Pharmakotherapie pathologischen aggressiven und autoaggressiven Verhaltens [Pharmacotherapy of pathological and aggressive behaviour]. In W Pöldinger and W Wagner, eds, Aggression, Selbstaggression, Familie und Gesellschaft [Aggression, self-aggression, family and society], pp. 121–134. Springer, Berlin, Heidelberg, New York.

Müller-Oerlinghausen B and Berghofer A (1999). Antidepressants and suicidal risk. Journal of Clinical Psychiatry, **60**, 94–99.

Oquendo MA, Malone KM, Ellis SP et al. (1999). Inadequacy of antidepressant treatment for patients with major depression who are at risk for suicidal behavior. American Journal of Psychiatry, **156**, 190–194.

Paykel ES (2001). Impact of public and general practice education in depression: evaluation of the defeat depression campaign. Psychiatria Fennica, **32**, 51–61.

Paykel ES, Hart D, Priest RG (1998). Changes in public attitudes to depression during the Defeat Depression Campaign. British Journal of Psychiatry, **173**, 519–522.

Paykel ES, Tylee A, Wright A et al. (1997). The Defeat Depression Campaign: psychiatry in the public arena. American Journal of Psychiatry, **154**, 59–65.

Perlis RH (2007). Treatment of bipolar disorder: the evolving role of atypical antipsychotics. American Journal of Managed Care, **13**, S178–S188.

Perlis RH, Baker RW, Zarate CA Jr et al. (2006). Olanzapine versus risperidone in the treatment of manic or mixed States in bipolar I disorder: a randomized, double-blind trial. Journal of Clinical Psychiatry, **67**, 1747–1753.

Pfeiffer-Gerschel T (2007). Veränderungen der Verordnungen von Antidepressiva durch niedergelassene Haus- und Fachärzte im Rahmen des 'Nürnberger Bündnisses gegen Depression'. University of Munich, Munich, online dissertation, http://www.edoc.ub.uni-muenchen.de/6619.

Rihmer Z (2001). Can better recognition and treatment of depression reduce suicide rates? A brief review. European Psychiatry, **16**, 406–409.

Rihmer Z (2004). Decreasing national suicide rates—fact or fiction? World Journal of Biological Psychiatry, **5**, 55–56.

Rix S, Paykel ES, Lelliott P et al. (1999). Impact of a national campaign on GP education: an evaluation of the Defeat Depression Campaign. British Journal of General Practice, **49**, 99–102.

Rutz W, von Knorring L, Walinder J (1992). Long-term effects of an educational program for general practitioners given by the Swedish Committee for the Prevention and Treatment of Depression. Acta Psychiatrica Scandinavica, **85**, 83–88.

Schrauzer GN and Shrestha KP (1990). Lithium in drinking water and the incidences of crimes, suicides, and arrests related to drug addictions. Biological Trace Element Research, **25**, 105–113.

Soler J, Pasqual JC, Campins J et al. (2005). Double-blind, placebo-controlled study of dialectical behavior therapy plus olanzapine for borderline personality disorder. American Journal of Psychiatry, **162**, 1221–1224.

Spivak B, Shabash E, Sheitman B et al. (2003). The effects of clozapine versus haloperidol on measures of impulsive aggression and suicidality in chronic schizophrenia patients: an open, non-randomized, 6-month study. Journal of Clinical Psychiatry, **64**, 755–760.

Stone MB and Jones ML (2006). Clinical Review: Relationship Between Antidepressant Drugs and Suicidality in Adults. Available at http://www.fda.gov/OHRMS/DOCKETS/AC/06/briefing/2006–4272b1–01-FDA.pdf.

Storosum JG, van Zwieten BJ, van den BW et al. (2001). Suicide risk in placebo-controlled studies of major depression. American Journal of Psychiatry, **158**, 1271–1275.

Tandon R, Belmaker RH, Gattaz WF et al. (2008). World Psychiatric Association Pharmacopsychiatry Section statement on comparative effectiveness of antipsychotics in the treatment of schizophrenia. Schizophrenia Research, **100**, 20–38.

Teicher MH, Glod CA, Cole JO (1993). Antidepressant drugs and the emergence of suicidal tendencies. Drug Safety, **8**, 186–212.

Thies-Flechtner K, Muller-Oerlinghausen B, Seibert W et al. (1996). Effect of prophylactic treatment on suicide risk in patients with major affective disorders. Data from a randomized prospective trial. Pharmacopsychiatry, **29**, 103–107.

Tondo L, Hennen J, Baldessarini RJ (2001). Lower suicide risk with long-term lithium treatment in major affective illness: a meta-analysis. *Acta Psychiatrica Scandinavica*, **104**, 163–172.

Tylee A, Gastpar M, Lepine JP *et al.* (1999a). DEPRES II (Depression Research in European Society II): a patient survey of the symptoms, disability and current management of depression in the community. DEPRES Steering Committee. *International Clinical Psychopharmacology*, **14**, 139–151.

Tylee A, Gastpar M, Lepine JP *et al.* (1999b). Identification of depressed patient types in the community and their treatment needs: findings from the DEPRES II (Depression Research in European Society II) survey. DEPRES Steering Committee. *International Clinical Psychopharmacology*, **14**, 153–65.

Ursano RJ, Bell C, Eth S *et al.* (2004). Practice guideline for the treatment of patients with acute stress disorder and posttraumatic stress disorder. *American Journal of Psychiatry*, **161**, 3–31.

Wasserman D (2006). *Depression: The Facts*. Oxford University Press, Oxford.

Zanarini MC and Frankenburg FR (2001). Olanzapine treatment of female borderline personality disorder patients: a double-blind, placebo-controlled pilot study. *Journal of Clinical Psychiatry*, **62**, 849–854.

# CHAPTER 55

# Severe anxiety and agitation as treatment modifiable risk factors for suicide

Jan Fawcett

## Abstract

This chapter focuses on the presence of symptoms of severe anxiety and agitation in depressed patients, as an indicator of heightened suicide risk and a target for treatment to reduce suicide risk. Published evidence demonstrates that from 33–70 per cent of suicides occur in individuals in active treatment by mental health professionals. Clinicians who treat depressed patients who are at high chronic risk for suicide based on prior ideation or attempts, or patients with severe depressive illness who have not admitted suicidal ideation, or given history of prior attempts face a dilemma, since roughly half of patients who complete a suicide have not made previous attempts. Severe anxiety and agitation, often comorbid with depression, are modifiable suicide risk factors if recognized and treated.

## Introduction

While there are many factors that can lead to suicide, and clinical research has pointed out many chronic risk factors for suicide, there is relatively little information to guide the clinician in determining risk factors for suicide in hours, days or weeks from a present assessment.

There is also limited guidance as to what can be done from the standpoint of treatment to reduce the acute risk of suicide, since in many cases patients determined to be at acute risk cannot be hospitalized because of their refusal of hospitalization, and the absence of evidence that would render them capable of being involuntarily hospitalized by most legal standards. Not infrequently, these same patients refuse electroconvulsive therapy (ECT), which can be very helpful in an acutely ill suicidal depressed patient.

While it is standard of care to inquire of a patient about suicidal thoughts or plans, there is ample evidence that denied suicidal ideation is not a useful predictor of acute suicide risk since denial of intent and the non-reporting of suicide ideation is very common prior to suicide; and suicide is common after patients have 'contracted for safety'. (Fawcett et al. 1990; Isometsa et al. 1995; Gladstone et al. 2001). As described, a classic study examining suicidal ideation among 134 suicides, 69 per cent had communicated the suicide ideation within a year of suicide, 60 per cent and 50 per cent to spouses and friends, respectively; however, only 18 per cent approached a helping professional regarding the suicide ideation (Robins 1981; Fawcett 2001). In the absence of a suicide plan and stated intent, the presence of suicidal ideation alone may not be a useful indicator of acute suicide risk. However, it may be an indicator of chronic high risk for suicide. There is, conversely, emerging evidence that psychic anxiety, agitation and panic attacks can be vital markers in identifying those who are at acute suicidal risk (Fawcett 2001).

## Clinical factors associated with acute high risk of suicide

The presence of severe psychic anxiety, panic attacks and/or agitation in a depressed patient can be a helpful indicator of acute suicide risk. This was initially noted in the National Institute of Mental Health (NIMH) collaborative study of major affective disorders: 954 patients (of which about 85 per cent had been hospitalized) were enrolled in a follow-up study and completed the SADS (Schedule for Affective Disorders and Schizophrenia) interview and then followed at 6-month intervals for 5 years and at yearly intervals for an additional 5 years while receiving treatment as usual. After 10 years of follow-up, 34 patients had completed suicide, 13 dying from suicide over the first year of follow-up. These patients were compared with the majority of patients who continued in the study.

The initial findings were vexing in that no differences were found between the patients who completed suicide and the majority of patients in the severity of suicidal ideation recorded, the number of past or recent suicide attempts, and the severity of hopelessness experienced at the baseline episode of depression. When the sample was examined by separating the first year of follow-up from the subsequent 9 years of follow-up, some interesting findings emerged. In the first year, there was no relationship between the outcome of suicide and severity of ideation, frequency of past or recent attempts, or severity of hopelessness, but there was significantly increased severity of psychic anxiety, presence of panic attacks, and severity of insomnia as well as moderate alcohol abuse in the patients who committed suicide. Only in years 2–10 was there evidence of increased severity of suicidal ideation, prior attempts, and hopelessness significantly correlating with suicide (Fawcett et al. 1990).

Anxiety symptoms were rated on the Schedule for Affective Disorders and Schizophrenia (SADS-C) scales for psychic anxiety and panic attacks (Clayton *et al.* 1991). The psychic anxiety rating, depending on both severity and waking time spent experiencing anxiety, were rated on levels of severity and those at a 5 rating (severe anxiety) were counted. The presence of anxiety in major affective disorders is not uncommon, with up to 65 per cent of patients with major depression scoring moderate level anxiety on the SADS, but as shown by Clayton *et al.* (Fawcett and Kravitz 1983) the additive anxiety scores across a sample of 327 patients from the NIMH collaborative depression study (including only patients diagnosed with primary major depression) showed a range of severity of patients diagnosed with primary major depression. This sample, which was chosen to rule out patients with primary anxiety disorders, shows that patients with very high composite anxiety scores comprise about 10 per cent of the group. The number of patients within the highest 20 per cent of summary (overall severity) anxiety scores amounts to less than 5 per cent of the patients in the sample. This illustrates that a very small proportion of patients were found with the severity of anxiety symptoms, which would suggest increased acute suicide risk.

A study of inpatient records of 76 inpatients, who committed suicide in the hospital or within days of hospital discharge, found that while 77 per cent had recorded denials of suicidal ideation as their last recorded communication and 27 per cent had contracted for safety, 67–79 per cent were found to have notes in the record indicating severe anxiety, agitation or both in their records with in 7 days of their suicide, another 20 per cent were rated as 4-moderate-very anxious on the SADS-C (Busch *et al.* 2003).

An earlier case report of three patients who experienced worsening depression and anxiety following the initiation or increase of their fluoxetine dose presented reports of two patients that made potentially lethal attempts by jumping, which by happenstance, did not result in death, but significant injury. One stated 'it was not the depression, but the anxiety that made me want to end my life', while the other patient said that he felt like he was jumping out of his skin and could not tolerate it any longer (Rothschild and Locke 1991).

A study of 100 patients seen in a city hospital emergency room for suicide attempts severe enough to require medical or psychiatric admission found that 90 per cent of the patients described symptoms of severe anxiety within a month of their attempt, while 80 per cent had made 'no-harm contracts' with their therapist (Hall *et al.* 1999).

## Subsequent studies of anxiety and anxiety disorders in various groups

Two studies of prison suicides list anxiety/agitation as a major clinical feature related to suicide. The first, a psychological autopsy study of forty prisoners who had received mental health treatment, found that factors associated with suicide included substance abuse, prior suicide attempts, mental health treatment prior to incarceration, recent 'bad news', recent disciplinary action, and *manifestation of agitation and or anxiety* (Kovasznay *et al.* 2004). It is worth noting here that agitation/anxiety was the only clinical sign noted. The second study reviews all seventy-six suicides that occurred between 1993 and 2001 in the New York State Department of Correctional Services prisons that had some contact with mental health services during their incarceration. This study noted that

'70 per cent displayed agitation or anxiety prior to suicide' and '48 per cent had a behavioural change' (Way *et al.* 2005). A third study investigated suicidal ideation in prisoners and found that a family history of suicidal behaviour, history of psychiatric hospitalization and symptoms of anxiety and depression were independent risk factors for suicidal ideation in prisoners (Lekka *et al.* 2006).

In a study of clinical correlates of anxious depression among elderly patients with depression (Jeste *et al.* 2006), 352 patients aged 59 or older with major depression were studied. The findings showed that 42 per cent of patients showed lifetime anxiety and that *patients with anxious depression were younger, and had greater suicide ideation*. The data clearly demonstrated that co-morbid anxiety disorders amplify the risks of suicide attempts in persons with mood disorders. A study of 20 medically treated suicide attempters and 20 healthy controls (Titelman *et al.* 2004) found that the suicide attempters were anxious.

In a study conducted by Boden and colleagues (2007), they examined anxiety disorders and suicidal behaviours among adolescence and young adults. Data was collected from a 25-year longitudinal study with over 1000 participants from the Christchurch Health and Development Study (CHDS). The results showed that anxiety disorders were strongly associated with suicidal ideation and attempts. Any anxiety disorder (e.g. phobia, generalized anxiety disorder and panic disorder) increased the odds of suicide ideation by 7.96 times (95 per cent CI 5.69–11.13) and suicide attempt rates by 5.85 times (95 per cent CI 3.66–9.32), respectively. The authors also found that the rates of suicidal behaviour increased with the number of anxiety disorders present.

In a study among university students, Eisenberg and associates (2007) examined 2843 students (response rate 56.6 per cent) for prevalence and correlates of depression, anxiety and suicidality. The findings estimated the prevalence of any depressive or anxiety disorder was 15.6 per cent and 13.0 per cent for undergraduates and graduates, respectively. Suicide ideation during the past 4 weeks was reported by 2 per cent of all students.

Sareen and colleagues (2005a) pursued the question whether anxiety disorders are independently associated (i.e. after adjusting for comorbid mental disorders) with suicidal ideation and attempts. The investigators adjusted for sociodemographic factors and all other mental disorders assessed in the survey of 7076 patients at baseline, and 4796 patients in terms of future suicidal ideation and attempts. They found that the presence of any anxiety disorder was associated with an elevated risk for suicidal ideation: odds ratio (OR) = 2.29 and suicide attempts (OR = 2.48). Further analyses indicated that the presence of anxiety, together with any mood disorder, was associated with suicide attempts more often than in the presence of a mood disorder alone. This study demonstrates that a pre-existing anxiety disorder is an independent risk factor for the subsequent onset of suicidal ideation and attempts, and that comorbid anxiety disorders amplify the risk for suicide attempts in patients with mood disorders. The same group (Sareen *et al.* 2005b), studied a sample of 5877 patients with 754 patients with suicidal ideation and 259 patients with a suicide attempt in terms of the presence of specific anxiety disorders. They found that post-traumatic stress disorder (PTSD) was the only anxiety disorder associated with elevated rate of suicidal ideation (OR = 2.79, p < 0.01) and suicide attempts (OR = 2.67, p < 0.01).

A number of studies reviewed show a consistent association of suicidal ideation, suicide attempts, and suicide in patients with anxiety symptoms, anxiety disorders, and agitation associated with mood and other psychiatric disorders (Hawgood and De Leo 2008). Similarly, Chioqueta and Stiles (2003) reported that the assessment of anxiety-level symptoms in patients with depressive episodes has special relevance in evaluating suicide risk, indicating the importance of measuring the severity of the anxiety symptoms in order to better understand potential acute suicide risks. Unfortunately, most of the studies were not designed to measure the *severity of the anxiety symptoms* as was noted above by Fawcett and colleagues (Fawcett and Kravitz 1983; Fawcett *et al*. 1990; Fawcett 2001), and Hall *et al*. (1999).

Comorbid anxiety is associated with a higher risk of suicide along with substance and alcohol abuse, family history of suicide, depression recurrence, seasonal effects, rapid cycling and a history for hospitalizations (Dunner 2004). Data from the first 500 patients of the Systematic Treatment Enhancement Program for Bipolar Disorder (STEP-BD) programme showed that lifetime comorbid anxiety disorders were associated with a greater likelihood of suicide attempts. It was found that although substance abuse disorders were particularly prevalent among patients with anxiety disorders, comorbid anxiety appeared to exert an independent deleterious effect on functioning, including history of suicide attempts (odds ratio = 2.45) (Simon *et al*. 2004).

The association of anxiety comorbidity with increased rates of suicidal ideation, suicide attempts and suicide in bipolar patients has been reported (Keller 2006; Simon *et al*. 2006). In a more recent study, Simon and colleagues (2007) investigated the link between comorbid anxiety symptoms in bipolar patients and suicidal ideation and behaviour. The authors examined ninety-eight bipolar patients for a range of anxiety symptoms: panic, phobic avoidance, anxiety sensitivity, and worry and fear of negative evaluation. Using the SBQ (Suicide Behaviours Questionnaire) as a measuring instrument, the results showed that each anxiety dimension (except for worry and fear of negative evaluation) as being associated with a greater SBQ score and rumination. The authors concluded that increased ruminations may play a role in the association between anxiety and suicidal behaviour. Accordingly, anxiety comorbidity with bipolar disorder modestly increases risk for suicide behaviour. Another study noted similar results on comorbid anxiety and suicide risk. Gonda and colleagues (2007) reported that anxiety and depression moderately increases suicide risk, however, anxiety–depression comorbidity increases suicidal risks dramatically. Across all of these studies, it is of note that the anxiety comorbidity is often the only clinical factor mentioned as associated with suicide or suicide attempts, in the midst of a list of historical factors such as substance abuse, prior suicide attempts, and prior hospitalizations.

For the clinician, assessment of severity of anxiety symptoms may be the most informative in terms of the acute risk for suicide. The implications of these studies are that assessment of the severity of anxiety symptoms should be an element of a clinical suicide assessment, and present severe anxiety symptoms can be addressed by the clinician, since anxiety is a treatment modifiable risk factor for suicide.

## Implications for management of acute suicide risk

The above findings, along with clinical experience, suggests that the recognition and aggressive treatment of severe psychic anxiety,

panic attacks and insomnia could reduce the likelihood of suicide in some patients.

There are, of course, no controlled studies showing that any treatment will reduce suicide in acutely suicidal depressed patients. However, there is evidence showing that short-term therapy with clonazepam added to SSRI treatment will enhance therapeutic response, including anxiety symptoms and insomnia over the first 6 weeks of treatment (Londberg *et al*. 2000). Atypical antipsychotic medications have also been effective in reducing anxiety and suicidal behaviour. Sharma (2003) reported significant improvement in the incidence of suicidal behaviour in patients with mood disorders with the use of the atypical antipsychotic drug clozapine. ECT also appears to be acutely beneficial for suicidality.

It has been reported that other atypical antipsychotic medications, olanzapine and quetiapine will reduce suicidal ideation as well as anxiety within 4–7 days of treatment (McIntyre and Katzman 2003; Houston *et al*. 2003; Thase *et al*. 2006). Fawcett (2001) states that other medications, e.g. anxiolytic agents (benzodiazepines), reduce high-risk characteristics of suicidality, i.e. panic, anxiety, and agitation, effectively. In addition, anticonvulsant medication (e.g. divalproex) can be used to reduce agitation. Fawcett adds that aggressive treatments, similar to the above-mentioned, can be life-saving for those with severe anxiety and ultimate acute suicide risk.

This is important because it has been shown that antidepressant treatment alone does not reduce suicide compared to placebo over eight weeks of treatment in FDA studies (Khan *et al*. 2003), even though several studies have shown a reduction in suicidal ideation with SSRI treatment. Antidepressant treatment alone cannot be relied upon to decrease suicide risk in the short term. Treatment with antidepressant medications, lithium, and antipsychotic medications alone or in combination for at *least 6 months*, show a 2.5 times reduction in suicide risk with combination treatment being the most effective in reducing deaths (Angst *et al*. 2002, 2005).

It is clear that a portion of patients who commit suicide do not show increased anxiety/agitation prior to their suicide or that it is masked. For example, one such patient was obtaining short-acting benzodiazepines secretly from a second doctor who was not aware that he was in treatment for depression, unbeknown to his treating psychiatrist, resulting in his taking double the dose of benzodiazepines prescribed by a physician and probably masking severe anxiety symptoms. This patient shot himself two weeks after he stopped all anxiolytic medication and began consuming alcoholic beverages. Based on clinical experience, patients who do not fully recover from depression with treatment and make elaborate plans over time to commit suicide may not exhibit signs and symptoms of severe anxiety/agitation prior to suicide and give no clinical signs of distress while they deny any plan. There is no available evidence at this time concerning the proportion of detectable severe anxiety prior to suicide. Based on the evidence reviewed here and clinical experience, the present estimate would be that at least 50 per cent of suicidal depressed patients (including outpatients) may show potentially detectable clinical risk factors of severe anxiety/agitation (70 per cent for inpatients and prisoners), if they are carefully assessed for anxiety symptoms by an alert clinician.

Utilization of the findings of Coryell and Young (2005) could be helpful in some of these cases. These investigators found that a rating of severe or very severe on the suicide tendencies scale of the Schedule for Affective Disorders and Schizophrenia (SADS-C) predicted subsequent suicide to a greater extent than a history of past suicide attempts alone. The additional information provided by the Suicidal Tendencies Scale is a history of mental or behavioural rehearsal of a suicide plan, which may occur in the absence of a suicide attempt. This seems to add predictive power compared with a history of prior attempts alone. An application of the suicidal tendencies ratings in seven cases of inpatient suicide illustrated that patients had a severe (5–6) suicidal tendencies rating (5 in the past and 2 prior to admission). In each case, their rating based on patient report showed declining scores to a level of 2 or mild risk as the last rating prior to their suicide (Busch and Fawcett 2004). This suggests that a past history of severe suicidal tendencies may be a more sensitive indicator of present risk during an affective recurrence than what is presented by the patient concerning their current suicide risk state. Patients may be more open about their past suicidal behaviour than they are likely to be candid about their current level of suicidal tendencies. Thus, high past suicidal tendency ratings in a patient suffering from recurring depression may be a useful guide to the patients current risk, irrespective of their report of their present status. This history, if taken into account, may result in much more probing assessment for evidence of acute suicide risk by a clinician.

## Conclusion

Suicide is difficult, but not always impossible, to prevent in a patient. It is hoped that this discussion may result in a few suicides being prevented by clinicians being alert to the presence of anxiety and agitation symptoms in suicidal persons. Anxiety and agitation in suicidal persons requires a viligant and adequate treatment. The clinician remains in great need of data that will permit a more accurate assessment of acute suicide risk. It is hoped that future research will provide more such information.

## References

Angst F, Stassen HH, Clayton PJ et al. (2002). Mortality of patients with mood disorders: follow up over 34–38 years. Journal of Affective Disorders, 68, 167–181.

Angst J, Angst F, Gerber-Werder R et al. (2005). Suicide in 406 mood-disorder patients with and without long term medication: a 40 to 44 years follow-up. Archives of Suicide Research, 9, 279–300.

Boden JM, Fergusson DM, Horwood LJ (2007). Anxiety disorders and suicidal behaviours in adolescence and young adulthood: findings from a longitudinal study. Psychological Medicine, 37, 431–440.

Busch KA and Fawcett J (2004). A fine-grained study of inpatients who commit suicide. Psychiatric Annals, 345, 11–18.

Busch KA, Fawcett J, Jacobs DG (2003). Clinical correlates of inpatient suicide. Journal of Clinical Psychiatry, 64, 14–19.

Chioqueta AP and Stiles TC (2003). Suicide risk in outpatients with specific mood and anxiety disorders. Journal of Crisis Intervention and Suicide, 24, 105–112.

Clayton PJ, Grove WM, Coryell W et al. (1991). Follow-up and family study of anxious depression. American Journal of Psychiatry, 148, 1512–1517.

Coryell W and Young EA (2005). Clinical predictors of suicide in primary major depressive disorder. Journal of Clinical Psychiatry, 66(, 412–417.

Dunner DL (2004) Correlates of suicidal behaviour and lithium treatment in bipolar disorder. Journal of Clinical Psychiatry, 65, 5–10.

Eisenberg D, Gollust SE, Golberstein E et al. (2007). Prevalence and correlates of depression, anxiety, and suicidality among university students. American Journal of Orthopsychiatry, 77, 534–542.

Fawcett J (2001). Treating impulsivity and anxiety in the suicidal patient. Annals of the New York Academy of Sciences, 932, 94–102.

Fawcett J and Kravitz HM (1983). Anxiety syndromes and their relationship to depressive illness. Journal of Clinical Psychiatry, 44, 8–11.

Fawcett J, Scheftner WA, Fogg L et al. (1990). Time-related predictors of suicide in major affective disorder. American Journal of Psychiatry, 147, 1189–1194.

Gladstone GL, Mitchell PB, Parker G et al. (2001). Indicators of suicide over 10 years in a specialist mood disorders unit sample. Journal of Clinical Psychiatry, 62, 945–951.

Gonda X, Fountoulakis KN, Kaprinis G et al. (2007). Prediction and prevention of suicide in patients with unipolar depression and anxiety. Annals of General Psychiatry, 6, 23.

Hall RC, Platt DE, Hall RC (1999). Suicide risk assessment: a review of risk factors for suicide in 100 patients who made serious suicide attempts. Evaluation of suicide risk in a time of managed care. Psychosomatics, 40, 18–27.

Hawgood J and De Leo D (2008). Anxiety disorders and suicidal behaviour: an update. Curr Opin Psychiatry, 1, 51–64.

Houston JP, Ahi J, Meyers AL et al. (2006). Reduced suicidal ideation in bipolar I disorder mixed-episode patients in a placebo-controlled trial of olanzapine combined with lithium or placebo. Journal of Clinical Psychiatry, 67, 251–259.

Isometsa ET, Heikkinen ME, Marttunen MJ et al. (1995). The last appointment before suicide: is suicide intent communicated? American Journal of Psychiatry, 152, 919–922.

Jeste ND, Hays JC, Steffens DC (2006). Clinical correlates of anxious depression among elderly patients with depression. Journal of Affective Disorders, 90(1), 37–41.

Keller MH (2006). Prevalence and impact of comorbid anxiety and bipolar disorder. Journal of Clinical Psychiatry, Suppl. 1, 1–7.

Khan A, Khan S, Kolts R et al. (2003). Suicide rates in clinical trials of SSRIs, other antidepressants, and placebo: analysis of FDA reports. American Journal of Psychiatry, 160, 790–792.

Kovasznay B, Miraglia R, Beer R et al. (2004). Reducing suicides in New York State correctional facilities. Psychiatric Quarterly, 75, 61–70.

Lekka NP, Argyrious AA, Beratis S (2006). Suicidal ideation in prisoners: risk factors and relevance to suicidal behaviour. A prospective case control study. European Archives of Psychiatry and Clinical Neuroscience, 256, 87–92.

Londberg PD, Smith WT, Glaudin V et al. (2000). Short-term cotherapy with clonazepam and fluoxetine; anxiety, sleep disturbance and core symptoms of depression. Journal of Affective Disorders, 61, 73–79.

McIntyre R and Katzman M (2003). The role of atypical antipsychotics in bipolar depression and disorders. Bipolar Disord, 2, 20–35.

Robins E (1981). The Final Months: A Study of the Lives of 134 Persons who Committed Suicide. Oxford University Press, New York. Cited in J Fawcett (2001) Treating impulsivity and anxiety in the suicidal patient. Annals of the New York Academy of Sciences, 932, 94–102.

Rothschild AJ and Locke CA (1991). Reexposure to fluoxetine after serious suicide attempts by three patients: the role of akathisia. Journal of Clinical Psychiatry, 52, 491–493.

Sareen J, Cox BJ, Afifi TO et al. (2005a). Anxiety disorders and risk for suicidal ideation and suicide attempts: a population-based longitudinal study of adults. Archives of General Psychiatry, 62, 1249–1257.

Sareen J, Houlahan T, Cox BJ et al. (2005b). Anxiety disorders associated with suicidal ideation and suicide attempts in the National Comorbidity Study. Journal of Nervous and Mental Disease, 193, 450–454.

Sharma V (2003). Atypical antipsychotics and suicide in mood and anxiety disorders. Bipolar Disorders, 2, 48–52.

Simon NM, Otto MW, Wisniewski SR et al. (2004). Anxiety disorder comorbidity in bipolar disorder: data from the first 500 STEP-BD participants. American Journal of Psychiatry, 161, 2222–2229.

Simon NM, Pollack MH, Ostacher MJ *et al.* (2007). Understanding the link between anxiety symptoms and suicidal ideation and behaviours in outpatients with bipolar disorder. *Journal of Affective Disorders*, **97**, 91–9.

Thase ME, Macfadden W, Weisler RH *et al.* and the BOLDER II Study Group (2006). Efficacy of quetiapine monotherapy in bipolar I and II depression: a double-blind, placebo-controlled study (the BOLDER II study). *Journal of Clinical Psychopharmacology*, **26**, 600–609.

Titelman D, Nilsson A, Estari J *et al.* (2004). Depression, anxiety, and psychological defense in attempted suicide: a pilot study using PORT. *Archives of Suicide Research*, **8**, 239–249.

Way BB, Miraglia R, Sawyer DA *et al.* (2005). Factors related to suicide in New York state prisons. *International Journal of Law and Psychiatry*, **28**, 207–221.

# CHAPTER 56

# Cognitive treatment of suicidal adults

Jan Beskow, Paul Salkovskis and
Astrid Palm Beskow

## Abstract

The progress of cognitive psychotherapy is accounted for by a systematic use of phenomenology, theory, laboratory research, and clinical studies. Effect studies of problem-solving, interpersonal therapy (which has many traits in common with cognitive psychotherapy), treatment of depression for suicide prevention and a cognitive psychotherapy method especially for treatment of suicide attempters are reviewed. The use of metaphors opens new possibilities. Step by step the researchers approach the suicidal individual's own formulations about their suicidality, developing the language of suicidality. Generally increased problem-solving capacity, more intensive outreach activities, an invitation to the patient to participate more actively in the analysis of their own problems and efforts to ameliorate the feelings of shame and guilt are all efforts to deal with painful interpersonal problems. A growing amount of evidence links these cognitions, emotions and behaviours to attachment problems in early life.

## Introduction

The suicidal person is slowly emerging out of the realm of taboo and the strong prejudices against open communication in which they were trapped for centuries. The suicidal person is emerging as a person in their own right, speaking independently and subsequently leading to genuine understanding of the suicidal process. As part of this progress, cognitive psychotherapy has contributed with the objective of recognizing the patient and the therapist as two researchers of equal value trying to solve a pressing problem, important for the survival of the client. One of the prime reasons for the rapid progress and excellent treatment results in cognitive psychotherapy is the use of the *normalcy theory* of emotion and emotional problems (rather than a theory of pathology). Like anxiety and despondency, suicidal ideation is considered a normal phenomenon with survival value, as well as the potential risk for deterioration into destructive pathology. Such a normalization makes it easier for the suicidal person to accept and talk about suicidal thoughts. Furthermore, the advancement of cognitive psychotherapy is due in part to the systematic use of phenomenology, theory, laboratory research, and outcome studies designed to develop more effective treatments. The aim is to create more

specific models in the context of Empirically Grounded Clinical Interventions (EGCI), an example of the scientist practitioner model (Salkovskis 2002). The strategy involves detailed clinical observation, theoretically driven and clinically relevant experimental studies and attention to treatment outcome. The model has been formulated as a way of understanding the rapid evolution of cognitive psychotherapy. However, it can fruitfully be used for the purpose of understanding the clinical process of cognitive therapy through *collaborative empiricism*, which implies a close collaboration between the clinician and the patient, setting up goals, evaluating outcomes, and adjusting their strategies together with regard to whether the patient is improving as expected or desired. It has been a challenge to use these principles in order to understand, develop and evaluate treatment strategies within the broad and complex area of suicidal behaviour. The outline provided in this chapter will show the long journey of developing treatment strategies, filled with disappointments along with several promising results.

## Outcomes of different strategies

In 1998, Hawton *et al.* conducted a meta-analysis of twenty randomized controlled trials (RCTs). They reviewed the effectiveness of psychosocial and drug treatments of a total of 2452 patients who had deliberately harmed themselves (self-poisoning or self-injury) divided into 10 groups of treatment strategies. The inclusion criteria were self-poisoning or self-injury shortly before the trial; participants were randomly assigned to treatment and control groups, with repeat of deliberate self-harm as the *primary outcome criterion*. Most of the trials used standard care as the comparison. The results were generally disappointing. The synthesis of results from the meta-analysis revealed no clinically significant improvements, either in the general sample or in the specific subgroups. The authors concluded that there was insufficient evidence on which to base firm recommendations about the most effective forms of treatment for patients who deliberately harmed themselves. Some promising results were, however, found for problem-solving therapy (Hawton *et al.* 1987; Salkovskis *et al.* 1990; McLeavey *et al.* 1994), depot flupenthixol (Montgomery *et al.* 1979), dialectic behaviour therapy (DBT) (Linehan *et al.* 1991; Linehan 1993) and for the provision of an emergency contact card in addition to standard care. There was no evidence that antidepressants were generally effective for these patients. The authors recommended that researchers design studies in which the statistical power is assessed in advance, probably leading to larger samples, and that they maximize the treatment effects through assertive reminders for poorly compliant patients.

## Problem-solving therapy

It is a well-known fact that suicidal people have a lot of problems or, seen from another angle, that they are psychosocially deprived. It is self evident that an increase in problem-solving capacity may first reduce the burden of unsolved problems and, second, reduce suicidal feelings. An experimental study (Schotte and Clum 1982) supported this idea theoretically. When comparing university students with and without suicidal ideation, the authors found that during life-stress, poor problem-solving subjects had significantly higher suicidal intent than other students. There is also considerable consensus regarding how to teach patients such strategies (Hawton et al. 1989; Heard 2000; Salkovskis 2001; Hawton and James 2005; Reinecke 2006). The patient can usually be motivated for the treatment when they understand how their low problem-solving capacity causes repeated failures to reach subjectively desirable goals, thus causing disappointment and psychological distress. A strategy involving a reduction of problems into small manageable steps is designed through problem listing, prioritizing the most important problem, brainstorming on possible solutions, selection of the most appropriate way to tackle the problems, identifying the first steps as well as psychological obstacles and monitoring the whole process. Every difficulty met by the patient during the process is reframed as a learning opportunity. The patient is also trained in generalizing their advances to new situations. This procedure thus introduces rational thinking to the client, helping them to separate themself from the problems. However, Williams (2001) noted that 'unsurprisingly', patients with less severe problems tend to show the largest response to problem-solving therapy.

In a new meta-analysis of five of the studies with problem-solving strategies in the study mentioned above, and one new study (Townsend et al. 2001), it was demonstrated that even if a group analysis of reduced repetition rate did not show significant improvement, the *secondary outcome criteria* significantly improved, in comparison with treatment as usual. They found improvements not only of their problems (OR = 2.31; 95 per cent CI 1.29 to 4.13) but also of their scores for depression (standardized mean difference = −0.36; 95 per cent CI −0.61 to −0.11) and hopelessness (weighted mean difference = −3.2; 95 per cent CI −4.0 to −2.41). Salkovskis et al. (1990) also found evidence of an effect on the rates of repetition over the 6 months after treatment. The relationship between problem-solving deficits and suicidality appear to be complex. Experimental studies have further elucidated this phenomenon. The major burden of problems is attributed to personal conflicts. The skills to solve such problems can be measured by the Means–Ends Problem-Solving Procedure (MEPS) (Platt et al. 1975). Using this method, Mitchell and Madigan (1984) were able to show that people who were depressed scored lower than those who were not depressed. Schotte et al. (1990) used the same method in a short-term, longitudinal study of 36 patients hospitalized for 'suicide observation', 39 per cent of whom were admitted for a suicide attempt and 22 per cent for reported past attempts. The researchers found marked improvements within one week in depressive symptoms: the number of patients with Beck Depression Inventory (BDI) scores over 21 decreased from 78 to 11 per cent, and also in states of anxiety and hopelessness. The changes were associated with improvements in interpersonal problem-solving skills. Such deficits thus seem to be concomitant with other symptoms (states of vulnerability) rather than a relative stable cause of depression, hopelessness and suicide intent (vulnerability traits).

Williams et al. (2005) also used the MEPS instrument in a study of three groups of participants (N = 34); one with no history of depression, one with previous history of depression without suicidality, and one with a previous depression combined with suicidal ideation and behaviour. Low mood was brought about among the participants through sad music and the reading of sentences with sad content. In the last group, the suicidal thoughts of the patients were activated and their capacity to solve interpersonal problems decreased. These results support the hypothesis of low problem-solving deficit as a state as opposed to a trait phenomenon. It also points out that suicidal ideas may be present without concomitant depression.

In a European multi-centre study (N = 386 medically treated deliberately self-harming [DSH] patients) McAuliffe et al. (2006) found that passivity and avoidance of problems (coupled with low self-esteem) was the most frequent factor associated with repetition of deliberate self-harm. They concluded that intensive therapeutic input and follow-up are required.

## Broader applications of cognitive psychotherapy

An advantage of problem-solving therapy for suicidal patients is that it is brief, and therefore cheap. The same idea, along with a broader foundation in cognitive theory leading to an multitude of intervention strategies, was used in the PROMACT study, a multi-centre study of 480 patients with recurrent episodes of deliberate self-harm but with no substance use disorder (Tyrer et al. 2003a, b). The patients were randomly assigned to a Manual-Assisted Cognitive Behavioural Therapy (MACT), or to treatment as usual. The patients were sent a 70-page booklet by mail and offered up to 7 sessions of cognitive behaviour therapy. There were no differences in baseline characteristics. The follow-up period was 12 months. The results from the above study were also disappointing. There were no significant differences in either repetition rates of deliberate self-harm, or on secondary outcome criteria such as clinical diagnosis, risk of parasuicide, self-rated anxiety, depressive symptoms or other parameters. The figures however were more favourable at 12 months than at baseline in both groups. A cost-effectiveness evaluation indicated the superiority of MACT over treatment as usual (Byford et al. 2003). The negative results in the previous study may be due to several weaknesses that will be discussed below (Hawton and Sinclair 2003; Arensman et al. 2004 including a reply by Tyrer et al. 2004).

First, patients who did not show up to the first appointment for treatment were offered only one second appointment with no further contact or home visit. Several other studies of patients with deliberate self-harm showing significant differences between experimental and control groups have used a more active approach to the patients (Salkovskis 1990; Guthrie et al. 2001; Brown et al. 2005). This is also true for a few studies with home visits by a nurse or mental health worker but without psychotherapy

(Welu 1977; van Heeringen 1995). Second, the internal drop-out from the therapy was high. Only 60 per cent of the MACT group used both the 70-page booklet and the sessions, 2 per cent did not use the booklet and 38 per cent did not show up at all for the sessions. Third, the group differences were reduced as the MACT therapists were not well-trained cognitive therapists but ordinary hospital staff with short training. On the other hand, the treatment as usual included psychological treatment in various degrees, such as problem-solving approaches and dynamic psychotherapy.

## Interpersonal therapy

Interpersonal problems may be perceived as a major cause of suicidal problems. As a treatment tradition especially focusing on such problems, interpersonal therapy was primarily used in the treatment of depression and focused on the relationship between the onset of depressive symptoms and the patients' current interpersonal problems (Klerman and Weissman 1989). Such manual-based, focused and active interventions are similar to cognitive therapy, which is clearly demonstrated in the reference lists. It thus seems adequate to discuss it here.

A randomized controlled study (Guthrie et al. 2001) offering interpersonal therapy to patients after deliberate self-poisoning (N = 119) yielded interesting results. The therapy in the intervention group (N = 58) was based on a model by Hobson (1985), and manualized by Shapiro and Startup (1990). The therapy was offered within one week, delivered by nurse therapists in the patient's home, and proceeded for a four week duration. Its focus was to identify and help resolve interpersonal difficulties which caused or exacerbated psychological distress. The control group (N = 61) was offered treatment as usual mostly, by their GPs, that did not include psychological therapy. The two groups were similar in terms of baseline characteristics with the exception of marital status. At the 6 months follow-up the self-reported subsequent episodes of self-harm were lower in the intervention group (9 vs 28 per cent, p = 0.009), and the differences in scores on the Beck scale for suicidal ideation were significantly lower, after a correction for marital status (p = 0.027). The patients' satisfaction with the therapy was significantly greater in the intervention group. The good results were obtained in spite of the fact that only 35 patients participated in all 4 sessions, and 50 patients in more than 2 sessions.

The strengths of the study discussed by the authors are the RCT design and the use of a method that previously has shown good results in treatment of other disorders (Guthrie et al. 1991; Shapiro et al. 1995). The good results may partly be due to the rapid intervention in the participants' home, the focus on interpersonal problems eliciting psychological distress, and the clear differences between intervention and control group. The limitation was that the rate of self-harm at follow-up was based on self-reports, data which is usually weaker than hospital admissions. On the other hand the broader range of self-harm in self-reports includes events that are often neglected in other studies.

## New ways of understanding and treating depression

The dominant hypothesis in psychiatry concerning the origin of suicidality starts from the fact that mental disorders, especially depression, are important risk factors. In the classification of psychiatric disorders, the DSM-IV (American Psychiatric Association 1994), suicidal ideation and acts are presented as symptoms of depression. It is a clinical and scientific fact that suicidal thoughts often vanish after effective treatment of a depressive episode. Adequate treatment of depressive disorders is generally accepted as an effective method for suicide prevention.

Aaron Beck observed the importance of cognitions in the development of depression. He enriched the understanding of the field with many new mediating factors. Dysfunctional thinking, especially always interpreting experiences in a negative way (habitual negative thinking) may lead to a de-evaluation of the self and feelings of helplessness, hopelessness and perception of a black future. Other 'thinking errors' are for instance the claim to understand other persons' thoughts without asking them (mind-reading), taking everything too personally (personalization) and overgeneralizing the importance of negative, subjective experiences (Beck 1967; Clark et al. 1999). These factors may start vicious spirals leading to more and more severe depression. In experiments using a number of new scales it was possible to demonstrate, quantitatively, the interaction of such factors in the development of depression, and their importance for creating and maintaining suicidal thoughts and plans. Based on these and other assumptions, a wealth of cognitive techniques have been developed for the treatment of depression. In numerous studies those methods have been shown to be as effective as drugs in the treatment of depression and anxiety disorders. Cognitive psychotherapy is therefore now accepted as a powerful treatment tool.

Maladaptive thinking (dysfunctional assumptions and attitudes) was typically thought to be elicited by very persistent dysfunctional schemas, i.e. dysfunctional meaning-making structures of cognition, assumed to have a neuronal basis but modified by personal experiences. They could be activated by even small internal and external stimuli and then accepted as true reality. In the therapy situation they could be disclosed by a close observation of the automatic thoughts they give rise to. The dysfunctional assumptions and attitudes could be measured by the Dysfunctional Attitude Scale (Weissman and Beck 1978). If such attitudes were of importance for the relapse of depression, they would be persistent during healthy phases as well. However, Ingram et al. (1998), analysing many such studies, found that this was not the case. The hypothesis that persistent cognitive structures elicit mood changes through dysfunctional coping with external stimuli was then replaced by the counter-hypothesis that even small moments of sad mood could elicit memory biases in the direction of remembering more negative and less positive events. Dysfunctional thinking styles thus existed only under the influence of a sad mood. Nevertheless, they could result in vicious circles leading to a relapse into depression. This 'differential activation hypothesis' (Teasdale 1988) was supported in studies of experimentally induced sad mood. These findings highlight the importance of even brief moments of sad feelings for eliciting depression and suicidality. As a consequence, the training of attention or 'mindfulness' in order to understand and cope with moments of sad mood and negative memory bias, was shown to be useful in reducing the relapse frequency in depression. Such awareness could break the development toward rapidly recurring depressions elicited by even lesser strains (Williams et al. 2000; Segal et al. 2002).

## More carefully elaborated cognitive therapy for suicide attempters

Cognitive psychotherapy involves supporting the client with new concepts, new knowledge and new techniques, adapted to their actual personal needs, and immediately useful in their efforts to change their behaviour. Recently, a manual, specifically for suicide attempters, has been developed (Brown *et al.* 2002, 2006, Henriques *et al.* 2003; Berk *et al.* 2004) and tested in a randomized controlled trial (Brown *et al.* 2005). Ten sessions of cognitive therapy were given to 60 patients who hade attempted suicide and whose suicidal intention still persisted, according to the Suicidal Intent Scale. The intervention group was compared with 60 patients in a control group offered treatment as usual. There were no significant differences in demographic and psychiatric baseline variables. Among the participants 77 per cent had major depressive disorder, 68 per cent substance use disorder, and 85 per cent more than one diagnosis. The cumulative attrition rate at the 18 months follow-up was 25 per cent for the cognitive therapy group and 34 per cent for the treatment as usual group (p = 0.045). The therapists' adherence to the manual was controlled, and divergences were discussed.

The primary aim of the trial, was to decrease the risk of recurrent suicidal acts. Thoughts, images and basic assumptions, activated immediately before the attempt, were identified. Specific strategies to deal with such manifestations were worked out. Attention was also directed to coping with stressful situations and more general vulnerability factors, such as feelings of hopelessness, poor impulse control, low problem-solving capacity, non-compliance during the treatment and social isolation. Towards the end of treatment patients were helped to devise strategies to deal with acute suicidal ideation and intent. After 18 months, 13 (24.1 per cent) in the cognitive group, and 23 (41.6 per cent) in the control group made at least one more suicide attempt (p = 0.49). The probability of repeated suicide attempt was 50 per cent lower in the cognitive group (hazard ratio 0.51; 95 per cent CI, 0.26–0.997). Some secondary measures, the severity of self-reported depression and of hopelessness, were also reduced. Interestingly, suicidal ideation was not significantly reduced.

The strengths of this well-designed and conducted study is its specificity: targeting the suicidal mode as it expressed itself immediately before the act, the inclusion of patients with different psychiatric disorders, including a high percentage of substance use disorders, special study case managers following the patients and making contact when necessary, as well as the creation of action plans for avoiding further suicide attempts at the end of the therapy. The study showed that relatively brief interventions may give positive results, even if the result of the main criterion, a reduced frequency of recurrent attempts, was just on the border of significance. The therapeutic concentration on the acute suicidal episodes is the principal interesting aspect of the study above. Such episodes are usually time-limited, as it is often very time-limited. Thus there are important differences in the risk pattern between a baseline suicide risk and the acute episode (Brown *et al.* 2002; Berk *et al.* 2004; Brown *et al.* 2005; Rudd 2006), requiring a risk analysis in two steps. The suicidal episode is determined by strong rapid influences in a short time, accompanied by a loss of control. It seems likely that the probabilistic perspective is especially useful in terms of acute episodes, with its higher speed in the interaction between the person and the environment.

In these respects, they are similar to accidents (Beskow 1983; Clarke and Lester 1989; Reason 2006).

## An evolution-based model

It is popularly believed that suicidal ideation and acts are primarily a form of communication, a cry for help. On the contrary, Williams (2001) and Williams and Pollock (2000) suggested that suicidality primarily emerges from real suffering, eliciting a cry of pain, with communication only as a secondary effect. The inspiration for the model came from ethological research on the reactions of birds to losing a fight over territorial boundaries (Gilbert 1989). The defeated bird lowers its wings and head and retreats; it looks 'depressed' or 'shamed'. Submission saves its life. When there is no place to identify a new territory, the 'depression' continues and the bird becomes easy prey to predators. In humans, theoretically, the same situation occurs when there is no chance for either flight or fight, and where submission is the only available reaction mode. The pain is caused by both feelings and images of being 'defeated', 'closed in' in a trap with 'no way out'. It is then impossible to go on with life. These three components have been elaborated in theory and studied experimentally. Psychological measures and cognitive treatment strategies have been developed.

The feeling of being *defeated* can arise from both external and internal circumstances. Numerous situations in the family, at school and at work can both elicit and maintain feelings of worthlessness, uselessness and powerlessness, giving rise to feelings of being a loser. These feelings may, however, to a considerable extent, be a product of the person's own constructive processes (Ellis 2006; Neimeier and Winter 2006) and may be maintained by dysfunctional schemas, such as negative thinking. Moreover feelings of shame, humiliation and weakness act as a barrier to peers and family, leading to a downward spiral of increased loneliness and a sense of not belonging. Such feelings are also present in exhaustion reactions, with a wish to rest, to be alone and to be sheltered from further painful stimuli. Other types of distorted or biased thinking may add to the negative experience, resulting in feelings of extreme pain. Early in the process, where escape potential is threatened but not yet eliminated, escape attempts will be characterized by high levels of activity, anger and 'protest'. Later in the process the person may feel totally closed in. These feelings may originate from a safety-seeking behaviour with avoidance of specific and concrete experiences, images and descriptions, that evoke strong feelings and a preference for interpreting them by use of general images and descriptions. It has been understood as the construction and use of over-generalized memories (OGM) (Williams and Broadbent 1986; Williams 2001; Williams and Pollock 2001). In these efforts the patients unfortunately also lose the positive feelings necessary for close human relations and for feelings of a meaningful life. Their life will be colourless, silent, numb and odourless. The patient says: 'I am alone', 'I no longer feel alive'. These are the walls of the trap. The experience of a positive future is essential for the feeling of hope and the will to live. Asking patients and controls to describe events that might happen to them within one day, one week etc. up to ten years from now has shown that depressive/suicidal persons anticipate more difficulties, but especially fewer positive events in the future, and that these are correlated with a greater degree of hopelessness (MacLeod *et al.* 1993). A totally dark future informs us that there is no way out of the trap and the ongoing pain.

The possibility of suicide may then be perceived as the least unattractive option.

The psychological model above has recently been tested (O'Connor 2003) in a cross-sectional comparison between 30 patients admitted for deliberate self-harm and 30 controls from the same emergency wards, matched for age, sex and marital status. The escape potential was a composite score of two items, assessing escapability and controllability of 'the most stressful life event that they had experienced in the last six months', and it was assessed on 5-point Likert scales. The defeat scale consisted of four items measuring the degree to which their most stressful recent life event led to feelings of defeat, rejection, loss and failure. The possibility of rescue was operationalized in terms of availability of social support, measured by an 18 item multidimensional instrument. The result gave support to 'the cry for pain' model. Furthermore, the feelings of entrapment in the parasuicidal group were associated with intrusive thinking more frequently than the controls, a characteristic trait in depression. The model can readily be used in psychotherapy and also be the starting point for further scientific development.

## Suicidal images as a refuge

The normality perspective which has been so fruitful within cognitive psychotherapy implies that suicidal images may sometimes be functional, even life-saving. To accept suicide as a way out of the trap may ameliorate the pain and make further living possible.

'During the assault I felt myself first dying and then dead. However, I was not afraid that they would kill me. At home one hour later I looked at myself in the mirror. There was only an empty shell looking at me, a living dead. In that moment I said: "I will fix this as long as I can. When (not if) I can't fix it any more, I will take my life." I will never tell anyone.'

'These thoughts were not the result of pondering the situation but emerged suddenly as a completed decision. These suicidal images however were only linked to carrying it through to a small degree. The thought of suicide was "my place of refuge", comforting knowledge that there was a way out, a way I might take or escape. In the time immediately after, the suicidal images were "good" for me ....

I felt as if I would literally die of shame. I used the whole night in efforts to clean myself. Later the shame spread like a mist over my whole life. At first it lay there as a thick carpet but slowly it penetrated everything.'

Those lines summarize part of an interview with a 34-year-old woman made 14 years after she had been subject to violent sexual assaults (Vea 2006 and personal communication). She tells us about unexpected, sudden and strong emotions that threatened her mental life and about her intensive struggle to master them with rapid cognitions and firm decisions. She lost against her assailants and was consequently overwhelmed by shame and captured in a cage with no way out.

Interestingly, the idea of taking her life emerged immediately and spontaneously. It functioned as a refuge from the intolerable pain, thus underlining that suicidality sometimes may be an adaptive cognitive structure emerging instantly and that depressive symptoms may come later. Williams *et al.* (2006) have shown that in recurrent depressive disorder, suicidal ideas have a much higher consistency compared to the broad variations of other depressive symptoms. They are consistent with the relative ease of achieving changes in symptoms of depression measured by traditional scales compared to changes in cognitive functioning and self-esteem (Grawe 2007). The importance of traumatic experiences for the development of suicidality is now increasingly acknowledged (Meichenbaum 2006). It seems as if the first suicidal episode is often elicited by strong psychosocial strain, but that later episodes are much more easily elicited owing to an increase in vulnerability, just as is the case in depression.

Grasping the rapid images, thoughts, and behaviours of the patient requires an open collaboration on equal terms. However, this type of therapeutic alliance is still not in use everywhere, as noted by a working group of distinguished experts (Michel *et al.* 2002).

'The working group agreed that current mental health practice often does not take into account the subjective experience of patients attempting suicide, and that contemporary clinical assessments of suicidal behaviour are more clinician-centred than patient-centred. The group concluded that clinicians should strive for a shared understanding of the patient's suicidality, and that interviewers should be more aware of the suicidal patient's inner experience of mental pain and loss of self-respect.'

Michel *et al.* (2002, p. 424)

In order to do that the therapist must be prepared to receive and keep the pain of the patient and have a network for their own support.

## Attachment

The trap model summarizes the deep sense many suicidal people have of living in ultimate isolation or rejection. These feelings may be influenced by early acquired schemas. Bowlby's attachment theory maintains that dysfunctional inner 'working models' of the self and the environment develop as a function of the experiences the child has in their family, and may be the result of rejection by parental attitudes (Bowlby 1980). The importance of attachment in borderline states has been further developed by for example Fonagy *et al.* (1995) and in suicidal behaviour by Adam and colleagues (1996).

Studying therapy-refractory affective disorders with retrospective life-charts, Ehnvall *et al.* (2005, 2008) investigated if perception of themselves as being rejected/neglected by either parent in their childhood influenced the respective patients' depressive disorder and the number of suicide attempts. The subjects who felt unwanted had significantly more days of depressive illness, higher percentage of total days in illness over their lifetime and a higher number of illness days per episode. Female patients had a twofold greater chance of making at least one lifetime suicide attempt. Females reporting higher levels of rejection/neglect reported a greater number of lifetime suicide attempts. These findings could not be explained by mood-congruent recall.

From the adult perspective, there is a growing interest in how suicidal people express themselves (Beskow *et al.* 2005). This interest has led to observations of vicious circles between criticism, e.g. shame and guilt, and consolation, e.g. too much eating and drinking (Firestone 2006). Rudd *et al.* (2001) and Rudd (2006) noted these vicious cycles, and also demonstrated that some schemas are specific to suicidality and quite different from those routinely associated with depression, such as: 'I'm worthless and don't deserve to live' expressing the core belief of unlovability; 'I can't fix this problem and should just die' (helplessness); 'I'd rather die than feel this way' (poor distress tolerance) and 'everyone would be better off if I were dead' (perceived burdenness). A cascade of such themes can rapidly elicit a life-threatening situation for the patient. These verbal expressions may be seen as expressions of painfully frustrated basic needs of attachment, pleasure/avoidance of pain, self-enhancement and orientation/control (Grawe 2007). Probably these needs will best be provided for by a positive approach, opening the window for positive psychotherapy (Wingate *et al.* 2006).

## Conclusions

During the development of cognitive psychotherapy, the understanding of suicidality has changed profoundly from primarily a symptom of depression (a pathological perspective) to the result of a complex interaction of many cognitive, emotional and behavioural structures (a normal and systemic perspective). The suicidal process may be seen as a cognitive process of its own, separated from, but interacting with, depressive processes. All those structures interact in a very complex way on different levels of personality organization. They may primarily be functional coping strategies, such as avoidance of experienced harmful situations in personal relations, but later they may change toward dysfunction with increasing difficulties in solving interpersonal problems. The pain before a self-destructive act is often expressed in a vivid inner debate concerned with the questions of belonging or not belonging and the meaning of one's own life, often sandwiched in with an elaboration and evaluation of different methods of self-destruction.

Cognitive therapy, increased problem-solving capacity, outreach activities and an invitation to the patient to take a more participative role in the analysis of their own problems (features which have been successful for patients with other mental disorders, for example schizophrenia), as well as efforts to ameliorate the feelings of shame and guilt so essential in the 'cry for pain' model, are all efforts to deal with painful interpersonal problems and how they can be solved. A growing amount of evidence links these cognitions, emotions and behaviours to attachment problems in early life. Looking at suicidality from the point of view of frustrated, basic needs, the efforts to treat suicidal people may at this time be perceived as preliminary, identified parts of a support system, which eventually will become almost as differentiated and complex as suicidality itself.

## References

Adam KS, Sheldon-Keller AE and West M (1996). Attachment organization and history of suicidal behavior in clinical adolescents. *Journal of Consulting and Clinical Psychology*, **64**, 262–272.

American Psychiatric Association (1994). *Diagnostic and Statistical Manual of Mental Disorders*, 4th edn. American Psychiatric Association, Washington.

Arensman E, McAuliffe C, Corcoran P *et al.* (2004). Correspondence. *Psychological Medicine*, **34**, 1143–1146.

Beck AT (1967). *Depression: Causes and Treatment.* University of Pennsylvania Press, Philadelphia.

Berk MS, Henriques GR, Warman DM *et al.* (2004). A cognitive therapy intervention for suicide attempter: an overview of the treatment and case examples. *Cognitive Behavioral Practice*, **11**, 265–277.

Beskow J (1983). Longitudinal and transactional perspectives on suicidal behaviour. Experiences of suicide prevention in Sweden. In K Achté, K Nieminen, J Vikkula, eds, *Suicide Research II. Proceedings of the Symposium on Suicide Research by the Yrjö Jahnsson Foundation,* pp. 55–64. Psychiatrica Fennica 1982, suppl, Helsinki.

Beskow J, Palm Beskow A, Ehnvall A (2005). *Language of suicide.* [Suicidalitetens språk.] Studentlitteratur, Lund.

Bowlby J (1980). *Attachment and Loss: Loss, Sadness and Depression.* Hogarth Press, London.

Brown GK, Henriques GR, Ratto C *et al.* (2002). *Cognitive Therapy Treatment Manual for Suicide Attempters.* University of Pennsylvania, Philadelphia.

Brown GK, Jeglic E, Henriques GR *et al.* (2006). Cognitive therapy, cognition, and suicidal behaviour. In T Ellis, *Cognition and Suicide. Theory, Research and Therapy*, pp. 53–74. American Psychological Association, Washington.

Brown GK, Ten Have T, Henriques GR *et al.* (2005). Cognitive therapy for the prevention of suicide attempts. A randomized controlled trial. *JAMA*, **294**, 563–570.

Byford S, Knapp M, Greenshields J *et al.* (2003). Cost-effectiveness of brief cognitive behaviour therapy versus treatment as usual in recurrent deliberate self-harm: a rational decision-making approach. *Psychological Medicine*, **33**, 977–986.

Clark D, Beck AT, Alford B (1999). *Scientific Foundations of Cognitive Theory and Therapy of Depression.* John Wiley & Sons, New York.

Clarke R and Lester D (1989). *Suicide: Closing the Exits.* Springer-Verlag, New York.

Ehnvall A, Palm-Beskow A, Beskow J *et al.* (2005). Perception of rearing circumstances relates to course of illness in patients with therapy-refractory affective disorders. *Journal of Affective Disorders*, **86**, 299–303.

Ehnvall A, Parker GB, Hadzi-Pavlovic D *et al.* (2008). Perception of rejecting and neglectful parents in childhood relates to lifetime suicide attempts for females – but not for males. *Acta Psychiatrica Scandinavica*, **117**, 50–56.

Ellis T (2006). Introduction. In T Ellis, *Cognition and Suicide. Theory, Research and Therapy*, pp. 3–9. American Psychological Association, Washington.

Firestone L (2006). Suicide and the inner voice. In T Ellis, *Cognition and Suicide. Theory, Research and Therapy*, pp. 146–169. American Psychological Association, Washington.

Fonagy P, Steele H, Steele M *et al.* (1995). Attachment, the reflective self, and borderline states. The predictive specificity of the adult attachment interview and pathological emotional development. In S Goldberg, R Muir and J Kerr, eds, *Attachment Theory: Social Developmental and Clinical Perspectives,* pp. 233–278. Analytic Press, Hilsdale, New Jersey.

Gilbert P (1989). *Human Nature and Suffering.* Lawrence Erlbaum Associates, Hove and London.

Grawe K (2007). *Neuropsychotherapy. How the Neurosciences Inform Effective Psychotherapy.* Lawrence Erlbaum Associates, London.

Guthrie E, Creed F, Dawson D *et al.* (1991). A controlled trial of psychological treatment for the irritable bowel syndrome. *Gastroenterology*, **100**, 450–457.

Guthrie E, Kapur N, Mackway-Jones K *et al.* (2001). Randomised control trial of brief psychological intervention after deliberate self-poisoning. *British Medical Journal*, **323**, 1–5.

Hawton K and James A (2005). Suicide and deliberate self harm in young people. *British Medical Journal*, **330**, 891–894.

Hawton K and Sinclair J (2003). The challenge of evaluating the effectiveness of treatments for deliberate self-harm. *Psychological Medicine*, **33**, 955–58.

Hawton K, Arensman E, Townsend E *et al.* (1998). Deliberate self-harm: systematic review of efficacy of psychosocial and pharmcological treatments in preventing repetition. *British Medical Journal*, **317**, 441–447.

Hawton K, McKeown S, Day A *et al.* (1987). Evaluation of out-patient counselling compared with general practitioner care following overdoses. *Psychological Medicine*, **17**, 751–761.

Hawton KA, Kirk J, Clark DM (eds) (1989). *Cognitive Behaviour Therapy for Psychiatric Problems. A Practical Guide.* Oxford University Press, Oxford.

Heard HL (2000). Psychotherapeutic approaches to suicidal ideation and behaviour. In K Hawton and K van Heeringen, eds, *The International Handbook of Suicide and Attempted Suicide,* pp. 503–518. John Wiley & Sons, New York.

Henriques GR, Beck AT, Brown GK (2003). Cognitive therapy for adolescent and young adult suicide attempters. *Behaviour Scientific Law,* **46**, 1258–1268.

Hobson RF (1985). *Forms of Feeling.* Tavistock Publications, London.

Ingram RE, Miranda J, Segal ZV (1998). *Cognitive Vulnerability to Depression.* Guilford Press, New York.

Klerman GL and Weissman MM (1989). *Interpersonal Psychotherapy of Depression.* Basic Books, New York.

Linehan MM (1993). *Cognitive-behavioral Treatment of Borderline Personality Disorder.* Guilford Press, New York.

Linehan MM, Armstrong HE, Suarez A *et al.* (1991). Cognitive-behavioural treatment of chronically parasuicidal borderline patients. *Archives of General Psychiatry,* **48**, 1060–1064.

MacLeod AK, Rose GS, Williams JMG (1993). Components of hopelessness about the future in parasuicides. *Cognitive Therapy and Research,* **17**, 441–455.

McAuliffe C, Corcoran P, Keeley HS *et al.* (2006). Problem-solving ability and repetition of deliberate self-harm: a multicenter study. *Psychological Medicine,* **36**(1), 45–55.

McLeavey BC, Daly RJ, Ludgate JW *et al.* (1994). Interpersonal problem-solving skills training in the treatment of self-poisoning patients. *Suicide and Life-threatening Behaviour,* **24**, 382–394.

Meichenbaum D (2006). Trauma and suicide: a constructive narrative perspective. In T Ellis, *Cognition and Suicide. Theory, Research and Therapy,* pp. 333–353. American Psychological Association, Washington.

Michel K, Maltsberger JT, Jobes DA *et al.* (2002). Case study. Discovering the truth in attempted suicide. *American Journal of Psychotherapy,* **56**, 424–437.

Mitchell JE and Madigan RJ (1984). The effects of induced elation and depression on interpersonal problem-solving. *Cognitive Therapy and Research,* **8**, 277–285.

Montgomery SA, Montgomery DB, Jayanthi-Rani S *et al.* (1979). Maintenance therapy in repeat suicidal behaviour: a placebo controlled trial. *Proceedings of 10th International Congress for Suicide Prevention and Crisis Intervention,* pp. 227–229. IASP Congress, Ottawa.

Neimeier RA and Winter DA (2006). To be or not to be: personal constructions of the suicidal choice. In T Ellis, *Cognition and Suicide. Theory, Research and Therapy,* pp. 149–169. American Psychological Association, Washington.

O'Connor RC (2003). Suicidal behaviour as a cry of pain: test of a psychological model. *Archives of Suicide Research,* **7**, 297–308.

Platt J, Spivack G, Bloom W (1975). *Manual for the Means–Ends Problem-Solving Procedure (MEPPS): A Measure of Interpersonal Problem-solving Skill.* Hahnemann Medical College and Hospital, Philadelphia.

Reason J (2006). *Human Error,* 17th edn. Cambridge University Press, Cambridge.

Reinecke MA (2006). Problem-solving: a conceptual approach to suicidality and psychotherapy. In T Ellis, *Cognition and Suicide. Theory, Research and Therapy,* pp. 237–260. American Psychological Association, Washington.

Rudd MD (2006). Fluid vulnerability theory: a cognitive approach to understanding the process of acute and chronic suicide risk. In T Ellis, *Cognition and Suicide. Theory, Research and Therapy,* pp. 355–368. American Psychological Association, Washington.

Rudd MD, Joiner T, Rajab MH (2001). *Treating Suicidal Behavior. An Effective, Time-limited Approach.* The Guilford Press, London.

Salkovskis PM (2001). Psychological treatment of suicidal patients. In D Wasserman, ed., *Suicide—An Unnecessary Death,* pp. 161–172. Martin Dunitz, London.

Salkovskis PM (2002). Empirically grounded clinical interventions: cognitive-behavioural therapy progresses through a multidimensional approach to clinical science. *Behavioural and Cognitive Psychotherapy,* **30**, 3–9.

Salkovskis PM, Atha C, Storer D (1990). Cognitive-behavioural problem-solving in the treatment of patients who repeatedly attempt suicide. A controlled trial. *British Journal of Psychiatry,* **157**, 871–876.

Schotte DE and Clum GA (1982). Suicide ideation in a college population: a test of a model. *Journal of Consulting and Clinical Psychology,* **50**, 690–696.

Schotte DE, Cools J, Payvar S (1990). Problem-solving deficits in suicidal patients. Trait vulnerability or state phenomenon? *Journal of Consulting and Clinical Psychology,* **58**, 562–564.

Segal ZV, Williams JMG, Teasdale JD (2002). *Mindfulness-based Cognitive Therapy for Depression. A New Approach to Preventing Relapse.* The Guilford Press, New York.

Shapiro DA and Startup MJ (1990). *Raters´ Manual for the Sheffield Psychotherapy Rating Scale.* MRC/ESRC Social and Applied Psychology Unit, University of Sheffield (Memo No. 1154), Sheffield.

Shapiro DA, Rees A, Barkham M *et al.* (1995). Effects of treatment duration and severity of depression on the maintenance of gains following cognitive-behavioral therapy and psychodynamic-interpersonal psychotherapy. *Journal of Clinical and Consulting Psychology,* **63**, 378–387.

Teasdale JD (1988). Cognitive vulnerability to persistent depression. *Cognition and Emotion,* **2**, 247–274.

Townsend E, Hawton K, Altman DG *et al.* (2001). The efficacy of problem-solving treatments after deliberate self-harm: meta-analysis of randomized controlled trials with respect to depression, hopelessness and improvement in problems. *Psychological Medicine,* **31**, 979–988.

Tyrer P, Jones V, Thompson S *et al.* (2003b). Service variation in baseline variables and prediction of risk in a randomised controlled trial of psychological treatment in repeated parasuicide: the POPMACT study. *International Journal of Social Psychiatry,* **49**, 58–69.

Tyrer P, Thompson S, Schmidt U *et al.* (2003a). Randomized controlled trial of brief cognitive behaviour therapy versus treatment as usual in recurrent deliberate self-.harm: the POPMACT study. *Psychological Medicine,* **33**, 969–976.

Tyrer P, Schmidt U, Davidson K *et al.* (2004). Correspondence. *Psychological Medicine,* 34, 1144–1146.

Van Heeringen C, Jannes S, Buylaert W *et al.* (1995). The management of non-compliance with referral to out-patient aftercare among attempted suicide patients: a controlled intervention study. *Psychological Medicine,* **25**, 963–970.

Vea I (2006). Godt liv med schizofreni. Dødelig skam. [Good life with schizophrenia. Deadly shame.] *Suicidologi,* **11**, 19–20. Published with permission from the editor of *Suicidology.*

Wasserman D (ed.) (2001). *Suicide—An Unnecessary Death.* Martin Dunitz, London.

Weissman M and Beck AT (1978). Development and validation of the Dysfunctional Attitude Scale. Paper presented at the meeting of the Association for Advancement of Behaviour Therapy, Chicago.

Welu TC (1977). A follow-up program for suicide attempters: evaluation of effectiveness. *Suicide and Life-Threatening Behavior,* **7**, 17–30.

Williams JMG, Barnhofer T, Crane C *et al.* (2005). Problem solving deteriorates following mood challenge in formerly depressed patients with a history of suicidal ideation. *Journal of Abnormal Psychology,* **114**, 421–431.

Williams JMG, Crane C, Barnhofer T *et al.* (2006). Recurrence of suicidal ideation across depressive episodes. *Journal of Affective Disorders,* **91**, 189–194.

Williams JMG, Teasdale JD, Segal ZV *et al.* (2000). Mindfulness-based cognitive therapy reduces overgeneral autobiographical memory in formerly depressed patients. *Journal of Abnormal Psychology*, **109**, 150–155.

Williams M (2001). *Suicide and Attempted Suicide. Understanding the Cry of Pain*. Penguin Books, London, 1st edition 1997.

Williams M and Broadbent K (1986). Autobiographical memory in suicide attempters. *Journal of Abnormal Psychology*, **95**, 144–149.

Williams M and Pollock L (2000). The psychology of suicidal behaviour. In K Hawton and K van Heeringen, eds, *The International Handbook of Suicide and Attempted Suicide*, pp. 79–93. John Wiley & Sons, New York.

Williams M and Pollock L (2001). Psychological aspects of the suicidal process. In K van Heeringen, ed., *Understanding Suicidal Behavior. The Suicidal Process Approach to Research, Treatment and Prevention*, pp. 76–93. John Wiley & Sons, Chichester.

Wingate LRR, Burns AB, Gordon KH *et al.* (2006). Suicide and positive cognitions: positive psychology applied to the understanding and treatment of suicidal behaviour. In T Ellis, *Cognition and Suicide. Theory, Research and Therapy,* pp. 262–283. American Psychological Association, Washington.

# CHAPTER 57

# Dialectical behaviour therapy for suicidal individual

## The international perspective

Barbara Stanley and Beth S Brodsky

## Abstract

Dialectical behaviour therapy (DBT) is an outpatient, cognitive behavioural treatment shown to reduce self-injury and suicidal behaviour in individuals with borderline personality disorder (BPD). In this chapter, we review the basic principles of the DBT approach to the treatment of suicidal individuals, and the status of DBT treatment and research from an international perspective. The diagnostic criteria for BPD (developed and validated in the US) have been found to be applicable to and prevalent among various populations worldwide. The efficacy of DBT in reducing suicidal behaviour in individuals with BPD has led to its widespread adaptation in clinical settings all over the world. International clinical research teams are conducting randomized clinical trials to further test DBT's efficacy in reducing suicidal behaviour and associated symptomatology in borderline populations.

## Introduction

### What is borderline personality disorder?

Recurrent suicidal behaviour and non-suicidal self-injury is a hallmark of borderline personality disorder (BPD), and one of the most difficult aspects of BPD to treat. Dialectical behaviour therapy (DBT) is an outpatient, cognitive behavioural treatment shown to reduce self-injury and suicidal behaviour in this population (Linehan et al. 1993, 2006).

In the US, both suicidal and non-suicidal self-injurious behaviour among individuals with BPD is responsible for a high percentage of both outpatient and inpatient mental health service utilization (Sansone et al. 2005). Until recently, very few mental health treatments, either psychosocial or psychopharmacological, have been effective in treating the symptoms of BPD. The preliminary reports of the efficacy of DBT have stimulated an interest in DBT both across the US and internationally. In this chapter, we will review the basic principles of the DBT approach to the treatment of suicidal individuals, and the status of DBT treatment and research from an international perspective.

## Prevalence

How prevalent is BPD in other countries outside the US? A personality disorder is defined in the *Diagnostic and Statistical Manual of Mental Disorders* (APA 2000) as 'an enduring pattern of inner experience and behaviour that deviates markedly from the expectations of the individual's culture' and therefore, personality disorder is by definition a cultural concept. Paris (1996, 1998) suggested, based on cross-cultural differences in the prevalence of symptoms such as suicidal behaviour, non-suicidal self-injury and completed suicide, that BPD is more frequent in modern than traditional societies. Traditional societies are characterized by slow rates of social change, intergenerational continuity, family and community cohesion, and clear social roles. The aspects of modern culture that would contribute to BPD pathology include a societal emphasis on autonomy, along with less clear social roles that result in reduced support and reference points for identify formation, and decreased family and community cohesion, which can result in destabilization and disintegration of family supports. Paris (1996) hypothesizes that social protective factors of the traditional societies in developing countries suppress the development of borderline traits into a diagnosable disorder.

## BPD on different continents

There are very few systematic epidemiological studies of BPD. The prevalence of BPD in the United States (APA 2000) is estimated to be about 2 per cent of the general population. In a community sample in Oslo, Norway, the prevalence of BPD was 0.7 per cent (Torgersen 2001). Kroll et al. (1982) investigated whether the BPD diagnosis 'exists' in Britain and found that the DSM criteria for BPD (developed and validated in the US) were applicable to and prevalent within an inpatient population in Britain. In the first clinical study of BPD in Asia, Moriya et al. (1993) used the Diagnostic Interview for Borderlines to diagnose 85 Japanese female outpatients and found that 38 per cent met criteria for BPD. The authors concluded that BPD exists in Japan, although the incidence of substance-use disorders is significantly lower than in American BPD populations, and that the Japanese patients were more likely than Americans to live at home and, thus, 'maintain stormy and masochistic relationships with their parents'. Ikuta et al. (1994) compared American and Japanese outpatients and found that the Japanese patients who meet criteria for BPD were basically identical to the American BPD patients. Within the US, Chavira et al. (2003) reported that in treatment-seeking samples, individuals from different ethnicities may present with different types of personality pathology. They found disproportionately higher rates of BPD in Latino participants than in Caucasian and African-American participants. These studies indicate that the diagnosis of BPD can be made cross-culturally and, therefore, treatments for BPD ought to be tested across ethnicities and cultures. To date, DBT has been of interest to and adopted, for the most part, by modern, Westernized countries. The most intensive research in DBT is taking place in the United States, Germany, and the Netherlands. Seven well-controlled randomized clinical trials of DBT have been conducted across four independent research teams (Lynch *et al.* 2006). Other research and clinical programmes exist in Spain, the United Kingdom, Canada, Switzerland, Sweden, and Australia.

## What is dialectical behaviour therapy?

DBT was designed to reduce self-mutilation and suicidal behaviour in the most severe subgroup of the BPD patient population. The treatment aims to provide increased support for patients to stay safe from self-harm on an outpatient basis. In addition to providing for the patient, dialectical behaviour therapy provides support for the therapist working with the chronically suicidal outpatient. DBT was developed by psychologist Marsha M. Linehan (1993), who has provided empirical evidence of its effectiveness in reducing self-injurious and suicidal behaviour in individuals with BPD in the United States. Evidence regarding the actual mechanisms of change in dialectical behaviour therapy is just beginning to emerge, exposing the utility of such therapy in reducing treatment-resistant behaviours within a diagnostic group traditionally difficult to engage and maintain in treatment. According to Lynch *et al.* (2006) DBT's emphasis on mindfulness, validation, targeting, dialectics and chain analysis which are mechanisms of change that 'reduce ineffective action tendencies linked with dysregulated emotions' in individuals with BPD. These mechanisms (which will be described below) arise from the unique dialectic philosophy that underlies the theory and application of DBT, combined with a comprehensive yet straightforward set of cognitive behavioural interventions.

### The dialectic philosophy

The dialectic approach distinguishes dialectical behaviour therapy from behavioural and cognitive behavioural approaches to the treatment of borderline personality disorder, and informs DBT theory and intervention technique. From a DBT perspective, exclusive focus on change in standard behaviour therapy is experienced as invalidating by traumatized or rejection-sensitive individuals, and can result in early drop out or resistance to change within the treatment. However, ignoring the need for change is just as invalidating, in that it does not take the problems and negative consequences of the patient's behaviour seriously. Disregarding the patient's need for change can lead to hopelessness and suicidality. The dialectic strategy aims to introduce acceptance of whatever is valid about the individual's current behaviours and viewing these behaviours as the patient's best efforts to cope with unbearable pain. This acceptance and validation is balanced with change strategies. Change is achieved in the tension and resolution of the essential conflict between acceptance of the individual as they are right now and the demand for change. Patient motivation is enhanced through validation and a non-judgemental stance with emphasis on problem-solving. Therapist motivation is enhanced by acknowledging the responsibility of the patient, as well as by validating the need for therapist support. Validation is a core intervention, in which the therapist recognizes the pain and difficulty of making changes, and places emphasis on understanding the valid aspects of a patient's feelings and experience.

## Individual sessions

In outpatient dialectical behaviour therapy, patients attend at least one individual therapy session of one to one-and-a-half hours each week. The individual therapy session is structured by a number of behavioural techniques. First, patient and therapist work together to identify the target behaviours that the patient wants to change. The patient keeps a daily record of target behaviours, level of misery and suicidal ideation in a so-called diary card (Linehan 1993). Therapist and patient review the diary card together and use it to create an agenda for each session. If the patient has engaged in self-injury during the week, a behavioural analysis (described below) is required. In the absence of self-destructive behaviour, other therapy-interfering behaviour is highlighted and subject to behavioural analysis. In the absence of either self-injury or therapy-interfering behaviour, the patient can choose to address an issue that interferes with their quality of life, such as interpersonal or vocational difficulties.

A major change in technique used in such individual sessions is the step-by-step behavioural (chain) analysis of self-injurious or therapy-interfering behaviour. DBT takes a dialectical approach to behavioural analysis; the vulnerability the patient brings to the situation is identified alongside the precipitating event and the reinforcing consequences of the self-injurious behaviour. The positive consequences for the patient, such as immediate relief from unbearable emotional pain, is highlighted and validated. The patient and therapist then collaborate in reconstructing the series of events (thoughts, feelings, actions and environmental events) that lead to the self-injury. The therapist asks for as much detail as possible, and weaves solutions and alternative ways of conduct used by the patient, into the thread of analysis.

The DBT individual session differs somewhat from other cognitive behaviour treatments in that the therapist insists on behavioural change and problem-solving, balanced with validation of the feelings and positive consequences associated with unskilful behaviours. The focus of DBT intervention is emotion regulation and behavioural change. Although cognitions are also targeted in DBT, they are not the main focus of treatment, as they are in Beck's cognitive therapy for borderline personality disorder, in which the primary target is the 'dysfunctional beliefs' and cognitive distortions of the suicidal individual (Wenzel *et al.* 2006). The individual therapy session and relationship with the therapist is where patients are given direct guidance in how to incorporate skills into their lives. In addition, the individual therapist conducts skills coaching in order to provide the necessary support for the learning of new behaviours. Patients are encouraged to call or page individual therapists between sessions when they are fighting urges to self-injure and need help in implementing an alternative behaviour. During these phone contacts, the therapist and patient decide upon a number of proficient ways of handling the current stressful situation.

## Validation

The behavioural analysis, skills training, and phone coaching are all therapeutic interventions that aim at changing behaviour. All of these change-oriented techniques are balanced in DBT by an equal emphasis on validation: the validation of the patient, their feelings, and any thoughts or behaviours that can be considered valid. Validation is an explicit strategy in DBT for the purposes of enhancing motivation (in both patient and therapist) and for teaching patients to self-validate. As such, it is only effective if the therapist is completely honest. There are certain aspects of any therapy that involve validation, such as the therapist being on time, listening and paying attention, treating the patient with respect, and accurately reflecting back to the patient what they have heard. Most therapies also involve accurate interpretation, which is usually experienced by the patient as extremely validating. DBT expands the concept of validation, focusing on historical validation, where the therapist understands current unskilful cognitions and behaviours within the context of past experience. Biological validation takes the genetic and biological aspects of emotion dysregulation into account when unskilful behaviours are reviewed and targeted. In DBT, the therapist is trained to identify and highlight any aspects of unfit behaviour that seem to be a normal reaction that most people would have to a given event or situation. In the highest level of validation, called radical genuineness, a DBT therapist shares their own difficult experience with the patient in a non-judgemental manner, with the implicit understanding that the patient is an equal, and can handle receiving feedback that is given honestly and in the spirit of wanting to help the patient and/or protect the therapeutic relationship. In DBT, therapists repeatedly validate emotional pain and the difficulty of having to change.

## Skills training

The teaching of skilful behaviours with which to replace the maladaptive ones is a major component of DBT. A weekly skills group serves to introduce and teach the concepts of skills, and provides an opportunity to interact with other patients who are also gathering skills. The four modules of skills target the four areas of dysregulation in patients with borderline personality disorder: mindfulness skills addressing cognitive dysregulation, distress tolerance skills for behavioural dysregulation, interpersonal effectiveness, and finally, emotion regulation skills. Mindfulness, based on a Zen Buddhist philosophy, is the core skill enhancing self-acceptance, and behavioural and emotional regulation. Patients are taught how to mindfully focus their attention on the present moment, to observe and describe without judgement.

## Inter-session coaching and the consultation team

As a behavioural therapy, DBT utilizes and promotes the technique of *in vivo* skills coaching. The individual therapist plays the role of a skills coach, both within and between sessions. Between-session contact is encouraged to give the therapist the opportunity to coach the patient in using skilful behaviours learned during individual or group sessions in the actual moment in which the patient needs to use the newly learned behaviour. Therapist availability for coaching is also aimed at reducing the reinforcement that can result from being available only in a suicidal crisis, thus expanding the opportunity for increased therapist contact in response to skilful help-seeking behaviour. Phone contacts are focused and limited to skills-coaching and relationship repair. DBT therapists need to be available between sessions to support skills acquisition, however, they also need to understand the limits of their availability and are obliged to communicate these to the patient. Therapists meet with a peer consultation team on a weekly basis in order to obtain support for identifying and observing their limits, and to maintain a non-judgemental stance and a therapeutic balance between validation and change. Team members are also available to each other for consultation and support when a therapist is struggling with a patient's suicide risk.

In summary, the individual DBT therapist uses behavioural analysis and contingency management (attending to the reinforcing consequences of behaviours) balanced with validation strategies to decrease self-injury and non-skilful behaviours in the patient. The skills-training component of DBT complements the individual session through the teaching and reinforcement of skilful behaviours.

# Empirical studies of DBT: the US perspective

In randomized clinical trials comparing one year of outpatient dialectical behaviour therapy treatment to 'treatment as usual' (TAU) in the community, Linehan demonstrated that BPD individuals receiving DBT had significantly larger decreases in parasuicidal behaviours, fewer inpatient hospitalizations, and a lower drop-out rate than those in the TAU condition at the completion of one year of treatment (Linehan et al. 1993). In a two-year randomized controlled trial of DBT versus 'therapy by experts' in the community (Linehan et al. 2006), subjects receiving DBT were significantly less likely to make a suicide attempt, required less hospitalization for suicidal ideation and had lower medical risk associated with suicide attempts and non-suicidal self-injury.

Randomized clinical trials designed to replicate Linehan's initial findings as well as to further investigate DBT's efficacy in reducing self-injury and suicidal behaviour in individuals with BPD are being conducted at six sites around the world. In the United States, Linehan's group at the University of Washington in Seattle continues to study DBT's efficacy with BPD individuals as well as within other diagnostic groups such as people with substance abuse. In New York, randomized clinical trials comparing DBT with other psychosocial and psychopharmacological interventions for individuals with BPD are currently being conducted at Columbia University, New York Presbyterian Hospital, Weill Medical College of Cornell University (Clarkin et al. 2004), and Mount Sinai Hospital. Stanley et al. (2007) conducted a DBT 6-month open trial in individuals with BPD and found that suicidality and self-injury urges decreased over time.

# International studies of DBT

In Germany, a number of clinical researchers have adapted and studied DBT for inpatients. Bohus et al. (2000) have hypothesized that the course of outpatient DBT therapy could be accelerated and improved by an initial 3-month DBT inpatient stay. In one of their studies at the University of Freiburg, 31 female patients meeting criteria for borderline personality disorder were placed into a 3-month DBT inpatient trial, while 19 others had been placed on a waiting list and received treatment as usual in the community. The inpatient DBT group showed significantly greater decreases in measures of depression, anxiety, interpersonal functioning, social adjustment, global psychopathology and self-mutilation than did the outpatient TAU group. In a later study, in which twenty-four of these inpatient DBT patients were followed one month after discharge, their decreased ratings in psychopathology and self-injury were maintained compared to their initial baseline ratings upon admission. In another inpatient DBT efficacy study in Braunschweig, Germany (Kroger *et al.* 2005), fifty consecutively admitted individuals with BPD and with high axis I comorbidity showed significant reductions in BPD psychopathology at post-treatment and follow-up.

Comprehensive clinical trials comparing outpatient DBT to TAU have been conducted in the Netherlands. Verheul and colleagues (van den Bosch *et al.* 2002; Verheul *et al.* 2003) have randomly assigned 58 women with BPD, with or without substance-use, to either 52 weeks of DBT or TAU. Those assigned to DBT had significantly greater reductions in suicidal behaviour and impulsivity. At a follow-up assessment, 6 months after the discontinuation of DBT (van den Bosch *et al.* 2005), the benefits of DBT over TAU in terms of decreased suicidal and impulsive behaviours, as well as in alcohol use, were sustained. There were no differences between the two treatment conditions in patients using drugs. These researchers propose that DBT should be 'multi-targeted' within the BPD/substance-use population, to address a number of impulsive behaviours including suicidal and self-injurious behaviours, binge eating and substance use.

A double-blind, placebo-controlled study of dialectical behaviour therapy combined with olanzapine treatment for borderline personality disorder patients has been conducted in Barcelona, Spain by Soler *et al.* (2005). Sixty patients with BPD received DBT and were randomly assigned to receive olanzapine or a placebo. The active medication group who also received DBT showed the most improvement in symptoms of anxiety, depression and impulsive/aggressive behaviour, and also displayed lower drop out rates. The research team did not report any findings related to suicidal or self-injurious behaviours.

Pilot DBT programmes to treat female prisoners with BPD are being implemented by the International Centre for Research in Forensic Psychology at the Department of Psychology at the University of Portsmouth, United Kingdom. In the year long-treatment programme offered to 30 women in three British prisons for women, 33 per cent voluntarily dropped out and a total of 16 completed the programme. A reduction of deliberate self-harm was observed, and the vast majority of those who completed the programme showed improvements in various psychopathology measures.

A short-term intensive DBT treatment for outpatients with BPD in crisis is being studied at the Hôpitaux Universitaires de Genève in Chêne-Bourg, Switzerland (Bernhardt *et al.* 2005). The treatment consists of three weeks of individual therapy sessions, group skills training and team consultation. Over a 2-year study period, 87 individuals were admitted to the programme, of which 82 per cent completed it and 18 per cent dropped out. Patients showed significant improvement in scores on the Beck Depression Inventory (BDI) and the Beck Hopelessness Scale (BHS). Measures of self-injury and suicidal behaviour were not reported.

Clinical settings that emphasize the DBT approach to the treatment of suicidal behaviour are emerging in various countries. At the Karolinska Institute in Stockholm, Sweden, a small study investigated patients' and therapists' perceptions of DBT treatment. Patients regarded the DBT therapy as life-saving, and both patients'

and therapists' reports were concordant regarding the understanding, respect and confirmation the therapy provided, along with the cognitive and behavioural skills it offered (Perseius *et al.* 2003). Bernhardt *et al.* (2005) report on a unique inpatient acute crisis intervention implemented in Kiel, Germany, using DBT and skills training to focus on improved stress-tolerance and aiming at a fast reintegration into outpatient DBT treatment.

## Conclusion and directions for further research

In summary, the efficacy of DBT in reducing suicidal behaviour in individuals with BPD has led to its widespread adaptation in clinical settings all over the world. International clinical research teams are conducting randomized clinical trials to further test DBT's efficacy in reducing suicidal behaviour and associated symptomatology in borderline populations. Further research will yet have to establish the applicability of DBT to target groups outside the one on which it has primarily been tested until now, i.e. North-American Caucasian suicidal females with BPD. The efficacy of DBT in suicidal individuals with co-occurring substance and alcohol use disorders needs to be tested. There have been no trials ascertaining its applicability and results pertaining to males in general and Latino populations in the United States. DBT applicability to Latinos is particularly important to evaluate considering the high incidence of BPD in this population.

Two other areas for further research on DBT are important: What alterations would make the treatment more accessible to therapists yet still as effective; and what are the 'active ingredients' of DBT that lead to change? Questions such as whether the treatment can be shortened and maintain its efficacy need to be propounded. Furthermore, are the consultation team, skills training, inter-session coaching and all the techniques described in the individual therapy 'mandatory minimums'? In conclusion, although clinically DBT has been adapted to treat various behavioural disorders and altered it in various ways, further empirical research is needed.

## References

APA (American Psychiatric Association) (2000). *Diagnostic and Statistical Manual of Mental Disorders*, 4th edn, text revision. American Psychiatric Publishing Inc., Arlington.

Bernhardt K, Friege L, Gerok-Falke K *et al.* (2005). In-patient treatment concept for acute crises of borderline patients on the basis of dialectical-behavioural therapy. *Psychotherapie Psychosomatik, Medicinische Psychologie*, **55**, 397–404.

Bohus M, Haaf B, Stiglmayr C *et al.* (2000). Evaluation of inpatient dialectical-behavioural therapy for borderline personality disorder—a prospective study. *Behaviour Research and Therapy*, **38**, 875–887.

Chavira DA, Grilo CM, Shea MT *et al.* (2003). Ethnicity and four personality disorders. *Comprehensive Psychiatry*, **44**, 483–491.

Clarkin JF, Levy KN, Lenzenweger MF *et al.* (2004). The Personality Disorders Institute/Borderline Personality Disorder Research Foundation randomized control trial for borderline personality disorder: rationale, methods, and patient characteristics. *Journal of Personality Disorder*, **18**, 52–72.

Ikuta N, Zanarini MC, Minakawa K *et al.* (1994). Comparison of American and Japanese outpatients with borderline personality disorder. *Comprehensive Psychiatry*, **35**, 382–385.

Kroger C, Schweiger U, Sipos V *et al.* (2005). Effectiveness of dialectical behaviour therapy for borderline personality disorder in an inpatient setting. *Behaviour Research and Therapy*, **44**, 1211–1217.

Kroll J, Carey K, Sines L *et al.* (1982). Are there borderline in Britain? A cross-validation of US findings. *Archives of General Psychiatry*, **39**, 60–63.

Linehan MM (1993). *Skills Training Manual for Treating Borderline Personality Disorder*. Guilford, New York.

Linehan MM, Comtois KA, Murray AM *et al.* (2006). Two-year randomized controlled trial and follow-up of dialectical therapy vs therapy by experts for suicidal behaviours and borderline personality disorder. *Archives of General Psychiatry*, **63**, 757–66.

Linehan MM, Heard HL, Armstrong HE (1993). Naturalistic follow-up of a behavioural treatment for chronically parasuicidal borderline patients. *Archives of General Psychiatry*, **50**, 971–974.

Lynch TR, Chapman AL, Rosenthal MZ *et al.* (2006). Mechanism of change in dialectical behaviour therapy: theoretical and empirical observation. *Journal of Clinical Psychology*, **62**, 459–480.

Moriya N, Miyake Y, Minakawa K *et al.* (1993). Diagnosis and clinical features of borderline personality disorder in the east and west: a preliminary report. *Comprehensive Psychiatry*, **34**, 418–423.

Paris J (1996). Cultural factors in the emergence of borderline pathology. *Psychiatry*, **59**, 185–192.

Paris J (1998). Personality disorders in sociocultural perspective. *Journal of Personality Disorder*, **12**, 289–301.

Perseius KI, Ojehagen A, Ekdahl S *et al.* (2003). Treatment of suicidal and deliberate self-harming patients with borderline personality disorder using dialectical behavioural therapy: the patients' and the therapists' perceptions. *Archives of Psychiatric Nursing*, **17**, 218–227.

Sansone RA, Songer DA, Miller KA (2005). Childhood abuse, mental healthcare utilization, self-harm behaviour, and multiple psychiatric diagnoses among inpatients with and without a borderline diagnosis. *Comprehensive Psychiatry*, **46**, 117–120.

Soler J, Pascual JC, Campins J *et al.* (2005). Double-blind, placebo-controlled study of dialectical behaviour therapy plus olanzapine for borderline personality disorder. *American Journal of Psychiatric*, **162**, 1221–1224.

Stanley B, Brodsky B, Nelson JD *et al.* (2007). Brief Dialectical Behaviour Therapy (DBT-B) for suicidal behaviour and non-suicidal self-injury. *Arch Suicide Res*, **11**, 337–341.

Torgersen S, Kringlen E, Cramer V (2001). The prevalence of personality disorders in a community sample. *Archives of General Psychiatry*, **58**, 590–596.

Van den Bosch LM, Koeter MW, Stijnen T *et al.* (2005). Sustained efficacy of dialectical behaviour therapy for borderline personality disorder. *Behaviour Research and Therapy*, **43**, 1231–1241.

Van den Bosch LM, Verheul R, Schippers GM *et al.* (2002). Dialectical behaviour therapy of borderline patients with and without substance use problems. Implementation and long term effects. *Addictive Behaviours*, **27**, 911–923.

Verheul R, Van Den Bosch LM, Koeter MW *et al.* (2003). Dialectical behaviour therapy for women with borderline personality disorder: 12-month, randomised clinical trial in The Netherlands. *The British Journal of Psychiatry*, **182**, 135–140.

Wenzel A, Chapman JE, Newman CF *et al.* (2006). Hypothesized mechanisms of change in cognitive therapy for borderline personality disorder. *Journal of Clinical Psychology*, **62**, 503–516.

# CHAPTER 58

# The psychological and behavioural treatment of suicidal behaviour

## What are the common elements of treatments that work?

M David Rudd, Ben Williams and David RM Trotter

## Abstract

This chapter provides a review of all currently available clinical trials targeting suicidal behaviour. In contrast to some previous available reviews, the focus of the current chapter is on identifying *common elements* of treatments that work. More specifically, we attempted to answer the question, what do treatments that work have in common? A number of psychological treatments have emerged as effective or potentially effective at reducing suicidal behaviour (i.e. suicide attempts). There now appear to be a number of identifiable core elements for treatments that have proven effective at reducing suicide attempts, all with direct and meaningful implications for day to day clinical practice. We also point out limitations in current science, including problematic follow-up periods and questions about the high-risk nature of some study samples.

## Understanding and acknowledging the problem

Despite considerable disparity in observable rates, it is reasonable to say that suicidality (broadly defined, including death, attempts—single and multiple—and ideation) is a serious and persistent public health problem. Efficacious and effective treatments, both biological and psychological in orientation, are desperately needed. This chapter will summarize some of the current work from the psychological and behavioural perspective. To date, we have been able to identify fifty-three clinical trials targeting suicidality, with the majority (N = 28, 53 per cent) being cognitive-behavioural in orientation. When we say clinical trails, we mean only those studies that included both a treatment and control (or comparison) group; randomization was not an essential element. If randomization was included as a criterion it would have reduced the total number by almost half. For the sake of parsimony, only those studies deemed effective will be mentioned and considered below. However, all currently available studies, including those with negative or equivocal

results are included in Table 58.1 (at the end of this chapter). For the most part, it is most accurate to refer to equivocal results, that is, comparable findings across treatment and control conditions. We are unaware of any treatment that actually proved potentially harmful in contrast to treatment as usual or other control treatment conditions.

## Understanding treatment targets and impact

The focus of the chapter is on clinical trials that utilized a psychological and/or behavioural approach to treating suicidality. As mentioned, we were able to identify a total of fifty-three, with the majority (53 per cent) being cognitive behavioural therapy (CBT) in orientation. When considering treatment for suicidality, it is important to consider the broad variability in both the patient populations targeted (i.e. those exhibiting ideation, having made attempts, or those having made multiple attempts) and treatment goals (i.e. reduction of suicidal thinking, attempts, and/or related symptomatology). As is apparent, the possible permutations across targeted groups and outcomes are considerable, adding to the complexity in interpreting results and identifying *effective* treatments. A problem that has persisted across studies is the exclusion of high-risk cases, with Linehan (1997) estimating that 45 per cent of treatment efficacy trials excluded high-risk patients. Accordingly, we will make a distinction in the severity of the targeted patient population, along with treatment goals, in the discussion to follow.

When talking about treatment outcome for suicidality, we can ask two critical questions. First, what treatments work? And second, what do they have in common that might help us understand why they work? Although dismantling studies are yet to be conducted that would definitely answer these questions, we do have enough data to engage in informed discussion. We do not have adequate data to answer the question about whether or not psychological treatment has enduring impact, that is, that treatment effects will

**Table 58.1** Treatment outcome studies targeting suicidality

| Study | Total patients (cumulative drop-out rate), N (N) | Inclusion/exclusion criteria | Follow-up period, months | Suicide attempts by condition, N (%) |
|---|---|---|---|---|
| Chowdhury et al. 1973 | E: 113<br>C: 84 | **Inclusion:** repeat suicide attempters admitted to poisoning treatment centre<br>**Exclusion:** individuals at high risk of parasuicide to present ethnical concern | 6 | E 17 (24) $_p$ *<br>C 19 (23) $_p$ * |
| Termansen and Bywater 1975 | $E_1$: 57 (12)<br>$E_2$: 57 (24)<br>$E_3$: 50 (18)<br>C: 38 (20) | **Inclusion:** attempted suicide admissions, with suicide defined as 'any act of self-injury, regardless of its seriousness, which was motivated by self-destructive tendencies'<br>**Exclusion:** patients with no initial or final assessment | 3 | $E_1$: 1 **<br>$E_2$: 2 **<br>$E_3$: 7 **<br>C: 2 ** |
| Welu 1977 | E 63 (1)<br>C 57 | **Inclusion:** suicide attempters, defined by any non-fatal act of self-damage inflicted with self-destructive intention, however vague and ambiguous; residing in catchment area for community mental health centre; brought to the hospital emergency room<br>**Exclusion:** under 16 years of age; students living in college or university housing; persons with usual residence of care-giving institution; individuals institutionalized at the time of the suicide attempt | 4 | E 3 *<br>C 9 * |
| Gibbons et al. 1978 | E 200 (19 per cent)<br>C 200 (22 per cent) | **Inclusion:** at least 17 years of age; episode of deliberate self-poisoning; defined geographical area<br>**Exclusion:** formal psychiatric illness requiring immediate psychiatric treatment; immediate suicide risk; continuing treatment with psychiatrist or social worker seen within 2 weeks | 12 | E (13.5)* $_P$<br>C (14.5)* $_P$ |
| Hawton et al. 1981 | E: 48 (5)<br>C: 48 (15) | **Inclusion:** 16 or older; giving informed consent; registered with general practitioner; live within 15 miles of hospital; suitable for outpatient care; admitted to Oxford following an overdose; not in need of formal psychiatric or specialist facilities (i.e., inpatient care or rehabilitation) care; not in current care (social work, probation, psychologist, or other professional); agreeable and willing to receive care | 12 | E (10) $_{SH}$ **<br>C (15) $_{SH}$ ** |
| Liberman and Eckman 1981 | E: 12<br>C: 12 | **Inclusion:** repeated suicide attempters (at least one previous attempt in preceding 2 years); referred to 10-day inpatient programme by psychiatric emergency team, local community mental health services, or hospital emergency room physician<br>**Exclusion:** psychotic patients; organic brain syndrome; currently addicted to alcohol or drugs | 24 | E: 2 *<br>C: 5 *<br>11 total attempts |
| Patsiokas and Clum 1985 | E 1: 5<br>E 2: 5<br>C: 5 | **Inclusion:** patients in psychiatric inpatient ward; admitted for suicide attempt<br>**Exclusion:** diagnosis of psychosis, alcoholism, or drug abuse | none | Not specified |
| Hawton et al. 1987 | E 41 (11)<br>C 39 4) | **Inclusion:** episode of overdose; at least 16 years of age; give informed consent; registered with GP; living within 15 miles of the hospital; suitable for outpatient counselling (as determined by hospital counsellors)—continuing problems willing to tackle with help of counsellors; not in need of formal psychiatric care or specialist facilities; not in current care of psychiatric services, social worker, probation officer, psychologist, or professional agency; agreeable to assessment with counsellors; willing to accept after care | 9 | E 3 (7.3)*<br>C 6 (15.4) * |
| Torhorst et al. 1988 | E 1: 40<br>E 2: 40 | **Inclusion:** suicide attempt by intoxication; first parasuicide; repeated parasuicide<br>**Exclusion:** psychosis; continuing psychotherapeutic treatment elsewhere; inpatient psychiatric therapy of non-psychotic condition; drug overdose; lack of understanding of language; too long a travel time to outpatient centre | 3, 12 | E 1: (22.5) **<br>E 2: (22.5) **<br>Only 2 attempts after 3 months, varies by treatment compliance |
| Lerner and Clum 1990 | E: 9<br>C: 9 | **Inclusion/Exclusion:** aged 18–24; currently experiencing 'clinically significant' suicide ideations, as defined as a score of 11 or more on Modified Scale for Suicidal Ideations (MSSI); no signs of psychosis or substance abuse | 3 | Not specified |

**Table 58.1** (Continued) Treatment outcome studies targeting suicidality

| Study | Total patients (cumulative drop-out rate), N (N) | Inclusion/exclusion criteria | Follow-up period, months | Suicide attempts by condition, N (%) |
|---|---|---|---|---|
| Salkovskis et al. 1990 | E 12 (0) <br> C 8 (0) | **Inclusion:** aged 16–65; fixed abode within hospital boundary; not in need of immediate psychiatric treatment; not psychotic of suffering from organic illness; meet two or more of the following: previous suicide attempts; antidepressants taken as overdose; score of 4 or higher on Bugless and Horton (1974) risk of repetition scale | 12 | E 0 <br> C 3 * <br> 4 ** |
| Waterhouse and Platt 1990 | E 27 <br> C 25 | **Inclusion:** parasuicides, defined as non-fatal act in which an individual deliberately ingests a substance in excess of any prescribed or generally recognized therapeutic dosage, with no immediate medical or psychiatric treatment needs <br><br> **Exclusion:** parasuicides using methods other than self-poisoning; under 16 years of age; no fixed abode; living further than 16 miles from city; current psychiatric inpatient; self-discharges from hospital; direct referral to medical ward/bypassing casualty department | 16 weeks | Not specified |
| Linehan et al. 1991 | E 32 (10) <br> C 31 (9) | **Inclusion:** score of 7 on Diagnostic Interview for Borderlines; meet criteria for DSM-III diagnosis of BPD; at least 2 incidents of parasuicide in past 5 years, with at least one occurring within the past 8 weeks; aged 15–45; agreed to study conditions <br><br> **Exclusion:** meet DSM-III criteria for schizophrenia, bipolar disorder, substance dependence, or mental retardation | 12 | E $(63.6)_p$ * <br> C $(95.5)_p$ * |
| Allard et al. 1992 | E 76 (13) <br> C 74 (11) | **Inclusion:** seen by emergency department after concrete suicide attempt; residing within psychiatric catchment area; speak French or English <br><br> **Exclusion:** no fixed address or expecting to move; already in the care of institution responsible for follow-up; physical handicap preventing attendance; inability for informed consent; sociopathy with physical threat to hospital personnel; attempt not occurring within one week | 24 | E 22 (35)* <br> C 19 (30)* |
| Klingman and Hochdorf 1993 | E 116 <br> C 121 | **Inclusion:** 8th grade students | 12 weeks | Not specified |
| Morgan et al. 1993 | E 101 (0) <br> C 111 (0) | **Inclusion:** reside within hospital catchment area; no previous history of non-fatal deliberate self-harm | 12 | E: 5 $(4.95)_{SH}$ * 7 ** <br> C: 12 $(10.81)_{SH}$ * <br> 15 ** |
| McLeavey et al. 1994 | E 19 (2) <br> C 20 (4) | **Inclusion:** aged 15–45; no history of psychosis, mental retardation, or organic cognitive impairment; engaged in intentional self-poisoning; not in need of inpatient or day-patient car for psychiatric illness and/or suicidal risk; IQ of at least 80 on Mill Hill Vocabulary Scale | 12 | E $(10.5)_{SH}$ * <br> C $(25)_{SH}$ * |
| Cotgrove et al. 1995 | E 47 <br> C 58 | **Inclusion:** aged 16 or below; suicide attempt, including deliberate self-injury and deliberate-self poisoning | 12 | E 3 (6)* <br> C 7 (12)* |
| van Heeringen et al. 1995 | E 258 (62) <br> C 258 (63) | **Inclusion:** at least 15 years of age; live in Gent or suburbs; suicide attempters defined as deliberate self-poisoning and deliberate self-injury <br><br> **Exclusion:** patients in need of inpatient medical treatment | 12 | E 21(10.7) * <br> C 34 (17.4) * |
| Rudd et al. 1996 | E 181 (38) <br> C 121 | **Inclusion:** individuals who made an attempt precipitating referral; individuals with mood disorder and concurrent ideation, to include mixed symptomatology and adjustment disorder diagnoses; those abusing alcohol episodically with concurrent ideation <br><br> **Exclusion:** substance dependence or chronic abuse requiring separate treatment; psychotic component to presentation; diagnosable thought disorder; personality disorder diagnosis making outpatient group participation ineffective, disruptive, or inappropriate | 24 | Not specified |

**Table 58.1** (Continued) Treatment outcome studies targeting suicidality

| Study | Total patients (cumulative drop-out rate), N (N) | Inclusion/exclusion criteria | Follow-up period, months | Suicide attempts by condition, N (%) |
|---|---|---|---|---|
| van der Sande et al. 1997 | E 140 (33 per cent) C 134 (63 per cent) | **Inclusion:** at least 15 years of age; attending Utrecht University Hospital for somatic treatment following suicide attempt<br><br>**Exclusion:** habitual self-harm activities (e.g., wrist-cutting or using excessive amounts of substances); accidental overdose; inability to understand and write Dutch; reside outside of hospital catchment area; psychiatric hospitalization; imprisonment; acute psychosis; drug or alcohol addiction; recurrent consultations with liaison psychiatrist; suicide attempters receiving experimental treatment during pilot phase | 12 | E 24 ** C 20 ** |
| Harrington et al. 1998 | E 85 C 77 (33 total) | **Inclusion:** age 16 or younger; diagnosed with deliberate self-poisoning; consent from legal guardian<br><br>**Exclusion:** other forms of self-harm (e.g., cutting or attempted hanging); social situations precluding family intervention; clinical or psychiatric contraindication; cases in which it was not clear if deliberate | 6 | Not specified |
| Evans et al. 1999 | E 417 C 410 | **Inclusion:** adult inpatients following deliberate self-harm; referred for routine psychiatric evaluation<br><br>**Exclusion:** individuals normally residing outside of catchment area; individuals who met the following clinical criteria meaning they were unlikely to use the intervention appropriately, placing themselves or others at risk; 3 or more contacts in past 6 months but failing to engage with psychiatric services; presenting unacceptable type or degree of aggression within previous 6 months; individuals inappropriately using alcohol or drugs leading to repetitive presentation in intoxicated state resulting in aggression or inability to engage in treatment | 6 | 0 DSH repeats: E: 347 C: 351 1 DSH repeats: E: 46 C: 32 2 or more DSH repeats: E: 24 C: 27 2 suicides in experimental group 3 suicides in control group |
| Evans et al. 1999 | E 18 (0) C 16 (2) | **Inclusion:** episode of deliberate self harm; aged 16–50; personality disturbance within flamboyant personality cluster; histrionic or emotionally unstable; at least one previous episode of deliberate self-harm within previous year<br><br>**Exclusion:** primary ICD-10 diagnosis within the organic, alcohol or drug dependence, or schizophrenia groups | 6 | E 10 (56) * C 10 (71) * |
| Linehan et al. 1999 | E 12 (5) C 16 (8) | **Inclusion:** women aged 15–45; met criteria for BPD on both PDE and SCID-II; met criteria for substance use disorder for opiates, cocaine, amphetamines, sedatives, hypnotics, anxiolytics, or polysubstance use disorder on SCID<br><br>**Exclusion:** met criteria for schizophrenia; another psychotic disorder, or bipolar mood disorder on SCID; mental retardation as assessed by Peabody Picture Vocabulary Test-Revised | 16 | Not specified |
| Turner 2000 | E 12 (4) C 12 (6) | **Inclusion:** patients initially treated in local hospital emergency services for suicide attempts; meet diagnostic criteria for BPD; not meet exclusionary diagnosis; give written informed consent; accept random assignment to treatment<br><br>**Exclusion:** schizophrenia; schizoaffective disorder; bipolar disorder; organic mental disorders; mental retardation; in need of inpatient drug or alcohol treatment | 12 | Not specified |
| Koons et al. 2001 | E 14 (4) C 14 (4) | **Inclusion:** honourably discharged women veterans; met criteria for DMS-III-R BPD<br><br>**Exclusion:** schizophrenia; bipolar disorder; substance dependence; antisocial personality disorder | 6 | E: (10)* SH, including suicide C: (20)* SH, including suicide |

**Table 58.1** (Continued) Treatment outcome studies targeting suicidality

| Study | Total patients (cumulative drop-out rate), N (N) | Inclusion/exclusion criteria | Follow-up period, months | Suicide attempts by condition, N (%) |
|---|---|---|---|---|
| Guthrie et al. 2001 | E 58 (11) C 61 (13) | **Inclusion:** presenting with episode of deliberate self-poisoning; able to read and write English; live within hospital catchment area; registered with a GP; not in need of inpatient treatment<br><br>**Exclusion:** living outside catchment area; not approached by emergency staff; discharged self without being seen; too physically/psychiatrically unwell; no fixed abode; not registered with GP | 6 | E 5 (9)$_{SH}$ * C 17 (28)$_{SH}$ * |
| Wood et al. 2001 | E 32 (1) C 31 (0) | **Inclusion:** aged 12–16; referred to child and adolescent mental health service following deliberate self-harm incident; incident of deliberate self-harm at least once over the previous year; deliberate self-harm defined as any intentional self-inflicted injury, irrespective of the apparent purpose of the act<br><br>**Exclusion:** accidental overdose of recreational drugs or alcohol; judged as too suicidal for ambulatory care; could not attend groups given current situation (e.g., incarceration); psychiatric diagnosis; unlikely to benefit from group intervention (e.g., learning problems) | 6 | E 50 $_{SH}$ ** C 47 $_{SH}$ ** |
| Motto and Bostrom 2001 | E 389 C 454 | **Inclusion:** Patients admitted to psychiatric inpatient unit following depressive or suicidal state | 15 years | E 25 (death by suicide) C 27 (death by suicide) |
| Raj et al. 2001 | E: 20 C: 20 | **Inclusion:** individuals with first or second attempted suicide by overdose of drugs or pesticides; aged 16–50; anxiety, depression (without psychotic symptoms), or adjustment disorder<br><br>**Exclusion:** score of less than 20 on MMSE; psychosis; dysthymia; bipolar affective disorder; obsessive–compulsive disorder; eating disorder; alcohol dependence or abusing other psychoactive substances; personality disorders; previous psychological intervention | 3 | E: 0 C: 1* |
| Wood et al. 2001 | E: 32 (1) C: 31 (0) | **Inclusion:** aged 12–16; referred for treatment following incident of deliberate self-harm, defined as any intentional self-inflicted injury, irrespective of the apparent purpose of the act; at least one other deliberate self-harm incident during previous year<br><br>**Exclusion:** judged to be too suicidal for ambulatory care; current situation meant they could not attend groups (e.g., incarcerated); psychotic disorder; unlikely to benefit from group intervention (e.g., learning problems) | 7 | E: 2 (6)* $_{SH}$ C: 10 (32)* $_{SH}$ |
| Bennewith et al. 2002 | E 964 C 968 | **Inclusion:** patients with episode of self-harm; self-harm defined as deliberate and non-fatal act done in the knowledge that it is potentially harmful/excessive (as in drug overdose)<br><br>**Exclusion:** alcohol overdose (unless act of self-harm or suicide); illicit drug overdose (unless act of self-harm or suicide); less than 16 years of age; no fixed abode; imprisoned request for no one to be informed of the episode; deliberate self-harm in response to psychotic hallucination or delusion; managed entirely by primary care | 12 | E 211 (21.9) $_{SH}$ * C 189 (19.5) $_{SH}$ * |
| Cedereke et al. 2002 | E 107 (18) C 109 (20) | **Inclusion:** suicide attempt; living within hospital catchment area | 12 | E 14 (17) * 26 ** C 15 (17) * 27 ** |
| Clarke et al. 2002 | E 220 C 247 | **Inclusion:** episode of deliberate self-harm; deliberate self-harm defined as non-fatal act in which an individual deliberately causes self-injury or ingests a substance in excess of the therapeutic dose; adult residents of geographical area<br><br>**Exclusion:** less than 16 years of age; individuals aged 16–19 in full-time secondary education; overdose from recreational or problematic alcohol and/or drug use | 12 | E 19 (9) $_{SH}$ readmission * C 25 (10) $_{SH}$ readmission * |

**Table 58.1** (Continued) Treatment outcome studies targeting suicidality

| Study | Total patients (cumulative drop-out rate), N (N) | Inclusion/exclusion criteria | Follow-up period, months | Suicide attempts by condition, N (%) |
|---|---|---|---|---|
| Nordentoft et al. 2002 | E: 156 (35) C: 148 (42) | **Inclusion/Exclusion:** aged 18 to 45; legal residence in catchment area; diagnosis of schizophrenia, schizotypal disorder, delusional disorder, acute or transient psychosis, schizoaffective psychosis, induced psychosis, or unspecified non-organic psychosis according to ICD-10; exposure to antipsychotic medication never exceeding 12 weeks of continuous medication in antipsychotic dosage; absence of mental retardation (learning disability), organic mental disorder, and psychotic condition because of acute poisoning or a withdrawal state; familiarity with Danish language; written informed consent | 12 | E: 1 suicide E: 18 (12) * C: 13 (10.4)* |
| Rathus and Miller 2002 | E: 29 C: 82 | **Inclusion:** adolescent outpatient admissions; inclusion for DBT (must have both): suicide attempt within last 16 weeks (defined as self-harm with the intent to die); diagnosis of borderline personality disorder or minimum of 3 borderline personality features **Inclusion to TAU:** those meeting either criteria A or B for DBT, but not both | | |
| Spirito et al. 2002 | E 36 (7) C 40 (6) | **Inclusion:** aged 12–18; receiving medical care at children's hospital following suicide attempt; suicide attempt defined as any intentional self-injury, regardless of lethality, as attempt to harm or kill oneself | 3 | Not specified |
| Meltzer et al. 2003 | E 490 (192) C 490 (187) | **Inclusion:** women; aged 18–65; DSM-IV diagnosis of schizophrenia or schizoaffective disorder; considered to be at high risk for committing suicide, defined as any one of the following: history of previous attempts or hospitalizations in previous 3 years; moderate to severe current suicidal ideation with depressive symptoms; command hallucinations for self-harm within 1 week | 12 | E: 34 C: 55 |
| Power et al. 2003 | E 31 (10) C 25 (4) | **Inclusion:** acutely suicidal youth with severe mental illness; score between 4 and 7 on Expanded Version 4 of Brief Psychiatric Rating Scale (BPRS) suicidality subscore, with 4 equating a 'suicidal thoughts frequent, without intent or plan' and 7 equating 'a specific suicidal plan and intent or suicide attempt'; agreement to participate **Exclusion:** attended service for more than 1 year | 6 | E: 1 suicide C: 1 suicide |
| Tyrer et al. 2003 | E 239 (40) C 241(38) | **Inclusion:** episode of self-harm; previous episode; informed written consent; do not require in-patient psychiatric treatment **Exclusion:** psychotic disorder; bipolar disorder; primary diagnosis of substance dependence | 12 | E (39) $_p$ C (46) $_p$ |
| Verheul et al. 2003 | E 27 (3) C 31 (8) | **Inclusion:** women aged 18–70; borderline personality disorder; no restriction on referral source; were able to find or had a referral source willing to provide 12 months treatment **Exclusion:** DSM-IV diagnosis of bipolar disorder or chronic psychotic disorder; insufficient command of Dutch language; severe cognitive impairments | 12 | E: 2 (7) * C: 8 (26) * Self-mutilation E: 8 (35) * C: 13 (57) * |
| Katz et al. 2004 | E: 32 (6) C: 30 (3) | **Inclusion:** aged 14–17; suicide attempt or suicidal ideation severe enough to warrant psychiatric admission; adolescent agreed to stay in the hospital for brief treatment **Exclusion:** mental retardation; psychosis; bipolar affective disorder; severe learning disabilities | 12 | Total hospitalizations E: 6 C: 6 Total ER visits E: 8 C: 14 Total incidents in hospital E: 2 C: 10 |

**Table 58.1** (Continued) Treatment outcome studies targeting suicidality

| Study | Total patients (cumulative drop-out rate), N (N) | Inclusion/exclusion criteria | Follow-up period, months | Suicide attempts by condition, N (%) |
|---|---|---|---|---|
| March et al. 2004 | $E_1$ 109 (18)<br>$E_2$ 111 (24)<br>$E_3$ 107 (17)<br>C 112 (23) | **Inclusion:** aged 12–17; ability to receive care as outpatient; primary DSM-IV diagnosis of MDD; written consent from patient and at least one parent; Children's Depression Rating Scale-Revised (CDRS-R) total score of 45 or higher; not taking antidepressants; depressive mood in at least 2 of 3 contexts (home, school, among peers) for at least 6 weeks prior<br><br>**Exclusion:** ccurrent or past diagnosis of bipolar disorder, severe conduct disorder, current substance abuse or dependence, pervasive developmental disorder(s), thought disorder; concurrent treatment with psychotropic medication or psychotherapy outside study; 2 failed SSRI trials; poor response to clinical treatment containing CBT for depression; intolerance of fluoxetine; confounding medical condition; non-English speaking patient or parent; pregnancy or refusal to use birth control; hospitalization for dangerousness to self or others within 3 months of consent; deemed 'high risk' because of a suicide attempt requiring medical attention within 6 months, clear intent or an active plan to commit suicide, or suicidal ideation with disorganized family unable to guarantee adequate safety monitoring | 12 weeks | Total adverse events: 33 (7.5)*<br>$E_1$: 13 (11.9)<br>$E_2$: 5 (4.5)<br>$E_3$: 107 (8.4)<br>C: 6 (5.4)<br>Total suicide-related adverse events: 24 (5.5)*<br>$E_1$: 9 *8.26)<br>$E_2$: 5 (4.50)<br>$E_3$: 6 (5.61)<br>C: 4 (3.57) |
| Brown et al. 2005 | E 60 (15)<br>C 60 (20) | **Inclusion:** suicide attempt, defined as a potentially self-injurious behavior with a non-fatal outcome for which there is evidence, either explicit or implicit, that the individual intended to kill himself or herself, within 48 hours prior to evaluation in emergency department; age 16 or older; English-speaking; able to complete baseline assessment; able to provide at least 2 verifiable contacts for tracking; ability to give informed consent<br><br>**Exclusion:** medical disorder preventing outpatient treatment | 18 | E 13 (24.1)*<br>C 23 (41.6)* |
| Donaldson et al. 2005 | E 15<br>C 16<br>(8 total) | **Inclusion:** adolescents aged 12–17; admitted to emergency department or inpatient unit following suicide attempt; suicide identified as any intentional, non-fatal self-injury, regardless of medical lethality with intent to die<br><br>**Exclusion:** primary inclusion other than English; psychosis indicated on mental status examination; intellectual functioning precluding outpatient psychotherapy | 6 | E 4 (26.7) *<br>C 2 (12.5) * |
| Evans et al. 2005 | E 417<br>C 410 | **Inclusion:** patients admitted to hospital for self-harm | 12 | E 90 (21.6) $_{SH}$ *<br>C 77 (18.8) $_{SH}$ * |
| Nordentoft et al. 2005 | E: 362 (149)<br>C: 39 (19) | **Inclusion:** inhabitants in Copenhagen or Frederiksberg municipality; aged 16–40; severe suicidal thoughts or incidents of attempted suicide; understand and willing to give informed consent<br><br>**Exclusion:** psychotic illness; intravenous drug abuse | 12 | 3 suicides in experimental group<br>E: 213 (7)*<br>C: 21 (33.3)* |
| Rhee et al. 2005 | $E_1$ (16, 50 per cent)<br>$E_2$ (10, 37 per cent)<br>C (15 per cent)<br>Total: 85 | **Inclusion:** callers from telephone crisis hotline; currently not in therapy; currently at no or low risk for suicide; no indications for psychiatric referral due to severe impairment of functioning or psychotic symptoms; no indications for hospitalization or police intervention; expressed interest in beginning psychotherapy<br><br>**Exclusion:** medium or high risk for suicide | 6 weeks | Not specified |
| van den Bosch et al. 2005 | E 27<br>C 31 | **Inclusion:** female; aged 18–65; DSM-IV diagnosis of BPD according to SCID-II<br><br>**Exclusion:** DSM-IV diagnosis of bipolar disorder or chronic psychotic disorder; insufficient command of Dutch language; severe cognitive impairments | 18 | During 12-month study<br>E: (7)*<br>C: (26)*<br>During 26-week follow-up<br>E: 1 (4)*<br>C: 6 (19)* |

**Table 58.1** (Continued) Treatment outcome studies targeting suicidality

| Study | Total patients (cumulative drop-out rate), N (N) | Inclusion/exclusion criteria | Follow-up period, months | Suicide attempts by condition, N (%) |
|---|---|---|---|---|
| Linehan *et al.* 2006 | E: 52 (16) C: 49 (35) | **Inclusion:** women; aged 18–45; met criteria for BPD; current and past suicidal behaviour defined as at least 2 suicide attempts or self-injuries in the past 5 years, with at least 1 in the past 8 weeks **Exclusion:** lifetime diagnosis of schizophrenia, schizoaffective disorder, bipolar disorder, psychotic disorder NOS, or mental retardation; seizure requiring medication; mandate to treatment; need for primary treatment for another debilitating condition | 24 | E: (23.1) ** C: (46)** |
| Tarrier *et al.* 2006 | | **Inclusion/Exclusion:** either first or second admission (within 2 years of a first admission) to inpatient or day patient unit for treatment of psychosis; DSM-IV criteria of schizophrenia, schizophreniform disorder, schizoaffective disorder, delusional disorder, or psychosis NOS; Positive psychotic symptoms for 4 weeks or more; score of 4 or more (moderate to extreme) on PANSS target item for either delusions or hallucination; no substance misuse; psychotic symptoms not caused by organic disorder | 18 | E: 0 C: 3 deaths by suicide |
| Weinberg *et al.* 2006 | E: 15 C: 15 | **Inclusion:** females; borderline personality disorder; aged 18–40; history of repetitive DSH, with at least one episode during past month **Exclusion:** comorbid psychotic disorder; bipolar I disorder; substance dependence score of 9 or higher on Beck Hopelessness Scale describing concrete immediate suicide plan | 8 | Frequency E: 1.98 $_{SH}$ C: 6.69 $_{SH}$ |

E, experimental condition; C, control condition; $_p$ parasuicide; $_{SH}$ deliberate self-harm; * total repeat attempters; ** total repeat attempts.

last for many years. To date (among the fifty-three trials identified), the longest follow-up available is 24 months with the average being 10 months. Clearly, such limited follow-up timeframes are inadequate to address questions about enduring impact. It could actually be argued that current data only indicate that psychological and behavioural treatments can *delay* suicide.

Perhaps the primary contribution this chapter can make is to identify *common elements* across treatment trials that are associated with positive outcomes. More specifically, can we identify similarities across treatments demonstrated to be effective? This would help distil existing findings into clear, concise and usable recommendations for day to day clinical practice. By comparison to other problems targeted in the medical literature, a total number of fifty-three for treatment outcome studies is indeed very small. Accordingly, it is important to look for similarities across trials in an effort to focus resources in the areas that hold the most promise for effective treatment and intervention. There is little question that more difficult and elaborate questions can be asked of the treatment literature (cf. Rudd *et al.* 2004), but at this point, we simply do not have adequate data to answer them.

Somewhat in opposition to the current chapter and our emphasis on identifying what actually works in treatment, it is important to note that a recent meta-analysis concluded that 'results do not provide evidence that additional psychosocial interventions following self-harm have a marked effect on the likelihood of subsequent suicide' (Crawford *et al.* 2007, p. 11). As has been mentioned elsewhere (Rudd 2007), there are a number of confounds that limit the accuracy of their conclusion, but two are at the heart of the problem. First, the interventions included in the meta-analysis were not developed nor intended to reduce suicide rates, rather they targeted suicide attempts and associated symptoms such as suicidal

ideation, hopelessness, and depression. Second, it is also arguable that the studies included are not actually amenable to a meta-analytic approach given variable inclusion/exclusion criteria and treatment targets, with the net outcome being that the meta-analysis inappropriately assumed *intervention* and *treatment* studies were comparable, along with including samples of highly disparate ages, ranging from age 12 to over 50. Rudd (2007) provides a detailed list of identifiable confounds that corrupt the conclusions offered by Crawford *et al.* (2007).

## Previous reviews of psychological and behavioural treatments

There are a number of comprehensive reviews already available in the literature, including Gunnell and Frankel (1994), Hepp *et al.* (2004), Linehan (1997), Rudd (2006), and several previous meta-analyses that are methodologically sound (van der Sande *et al.* 1997; Hawton *et al.* 1998, 2005). These reviews include in-depth discussion of methodological problems and limitations across studies. We are not going to repeat what is available elsewhere, rather we will critique available studies in an effort to answer the two questions raised earlier: What psychological treatments work in reducing suicidality?, and are there *common elements* that can be identified across studies that can be integrated into clinical practice?

## Identifying treatments that work

As mentioned above, it is important to think about not just the nature of the treatment and the sample targeted (e.g. high versus low risk), but also treatment goals (e.g. reduction in suicide attempts, suicidal ideation, or associated symptoms such as depression, hopelessness, anxiety). Given the variable nature of symptomatology associated with suicide risk, particularly suicidal ideation, the best and most accurate marker of lower risk following treatment is a reduction in suicide attempts during the follow-up period (cf. Rudd *et al.* 2004). If we focus specifically on what treatments are effective at reducing suicide attempts and also do not have serious or disqualifying methodological problems, the list is relatively short, including nine studies with a CBT focus or orientation (Salkovkis *et al.* 1990; Linehan *et al.* 1991; McLeavey *et al.* 1994; Nordentoft *et al.* 2002; Linehan *et al.* 2004; Brown *et al.* 2005; van den Bosch *et al.* 2005; Koons *et al.* 2001, 2006). It would appear that CBT approaches are emerging as a frontrunner when it comes to effective treatments for suicidality. Only two other treatments (Guthrie *et al.* 2001; Wood *et al.* 2001) have proven effective at lowering subsequent suicide attempt rates. Guthrie *et al.* (2001) demonstrated that brief in-home interpersonal psychotherapy was more effective than treatment as usual at reducing subsequent suicide attempts. The follow-up period for this study was only 6 months. Similarly, Wood *et al.* (2001) found that *developmental group therapy* was more effective at reducing suicide attempts in comparison to treatment as usual for adolescents. It is important to remember, though, that a number of other treatments have been demonstrated to reduce associated symptoms such as depression, anxiety, hopelessness and features of suicidal thinking (e.g. specificity and intensity). As was mentioned before, though, the *variable nature* of associated symptoms like suicidal ideation, depression, and hopelessness significantly limit their utility as outcome measures.

## Are there common elements that work?

As mentioned above, an important question is whether or not there are identifiable *common elements* across treatments that work at reducing subsequent suicide attempt rates? Among the studies referenced above, a review of these studies supports several conclusions about common elements, techniques and interventions:

### Theoretical models easily translated to clinical work

All of the treatments have clearly articulated well-defined and understandable theoretical models that are embedded in empirical research. The theoretical models also have common elements, as might be expected for CBT-oriented treatments. They all identify cognitions, emotional processing and associated behavioural responses as critical to understanding motivation to die, associated distress (and symptoms) and ultimately changing the suicidal process. Patients find the models easy to understand, distilling them down to thoughts, feelings and behaviours that are associated with suicide risk and hopelessness. In short, these treatments have made it easy to sit down with a patient and *explain in understandable language why they have tried or are thinking about killing themselves.* This is an important consistency across effective treatments and prompts a number of important questions. When a treatment model is simple, straightforward, and easy to understand, does it facilitate hope, improve motivation and result in better compliance? If so, the net outcome would be enhanced skill development, reduced symptom severity, and fewer subsequent suicide attempts.

### Treatment fidelity

In all of the treatments referenced above, treatment fidelity was a critical factor. This translates to clinicians being trained to a target standard of competence and supervised throughout (with variable formats). For the most part, the treatments were manual-driven, with a clear sequence and hierarchy of treatment targets, with a reduction of suicidal behaviour as a central and *primary* focus. Rather than focus on peripheral or associated symptoms, effective treatments target suicidality specifically. Effective psychological and behavioural treatments view suicidality as, at least to some degree, independent of diagnosis. Targeting suicidal behaviour as a treatment outcome clearly seems to lend itself to positive changes in subsequent attempt rates. What is also clear is that all four studies conceptualized the treatment of suicidality as requiring unique competencies, consistent with the recent movement to identifiable core competencies in the assessment, management and treatment of suicidality (Suicide Prevention Resource Center 2006).

### Compliance

Effective treatments also targeted treatment compliance in specific and consistent fashion. More specifically, all had speific interventions and techniques that targeted poor compliance and motivation for treatment. Treatment is only effective if the patient is active, involved and invested. It is clear from effective treatments that compliance with care needs to be a central and primary focus, with clear plans about *what to do* if non-compliance emerges. Just as suicidal behaviour needs to be a primary target, motivation and investment in care is important. When motivation, investment, and involvement drop, they need to become a primary treatment target until effectively resolved.

### Targeting identifiable skills

Consistent with easy to understand theoretical models of suicidality driving the treatment process, effective treatments targeted clearly identifiable skill sets (e.g. emotion regulation, anger management, problem-solving, interpersonal relationships, cognitive distortions). In these treatments, patients understood what was 'wrong' and 'what to do about it' in order to reduce suicidal thinking and behaviours. They also had the opportunity to practice and build skill sets over time.

### Personal responsibility

Consistent with each of the above points, effective treatments emphasized self-reliance, self-awareness, self-control and issues of personal responsibility. Effective treatments are clear in the goal that if patients developed appropriate skills, the distress and upset tied to early events would diminish and associated suicidal urges would as well. Consistent with this goal, patients assumed a considerable degree of personal responsibility for their care, including crisis management. Again, this is consistent with the issue of improved compliance and motivation for care. Although there are a range of models available for facilitating compliance and crisis management, but we would encourage clinicians to consider use of the 'commitment to treatment agreement' (cf. Rudd *et al.* 2006).

### Easy access to treatment and crisis services

Effective treatments emphasize the importance of crisis management and access to available emergency services during and after treatment, with a clear plan of action being identified. Additionally, effective treatments more often than not dedicated time to practising the skills sets necessary to effective crisis management, with patients learning to identify what characterizes a 'crisis or emergency', using a 'safety' or 'crisis management plan' and learning to use these services in judicious and appropriate fashion.

# Conclusions

As other reviews have made clear (cf. Gunnell and Frankel 1994; Linehan 1997; Hepp *et al.* 2004; Rudd 2006), a reasonable database is starting to emerge to answer the question about what works in the treatment of suicidality. What has also emerged are some readily identifiable *common elements* that have important and concrete implications for day to day clinical practice with suicidal patients, not to mention provide a solid foundation for future dismantling studies that can answer the relatively simple questions in more definitive fashion.

## References

Allard R, Marshall M, Plante MC (1992). Intensive follow-up does not decrease the risk of repeat suicide attempts. *Suicide and Life-Threatening Behavior*, **22**, 303–314.

Bennewith O, Stocks N, Gunnell D *et al.* (2002). General practice-based intervention to prevent repeat episodes of deliberate self harm: cluster randomised controlled trial. *British Medical Journal*, **32**, 1254–1257.

Brown GK, Have TT, Henriques GR *et al.* (2005). Cognitive therapy for the prevention of suicide attempts: a randomized controlled trial. *Journal of the American Medical Association*, **294**, 563–570.

Cedereke M, Monti K, Ojehagen A (2002). Telephone contact with patients in the year after a suicide attempt: does it affect treatment attendance and outcome? A randomised controlled study. *European Psychiatry*, **17**, 82–91.

Chowdhury N, Hicks RC, Kreitman N. (1973). Evaluation of an after-care service for parasuicide (attempted suicide) patients. *Social Psychiatry*, **8**, 67–81.

Clarke T, Baker P, Watts C *et al.* (2002). A randomized controlled trial of nurse-led case management versus routine care only. *Journal of Mental Health*, **11**, 167–176.

Cotgrove A, Zirinsky L, Black D *et al.* (1995). Secondary prevention of attempted. suicide in adolescence. *Journal of Adolescence*, **18**, 569–577.

Crawford MJ, Thomas O, Khan N *et al.* (2007). Psychosocial interventions following self-harm: A systematic review of their efficacy in preventing suicide. *The British Journal of Psychiatry*, **190**, 11–17.

Donaldson D, Spirito A, Esposito-Smythers C (2005). Treatment for adolescents following a suicide attempt: results of a pilot trial. *Journal of American Academy for Child and Adolescent Psychiatry*, **44**, 113–120.

Evans J, Evans M, Morgan H *et al.* (2005). Crisis card following self-harm: 12-month follow-up of a randomized controlled trial. *British Journal of Psychiatry*, **187**, 186–187.

Evans MO, Morgan HG, Hayward A *et al.* (1999). Crisis telephone consultation for deliberate self-harm patients: Effects on repetition. *British Journal of Psychiatry*, **175**, 23–27.

Gibbons JS, Butler J, Unrwin P *et al.* (1978). Evaluation of a social work service for self-poisoning patients. *British Journal of Psychiatry*, **133**, 111–118.

Gunnell D and Frankel S (1994). Prevention of suicide: aspirations and evidence. *British Medical Journal*, **308**, 1227–1233.

Guthrie E, Navneet K, Moorey J *et al.* (2001). Randomized controlled trial of brief psychological intervention after deliberate self-poisoning. *British Medical Journal*, **323**, 135–138.

Harrington R, Kerfoot M, Dyer E *et al.* (1998). Randomized trial of a home-based family intervention for children who have deliberately poisoned themselves. *Journal of American Academy of Child and Adolescent Psychiatry*, **37**, 512–518.

Hawton K, Arensman E, Townsend E *et al.* (1998). Deliberate self-harm: systematic review of efficacy of psychosocial and pharmacological treatment in preventing repetition. *British Medical Journal*, **317**, 441–447.

Hawton K, Bancroft J, Catalan J *et al.* (1981). Domiciliary and out-patient treatment of self-poisoning patients by medical and non-medical staff. *Psychological Medicine*, **11**, 169–177.

Hawton K, McKeown S, Day A *et al.* (1987). Evaluation of out-patient counselling compared with general practitioner care following overdoses. *Psychological Medicine*, **17**, 751–761.

Hawton K, Townsend E, Arensman E *et al.* (2005). Psychosocial and pharmacological treatments for deliberate self-harm. *The Cochrane Library*, **3**.

Hepp U, Wittmann L, Schnyder U *et al.* (2004). Psychological and psychosocial interventions after attempted suicide. *Crisis*, **25**, 108–117.

Katz LY, Cox BJ, Gunasekara S *et al.* (2004). Feasibility of dialectical behavior therapy for suicidal adolescent inpatients. *Journal of American Academy for Child and Adolescent Psychiatry*, **43**, 276–282.

Klingman A and Hochdorf Z (1993). Coping with distress and self harm: the impact of a primary prevention program among adolescents. *Journal of Adolescents*, **16**, 121–140.

Koons CR, Chapman AL, Betts BB *et al.* (2006). Dialectical behavior therapy adapted for the vocational rehabilitation of significantly disabled mentally ill adults. *Cognitive and Behavioral Practice*, **13**, 146–156.

Koons CR, Robins CJ, Tweed JL *et al.* (2001). Efficacy of dialectical behavior therapy in women veterans with borderline personality disorder. *Behavior Therapy*, **32**, 371–390.

Lerner MS and Clum GA (1990). Treatment of suicide ideators: a problem solving approach. *Behavior Therapy*, **21**, 403–411.

Liberman RP and Eckman T (1981). Behavior therapy vs insight-oriented therapy for repeated suicide attempters. *Archive of General Psychiatry*, **38**, 1126–1130.

Linehan M (1997). Behavioral treatments of suicidal behaviors: definitional obfuscation and treatment outcomes. *Annals of the NY Academy of Sciences*, **836**, 302–328.

Linehan MM, Armstrong HE, Suarez A *et al.* (1991). Cognitive-behavioral treatment of chronically parasuicidal borderline patients. *Archives of General Psychiatry*, **48**, 1060–1064.

Linehan MM, Comotois KA, Korslund KE (2004). Dialectical behavior therapy versus non-behavioral treatment by experts in the community: clinical outcomes. JR Koum and N Lindenboim (Chairs). Symposium conducted at the 112th Convention of the American Psychological Association, Honolulu.

Linehan MM, Comtois KA, Murray AM *et al.* (2006). Two-year randomized controlled trial and follow-up of dialectical behavior therapy vs therapy by experts for suicidal behaviors and borderline personality disorder. *Archives of General Psychiatry*, **63**, 757–766.

Linehan MM, Schmidt H 3rd, Dimeff LA *et al.* (1999). Dialectical behavior therapy for patients with borderline personality disorder and drug-dependence. *American Journal of Addiction*, **8**, 279–292.

March J, Silva S, Petrycki S *et al.* (2004). Fluoxetine, cognitive-behavioral therapy, and their combination for adolescents with depression. *Journal of the American Medical Association*, **292**, 807–820.

McLeavy BC, Daly RJ, Ludgate JW *et al.* (1994). Interpersonal problem-solving skills training in the treatment of self-poisoning patients. *Suicide and Life-Threatening Behavior*, **24**, 382–394.

Meltzer Y, Alphs L, Green AI *et al.* (2003). Clozapine treatment for suicidality in schizophrenia: International Suicide Prevention Trial (InterSePT). *Archives of General Psychiatry*, **60**, 82–91.

Morgan HG, Jones E, Owen J (1993) Secondary prevention of non-fatal deliberate self-harm. The Green Card Study. *British Journal of Psychiatry*, **163**, 111–112.

Motto JA and Bostrom AG (2001). A randomized controlled trial of postcrisis suicide prevention. *Psychiatric Services*, **52**, 828–833.

Nordentoft M, Branner J, Drejer K *et al.* (2005). Effect of a Suicide Prevention Centre for young people with suicidal behaviour in Copenhagen. *European Psychiatry*, **20**, 121–128.

Nordentoft M, Jeppesen P, Abel M *et al.* (2002). OPUS study: suicidal behaviour, suicidal ideation and hopelessness among patients with first-episode psychosis. One-year follow-up of a randomised controlled trial. *British Journal of Psychiatry*, **181**, 97–106.

Patsiokas AT and Clum GA (1985). Effects of psychotherapeutic strategies in the treatment of suicide attempters. *Psychotherapy*, **22**, 281–290.

Power PJR, Bell RJ, Mills R *et al.* (2003). Suicide prevention in first episode psychosis: the development of a randomised controlled trial of cognitive therapy for acutely suicidal patients with early psychosis. *Australian and New Zealand Journal of Psychiatry*, **37**, 414–420.

Raj MA, Kumaraiah V, Bhide AV (2001). Cognitive-behavioural intervention in deliberate self-harm. *Acta Psychiatrica Scandinavica*, **104**, 340–345.

Rathus JH and Miller Al (2002). Dialectical behavior therapy adapted for suicidal adolescents. *Suicide and Life-Threatening Behavior*, **32**, 146–157.

Rhee WK, Merbaum M, Strube MJ *et al.* (2005). Efficacy of brief telephone psychotherapy with callers to a suicide hotline. *Suicide and Life-Threatening Behavior*, **35**, 317–328.

Rudd MD (2006). An update on the psychotherapeutic treatment of suicidal behavior. In J Trafton and W Gordon, eds, *Best Practices in the Behavioral Management of Chronic Disease*, p. 4. Institute for Brain Potential, California.

Rudd MD (2007). Inaccurate conclusions based on limited data. *The British Journal of Psychiatry*, **190**, (Letters to the Editor, online version): Accessed at: http://bjp.rcpsych.org/cgi/eletters?lookup=by_dateanddays=30

Rudd MD, Joiner TE, Rajab H (1996). Help negation after acute suicidal crisis. *Journal of Consulting and Clinical Psychology*, **63**, 499–503.

Rudd MD, Joiner TE, Rajab H (2004). *Treating Suicidal Behavior*, 2nd edn. Guilford Press, New York.

Rudd MD, Mandrusiak M, Joiner TE (2006). The case against no-suicide contracts: The Commitment to Treatment statement as an alternative for clinical practice. *Journal of Clinical Psychology: In Session*, **62**, 243–251.

Salkovkis PM, Atha C, Storer D (1990). Cognitive-behavioral problem solving in the treatment of patients who repeated attempt suicide: a controlled trial. *British Journal of Psychiatry*, **157**, 871–876.

Spirito A, Boergers J, Donaldson D *et al.* (2002). An intervention trial to improve adherence to community treatment by adolescents after suicide attempt. *American Academy for Child and Adolescence Psychiatry*, **41**, 435–442.

Suicide Prevention Resource Center (2006). *Assessing and Managing Suicide Risk: Core Competencies for Mental Health Professionals.* Newton, Massachusetts.

Tarrier N, Haddock G, Lewis S *et al.* (2006). Suicide behaviour over 18 months in recent onset schizophrenic patients: the effects of CBT. *Schizophrenia Research*, **83**, 15–27.

Termansen PE and Bywater C (1975). S.A.F.E.R.: a follow-up service for attempted suicide in Vancouver. *Canadian Psychiatric Association Journal*, **20**, 29–34.

Torhorst A, Möller HJ, Kurz A *et al.* (1988). Comparing a 3-month and a 12-month-outpatient aftercare program for parasuicide repeaters. In HJ Möller, A Schmidtke and R Welz, eds, *Current Issues of Suicidology*, pp. 419–424. Springer-Verlag, Berlin.

Turner RM (2000). Naturalistic evaluation of dialectical behavior therapy-oriented treatment for borderline personality disorder. *Cognitive and Behavioral Practice*, **7**, 413–419.

Tyrer P, Thompson S, Schmidt U (2003). Randomized controlled trial of brief cognitive behaviour therapy versus treatment as usual in recurrent deliberate self-harm: the POPMACT study. *Psychological Medicine*, **33**, 969–976.

Van den Bosch LM, Koeter MW, Stijnen T *et al.* (2005). Sustained efficacy of dialectical behavior therapy for borderline personality disorder. *Behavior Research and Therapy*, **43**, 1231–1241.

Van der Sande R, van Rooijen L, Buskens E *et al.* (1997). Intensive inpatient and community intervention versus routine care after attempted suicide: a randomized controlled intervention study. *British Journal of Psychiatry*, **171**, 35–41.

Van Heeringen C, Jannes C, Buylaert W *et al.* (1995). The management of non-compliance with referral to out-patient after-care among attempted suicide patients: a controlled intervention study. *Psychological Medicine*, **25**, 963–970.

Waterhouse J and Platt S (1990). General hospital admission in the management of parasuicide. A randomised controlled trial. *British Journal of Psychiatry*, **156**, 236–242.

Weinberg I, Gunderson JG, Hennen J *et al.* (2006). Manual assisted cognitive treatment for deliberate self-harm in borderline personality disorder patients. *Journal of Personality Disorders*, **20**, 482–492.

Welu TC (1977). A follow-up program for suicide attempters: evaluation of effectiveness. *Suicide and Life-Threatening Behavior*, **7**, 17–20.

Verheul R, Van Den Bosch LM, Koeter MW *et al.* (2003). Dialectical behaviour therapy for women with borderline personality disorder: 12-month, randomised clinical trial in The Netherlands. *British Journal of Psychiatry*, **182**, 135–140.

Wood A, Trainor G, Rothwell J, Moore J *et al.* (2001). Randomized trail of group therapy for repeated deliberate self-harm in adolescents. *Child and Adolescent Psychiatry*, **40**, 1246–1253.

# CHAPTER 59

# Family psychoeducation with suicide attempters

Edward J Dunne

## Abstract

Inappropriate or inadequate treatment in emergency treatment settings frequently leads to failures to adhere to after-care prescriptions and an increase in subsequent suicidality. Working collaboratively with the patient and the family can increase compliance and reduce risk. An intervention based on the family psychoeducation model developed to treat serious mental illnesses is described. A rationale for using this model is presented, which stems from the high rate of mental illness diagnoses in psychological autopsies of completed suicides. Sequential tasks for the clinician are presented. 'Joining' as a collaborative technique with both the patient and the family is described. Specific guidelines for the family to reduce potential for further harm are suggested.

## Introduction

Suicidal thoughts, suicide attempts, and completed suicides are all both individual and systemic events. Every completed suicide hurls surviving family and loved ones into a protracted and problematic grieving period (Dunne 1992). In the past quarter century, it has become increasingly apparent that many of these survivors need special attention if they are to successfully negotiate the tasks of grieving. Considerably less is known about the consequences for a family of loved one's repeated attempts to end their own life. During this same time period, it has also become clear that treatment of people with major mental illnesses stands the best chance of a positive outcome if the family is actively engaged in the treatment (McFarlane and Dunne 1991).

As with the trend in physical medicine, in which family members of cancer and heart patients are involved in the after care, family pychoeducation has spread from its original application to people with schizophrenia, to individuals with bipolar disorder, major depression, substance abuse, and persons diagnosed with borderline personality disorder (McFarlane 2002). These studies aptly demonstrate the wisdom of involving families in treatment of these disorders as a means of reducing symptoms and avoiding relapse.

It would then seem natural that suicide prevention, particularly after a suicide attempt, would find increased success if the family of the attempter were involved in after care. Unfortunately, with a very few notable exceptions (Rotheram-Borus et al. 1996; Greenfield et al. 2002), this is not routinely the case. Clinicians in both psychiatric emergency settings, inpatient and outpatient facilities frequently see the family as merely a source of information about things the patient will not discuss or does not remember. They can go so far as to criticise the family for their pre-episode behaviour, for example failing to respond to what now are evident signs of suicidal thinking or 'early warning signs'.

If the person who attempts suicide is hospitalized, all too often the family is included only in discharge planning as it becomes evident that the patient will be returned to the community with the family acting as the de facto caretakers, providing the majority of the surveillance and monitoring of the patient. They are only infrequently coached about effective ways of performing their role. Keeping the family excluded from the beginning, and then expecting them to implement the after care part of the treatment plan will result in the family's either performing the role poorly or rejecting it with a concomitant increase in suicidal risk. What follows is a rationale for using the family pychoeducation model in preventing future attempts of suicidal people.

## Family psychoeducation in the treatment of mental illness

It is important at the outset to understand what family pychoeducation is. Anderson and colleagues (1986) view family pychoeducation as a tripartite collaboration among equals, which encompasses the person with the diagnosis, their 'family', and the clinician. The word family is placed in quotation marks because it represents, in this context, not merely those individuals who are biological relatives of the patient, but also includes people who have close personal ties to him or her, and who are likely to be sources of support or who will need to change their routine way of relating to the patient to allow for recovery. In this collaboration, each entity has a distinct role to play in the shared enterprise of defeating the illness. Thus, the patient's role is to identify symptoms and sources of stress, and to report them as accurately as possible to the family and clinician. The patient is also expected to report accurately on participation in the after care prescribed, including medications. The family's role is to supplement this reporting by explicating symptoms if the patient fails to identify and to report on prodromal symptoms. The clinician is, at the outset, the educator for the family and the patient in all that is known about the present illness, and what can be done to alleviate it. Additionally, the clinician, as a neutral third party, serves to help resolve conflicts between the patient and the family. Finally, the clinician leads the family and the patient in a highly structured problem-solving exercise directed initially towards symptom reduction, and eventually towards social and vocational rehabilitation.

Anderson *et al.* place great emphasis on the relationships between, and among, all parties as key to the success of the treatment. They point out that families have to be engaged from a position of collaboration as equal partners with the clinician. This stance is in direct opposition to the more usual hierarchical relationships that typify most people's expectations (and experience) of the mental health system. Likewise, in this endeavour, the clinician must work to gain the patient's trust in order to gain permission to involve the family (if the patient is an adult) and if the patient is to cooperate. The technique of doing this is formally known as 'joining' with the family and the patient, and it is accomplished in a prescribed manner through a variety of behaviours on the clinician's part, which are directed at breaking down the traditional 'doctor–patient' relationship. It is absolutely essential to the success of this treatment that such joining take place both with the family and with the patient, since, eventually, all parties must be convinced that the clinician is there for them as a powerful ally against the re-emergence of symptoms.

The next step is to provide the family and the patient with as much information about the illness as they can reasonably handle. In this model, the psychobiological underpinnings of the diseases under consideration are usually emphasized over more purely psychological or psychosocial theories. It has been found that a key step in getting the family to collaborate in the treatment is to de-stigmatize the illness, and thereby the family and the patient. This is best accomplished by avoiding blaming the family for the patient's illness, and requires recognizing that even, if eventually, not useful or even harmful, the efforts of the family in the past have been motivated by concern for the patient. Likewise, the patient's past troublesome behaviours are attributed to the illness itself, and not to deliberately hurtful motives. In an atmosphere of increasing trust, both family and patient can join with the clinician in overcoming the illness.

## Family psychoeducation in the case of suicide attempts

The question of appropriate discharge planning for suicide attempters is one that continues to vex clinicians and other caregivers. On the one hand, attempters are frequently unwilling to admit the seriousness of their situation, and may even be in denial about their lethal intent. They frequently advocate for limited after care as a way of 'putting all this behind' them and avoiding the stigma of mental illness. Likewise, they often resist involving their families in treatment, either because they do not want to burden them (feeling too inadequate to deserve special attention) or because they see their family as at least one of the sources of their difficulties. In addition, they often have an acute embarrassment about the attempt and are reluctant to share their feelings and thoughts with other family members. These tendencies increase the further the attempter is from the episode, that is, as they stabilize and begin to recover.

In similar fashion, the families of attempters also frequently advocate for limited after care as a way of avoiding the stigma associated

with mental illness and suicide attempts, both for their ill family member and for themselves. Often, they have been burdened by the patient's behaviour prior to the attempts, which frequently include aggression, destructiveness, withdrawal, or acts of physical self-harm. Frequently, they have been the persons directly responsible for maintaining the patient's safety as they moved into a suicidal phase, but before actual suicidal behaviours emerged. Hence, they are often exhausted and demoralized after a suicide attempt is made, and may no longer trust their competence to keep their loved one alive. In some instances, they too are in denial about the seriousness of the attempt, dismissing it as an attention-getting device. And as is true of the patient, the further they are from the episode, the more reluctant they become about being involved.

These factors would argue for prompt and early engagement of the family and the patient in an effort to attach the patient to the appropriate after care following a suicide attempt. It is generally reported that less than one half of all attempters keep their first appointment following discharge from emergency treatment (O'Brien *et al.* 1987; Sakinofsky and Roberts 1990; Moller 1990). This is a serious treatment failure considering the number of completed suicides who were attempters in the past.

Many health care systems are prohibited from disclosing medical and psychiatric information about an adult patient to anyone without the express permission of the patient, except in instances when the patient is an imminent danger to himself or to others. Unfortunately, all too often clinicians and other care-staff either misinterpret the meaning of these statutes to support not contacting the family, or use them to avoid making the extra effort it takes to get the patient's permission to involve the family. It can be argued that all persons who have made an attempt to end their own lives of sufficient severity as to require emergency treatment are, and remain, for some time thereafter, an imminent danger to themselves, and thus the family can be contacted even absent permission. It is also true that when the clinician takes sufficient time to elaborate the reasons for including the family, most patients eventually agree. Patients' negative attitudes towards involving family can be overcome if the clinician has time to build a relationship with the patient, and to understand the basis of the attitude. The clinician may also need time to convince the patient that family can be helpful for rehabilitation or treatment purposes. In the majority of cases, given sufficient time for this kind of intervention, it is possible to persuade the patient to involve family in the treatment and rehabilitation process without breaking existing rules and laws in the health care systems.

If applied to the treatment of suicide attempters, the family psychoeducational model would require engagement of both the patient and the family at the earliest possible juncture. Rotheram-Borus and colleagues (1996) were able to achieve remarkably high treatment adherence rates in a post-attempt intervention by actually contracting with the patient and the family, while the patient was still in the emergency room (ER). In this instance, the attempters were all adolescents necessitating face-to-face contact with the parents prior to discharge from the ER. This provided an extra bit of leverage and helped the clinician begin the joining process immediately. In the case of adult attempters, no such requirement for family involvement is usually the case. To overcome this disadvantage, it is recommended that the patient be admitted to the general hospital, or to an inpatient psychiatric service for at least 24 hours after presenting to the ER, depending on how much physical harm the attempter has suffered. The following is a series of steps which can ensure maximum safety and aftercare treatment compliance in the event of a suicide attempt.

# Programme for implementing family psychoeducation in the event of a suicide attempt

## Step 1: Hospitalize all attempters regardless of lethality of the attempt for no less than 24 hours whenever possible

This allows time for a thorough psychiatric evaluation outside of the time constraints, usually present in emergency room settings, and facilitates efforts to engage the family in aftercare. It also gives time for an assessment of the family as a resource, and the likelihood of providing a safe environment for the patient after discharge. ER staff need to overcome their reluctance to 'label' the patient, and insist on a thorough psychiatric exam before discharge. If general hospital admission is required, the family should optimally be contacted by the outpatient clinician who will work with the patient after discharge. Inpatient clinicians can initiate the family contact once the patient is in their care, but every effort should be made to involve the outpatient clinicians as quickly as possible, since it is they who will ultimately have responsibility for the patient's safety and treatment.

## Step 2: Join with the patient

The clinician's first task is to join with the patient in such a way as to promote the establishment of trust between them. This, in turn, allows the clinician to recommend engaging the family in the after care planning. To accomplish this, the clinician must negotiate several issues with the patient. First, the patient needs to be educated about suicidal thoughts and behaviours, particularly as they relate to the broad spectrum of mental illnesses. This must be accomplished in the context of joining, in order to establish a collegial rapport and foster trust. Thus, the clinician should blame the illness rather than the patient, while empathizing with the recent feelings of despair and helplessness. The link between these feelings and depression, in particular, should be drawn. It is important for the clinician to validate other common emotions associated with a suicide attempt such as shame, guilt, and anger, and aim to reassure the patient that, with treatment, these emotions need not again overwhelm them. Likewise, the clinician should help the patient turn away from blaming others for his or her actions, suggesting that, ultimately, the blame rests with the illness.

A short explanation of the psychobiology of mental illnesses and their neurological underpinnings should be presented in order to help the patient understand the nature of their illness and the steps needed to recover from it. Next, the clinician must educate the patient that research has clearly demonstrated that patient safety and recovery are most likely achieved when the patient's social network is involved, and it is for that reason that the clinician seeks permission to involve other people, particularly family members.

A further step is to clearly outline to the patient what the intervention would look like—that it is collaboration for safety and recovery, not an opportunity to blame and shame. Next, the clinician should carefully delineate the patient's social network, identifying with the patient who would be likely to participate in such an endeavour and how they may be contacted. It is important that the clinician offers to make the contact, rather than leaving it up to the patient.

Finally, the clinician should begin to reach out to the family as agreed to by the patient. The goals of the initial joining session are to:

1   Help the patient understand the seriousness of the situation;

2   To separate illness from the person;

3   Identify problems which might interfere with after care;

4   Explore multiple solutions to the immediate problem;

5   Secure an agreement to include family members in after care; and

6   Delineate a treatment plan.

Naturally, all this must also be in tune with the physical and psychological condition of the patient as well.

## Step 3: Contact and joining with the family

After securing an agreement to after care involving the family, the next step is to contact and join with those family members identified by the patient as important to safety and recovery. If feasible, this should be accomplished during the initial interview, either in person with the people who accompanied the patient to the emergency room, or by phone if necessary. This initial contact with the patient's family represents the first step in joining with them, which is crucial to a successful outcome. It is critical that the clinician approaches the family from a collegial point of view. The failure to engage families in treatment can almost always be attributed to their detection of underlying attitudes of judgement or blame on the part of treatment personnel. In fact, many of the early family-based interventions for attempters suffered from an excessive pathologizing of the family with such family descriptors as 'disorganized' (Pfeffer 1990), and 'unbalanced' (Frances and Pfeffer 1987).

Here, the goals are similar, and the clinician's approach matches that described in joining with the patient: that is he/she is collegial, frank but optimistic, and supportive of the family's emotional responses to the crisis. The education of the family includes the information shared with the patient about the psychobiology of mental illness, and the relationship between them and suicidal thoughts and behaviours. The clinician helps to de-mystify mental illness and suicide by describing them in objective, non-blaming terms. Prejudices that the family may hold regarding suicide (attention-getting, trying to manipulate us, etc.) are gently challenged.

Next, the clinician must assist the family is making a realistic survey of the safety of the home environment, in terms of access to lethal means, and to develop an action plan to eliminate as many potential sources of self-harm as possible. Following this, the family is helped to recall the days leading up to the attempt in order to expose any prodromal indicators, which had gone undetected at the time or whose meaning was unclear.

Whatever the elements of the after care plan (family psychoeducation, psychotherapy, medication, etc.), the family should be informed about its details and procedures and enlisted to assist in ensuring strict compliance. An action plan, which increases the safety of the patient, is developed. As was true in the case of joining with the patient, the clinician should help the family identify others who might be of assistance in implementing the treatment plan. The clinician must offer round-the-clock accessibility, either to herself or her team in the event of future emergencies. The family should be encouraged to contact the clinician even if they are uncertain about the severity of the situation, since the clinician should be engaged with the family in helping assess what is happening and what action, if any, should be taken.

## Step 4: Devise and implement an after-care plan

After care for suicide attempters must address two distinct issues: immediate short-term safety and avoidance of subsequent attempts. Ensuring immediate safety will, particularly, involve the family since, in most cases, they become the after care monitors. Thus, the family needs to be educated about prodromal signs of suicide, as well as being helped to develop communication skills, which will promote confidence and trust. Likewise, they need to be knowledgeable about the ancillary treatment(s) their family member is engaged in (medication, CBT, etc.), so that they can serve as effective observers of treatment compliance. Longer-term objectives include the avoidance of relapse through the development of skills and attitudes, which counter despair and hopelessness. Actively engaging the family with the patient in a psychoeducational setting can be effectively used to accomplish these objectives. The use of problem-solving is especially helpful since it 'objectifies' the issues and helps avoid high emotionality and conflict. Family psychoeducation, in this context, may consist of 4–8 meetings with the patient and the family spread out over several weeks, while the patient is simultaneously being seen by an individual therapist. The purpose of these meetings is to assure compliance with all aspects of the after care plan, and to keep the family informed as to the mental status of the patient *vis-à-vis* current suicide risk. The clinician makes it clear that the material discussed with the family involves issues of safety and not the content of therapy sessions, which do not directly relate to this. If substantial risk remains, the clinician helps the family review the safety plans they have in effect and suggests revisions when necessary or appropriate. The family and the patient should be informed that the early stages of convalescence from a suicide attempt may include the return of suicidal thoughts, so as to normalize the occurrence of such thoughts and prepare everyone for them. At the same time, the clinician holds out the hope that, with continued participation in treatment, the danger will subside and the family can resume normal functioning.

As in most psychoeducational endeavours, clear and consistent guidelines for both the family and the patient help reduce conflict and tension in the early stages of recovery. The family guidelines (see Table 59.1), adapted from McFarlane (2002) and Anderson *et al.* (1986) are specific to suicide attempts and might be used in addition to whatever other guidelines are suggested by the psychiatric diagnosis.

In the ideal situation, the patient and the family would continue to work together with the clinician to solve problems, the recovery from this episode encounters, and to work proactively to promote a healthy adjustment and avoid future episodes. The clinician takes the lead in helping the patient and the family identify potentially troublesome situations and engages them in formal problem-solving, as described by McFarlane (2002). Initially, the focus will be on issues of safety, but gradually, the focus will shift to resolving issues which impede communication among family members, and which keep recovery moving forward. Directly engaging the family in a collaborative process which taps into their experience with the

**Table 59.1** Family guidelines in the aftermath of a suicide attempt

*Go slow*. Safety and recovery take time. Give the suicidal person the time they need.

*Keep to the plan*. Check out any changes in the safety and recovery plan with the clinician before enacting them.

*Be aware of medications*. Take all prescribed medicines. Do not keep unused medications. Dispose of them safely.

*Keep a safe house*. Secure all firearms, prescription medications, car keys, sharp instruments, ropes, and poisons. Put up with the temporary inconvenience this may entail. Keep the clinician informed of any changes in the situation.

*Don't ignore changes*. Report prodromal signs of depression, suicidal communication or of an attempt.

*Be alert*. Anticipate and monitor behaviour and feelings around stressful events, especially those which involve personal or interpersonal disappointments.

*Avoid conflict*. Refer your disagreements to the clinician for problem-solving.

*Be low key*. Lower the emotional tone in the household.

*Know how to get help*. Keep emergency contact numbers public and available.

*Be available to listen*. Be ready to be shut out. Keep communications open.

patient provides them with knowledge and skills about preventing suicide, increases communication between them and their family member, and greatly enhances the likelihood of after care treatment compliance and the avoidance of subsequent attempts.

## Conclusion

Completed suicides of people who have made an attempt in the past suggests a failure in after care, which can often be traced back to the decisions and behaviours of the clinicians and care-staff who handled the initial attempt. Sufficient evidence now exists to demonstrate the efficacy of involving the family in the treatment of a variety of physical and psychiatric disorders, to allow the supposition that involvement of the family after a suicide attempt is likely to reduce not only immediate danger, but also improve after care treatment adherence and reduce the likelihood of subsequent attempts. The family psychoeducation model is a means of involving the family in a way which is respectful of their strengths and sensitive to the needs of the patient. Implementing such an intervention requires the clinician to make an effort to work in a collaborative way, with both the patient and the family, preferably prior to discharge from the emergency treatment setting.

## References

Anderson CM, Reiss J, Hogarty G (1986). *Schizophrenia and the Family: A Practitioner's Guide to Psychoeducation and Management*. Guilford, New York.

Dunne EJ (1992). Following a suicide: postvention. In B Bongar, ed., *Assessment, Management, and Treatment of Suicide: Guidelines for Clinical Practice*, pp. 221–234. Oxford University Press, Oxford.

Frances A and Pfeffer CR (1987). Reducing environmental stress for a suicidal ten-year-old. *Hospital and Community Psychiatry*, **38**, 22–24.

Greenfield B, Larson C, Hechtman L *et al.* (2002). A rapid-response outpatient model for reducing hospitalization rates among suicidal adolescents. *Psychiatric Services*, **53**, 1574–1579.

McFarlane WR (2002). *Multifamily Groups in the Treatment of Severe Psychiatric Disorders*. Guilford, New York.

McFarlane WR and Dunne EJ (1991). Family psychoeducation and multi-family groups in the treatment of schizophrenia. *Directions in Psychiatry*, **11**, 2–7.

Moller HJ (1990). Evaluation of aftercare strategies. In G Ferrari, M Bellini and P Crepet, eds, *Suicidal Behaviour and Risk Factors*, pp. 39–44. Monduzzi Editore, Bologna.

O'Brien G, Holton AR, Hurren K et al. (1987). Deliberate self-harm and predictors of out-patient attendance. *Brittish Journal of Psychiatry*, **150**, 246–247.

Pfeffer CR (1981). The family system of suicidal children. *American Journal of Psychotherapy*, **35**, 330–341.

Rotheram-Borus MJ, Piacentini J, Miller S *et al.* (1996). Toward improving treatment adherence among adolescent suicide attempters. *Clinical Child Psychology and Psychiatry*, **1**, 99–106.

Sakinofsky I and Roberts RS (1990). Why parasuicides repeat despite problem resolution. *The British Journal of Psychiatry*, **156**, 399–405.

# CHAPTER 60

# The role of paintings in suicide treatment and prevention

Thomas Bronisch and Flora von Spreti

## Abstract

The theme 'suicide' in paintings mirror social, cultural, religious and philosophical stances to suicide. However, behind these more public aspects of the artist's work there is often a personal meaning for the artist as well. The motives and interests of the artists go beyond the theme of suicide. An important factor in suicidal behaviour is a depressive mood or a depressive disorder. However, the depressive mood as well as the underlying manic-depressive illness of some artists may also be seen as an important prerequisite for their creativity. Despite the importance of suicidality in art and that art therapy is well-established for treating patients in psychiatry and psychotherapy, only a small body of empirical literature about the role of art therapy in depressed and suicidal patients exists today. In paintings and sculptures of art therapy, done by patients primarily reflect the inner experiences of their illness and biography. Art therapy can help the patient to alleviate self-destructive ways of acting.

## Introduction

Suicidal behaviour is an important existential phenomenon that has been reflected in art, especially in paintings. Art has also been used for the purpose of diagnostics and therapy of such behaviour.

An attempt is made in this chapter to discuss this relation between paintings and suicidal behaviour, giving some examples of suicidal behaviour depicted in Western European paintings and mainly focusing on art therapy.

There is no way to find out whether there are suicides among the buried of the Stone Age, or if the makers of stone tools ever directed such utensils against themselves (van Hooff 2000). Furthermore, there are no reports on arts and suicide in the pre-antiquity era. However, suicide is a common theme in Western art, at least since the time period known as classical antiquity (van Hooff 1990). The role of paintings in suicide prevention can be approached from numerous angles:

◆ Can suicide presented in paintings reflect the zeitgeist, and particularly the cultural and intellectual climate of a particular era?

◆ Can paintings of suicidal artists tell us something about the suicidal process?

◆ Can art be used as a diagnostic tool for suicidality?

◆ Can art be used as therapy for suicidality?

◆ Can art spontaneously intervene with the suicidal process?

## Suicide in paintings: a concise historical outline

First, a brief introduction of how suicidality has been presented in paintings during the history of what has been lately referred to as Western art. Throughout all historical epochs, art has reflected on different aspects of suicidality (Brown 2001). Brown asserts that 'if images of suicide say one thing above all, it is that this strange death has never had a fixed meaning' (2001, p. 221). Art reflects—reflected—the cultural, philosophical, religious and sociological mainstream in the history of mankind. Van Hooff (2000) divided the history of suicide into antiquity, the middle ages, early modern time (fifteenth to seventeenth century), eighteenth century, nineteenth century and finally modern times (twentieth century).

### Antiquity

In classical antiquity, self-killing was not 'gambling with death' by taking a handful of pills. In the Greco-Roman world, self-killing was typically seen as a deliberate, resolute, and heroic act (van Hooff 1994). The most common Greek and Latin terms for suicide express this idea: self-killing was referred to as voluntary death, in Greek *hekousios thanatos* and in Latin *mors voluntari*. The prototype of ancient suicide is Ajax. After the death of Achilles in the Trojan War, a controversy arose among the Greek heroes as to whom Achilles' armour should be adjudged. Ulysses won the contest. The fatal blow to his honour made it impossible for Ajax to face his comrades any longer. He thrust himself on his sword, as can be seen in a black-figure krater, a vase which was used to mix wine and water, which has been attributed to Exekias 540 BCE (van Hooff 2000). Shame was the dominant motive for killing oneself during antiquity. However, van Hoof (1990) during his study of sculptures, paintings, epitaphs, historical reports and myths, discovered a wide range of motives for suicide in classical antiquity: *conscientia* (consciousness of guilt), *desperatio* (seeing no exit during times of acute distress), *devotio* (sacrificing ones' life for the benefit of the community), *dolor* (mourning over the loss of a partner), *exsecratio* (cursing of an enemy), *fides* (loyalty of a wife or a subordinate), *furor* (frenzy), *iactatio* (demonstration of a philosophical contempt of death), *inpatientia* (unbearable bodily suffering), *necessitas* (enforced self-killing), *pudor* (shame) and *taedium vitae* (being fed up with life).

## The Middle Ages (*c.* fifth–fifteenth centuries)

The Middle Ages across most of Europe were dominated by the Christian view of suicide as sin. The most prominent articulation of this view was made by St Augustine in *De Civitate Dei* (Aurelius Augustinus 400) equating suicide (self-murder) with homicide (Minois 1995; Murray 1998).

Judas Iscariots' suicide was the final proof of that he completely rejected God's grace, whereas the robber who was crucified next to Christ was redeemed and entered paradise together with the Saviour. Some unknown artists depict the death of Judas in churches (Brown 2001). As a further example, the Italian painter Giotto shows the '*desperacio*' hanging him- or herself while the devils flutter around on the wall of the Arena Chapel in Padua (*c.* 1305) (van Hooff 1994).

## Early modern times (sixteenth and seventeenth centuries)

Early modern times, including what has commonly been referred to as the Reformation, Renaissance and Baroque, brought about the development of schools of thought accentuating individualism. Moreover, renewed dialogue with Greek and Roman philosophy resulted in a greater respect for the dignity and complexity of human beings (van Hooff 2000; see also MacDonald and Murphy 1990). Lucretia's suicide, an act to avoid rape and desecration, was deemed both an honourable deed and a crime. St Augustine presented Lucretia's suicide as an example of sin in *De Civitate Dei* (400), but by early modern times, her deed was seen as honourable. This discussion was reflected and replicated in numerous paintings by artists in the Renaissance such as Lucas Cranach the Elder (Bronisch 2002).

## Eighteenth century

The eighteenth century is known as the Age of Reason, and for the first time since antiquity, suicide comes to represent the right to take leave of life. Furthermore, suicide was being accepted as a psychological illness in case of melancholia (MacDonald and Murphy 1990).

Suicide's romantic edge was reinforced by the novel *Young Werther's Sufferings*, written by the German poet Goethe in 1774, but not directly depicted as far as we know. However, there are paintings concerning the suicide of other young men, such as the painting of the young poet Chatterton's suicide by Henry Wallis (1856) in England, or the young martyr by Paul Delaroche (1855) in France one century later. The paintings mirror the change in attitudes toward suicide in early modern times and reflect the image of romantic suicide. This international trend was a consequence of the secularization in agreement with the emerging philosophy of enlightenment and acknowledgement of the importance of the individual. 'It culminates in a pivotal period of change wherein death itself was secularized, and after which a rash of suicidal imagery emerged alongside a neo-Gothic art which attempted to bring back the spiritual' (Brown 2001, p. 126).

## Nineteenth century

The growing acceptance of suicide as one possibility of ending one's life led to the development of sociological discussions on suicide (see Anderson 1987), of which Emile Durkheim's sociological treatise about suicide is the most well-known: *Le Suicide* (1897). The 'moloch of metropolis' (van Hoof 2000) is demonstrated by several illustrations of suicide in the city, for example, Camille Pissaro's *Le Pendu* made between 1889–1890 (Brown 2001).

## Twentieth century

The twentieth century finally tries to document suicide without a moral, ethical and philosophical evaluation, as presented by Andy Warhol in his 'Death Series' (Andy Warhol, *Purple Jumping Man*, detail 1965). Moreover, abstract paintings are given titles and meanings connected to suicidality, for example, works by Man Ray and Paul Klee (Brown 2001).

# Depression and suicide in artists

Accounts reveal suicidal behaviour of specific artists beginning in the antiquity up to modern times. However, the question arises whether art really can be used as a diagnostic tool for discovering suicidality in an individual? As mentioned above, art can reflect the zeitgeist of an epoch. What could we learn on an individual level from the paintings of artists who were depressed and committed suicide?

## Depression in artists

Depression is a pathfinder for suicidal tendencies (Bronisch 2003). The physiognomy of depressives has been widely depicted by artists, for example by Hans Baldung Grien in his picture *Saturn*, showing the pronounced nasolabial folds described by Veraguth as indicative for melancholia. The painting *The lonely souls* by Ferdinand Hodler depicts four men with loosely sunken heads, hanging shoulders and the shrunk figure of the typically depressed (Pöldinger 1986).

Joan Miró, referring to his depressions, described in letters, interviews, and articles how they affected his art (Schildkraut and Hirshfeld 1995). He became most influential for the New York School of abstract expressionist painters (see below). In regard to painters in modern times, Bernard Buffet, Vincent van Gogh, Arshile Gorky, Ernst Ludwig Kirchner, Wilhelm Lehmbruck, and Mark Rothko are well-known examples. Most of these artists are reported to have been suffering from severe depression: Vincent van Gogh was diagnosed with temporal lobe epilepsy which produced, at times, schizophrenic-like episodes with hallucinations and depression (Finkelstein 1971). His family was heavily burdened with psychosis and recurrent depression (Jamison 1993). His suicide was probably a result of deep depression, however, there still remains controversy on this matter (Maire 1971). The German expressionist Ernst Ludwig Kirchner had severe depression (Grote *et al.* 2000). The painters of the New York School of abstract expressionism, Arshile Gorky and Mark Rothko, suffered from depression (Schildkraut and Hirshfeld 1994). Bernard Buffet was struck by Parkinson's disease and additionally endured depression (Grote *et al.* 2000). Jamison (1989a) found in her research that 38 per cent of contemporary visual artists had histories of severe mood swings. Furthermore, alcoholism or alcohol abuse was found in many painters (Schildkraut *et al.* 1994).

There is no doubt that periods of severe depression and desperation are mirrored in the paintings of Vincent van Gogh (Maire 1971). Van Gogh and Ernst Ludwig Kirchner used gloomy motifs and furnished them with dark colours. The abstract paintings of Mark Rothko demonstrate dark colours (Schildkraut *et al.* 1994), and some authors (Ravin *et al.* 1978) interpret his latest paintings as suicide notes. However, even in conjunction with a psychiatric, especially depressive illness, the artist tries to work through the inner experiences, so that the work of art goes beyond their personal existence. The inner experience of psychiatric illness and life experiences must be seen as a source for the general meaning of the artist's paintings and sculptures.

## Suicide in artists

Epidemiological research, as well as reports on famous artists about the frequencies of suicide in artists, especially in painters, reveals an elevated rate (Juda 1949; Andreasen 1978; Jamison 1989a; Schildkraut *et al.* 1994; Stack 1996, 1997; Lester 1998). Furthermore, Juda (1949), Andreasen (1987), Jamison (1989b), and Schildkraut *et al.* (1994) reported higher suicide rates in painters and other artists; however, Preti and Motto (1999) reported a lower rate as compared to the general population. Reasons for the higher rates in depression may be psychoneurotic qualities such as hypersensitivity, rapidly changing emotions, and inner depressive experiences that may have positive effects on artistic creation (Juda 1949; Jamison 1989a), but they also increase the odds of suicide (Schildkraut *et al.* 1994). Furthermore, even among notable artists, many if not most 'creative products' are rejected. These frequent rejections, involving highly personal products such as paintings, are difficult to deal with. Rejection and performance below one's potential are often a precursor to suicide among artists (Lester 1993).

## Depression as a productive but dangerous tool for artistic creativity

Are there therapeutic effects of art making? By analysing the abstract expressionists of the New York School, Schildkraut *et al.* (1994) posit that:

> Depression inevitably leads to a turning inward and to the painful re-examination of the purpose of living and the possibility of dying. Depression may have been particularly destructive at a personal level; yet, for instances such as those … depression in the artist may be of adaptive value to society at large.
>
> Schildkraut *et al.* (1994, p. 487)

Juda (1949) investigated 294 highly gifted creative German personalities from 1650 to 1900. They were divided into two main groups, 113 artists and 181 scientists: the subgroup of the artists included 12 architects, 18 sculptors, 37 poets, 20 painters and 26 musicians (composers only). She reported on personality disorders (psychoneurotic individuals and psychopaths) and maintained 'how delicately the psychic equilibrium of highly gifted artists is balanced with its counter play of high-geared sensitivity and deep emotions, and the driving force of creative ideas and the subconscious repercussions' (1949, p. 298).

Fifty years later, Jamison (1989b) asked forty-seven British playwrights, novelists, biographers and artists questions about their respective histories, if any, of affective illnesses, possibly treated and investigated. Inquiry into whether any behavioural, cognitive and mood change with diurnal and seasonal patterns correlated with their periods of creative work and its intensity was made. About one-third of the writers and artists reported histories of severe mood swings, essentially cyclothymic in nature, and a quarter reported histories of extended elated mood states. Virtually all subjects (89 per cent) reported having experienced intense, highly productive and creative episodes. When the subjects were asked specifically about the importance of very intense feelings and moods on the development and execution of their work, 90 per cent stated that such moods and feelings were either integral or necessary (60 per cent) or very important (30 per cent). The treatment rate for affective illness (38 per cent) was strikingly high in this sample of outstanding British writers and artists. Jamison stated that:

> For writers and artists, who draw so deeply from their lives and emotions for their work, the wide range and intensity, fluctuation and variability of emotional experience brought about mood disorders which can work to the advantage, as well as disadvantage of original composition.
>
> Jamison (1989b, p. 131)

Furthermore, Richards *et al.* (1988) found significantly increased creativity in manic-depressive and cyclothymic patients, as well as their normal first-degree relatives, when compared with control subjects. Navratil (2002) suggests that mixed manic-depressive states in the modern sense of a cyclothymia predisposes to creativity in arts (see also Goodwin and Jamison 1990).

## Art as a diagnostic and therapeutic tool in depressed and suicidal patients

'The function of art is to acquaint the beholder with something he has not known before' (Langer 1953, p. 22). Having explored the relationship of artist and their paintings to depression and suicidality, we proceed to our patients.

### Characteristics of drawings of depressed patients

Drawings as diagnostic and therapeutic tools were first used in France (Simon 1972) and Germany (Mohr 1906). The first comprehensive English review was undertaken by Anastasi and Foley (1941). Cohen *et al.* (1988) developed a comprehensive assessment checklist, a drawing analysis form, the so-called Drawing Diagnostic Series (DDS). The following criteria were assessed in their study: colour type, blending, idiosyncratic colour, line/shape, integration, abstraction, representational, enclosure, groundline, people, animals, inanimate objects, abstract symbols, word inclusion, landscape, line quality/pressure, line length, movement, space usage, tree, tilt, and unusual placement. Stylistic changes in paintings of chronic depressed patients are considered as possible indicators for suicidal despair and as an expression for need of increased support by the therapist (Simon 1972). In art therapy, it is possible to detect depressive tendencies, and depression, is a pathfinder for suicidal tendencies (Bronisch 2003). There are many descriptions of formal and symbolic characteristics of drawings of depressed patients that give hints for the diagnosis of depression.

Miljkovitch de Heredia and Miljkovitch (1998) performed a controlled study, whereby twenty-six patients with major depression and twenty-six controls were asked to make a 'funny' and a 'sad' drawing, which were respectively scored on twenty-two variables describing their formal aspects and contents. In a stepwise discriminant analysis, the significant differences found primarily concerned the formal characteristics: the depressed patients' drawings were drawn in dark colours, often brown or purple, and traced in shaky lines. The patients with depression were less able than the participants in the control group to make 'funny' drawings that did not ressemble 'sad' ones. They had limited freedom in their drawing abilities that could be related to psychomotor inhibition, lack of interest for the outer world, and feelings of loneliness, which are part of the depressive syndrome. They tended to make small drawings, close to the edge of the page, with few colours (often only one), and there were rarely any light or warm ones. They drew few elements, few living beings, few humans (often none or only one), with merely a head rather than the whole body. To express fun they used a small range of colours, pictured one person, rather than a get-together, and were less fanciful (drew fewer incongruities) than the control participants. Themes and contents such as death, loss or separation, or a grave, which may seem typical of a depressive disorder, did not actually distinguish depression group drawings from control group drawings.

Cohen *et al.* (1988) developed a standardized approach for types of drawings and evaluation of drawings (see DDS above). An explorative study with patients in a psychiatric hospital as well as with a healthy control group was performed. The patients were diagnosed according to DSM-III as dysthymia, major depression and schizophrenia. All the participants had to draw three different pictures: a 'free' picture (i.e. without any instruction about the topic), a picture of a tree and a picture of how one is feeling, using lines, shapes and colours. Each picture had to be done within 15 minutes. The standardized evaluation showed an unusual placement on the page in both the 'free' and tree pictures among the depressives, a variable that showed up in no other diagnostic groups. The depressed patients sample lacked landscape in the tree picture, whereas dysthymics were predicted by the presence of landscape in the tree picture. Other characteristics of the pictures of the depressed patients were presence of a water scene in the 'feeling picture' and, somewhat less often, the absence of words in the 'free' picture.

Wadeson (1971) studied the pictures produced by ten hospitalised depressed patients. Pictures made on days when depression was high were compared with pictures produced by the same patients when depression was low. During pronounced depression the patients' pictures revealed less colour used, more empty space, and less investment of effort than during weaker depression. Though not of statistical significance, there was a trend toward the pictures being more constricted and more meaningless during more severe depression. Furthermore, gloomy colours could be indicative of a depressed mood, especially changes in colours. Contents of the paintings could suggest suicidality such as themes touching on death and dying. Finally, comments of the patients about their paintings were indicative of suicidality. Halbreich *et al.* (1980) presented three cases of subconscious premonition of death. In these three patients, premonition was expressed by means of painting. This might have been meaningless to the subject, but illuminative to an experienced and alert psychotherapist. Wadeson and Carpenter (1976) comparing patients with schizophrenia, bipolar and unipolar disorder, could not find different styles of drawing between the three different diagnostic groups when controlled for age. The conclusion was that pictorial characteristics are not closely associated with diagnosis, and that a considerable diagnostic group variability and between group-overlap exists.

## Art as a tool for detecting suicidality in depressed patients

Art therapy can provide one avenue of communication for depressed patients. Paintings may facilitate the expression of suicidal feelings of the depressed since they often have difficulties in verbalising feelings. Wadeson (1975) and Wadeson and Carpenter (1976) investigated 93 patients who were participating in art therapy during an 8-year period. Of these sixteen, 67 per cent had earlier made suicide attempts or gestures from which five had almost died; four others eventually did kill themselves, two shortly after making a suicidal picture, and two a long time after their discharge from the hospital. Wadeson (1975) collected suicidal artwork, consisting of fifty-six pictures and two works in clay, which were amassed during the 8-year period. This collection includes only those works that the individual patient associated with suicidal ideation or made just before or after a suicide attempt. The author found the following themes to be present in the paintings: hopelessness, self-hatred, being harmful to others, isolation, and anger.

## Art therapy for depressive and suicidal patients

Art therapy for suicidal patients always has to consider the manifest or underlying depression or depressive tendencies of the patients as well as the typical emotional and cognitive characteristics of the depressive state.

## Art therapy in depressives

Von Spreti (2005) emphasizes three portable pillars of the art therapists' understanding of their work. The first pillar is the ingrained conviction that creation in art yields creative pleasure and knowledge for nearly all humans, during all times, but especially in times of illness and trouble relief. The second pillar is the curiosity of human beings voiced through the multiplicity of human expression. The third pillar of the therapeutic stance could be humour. Spaniol (2003) observed in art therapy that in adults with severe mental illness, such as schizophrenia and severe depression, the therapists' attitude is even more essential than what she or he says or does. The authentic and sincere engagement with people, and the art materials themselves, are the basic curative elements in art therapy with this population. Assel and Popovici-Wacks emphasize that 'therapists are still biased in their view that the depressed patient is *non-creative, non-communicative*' (1989, p. 223), and is slowed or even inhibited by the illness. In fact, the opposite is true: the patient seeks to find other ways to communicate and express their feelings; by doing so, they revive the archaic, inborn pictorial language, which precedes the spoken and written word in the history of human kind, and in the development of each and every individual.

In our society, non-verbal communication is a neglected or forgotten way of communication. Furthermore, this kind of communication seems to be loaded with the connotation of inferiority and primitivism. Forrest (1978) observed that patients can easily overcome the language barrier and give self-disclosure by non-verbal expression, such as painting and drawing, especially of suicidal tendencies. It is much easier for the depressed patient to paint than to talk or write; by painting, they are able to overcome the inhibition of depression, guilt feelings, self-accusations and self-depreciation. Spontaneous painting sublimates their anger, anxiety and auto-aggressiveness, and restores their self-esteem and dignity. These emotions are all positive factors stimulating and enabling the creativity of depressed patients, who—until now—have mistakenly been deemed passive, inactive, non-creative and non-productive. If the therapist can activate the depressed patient into a creative patient, the treatment can be helpful in aiding their quick recovery (Assel and Popovici-Wacks 1989). Art therapy enables the depressed patient to discover their creative abilities, expressing thoughts in paintings and sculptures, and to get in contact with others. Therefore, art therapy paves the way for relieving energy and leads to new areas of interest and activity away from the depression. Art exercises are directed at helping the patient to find strength and self-worth through the discovery of their own artistic expression (Robbins 1987).

## Art therapy as intervention within the suicidal process

Art therapy tries to make a spontaneous intervention in the suicidal process. Creative activity in depressed patients consists of the following aspects: proof of the patients' vitality and *raison d'être*; mastery of copying aggression, auto-aggression and anger; sublimation of anxiety; fastening positive transference and establishing a therapeutic alliance and 'emotional dialogue'; a transitional substitutional object replacing the 'lost', new reality with equilibrium and homeostasis; preserving intellectual abilities and activities of daily life; providing creative experience and satisfaction; identifying suicidal clues and ideation; making an alternative channel of communication available; providing aesthetic and cathartic experiences; and improving the cognitive triad (Assael and Popovici-Wacks 1989).

Of special interest is the fact that in some spontaneous paintings, as in prophetic dreams, the suicidal patient unconsciously and/or unwillingly 'prophesies' and communicates their prediction of death. Through their painting, some suicidal patients communicate spontaneously, unwillingly and subconsciously, their plans for suicide (Assael and Popovici-Wacks 1989).

Wadeson (1975) studied a collection of suicidal artwork, consisting of fifty-six pictures and two works in clay from patients hospitalized for mania and depression seen in art therapy at the National Institute of Health's Clinical Center in Bethesda. The patient's comments on their production were recorded. Wadeson found that artwork had important communicative and cathartic value for the patient and was especially significant to the staff for predicting possible suicidal behaviour.

Hetero-aggression, auto-aggression and anger are important aspects of suicidality and may be alleviated during the process of painting. In some instances picture-making may well have replaced self-destructive ways of acting on such feelings and facilitated the patients' own exploration and understanding of their suicidal wishes.

The Dutch psychiatrist Piet Kuiper (2002) gives a very impressive description of a severe psychotic depression with auto- and hetero-aggressive tendencies. Kuiper describes overcoming the worst episodes of depression and of self-destructiveness by painting in the frame of non-pharmacological inpatient and outpatient treatment measures. Painting was a very important possibility for working through the distressing experiences during the illness, especially in the period of recovery.

# Case reports

### Case report 1

A 30-year-old female patient has been discharged of her own will after an inpatient stay of 7 months. At first, she had been treated in a closed ward, and later in an open ward of a psychiatric hospital. She was living alone and was dependent on her parents because of her chronic depressive illness. Earlier she had worked as a social worker.

At her last session with her psychiatrist, she assured him that she was convinced that suicide would not be the solution to her problems and promised to get in contact with the hospital in case of suicidal ideation. Additionally, she concluded an agreement for two visits per week at the outpatient department with the same psychiatrist who knew the patient and whom she trusted. However, two weeks after discharge the patient took an overdose of antidepressants and died.

The patient made paintings at home when on leave from the clinic, during the last weeks of her inpatient stay, and they were discovered after her suicide. Furthermore, a suicide note written to her art therapist was found in the patient's home. Before discharge, the patient admitted in the sessions with her art therapist that, for the time being, no actual suicide wish existed, but in case of problems after the discharge from the clinic, suicide would be her very last resort. Psychotherapy individually and in groups as well as case management over several years could apparently not curb overwhelming and yearning idealized death wishes. The immediate trigger for suicide after discharge seemed to be the announcement of her boss that she could not return to her old workplace after the two months of occupational therapy. This announcement, in itself, seemed to be sufficient for her to indulge in death wishes.

### The mother

After the death of the daughter, the mother came to regular sessions with the art therapist. She asserted that she could better understand her daughter and could be closer to her when watching and speaking about the paintings. She reported that she had felt alienated from her daughter from early childhood until her death. During one of the first sessions with the art therapist, she suddenly, and unexpectedly, asked if the therapist likes to live. The mother seemed amazed at the art therapist's positive reply. She herself had never experienced life as joyful but rather as painful. The only reason for not having committed suicide was that she did not want to bring shame on the family. Therefore, she could completely understand her daughter having fulfilled her wishes and been freed from anguish.

### The daughter

The patient was reared in a middle-class family. The father was a government official, the mother a teacher, who since the birth of her daughter was a housewife. Since she was 8 years old, the daughter spent the greater part of her days on a farmyard with horses close to the apartment of her parents. Her mother told the art therapist that riding was her daughter's greatest pleasure. However, the parents forbade her to ride at the age of 13 because of decreasing performance at school. The daughter was obedient. However, she developed a severe eating disorder during puberty and made her first suicide attempt at the age of 14.

When hospitalized, the patient participated in daily art therapy, and the preferred subject of her drawings were horses. Because of her talent, she received appreciation for her paintings. An enduring and trustful relationship developed between the patient and art therapist.

## Description and interpretation of the paintings

The horse presented in Figure 60.1 as 'my horse' can be considered as an object of yearning for tenderness, sensuality, and closeness, and at the same time, the symbol of her self. The horse is directed to the left side of the painting, which is often associated with the meaning of regression, the past, one's mother and introversion (see below for the theoretical implications for art therapy).

In Figure 60.2, a horse is running on a red path to the entrance of a tunnel. The picture reflects threat and no escape with its strong polarity of colours. The red colour of the path is reminiscent of blood. The light in the gorge is yellow and the horse is white, giving the impression of being without a body. Such a horse with empty eye sockets, and seemingly scorning mouth, was referred to by the patient as the 'ghost of life'. Already in this painting one gets the impression that the animal is driven by an invisible force (maybe the 'ghost of life') to the yellow gorge as if there is no other choice, even if it leads to danger and ruin.

Finally, what is almost certainly the last picture of the patient, probably painted shortly before the suicide (Figure 60.3). It represents the same scene as painted in Figure 60.2. However, the white horse has already entered the bright fiery opening of the gorge—maybe the entrance of a cave. The head of the horse is not visible any more. The so-called 'ghost of life' is only present as a half circle spot at the right upper edge of the canvas. The painting gives the impression that the animal has come from the threatening, dark and cold through a path of pain and blood and reached its yearning, a shelter, albeit uncertain. It gives the impression of a last dangerous regression back to the burning body of mother earth.

This case report demonstrates that the treatment of chronic suicidality cannot always be successful. Even after an inpatient's treatment, where symptoms of auto- and hetero-aggressiveness have apparently diminished, nobody can be sure that the patient will not fall back into suicidality after being exposed to conflicts and difficult life situations. The suicide of this patient could not be prevented despite transient stabilization and close after care. Perhaps we have to understand and accept suicide as a possibility for escape from an unbearable conflict combined with a deep fear of life. Pictures two and three, could post hoc be interpreted as a demonstration of a fateful suicidal dynamic.

## The theoretical framework of art therapy for Case 1

The ambivalence of the presentation, i.e. the coexistence of messages with depressive (black colour) and aggressive (red colour) elements, reveals the inner atmosphere of the patient (see Figures 60.2 and 60.3). The polarity of opposite feelings is visible within the picture as well as noticeable for the observer. The severe inner tension of the painter is evident: the intolerability of the opposite affects can be experienced in a situation where severe depression coincides with strong aggression. Intolerable ambivalent affect and unresolved conflict generates paralysis, and suicide seems to be the only way out in a last impulsive action. The aggression

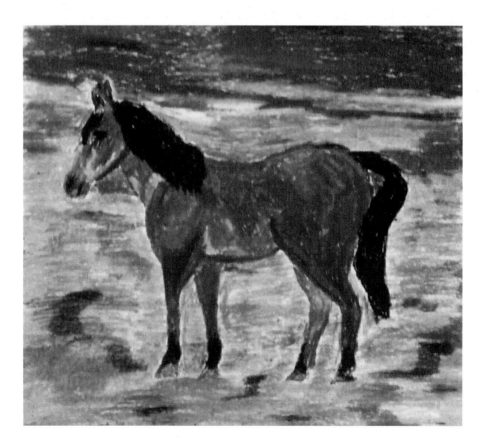

**Fig. 60.1** My horse. (See also colour section.)

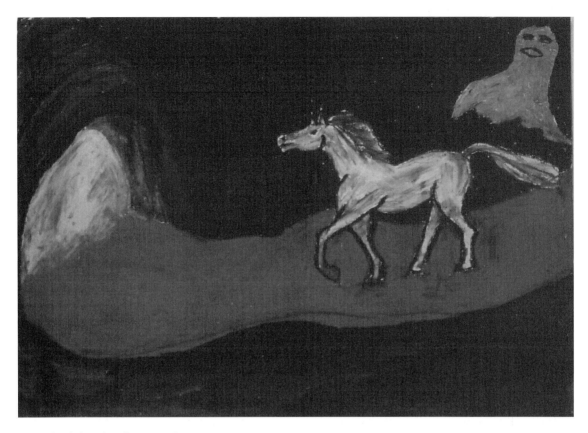

**Fig. 60.2** Horse on red path. (See also colour section.)

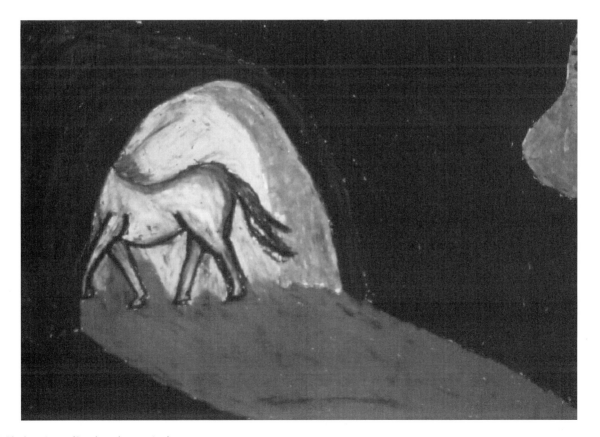

**Fig. 60.3** The last picture. (See also colour section.)

of the patient is expressed as archaic rage against the self, which is primarily directed against a disappointing and refusing early relationship.

The surface of a picture serves as a dimension of real 'life space'. The canvas gives the opportunity of unfolding space in the sense of unfolding of possibilities and future, i.e. of life. In contrast, space narrowness can be interpreted as the loss of possibilities and future (Fuchs 2002). The space distribution of a picture has its own meaning: the lower left side of a painting could be interpreted as regression, retardation and fixation, the left middle side could be dedicated to the past, one's mother and introversion, and the upper left side could stand for emptiness and nothingness, but also for yearning, the cosmos and retreat. In contrast, the upper right side could be associated with aim, zenith, end and death, the lower right side with earth, hell, decay and the material. However, the context for the development of the painting has to be considered, and these interpretations of space are taken cautiously.

### Case report 2

'I can exactly observe what there is outside behind the walls of my house, however nobody can see me. There are cannons that I can shoot outward if somebody is trying to conquer my castle. However, nobody will look for me because nobody will miss me. Anyway, the castle will blast itself if somebody is trying to come too close to me.' This is the account of an 18-year-old, but younger looking, female patient about her picture performed during art therapy (see Figure 60.4, Edifice). The girl suffered from a severe depressive episode in the frame of a pronounced personality disorder with borderline traits. She had undertaken several serious suicide attempts

before admission to an acute psychiatric ward. Her inpatient stay was for a long time overshadowed by her suicidality. The patient could not communicate her inner feelings, being nearly mute. Therefore, the background for her suicidality remained completely uncovered. The way to understanding her inner conflicts was paved only through painting. The spare commentaries of this young girl about her artistic products revealed progressively an impressive portrait of her personal landscape. At a first glimpse, a severe conflict between closeness and distance unfolded.

### Biography

The patient's parental home, where she was reared, was fervently Christian. She suffered as a toddler from neurodermatitis, and additionally, since the age of six, from asthma bronchialis. These illnesses lead to several inpatient treatments and stays in nursing homes with separation from her parents. Nearly the whole school time was spent in boarding schools, and only during vacations, depending on her health status, could she be at home. Both parents were heavily engaged in social activities and not very much concerned with her. Nevertheless, both parents contended that there was no lack of parental care: 'our daughter has always had all that seemed to be necessary'. The fact that their daughter was a very fragile, anxious and shy person was seen as an inherited character trait rather than coined by early childhood illnesses and family surroundings.

### Description and interpretation of the paintings

This painting, the Edifice, performed during art therapy (Figure 60.4) contained an ambivalent message. The dark tones of the picture show a grey edifice before a dark background. The grey

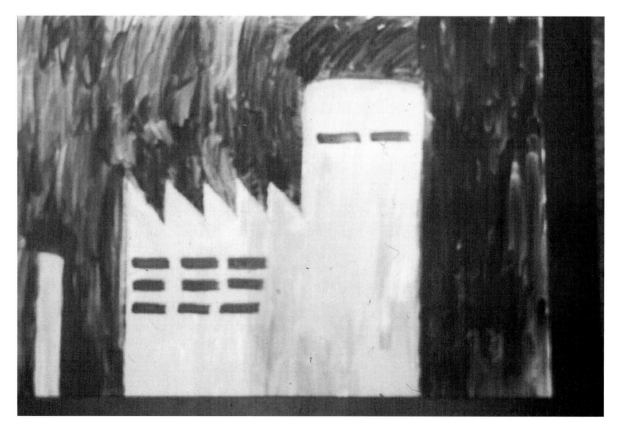

**Fig. 60.4** Edifice. (See also colour section.)

uniform façade with no door is interrupted by horizontal tiny dark holes on the left side in the upper two thirds. The façade ends with five sharp spikes. On the right side, the edifice is soaring to a tower. Again, in the upper half are two tiny side-by-side holes. On the left side, a small high structure with the same grey tone, not connected with the edifice, is growing from the brink of the picture to the top.

The black and grey tone of the picture depicts a gloomy atmosphere and conveys to the observer a feeling of hopelessness and void. In contrast to this, the representation of the edifice is signalling a threat by the aggressive, fixed and hostile exerting characteristics of the form. The sharp spikes remind the observer of the back of dangerous reptiles. The polished, bare and non-surmountable walls, holes as vision slits or arrow slits, on the right side of the edifice resemble hostile or controlling eyes. They convey anxiety and apprehension that together with the chimneys resemble crematoria.

Some days after painting the edifice, the patient painted a perspective delineated path in yellow and dark brown, which ends in a formation looking like a tunnel (see Figure 60.5, The tunnel). This path leads directly to a half-round light spot, which could be imagined as an exit out of the tunnel. A small black figure is guided on the yellow path to the light spot. There seems to be no way out of this path, because the dark blue of the background gives the observer the impression of the endlessness of the universe. The small black figure would fall in the abyss of loneliness if leaving this path.

The patient could genuinely distance herself from suicidal ideas after a while. A major contribution was her ability to transfer inner imagination adequately to the paintings. Furthermore, the antidepressant medication alleviated the depression. Finally, the therapeutic relationship, coined by the positive transference to the art therapist, the continuity of a daily therapeutic group and last, but not least, the confidential relationship with the psychiatrist enabled her to successfully overcome depression and suicidal tendencies.

## Theoretical implications for art therapy for Case 2

Pronounced polarity in paintings during art therapy can be an indication for auto- or hetero-destructive decisions, which can be seen in Figure 60.5. Polarity of colours such as the deepest dark and brightest light (e.g. black and yellow) may also point in this direction. These types of colours mirror the seemingly unresolvable conflict between a non-acceptable deficient state, and the yearning for an unrealistic ideal of eternal happiness. The desire of an idealized state of happiness, together with wishes for fusion, is transferred to the realm of the other world, since the state is not reachable in the reality of life. Black is the colour of mourning, hopelessness, anxiety and death, whereas red the colour of blood, the symbol of love, pain, and rage.

The pictures of the patient changed considerably in their formal and substantial expression during the course of art therapy, consisting of two hours group therapy twice a day at the closed ward. The rigidity, destructiveness and aggressiveness vanished. The language of the pictures, coined by rigid grandiose ideas, receded in favour of unfulfilled needs for love, protection and safety. This was impressively depicted in a picture several weeks after admission (see Figure 60.6). The patient could, with her picture, offer a

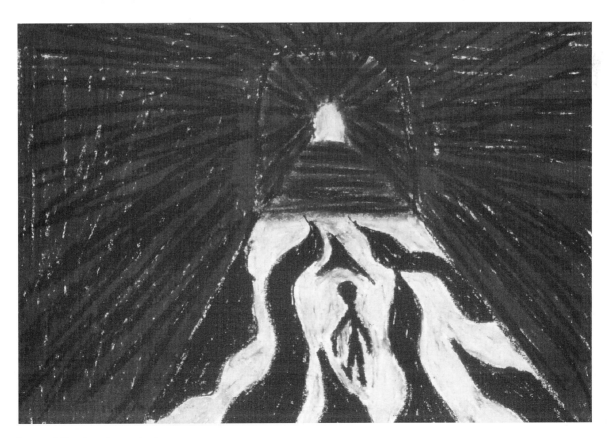

**Fig. 60.5** The tunnel. (See also colour section.)

non-verbal communication and, therefore, a first cautious contact with her significant others. The inclusion of a third person is of particular importance: it is authentic toward her inner self and an expression of the self outward, since the work is not only standing for itself but refers to an observer (Resch 2002).

Under the empathetic and holding stance of the therapist, the patient experiences her inner loneliness as a necessary prerequisite for the creative process (Niederland and Englewood 1997). With her imagination, the patient starts working on paper and develops a dialogue with her inner world. Therefore, the patient can work in this 'progressive loneliness' with her opposite inner strivings. The picture is the stage where the patient can experience herself as an acting person: the permission for loneliness is also the permission for autonomy (Klosinski 2000). The creative description of the inner conflict enables the patient to overcome rigid structures and to extend the space for painful feelings in order to finally accept them. She can mould her own reality with her distant position. The patient is not exclusively bound by the power of the negative one-sided memories in regard to her deficits. All these interpretations are only valid in the frame of a clear-cut clinical picture of a psychiatric illness. Pictures outside this context may have different meanings, and conclusions should not be drawn as presented here.

## Conclusions

The theme 'suicide' in paintings mirror social, cultural, religious and philosophical stances to suicide. However, behind these more public aspects of the artist's work is always an individual meaning for the artist. Motives and interests of the artists go beyond the theme of suicide. For instance, the theme of the death of Lucretia, often adopted by Renaissance artists, was the focus of their attention because of the naked female body (Bronisch 2002).

The most important precipitant for suicidal behaviour, in general, is a depressive mood or disorder (Bronisch 2003). Paintings of suicidal artists may post hoc be interpreted as indicators of a severe depression, such as the last paintings of Mark Rothko before he committed suicide (Schildkraut *et al.* 1995). However, the depressive mood as well as the underlying manic-depressive illness of some artists may also be seen as an important prerequisite for their creativity (Jamison 1993). Lastly, the depressive illness, or the depressive mood of the artist, primarily serves as a circumstance for their artwork, which goes beyond the personal experiences of the artist. In contrast to the artist, the paintings and sculptures of art therapy patients primarily reflect the inner experiences of their illness and biography. Taking the literature on art and depression in consideration, there is no doubt that specific—formal—aspects are represented in paintings of depressed artists and patients. The analysis of the patients' pictures during episodes of depression reveal less colour used, more empty space, less investment of effort or less complete, and more depressive affect or no effect at all compared to episodes where the patients are less depressed. Furthermore, there is a trend toward the pictures being more constricted than when less depressed. Gloomy colours could be indicative of a depressed mood, especially changes in colours.

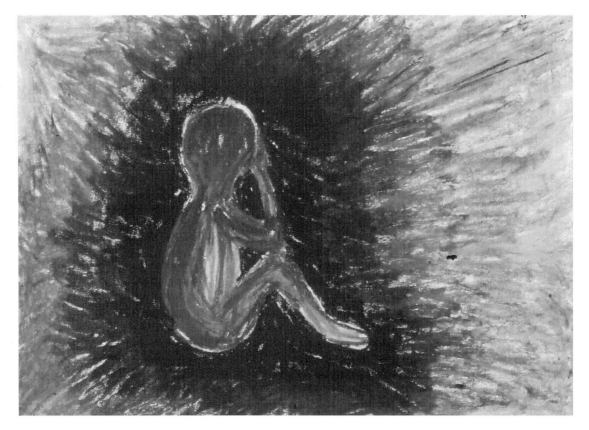

**Fig. 60.6** Safe? (See also colour section.)

Content of paintings could suggest suicidality, such as themes touching on death and dying. Comments of the patients on their paintings seem to be very important (Wadeson 1971).

Patients can easily overcome language barriers and give self-disclosure through non-verbal expression such as painting and drawing, especially concerning suicidal tendencies (Forrest 1978). In some spontaneous paintings, as in prophetic dreams, the suicidal patients create unconscious and unwilling 'prophesies' and communicate their prediction of death (Assael and Popovici-Wacks 1989). Art therapy in depressive patients releases energy and leads to new areas of interest and activity away from depression. Art exercises are directed at helping the patient to find strength and self-worth through the discovery of their artistic expression (Robbins 1987). Aggression, auto-aggression and anger are important aspects of suicidality, and may be alleviated during the process of painting. In some instances, picture-making may well have replaced self-destructive ways of acting on such feelings and facilitates the patients' own exploration and understanding of their suicidal wishes (Wadeson 1975).

## References

Anastasi A, Foley JP (1941). A survey on artistic behavior in the abnormal: IV experimental investigations. *The Journal of General Psychology*, **25**, 137–237.

Anderson O (1987). *Suicide in Victorian and Edwardian England*. Clarendon Press, Oxford.

Andreasen NC (1978). Creativity and psychiatric illness. *Psychiatric Annals*, **8**, 113–119.

Andreasen NC (1987). Creativity and mental illness: prevalence rates in writers and their first degree relatives. *American Journal of Psychiatry*, **144**, 1288–1292.

Assel M and Popovici-Wacks M (1989). Artistic expression in spontaneous paintings of depressed patients. *Israel Psychiatry and Related Sciences*, **26**, 223–243.

Aurelius Augustinus (400). De Civitate Dei I, Summa Theologica, II-III, 1271/73. In JWC Wand, ed. and trans. (1963). *City of God*. Oxford University Press, London.

Bronisch T (2002). Eros und Thanatos. Liebe und Sünde. Die Darstellung der Lucretia in der Malerei der Renaissance [Eros and Thanatos. Love and sin. The depiction of Lucretia in the paintings of the Renaissance]. In MP Heuser, HP Kapfhammer, HJ Möller *et al.*, eds, *Die Sünde … von der Schuld zum Wahn, von der Sühne zur Therapie*, pp. 75–80. VIP Verlag, Insbruck.

Bronisch T (2003). Depression and suicidal behaviour. Letter to the editors. *Crisis*, **24**, 179–180.

Brown RM (2001). *The Art of Suicide*. Books, London.

Cohen BM, Hammer JS, Singer S (1988). The diagnostic drawing series: a systematic approach to art therapy evaluation and research. *The Arts in Psychotherapy*, **15**, 11–21.

Durkheim, E (1897). *Le Suicide*. In JA Spading, and G Simpson, trans. (1952). [The Suicide]. Routledge and Kegan Paul, London.

Finkelstein HA (1971). Van Gogh's suicide. *JAMA*, **218**, 1832.

Forrest G (1978). An art therapists' contribution to the diagnostic process. *American Journal of Art Therapy*, **17**, 99–105.

Fuchs T (2002). Der Raum in der Kunsttherapie [The space in art therapy]. In R Hampe, P Martius, D Ritsch, F von Spreti, eds, *Generationenwechsel*, pp. 21–33. Universität Bremen, Bremen.

Goodwin F and Jamison KR (1990). *Manic Depressive Illness*, pp. 332–367. Oxford University Press, Oxford, New York.

Goethe JW (1774). *Das Leiden des Jungen Werther* [The diary of a self-murderer]. In A Stanley, trans. (2004) [The sorrows of young Werther]. Dover Publications, Mineola.

Grote G, Völkel M, Weyershausen K (2000). *Das Lexikon der prominenten Selbstmörder*. Lexikon Verlag.

Halbreich U, Assael M, Driefus D (1980). Premonition of death in painting. *Confinia Psychiatrica*, **23**, 74–81.

Jamison KR (1989a). *Touched with Fire: Manic-depressive Illness and the Artistic Temperament*. Free Press, New York.

Jamison KR (1989b). Mood disorders and patterns of creativity in British writers and artists. *Psychiatry*, **52**, 125–134.

Jamison KR (1993). *Touched with Fire*, pp. 234. The Free Press, New York.

Juda A (1949). The relationship between highest mental capacity and psychic abnormalities. *American Journal of Psychiatry*, **106**, 296–307.

Klosinski G (2000). Zur Bedeutung der Kunst und Gestaltungstherapie für die Psychiatrie und Psychotherapie am Beginn eines neuen Jahrtausends [The importance of art therapy for psychiatry and psychotherapy at the beginning of a new millenium]. *Zeitschrift für Musik- und Kunsttherapie*, **11**, 179–186.

Kuiper P (2002). *Seelenfinsternis. Die Depression eines Psychiaters* [Darkness of souls. The depression of a psychiatrist]. Frankfurt am Main: S. Fischer, 4. Auflage. German translation of the Dutch version: Ver heen; Verslag van een depressie. Gravenhage Netherlands: SDU uitgeverij (1988).

Langer S (1953). *Feeling and Form: A Theory of Art*, pp. 22. Routledge and Kegan Paul, London.

Lester D (1993). *Suicide in Creative Women*. Comac Nova Science Publishers, New York.

Lester D (1998). Suicide in eminent persons. *Perceptual and Motor Skills*, **87**, 90.

Mac Donald M and Murphy TR (1990). *Sleepless Souls. Suicide in Early Modern England*. Clarendon Press, Oxford.

Maire FW (1971). Van Gogh's suicide. *JAMA*, **217**, 938–939.

Miljkovitch de Heredia RM and Miljkovitch I (1998). Drawings of depressed inpatients: intentional and unintentional expression of emotional states. *Journal of Clinical Psychology*, **54**, 1029–1042.

Minois G (1999). *History of Suicide: Voluntary Death in Western Culture*. Johns Hopkins Press, Baltimore.

Mohr F (1906). Über Zeichnungen von Geisteskranken und ihre diagnostische Verwertbarkeit [The sketchesof the insane and their diagnostic utilization]. *Journal für Psychologie und Neurologie*, **7**, 99–140.

Murray A (1998). *Suicide in the Middle Ages*, Volume I. Oxford University Press, Oxford.

Navratil L (2002). Johann Hausers Leichenwagen. Über manisch-depressive Mischzustände und ihre Spiegelungen in Bildern und Gedichten [Johann Hauser's hearse. About manic depressive mixed states and their mirroring in paintings and poems]. *Fundamenta Psychiatrica*, **16**, 144–146.

Niederland WG and Englewood NJ (1979). Psychoanalytische Überlegungen zur künstlerischen Kreativität [Psychoanalytic considerations about artistic creativity]. *Psyche*, **4**, 329–354.

Pöldinger W (1986). The relation between depression and art. *Psychopathology*, **19**, 263–268.

Preti A and Miotto P (1999). Suicide among eminent artists. *Psychological Reports*, **84**, 291–301.

Ravin JG, Hartman JJ, Fried RI (1978). Mark Rothkos' paintings—suicide notes? *The Ohio State Medical Journal*, **74**, 78–79.

Resch F (2002). Kunst spielt eine Rolle [Art plays a role]. In T Fuchs, I Jadi, B Brand-Claussen *et al.*, eds, *WahnWeltBild. Die Sammlung Prinzhorn. Beiträge zur Museumseröffnung*, pp. 349–358. Springer, Heidelberg.

Richards RL, Kinney DK, Lunde I *et al.* (1988). Creativity in manic-depressives, cyclthymes, and their normal first-degree relatives: a preliminary report. *Journal of Abnormal Psychology*, **97**, 281–288.

Robbins A (1987). An object relations approach to art therapy. In AJ Rubin, ed., *Approaches to Art Therapy. Theory and Technique*, pp. 63–74. Bruner-Maazel, New York.

Schildkraut JJ, Hirshfeld AJ, Murphy JM (1994). Mind and mood in modern art II: depressive disorders, spirituality, and early deaths in the abstract expressionist artists of the New York School. *American Journal of Psychiatry*, **151**, 482–488.

Schildkraut JJ and Hirshfeld AJ (1995). Mind and mood in modern art I: Miró and 'Melancholie'. *Creativity Research Journal* **8**, 139–156.

Simon R (1972). Pictorial styles of the habitually depressed. *International Journal of Social Psychiatry*, **18**, 146–152.

Spaniol S (2003). Art therapy with adults with severe mental illness. In CA Malchiodi, ed., *Handbook of Art Therapy*, pp. 268–280. The Guilford Press, New York, London.

Stack S (1996). Gender and suicide risk among artists: a multivariate analysis. *Suicide and Life-Threatening Behavior*, **26**, 374–379.

Stack S (1997). Suicide among artists. *The Journal of Social Psychology*, **137**, 129–130.

Van Hooff AJL (1990). *From Autothanasia to Suicide. Self-killing in Classical Antiquity*. Routledge, London and New York.

Van Hooff AJL (1994). Icons of ancient suicide: self-killing in classical art. *Crisis*, **15**, 179–186.

Van Hooff AJL (2000). A historical perspective on suicide. In RW Maris, AL Berman and MM Silverman, eds, *Comprehensive Textbook of Suicidology*, pp. 96–123. The Guilford Press, New York and London.

Von Spreti F (2005). Himmelhoch und Dämmergrau. Kunsttherapie bei Depression [High as the heaven and grey as the dawn. Art therapy in depression]. In F von Spreti, M Martius and H Förstl, *Kunsttherapie bei psychischen Störungen*, pp. 81–106. Elsevier, Urban and Fischer, München.

Wadeson H (1971). Characteristics of art expression in depression. *Journal of Nervous and Mental Disease*, **153**, 197–204.

Wadeson H (1975). Suicide: expression in images. *American Journal of Art Therapy*, **14**, 75–82.

Wadeson H and Carpenter WT (1976). A comparative study of art expression of schizophrenic, unipolar depressive, and bipolar manic-depressive patients. *The Journal of Nervous and Mental Disease*, **162**, 334–344.

# Health Care Strategies: Treatment Settings for Adults

# CHAPTER 61

# Crisis hotlines

Madelyn S Gould and John Kalafat[†]

## Abstract

This chapter reviews the evidence of the effectiveness of telephone crisis services ('hotlines') as a suicide prevention strategy. Hotlines are a ubiquitous source of help internationally, but the evidence for their effectiveness is equivocal. Recent research provides support for crisis hotlines' role in reducing callers' crisis and suicidal states, bearing in mind the lack of control conditions. However, studies have also raised concerns about the extent and quality of suicide risk assessments and crisis interventions by hotline staff. A particular challenge is making hotline services attractive to youth. These concerns have prompted current efforts to enhance risk assessments, training and outreach strategies in telephone crisis centres.

Crisis hotlines are ubiquitous sources of help worldwide. A rationale for the role of crisis hotlines in suicide prevention is that suicidal behaviour is often associated with a crisis (Mishara and Daigle 2000). The psychological autopsy research generally supports the association of stressful life events, such as interpersonal losses and legal or disciplinary problems, with suicide (Runeson 1990; Brent *et al.* 1993; Gould *et al.* 1996). Furthermore, suicide is usually contemplated with psychological ambivalence—surviving suicide attempters often report that the wish to die coexisted with wishes to be rescued and saved (Shaffer *et al.* 1988). This can result in a 'cry for help', which can be addressed by those with special training (Litman *et al.* 1965). Lastly, crisis services may provide relief to an individual who is in the 'final common pathway to suicide' (Shaffer *et al.* 1988) by providing the opportunity for immediate support at these critical times. The goal of crisis hotlines is to prevent deleterious outcomes for callers by reducing their current crisis and/or suicidal states and identifying alternate coping approaches, including referrals to formal and/or informal community resources. Crisis hotlines have the practical advantage of providing temporally, financially, and geographically accessible services.

## Evaluation of hotlines

Despite the strong theoretical and practical justification as a suicide prevention strategy, hotlines' empirical effectiveness has yet to be

demonstrated unequivocally. Evaluations of telephone crisis services have included caller feedback/satisfaction, rates of follow-up with referrals, assessments of helping processes and proximal outcomes (changes in caller crisis or suicidal status), and assessments of distal outcomes consisting of changes in community suicide rates.

Early process evaluations of telephone counselling interventions focused on helper (i.e. counsellor)-offered empathy, warmth, and genuineness (Rogers 1957), which are representative of helping approaches of many telephone crisis centres to this day. Studies found moderate levels of these conditions (as rated on simulated calls and role plays), variations between centres, and increased levels associated with training and experience (Bleach and Claiborn 1974; Caruthers and Inslee 1974; France 1975; O'Donnell and George 1977; Kalafat *et al.* 1979). However, the relationship between these conditions and call outcomes was not assessed.

A consensus among crisis hotlines has evolved around a 4–6-step problem-solving intervention model first adopted by the Los Angeles Suicide Prevention Center (Farberow *et al.* 1968), and consisting of establishing rapport; defining the problem(s) including assessing risk for suicide; exploring affect (including reducing anxiety and other affects that attenuate problem solving); exploring callers' coping repertoires; and developing alternatives for addressing the problem, i.e. a specific plan of action and/or referral to informal or formal resources. Studies have employed silent monitoring of (listening to) calls to crisis hotlines to assess the presence and timing of the components of the helping model, and have examined their relationships to caller outcomes through follow-up calls to callers (Echterling *et al.* 1980; Echterling and Hartsough 1989; Young 1989). The presence and timing of these helping components were related to positive caller feedback and outcomes such as relief of distress, increased confidence, and emotional awareness. None of these process evaluations employed control conditions.

A measure of the distal effect of telephone crisis services has entailed the assessment of suicide rates in communities served by the centres. Studies examining the impact of crisis hotlines on mortality have largely employed ecological designs that have compared the suicide rates in areas with and without a crisis programme or in areas before and after the introduction of a crisis program. Several studies (Wiener 1969; Lester 1973, 1974; Barraclough *et al.* 1977; Bridge *et al.* 1977; Jennings *et al.* 1978; Riehl *et al.* 1988), including a meta-analysis (Dew *et al.* 1987) found no significant effects of

---

† In Memoriam. This chapter, prepared in tribute to Dr John Kalafat, is an adaptation and update of our earlier papers.

hotlines on suicide rates. A significant effect of Samaritan suicide prevention programmes in England was found by Bagley (1968), but the results were not replicated by other researchers using more elaborate and accurate statistical techniques (Barraclough *et al.* 1977; Jennings *et al.* 1978). More recently, Lester (1997) conducted a meta-analysis of fourteen studies on the relationship of suicide prevention centres to suicide rates. While the results of individual studies did not always reach statistical significance, Lester found a significant overall preventive effect. Leenaars and Lester (2004) reported two studies on the number of suicide prevention centres in ten Canadian provinces and two territories. The first assessed the relationship between the density of centres in 1985 and age-adjusted suicide rates for 1985–1989 and found no significant preventive impact. The second assessed the relationship between the density of centres in 1994 and age-adjusted suicide rates for 1994–1998 and found negative correlations between presence of centres and change in the suicide rates for eight of the twelve correlations. That is, the more centres, the lower the suicide rates. When the Yukon and Northwest territories were excluded, the correlation coefficients 'approached or reached statistical significance'. They concluded that this indicated 'a preventive impact, though weak, of suicide prevention centres on suicide in Canada' (Leenaars and Lester 2004, p. 67). However, caution is advised against the use of the term 'impact', as the authors correctly note that the study was correlational and did not take into account changes in other social variables over the period. Moreover, these broad measures of community suicide rates did not consider the populations reached by crisis services, the majority of which have been white female callers. Miller *et al.* (1984) examined race-sex-age-specific suicide rates in US counties with and without, and before and after, the introduction of a suicide prevention programme. A significant reduction in the suicide rate in young white females was found, but no evidence of an impact in other population groups emerged.

It is difficult to draw conclusions about the effectiveness of crisis centres from studies of the relationship between the presence of suicide prevention/crisis centres and community suicide rates without a consideration of a complementary evaluation of proximal outcomes among crisis centre users. One means to evaluate proximal outcomes is through silent monitoring of calls (Mishara and Daigle 1997). Mishara and Daigle (1997) listened to 617 telephone calls from suicidal callers to two Canadian suicide centres. Immediate or proximal effects on the reduction of depressive mood and in suicidal urgency were linked to specific intervention styles, most notably a Rogerian style that consisted of non-directive and empathetic responses. King *et al.* (2003) rated 100 taped suicide calls to Kids Help Line in Australia. Significant decreases in suicidality and significant improvements in the mental state of youth were observed during the course of the call. Recently, Mishara *et al.* (2007a, b) monitored 2611 calls to 14 crisis lines in the Hopeline network, observing counsellor behaviours, caller characteristics, and changes during the calls. Among the authors' conclusions were that centre directors' descriptions of what counsellors did was not necessarily an accurate description of what was observed by the monitors; centres varied greatly in the nature and quality of the telephone help they provided; empathy and respect were desired counsellor qualities; and a supportive approach, good contact and collaborative problem-solving were intervention styles that related to better call outcomes. Lastly, while callers appeared to be helped in a significant numbers of calls and some lives may have been saved, counsellors did not consistently evaluate suicide risk, and when evaluations were conducted they were usually incomplete.

Another recent assessment of proximal outcomes was conducted by the current authors (Kalafat *et al.* 2007; Gould *et al.* 2007). Eight crisis hotlines across the US were engaged in the study of outcomes associated with adult suicidal (N = 1085) and non-suicidal crisis (N = 1617) callers. The study employed callers' own ratings of their mental state and suicidality, in response to a standardized set of inquiries by the crisis counsellors at the beginning and end of the call, to assess the immediate proximal effect of the crisis intervention. A follow-up assessment, two to four weeks later, was also conducted to assess the duration of an effect and the telephone intervention's impact on future suicidal risk and behaviour. A key finding was that there were significant reductions in callers' self-reported crisis and suicide states from the beginning to the end of the calls; however, without a control group, these effects cannot be definitively attributed to the crisis intervention. Other notable findings were that seriously suicidal individuals were calling telephone crisis services; 11.6 per cent of suicidal callers reported at follow-up that the call prevented them from harming or killing themselves; a caller's intent to die at the end of the call was the most potent predictor of suicidality at follow-up; and, of the callers who were rated as *non-suicidal* crisis callers by crisis staff, 12 per cent reported at follow-up that they were either feeling suicidal during or since their calls to the centre. While providing some support for the clinical effectiveness of the crisis centres, the results also raised a concern about the adequacy of suicide risk assessments conducted by some crisis centre staff.

Current priorities of the National Suicide Prevention Lifeline (NSPL), the national network of hotlines in the United States, include the development and dissemination of evidence-based risk assessment standards and guidelines, and training for network crisis centres (Joiner *et al.* 2007). The Living Works' Applied Suicide Intervention Skills Training (ASIST; http://www.livingworks.net), an internationally disseminated programme designed as 'suicide first-aid' has been chosen as a gatekeeper training programme that could be adapted to crisis hotlines. ASIST trainers and NSPL training personnel have recently collaborated on the ASIST adaptation for this context. The ASIST programme has been field-tested in a variety of settings where pre-post differences in attitudes and knowledge have been examined (Turley *et al.* 2000; Guttormsen *et al.* 2003; Pearce *et al.* 2003, Silvola *et al.* 2003) but to date, there has been no controlled study of its effectiveness. A randomized control trial of ASIST in the context of telephone crisis counselling is currently being conducted by the chapter's first author.

## Hotline utilization and effectiveness among adolescents

Recent evidence indicates that youth who use hotlines are helped by them (King *et al.* 2003); however, service utilization surveys of adolescents indicate that, despite high awareness of hotlines and high satisfaction ratings among those who do contact hotlines, adolescents access them infrequently (Slem and Colter 1973; King 1977; Barnes *et al.* 2001; Gould *et al.* 2006) and less often than they access other help sources (Offer *et al.* 1991; Vieland *et al.* 1991; Beautrais *et al.* 1998). Furthermore, negative attitudes among adolescents are stronger toward hotlines than they are toward other sources of help (Gould *et al.* 2006). Unfortunately, adolescents who identify themselves as in need of help by virtue of impaired functioning or feelings of hopelessness have particularly negative attitudes toward hotlines (Gould *et al.* 2006). If hotline services are going to increase utilization among adolescents they must work to promote a specific function that can be provided to adolescents in a manner that fits with an adolescent's sense of their needs and is compatible with a teenager's lifestyle. The Internet is one potential avenue for enhancing access to crisis services by youth. Teenagers have been found to be as likely to access the Internet for help as they are to see a school counsellor or mental health professional (Gould *et al.* 2002), and findings highlight the substantially greater popularity of this medium over telephone crisis services (Gould *et al.* 2006). It behooves hotline advocates to take advantage of the Internet's growing accessibility and teenagers' propensity to use it as a means to obtain help.

## Conclusion

Crisis/suicide hotlines' potential to serve vulnerable individuals in crisis makes it a valuable suicide prevention strategy. Research provides some support for crisis hotlines' role in reducing crisis and suicidal states in youth and adult callers, bearing in mind the lack of control conditions. On the other hand, studies have raised concerns about the extent and quality of suicide risk assessments and crisis interventions by hotline staff—highlighting the need for improved training of crisis counsellors.

Among youth, the low utilization of hotlines and the negative attitudes toward them is particularly distressing. Efforts are continuing to optimize hotlines' effectiveness and outreach to suicidal individuals of all ages.

## References

Bagley C (1968). The evaluation of a suicide prevention scheme by an ecological method. *Social Science and Medicine*, **2**, 1–14.

Barnes LS, Ikeda RM, Kresnow M (2001) Help-seeking behavior prior to nearly lethal suicide attempts. *Suicide and Life-Threatening Behavior*, **32**, 68–75.

Barraclough BM, Jennings C, Moss JR (1977). Suicide prevention by the Samaritans: a controlled study of effectiveness. *The Lancet*, **1**, 237–238.

Beautrais AL, Joyce PR, Mulder RT (1998). Psychiatric contacts among youths aged 13 through 24 years who have made serious suicide attempts. *Journal of the American Academy of Child and Adolescent Psychiatry*, **37**, 504–511.

Bleach G and Claiborn WL (1974). Initial evaluation of hotline telephone crisis centers. *Community Mental Health Journal*, **4**, 387–394.

Brent DA, Perper JA, Moritz G *et al.* (1993). Stressful life events, psychopathology and adolescent suicide: a case control study. *Suicide and Life-Threatening Behavior*, **23**, 179–187.

Bridge TP, Potkin SG, Zung WW *et al.* (1977). Suicide prevention centers: ecological study of effectiveness. *Journal of Nervous and Mental Disease*, **164**, 18–24.

Caruthers JE and Inslee L J (1974). Level of empathic understanding offered by volunteer telephone services. *Journal of Counseling Psychology*, **21**, 274–276.

Dew AM, Bromet EJ, Brent D *et al.* (1987). A quantitative literature review of the effectiveness of suicide prevention centers. *Journal of Consulting and Clinical Psychology*, **55**, 239–244.

Echterling LG and Hartsough DM (1989). Phases of helping in successful crisis telephone calls. *Journal of Community Psychology*, **17**, 249–257.

Echterling LG, Hartsough DM, Zarle TH (1980). Testing a model for the process of telephone crisis intervention. *American Journal of Community Psychology*, **8**, 715–725.

Farberow NL, Heilig SM, Litman RE (1968). *Techniques in Crisis Intervention: A Training Manual.* Suicide Prevention Center, Inc., Los Angeles.

France K (1975). Evaluation of lay volunteer crisis telephone workers. *American Journal of Community Psychology*, **3**, 197–219.

Gould MS, Fisher P, Parides M *et al.* (1996). Psychosocial risk factors of child and adolescent completed suicide. *Archives of General Psychiatry*, **53**, 1155–1162.

Gould MS, Greenberg T, Munfakh JLH *et al.* (2006). Teenagers' attitudes about seeking help from telephone crisis services (hotlines). *Suicide and Life-Threatening Behavior*, **36**, 601–613.

Gould MS, Munfakh JLH, Lubell K *et al.* (2002). Seeking help from the internet during adolescence. *Journal of the American Academy of Child and Adolescent Psychiatry*, **41**, 1182–1189.

Gould MS, Kalafat J, Munfakh JLH *et al.* (2007). An evaluation of crisis hotline outcomes, Part II: suicidal callers. *Suicide and Life-Threatening Behavior*, **37**, 338–352.

Guttormsen T, Hoifodt TS, Silvola K *et al.* (2003). Applied suicide intervention skills training—an evaluation. *Tidsskrift for Norske Laegeforening*, **123**, 2284–2286.

Jennings C, Barraclough BM, Moss JR (1978). Have the Samaritans lowered the suicide rate? A controlled study. *Psychological Medicine*, **8**, 413–422.

Joiner T, Kalafat J, Draper J *et al.* (2007). Established standards for the assessment of suicide risk among callers to the National Suicide Prevention Lifeline: a background paper. *Suicide and Life-Threatening Behavior*, **37**, 353–365.

Kalafat J, Boroto DR, France K (1979). Relationships among experience level and value orientation and the performance of paraprofessional telephone counselors. *American Journal of Community Psychology*, **7**, 167–180.

Kalafat J, Gould MS, Munfakh JLH *et al.* (2007). An evaluation of crisis hotline outcomes, Part I: non-suicidal crisis callers. *Suicide and Life-Threatening Behavior*, **37**, 322–337.

King GD (1977). An evaluation of the effectiveness of a telephone counseling center. *American Journal of Community Psychology*, **5**, 75–83.

King R, Nurcombe R, Bickman L *et al.* (2003). Telephone counseling for adolescent suicide prevention: changes in suicidality and mental state from beginning to end of a counseling session. *Suicide and Life-Threatening Behavior*, **33**, 400–411.

Leenaars AA and Lester D (2004). The impact of suicide prevention centers on the suicide rate in the Canadian provinces. *Crisis*, **25**, 65–68.

Lester D (1973). Prevention of suicide. *Journal of the American Medical Association*, **225**, 992.

Lester D (1974). Effect of suicide prevention centers on suicide rates in the United States. *Health Services Reports*, **89**, 37–39.

Lester D (1997). The effectiveness of suicide prevention centers. *Suicide and Life-Threatening Behavior*, **27**, 304–310.

Litman RE, Farberow NL, Shneidman ES *et al.* (1965). Suicide prevention telephone service. *Journal of the American Medical Association*, **192**, 107–111.

Miller HL, Coombs DW, Leeper JD *et al.* (1984). An analysis of the effects of suicide prevention facilities on suicide rates in the United States. *American Journal of Public Health*, **74**, 340–343.

Mishara BL, Chagnon F, Daigle M *et al.* (2007a). Which helper behaviors and intervention styles are related to better short term outcomes in telephone crisis intervention? Results from a silent monitoring study of calls to the U.S. 1–800-SUICIDE network. *Suicide and Life-Threatening Behavior*, **37**, 291–307.

Mishara BL, Chagnon F, Daigle M *et al.* (2007b). Comparing models of helper behavior to actual practice in telephone crisis intervention: a silent monitoring study of calls to the U.S. 1–800-SUICIDE network. *Suicide and Life-Threatening Behavior*, **37**, 308–321.

Mishara BL and Daigle M (1997). Effects of different telephone intervention styles with suicidal callers at two suicide prevention centers: an empirical investigation. *American Journal of Community Psychology*, **25**, 861–855.

Mishara BL and Daigle M (2000). Helplines and crisis intervention services: challenges for the future. In D Lester, ed., *Suicide Prevention: Resources for the Millennium*, pp. 153–171. Brunner-Routledge, Philadelphia.

O'Donnell JM and George K (1977). The use of volunteers in a community mental health center emergency and reception service: a comparative study of professional and lay telephone counseling. *Community Mental Health Journal*, **1**, 3–12.

Offer D, Howard KI, Schonert KA, Ostrov E (1991). To whom do adolescents turn for help? Differences between disturbed and non-disturbed adolescents. *Journal of the American Academy of Child and Adolescent Psychiatry*, **30**, 623–630.

Pearce K, Rickwood D, Beaton S (2003). Preliminary evaluation of a university-based suicide intervention project: impact on participants. *Australian e-Journal for the Advancement of Mental Health*, **2**, 1–11.

Riehl T, Marchner E, Moller HJ (1988). Influence of crisis intervention telephone services ('Crisis Hotlines') on the suicide rate in 25 German cities. In HJ Moller, A Schmidtke and R Welz, eds, *Current Issues of Suicidology*, pp. 431–436. Springer-Verlag, Berlin.

Rogers CR (1957). The necessary and sufficient conditions of therapeutic personality change. *Journal of Consulting Psychology*, **21**, 95–103.

Runeson B (1990). Psychoactive substance use disorder in youth suicide. *Alcohol*, **25**, 561–568.

Shaffer D, Garland A, Gould M *et al.* (1988). Preventing teenage suicide: a critical review. *Journal of the American Academy of Child and Adolescent Psychiatry*, **27**, 675–687.

Silvola K, Hoifodt TS, Guttormsen T *et al.* (2003). Applied suicide intervention skills training. *Tidsskrift for Norske Laegeforening*, **123**, 2281–2283.

Slem CM and Cotler S (1973). Crisis phone services: evaluation of a hotline program. *American Journal of Community Psychology*, **1**, 219–227.

Turley B, Pullen L, Thomas I *et al.* (2000). *Living Works Applied Suicide Intervention Skills Training (ASIST). A Competency-based Evaluation*, pp. 1–6. Lifeline Australia Inc., Melbourne.

Vieland V, Whittle B, Garland A *et al.* (1991). The impact of curriculum-based suicide prevention programs for teenagers: an 18-month follow-up. *Journal of the American Academy of Child and Adolescent Psychiatry*, **30**, 811–815.

Wiener IW (1969). The effectiveness of a suicide prevention program. *Mental Hygiene*, **53**, 357–363.

Young R (1989). Helpful behaviors in the crisis center call. *Journal of Community Psychology*, **17**, 70–77.

# CHAPTER 62

# Treatment of attempted suicide and suicidal patients in primary care

Zoltán Rihmer and Wolfgang Rutz

## Abstract

Although suicidal behaviour is a rare event in society in general, it is very common among psychiatric patients who contact their general practioner (GP) before the suicide event. The most common current psychiatric diagnosis among suicide victims and attempters is major depressive episode (56–87 per cent). The current prevalence of major depressive episodes in GP practice is around 10 per cent, but at least half of these cases are not recognized and treated adequately by GPs. Successful acute and long-term treatment of depression significantly reduces the risk of suicidal behaviour. Given that more than half of all suicide victims contact their GPs within four weeks before their death, GPs play an important role in suicide prevention. Several large-scale community studies demonstrate that education of GPs on the diagnosis and appropriate pharmacotherapy of depression, particularly in combination with psychological interventions and public education, improve the identification and treatment of depression and reduces the frequency of suicidal behaviour in the areas served by trained GPs.

## Introduction

Suicide, an 'unnecessary death', the expression coined by Wasserman (Wasserman 2001), is among the most tragic events in human life, causing serious distress among relatives and friends as well as imposing a great economic burden on society as a whole. Although suicide attempts, and particularly completed suicides, are relatively rare events in the community, in many countries they exceed the number of traffic accidents. About 10–18 per cent of adults across diverse regions of the world, including western and central Europe, North America and the Far East, report lifetime suicidal ideation, and 3–5 per cent have made at least one suicide attempt at some point in their life (Kessler *et al.* 1999; Weissman *et al.* 1999; Szádóczky *et al.* 2000; Bertolote *et al.* 2005). Suicidal ideation, suicide attempt and completed suicide are three different, but greatly overlapping features. Previous suicide attempt and current major depression are the two best predictors of future suicide, and the vast majority of suicide attempters/completers come from a population of people with current suicidal ideation, particularly in the presence of untreated major depression (Kessler *et al.* 1999; Rihmer *et al.* 2002; Goldney *et al.* 2003). More than one-third of suicide victims have at least one previous suicide attempt, and the first suicide attempt (even if the method used is non-violent or non-lethal) significantly increases the risk of completed suicide during the next 10–15 years (Isometsa and Lönnqvist 1998; Hawton and van Heeringen 2000; Wasserman 2001; Suokas *et al.* 2001; Rihmer *et al.* 2002; Suominen *et al.* 2004). This is partly due to the fact that repeating suicide attempters frequently switch their method from non-violent to violent or from non-lethal to lethal methods (Rihmer *et al.* 1995; Isometsa and Lönnqvist 1998).

Suicide attempts are common among psychiatric patients who contact different levels of health care, particularly a few weeks or months before the suicide or suicide attempt (Isometsa *et al.* 1994a, 1995; Michel *et al.* 1997; Pirkis and Burgess 1998; Andersen *et al.* 2000; Rihmer *et al.* 2002; Fekete *et al.* 2004; Qin and Nordentoft 2005). In spite of the fact that suicidal behaviour is a relatively rare event in the primary care practice, but considering that depression is very common among completed suicides, depression and suicidality should be taken very seriously by general practitioners. In a given region, where the suicide rate is 20/100,000, a GP with a list of 2000 patients would be likely to have one completed suicide in every 2–3 years, but the yearly number of people with suicide attempts, current suicidal ideation and with current major depression would be 4–8, 40–50, and 160–200 respectively (Lecrubier 1998; Gunnel *et al.* 2004; Berardi *et al.* 2005; Rihmer and Angst 2005a, b).

## Suicide risk and protective factors detectable in primary care

Suicidal behaviour is neither a normal response to the levels of stress experienced by most people, or a standard consequence of major mental disorders. Suicide is a very complex, multicausal human behaviour with several biological as well as psychosocial, existential and cultural components. It is also associated with a number of psychiatric–medical (e.g, major mental) disorders, psychosocial (e.g, adverse) life situations, and demographic (e.g, gender, age)

**Table 62.1** Lifetime and current suicide risk factors

| Lifetime risk factors | Current acute risk factors |
|---|---|
| History of: | Current |
| Depressive/bipolar disorder | Major (severe) depression: |
| Substance use disorders | ◆ agitation/anxiety/insomnia |
| Schizophrenia | ◆ hopelessness |
| Anxiety disorders | ◆ comorbid anxiety/substance use and severe medical disorders |
| Prior suicide attempt | ◆ hospital discharge |
| Family history of suicide | ◆ suicide thoughts |
| Childhood negative life events | ◆ psychosocial stressors |
| Isolation/living alone | (loss-events, financial disaster) |
| Unemployment | ◆ spring/early summer |
| Male gender, old age | |

suicide risk factors of varying prognostic utility (Rihmer *et al.* 2002). Although the statistical relationship between the different psychosocial and demographic risk factors and suicidal behaviour is well documented, they have limited value in predicting suicide in individual cases. However, since suicide and attempted suicide is very rare in the absence of current major psychiatric disorders, psychiatric–medical suicide risk factors, particularly current major depression with a prior suicide attempt are the most powerful and clinically useful predictors of suicidal behaviour, especially in the presence of psychosocial and demographic risk factors (Beautrais *et al.* 1996; Shah and De; 1998; Wasserman *et al.* 1998; Hawton and van Heeringen 2000; Wasserman 2001; Rihmer *et al.* 2002; Balázs *et al.* 2003; Goldney *et al.* 2003; Tylee and Rihmer 2004; Rihmer 2005). The classification of suicide risk factors in terms of their duration are shown in Table 62.1. Lifetime (permanent) suicide risk factors result in high-risk groups, while current (acute) suicide risk factors create high-risk situations (Wasserman 2001; Rihmer *et al.* 2002; Tylee and Rihmer 2004), and when a high-risk period occurs in a high-risk person, the chance of suicide increases markedly.

Notwithstanding the fact that more than two-thirds of suicide victims and attempters have current major depression and up to 66 per cent of them contact their GPs within four weeks before the suicidal act the rate of pharmacotherapy with antidepressants and/or mood stabilizers in depressed suicidal patients is less than 20 per cent and thus disturbingly low (Rihmer *et al.* 1990; Beautrais *et al.* 1996; Marzuk *et al.* 1996; Pirkis and Burgess 1998; Oquendo *et al.* 1999; Andersen *et al.* 2000; Hawton and van Heeringen 2000; Henriksson *et al.* 2001; Wasserman 2001; Luoma *et al.* 2002; Rihmer *et al.* 2002; Balázs *et al.* 2003; Fekete *et al.* 2004). The same applies to short term psychological treatments effective in therapy of depression. This is a direct reflection of the well-documented fact that only a minority of depressed patients are recognized by their GPs in primary care and fewer still are adequately treated (Tylee *et al.* 1993; Lecrubier 1998; Davidson and Meltzer-Brody 1999; Berardi *et al.* 2005).

In contrast to the numerous suicide risk factors, only a few factors are known to have protective effects. Good family support as well as social significance, good life mastery skills, a sense of coherence and meaningfulness in life, pregnancy, the post-partum period,

having children, holding strong religious beliefs, together with appropriate medical care are traditionally cited as protective factors. It is important to note, that in spite of the fact that the post-partum period is regarded statistically as a protective factor, it may in individual patients, particularly in the cases of 'post-partum blue' and postnatal depression, increase the suicide risk (Appleby *et al.* 1999; Hawton and van Heeringen 2000; Malone *et al.* 2000; Wasserman 2001; Rihmer *et al.* 2002; Rihmer 2005). In the everyday clinical practice, however, the presence of one or more suicide risk factors is more important than the lack of protective ones. Given the very high proportion of current major mental disorders among people with suicidal behaviour, in the early 1980s Khuri and Akiskal (1983) considered that much of the putative psychosocial and demographic suicide risk factors were not modifiable in the frame of individual health care. Consequently, they proposed that suicide prevention should focus on the treatable contributory psychiatric disorders involved in such behaviour. On an aggregate level, however, organization and societal changes, e.g. the improvement of a primary health care system, empowerment strategies in the workplace and community, or the alleviation of unpredictability and stressful transitions in a society seem to reduce increased suicide figures (Rutz 2006).

## Depressive and related disorders in primary care

Unipolar and bipolar major depressive episodes, the most common current diagnoses of suicide victims and attempters are among the most frequent psychiatric illnesses in the community and in a variety of clinical settings. In addition to their frequent and serious complications (suicidal behaviour, secondary substance use disorders etc.) they are strongly associated with limitations in well-being and daily functioning that are equal to or greater than those of several chronic medical disorders (Davidson and Meltzed-Brody 1999; Rihmer and Angst 2005a, b). About two-thirds of patients with unipolar depression and bipolar disorder have comorbid anxiety disorder(s), and/or substance use disorders, and around one-third of them have one or more serious medical illness, and as it has been reported that these comorbid conditions increase the risk of suicidal behaviour (Davidson and Meltzer-Brody 1999; Tondo *et al.* 1999; Wasserman 2001; Hawton and van Heeringen 2000; Rihmer *et al.* 2002; Rihmer 2005; Rihmer and Angst 2005a; Wasserman 2006). Anxiety disorders also lead to risk of suicidal behaviour, but they are often associated with an elevated risk of subsequent major depression and suicidality particularly among untreated patients (Goodwin and Olfson 2001; Rihmer *et al.* 2002).

Less than half of all depressed patients in the community seek medical help. The majority of the ones who do consult their GPs however, are not adequately diagnosed and treated; which is to a large extent due to many GPs still widespread difficulties in recognizing and monitoring depression, despite the last decades great diagnostic and therapeutic achievements in the field (Lecribier 1998; Lerrubier and Hergueta 1998; Davidson and Meltzer-Brody 1999; Tylee 1999; Lecrubier 2001; Berardi *et al.* 2005; Wasserman 2006). Several European and North American studies have confirmed this by demonstrating that the current prevalence of DSM-III/DSM-IV or ICD-10 major depression in the primary care practice is around 8–10 per cent (range 4–18 per cent), but the majority of depressed patients are not recognized by their GPs and the rate of adequate antidepressive pharmacotherapy among identified depressives was less than 20 per cent (Spitzer *et al.* 1994; Lecrubier 1998; Davidson and Meltzer-Brody 1999; Christensen *et al.* 2001; Wittchen *et al.* 2001; Ansseau *et al.* 2004; Szádóczky *et al.* 2004; Al Windi 2005; Berardi *et al.* 2005). The WHO Collaborative Study, Psychological Problems in General Health Care, conducted in 1991 on more than 25,000 primary care patients in 14 countries from 4 continents found that on the whole, approximately 50 per cent of the patients with an ICD-10 diagnosis of major depressive episode were recognized as suffering from some kind of mental disorder by their GPs, but only 15 per cent of major depressives were recognized as having depression, and fewer than half of them were prescribed antidepressants for their depression (Lecrubier 1998, 2001; Lecrubier and Hergueta 1998). Studies from some European countries and from the USA, performed 5–10 years later, reported much higher rates of recognition and treatment of depression in primary care practice: 62–85 per cent of the depressed cases were recognized by the GPs and 33–50 per cent of them were treated with antidepressants (Wittchen *et al.* 2001; Lecrubier 2001; Simon and von Korff 1995; Berardi *et al.* 2005). These findings indicate that the situation does appear to be improving as a consequence of steadily increasing awareness of depression and development of better treatment strategies in primary care.

Most patients with depression consult their GPs mainly for somatic reasons, either because of their somatic comorbidity or because of the predominant somatic symptom because they do not 'believe' or understand they solely have a depression (Tylee *et al.* 1993; Davidson and Meltzer-Brody 1999; Tylee 1999; Lecrubier 2001; Tylee and Rihmer 2004). This is particularly important, since major depression is frequently associated with chronic physical disorders (cardiovascular diseases, hypertension, stroke, cancer, epilepsy, Parkinson's disease, HIV infection/AIDS, etc.), which further increase the suicide risk (see Chapter 40 in this book). The 1-year prevalence of severe major depression in individuals with two or more chronic physical disorders is fourfold higher (12 per cent) than in persons without such conditions (3 per cent) (Kessler *et al.* 1997), but paradoxically, primarily depressed patients with significant somatic comorbidity remain unrecognized in primary care (Tylee *et al.* 1993; Davidson and Meltzer-Brody 1999; Stoppe *et al.* 1999; Tylee 1999; Lecrubier 2001).

Another cause for somatization, however, especially in males, is the common alexithymic incapacity of men to recognize and realize their own depressive symtoms in a self-reflective way, to feel and show weakness and to ask for help, resulting in the tendency of many depressed males to seek primary health care for downplayed somatic symtoms (Möller-Leimkühler 2002). Several factors, relating to both patients and doctors, are likely to influence the recognition of major depression in primary care. Patient factors associated with non-recognition include: comorbid psychiatric (anxiety, substance abuse and personality) disorders, comorbid (mostly chronic) medical disorders, low degree of disability, less severe depressions, predominantly somatic symptom presentation (pains, paresthesias, anorexia, weight loss, etc.), male gender, younger or older age, and married status. On the other hand, high-level disability, lack of comorbid psychiatric and medical disorders, more severe depression, higher number of depressive symptoms, presenting depression predominantly with psychological symptoms (depressed mood, poor concentration, fatigue, psychomotor retardation), middle age-range, female gender and separated or divorced marital

status increases the chance of correct identification (Tylee *et al.* 1993; Rutz *et al.* 1995, 1997; Lecrubier 1998; 2001; Stoppe *et al.* 1999; Tylee 1999; Wittchen *et al.* 2001; Szádóczky *et al.* 2004).

Although many depressed patients report somatic symptoms and there is a permanent pressure in primary care not to miss organic disorders leading to suffering and death, it should be taken into account that untreated or inadequately treated depression can be highly dangerous, leading to dramatic suffering in the individual and their family and that this disorder is in fact among the most successfully treatable illnesses in medicine. Despite improvements in the last decade, the recognition of depression in primary care is still far from the ideal (Lecrubier 2001; Wittchen *et al.* 2001; Berardi *et al.* 2005). Physician factors related to poor recognition of depression are: lack of experience, insufficient or suboptimal knowledge about the symptoms, prejudices about mental illness, lack of postgraduate psychiatric training, insufficient interview skills, lack of cooperation with psychiatrists, and low level of empathy (Rutz *et al.* 1997; Tylee 1999; Lecrubier 2001; Thompson 2001; Wittchen *et al.* 2001). There is also evidence suggesting that specific organizational interventions and postgraduate training programmes improve the recognition and treatment of depression in primary care (Butler *et al.* 1997; Rutz *et al.* 1997; Appleby *et al.* 2000; Thompson 2001; van Oss *et al.* 2002; Gilbody *et al.* 2003; Hegerl *et al.* 2006; Mann *et al.* 2005; Szántó *et al.* 2007). Short screening-instruments (e.g, Shortened Beck Depression Inventory, Zung Self-Rating Depression Scale, the WHO 5 Well-Being Scale, the depression module of the Primary Care Evaluation of Mental Disorders [PRIME-MD], the Mini International Neuropsychiatric Interview [MINI], the Geriatric Depression Scale and the General Health Questionnaire), some of them designed specifically for primary care (Davidson and Meltzer-Brody 1999; Lecrubier 2001; Parashos *et al.* 2002; Szádóczky *et al.* 2004) are also helpful, but they do not replace a well-performed clinical interview.

While the majority of the literature on suicide in primary care focuses on unipolar major depression, less attention is paid to bipolar disorder, the point prevalence of which is between 1–2 per cent in the GP practice (Spitzer *et al.* 1994; Szádóczky *et al.* 1997; Ansseau *et al.* 2004; Das *et al.* 2005). Since the depressive episode of bipolar disorder carries an even higher risk of suicide than unipolar major depression, and because the vast majority of hypomanic and manic patients also become depressed (Rihmer 2005; Rihmer and Angst 2005b; Wasserman 2006), patients with history of hypomania and mania, particularly in the presence of current depression, should be considered as persons at very high risk of suicide.

## The suicidal patient in primary care

Suicidal behaviour in major mood disorder patients occur mostly during major depressive episodes (79–89 per cent), less frequently in the frame of dysphoric (mixed) mania (11–20 per cent), but practically never during euphoric mania and euthymia (0–1 per cent) (Isometsa *et al.* 1994b; Tondo *et al.* 1999). This suggests that suicidal behaviour in mood disorder patients is a state-dependent phenomenon, indicating the crucial role of recognition and treatment of depression in suicide prevention (Khuri and Akiskal 1983; Rihmer *et al.* 2002; Mann *et al.* 2005; Wasserman 2006). Since up to 66 per cent of suicide victims contact their GPs 4 weeks before their death (Isometsa *et al.* 1995; Pirkis and Burgess 1998; Andersen *et al.* 2000; Luoma *et al.* 2002), it is very likely that at these visits the vast majority of the patients are definitely depressed, and most of them have one or more comorbid psychiatric and/or medical disorder. Alcohol also plays an important role in suicidal behaviour (Rutz *et al.* 1995, 1997; Wasserman *et al.* 1998; Tondo *et al.* 1999; Wasserman 2001, 2006). Men who are depressed tend to act out and resort to alcohol and it may be that they mask their depression in this way (Angst *et al.* 2002; Rutz *et al.* 1995, 1997; Wasserman 2006). The results of the Swedish Gotland Study showed that the clinical picture of suicidal, depressed men is often masked by aggressive, impulsive and abusive behaviour (so-called male depressive syndrome), and that these men are better known to legal and social welfare agencies than to their GPs (Rutz *et al.* 1995, 1997).

Both specific acute psychiatric features (psychomotor agitation, insomnia, hopelessness, guilt etc) and adverse psychosocial factors (permanent adverse life situations, acute negative life events) play a significant role in triggering the actual suicidal behaviour (Hawton and van Heeringen 2000; Malone *et al.* 2000; Wasserman 2001; Rihmer *et al.* 2002; Mann 2004; Mann *et al.* 2005; Rihmer 2005). The complex interaction between these personality, psychiatric and psychosocial factors in suicidal behaviour is best explained by the stress–diathesis model for suicidal behaviour (Mann 2004), where the stressors include acute psychiatric disorder and negative life events ('state'), and the diathesis includes aggressive, impulsive and pessimistic personality features ('trait'). Both pessimism and aggressivity/impulsivity may be amenable to cognitive/behavioural therapy and pharmacotherapy, like SSRI antidepressants and lithium (Mann 2004).

As stated above, GP contact is very common before suicide: 47–73 per cent of suicide victims visit their GPs 3 months before their death, and 34–66 per cent and 20–40 per cent also do so in the last 4 weeks and in the last week, respectively (Ismometsa *et al.* 1995; Pirkis and Burgess 1998; Andersen *et al.* 2000; Luoma *et al.* 2002). Recent GP contact is particularly frequent among elderly suicide victims, as up to 90 per cent are reported to have seen their GPs in the preceding 3 months and up to 50 per cent in the last week (Shah and De 1998; Luoma *et al.* 2002). The rate of suicide victims without any recent medical contact is higher in males and in younger persons. Compared to non-suicidal primary care patients, suicide victims visit their GPs three times more frequently (Rutz *et al.* 1995, 1997; Isometsa *et al.* 1994a; Pirkis and Burgess 1998; Andersen *et al.* 2000; Luoma *et al.* 2002). In addition, the number of GP visits increases significantly before the suicidal act both among completed suicides (Appleby *et al.* 1996; Andersen *et al.* 2000) and suicide attempters (Michel *et al.* 1997; Fekete *et al.* 2004). However, among those with medical contact, the frequency of persons who communicate explicitly their intention to commit suicide is only around 20 per cent, and it is particularly rare in primary care (11 per cent) and in other (non-psychiatric) specialist settings (6 per cent). At the last GP contact, female suicide victims communicate their suicide intent almost twice as frequently as males (17 vs 10 per cent), and suicide victims with past history of suicide attempt report suicidal ideation more frequently than those without such history (Isometsa *et al.* 1994a, 1995). One study found that 18 per cent of the suicide victims visited GPs on the last day of their life, but the topic of suicide was discussed in only 21 per cent of these cases (Isometsa *et al.* 1995). Similarly low figures of communication of suicidal intent have also been reported for suicide attempters (Fekete *et al.* 2004). On the other hand, however, it has

also been reported that only 3 per cent of the GPs asked about suicidal ideation at least in old-age depressed patients (Stoppe *et al.* 1999; Wasserman 2001).

Discussing the possibility of suicidal behaviour with the patient and family members as a common but preventable complication of acute severe mental disorders is particularly important, given that there is a general consensus that asking questions about suicidal ideation and past suicide attempts does not trigger suicide (Hawton and van Heeringen 2000; Gould *et al.* 2005). This is particularly true if such a discussion is accompanied by an explanation that suicidal behaviour in psychiatric patients is a 'state-dependent' phenomenon, that depressive disorders can be successfully treated, and that suicidal ideation/wishing to die will vanish after (or even before) the recovery from depression. This is beneficial, as many patients think they are alone or unique in their suicidal ideas. Leaflets, posters, and fliers left in the waiting room indicating the main symptoms and dangers of depression as well as information on good prognosis of treatment may prompt people to ask for help. Short screening instruments, like the Beck Scale for Suicide Ideation (an interview-rated 19-item scale) and the Beck Hopelessness Scale (a 20-item self-reported questionnaire) are useful in clinical practice for detecting actual suicide risk (Hawton and van Heeringen 2000; Wasserman 2001) (see also Chapter 41 in this book). Yet no one screening instrument can replace the optimal doctor–patient relationship, including asking the right questions at the right time, accompanied by a highly professional and empathic atmosphere. Asking simple questions ('what do you think about the future?', 'do you feel that life is not worth living?', etc.) can easily facilitate further, more deep and honest discussion on the topic of suicide.

The risk of suicide is extremely high a few days and weeks after the discharge from inpatient psychiatric departments, particularly in the case of unplanned discharge and in patients with short hospital stay and with a high number of previous hospitalizations (Appleby *et al.* 1999; Hawton and van Heeringen 2000; Wasserman 2001; Qin and Nordentoft 2005). Therefore, GPs should be alert when a patient discharged from the psychiatric clinic seeks help.

The most characteristic clinical, psychosocial, and demographic features of the acutely suicidal patient in primary care are listed in Table 62.2.

## Prevention of suicide in primary care

Prevention of suicide in primary care is possible. Self-destructive behaviour usually does not occur in the very early stages of the depression and this allows enough time to make a precise diagnosis and to start appropriate treatment. Several studies from Europe, the United States and Australia showed that depression-training for GPs improved recognition of depression, including detection of current suicidal ideation, and increased treatment of depression, while a few others from the United Kingdom, the United States and Brazil found no positive effects (Mann *et al.* 2005; Nutting *et al.* 2005; Szántó *et al.* 2007). Since no one study reported the opposite (i.e. decreasing recognition and worsening treatment after the GP education), specific training and organizational interventions remain the only possibilities to make further progress on this field. However, improved primary care education in isolation does not have any significant long-term effect, and only complex educational and organizational interventions that incorporate continuous clinician education, an enhanced role of nurses

**Table 62.2** Most characteristic features of acutely suicidal patients in primary care

| Clinical features | Psychosocial features | Demographic features |
|---|---|---|
| Severe depression (agitation, anxiety, insomnia, hopelessness, guilt) | Acute psychosocial stressors (loss-events, acute major financial problems) Isolation/living alone Gun/poison at home | Male gender Old age (both genders) Young males Spring/early summer |
| Acute/chronic alcohol/ drug problems | | |
| Severe comorbid medical disorder(s) | | |
| Wish to die, suicide ideas, suicide plan, suicide gestures | | |
| Recent discharge from inpatient psychiatric department (short hospital stay, high number of prior hospitalizations, unplanned discharge) | | |

and social workers, as well as high level of integration between primary and secondary (psychiatric) care (consultation-liaison) are beneficial. Education should be well-focused, relatively short and interactive, include written materials, lectures, seminars, video demonstrations, and small-group discussions (Butler *et al.* 1997; Rutz *et al.* 1997; Schulberg *et al.* 1998; Appleby *et al.* 2000; Thompson 2001; Gilbody *et al.* 2003; Mann *et al.* 2005; Szanto *et al.* 2007).

The first example for the significant role of GPs in suicide prevention comes from the Swedish Gotland Study. Rutz *et al.* demonstrated that after a short intensive postgraduate training for GPs on the island of Gotland on the diagnosis and treatment of depression, the suicide rate and the rate of hospital admissions for depression declined significantly and antidepressant prescription increased markedly a few years after the training (Rutz *et al.* 1995, 1997). The rate of depressive suicides among all suicides decreased significantly after the training, indicating that the decline in suicide mortality after the education resulted directly from a robust decrease in depressive suicides, and suggesting that this result might not be caused by random fluctuation (Rihmer *et al.* 1995). However, the decline in depressive suicides after the training was almost entirely the result of a decrease in female depressive suicides, whereas male suicidality was almost unchanged. Few suicidal males were known to the local medical services, although many of these people were known to the police and social welfare services. These favourable effects faded in a few years and repeated education again led to another decrease in suicides, again mainly in females (Rutz *et al.* 1995, 1997).

Improved management of depression requires not only better recognition and treatment skills from the doctors, but also good compliance from the patients, since non-adherence to antidepressant therapy is one of the most common major causes of treatment failure. About one-third of patients stop taking antidepressants during the first 4 weeks of therapy, and around half of them take them until the end of the third month (Lin *et al.* 1995). The better side-effect profile and less toxic nature of SSRIs and other new

antidepressants, and the recently increasing practice of GPs preferring these drugs over tricyclic antidepressants, is also beneficial for improving the quality of care and reducing the risk of death in the case of overdose (Lin *et al.* 1995; Butler *et al.* 1997; Donoghue 1998; van Os *et al.* 2002). Using simple psycho-educational messages (i.e. why, how, and how long to take antidepressants and what to do in the case of side-effects, to optimize the clinical response) both in oral and written form increases the adherence to antidepressant therapy (Lin *et al.* 1995). Psychological treatments of depression should also be available in the GP's office or in adjunction to it (Wasserman 2006).

Treatment of depression in primary care should follow international and national guidelines established (Schulberg *et al.* 1998; van Os *et al.* 2002; Wasserman 2006). In contrast to recent concerns on the 'suicide-provoking potential' of antidepressants, it is evident that antidepressants and mood stabilizers, like lithium, carbamazepine, valproate and others treat depression effectively and decrease suicidality markedly among unipolar and bipolar depressives (Yerevanian *et al.* 2004; Akiskal *et al.* 2005; Simon *et al.* 2006). However, since antidepressant monotherapy, unprotected by mood stabilizers in bipolar depression, sometimes induces agitation, excitement (and rarely also auto- and hetero-aggressive behaviour) in the first few days or weeks of treatment, all depressive patients should be carefully checked for bipolarity and followed closely in the fist 1–3 weeks of the therapy (Akiskal *et al.* 2005). Anxiety, agitation or insomnia should always be controlled with concomitant use of high-potency benzodiazepines, which hasten the clinical response if combined with antidepressants (Furukawa *et al.* 2001). Regular after care with fixed appointments is highly recommended, particularly for those patients with previous suicide attempts. Psychological support should be available for suicidal depressed patients. This is important, since the actual clinical picture immediately after suicide attempt is often misleading, due to the cathartic effect of self-aggression, resulting in a short-lived but sometimes marked improvement of the depression (Jallade *et al.* 2005). This can also serve as one of the explanations why some health care workers misinterpret suicide attempts as manipulative acts.

Patients with acute suicidal danger usually need inpatient treatment even of an involuntary nature. In the case of severe agitation or anxiety prompt anxiolysis with benzodiazepines and close observation before and during transportation to the hospital is highly recommended. After an open discussion with the patient and relatives, involuntary admission is rarely needed. It should be explained that hospitalization is for and not against the patient's best interests. When acute hospitalization is not indicated, a close observation by family members and removing possible means of suicide (i.e, guns, drugs, pesticides, car key etc.) as well as consultation with a local outpatient psychiatrist is advised. GPs should work in close and permanent collaboration with the local mental health services. Outpatient psychiatric consultation is also helpful in the cases of differential-diagnostic problems, treatment resistance and comorbid substance use disorder regardless of whether the patient is suicidal or not. If long-term/prophylactic pharmacotherapy is needed (bipolar disorder, recurrent unipolar major depression) the GP may direct the patient to a psychiatrist for optimizing the therapy (Hawton and van Heeringen 2000; Wasserman 2001; Tylee and Rihmer 2004). The most frequent reasons of outpatient consultation and inpatient admission are shown in Table 62.3.

**Table 62.3** When to refer primary care patients to mental health services?

| Outpatient psychiatric care | Inpatient psychiatric admission |
| --- | --- |
| Recent suicide attempt | Acute suicidal danger |
| Treatment-resistant depression | Extreme severe (psychotic, catatonic |
| Differential diagnostic problem | negativistic) depression |
| Comorbid substanceuse disorders | Manic episode |
| Noncompliance with the treatment | Acute psychosis |
| Severe personality disorder | Severe comorbid medical disorder |
| Hypomanic episode | |
| Newly recognized bipolar disorder | |

# Conclusion

Suicide prevention in primary care is not an easy task, but it is possible, as general practitioners are key persons in suicide prevention. GPs are the first to meet depressed patients and should be trained in diagnostics and up to date use of antidepressants. Although, until now, specific depression-targeted psychotherapies exceed the frame of primary care, psycho-education and supportive psychotherapy is needed and it is essential to offer this kind of treatment in primary care settings. Regardless, GPs should have knowledge and collaboration with facilities offering psychological treatments. If every second suicide in primary care could be prevented this would mean that the suicide rate of a given area would drop by one-third.

# References

Akiskal HS, Benazzi F, Perugi G et al. (2005). Agitated 'unipolar' depression re-conceptualized as a depressive mixed state: implications for the antidepressant-suicide controversy. *Journal of Affective Disorders*, **85**, 245–258.

Al Windi A (2005). Depression in the general practice. *Nordic Journal of Psychiatry*, **59**, 272–277.

Andersen UA, Andersen M, Rosholm JU et al. (2000). Contacts to the health care system prior to suicide: a comprehensive analysis using registers for general and psychiatric hospital admissions, contacts to general practitioners and practising specialists and drug prescriptions. *Acta Psychiatrica Scandinavica*, **102**, 126–134.

Angst J, Gamma A, Gastpar M et al. (2002). Gender differences in depression. Epidemiological findings from the European DEPRES I and DEPRES II studies. *European Archives of Psychiatry and Clinical Neuroscience*, **252**, 201–209.

Ansseau M, Dierick M, Buntinkx F et al. (2004). High prevalence of mental disorders in primary care. *Journal of Affective Disorders*, **78**, 49–55.

Appleby L, Amos T, Doyle I et al. (1996). General practitioners and young suicides. A preventive role for primary care. *British Journal of Psychiatry*, **168**, 330–333.

Appleby L, Dennehy JA, Thomas CS et al. (1999). Aftercare and clinical characteristics of people with mental illness who committ suicide: a case–control study. *Lancet*, **353**, 1397–1400.

Appleby L, Morriss R, Gask L et al. (2000). An educational intervention for front-line health professionals in the assessment and management of suicidal patient. The STROM Project. *Psychological Medicine*, **30**, 805–812.

Balázs J, Lecrubier Y, Csiszér N et al. (2003). Prevalence and comorbidity of affective disorders in persons making suicide attempts in Hungary: importance of the first depressive episode and of bipolar II diagnoses. *Journal of Affective Disorders*, **76**, 113–119.

Bertolote JM, Fleischmann A, De Leo D et al. (2005). Suicide attempts, plans, and ideation in culturally diverse sites: the WHO SUPRE-MISS community survey. *Psychological Medicin*, **35**, 1457–1465.

Butler R, Collins E, Katona C et al. (1997). Does a teaching programme improve general practitioners' management of depression in the elderly? *Journal of Affective Disorders*, **46**, 303–308.

Beautrais AL, Joyce PR, Mulder RT et al. (1996). Prevalence and comorbidityof mental disorders in persons making serious suicide attempts: a case–control study. *American Journal of Psychiatry*, **153**, 1009–1014.

Berardi D, Menchetti M, Cevenini N et al. (2005). Increased recognition of depression in primary care. *Psychotherapy and Psychosomatics*, **74**, 225–230.

Christensen O, Bundgaard S, Bech P (2001). Prevalence of clinical (major) depression in general practice using the DSM-IV version of PRIME-MD. *International Journal of Psychiatry in Clinical Practice*, **5**, 49–54.

Das AK, Olfson M, Gameroff MJ et al. (2005). Screening for bipolar disorder in a primary care practice. *JAMA*, **293**, 956–963.

Davidson JRT and Meltzer-Brody SE (1999). The underrecognition and undertreatment of depression: what is the breadth and depth of the problem? *Journal of Clinical Psychiatry*, **60**, 4–9.

Donoghue J (1998). Sub-optimal use of tricyclic antidepressants in primary care. *Acta Psychiatrica Scandinavica*, **98**, 429–431.

Fekete S, Osvath P, Michel K (2004). Contacts with health care facilities prior to suicide attempts. In D De Leo, U Bille-Brahe, A Kerkhof et al., eds, *Suicidal Behaviour. Theories and Research Findings*, pp. 303–313. Hogrefe and Huber Publishers, Göttingen.

Furukawa TA, Steiner DL, Young LT (2001). Is antidepressant–benzodiazepine combination therapy clinically useful? A meta-analytic study. *Journal of Affective Disorders*, **65**, 173–177.

Gilbody S, Whitty P, Grimshaw J et al. (2003). Educational and organizational interventions to improve the management of depression in primary care. *JAMA*, **289**, 3145–3151.

Goldney RG, Dal Grande E, Fisher LJ et al. (2003). Population-attributable risk of major depression for suicidal ideation in a random and representative community sample. *Journal of Affective Disorders*, **74**, 267–272.

Goodwin R and Olfson M (2001). Treatment of panic attack and the risk of major depressive disorder in the community. *American Journal of Psychiatry*, **158**, 1146–1148.

Gould MS, Marrocco FA, Kleinman M et al. (2005). Evaluating iatrogenic risk of youth suicide screening programs. A randomized controlled trial. *JAMA*, **293**, 1635–1643.

Gunnel D, Harbord R, Singleton N et al. (2004). Factors influencing the development and amelioration of suicidal thoughts in the general population. *British Journal of Psychiatry*, **185**, 385–393.

Hawton K, and van Heeringen K (eds) (2000). *International Handbook of Suicide and Attempted Suicide*. John Wiley and Sons, Chichester.

Hegerl U, Althaus D, Schmidtke et al. (2006). The alliance against depression: 2-year evaluation of a community-based intervention to reduce suicidality. *Psychological Medicine*, **36**, 1225–1234.

Henriksson S, Boethius G, Isacsson G (2001). Suicides are seldom prescribed antidepressants: findings from a prospective prescription database in Jamtland county, Sweden. *Acta Psychiatrica Scandinavica*, **103**, 301–306.

Isometsa ET, Aro HM, Henriksson MM et al. (1994a). Suicide in major depression in different treatment settings. *Journal of Clinical Psychiatry*, **55**, 523–527.

Isometsa ET, Henriksson MM, Aro HM et al. (1994b). Suicide in bipolar disorder in Finland. *American Journal of Psychiatry*, **151**, 1020–1024.

Isometsa ET and Lönnqvist JK (1998). Suicide attempts preceding completed suicide. *British Journal of Psychiatry*, **173**, 531–533.

Ismometsa ET, Heikkinen ME, Marttunen MJ et al. (1995). The last appointment before suicide: is suicide intent communicated? *American Journal of Psychiatry*, **152**, 919–922.

Jallade C, Sarfati Y, Hardy-Baylé MC (2005). Clinical evolution after self-induced or accidental traumatism: a controlled study of the extent and the specificity of suicidal crisis. *Journal of Affective Disorders*, **85**, 283–292.

Kessler RC, Zhao S, Blazer DG *et al.* (1997). Prevalence, correlates, and course of minor and major depression in the National Comorbidity Survey. *Journal of Affective Disorders*, **45**, 19–30.

Kessler RC, Borges G, Walters EE (1999). Prevalence and risk factors for lifetime suicide attempts in the National Comorbidity Survey. *Archives of General Psychiatry*, **56**, 617–626.

Khuri R and Akiskal HS (1983). Suicide prevention: the necessity of treating contributory psychiatric disorders. *Psychiatric Clinics of North America*, **6**, 193–207.

Lecrubier Y (1998). Is depression under-recognised and undertreated? *International Clinical Psychopharmacology*, **13**, 3–6.

Lecrubier Y (2001). Improved ability to identify symptoms of major depressive disoder (MDD) in general practice. *International Journal of Psychiatry in Clinical Practice*, **5**, 3–10.

Lecrubier Y and Hergueta T (1998). Differences between prescription and consumption of antidepressants and anxiolytics. *International Clinical Psychopharmacology*, **13**, 7–11.

Lin EHB, von Korff M, Katon W *et al.* (1995). The role of the primary care physician in patients' adherence to antidepressant therapy. *Medical Care*, **33**, 67–74.

Luoma JB, Martin CE, Pearson JL (2002). Contact with mental health and primary care providers before suicide: a review of the evidence. *American Journal of Psychiatry*, **159**, 909–916.

Malone KM, Oquendo MA, Haas GL *et al.* (2000). Protective factors against suididal acts in major depression: Reasons for living. *American Journal of Psychiatry*, **157**, 1084–1088.

Mann JJ (2004). Searching for triggers of suicidal behavior. *American Journal of Psychiatry*, **161**, 395–397.

Mann JJ, Apter A, Bertolote J *et al.* (2005). Suicide prevention strategies. A systematic review. *JAMA*, **294**, 2064–2074.

Marzuk PM, Tardiff K, Leon AC *et al.* (1996). Use of prescription psychotropic drugs among suicide victims in New York City. *American Journal of Psychiatry*, **152**, 1520–1522.

Michel K, Runeson B, Valach L *et al.* (1997). Contacts of suicide attempters with GPs prior to the event: a comparison between Stockholm and Bern. *Acta Psychiatrica Scandinavica*, **95**, 94–99.

Möller-Leimkühler AM (2002). Barriers to help-seeking by men: a review of socio-cultural and clinical literature with particular reference to depression. *Journal of Affective Disorders*, **71**, 1–9.

Nutting PA, Dickinson LM, Rubenstein LV *et al.* (2005). Improving detection of suicidal ideation among depressed patients in primary care. *Annals of Family Medicine*, **3**, 529–536.

Oquendo MA, Malone KM, Ellis SP *et al.* (1999). Inadequacy of antidepressant treatment for patients with major depression who are at risk of suicidal behavior. *American Journal of Psychiatry*, **156**, 190–194.

Parashos IA, Stamouli S, Rogakou E *et al.* (2002). Recognition of depressive symptoms in the elderly: what can help the patient and the doctor. *Depression and Anxiety*, **15**, 111–116.

Pirkis J and Burgess P (1998). Suicide and recency of health care contacts. *British Journal of Psychiatry*, **173**, 462–474.

Qin P and Nordentoft M (2005). Suicide risk in relation to psychiatric hospitalization. *Archives of General Psychiatry*, **62**, 427–432.

Rihmer Z, Barsi J, Arató M *et al.* (1990). Suicide in subtypes of primary major depression. *Journal of Affective Disorders*, **18**, 221–225.

Rihmer Z, Rutz W, Pihlgren H (1995). Depression and suicide on Gotland. An intensive study of all suicides before and after a depression-training programme for general practitioners. *Journal of Affective Disorders*, **35**, 147–152.

Rihmer Z, Belső N, Kiss K (2002). Strategies for suicide prevention. *Current Opinion in Psychiatry*, **15**, 83–87.

Rihmer Z (2005). Prediction and prevention of suicide in bipolar disorders. *Clinical Neuropsychiatry*, **2**, 48–54.

Rihmer Z and Angst J (2005a). Mood disorders: epidemiology. In Sadock BJ and Sadock VA, eds, *Kaplan and Sadock's Comprehensive Textbook of Psychiatry*, 8th edn, pp. 1575–1582. Lipincott Williams and Wilkins, Philadelphia,

Rihmer Z and Angst J (2005b). Epidemiology of bipolar disorder. In S Kasper and RMA Hirschfeld, eds, *Handbook of Bipolar Disorder*, pp. 21–35. Taylor and Francis, New York.

Rutz W, von Knorring L, Pihlgren H *et al.* (1995). Prevention of male suicides: lessons from Gotland study. *Lancet*, **345**, 524.

Rutz W, Waliner J, Knorring L *et al.* (1997). Prevention of depression and suicide by education and medication: impact on male suicidality. An update from the Gotland study. *International Journal of Psychiatry in Clinical Practice*, **1**, 39–46.

Rutz W (2006). Social psychiatry and public mental health: present situation and future objectives. Time for rethinking and renaissance? *Acta Psychiatrica Scandinavica*, **Suppl. 429**, 95–100.

Schulberg HC, Katon W, Simon GE *et al.* (1998). Treating major depression in primary care practice. An update of the Agency for Health Care Policy and Research Guidelines. *Archives of General Psychiatry*, **55**, 1121–1127.

Shah A and De T (1998). Suicide in the elderly. *International Journal of Psychiatry in Clinical Practice*, **2**, 3–17.

Simon GE and von Korff M (1995). Recognition, management, and outcomes of depression in primary care. *Archives of Family Medicine*, **4**, 99–105.

Simon GE, Savarino J, Operskalski B *et al.* (2006). Suicide risk during antidepressant treatment. *American Journal of Psychiatry*, **163**, 41–47.

Spitzer RL, Williams JBW, Kroenke K *et al.* (1994). Utility of a new procedure for diagnosing mental disorders in primary care. The PRIME-MD 1000 Study. *JAMA*, **272**, 1749–1756.

Stoppe G, Sandholzer H, Huppertz C *et al.* (1999). Family physicians and the risk of suicide in the depressed elderly. *Journal of Affective Disorders*, **54**, 193–198.

Suokas J, Suominen K, Isometsa ET *et al.* (2001). Long-term risk factors for suicide mortality after attempted suicide—findings of a 14-year follow-up study. *Acta Psychiatrica Scandinavica*, **104**, 117–121.

Suominen K, Isometsa ET, Suokas J *et al.* (2004). Completed suicide after a suicide attempt: a 37-year follow-up study. *American Journal of Psychiatry*, **161**, 563–564.

Szádóczky E, Rihmer Z, Papp Z *et al.* (1997). The prevalence of affective and anxiety disorders in primary care practice in Hungary. *Journal of Affective Disorders*, **43**, 239–244.

Szádóczky E, Vitrai J, Rihmer Z *et al.* (2000). Suicide attempts in the Hungarian adult population. Their relation with DIS/DSM-III-R affective and anxiety disorders. *European Psychiatry*, **15**, 343–347.

Szádóczky E, Rózsa S, Zámbori J *et al.* (2004). Anxiety and mood disorders in primary care practice. *International Journal of Psychiatry in Clinical Practice*, **8**, 77–84.

Szántó K, Kalmar S, Hendin H *et al.* (2007). A suicide prevention program in a region with a very high suicide rate. *Archives of General Psychiatry*, **64**, 914–920.

Thompson C (2001). Managing major depression: improving the interface between psychiatrists and primary care. *International Journal of Psychiatry in Clinical Practice*, **5**, 11–18.

Tondo L, Baldessarini RJ, Hennen J (1999). Suicide attempts in major affective disorder patients with comorbid substance use disorders. *Journal of Clinical Psychiatry*, **60**, 63–69.

Tylee A (1999). Depression in the community: physician and patient perspective. *Journal of Clinical Psychiatry*, **60**, 12–16.

Tylee AT, Freeling P, Kerry S (1993). Why do general practitioners recognize major depression in one woman patient yet miss it in another? *The British Journal of General Practice*, **43**, 327–330.

Tylee A and Rihmer Z (2004). Suicide and attempted suicide. In R Jones, N Britten, L Culpepper *et al.*, eds, *Oxford Textbook of Primary Medical Care, vol. 2, Clinical Management*, pp. 959–962. Oxford Unniversity Press, Oxford and New York.

van Os TWDP, van den Brink RHS, Jenner JA *et al.* (2002). Effects on depression pharmacotherapy of a Dutch general practitioner treating program. *Journal of Affective Disorders*, **71**, 105–111.

Wasserman D, Varnik A, Dankowicz M *et al.* (1998). Suicide-preventive effects of perestroika in the former USSR: the role of alcohol restriction. *Acta Psychiatrica Scandinavica*, **Suppl. 394**, 1–44.

Wasserman D (ed.) (2001). *Suicide—An Unnecessary Death*. Martin Dunitz, London.

Wasserman D (2006). *Depression: The Facts*. Oxford University Press, Oxford.

Weissman MM, Bland RC, Canino GJ *et al.* (1999). Prevalence of suicide ideation and suicide attempts in nine countries. *Psychological Medicine*, **29**, 9–17.

Wittchen HU, Höfler M, Meister W (2001). prevalence and recognition of depressive syndromes in German primary care settings: poorly recognized and treated? *International Clinical Psychopharmacology*, **16**, 121–135.

Yerevaninan BI, Koek RJ, Feusner JD *et al.* (2004). Antidepressants and suicidal behaviour in unipolar depression. *Acta Psychiatrica Scandinavica*, **110**, 452–458.

# CHAPTER 63

# Treatment of suicide attempts and suicidal patients in psychiatric care

Lars Mehlum

## Abstract

No other known risk factor has such a high suicide prevention potential as a psychiatric disorder. However, to release this potential psychiatric care needs to be made more available to suicidal individuals, and there is a necessity to establish a continuity of care between hospital and outpatient treatment for patients who have been admitted after a suicide attempt. In this chapter important aspects of the psychiatric treatment of suicidal individuals are described. The importance of conducting systematic and repeated clinical risk assessments, providing treatments targeted at the patient's needs and instigating safety measures according to the actual risk level is re-inforced. Treatment standards should be kept high through continuous staff education measures, clinical supervision, adherence to written procedures, and should be improved through suicide review procedures whenever there has been a severe suicidal incident within the context of the clinical unit.

## Introduction

Psychiatric disorders are present in at least 90 per cent of suicides (Cavanagh *et al.* 2003), and in most cases patients are untreated at the time of death (Lonnqvist *et al.* 1995). The strong association between suicide, attempted suicide and psychiatric disorders makes effective psychiatric treatment and care central components to suicide prevention (Mann *et al.* 2005). A major problem is, however, that most of the treatments we currently rely upon in clinical practice have not yet demonstrated their effectiveness in preventing suicide. One reason for this is that suicidal individuals have often been excluded from clinical trials on treatment efficacy due to ethical, legal and practical considerations. Since suicide remains the most serious outcome of mental disease, it is essential that we find ways of overcoming these research obstacles in order to provide a set of evidence-based treatments adapted to the specific needs for different groups of suicidal patients. Data from Danish registers have demonstrated that the population-attributable risk (PAR)—the proportion of suicides *in the population* that could be removed if the risk factor could be removed—for suicide associated with lifetime psychiatric hospitalization is about 40 per cent (Qin *et al.* 2003). No other known risk factor has such a strong PAR.

Furthermore, as demonstrated in the systematic literature review by Pirkis and Burgess (1998) perhaps as many as 40 per cent of individuals in the general population who died by suicide had undergone inpatient psychiatric care less than one year before their death. Accordingly, this chapter will place its emphasis on the situation of patients in psychiatric hospital care and describing aspects of such care relevant to suicide prevention.

## Psychiatric care: indispensable yet often inaccessible

According to estimates by Bertolote *et al.* (2003) as many as 165 000 lives could possibly be saved worldwide annually if adequate psychiatric treatment for major psychiatric disorders were provided. In large parts of the world, particularly developing countries, there is a profound lack of mental health resources. There is a scarcity of hospital facilities, community mental health centres and adequately trained mental health workers. Even in many so-called developed countries of North America and Europe, not enough psychiatric treatment resources are available to populations that seem to have become increasingly in need of them. The downsizing and closing of psychiatric hospitals in many countries have made things worse since not enough outpatient facilities have been established to compensate for such cutbacks. A study by Hansen and co-workers of downsizing of psychiatric inpatient facilities in Norway suggested an association between the downsizing and a subsequent substantial increase in suicide rates of the patient population in the relevant catchment areas (Hansen *et al.* 2001).

There is clearly a need to strengthen psychiatric services in most countries. Equally important is to carefully plan services in order to make them more optimally available. Whereas many developed countries are in the process of strengthening community mental health services, some countries—for example many European countries in transition—have retained a nearly totally hospital-based psychiatric care. Yet, in the Baltic States for example, most patients with mental disorders, such as depression, will never encounter hospital psychiatrists. Still, there are general practitioners who have generally not received sufficient training in the treatment of common psychiatric disorders and suicidality. From a suicide preventive perspective, it is of the utmost importance to resolve the problems of access to psychiatric treatments in all regions of the world.

## Emergency psychiatric care

Suicidal ideation or behaviour is frequently seen in patients seeking emergency psychiatric care. Such care is differently organized across the world. Frequently, however, the suicide attempter will require crisis intervention at a general hospital or in an emergency room. Working with patients in suicidal crises, clinicians are faced with three important challenges: (a) to protect the patient against the danger of suicide or irreversible injury; (b) to reduce the patient's profound feeling of hopelessness and despair; and (c) to elevate the patient's subjective experience of quality of life. Essential to the first challenge is to conduct a systematic clinical assessment of suicide risk. Specific questionnaires and interviews have been developed for the purpose of evaluating suicide intent and suicide risk (Beck *et al.* 1974; Mieczkowski *et al.* 1993), but since they have so far not been able to predict suicide more effectively than clinical evaluations, the clinical interview remains the gold standard in suicide risk assessment. This includes a psychiatric examination, in which adequate history is taken, psychiatric symptoms are recorded and the patient's current suicidal ideation and intent is evaluated. For a detailed description of the assessment interview see Chapter 43 and 44 in this volume. The psychiatric consultation should provide information necessary for treatment planning and it should also serve as a clinical intervention focusing on the patient's most critical problems and psychological needs. To establish a therapeutic alliance is of the utmost importance for successful treatment of patients in suicidal crises. While patients must get the opportunity to recover from their medical condition, e.g. the intoxication, and to rest in an atmosphere of kindness and reassurance, most patients will also need to express, with the therapists help, their problems and emotions verbally. Emotions such as hopelessness, feelings of guilt, shame, rage, abandonment and self-hatred are commonly seen in suicidal patients (Hendin *et al.* 2004) and may evoke countertransference reactions in the therapist (the arousal of the therapist's own repressed feelings through identification with the patient's experiences and problems, or through responding to the patient's expressions of love or hostility toward the therapist). In case of countertransference this must be dealt with properly through professional supervision. The therapists need to demonstrate that they accept and validate the *patient* but not necessarily the *suicidal behaviour*, and discuss problem-solving strategies other than suicide. Most patients will initially be in a state of emotional turmoil and chaos, and need help to get a better understanding of what has happened and why. Patients who have attempted suicide will often require treatment in an emergency room, and then be observed for the next 1–3 days in an acute medical ward according to their medical condition. After this, some patients will need further hospitalization, as discussed below. However, effective treatment of the majority of patients will, under most circumstances, be possible in an outpatient setting. Depending on the clinical picture there may be a need for follow-up of medication, referral for alcohol or drug rehabilitation and individual or family therapy. Some patients can rely on their family doctor as a coordinator of the different treatment components, but treatment delivered by the family doctor alone is seldom enough. To ask the patient

whether they have easy access to potentially toxic medication, other substances or guns that can be easily used for suicide, and to consequently have these removed from the patient's home before they are discharged from the hospital is an advisable and effective precaution (Kruesi *et al.* 1999). The patient and their family should furthermore be provided with written information about available crisis resources in case of rapid re-emergence of suicidal impulses; this has been demonstrated to reduce the risk of repetitive suicidal behaviour (Cotgrove *et al.* 1995).

It is recommended that treatment contact is continued in some form with most of these patients for the first year after the suicide attempt. Longitudinal studies have shown that patients treated for suicide attempts run a particularly high risk of completed suicide during the first year after their discharge (Hawton *et al.* 2003). Since many patients have a strong tendency to drop out of follow-up care, any measures that can motivate the patient and improve adherence to treatment will be important, and good results have been attained with several treatment compliance-oriented programmes for suicide attempters in emergency care (Rotheram-Borus *et al.* 1996; Koons *et al.* 2001; Guthrie *et al.* 2001; Spirito *et al.* 2002). A special chain of care programme for suicide attempters has been implemented as part of the Norwegian national strategy for suicide prevention (Norwegian Board of Health 1994), establishing a structured collaboration between general hospitals, emergency facilities and after-care providers (Mehlum 2000) resulting in a substantially improved level in the quality of care (Mork *et al.* 2001) and a decreased prevalence of rapid repetition of the suicide attempt (Dieserud *et al.* 1992).

## Hospitalization

Patients who have one or more of the following characteristics will usually need a prolonged psychiatric inpatient treatment: having made suicide attempts with a high degree of suicidal intent; having a continued wish/plan for suicide; having symptoms of a severe mental disorder such as severe major depression or psychosis and/ or alcohol or other substance use disorder; having poor impulse control or weak barriers against suicide; having poor social support; having experienced recent severe social stressors, loss or emotional trauma. The exception is patients with a pattern of repetitive episodes of suicide attempts and suicidal gestures and signs and symptoms of borderline personality disorder, for which extended hospitalization is not necessarily beneficial (Paris 2002). These patients' suicidality may actually intensify through what has been labelled as 'malignant regression' (Balint 1968). This may lead to escalating suicide threats, self-mutilating or suicidal behaviour and, as a consequence, extended admissions or, even worse, precipitating premature discharge or other angry rejection from the hospital staff. Except in cases of severe suicide risk and/or psychotic symptoms, these often chronically suicidal patients should preferably be treated in an outpatient setting where increased therapeutic support will often be necessary in situations of increased suicidal feelings and tendencies. Therapeutic support means both specific psychiatric interventions *and* psychosocial support from the clinician. Such support is essential to counteract the often profound feeling of hopelessness, abandonment and shame experienced by the suicidal patient. While providing such support, it is important to actively avoid teaching borderline patients that appropriate attention to their needs will only be provided when they show signs of suicidality; sadly, this is often the case in many busy clinical outpatient units. Hence, there is a strong need for carefully planned long-term outpatient treatment programmes for borderline patients with suicidal behaviour.

## Safety measures

Sometimes the patient refuses to be hospitalized. If in such cases there is imminent danger to the patient's life, involuntary commitment will often be necessary. When the patient is transferred to a psychiatric hospital there is a need to promote the establishment of a new therapeutic alliance through measures mentioned above. A clinical re-evaluation should be conducted immediately and according to this, all necessary safety measures should be undertaken. Necessary precautions such as placing the patient in a special observation unit, removing belts, razors and other dangerous objects among the patient's belongings should be undertaken. Control measures such as these have the potential of threatening the patient's personal integrity and should therefore be implemented with care and respect. In order to reduce the need of control measures over prolonged periods of time the staff may ask the patient to sign or to verbally agree to a 'no suicide' contract, in which the patient agrees not to harm himself for a specific limited time period and that they will contact the staff if their feelings or the situation changes.

Special observation units must be carefully designed to remove opportunities for hanging, jumping out of windows or other means that could be used for self-harm. Wards providing treatment for suicidal patients should be audited at least annually to ensure they comply with these requirements (Duffy *et al.* 2003). Equally important is that staff are adequately trained for the treatment and protection of these critically ill patients. In many hospitals there is, however, an unacceptable and potentially dangerous variation and confusion in terminology and practice regarding procedures for special observation and protection against suicide. For example, a psychiatrist in charge of the treatment may find it necessary to prescribe 'continuous observation' as a protective measure against suicide for a given patient and by this he expects the nursing staff to be close to the patient and not to lose sight of them even for a moment. The member of the nursing staff who receives the doctor's orders may, however, have been trained to use the term 'continuous observation' in a slightly different and less restrictive manner and this could imply a hazard to the patient's safety. Every treatment facility must therefore have a crystal clear observation policy in which newcomers are to be educated and to which all staff must adhere.

## Critical phases

Some phases and situations during the clinical course in suicidal patients are generally regarded as particularly dangerous with respect to completed suicide. One of these phases takes place within the first few days after admission when the patient's condition is often unstable, and should be met with increased levels of observation and protection. Some patients, e.g. young people with a diagnosis of schizophrenia, may become increasingly depressed after acknowledging the severity of the handicaps of their mental disorder (Bourgeois *et al.* 2004), or because of the seemingly irreversible consequences of the actions they may have undertaken during phases of psychosis or confusion.

Clinical experiences indicate that the risk of suicide could be increased in some patients during early phases of antidepressant medication, when in many instances a normalizing effect upon psychomotor inhibition symptoms precedes a normalizing of the depressed mood. The risk of fatal or non-fatal self-harm associated with the use of selective serotonin reuptake inhibitors (SSRI) seems, however, not to be different than for tricyclic antidepressants (Martinez *et al.* 2005), with a possible exception for those aged 18 years or younger.

Single case observations, but not clinical and epidemiological studies (Taiminen and Helenius 1994; King *et al.* 1995), have indicated that there may exist a clustering effect of suicidal behaviour among psychiatric inpatients. In the aftermath of an inpatient suicide, it would therefore be advisable to be alert to the possibility of contagious effects. Particularly important will be to provide adequate information about the incident to the other patients and to help them cope with grief and stress reactions.

When patients are in transition, either between treatment units, therapists, at home leaves or at discharge, there is a danger that they may react with increased suicide risk and that this risk is not detected because of the changes in therapists. To counteract this danger, it is advisable to conduct repeated evaluations of suicide risk before any major changes are made to the patient's treatment setting or to the protection level. Before free exit or home leave is permitted careful evaluation must be performed and the patient's family should be informed. For patients admitted due to suicidality, an evaluation of suicide risk should be conducted no more than 24 hours before discharge to see if the risk signs and symptoms have been adequately ameliorated. A classical type of risk situation may take place when the patient's therapist is unavailable, on leave or quits the job. As a therapist, one should not underestimate the protective effects against suicide that may arise from the patients' attachment; often an indispensable resource in the treatment. This important aspect of our contact with the patient should be addressed in case a temporal or permanent separation is up coming.

## Psychotherapeutic and pharmacological interventions

A description of specific treatments, both psychological and pharmacological are given in Part 9, Chapters 53–60 of this book.

# Ensuring adequate quality standards

Many of the treatments described in Part 9 of this book, and procedures reviewed in this chapter have been shown, in randomized controlled studies, to be efficacious in reducing suicidal ideation and/or behaviour. Whether they will prove to be equally effective in daily clinical practice will depend heavily upon our ability to keep up to adequate quality standards over time. Quality work will often require more resources. It is therefore a leadership responsibility to make necessary priorities and resource allocations and, if needed, to protect treatment programmes of good standards against budget cuts and the sometimes detrimental effects of reorganizing processes. It is absolutely necessary that all clinical staff in a wide range of mental health settings are adequately trained in suicide risk assessment, and in the essentials of treatment and protection of patients at risk of suicide during the different critical phases of their illness. This training must be regularly updated. Equally important is that all new staff are educated to comply with the unit's standards and procedures.

Probably only in an ideal world would we be able to prevent every patient suicide. When suicide does occur in the hospital setting, complex reactions arise among the other patients, the patient's family and the staff (Bartels 1987). Unless we respond constructively to the many challenges and needs that arise, there is risk that the suicide will lead to negative processes, both in the group of patients and among the staff (Brown 1987), and we will probably not be able to learn from what has happened. It is therefore essential that early emotional support is given to all those that have been affected by the suicide, especially the patient's family (Wolfersdorf et al. 2001), but also the fellow patients and to those staff members who were responsible for the patient's treatment (Hodgkinson 1987). This supportive work will follow common principles of crisis intervention bearing in mind the special burdens, risks and social stigma suicide survivors often carry over longer periods of time (Brown 1987; Ness and Pfeffer 1990). After necessary emotional support has been provided to those who have been directly affected by the suicide, it is important to review the incident critically in order to identify possible shortcomings or errors that may have been made in the treatment or protection of the patient. For such a purpose, many units find it useful to hold a review meeting in the aftermath of an inpatient suicide. In this meeting, the clinician in charge of the patient's treatment will first present a summary of the case: history, presenting problem, symptoms, diagnostic evaluations, treatments given, and observations made during the hospital stay. It is of particular importance to provide a detailed account of the last days and hours before the suicide. The rest of the involved staff members will then have the opportunity to make their own contribution in order to create a more complete picture of what happened and why. If possible, a review meeting should be chaired by the unit's clinical director and it is their task to clarify the purpose of the meeting and to make sure that painful, but necessary critical questions are raised about shortcomings and errors in the treatment at the same time as he must counteract tendencies of self-blaming or scapegoating (Wasserman 2001, Beskow et al. 1990). Last, but not least, it is important that the suicide review also includes an evaluation of the quality of the emotional and practical support provided by the treatment unit for the bereaved in the aftermath of suicide.

Most clinical units will find it useful to produce written procedures for many of the specific methods, standards, assessments, precautions or protective actions discussed in this chapter. These documents should be made as clear and explicit as possible and should be the basis for staff training and updating. It is necessary that these written procedures be revised at regular intervals. Local health authorities should also consider regularly auditing treatment units for suicidal patients.

## Conclusion

Suicide is the most serious outcome of mental disease and no other known risk factor has such a high prevention potential in relation to suicide as psychiatric disorders. While this underlines the important role played by psychiatric care facilities in suicide prevention, there is, however, a need to strengthen several aspects of the care of suicidal individuals. Psychiatric care needs to be made more available to the population in most countries and there is a need to establish a continuity of care between hospital and outpatient treatment for patients who have been admitted after a suicide attempt. Furthermore, the quality of care must be kept to high standards of clinical evaluations, treatments and safety measures through education of staff, clinical supervision and through adherence to written procedures and it should be improved through review procedures whenever there has been a severe suicidal incident during inpatient care by any of the patients.

## References

Balint M (1968). *The Basic Fault: Therapeutic Aspects of Regression.* Tavistock, London.

Bartels SJ (1987). The aftermath of suicide on the psychiatric inpatient unit. *General Hospital Psychiatry*, **9**, 189–197.

Beskow J, Runeson B, Åsgard U (1990). Psychological autopsies: methods and ethics. *Suicide and Life-Threatening Behaviour*, **20**, 307–323.

Brown HN (1987). The impact of suicide on therapists in training. *Comprehensive Psychiatry*, **28**, 101–112.

Beck AT, Schuyler D, Herman I (1974). Development of suicide intent scales. In AT Beck, HLP Resnick, D Lettiem et al., eds, *The Prediction of Suicide*, pp. 45–56. Charles Press, Philadelphia.

Bertolote JM, Fleischmann A, De Leo D et al. (2003). Suicide and mental disorders: do we know enough? *British Journal of Psychiatry*, **183**, 382–383.

Bourgeois M, Swendsen J, Young F et al. (2004). Awareness of disorder and suicide risk in the treatment of schizophrenia: results of the international suicide prevention trial. *American Journal of Psychiatry*, **161**, 1494–1496.

Cavanagh JT, Carson AJ, Sharpe M et al. (2003). Psychological autopsy studies of suicide: a systematic review. *Psychological Medicine*, **33**, 395–405.

Cotgrove A, Zirinsky L, Black D et al. (1995). Secondary prevention of attempted suicide in adolescence. *Journal of Adolescence*, **18**, 569–577.

Dieserud G, Andersen-Gott MSH, Egede Borg S (1992). *Selvmordsforsøk i Bærum 1984–88. Rapport om det oppfølgende arbeidet etter selvmordsforsøk i Bærum kommune* [Suicide attempts in Baerum 1984–88. Report on the follow-up programme for suicide attempters in the municipality of Baerum]. Bærum Kommune, Helseetaten, Bærum.

Duffy D, Ryan T, Purdy R (2003). *Preventing Suicide: A Toolkit for Mental Health Services*. National Institute of Mental Health, Leeds.

Guthrie E, Kapur N, Kway-Jones K et al. (2001). Randomised controlled trial of brief psychological intervention after deliberate self poisoning. *British Medical Journal*, **323**, 135–138.

Hodgkinson PE (1987). Responding to in-patient suicide. *British Journal of Medical Psychology*, **60**, 387–392.

Hansen V, Jacobsen BK, Arnesen E (2001). Cause-specific mortality in psychiatric patients after deinstitutionalisation. *British Journal of Psychiatry*, **179**, 438–443.

Hawton K, Zahl D, Weatherall R (2003). Suicide following deliberate self-harm: long-term follow-up of patients who presented to a general hospital. *British Journal of Psychiatry*, **182**, 537–542.

Hendin H, Maltsberger JT, Haas AP et al. (2004). Desperation and other affective states in suicidal patients. *Suicide and Life-Threatening Behaviour*, **34**, 386–394.

King CA, Franzese R, Gargan S et al. (1995). Suicide contagion among adolescents during acute psychiatric hospitalization. *Psychiatric Services*, **46**, 915–918.

Koons CR, Robins CJ, Tweed JL et al. (2001). Efficacy of dialectical behaviour therapy in women veterans with borderline personality disorder. *Behaviour Therapy*, **32**, 371–390.

Kruesi MJ, Grossman J, Pennington JM et al. (1999). Suicide and violence prevention: parent education in the emergency department. *Journal of the American Academy of Child and Adolescent Psychiatry*, **38**, 250–255.

Lonnqvist JK, Henriksson MM, Isometsa ET *et al.* (1995). Mental disorders and suicide prevention. *Psychiatry and Clinical Neuroscience,* **49**, 111–116.

Mehlum L (2000). The chain of care after attempted suicide—an essential feature of the Norwegian national strategy for suicide prevention. *Nordic Journal of Psychiatry,* **54**, 26–27.

Mann JJ, Apter A, Bertolote J *et al.* (2005). Suicide prevention strategies: a systematic review. *Journal of the American Medical Association,* **294**, 2064–2074.

Martinez C, Rietbrock S, Wise L *et al.* (2005). Antidepressant treatment and the risk of fatal and non-fatal self harm in first episode depression: nested case-control study. *British Medical Journal,* **330**, 389.

Mieczkowski TA, Sweeney JA, Haas GL *et al.* (1993). Factor composition of the Suicide Intent Scale. *Suicide and Life-Threatening Behaviour,* **23**, 37–45.

Mork E, Ekeid G, Ystgaard M *et al.* (2001). Psychosocial follow-up after parasuicide in Norwegian general hospitals. *Tidsskrift for den Norske Laegeforening,* **121**, 1038–1043.

Ness DEM and Pfeffer CRM (1990). Sequelae of bereavement resulting from suicide. *American Journal of Psychiatry,* **147**, 279–285.

Norwegian Board of Health (1994). *The Norwegian National Plan for Suicide Prevention.* Norwegian Board of Health, Oslo.

Paris J (2002). Chronic suicidality among patients with borderline personality disorder. *Psychiatric Services,* **53**, 732–742.

Pirkis J and Burgess P (1998). Suicide and recency of health care contacts. A systematic review. *British Journal of Psychiatry,* **173**, 462–474.

Qin P, Agerbo E, Mortensen PB (2003). Suicide risk in relation to socioeconomic, demographic, psychiatric, and familial factors: a national register-based study of all suicides in Denmark, 1981–1997. *American Journal of Psychiatry,* **160**, 765–772.

Rotheram-Borus MJ, Piacentini J, Van RR *et al.* (1996). Enhancing treatment adherence with a specialized emergency room program for adolescent suicide attempters. *Journal of the American Academy of Child and Adolescent Psychiatry,* **35**, 654–663.

Spirito A, Boergers J, Donaldson D *et al.* (2002). An intervention trial to improve adherence to community treatment by adolescents after a suicide attempt. *Journal of the American Academy of Child and Adolescent Psychiatry,* **41**, 435–442.

Taiminen TJ and Helenius H (1994). Suicide clustering in a psychiatric hospital with a history of a suicide epidemic: a quantitative study. *American Journal of Psychiatry,* **151**, 1087–1088.

Wasserman D (2001). The work environment for health care staff. In D Wasserman, ed., *Suicide—An Unnecessary Death,* pp. 237–242. Martin Dunitz Ltd, London.

Wolfersdorf M, Vogel R, Kornacher J *et al.* (2001). The aftermath of suicide of a psychiatric inpatient—experiences in psychiatric hospitals with relatives as suicide survivors. *Psychiatrische Praxis,* **28**, 341–344.

# CHAPTER 64

# A specialized inpatient unit for suicidal patients

## Advantages and disadvantages

Lil Träskman-Bendz and Charlotta Sunnqvist

## Abstract

In 1986, the Suicide Research Unit (SRU) in Lund, Sweden was established. The unit included a psychiatric inpatient facility specializing in suicidal behaviour until it closed down in 2001. Structured management based on research, scientific evidence and confidence-building measures was offered. The SRU also had a consultation liaison with somatic clinics, an outpatient facility, as well as a unit for the aftermaths of suicide. At SRU, a structured psychiatric diagnostics as well as an organized nursing concept with different levels of supervision and treatment planning were in use. Care included contacts with families and significant others. SRU also collaborated with child and adolescent psychiatry staff. In order to prevent further suicidal acts, a confidence-inspiring relationship with the patients was created at SRU. Strong empathy for suicidal patients, non-judgemental attitudes as well as acceptance of the various feelings of the patients were cornerstones of the care. Warning signs of suicidal behaviour were discovered and discerned.

## Introduction

A structured management is essential when taking care of patients after a suicide attempt. In order to prevent further suicidal acts, one important strategy is to create and maintain a confidence-inspiring relationship with the patient. During 1986–2001, the clinical organization of the Suicide Research Unit (SRU) in Lund, Sweden, included a consultation liaison with somatic clinics, an inpatient and outpatient facility, as well as a unit for the aftermaths of suicide. Continuous contact was kept with the department of forensic medicine. Research and development were integral to all the services offered. Professional structure, confidence-building measures and knowledge were the cornerstones of the organiztion. This structure had several advantages. In the year 2001, the SRU was closed, primarily due to economic cutbacks. The ward became a conventional general psychiatric facility. The university-affiliated part of the SRU is still active as is the philosophy concerning the care of suicidal patients.

## The specialized psychiatric ward

### A consultation liaison

A psychiatrist specializing in suicidology, and in many instances a social worker, were in charge of the consultation liaison with somatic clinics. Most psychiatric assessments of suicide attempters were performed in the medical intensive care unit as soon as the patient was able to communicate after a suicide attempt—usually within 12 hours. A structured assessment after a suicide attempt formed the basis for further investigations, assessments and care of the patient (Niméus et al. 2000; Holmstrand et al. 2006; Niméus et al. 2006). Apart from the diagnostic procedure and ratings, the assessment was based on a checklist of items, including information on previous suicidality, psychiatric and somatic diseases, substance use and social status. Suicide risk was estimated with help of the SAD PERSONS scale ([male] sex, [high] age, depression, previous suicide attempt, ethanol abuse, [ir]rational thinking, social support lacking, organized plan [to commit suicide], no spouse, [somatic] sickness) (Patterson et al. 1983) and suicidal intent with the Beck Suicide Intent Scale (SIS) (Beck et al. 1974a). The *Diagnostic and statistical manual of mental disorders* (American Psychiatric Association 1987) axis I for psychiatric diagnostics was used. In most cases, significant others were contacted and interviewed. After this evaluation, about 50 per cent of all suicide attempters were referred to an inpatient unit, which specialized in suicide attempters (Niméus et al. 2000). Acute suicidality combined with severe psychiatric morbidity, and/or a weak social network was often behind the decision for referral. A member of the nursing staff usually brought the patient to the ward. Admissions could sometimes be compulsory.

### The inpatient investigation

The psychiatric inpatient investigation of the suicidal patient and their family started immediately after arrival on the ward. A life history, including the family history of somatic and psychiatric conditions and suicidality, was collected. Comprehensive DSM III diagnostics were often performed by more than one psychiatrist.

The psychosocial situation was evaluated by a psychologist (Fribergh *et al.* 1992) and a social worker. The latter investigated the patient's social network (Magne-Ingvar *et al.* 1992). In the evaluation process, different kinds of rating scales were also used, such as the Suicide Assessment Scale (SUAS) (Stanley *et al.* 1986; Niméus *et al.* 2000, 2006), the Scale for Suicide Ideation (SSI) (Beck *et al.* 1988), the Hopelessness Scale (HS) (Beck *et al.* 1974b), the Comprehensive Psychopathological Rating Scale (CPRS), from which the Montgomery–Åsberg Depression Rating Scale (MADRS) was extracted (Montgomery and Asberg 1979). Temperament was also assessed by use of various questionnaires (Engstrom *et al.* 1996). From a biological point of view, the patient could be assessed concerning the regulation of stress-hormones and peptides, e.g. by use of the Dexamethasone suppression test (DST) (Westrin *et al.* 1997). Lumbar cerebrospinal fluid (CSF) offered information on, for example, monoamine metabolites (Träskman-Bendz *et al.* 1981).

## A structured nursing concept

### Levels of supervision

The patient always received an intensive and continuous nursing supervision at the medical intensive care unit, and this continued until the point of evaluation by a psychiatrist belonging to the SRU. On arrival in the ward, the staff always searched for and secured the patient's belongings for their own safety (Neilson and Brennan 2001). Professional supervision is a complex nursing procedure, involving both life-preserving actions and a good opportunity for building a nursing alliance (Duffy 1995; Cleary *et al.* 1999; Neilson *et al.* 2001; Sullivan *et al.* 2005; Vråle and Steen 2005). The main aim of surveillance is to reduce suicidal behaviour, to increase trust, to create hope, and to find alternative non-suicidal behaviour. Therefore, a vigilant inpatient nursing staff and good communication between the staff members were important requirements of nursing at the ward.

At the ward, the doctor usually prescribed the level of surveillance. In an emergency situation, however, a nurse could do so. A written record was always made in the patient's chart, and the patient was always verbally informed about the concerns, safety and rules of the ward. If a high level of surveillance (i.e. constraint) was prescribed, the patient was restricted to the ward environment, and thus not allowed to leave the ward as a safety precaution. After a new assessment of suicidality and an oral agreement with the patient, the surveillance was always terminated by a psychiatrist.

### Tightly scheduled observation

The nursing staff created this observation method in order to solve the problem of long-term continuous observation of patients showing signs of repeated self-injuries. This type of observation included a daily and well-structured schedule from 7 a.m. until 9.30 p.m. together with other patients and nursing staff (Table 64.1). The goal was to reduce anxiety and to divert thoughts of self-injury. Each day, the staff and the patient discussed the patient's behaviour, in order to help the patient find new skills to prevent self-harm. This special observation was prescribed by the psychiatrist and lasted for at least one week, or until the patient was able to make a 'no self-harm agreement' with the staff. Since the introduction of this concept of fighting self-harm, the number of days on continuous observation decreased by roughly 50 per cent as compared to the year before (Sunnqvist *et al.* 1996).

**Table 64.1** The unit's three different kinds of surveillance

| Continuous observation | Monitoring the patient all the time, and being sufficiently close to prevent them from self-harm and/or suicide (Duffy 1995). |
| --- | --- |
| 15 min. observation | The staff observes the patient's behaviour and mood (only observed during night) by talking to them every 15 min. |
| An alternative observation, following a strict schedule | An emergency period of time, where the patient follows a tight schedule at the ward in order to prevent repeated self-injuries. |

No suicides occurred inside the SRU. The unit rules concerning special observation were written very clearly and were agreed upon and understood by the staff. The rules were not flexible. This might be in contrast with policies of other units as described by Duffy (1995) and Vråle and Steen (2005). Our understanding is that the work by all staff members of the ward aimed at promoting the patients' responsibility for their own situation. The staff aimed at supporting and helping the patient *before* a self-injury, instead of afterwards, and wanted the patient to contact the staff when they felt suicidal or had suicidal thoughts. In the preventive work, the nursing staff used its knowledge about the suicidal process and was vigilant to signs, symptoms and feelings shown by the patients. The staff confronted and helped the patients each time they mentioned anything about suicide thoughts. If the staff intuitively felt that something was wrong, or if they didn't get eye contact with the patient, they again confronted the patient concerning their thoughts and feelings. The atmosphere at the ward was warm, gentle and supportive. Evaluations showed that the patients found it meaningful to make an agreement concerning their suicidality (Sunnqvist *et al.* 1996).

### Therapeutic alliance

It is a true challenge to help a person who does not want to live any more. The patient was always offered two contact persons, usually one nurse and one assistant nurse. The nursing staff used a humanistic view and a holistic existential psychiatric nursing model described by Hummelvoll and Bunch (1994). The humanistic view of a person means that the person is seen as a unique individual, i.e. an autonomous, rational, social and spiritual being with responsibilities for their choices and actions. The staff tried to understand, support, inform, guide and create a good, warm and kind atmosphere for all patients. The patients' coping strategies were assessed in different situations. In order to establish a good nursing relationship, the nursing staff used specialized care planning (Persson and Stenquist 1990; Sunnqvist 1990; Träskman-Bendz *et al.* 1991), which included elements like trusting, listening and focusing on the patient (Cleary *et al.* 1999; Langley and Klopper 2005).

### Care plan

Based on the care plan, the contact person(s) had at least two 45-minute conversations a week with the patients. Psychiatric nursing is a planned activity, and the work has a clear purpose, which in the case of nursing suicide-prone patients is to give hope for the future. The care plan supported and helped the nursing staff and the patient to get a structure, and also to make a tailor-made nursing plan for each patient (Samuelsson *et al.* 2000). It also offered opportunities to talk about the suicide attempt, formulate the patients' problems, and to work for a better situation by use of goals and preventive measures (McLaughlin 1999). The care plan dealt with the patient's qualities, strengths and patterns of coping.

### Nursing attitudes towards melancholia and borderline patients

In our view, we dealt with two extremes of patients, according to their psychiatric diagnoses: patients with major depressive disorder, melancholia, and those with a cluster B personality disorder. Patients with melancholia needed rest and no nursing demands until their antidepressive treatment showed effect. Then we tried to stimulate them to again become interested in their environment, e.g. family, work, and their own health. Patients with a personality disorder needed structured nursing from the very beginning. Usually, we made an every day schedule, including chores at the ward, but also outside. The aim was, in this case, to keep busy in order to reduce anxiety and self-destructive thoughts.

### Psychological tutorial and education

Twice a week, the nursing staff had a psychological tutorial, aimed at penetrating their own feelings and attitudes towards the suicidal patients. This proved extremely important for the nursing relationship (Hawton *et al.* 1981; Wolk-Wasserman 1987; Samuelsson *et al.* 1997, 2000). Negative or hopeless emotions among the nursing staff can be dangerous for a suicidal person (Rayner *et al.* 2004). If a contact person felt helpless in respect to a patient, the rules were to receive an immediate tutorial because of psychological transference reactions. The tutorial session also helped the nursing staff to perceive and follow the care plan and offered support concerning different cognitive techniques. The nursing staff was also educated in basic conversational and cognitive therapy, as well as continuous training education for suicide prevention (Samuelsson and Åsberg 2002; Ramberg and Wasserman 2004).

## The structure of the ward

The team work, composed of professionals from various backgrounds, served as the base of the ward. Everybody aimed at the same goal—the patient's recovery (Bauer and Hill 2000). Different opportunities and means of collaboration were employed, e.g daily reports from nurses to the psychiatrist about the patients' state of health. Twice a week, the psychiatrist held rounds in order to discuss the patients' treatment and/or further medical investigations. Sometimes we also took the opportunity to discuss an individual patient at a grand round. The aim was then to structure and discuss the treatment of the patient, usually together with invited after care personnel. During these different stages of collaboration, the contact person represented the views of the patient. The multilayered structure resulted in effective care and a breeding ground for a protective environment for suicidal patients (Sun *et al.* 2006).

### After care

The time after discharge from an inpatient unit is a critical point for a suicidal person (Jacobs 1999; Sullivan *et al.* 2005). Therefore, the staff got in touch with the outpatient unit well before the discharge of a patient. If the patient did not have any prior outpatient contact, such contact was established. Nursing and treatment discharge notes were written and sent to the after care facility as a summary of the inpatient process. Usually the patient got a copy of the nursing epicrisis, which contained information such as:

- Signals to be aware of;
- What to do when suicidal thoughts appear and are overwhelming;
- Ways to cope with suicidal thoughts;
- Who to call for help.

The staff of the ward also offered 24-hour telephone guidance if the patient needed help in a stressful situation, such as in times of suicidal thoughts, anxiety, crisis etc.

### Collaboration with family and/or significant others

The staff members of our specialized unit started collaboration with the patients' family and/or significant others in the psychiatric consultation situation (see above). A social worker or another staff member phoned or met a significant other after acceptance and choice of the patient. The information gathered from a significant other encompassed questions about their view of the patient's situation, the reasons for the suicide attempt, their perception concerning verbal and non-verbal suicidal communication, etc. The social worker also asked about the significant others' own mental and physical health, and if they needed any help (Magne-Ingvar *et al.* 1999a). Magne-Ingvar *et al.* (1999b) found that significant others can provide valuable additional information for the global assessment of the patient, and that they also need guidance and support themselves. The family and/or significant others were informed about the patient's treatment, provided that the patient gave permission.

### Collaboration between the ward and child and adolescent psychiatry

Many of our patients had children, and it was not unusual that children found a parent unconscious after a suicide attempt or lifeless after a suicide. The children might have heard verbal, direct and/or indirect suicidal threats. They had also lived together with a depressed and psychiatrically ill parent for a period of time. Therefore, we collaborated with the department of child and adolescent psychiatry. We could offer all patients with children below the age of 18 years family sessions, together with a child psychiatrist and a social worker of the ward. One aim was to identify risk factors concerning the children's mental health and to offer crisis intervention for the whole family. Many of the children showed one or more anxious and depressive symptoms, which often improved (Fridell-Johnsson *et al.* 1994).

When a suicide occurred during hospitalization (for example, when on leave), the ward psychiatrist and the head of the clinic were immediately contacted, so that an appraisal of the situation could be organized. The door of the ward was locked immediately, and the staff offered emotional debriefing. The patients were informed by the ward psychiatrist about the suicide as soon as possible. Immediately after this, all patients had a one on one debriefing with the staff, and their reactions were noted. After a few months, upon receiving police and forensic medical reports, the staff had a formal meeting. Then the signs and symptoms preceding the patient's death were analysed. The aim of this meeting was to learn from experience in order to prevent future suicides (Beskow 1979).

The retrospective meeting included the following points:

♦ The circumstances of the suicide (5 min);

♦ Life history of the patient (10 min);

♦ Problems, resources, relations (10 min);

♦ Nursing staff observations (10 min);

♦ The suicidal process: origin and development (10 min);

♦ Summary and implications (15 min).

### Support to significant others after a suicide

Significant others usually have more guilt reactions after a suicide than after a regular death. They generally try to find some explanation as to why their relative committed suicide, and they often don't get any support in their grief. The Suicide Research Centre in Lund started a unit to help and support significant others in their grief. Two social workers (psychotherapists) and a medical doctor offered significant others support and crisis intervention (Traskman-Bendz *et al.* 1999).

## Advantages and disadvantages with units for suicide attempters

In our opinion, SRU offered several advantages. We had the opportunity to develop a structured management of suicidal patients, based on confidence-building measures, knowledge and research. For example, we organized the nursing so that we were able to spend time communicating with the patients. We learned how to become non-judgemental and to accept the feelings of the patients, and also to feel empathy for their situation. These are important attitudes towards suicidal patients (McLaughlin 1999; Talseth *et al.* 1999; Sun *et al.* 2004). Our way of nursing also offered the possibility of discerning warning signs of suicidal behaviour (Clearly *et al.* 1999). The structured management and its cornerstones made the patient and their families believe in the future. Alongside gradually increasing knowledge and experience with suicidal persons as well as the development of new strategies, an alternative scheduled observation could be developed.

The disadvantages were few, but often marked. Preventing suicide and withstanding the patients' physical and emotional state were onerous duties. Suicidal thoughts, behaviour, and self-harm were often transmitted from one patient to another (Taiminen *et al.* 1998). Negative feelings were aroused both in the staff and in the patient group. The team continuously had to work hard to create a protective environment, and this could sometimes be experienced as very stressful for the staff. However, the grateful attitudes from the patients, when finally recovered, outweighed many disadvantages.

## Conclusion

Among other strategies to prevent further suicidal acts, one is to create and keep a confidence-inspiring relationship with the patient. SRU, which was based on research and gained knowledge, taught us to become non-judgemental, to accept feelings of the suicidal patients, to feel empathy for their situation, and to discern warning signs of suicidal behaviour. Structured management is essential when taking care of patients after a suicide attempt, and the ward's cornerstones made the patient and their family believe in the future.

### References

Bauer BB and Hill SS (2000). *Mental Health Nursing: An Introductory Text*. WB Saunders Company, Philadelphia.

Beck AT, Herman I, Schuyler D (1974a). Development of suicidal intent scales. In AT Beck, HPL Resnik and D Lettieri, eds, *The Prediction of Suicide*, pp. 45–56. Charles Press, Bowie.

Beck AT, Steer RA, Ranieri WF (1988). Scale for Suicide Ideation: psychometric properties of a self-report version. *Journal of Clinical Psychology*, **44**, 499–505.

Beck AT, Weissman A, Lester D *et al.* (1974b). The measurement of pessimism: The Hopelessness Scale. *J Consult Clin Psychol*, **42**, 861–865.

Beskow J (1979). Suicide and mental disorder in Swedish men. *Acta Psychiatrica Scandinavica*, **277**, 1–137.

Cleary M, Jordan R, Horsfall J *et al.* (1999). Suicidal patients and special observation. *Journal of Psychiatric and Mental Health Nursing*, **6**, 461–467.

American Psychiatric Association (1987). *Diagnostic and Statistic Manual of Mental Disorders III*. American Psychiatric Association, Washington.

Duffy D (1995). Out of the shadows: a study of the special observation of suicidal psychiatric in-patients. *Journal of Advanced Nursing*, **21**, 944–950.

Engstrom G, Nyman GE, Träskman-Bendz L (1996). The Marke-Nyman Temperament (MNT) Scale in suicide attempters. *Acta Psychiatria Scandinavica*, **94**, 320–325.

Fribergh H, Traskman-Bendz L, Ojehagen A, Regnell G (1992). The Meta-Contrast Technique—a projective test predicting suicide. *Acta Psychiatrica Scandinavica*, **86**, 473–477.

Fridell-Johnsson E, Eidevall-Wallin L, Miklos-Ljungberg J *et al.* (1994). Samarbete vuxenpsykiatri och barnpsykiatri efter ett självmordsförsök [Collaboration between general psychiatry and child–adolescence psychiatry services after a suicide attempt]. *Socialmedicinsk tidskrift*, **2–3**, 137–140.

Hawton K, Marsack P, Fagg J (1981). The attitudes of psychiatrists to deliberate self-poisoning: comparison with physicians and nurses. *British Journal of Medical Psychology*, **54**, 341–348.

Holmstrand C, Nimeus A, Traskman-Bendz L (2006). Risk factors of future suicide in suicide attempters—a comparison between suicides and matched survivors. *Nordic Journal of Psychiatry*, **60**, 162–167.

Hummelvoll JK and Bunch EH (1994). A holistic–existential model for psychiatric nursing. *Perspectives on Psychiatric Care*, **30**, 7–14.

Jacobs D (1999). *The Harvard Medical School Guide to Suicide Assessments and Interventions*. Josey Bass Inc, San Francisco.

Langley GC and Klopper H (2005). Trust as a foundation for the therapeutic intervention for patients with borderline personality disorder. *Journal of Psychiatric and Mental Health Nursing*, **12**, 23–32.

Magne-Ingvar U and Ojehagen A (1999a). Significant others of suicide attempters: their views at the time of the acute psychiatric consultation. *Social Psychiatry and Psychiatric Epidemiology*, **34**, 73–79.

Magne-Ingvar U and Ojehagen A (1999b). One-year follow-up of significant others of suicide attempters. *Social Psychiatry and Psychiatric Epidemiology*, **34**, 470–476.

Magne-Ingvar U, Ojehagen A, Traskman-Bendz L (1992). The social network of people who attempt suicide. *Acta Psychiaticaria Scandinavica*, **86**, 153–158.

McLaughlin C (1999). An exploration of psychiatric nurses´and patients´opinions regarding in-patient care for suicidal patients. *Journal of Advanced Nursing*, **29**, 1042–1051.

Neilson P and Brennan W (2001). The use of special observations: an audit within a psychiatric unit. *Journal of Psychiatric and Mental Health Nursing*, **8**, 147–155.

Niméus A, Hjalmarsson-Stahlfors F, Sunnqvist C *et al.* (2006). Evaluation of a modified interview version and of a self-rating version of the Suicide Assessment Scale. *European Psychiatry*, **21**, 471–477.

Niméus A, Alsen M, Traskman-Bendz L (2000). The suicide assessment scale: an instrument assessing suicide risk of suicide attempters. *European Psychiatry*, **15**, 416–423.

Montgomery SA and Asberg M (1979). A new depression scale designed to be sensitive to change. *British Journal of Psychiatry*, **134**, 382–389.

Patterson WM, Dohn HH, Bird J et al. (1983). Evaluation of suicidal patients: the SAD PERSONS scale. *Psychsomatics*, **24**, 343, 348–349.

Persson I and Stenqvist C (1990). *Utvärdering av Hummelvolls omvårdnadsplan ur ett patientperspektiv* (Evaluation of Hummelvolls caring plan from the patients point of view). Malmöhus Läns Landsting Vårdskola, Lund.

Ramberg IL and Wasserman D (2004). Benefits of implementing an academic training of trainers program to promote knowledge and clarity in work with psychiatric suicidal patients. *Archives of Suicide Research*, **8**, 331–343.

Rayner GC, Allen SL, Johnson M (2004). Countertransference and self-injury: a cognitive behavioural cycle. *Journal of Advanced Nursing*, **50**, 12–19.

Samuelsson M and Asberg M (2002). Training program in suicide prevention for psychiatric nursing personel enchance attitudes to attempted suicide patients. *International Journal of Nursing Studies*, **39**, 115–121.

Samuelsson M, Asberg M, Gustavsson JP (1997). Attitudes of psychiatric nursing personel towards patients who have attempted suicide. *Acta Psychiatrica Scandinavica*, **95**, 222–230.

Samuelsson M, Wiklander M, Asberg M et al. (2000). Psychiatric care as seen by the attempted suicide patient. *Journal of Advanced Nursing*, **32**, 635–643.

Stanley B, Träskman-Bendz L, Stanley M (1986). The Suicide Assessment Scale: a scale evaluating change in suicidal behaviour. *Psychopharmacological Bulletin*, 1, 200–205.

Sullivan AM, Barron CT, Bezmen J et al. (2005). The safe treatment of the suicidal patient in an adult inpatient setting: a proactive preventive approach. *Psychiatric Quarterly*, **76**, 67–83.

Sun F-K, Long A, Boore J et al. (2004). A theory for the nursing care of patients at risk of suicide. *Journal of Advanced Nursing*, **53**, 680–690.

Sun F-K, Long A, Boore J et al. (2006). Patients and nurses´ perceptions of ward environmental factors and support system in the care of suicidal patients. *Journal of Clinical Nursing* **15**, 83–92.

Sunnqvist C (1990). *Utvärdering av Hummelvolls omvårdnadsplan* (Evaluation of Hummelvolls caring plan). Vårdhögskolan (The Nursing School), Lund.

Sunnqvist C, Cedereke M, Adelmyr L et al. (1996). Quality assurance of nursing of suicidal patients. Lecture at the Sixth European Symposium on Suicide and Suicidal Behaviour in Lund, Sweden.

Taiminen TJ, Kallio-Soukainen K, Nokoso-Koivisto H et al. (1998). Contagion of deliberte self-harm among adolescent inpatients. *Journal of American Academy of Child and Adolescence Psychiatry*, **37**, 211–217.

Talseth A-G, Jacobsson L, Norberg A (1999). The meaning of suicidal psychiatric inpatients'experiences of being treated by pshysicians. *Journal of Advanced Nursing*, **34**, 96–106.

Träskman-Bendz L, Åsberg M, Bertilsson L (1981). Serotonin and noradrenaline uptake inhibitors in the treatment of depression-relationship to 5-HIAA in spinal fluid. *Acta Psychiatrica Scandinavia*, **290**, 209–218.

Träskman-Bendz L, Fribergh H, Magne-Ingvar U et al. (1991). Suicidforskningsenheten i Lund [The Lund suicide unit]. *Socialmedicinsk Tidskrift*, **1**, 10–12.

Träskman-Bendz L, Söderling H, Bohm K et al. (1999). Stödverksamhet till närstående vid självmord [Support services for significant others after a suicide]. *Socialmedicinsk Tidskrift*, **2**, 118–164.

Westrin Å, Engström G, Ekman R et al. (1997). Correlations between plasma-neuropeptides and temperament dimensions differ between suicidal patients and healthy controls. *Journal of Affective Disorders*, **49**, 45–54.

Wolk-Wasserman D (1987). Some problems connected with the treatment of suicide attempt patients: transference and countertransference aspects. *Crisis*, **1**, 69–82.

Vråle GB and Steen E (2005). The dynamics between structure and flexibility in constant observation of psychiatric inpatients with suicidal ideation. *Journal of Psychiatric and Mental Health Nursing*, **12**, 513–518.

# CHAPTER 65

# Physician-assisted suicide and euthanasia

## A medical and psychological perspective

Herbert Hendin

## Abstract

Until relatively recently it did not seem possible to relieve much of the suffering associated with serious or terminal illness. Depression associated with physical illness was assumed to be its natural and inevitable consequence. This mixture of assumptions and facts provided the impetus for the Dutch to begin to sanction assisted suicide and euthanasia more than a decade before the advances in palliative care of the last fifteen years.

This chapter examines the practice of assisted suicide and euthanasia in the Netherlands from a medical and psychological perspective: the Netherlands is the only country to have had extensive experience in giving legal sanction to both practices. From the same perspective, the chapter examines assisted suicide in the state of Oregon, which has had a decade of experience with legalized assisted suicide, and is the only state in the United States to have legalized the practice. The experience of Belgium and Switzerland, the two other countries that have given legal sanction to assisted suicide (Switzerland) or euthanasia (Belgium) is discussed briefly. Both countries appear to have been stimulated, at least in part, by the experience of the Netherlands and Oregon.

## Assisted suicide and euthanasia in the Netherlands

Legal sanction for assisted suicide and euthanasia began as a result of a series of cases involving the trials of doctors for performing euthanasia, which was a violation of the penal code in the Netherlands. A 1983 case eventually went to the Dutch Supreme Court. The Court's opinion supported an exception to the penal code when a doctor faces an irresolvable conflict between the law and his responsibility to help a patient whose irremediable suffering makes euthanasia necessary (Gomez 1991).

Over the next two decades the Netherlands moved from considering assisted suicide (preferred over euthanasia by the Dutch Voluntary Euthanasia Society) to giving legal sanction to both physician-assisted suicide and euthanasia, from euthanasia for terminally ill patients to euthanasia for those who are chronically ill, from euthanasia for physical illness to euthanasia for psychological distress, and from voluntary euthanasia to non-voluntary and involuntary euthanasia (Hendin *et al.* 1997). 'Non-voluntary' is the term used to describe euthanasia with patients not capable of requesting it; 'involuntary' is used to describe euthanasia with patients who did not request it but were capable of doing so.

According to the General Board of the Royal Dutch Medical Association (KNMG) (1994), it did not seem reasonable medically, legally, or morally to sanction only assisted suicide, thereby denying more active medical help in the form of euthanasia to those who could not effect their own deaths. Nor could the Dutch deny assisted suicide or euthanasia to the chronically ill who have longer to suffer than the terminally ill, or to those who have psychological pain not associated with physical disease. To do so would be a form of discrimination. Involuntary euthanasia is not legally sanctioned by the Dutch, but is excused as necessary to end suffering in patients who, for a variety of reasons, are not able or willing to choose to hasten death. Except for the legal sanction of euthanasia for mental suffering without physical illness, all the other expansions of the indications for euthanasia had taken place by 1990.

The Dutch courts had accepted the following guidelines formulated by the KNMG for the regulation of assisted suicide and euthanasia:

- The patient must make a well-considered, persistent voluntary request;
- The patient must be experiencing intolerable suffering that cannot be relieved;
- There must be consultation with a second physician; and
- All cases of physician-assisted suicide and euthanasia must be reported.

## Violation of the guidelines

Charges of abuse contributed to the Dutch government sanctioning examinations of assisted suicide and euthanasia by physicians in the Department of Public Health and Social Medicine at the Erasmus University in Rotterdam from 1990 and 1995. To obtain the information they needed, the investigators utilized large surveys of physicians as well as interviews with a representative smaller sample of physicians (Van Der Maas *et al.* 1992, 1996). These studies of the practice of assisted suicide and euthanasia were supported by the KNMG with the promise from the government that physicians would not be prosecuted for anything they revealed. This assurance enabled the disclosure of the many violations of the guidelines that were subsequently revealed. For example, over 50 per cent of physicians had suggested or felt free to suggest euthanasia to patients, which may compromise the voluntary nature of the process. The majority of Dutch cases were not reported, which made evaluation of the regulations impossible.

The most alarming concern to arise from the Dutch studies has been the documentation of cases in which patients who have not given their consent have their lives ended by physicians. The studies revealed that in about 1000 cases in each of the years studied, physicians admitted they actively caused death without the explicit consent of the patient. About a quarter of physicians stated that they had 'terminated the lives of patients without an explicit request' from the patient to do so and a third more could conceive of doing so.

The use of the word 'explicit' is somewhat inaccurate, since in half of these cases there was no request of any kind, and in the others there were mainly references to patients' earlier statements of not wanting to suffer.

The studies documented that cases classified as 'termination of the patient without explicit request' were a fraction of the non-voluntary and involuntary euthanasia cases. International attention had also centred on the 1350 cases (1 per cent of all Dutch deaths) in 1990 and the 1896 cases in 1995 (1.4 per cent of all Dutch deaths) in which physicians gave pain medication with the explicit intention of ending the patient's life. As reported by the physicians in the 1995 study, in more than 80 per cent of these cases (1537 deaths), no request for death was made by the patient. The Dutch investigators minimized the significance of the number of deaths without consent by explaining that the patients were incompetent. However, in the 1995 study, 21 per cent of the individuals classified as 'patients whose lives were ended without explicit request' were competent: in the 1990 study, 37 per cent were competent (Van Der Maas *et al.* 1992, 1996).

Physicians usually gave as the reason for not discussing the decisions with patients that they had previously had some discussion of the subject with the patient. Yet it is hard to understand how a physician would terminate the life of a competent patient on the basis of a previous discussion without checking what the patient felt currently.

An illustration presented to me as to why it was often necessary for physicians to end the lives of competent patients without their consent was the case of a nun whose physician ended her life a few days before she would have died because she was in excruciating pain, but her religious convictions did not permit her to ask for death (Hendin *et al.* 1997). In another documented case a Dutch patient with disseminated breast cancer who had rejected the possibility of euthanasia had her life ended because in the physician's words: 'It could have taken another week before she died. I just needed this bed' (Twycross 1995).

Since the government-sanctioned Dutch studies are primarily numerical and categorical, they do not examine the interaction of physicians, patients, and families that determines the decision for euthanasia. Other studies conducted in the Netherlands have indicated how voluntariness is compromised, alternatives are not presented, and the criterion of unrelievable suffering is bypassed. A few examples help to illustrate how this occurs:

A wife, who no longer wished to care for her sick, elderly husband, gave him a choice between euthanasia and admission to a home for the chronically ill. The man, afraid of being left to the mercy of strangers in an unfamiliar place, chose to have his life ended; the doctor, although aware of the coercion, ended the man's life (Ten Have and Kisma 1985).

A healthy 50-year-old woman who lost her son recently to cancer, refused treatment for her depression and said she would accept only help in dying. She was referred by the Dutch Voluntary Euthanasia Society to a psychiatrist who had requested referral of such cases and who assisted in her suicide within four months of her son's death. He told me that he had seen her for a number of sessions when she told him that if he did not help her she would kill herself without him. At that point, he did. He seemed on the one hand to be succumbing to emotional blackmail and on the other to be ignoring the fact that even without treatment, experience has shown that time alone was likely to have affected her wish to die (Hendin 1997). This last case had particular importance since it helped establish that mental suffering could be the justification for assisted suicide or euthanasia.

A Dutch physician who was filmed ending the life of a patient recently diagnosed with amyotrophic lateral sclerosis said of the patient: 'I can give him the finest wheelchair there is, but in the end it is only a stopgap. He is going to die and he knows it.' That death may be years away but a physician with this attitude may not be able to present alternatives to this patient. The patient in this case was clearly ambivalent about proceeding and wanted to put off the date for his death. This ambivalence was ignored by the doctor, who was supporting the desire of the patient's wife to move forward quickly. The doctor never saw the patient alone, permitted the wife to answer all questions for the patient about whether he wanted to die, and presented an exaggerated picture of the death that awaited him without euthanasia (Hendin 1995).

In *Appointment with Death*, a documentary film by the Dutch Voluntary Euthanasia Society that was intended to promote euthanasia, a 41-one-year-old artist was diagnosed as HIV positive. He had no physical symptoms but had been terrified by watching others suffer with them and wanted his physician's help in dying. The doctor compassionately explained to him that he might live for some years symptom-free. Despite this, over time the patient repeated his request for euthanasia. Although the doctor thought his patient was acting unwisely and prematurely, he rationalized that respect for the patient's autonomy required that he grant the patient's request.

Consultation in the case was pro forma; a colleague of the doctor saw the patient briefly to confirm his wishes. Although the primary doctor established that the patient was persistent in his request and competent to make the decision, thus meeting those criteria, he did not address the terror that underlay the patient's request, nor did he refer the patient to someone who could. This patient had clearly been depressed and overwhelmed by the news of his situation. Had his physician been able to deal with the psychological distress of this patient rather than only determining whether the patient met formal criteria regarding a request to die, this man would probably not have been assisted in suicide (Hendin 1997).

The last two cases surely needed a psychiatric consultation, but one was never considered. This is despite the fact that we know that most suicides and most of those who respond to terminal illness with a desire to hasten death are suffering from depression (Hendin and Klerman 1993). Only 3 per cent of Dutch patients requesting assisted suicide or euthanasia, however, are referred for psychiatric consultation (Groenewoud *et al.* 1997).

The Dutch like to point out that they have reduced their suicide rate from 14.3/100,000 in 1980 to 9.7 per cent in 2002 (a drop of 32 per cent). The drop is mainly in the age groups above 50 that contain almost 80 per cent of the assisted suicide and euthanasia cases. Medical illness plays an important role in 50 per cent of suicides over the age of 50 and in 70 per cent of those over the age of 60 (Mackenzie and Popkin 1990). However, the suicide rates would show a significant increase if the 400 to 500 cases of assisted suicide that occur each year were counted in the statistics. This increase would be even more profound if the several thousand cases of euthanasia were also included. Among an older population physical illness of all types is common, and many who have trouble coping with physical illness become suicidal.

The likelihood that patients would end their own lives if assisted suicide and euthanasia were not available to them is one of the justifications given by Dutch doctors for providing such help. Assisted suicide and euthanasia, originally proposed as a last resort, appear to be substitutes for the treatment of patients with physical illness and mental illness who become depressed and suicidal. In the process there is evidence that palliative care was also one of the casualties, while hospice care lagged behind that of other countries (Dorrepaal *et al.* 1989; Zylicz 1991, 1993; Matthews 1998; De Witt *et al.* 1999). Dutch deficiencies in palliative care have been attributed by Dutch palliative care experts to the easier alternative of euthanasia (Zylicz 1991, 1993).

## Change in the Netherlands

In 1998 there was a significant change in Dutch policy toward end-of-life care and its relation to assisted suicide and euthanasia. The Dutch government established six regional palliative care centres which were to integrate palliative care services within the Dutch health care system working with university hospitals and comprehensive cancer centres. Small regional networks were constructed within which palliative care services such as nursing homes, home care services, GPs, and hospitals could work closely together with consultation provided by the centres (Gordijn and Janssens 2004). The government initiative was a stimulus to non-governmental activities. Although previously there had been only a handful of hospices in the country, many more were now established. One that was already established, the Rosenheuvel at Arnhem, had already been educating physicians in palliative care. The KNMG now also instituted training programmes for physicians.

Education in palliative care has had an effect on a significant number of Dutch physicians. Physicians who were practitioners of and consultants on euthanasia cases have expressed the opinion that instead of starting with legalizing euthanasia, the Dutch should first have developed palliative care. A number have publicly expressed regrets for having previously euthanized patients because had they known then what they knew now, the euthanasia would not have been necessary. They recognize that many requests for euthanasia are in fact requests for relief from distress. Some have realized that when they provide that relief, instead of suggesting the possibility of euthanasia, the requests of patients for euthanasia disappear (Oostveen 2001; Gordijn and Janssens 2004).

The effects of education in palliative care appear to be reflected in subsequent government-sponsored studies of assisted suicide and euthanasia; a third study done in 2001 and a fourth study done in 2006. The rates for euthanasia in the four studies were 1.7 per cent of all deaths in 1990, 2.4 per cent in 1995, 2.6 per cent in 2001, and 1.7 per cent in 2005 (Van Der Heide 2007). The 2005 study was the first to show a reduction in euthanasia. The change should not be surprising since there was other evidence of the difference making palliative care available can have. The experience of Rozenheuvel hospice is impressive: 25 per cent of 571 patients seen in the ten years after it was established in 1994 entered the hospice with a request for euthanasia if suffering became unbearable (Gordijn and Janssens 2004). The assurance that patients received that they would not have to suffer unbearably, and the empathic care they actually received in a home-like environment were such that only two patients persisted in their request; they were transferred and were given euthanasia performed outside the hospice (Janssens *et al.* 1999).

A professional consensus is emerging in the Netherlands, and in most Western countries, that deep sedation is justified, even at the risk of causing death, when the patient is suffering unbearably and hopelessly and where standard therapeutic modalities that do not reduce consciousness are no longer effective. Sedation in such cases and generally improved palliative care appear to be contributing to the decrease in euthanasia. The number of cases of physician-assisted suicide has also diminished significantly but they had been dropping even earlier and that has to do with patient as well as physician preference. The percentage of cases in which patients' lives are ended without their having requested it remains unchanged and the Dutch investigators recognize it as an ongoing problem.

Changes in the reporting system have helped reduce the number of unreported cases. Physicians had maintained that fear of prosecution was the major reason for their not reporting cases. In 1998 the law was changed so that reported cases are not reviewed directly by public prosecutors but go first to regional review committees consisting of a lawyer, an ethicist, and a physician. In 2002, the Dutch Euthanasia Act gave physicians the added protection of a statute in addition to case law. The review committees still examine all reported cases, but only those that do not meet the requirements of prudent practice are subsequently reviewed by the public prosecutors. The number of unreported cases dropped to 20 per cent in 2005. The unreported cases are primarily those where patients' lives were ended without a specific request; those cases are almost never reported. Some researchers see the review committees as having an educational role for physicians. They would have greater possibility of playing this role if the physician member were required to be someone with palliative care training.

Despite the continuation of involuntary euthanasia, and the fact that the Dutch continue to ignore the role that depression plays in the euthanasia request, euthanasia has been reduced and there is reason for optimism. In addition to the Dutch investigators and the Dutch government, a gradually increasing segment of physicians appear to be becoming aware of the possibilities of palliative care. Even among physicians who are not opposed to euthanasia an increasing number are reluctant to perform it themselves and there is an even greater reduction in the number who are willing to end the lives of patients who have not requested it. As a result, a diminishing number of physicians are now performing a disproportionate number of cases (Onwuteaka-Phillipsen *et al.* 2003). It is not likely the Dutch will abandon their euthanasia policy, but it now seems likely that the pressure to improve care for incurably or terminally ill patients will grow from both opponents and supporters of euthanasia.

There is one caveat to this optimism. The KNMG has issued a report recommending that 'suffering from living' be included as a justification for euthanasia (Sheldon 2005). At present, doctors must follow a 2002 ruling by the Dutch Supreme Court that only a classifiable physical or mental condition constitutes the 'hopeless and unbearable suffering' that can justify a case of legal euthanasia. The leader of the KNMG report criticised the Court, maintaining that in half of the requests there was no classifiable disease. Since Dutch doctors make virtually no referrals to psychiatrists of patients requesting euthanasia, the KNMG is in no position to make such a claim.

Although the Dutch government does not seem inclined to act on this recommendation, a group of Dutch doctors and researchers are attempting to circumvent the law. They have written a book, available only through their website, describing how patients who wish to end their lives, but who do not meet the requirement of unbearable suffering, can do so by stopping eating and drinking and taking drugs to induce coma (Sheldon, 2008). The KNMG recommends the book, and the KNMG's ethics policy adviser states that doctors have a moral obligation to become involved in such cases. They do not specifically suggest that doctors prescribe the medication to induce coma, which is forbidden by law in these cases. The book's authors state that the book is not intended for young people who, if they feel suicidal, should seek professional help. Are older people who become depressed and suicidal not worth treating, even when we know that most of them respond well to treatment? As long as the Dutch government and courts do not embrace this fringe view, the work of this group should not be able to reverse the progress that is being made.

## Assisted suicide in Oregon

In 1997, five months after the US Supreme Court ruled that there was no right to assisted suicide in the Constitution but implied that states have the right to decide for themselves whether to permit or prohibit physician-assisted suicide, the Oregon Death with Dignity Act took effect. The law was passed by referendum with the assurance to Oregon voters that it had safeguards that ensure the care and protect the welfare of terminally ill patients. It was thought that Oregon would serve as a 'laboratory of the states', showing us how physician-assisted suicide (PAS) would work. None of this has occurred in part because the law was not written with that in mind and in large part because the Oregon Public Health Division (OPHD), charged with monitoring the law, has interpreted its mandate in an extremely restrictive manner.

OPHD limits its yearly reports to general epidemiological data and collects limited information from physicians who have prescribed lethal medication. Physicians who declined to prescribe the lethal medication, as well as nurses and social workers who cared for the patients, pharmacists who filled the prescriptions, and family members, are not interviewed. Not all the information collected is made public, and after a year all source documentation is destroyed.

The Oregon law seemed to require reasonable safeguards regarding the care of patients near the end of life, which include presenting patients with the option for palliative care; ensuring that patients are competent to make end-of-life decisions for themselves; limiting the procedure to patients who are terminally ill; ensuring the voluntariness of the request; obtaining a second opinion on the case; requiring the request to be persistent, i.e. made a second time after a two-week interval; encouraging the involvement of the next of kin; and requiring physicians to inform OPHD of all cases in which they have written a prescription for the purpose of assisted suicide.

Since the passage of Oregon's Death with Dignity Act, however, various sources—patients, families, health care professionals, physicians, nurses, social workers, chaplains, and advocacy groups—have supplied more detailed information that suggests that the implementation of the law has had unintended, harmful consequences for patients. Case studies and information provided by doctors, families, and other caregivers have documented that safeguards for the care and protection of terminally ill patients written into the Oregon law are being circumvented.

Addressing and correcting the situation would require more information than OPHD has been willing to obtain. Instead, based on the inadequate information it collects, OPHD has been issuing annual reports declaring that terminally ill Oregon patients are receiving adequate care. In its behaviour and actions, OPHD acts as the defender of the law rather than as protector of the welfare of terminally ill patients.

Although legalizing only assisted suicide and not euthanasia, Oregon's law differs from the Dutch in another major respect. Intolerable suffering that cannot be relieved is not a basic requirement for authorizing assisted suicide in Oregon as it has been in the Netherlands. A diagnosis of terminal illness with a prognosis of less than six months to live is considered a sufficient criterion. The presumption and stipulation in the Oregon law that a diagnosis of terminal illness is sufficient does not encourage physicians to inquire into the source of the medical, psychological, social, and existential concerns that usually underlie such a request, an inquiry that leads patients and physicians to have the kind of discussion that often leads to relief for patients and makes assisted suicide seem unnecessary. Nor are physicians asked or required by the Oregon law to make such an inquiry.

This shifts the focus from relieving the suffering of dying patients desperate enough to consider hastening death to meeting statutory requirements for assisted suicide. To satisfy statutory requirements physicians often go through the motions of offering palliative care, providing serious psychiatric consultation, or making an effort to protect those who are vulnerable.

## Palliative care in Oregon

When a terminally ill Oregon patient makes a request for assisted suicide, physicians must indicate that palliative care and hospice care are feasible alternatives. They are not required, however, to be knowledgeable about how to relieve either physical or emotional suffering in terminally ill patients. Without such knowledge the physician cannot present feasible alternatives. Most physicians lack such training. Even if they do, they are not required to refer patients requesting assisted suicide for consultation with a physician knowledgeable about palliative care. In only 13 per cent of the first 142 requests for assisted suicide after the Oregon law went into effect was a palliative care consultation recommended (Ganzini et al. 2003). We do not know how many of these recommendations were actually implemented.

The first case known to the public under the new law exemplified how pro forma was the presentation of the palliative care alternative. The patient, a woman in her mid-80s, was described as having metastatic breast cancer and was in a hospice programme. The patient's own doctor was not willing to assist in her suicide for reasons that were not specified. A second physician also refused on the grounds that she was depressed. Much of the information about the case came from an audiotape made by the physician who assisted in the suicide and played for the media the day after the patient's death by Compassion in Dying, the advocacy organization for assisted suicide that had referred the case to him. The physician subsequently published details about the case in a medical journal (Reagan 1999).

There is no indication that the physician was trying to find any feasible alternative to suicide. In the taped interview he follows the law's requirement, listing in three sentences other choices she could make:

> Doctor: There is, of course all sorts of hospice support that is available to you. There is, of course, chemotherapy that is available that may or may not have any effect, not in curing your cancer, but perhaps in lengthening your life to some extent. There is also available a hormone which you were offered by the oncologist—tamoxifen—which is not really chemotherapy, that would have some possibility of slowing or stopping the course of the disease for some period of time.
>
> Patient: Yes, I don't want to take that.
>
> Doctor: All right, that's pretty much what you need to understand (Hoover and Hill 1998).

During the taped remarks, the patient, referred to as Helen, expressed concern about being artificially fed, a concern that suggests greater vulnerability and uncertainty about her course of action than the physician perceives. He does not assure her that this need not happen in any case. He ignores the remark and instead asks a question designed to elicit a response about her desire to die (Foley and Hendin 1999).

The prescribing physician told a reporter from *The Oregonian* that he was struck by Helen's tenacity and determination. 'It was like talking to a locomotive. It was like talking to Superman when he's going after a train' (Hoover 1998). The fact that he describes her as like an unstoppable locomotive in her desire for death, even though she was not in great immediate distress, should in itself give him pause. Urgency that brooks no questioning in such a matter is often a sign of irrational motives.

The case raises disturbing questions. The physicians who evaluated the patient offered two contradictory sets of opinions about the appropriateness of her decision. The doctor performing the euthanasia made no effort to contact the two doctors who had a different opinion—one of whom knew her for some time and the other who considered that she was depressed.

OPHD's yearly progress reports contend that patients who requested assisted suicide were receiving adequate end-of-life care. Data from patient interviews, surveys of families of patients receiving end-of-life care in Oregon, surveys of physicians, and the data from the cases where information has been made available indicate otherwise. A study at the Oregon Health Sciences University indicated that there was a greater percentage of cases of inadequately treated pain in terminally ill patients since the Oregon law went into effect (Fromme 2004).

A report, *Means to a Better End*, of the Last Acts Program of the Robert Wood Johnson Foundation evaluated end-of-life care in all fifty states, and gave Oregon a mediocre grade. The Foundation and the Last Acts Program have no position on assisted suicide but have a strong commitment to improving end-of-life care.

The state received good marks for its use of advance directives, for not overusing intensive care units in ways that only prolong the dying process, and in training registered nurses in palliative care. Oregon did poorly on other measures utilized in the evaluations including: the large number of its nursing home residents in persistent pain, the small number of its hospitals providing hospice or palliative care, and the lack of state policies encouraging pain control and palliative care (Last Acts Organization 2002).

## Psychiatric evaluation not required by Oregon law

A psychiatric evaluation is the standard of care in all states outside of Oregon for patients who are preoccupied with suicide. Research establishing that most patients requesting assisted suicide are depressed, and that depression is the best predictor of the request for suicide, was done in the United States and Canada (Emanuel *et al.* 1996; Chochinov *et al.* 1998). Yet Oregon law does not require a psychiatric evaluation in assisted suicide cases even if the physician recognizes that the patient is depressed. Under the law, only if the physician believes the patient's depression is causing impaired judgement must the physician refer the patient to a licensed psychiatrist or psychologist.

The caveat about impaired judgement is strange since impaired cognitive function is one of the characteristics of depression; a rigid tendency to see only one possible solution (such as suicide) to their problems is also characteristic of individuals with the disorder (Hendin and Klerman 1993). In any case, studies have shown that physicians are not reliably able to diagnose depression, let alone to determine whether depression is impairing judgment (Murphy1975; Passik *et al.* 1998).

Not all of the factors justifying a psychiatric consultation centre on current depression. Many patients who request assisted suicide are doing so not because of current pain and distress but out of fear of what will happen to them—such as Helen's fear of artificial feeding. Such fears often derive from patients' past experiences with the death of those close to them (and this we later learned was true of Helen) so a history of these experiences should be part of any physician's evaluation of requests for assisted suicide. That evaluation must also reflect an awareness of risk factors for suicide, such as alcoholism, a past history of depression, a family history of depression and/or suicide, and, of course any prior suicide attempts.

Most suicide attempts also reflect a person's ambivalence about dying, and patients requesting assisted suicide show an equal ambivalence. Physicians inexperienced in dealing with suicidal patients tend to take requests to die literally and concretely, and may act on them while failing to hear this ambivalence.

A survey of Oregon psychiatrists revealed that most of those who are willing to evaluate a patient's competence for assisted suicide favour the practice, leading the investigators to conclude that 'a bias may be introduced into the competency evaluation' (Ganzini *et al.* 1996). Since the advocacy group, Compassion in Dying, was shepherding 75 per cent of the cases and the referrals, the likelihood of such bias would seem to be even greater.

Making the psychiatrists and psychologists gatekeepers, needed at times to establish a patient's capacity to make the decision for assisted suicide, strips the evaluation of meaning and makes it into a source of protection for doctors rather than patients. Joan Lucas, an Oregon patient with amyotrophic lateral sclerosis, attempted suicide. Paramedics were called to Joan's house but her children sent them away, explaining 'We couldn't let her go to the ambulance. They would have resuscitated her.'

Joan survived her attempt and was assisted in suicide eighteen days later by a physician who gave interviews about the case to an Oregon newspaper on condition of anonymity. He stated that after talking with attorneys and agreeing to help aid Joan in death, he asked Joan to undergo a psychological examination.

'It was an option for us to get a psychological or psychiatric evaluation,' the physician said. 'I elected to get a psychological evaluation because I wished to cover my ass. I didn't want there to be any problems.'

The doctor and the family found a cooperative psychologist who asked Joan to take the Minnesota Multiphasic Personality Inventory, a standard psychological test. Because it was difficult for Joan to travel to the psychologist's office, her children read the true–false questions to her at home. The family found the questions funny, and Joan's daughter described the family as 'cracking up over them'.

Based on these test results, the psychologist concluded that whatever depression Joan had was directly related to her terminal illness—a completely normal response. His opinion is suspect, the more so because while he was willing to give an opinion that would facilitate ending Joan's life, he did not feel it was necessary to see her first (Foley and Hendin 2002).

Without a proper professional psychiatric evaluation, it is not possible even to ascertain if a patient has impaired judgment that would make him or her not 'capable' of an 'informed decision' as required by Oregon law. Without such a consultation there is less likely to be an attempt made to understand and relieve the desperation, anxiety, and depression that underlie most requests for assisted suicide.

## Protecting physicians not patients

A concern with physician protection, rather than patient protection, pervades the Oregon experience. Physicians are exempt from the ordinary standards of care, skill, and diligence required of Oregon physicians in other circumstances (e.g. a physician's conduct in withdrawing life support). Instead, the physician is immunized from civil and criminal liability for actions taken in 'good faith' in assisting a suicide irrespective of community standards in other matters and even when the physician acts negligently. A physician could act negligently or even recklessly, but as long as the physician subjectively believed those actions were appropriate, the defence can prevail. A standard of 'negligence', which is customary in professional practices, provides objective guidelines for a particular procedure or the established and objective standards for good practice. If the intent of the assisted suicide law is to protect physicians from accountability for violating the statute's provision, the good faith standard is ideal. If the intent of the law is to provide protection for patients, the negligence standard would be appropriate (Foley and Hendin 2002).

## Ten years perspective on the Oregon law

Since the Oregon assisted suicide law was implemented, 292 Oregonians have used PAS and died during the nine years from 1997–2006; 456 received prescriptions to do so. Those who did not

use them either died of natural causes or were still living. Sixteen Oregonians used PAS in 1998 and that number has almost tripled, rising to 46 in 2006. The rate of PAS deaths to total deaths has gone from 5/10,000 of total deaths in the state in 1998 to 14.7/10,000 in 2006 (Oregon Department of Human Services 2007).

Some proponents have argued that the number per year is relatively low and indicates that the Oregon law is working well. OPHD staff and Oregon investigators, however, admit they have no way of knowing how many cases are not reported. If OPHD wished to know what is going on they would need to do as the Dutch have done and grant physicians immunity for anything they have done and then survey them with both questionnaires and in-person interviews. They would need to ask about euthanasia as well as assisted suicide.

The more physicians know about palliative care the less they favour assisted suicide and euthanasia; the less they know the more they favour them (Portenoy et al. 1997). The critical question is: Does it change the way they practice medicine? In the Netherlands, we have seen there is evidence it has. There is no comparable evidence of any sort from Oregon nor is there likely to be until OPHD is ready to undertake objective study of what is transpiring.

## Autonomy and control

The impetus for passage of the Oregon law was its use in relieving intractable symptoms such as pain, but it has evolved into providing an option for control; the issues then are behavioural, cultural, and sociological as much as they are psychological and medical. The most common reason that Oregon patients give for choosing assisted suicide is not pain but a need for control. Zbigniew Zylicz, the Dutch palliative care expert and researcher who has treated hundreds of such patients in a hospice, describes most as changing their minds when good palliative care is made available to them. A small group, however, remain inflexibly control-oriented not just about when and how they die, but in their closest personal relationships (Zylicz 2002). Oregon researchers have described a similar group whose inflexibility and dread of being dependent on others is such that palliative care has no appeal for them. This is seen by the Oregon researchers as an issue of autonomy that should be respected (Ganzini et al. 2003).

The need for control, however, is characteristic of most suicidal patients. They make conditions on life: 'I won't live without my wife', 'if I lose my looks, power, prestige, or health' or 'if I am going to die soon' (Hendin and Klerman 1993). Depression, often precipitated by discovering a serious illness, exaggerates the tendency to see life in black and white terms, but for most such people the need for control has been a dominant feature of their life. They don't tolerate needing to depend on other people very well. In any case, the good practice of medicine obliges doctors to relieve distress rather than to assume that hastening death is the only way to do so.

## The need for change

We are able to identify serious problems in the Oregon law, but nothing will be done to correct them until OPHD is willing to address them. Public impetus for change is difficult when the state's monitoring agent seems fearful of transparency.

The most glaring limitation in OPHD's monitoring and reporting is its collection of information only from physicians who have written a lethal prescription. OPHD needs to interview doctors who, for whatever reason, declined to prescribe lethal medication and nurses, social workers, or family who cared for patients. Without such information we have no idea of how many requests for assisted suicide there are each year, why some physicians declined while others agreed to proceed, or what transpired in any particular case.

Under the current monitoring system, Oregon physicians appear to have been given great power without being in a position to exercise it responsibly. They are expected to inform patients that alternatives are possible, without being required to be knowledgeable about such alternatives or to consult with someone who is. They are expected to evaluate patient decision-making capacity and judgement without a requirement for psychiatric expertise or consultation. They are expected to make decisions about voluntariness without having to see those close to the patient who may exert a variety of pressures, from subtle to coercive (Wasserman and Wasserman 1994). They are expected to do all of this without necessarily knowing the patient. Since physicians cannot be held responsible for wrongful deaths if they have acted in good faith, substandard medical practice is encouraged, physicians are protected from the consequences, and patients are left unprotected while believing they have acquired a new right.

## Impact of the Dutch and Oregon experience

A number or European countries are considering legalizing euthanasia but only Belgium has done so. Although influenced by the Dutch experience, the Belgium law, passed in 2002, only legalized euthanasia and not assisted suicide, probably because assisting in a suicide was never against the law in Belgium. When the Dutch Euthanasia Statute was enacted, also in 2002, two decades of case law had made clear how the law would be implemented. Belgium had no such case law experience with euthanasia, so there is debate as to what the law means and how it will be implemented and it is still too early to tell (Adams and Nys 2003).

In Switzerland euthanasia is punishable by law. The penal code, however, does not condemn assisted suicide whether carried out by a medical doctor or another person, provided it is not carried out for 'selfish' motives (Burkhardt et al. 2006). Only in the past decade, however, have Swiss associations extensively engaged in assisted suicide. An estimate of over 2000 people have been assisted in suicide, with many from foreign countries, mainly Germany and Great Britain, being assisted in everything from travel arrangements to funeral services (Nickerson 2006). Investigators from those countries have complained that Dignitas, the most prominent of these organizations, has put to death people who were neither dying nor terminally ill.

Other countries have no statutes prohibiting assisted suicide but they can prohibit the practice by other means. Sweden, for example, can prosecute those who facilitate a suicide as assisting in manslaughter. In England and in individual states in the United States, this can be done, as it was in the Netherlands until 2002, by case law.

In its landmark 1997 decision that there was no constitutional right to assisted suicide and upholding the laws in New York and the state of Washington prohibiting the practice, and in a more recent 2006 case dealing specifically with the Oregon law, the US Supreme Court seemed to imply that the states have a right to decide for themselves what they want to do unless Congress passes a specific law to the contrary. Since 1997, bills modelled after the Oregon law have been introduced in thirteen states. One, in the state of Washington has passed. Four states have instead passed statutes prohibiting assisted suicide and euthanasia. Most states already had such prohibitions. Two states had public initiatives that were turned down by voters aided by strong opposition from the state medical societies. People are only beginning to learn that, with well-trained doctors and nurses and good end-of-life care, it is possible to avoid the pain of the past experiences of many of their loved ones and to achieve a good death.

## Conclusion

The prohibition of assisted suicide is meaningful only if good palliative care is provided as the alternative. Without it autonomy is an illusion since the choice for patients becomes continued suffering or a hastened death. In rejecting a constitutional right to assisted suicide a majority of the US Supreme Court challenged the states to provide such care.

The World Health Organization has recommended that governments do not consider assisted suicide and euthanasia until they have demonstrated the availability and practice of palliative care for their citizens. All states and all countries have a long way to go to achieve that goal.

## References

Adams M and Nys H (2003). Comparative reflections on the Belgian euthanasia act 2002. *Medical Law Review*, **11**, 353–376.

*British Medical Journal* (2008). Woman is given go ahead to clarify law on assisted suicide. *BMJ*, **336**, 1394–1395.

Burkhardt S, La Harpe R, Harding TW et al. (2006). Euthanasia and assisted suicide: comparison of legal aspects in Switzerland and other countries. *Medical Science Law*, **46**, 287–295.

Chochinov HM, Wilson KG, Enns M et al. (1998). Depression, hopelessness, and ideation in the terminally ill. *Psychosomatics*, **39**, 366–370.

De Witt R, Van Dam F, Vielvoye-Kerkmeer A et al. (1999). The treatment of chronic cancer pain in a cancer hospital in the Netherlands. *Journal of Pain and Symptom Management*, **12**, 333–350.

Dorreppaal KL, Aaronson NK, Van Dam FSAM (1989). Pain experience and pain management among hospitalized cancer patients. *Cancer*, **63**, 593–598.

Emanuel EJ, Fairclough DL, Daniels ER et al. (1996). Euthanasia and physician-assisted suicide: attitudes and experiences of oncology patients, oncologists, and the public. *Lancet*, **347**, 1805–1810.

Foley K and Hendin H (1999). The Oregon report: don't ask don't tell. The *Hastings Center Report*, **29**, 37–42.

Foley K and Hendin H (2002). The Oregon experiment. In K Foley and H Hendin, eds, *The Case Against Assisted Suicide: For the Right to End-of-life Care*, pp. 144–174. Johns Hopkins University Press, Baltimore.

Fromme W, Tilden VP, Drach LL et al. (2004). Increased family reports of pain or distress in dying Oregonians: 1996–2002. *Journal of Palliative Medicine*, **7**, 431–442.

Ganzini L, Fenn DS, Lee MA et al. (1996). Attitudes of Oregon psychiatrists toward physician-assisted suicide. *American Journal of Psychiatry*, **153**, 1469–1475.

Ganzini L, Dobscha SK, Heintz RT et al. (2003). Oregon physicians' perceptions of patients who request assisted suicide and their families. *Journal of Palliative Medicine*, **6**, 381–190.

General Board of the Royal Dutch Medical Society (1994). Vision in euthanasia. In *Euthanasia and the Netherlands*, pp. 12–26. Royal Dutch Medical Association, Utrecht.

Gomez CF (1991). *Regulating Death: Euthanasia and the Case of the Netherlands*. Free Press, New York.

Gordijn B and Janssens R (2004). Euthanasia and palliative care in the Netherlands: an analysis of the latest developments. *Health Care Analysis*, **12**, 195–207.

Groenewoud JH, van der Maas PJ, van der Wal G *et al.* (1997). Physician-assisted death in psychiatric practice in The Netherlands. *New England Journal of Medicine*, **336**, 1795–1801.

Hendin H (1995). Selling death and dignity. *The Hastings Center Report*, **25**, 19–23.

Hendin H (1997). *Seduced by Death: Doctors, Patients, and Assisted Suicide*. W.W. Norton & Co., New York.

Hendin H and Klerman GL (1993). Physician-assisted suicide: the dangers of legalization, *American Journal of Psychiatry*, **150**, 143–145.

Hendin H, Rutenfrans C, Zylicz Z (1997). Physician-assisted suicide and euthanasia in the Netherlands: lessons from the Dutch. *Journal of the American Medical Association*, **227**, 1720–1722.

Hoover E (1998). Two deaths add new angle to debate. *Oregonian*, 27 March, A01.

Hoover E and Hill GH (1998). Two die using Oregon suicide law. *Oregonian*, 26 March, A01.

Janssens MJPA, Have T, Zylicz Z (1999). Hospice and euthanasia in the Netherlands: an ethical point of view. *Journal of Medical Ethics*, **25**, 408–412.

Last Acts Organization (2002). *Means to a Better End: A Report on Dying in America Today*. Robert Wood Johnson Foundation website http://www.rwjf.org/files/publications/other/meansbetterend.pdf

Mackenzie TB and Popkin M (1990). Medical illness and suicide. In SJ Blumenthal and D Kupfer, eds, *Suicide Over the Life Cycle: Risk Factors, Assessment, and Treatment of Suicidal Patients*, pp. 205–235. American Psychiatric Press, Washington.

Matthews H (1998). Better palliative care could cut euthanasia. *British Medical Journal*, **317**, 617.

Murphy GE (1975). The physician's responsibility for suicide: (1) an error of commission and (2) errors of omission, *Annals of Internal Medicine*, **82**, 301–309.

Nickerson C (2006). Suicide groups make Switzerland a final destination. *Boston Sunday Globe*, A 12.

Onwuteaka-Phillipsen BD, Van der Heide A, Koper D *et al.* (2003). Euthanasia and other end-of-life decisions in the Netherlands in 1990, 1995, and 2001. *Lancet*, **362**, 395–399.

Oostveen MS (2001). Voorvechters van de euthanasiepraktijk bezinnen zich. [Regrets: Proponents of euthanasia reorient themselves]. *NRC Handelsblad* (Dutch Newspaper), 10 November. English translation available at http://www.internationaltaskforce.org/holbors.htm.

Oregon Department of Human Services (2007). *Ninth Annual Report on the Oregon Death with Dignity Act*, http://egov.oregon.gov/DHS/ph/pas/ar-index.shtml.

Passik SD, Dugan W, McDonald MV *et al.* (1998). Oncologists' regulation of depression in their patients with cancer. *Journal of Clinical Oncology*, **16**, 594–1600.

Portenoy RK, Coyle N, Kash KM *et al.* (1997). Determinants of the willingness to endorse assisted suicide: a survey of physicians, social workers, and nurses. *Psychosomatics*, **277**, 284–285.

Reagan P (1999). Helen. *Lancet*, **353**, 1265–1267.

Sheldon T (2005). Dutch euthanasia law should apply to patients 'suffering through living', report says. *British Medical Journal*, **330**, 61.

Sheldon T (2008). Dutch doctors make advice on euthanasia available to public. *British Medical Journal*, **336**, 1394–1395.

Ten Have H and Kisma G (1985). *Geneskunde: Tusen droom en drama* [Medical science: between dream and drama]. Kok Agora, Kampen.

Twycross RG (1995). Where there us hope, there is life: a view from the hospice. In J Keown, ed., *Euthanasia Examined: Ethical, Clinical, and Legal Perspectives*, pp. 141–168. Cambridge University Press, Cambridge.

Van Der Heide A (2007). End-of-life practices in the Netherlands under the euthanasia act. *New England Journal of Medicine*, **356**, 1957–1965.

Van der Maas PJ, Van Delden JJM, Pijnenborg L (1992). *Euthanasia and Other Medical Decisions Concerning the End of Life*. Elsevier Science, Inc., New York.

Van der Maas PJ, Van der Wal G, Haverkate I *et al.* (1996). Euthanasia, physician-assisted suicide, and other medical practices involving the end of life in the Netherlands, 1990–1995. *New England Journal of Medicine*, **335**, 1609–1705.

Wasserman D and Wasserman J (1994). Danger of assisted suicide for patients with mental suffering. *Lancet*, **344**, 822–823.

Zylicz Z (1991). Euthanasia [Letter]. *Lancet*, **338**, 1150.

Zylicz Z (1993). The story behind the blank spot: hospice in Holland. *American Journal of Hospice and Palliative Care*, **10**, 30–32.

Zylicz Z (2002). Palliative care and euthanasia in the Netherlands. In K Foley and H Hendin, eds, *The Case Against Assisted Suicide: For the Right to End-of-life Care*, pp. 122–143. Johns Hopkins University Press, Baltimore.

# CHAPTER 66

# Education and awareness programmes for adults

## Selected and multilevel approaches in suicide prevention

Ulrich Hegerl, Sandra Dietrich, Tim Pfeiffer-Gerschel, Lisa Wittenburg and David Althaus

## Abstract

Awareness campaigns and multilevel intervention programmes from different countries and continents, their effects on suicidality, as well as limitations of these programmes, are presented and discussed.

Experiences from multilevel interventions, such as the Nuremberg Alliance Against Depression in Germany, show that awareness campaigns develop the strongest effect when combined with other measures to create a synergistic effect. Awareness campaigns draw the attention and interest of primary care providers to activities focusing on depression and suicidality, and make it easier for them to consult with patients with psychiatric diagnoses and motivate them concerning treatment, not least because awareness campaigns can contribute to improving community mental health knowledge. Finally, for those affected by depression or other mental disorders, public campaigns reduce the perceived stigma, thus, lessening the isolation which contributes to despair and suicide risk.

## Introduction

Psychiatric disorders are among the most relevant factors contributing to suicide worldwide. Other risk factors for suicide, in most Western countries, are old age, male gender, social conditions, availability of lethal means to commit suicide and general physical health status. Help-seeking behaviour, access to psychiatric treatment and public attitudes towards suicide are also relevant associated aspects (Mann 2002; Buck 2004; Gunnell *et al.* 2004; Jacobi *et al.* 2004; Bouch and Marshall 2005; Bernal *et al.* 2007). Many suicide prevention interventions only address one or two of these aspects. The effects of such interventions might be limited, and not strong enough to be detectable in the outcome evaluation (Althaus and Hegerl 2003). The implementation of multilevel and multifaceted suicide prevention interventions appears to be promising. Targeting many of the factors associated with suicidality simultaneously may not only have additive suicide preventive effects, but the effect may also be stronger due to synergy between the different interventions (Figure 66.1). Awareness and education campaigns are an important element of such multilevel intervention programmes.

In the following chapter, awareness and education campaigns, as well as multilevel intervention programmes from different countries and continents, and their effects on suicidality, will be

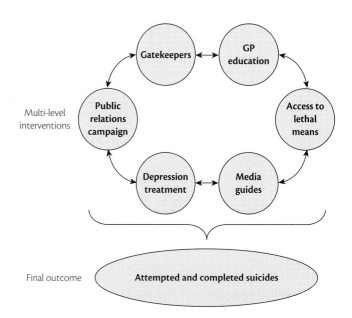

**Fig. 66.1** In multilevel and multifaceted suicide preventive interventions, an increased effectiveness can be expected due to synergistic effects between the different individual measures.

presented and discussed. Some of these campaigns address suicidality directly, e.g. the United States Air Force Suicide Prevention Programme, whereas others are targeting depressive disorders, e.g. beyondblue in Australia; Defeat Depression Campaign in Great Britain; European Alliance Against Depression (EAAD) and the German Alliance Against Depression.

## Education and awareness programmes for primary care physicians, general public and community or organizational gatekeepers

### Depression/awareness, recognition, treatment

In 1988, the National Institute of Mental Health (NIMH) launched the first major federally funded multiphase public and professional health information and education programme in the US: Depression/Awareness, Recognition, Treatment (D/ART) to improve the availability and quality of care for individuals suffering from affective disorders (Regier *et al.* 1988). A strong focus was put on raising awareness of depressive disorders among the general population and experts to educate both the public and professionals that depressive disorders are common, serious and treatable, and also to spotlight obstacles to improving depression recognition and treatment in primary care.

In close cooperation with regional partners, training materials, brochures and leaflets were produced and disseminated, advertisements were placed in newspapers and TV and training was offered in different languages, and used in the US to account for the heterogeneity of the population. Regional adaptations of the programme have been evaluated in several individual studies (e.g. O'Hara *et al.* 1996). O'Hara and colleagues evaluated 18 2-day clinical training programmes for professionals in Iowa, which were attended by 1221 participants (physicians, psychologists, social workers, and nurses) over a 3-year period. Evidence shows that participants' level of knowledge of depression significantly increased and a 6-month follow-up evaluation indicated a continued positive evaluation of the programme (O'Hara *et al.* 1996). The D/ART programme is not explicitly targeted at lowering suicidality, and to date, no systematic nationwide evaluation concerning this aspect has been conducted.

### Defeat Depression Campaign

An anti-stigma programme named Defeat Depression Campaign was implemented in the United Kingdom from 1992–1996, by the Royal College of Psychiatrists. It aimed to improve attitudes towards, and recognizing, depression on a national basis, supplemented by separate local and regional activities. The campaign addressed the problem on two levels: GPs were trained and offered support in diagnosis and treatment of depression. In addition, the general public was educated about depression through videos, flyers and brochures. Beside distributing information materials and delivering comprehensive training, a broad media campaign accompanied this programme. Due to a strong focus on primary care, the Defeat Depression Campaign also included the development of treatment guidelines, organization of case and consensus conferences, and the dissemination of training material, mainly for the field of primary care. During the programme, a noticeable improvement in awareness for depressive disorders,

and knowledge about neurobiological factors involved, could be observed (Paykel *et al.* 1997); however, it did not lead to a considerable and sustainable improvement in delivering care to affected patients (Rix *et al.* 1999).

Changes in prescribing rates of antidepressants were noted, the total number of prescriptions increased markedly from seven million in 1987 to about fifteen million in 1996 (Paykel 2001). National suicide rates were a key evaluating indicator during the Defeat Depression Campaign. Over the years of the campaign, suicide rates had fallen from 7.71/100,000 (1992) to 6.89/100,000 (1995) (Paykel 2001). However, the reduction in suicide rates cannot solely be attributed to the campaign (Rix *et al.* 1999; Paykel 2001). There are several other events that might have contributed to this effect. First, the introduction of the green paper 'The health of the nation: a strategy for health in England' in 1992, which also called for a 15 per cent reduction in the overall suicide rate, and a 33 per cent reduction in the suicide rate in the severely mentally ill (Hawton 1998), as an aim for the mental health services. Other factors that might have played a role are well-known fluctuations in suicide rates, and the introduction of new antidepressant drugs, with associated intensive marketing activity from the drug industry (Rix *et al.* 1999; Paykel 2001).

### Beyondblue

In 2000, the Australian government started a five-year initiative to prevent depression and respond effectively to it. The *beyondblue* initiative has five priority areas: community awareness and de-stigmatization, consumer and carer support, prevention and early intervention, primary care training and support, and applied research (Jorm *et al.* 2005). According to a first evaluation of this programme, an increase of public awareness and general recognition of the programme could be observed after three years of intervention (Hickie 2004; Jorm *et al.* 2005). A pre-existing national mental health policy and implementation plan, a substantial funding base and participation by key political, media and community leaders have probably contributed considerably to these short-term effects (Hickie 2004).

A major limitation in the evaluation of national strategies like beyondblue or the Defeat Depression Campaign is the absence of a control group, making it difficult to separate the effects of the intervention strategy from other influences, thus, making it impossible to know whether the observed changes would have occurred without the intervention. Jorm *et al.* (2005), for instance, attempted to overcome this by using the states that did not fund Beyondblue as a control group. They found that the 'high-exposure states' had a greater increase in belief in the helpfulness of several interventions than the control group. The 'high-exposure' states also showed a greater decrease in the belief that it is helpful to deal with depression alone. Jorm and colleagues concluded that beyondblue had a positive effect on some beliefs about depression treatment, most notably on counselling and medication, including the value of help-seeking in general.

### National Strategy for Suicide Prevention

In 2001, a National Strategy for Suicide Prevention (NSSP) was published in the US. Its aims were to promote awareness of suicide as a public health problem, to prevent premature deaths due to suicide across the lifespan, to reduce the rates of other suicidal behaviours, to reduce the harmful after-effects associated with suicidal behaviours and the traumatic impact of suicide on family and friends, to promote opportunities and settings to enhance resiliency, resourcefulness, respect, and interconnectedness for individuals, families, and communities. The aim of the strategy is to develop and implement community-based suicide prevention programmes, including training programmes for recognition of at-risk behaviour and delivery of effective treatment. Results of this initiative remain to be evaluated.

### United States Air Force Suicide Prevention Programme (AFSPP)

This approach to reducing the risk of suicide was first implemented in the United States Air Force in 1996, in response to the rise in the numbers of suicides between 1990 and 1995. Eleven initiatives were implemented, with the aim of strengthening social support, promoting development of effective social and coping skills, promoting awareness of the various risk factors related to suicide, reducing modifiable risk factors, enhancing factors considered protective, changing policies and norms to encourage effective help-seeking behaviours, and reducing the stigma related to help-seeking behaviour. The evaluation of AFSPP showed that the Air Force personnel exposed to the programme experienced a 33 per cent reduction of suicide risk compared with personnel prior to the implementation (Registry of Evidence-Based Suicide Prevention Programs 2005; Pflanz 2007). When the project began, suicides constituted the second leading cause of death in the Air Force, with an annual rate of 15.8/100,000. Since then, the suicide rate has declined (statistically significantly) to 5.6/100,000 in 1999. The suicide rates increased in 2000 and early 2001, but have declined again since April 2001, and have remained lower than rates prior to 1995. It must be noted that the suicide rates in the US also declined in the second half of the 1990s. This decline, however, is extremely small compared to that measured in the Air Force (The United States Air Force Medical Service 2002). As the Air Force community represents a select population, the generalizeability of these findings have been discussed (Knox *et al.* 2003).

### A look at Asia

Suicide prevention strategies, including public awareness campaigns, need to be shaped differently in Asia compared to Western countries, due to different cultural and social backgrounds. Compared to the West, self-poisoning with pesticides plays a far more important role in these regions than in Europe or Australia (Eddleston and Phillips 2004; Vijayakumar 2005), see also Chapter 17 in this book. In addition, compared to Western countries, higher suicide rates are found in rural, rather than urban areas, and more women than men die by their own hand in China for instance (Ji and Kleinman 2001).

For China, suicide is a major public health problem and it is gradually being recognized. Based on the results of a national case–control psychological post mortem study, Phillips and colleagues have drawn the conclusion that risk factors for suicide do not differ greatly between China and the West (Phillips *et al.* 2002). Furthermore, they suggest that suicide preventive programmes in China should also use a multilevel and multifaceted approach. This is supported by Motohashi and colleagues who conducted a community-based, multi-level intervention for suicide prevention in Japan, with the result of a decrease in suicide rates from 70.8/100,000 in 1999 to 34.1/100,000 in 2004 (Motohashi *et al.* 2007).

# Multilevel approaches to suicide prevention

## Choose Life

A 10-year National Strategy to reduce suicide in Scotland by 20 per cent by 2013 was launched in 2002. It is embedded into a complex national strategy to improve mental health and well-being in Scotland (http://www.wellontheweb.org). This two-phase plan (implementation phase 2003–2006, and evaluation, review and assessment phase 2006–2012) aims to improve early prevention and crisis response, engagement with the media, and adoption of an evidence-based approach (Mackenzie *et al.* 2007). The main aim is to set out a framework to achieve seven multifaceted objectives: early prevention and intervention, responding to immediate crisis, longer-term work to provide hope and support recovery, coping with suicidal behaviour and completed suicide, promoting greater public awareness and encouraging people to seek help early, supporting the media and knowing 'what works' to prevent suicide. The strategy addresses several levels by a variety of means, and among other things, includes a telephone advice line. Local actors such as the health service, councils and voluntary organizations are asked to jointly develop and implement local plans for suicide prevention. The outcome evaluation of this first phase mainly aims at evaluating the implementation process itself, rather than a possible impact on suicide rates, which is planned for later phases of the campaign.

The reduction in male suicide and undetermined deaths between 2002 (N = 673, rate = 34.1/100,000) and 2003 (N = 577, rate = 29.1/100,000) occurred when Choose Life had only been partially implemented, and perhaps may also be due to the influence of other factors, e.g. legislation restricting sales of paracetamol. In addition, in the absence of control data, there is a significant challenge in interpreting trends over time (MacKenzie *et al.* 2007). At the time of writing, the evaluation was still in progress.

# The Nuremberg Alliance Against Depression

The Nuremberg Alliance Against Depression, an intervention for suicide prevention, was implemented in the city of Nuremberg, Germany (population 500,000) in 2001 and 2002, with Würzburg (population 270,000) as the control region. The intervention approached the prevention of suicidality on four levels (see Figure 66.2).

## Level 1: cooperation with primary care physicians (GPs)

Twelve training sessions were carried out in Nuremberg over the two-year period. The course curriculum included diagnosis and treatment of depression, managing suicidality, guiding patients from screening to diagnosis to treatment, and using the WHO 5 Well-being Questionnaire as a screening tool.

GPs were also provided with two professionally produced videotapes. The first videotape informed GPs about the diagnosis and treatment of depression, the second video was intended to support the GPs in informing the individual patients about their disorder and its treatment.

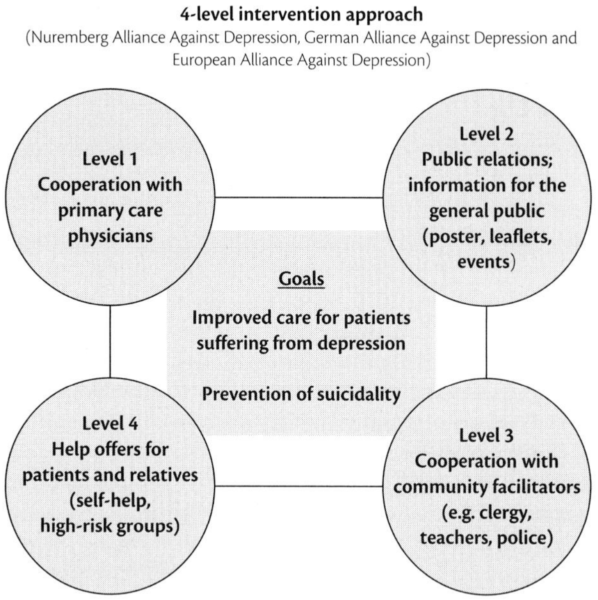

**4-level intervention approach**
(Nuremberg Alliance Against Depression, German Alliance Against Depression and
European Alliance Against Depression)

**Fig. 66.2** The four-level approach committed to improving the care of depressed people and the prevention of suicidality.

## Level 2: public relations campaign

A professional public relations campaign was established, including posters at public places, leaflets, information brochures and several public events. Additionally, a cinema spot was developed, a website was established and two prominent patrons supported the campaign (German Federal Minister for Family Affairs, Senior Citizens, Women and Youth and the Bavarian Minister of the Interior Affairs). Forty-three lectures and events for the general public were organized, 25,000 brochures and more than 100,000 leaflets were produced and distributed.

In addition, close cooperation with the media was established in order to avoid imitation suicides. A 14-item media guide was handed out to local media in Nuremberg, providing information how to report and how not to report suicide (Schäfer *et al.* 2006).

## Level 3: intervention with community facilitators

Eighty-four educational workshops were provided to important community facilitators, such as teachers, counsellors, priests, geriatric nurses, policemen, pharmacists and others. In the course of these workshops, more than 2000 individuals were trained how to recognize people with depression, and to influence depressed people to seek appropriate treatment.

## Level 4: intervention with high-risk groups

An emergency card was handed out to patients after a suicide attempt, containing a telephone number, which allowed easy access to professional help offered by a specialist 24 hours a day seven days a week (24/7). Several initiatives were started to establish new self-help activities and support existing self-help activities.

Evaluation of the intervention included data from a 1-year baseline study and from a control region. The only a priori defined primary outcome was the number of suicidal acts (fatal + non-fatal). This allowed a confirmatory statistical approach. Fatal and non-fatal suicidal acts were combined as a primary outcome,

because a power analysis revealed that even a population of 500,000 inhabitants is not sufficient to statistically detect a reduction in suicide rates of 20%.

During the two intervention years, the number of suicidal acts decreased by 24% in the intervention region, which was significantly more than the control region, where rates remained stable (Althaus *et al.* 2007). During the first intervention year, the lowest suicide rate ever measured was observed in Nuremberg, however, this number is still not outside of the 95% confidence interval of the preceding 12 years (95% –CI: 72.2–96.7) (Hegerl *et al.* 2006; Althaus *et al.* 2007). Interestingly, the reduction of suicidal acts was not a short-term effect, because an additional decrease was observed in the follow-up year after the 2-year intervention (–32% compared to the baseline year).

Furthermore, when analysing suicidal acts in terms of methods used, the strongest reduction (–47%) was observed for the five high-risk suicide methods (jumping from an extended height, hanging, suicide by firearms, drowning, being run over) (Hegerl *et al.* 2006; Althaus *et al.* 2007). This suggests that the reduction in suicidal acts observed in Nuremberg might be underestimated, because more attempted suicides, especially intoxications, may have been recognized after the awareness campaign.

Other evaluations have investigated the effects of the different interventions on the four levels, such as the effects of the media guide on news reporting about suicides, prescription rates of antidepressants or the effects of the public relations campaign in general.

Following the implementation of the 14-item media guide containing recommendations for appropriate, accurate and potentially helpful media coverage of suicide, suicide reports (N = 761, frequency, distribution and qualitative aspects) in three regional dailies (daily newspapers) in Nuremberg were compared (Schäfer *et al.* 2006). While there was a noticeable reduction in the number of articles on suicide (–26%) in two dailies, an increase in the number of suicide reports was found in the third newspaper, a famous German tabloid (+22%). Evaluation showed that more help-seeking information (telephone numbers, websites, self-help measures, etc.) was provided. One of the conclusions drawn from the evaluation was that the successful implementation of media guides on suicide reporting depends on the willingness of the main editors in charge to be engaged and willing to cooperate (Schäfer *et al.* 2006). Follow-up will show the long-term impact of the media guide on suicide reporting.

Changes in the prescription of antidepressants by practice-based doctors have also been analysed (Pfeiffer-Gerschel 2007). He compared the prescribed defined daily doses (DDD) in the intervention region and the rest of Bavaria (German federal state). After the first intervention year (2001), the prescribed DDD of all antidepressants increased by 15% in Nuremberg in comparison to the baseline year 2000; about 11,800 persons were treated with antidepressants in 2000 during the entire year, this number increased to 13,500 in 2001. This finding is statistically significant in comparison to the rest of Bavaria (increased by 8%). After the second intervention year, however, about 15% more antidepressants were prescribed, both in Nuremberg and the rest of Bavaria, as compared to 2000. It is noteworthy that prescriptions by neurologists increased significantly (+25% in 2001, +41% in 2002) as compared to the rest of Bavaria (+13% in 2001, +24% in 2002). Thus, with regard to prescription of antidepressants, the Nuremberg Alliance Against Depression mainly had an effect on practice-based neurologists.

The professional public relations campaign was evaluated based on the results of telephone surveys in 2000 and 2001, which assessed public beliefs and attitudes toward depression and suicidality (Hegerl *et al.* 2003). The evaluation revealed no major effects, e.g. the opinion that antidepressants are addictive was observed in 80% of the population before and, also, after the intervention (Althaus *et al.* 2002). This finding corresponds to experiences from other health campaigns: it is not too difficult to achieve awareness, but it is hard to change attitudes (Hegerl *et al.* 2003). There have been several spontaneous reports from depressed persons in Nuremberg stating that the campaign was very helpful, because they felt less stigmatized and able to speak more openly about their disorder. Finally, as Pfeiffer-Gerschel states, the interventions at the public relations level, self-help and cooperation with multipliers (see Figure 66.2), also encouraged more people with depression to seek professional help (Pfeiffer-Gerschel 2007). Therefore, we believe that the public relations campaign is still one of the most effective elements of the multilevel suicide prevention intervention. It seems to work by giving hope to those affected by psychiatric disorders, it motivates help-seeking behaviour and helps to overcome social isolation.

In conclusion, evaluation of the Nuremberg Alliance Against Depression has provided evidence that its four-level intervention concept and its materials are effective in the prevention of suicidality. The success of this multilevel intervention is most likely not only based on the effectiveness of the single intervention on all levels, but more on synergistic effects between them. This is in line with evidence derived from other fields of prevention, such as HIV prevention (UNAIDS 2006) and tobacco control (The World Bank 1999), which showed that tackling a public health problem on multiple levels and by multiple strategies is more effective than using one strategy on its own. Also, the WHO clearly advocates choosing a multifaceted approach in the prevention of mental disorders and suicidality (World Health Organization 2004).

## German Alliance Against Depression

Since 2002, the concept of the Nuremberg Alliance Against Depression has spread throughout Germany: 40 German regions and communities have initiated their own intervention programmes, and several more are planning to do so in the future (Hegerl and Schäfer 2007). Under the conceptual umbrella of the non-profit organization named German Alliance Against Depression, these regions share their knowledge and cooperate to improve the care of depressed and suicidal patients (http://www.buendnis-depression.de/). Results of this initiative remain to be evaluated.

## European Alliance Against Depression (EAAD)

Based on the Nuremberg intervention, the European Alliance Against Depression (EAAD) was formed in 2004 to disseminate this intervention method across Europe (http://www.eead.net/). The project combines the materials and methods of the Nuremberg Alliance Against Depression with the knowledge, experience, materials and networks of the partners in 17 European regions (Hegerl *et al.* 2004; Pfeiffer-Gerschel *et al.* 2007).

The European Commission presented the EAAD project as one of the most promising strategies in the area of mental health at the WHO European Ministerial Conference on Mental Health in Helsinki in 2005, and named it as a best practice example for improving mental health in Europe through community-based intervention (Hegerl *et al.* 2007). EAAD uses a bottom-up approach, i.e. starting from a regional model project and moving toward a national expansion of activities. Results of this initiative remain to be evaluated. Based on the EAAD concept, the European research project 'Optimised suicide prevention programmes and their implementation in Europe' (OSPI Europe, http://www.ospi-europe.com/) has been started in 2008 with the aim to optimize and evaluate community-based suicide prevention programmes in different European Countries.

## Conclusion: the role of awareness campaigns in suicide prevention

As outlined above, several regional and national awareness campaigns targeting suicidality directly or indirectly via depression, have been implemented and evaluated (Paykel *et al.* 1998; Regier *et al.* 1988; Paykel *et al.* 1997; Rix *et al.* 1999; Appleby *et al.* 2000; Hegerl *et al.* 2003; Hickie 2004; Green and Gask 2005; Morriss *et al.* 2005; Hegerl *et al.* 2006; Hegerl *et al.* 2007; Mackenzie *et al.* 2007; Pflanz 2007). Most of the awareness campaigns did not allow conclusions to be derived about the effectiveness of the interventions in preventing suicidality due to, for instance, the lack of a control region, or the lack of prospective studies of completed as well as attempted suicides. In addition, suicidality is linked to many other factors, such as socio-economic aspects, which are difficult to control in the evaluation.

However, there are good reasons to assume that awareness and education campaigns develop the strongest effect when integrated into a multilevel and multifaceted intervention programme. The goal should be to combine the awareness campaign with other measures in such a manner as to create synergistic effects. The experience from the Nuremberg Alliance Against Depression showed that a public awareness and education campaign makes it easier to get the attention and interest of primary care providers concerning Continuing Medical Education (CME) activities, which focus on depression and suicidality, and to get support from other community facilitators. Furthermore, a professional public campaign makes it easier for primary care providers to confront patients with psychiatric diagnoses and to motivate them concerning treatment, not least because awareness campaigns can contribute to improving community mental health knowledge. Finally, for those affected by depression or other mental disorders, the public campaign reduces the perceived stigma, thus lessening the isolation which contributes to despair and suicide risk.

## References

Althaus D and Hegerl U (2003). The evaluation of suicide prevention activities: state of the art. *World Journal of Biological Psychiatry*, **4**, 156–165.

Althaus D, Niklewski G, Schmidtke A *et al.* (2007). [Changes in the frequency of suicidal behaviour after a 2-year intervention campaign]. *Nervenarzt*, **78**, 272–282.

Althaus D, Stefanek J, Hasford J *et al.* (2002). [Knowledge and attitude of the general public regarding symptoms, etiology and possible treatments of depressive illnesses]. *Nervenarzt*, **73**, 659–664.

Appleby L, Morriss L, Gask L *et al.* (2000). An educational intervention for front-line health professionals in the assessment and management of suicidal patients (The STORM Project). *Psychological Medicine*, **30**, 805–812.

Bernal M, Haro JM, Bernert S *et al.* (2007). Risk factors for suicidality in Europe: results from the ESEMED study. *Journal of Affective Disorders*, **101**, 27–34.

Bouch J and Marshall JJ (2005). Suicide risk: structured professional judgement. *Advances in Psychiatric Treatment*, **11**, 84–91.

Buck A (2004). Suicide and self-harm. *Practice Nurse*, **28**, 64–68.

Eddleston M and Phillips MR (2004). Self-poisoning with pesticides. *British Medical Journal*, **328**, 42–44.

Green G and Gask L (2005). The development, research and implementation of STORM (Skills-based Training on Risk Management). *Primary Care Mental Health*, **3**, 207–213.

Gunnell D, Harbord R, Singleton N *et al.* (2004). Factors influencing the development and amelioration of suicidal thoughts in the general population: cohort study. *The British Journal of Psychiatry*, **185**, 385–393.

Hawton K (1998). A national target for reducing suicide. Important for mental health strategy as well as for suicide prevention. *British Medical Journal*, **317**, 156–157.

Hegerl U, Althaus D, Schmidtke A *et al.* (2006). The alliance against depression: 2-year evaluation of a community-based intervention to reduce suicidality. *Psychological Medicine*, **36**, 1225–1233.

Hegerl U, Althaus D, Stefanek J (2003). Public attitudes towards treatment of depression: effects of an information campaign. *Pharmacopsychiatry*, **36**, 288–291.

Hegerl U and Schäfer R (2007). Vom Nürnberger Bündnis gegen Depression zur European Alliance Against Depression (EAAD)— Gemeindebasierte Awareness-Kampagnen in Deutschland und Europa. [From the Nuremberg Alliance Against Depression to a European network (EAAD)—extending community-based awareness campaigns on national and European level]. *Psychiatrische Praxis*, **34**, S261–S265.

Hegerl U, Wittman M, Arensman E *et al.* (2007). The European Alliance Against Depression (EAAD): a multifaceted, community-based action programme against depression and suicidality. *World Journal of Biological Psychiatry*, **1**, 1–8.

Hegerl U, Wittmann M, Pfeiffer-Gerschel T (2004). Europaweites Interventions programm gegen Depression und Suizidalität. [European Alliance Against Depression]. *Psychoneuro*, **30**, 677–680.

Hickie I (2004). Can we reduce the burden of depression? The Australian experience with beyondblue: the national depression initiative. *Australasian Psychiatry*, **12**, S38–S46.

Jacobi F, Wittchen HU, Holting C *et al.* (2004). Prevalence, co-morbidity and correlates of mental disorders in the general population: results from the German Health Interview and Examination Survey (GHS). *Psychological Medicine*, **34**, 597–611.

Ji J and Kleinman A (2001). Suicide in contemporary China: a review of China's distinctive suicide demographics in their sociocultural context. *Harvard Review of Psychiatry*, **9**, 1–12.

Jorm AF, Christensen H, Griffiths KM (2005). The impact of beyondblue: the national depression initiative on the Australian public's recognition of depression and beliefs about treatments. *Australian and New Zealand Journal of Psychiatry*, **39**, 248–254.

Knox KL, Litts DA, Talcott GW *et al.* (2003). Risk of suicide and related adverse outcomes after exposure to a suicide prevention programme in the US Air Force: cohort study. *British Medical Journal*, **327**, 1376–1380.

Mackenzie M, Blamey A, Halliday E *et al.* (2007). Measuring the tail of the dog that doesn't bark in the night: the case of the national evaluation of Choose Life (the national strategy and action plan to prevent suicide in Scotland). *BMC Public Health*, **7**, 146–153.

Mann JJ (2002). A current perspective of suicide and attempted suicide. *Annals of Internal Medicine*, **136**, 302–311.

Motohashi Y, Kaneko Y, Sasaki H *et al.* (2007). A decrease in suicide rates in Japanese rural towns after community-based intervention by the health promotion approach. *Suicide and Life-Threatening Behaviour*, **37**, 593–599

Morriss R, Gask L, Webb R *et al.* (2005). The effects on suicide rates of an educational intervention for front-line health professionals with suicidal patients (the STORM Project). *Psychological Medicine*, **35**, 957–960.

O'Hara MW, Gorman LL, Wright EJ (1996). Description and evaluation of the Iowa Depression Awareness, Recognition, and Treatment Program. *American Journal of Psychiatry*, **153**, 645–649.

Paykel ES (2001). Impact of public and general practice education in depression. *Psychiatria Fennica*, **32**, 51–61.

Paykel ES, Hart D, Priest RG (1998). Changes in public attitudes to depression during the Defeat Depression Campaign. *British Journal of Psychiatry*, **173**, 519–522.

Paykel ES, Tylee A, Wright A *et al.* (1997). The Defeat Depression Campaign: psychiatry in the public arena. *American Journal of Psychiatry*, **154**, 59–65.

Pfeiffer-Gerschel T (2007). Changes in the prescription of antidepressants by practice-based physicians. Evaluation of the Nuremberg Alliance Against Depression. Unpublished Doctoral Thesis.

Pfeiffer-Gerschel T, Wittmann M, Hegerl U (2007). Die European Alliance Against Depression (EAAD). Ein europäisches Netzwerk zur Verbesserung der Versorgung depressiv erkrankter Menschen. [The European Alliance Against Depression. A European network targeting at effective care in community-based services for persons suffering from depressive disorders]. *Neuropsychiatrie*, **21**, 51–58.

Pflanz SE (2007). *Intervention Summary: United States Air Force Suicide Prevention Program*. http://www.nrepp.samhsa.gov/programfulldetails. asp?PROGRAM_ID=68#outcomes. Accessed 20 November 2007.

Phillips M, Yang G, Zhang Y *et al.* (2002). Risk factors for suicide in China: a national case–control psychological autopsy study. *Lancet*, **360**, 1728–1736.

Regier DA, Hirschfeld RM, Goodwin FK *et al.* (1988). The NIMH Depression Awareness, Recognition, and Treatment Program: structure, aims, and scientific basis. *American Journal of Psychiatry*, **145**, 1351–1357.

Registry of Evidence-Based Suicide Prevention Programs (2005). *US Air Force Program*. http://www.sprc.org/featured_resources/bpr/ebpp_ PDF/airforce.pdf. Accessed 20 November 2007.

Rix S, Paykel ES, Lelliott P *et al.* (1999). Impact of a national campaign on GP education: an evaluation of the Defeat Depression Campaign. *British Journal of General Practice*, **49**, 99–102.

Schäfer R, Althaus D, Brosius HB *et al.* (2006). Suizidberichte in Nürnberger Printmedien—Häufigkeit und Form der Berichterstattung vor und nach der Implementierung eines Medienguides. [Media coverage on suicide in Nuremberg's daily papers—frequency and form of the reporting before and during media intervention with guidelines]. *Psychiatrische Praxis*, **3**, 132–137.

The United States Air Force Medical Service (2002). *Air Force Suicide Prevention Program. A Population-based, Community Approach*. http:// www.jedfoundation.org/articles/AirForceSuicidePreventionProgram. pdf. Accessed 20 November 2007.

The World Bank (1999). *Curbing the Epidemic: Governments and the Economics of Tobacco Control*. The World Bank, Washington.

UNAIDS (2006). *UNAIDS Action Plan on Intensifying HIV Prevention 2006–2007*. http://data.unaids.org/pub/Report/2007/jc1218_ preventionactionplan_en.pdf. Accessed 20 November 2007.

Vijayakumar L (2005). Suicide and mental disorders in Asia. *International Review of Psychiatry*, **17**, 109–114.

World Health Organization (2004). *Prevention of Mental Disorders. Effective Interventions and Policy Options*. World Health Organization, Geneva.

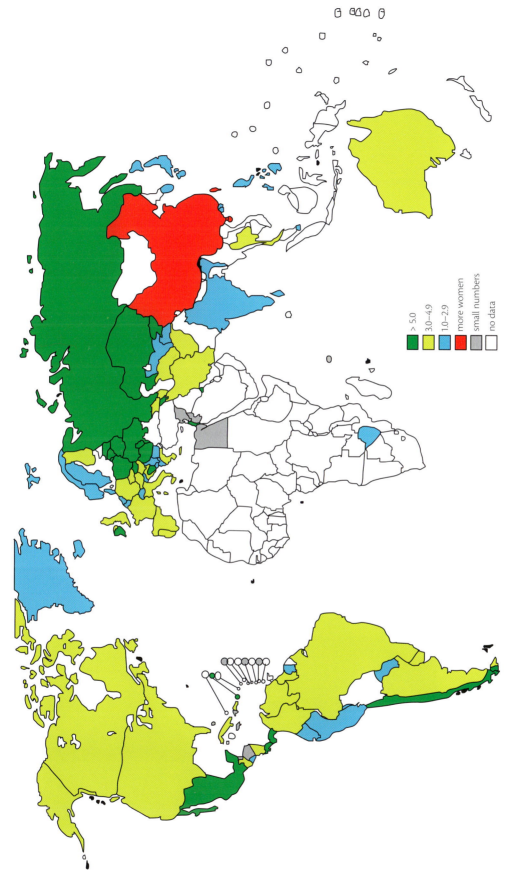

**Fig. 14.1** Proportion of suicide rates of men and women (most recent year available as of 2007: e.g. a proportion of three means that there are three times more men who commit suicide than women. Reproduced with permission from the WHO.

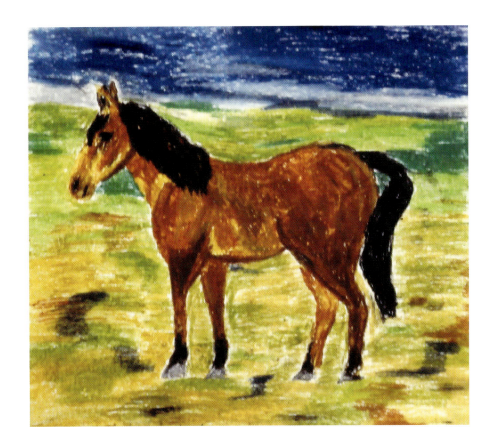

**Fig. 60.1** My horse.

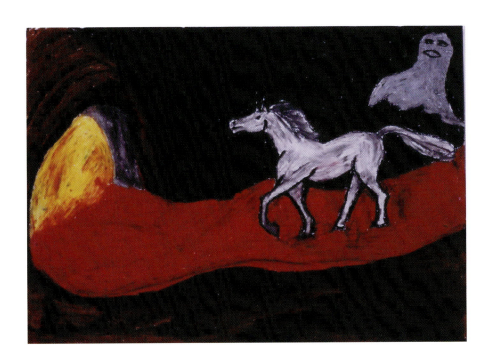

**Fig. 60.2** Horse on red path.

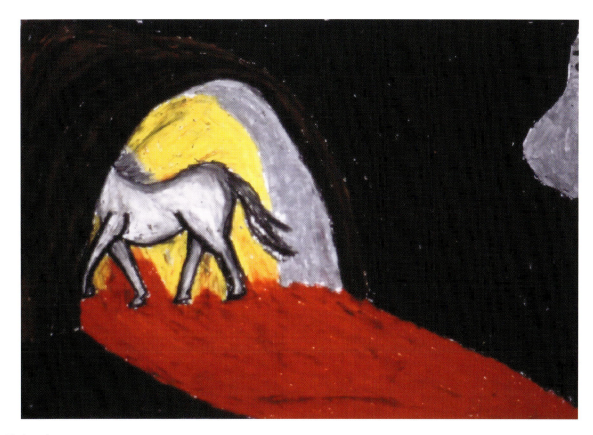

**Fig. 60.3** The last picture.

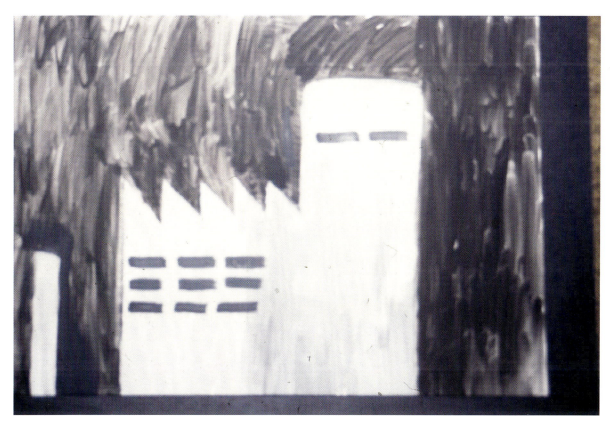

**Fig. 60.4** Edifice.

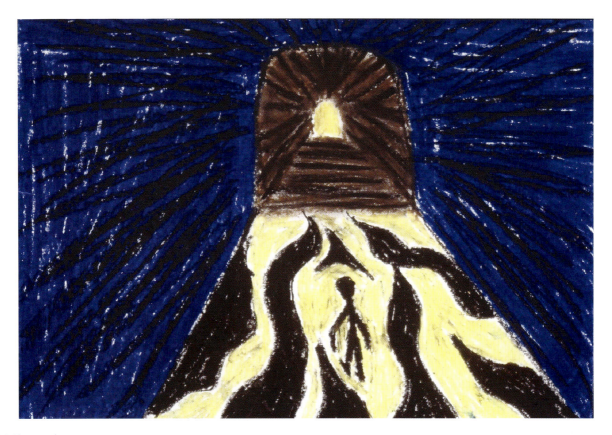

**Fig. 60.5** The tunnel.

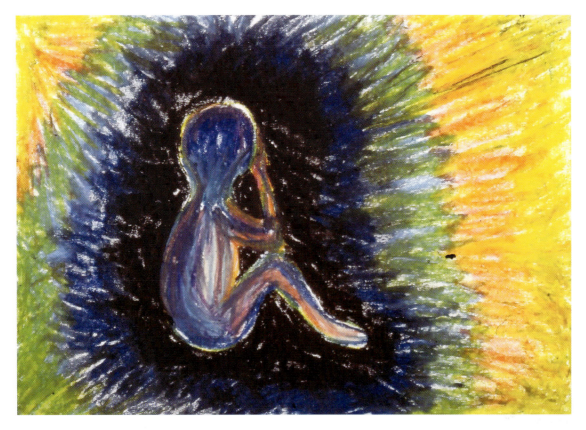

**Fig. 60.6** Safe?

# CHAPTER 67

# Suicide awareness and mental health among youth in the community

## Exposing dark secrets: what must be told

Christina W Hoven, Sam Tyano and
Donald J Mandell

## Abstract

In this chapter, we propose a strategy for increasing the likelihood of identifying youth who are experiencing serious emotional difficulties, which would place them at risk for suicide. Admittedly, current knowledge of the multiple causes of youth suicide remains incomplete, and the scant, currently available mental health resources to address this problem are generally woefully inadequate to meet the need. The situation is even worse in under-resourced environments throughout the world, where there is an acute lack of all mental health services for youth. New efforts are called for. Raising awareness of children's mental health among important youth stakeholders, parents, teachers, and youth themselves, and increasing help and treatment-seeking behaviours, holds out the potential to help reduce unnecessary deaths by suicide in youth.

## Introduction

Over the past four decades, the large productive and fertile opus of work carried out by research suicidologists has significantly advanced understanding of the multifaceted underpinnings of suicide, involving predisposing proclivities and associated neurobiological and genetic factors, history of mental illness, and other commonly identified risk factors established by conducting psychological autopsies of completed suicides (Ford *et al.* 1984; Shafii *et al.* 1984; Mann and Arango 1999). Prior suicide attempt, substance use, depression, bipolar disorder, and a pervasive sense of hopelessness, have all been found to be disproportionately represented in teen suicides (Ford *et al.* 1984; Shaffer 1988). Culture, race/ethnicity, religion and philosophical view of life's meaning also contribute to suicide vulnerabilities (Beautrais *et al.* 1996; Kleinman 2004; Timmermans 2005; Patel *et al.* 2006; Lee *et al.* 2007; WHO 2007; Yang *et al.* 2007). Yet, tempering this air of confidence over how we might benefit from what is known about these associated precursors to prevent suicides are bold data indicating our current failure to do so: to wit, while there are approximately 150,000 suicide attempts by teenagers

reported each year in New York State, and only 70 completed suicides, we have had but little success in identifying the 70 beforehand (Carpinello 2005). Bertolote *et al.* (2003) in a *British Journal of Psychiatry* editorial, asked: 'Do we know enough about the relationship of suicide and mental disorders?' continuing with a discussion of what we can say with confidence that we do know, and what we do not know.

Raising awareness about mental illness and related issues among youth has historically been viewed as inadvisable, even dangerous by creating a risk of improper labelling, based on misapplication of scant information by untrained individuals, thereby stigmatizing persons who only seem to fit little understood categorizations of mental disorder. Further, it has been feared that by raising issues of suicidal behaviour, it could, in consequence, spawn 'copycat' behaviour (Coleman 1987, 2005), and actually contribute to increased suicides (Shaffer *et al.* 1996). Gould *et al.* (2005), however, in a randomized control trial of suicide screening, which probed for suicidal ideation and behaviour, report no evidence of iatrogenic effects from suicide screening among high school students, and conclude that such screening is a safe component of youth suicide prevention efforts (Mann *et al.* 2005). Yet, one cannot ignore or turn a blind eye to the fact that copycat behaviour does indeed exist, especially after acts involving celebrities, or ones which gain international attention (Coleman 1987, 2005). Similarly, the popularity of committing suicide at a 'favourite' places such as San Francisco's Golden Gate Bridge are well-documented (Friend 2003), as well as instances of wearing black frocks in committing school shootings, copying the behaviour of the well-publicized Colorado shooting at Columbine High School (Coleman 2005).

Notwithstanding the advances that have been made in understanding precursors to suicide, we have seen that throughout the world the number of completed youth suicides, while decreasing in some countries and among select subpopulations, continues to increase in many countries (Moscicki 1999; Bertolote *et al.* 2003; Mittendorfer-Rutz *et al.* 2004). On five continents, youth suicide remains the third leading cause of mortality, following deaths from accidents and homicide (Moscicki 1999; Wasserman *et al.* 2005; WHO 2007). In response, efforts to stay the hand of those who would self-destruct must typically employ a spectrum of different approaches, and address this important, seemingly intractable problem in different ways and from different directions (Wasserman 2001).

## Difficulty detecting potential suicide completers

In a poignant examination of the difficulty of preventing a specific suicide, in *Autopsy of a Suicidal Mind,* Edwin Shneidman (Shneidman 2004) convincingly demonstrates the importance of conducting a psychological autopsy to glean the perspective of a number of individuals familiar with the life of a suicidal individual, so as to best understand why an untimely death happened, and more importantly, how it might have been prevented (Fisher and Shaffer 1984). Shneidman interviews relatives and close associates of the suicide victim: mother, father, elder brother, elder sister, lifelong best friend, ex-wife, current girlfriend, childhood psychotherapist, and current attending physician. In addition, he provides transcripts of these interviews, as well as the suicide note left by the deceased, for analysis and opinion to eight eminent suicidologists (Shneidman 2004). His, which is that of examining separate accounts, is reminiscent of the famous Japanese story *Rashomon*, where the telling of an event (an attempted rape and murder of the helpless husband) is remembered differently by each of the persons involved. Perspectives, after all, do differ, and a true picture often requires listening to more than a single point of view. Wasserman (Wolk-Wasserman 1986; Wasserman 2001) and Leenaars (Leenaars 2004) support this multiple-informant approach to revealing aspects of an individual who might be at risk for suicide.

Shneidman's (2004) account of a failure to prevent suicide in a carefully monitored person, who had had a history of prior attempts beginning at age 9 and a later suicide-related hospitalization, seems to augur against relying solely on professionals for information and intervention. While the victim and subject of Shneidman's book (Shneidman 2004) was himself a physician and lawyer, and presumably reasonably well-informed about suicide, there is a suggestion from those contributing information to his psychological autopsy that if their own unique and individual perspectives had been sought and shared with clinical staff, it might have been possible to prevent his specific suicide.

All too often, formal efforts designed to stem the tide of the increasing number of suicides are sorely under-funded and restricted to a one-dimensional focus, skirting the potential for a more effective, albeit more complex, comprehensive approach to suicide prevention. For example, Mann *et al.* (2005), suggest that a corrective approach involves better education of physicians about suicide as well as restricting access to lethal means: these are the best-known preventative methods, while public education, screening programmes, and media education are experimental and need more testing before implementation. While it is clear that more testing is good, it seems that so long as no known harm is involved, preventative methods through education are warranted. Methods of informing their youth about suicide have produced substantial evidence of efficacy (Gould *et al.* 2005) and should be used through expanded outreach (WHO 2007).

## Need for action

The greatest problem encountered in combating suicide is that it is extraordinarily difficult to successfully identify exactly which at-risk individuals who, without intervention, will be suicide completers (Beautrais *et al.* 1996; Pfeffer 2003; Timmermans 2005; Steele and Doey 2007). After all, only a minute fraction of youth who have experienced suicide ideation will actually become a suicide statistic (Carpinello 2005; Brezo *et al.* 2007). Further, while it is true that those who attempt suicide are at greater risk of dying by suicide, from an epidemiological point of view, attempted and completed suicide are considered to be quite different phenomena (Hawton and Heeringen 2000). What additional activities might be used to increase the chances that those youth who are most likely to choose to end their lives will be correctly identified, and their demise prevented?

Below, we describe a nine-country pilot study of mental health awareness campaigns, with suicide awareness issues embedded, offered in schools, simultaneously reaching out to students, teachers and parents—all key stakeholders of youth—who should also be allied in helping those they perceive to be at suicidal risk.

## A nine-country awareness campaign for youth pilot study on different continents

Based on the knowledge of worldwide deficiencies in understanding and addressing children's mental health needs, the World Psychiatric Association (WPA) developed a Presidential Program during 2002–2005 on Global Child Mental Health (initiated by WPA President at that time, under the leadership of Ahmed Okasha), a three-pronged initiative in 2002–2005 to address children's mental health, carried out in collaboration with the World Health Organization (WHO) represented by Norman Sartorius and the International Association of Child and Adolescent Psychiatry and Allied Professions (IACAPAP) represented by Myron Belfer. The Geneva Initiative in Psychiatry (GIP) supported the participation of the Azerbaijan and Georgian sites in the nine-country study at the same financial level as the seven WPA sponsored sites. This was the first major initiative by the WPA to specifically address mental health needs of children. Three multinational task forces were established to carry out the agenda: awareness (Sam Tyano, Israel, Chair), services (Peter Jensen, USA, Chair), and prevention (Helmut Renschmidt, Germany, Chair), with each task force functioning essentially independently. The mission of the awareness task force was to test ways of increasing knowledge of children's mental illness in general, while building on what had previously been learned from WHO's International Stigma Campaign (Sartorius and Schulze 2005).

The awareness task force took the position that, ethically, child mental health information should not be withheld, but shared with the public, especially key stakeholders, parents, teachers and the youth themselves. Further, it was agreed by the task force that it would challenge the approach of turning solely to child psychiatrists as the only reliable and acceptable professionals to be entrusted to advance child mental health. In under-resourced environments, this approach severely constricts public knowledge about child mental health, so that instead of helping to ameliorate mental health-related stigma, actually perpetuates it. With relying on so scarce a body of professionals, the worldwide shortage of child psychiatrists, an approach perpetuates failure to address the feelings of isolation and despair prevalent among youth, which, all too often, increases risk for suicide. Consequently, the awareness task force mandate was to develop child and adolescent mental health awareness campaigns, in order to increase the public's knowledge and understanding of child and adolescent mental illness and suicide. It was felt that this knowledge would open pathways of communication among essential stakeholders, so as to reach those at risk for self-destructive or suicidal behaviour. Clearly, this approach is consistent with the need to prepare the next generation with the appropriate understanding and knowledge they will need to confront the significant burden of mental illness in the future (WHO 2007). Enlisting key stakeholders: parents, teachers, as well as the youth themselves, is emblematic of the task force approach.

## Awareness campaign for youth: design and procedures

The awareness task force study was designed for and carried out in Armenia (Yerevan), Azerbaijan (Baku), Brazil (Porto Alegre), China (Shanghai), Egypt (Alexandria), Georgia (Tbilisi and Rustavi), Israel (North), Russia (Chernoprudsky), and Uganda (Kampala), each under the direction of a local psychiatrist, based on a pre- and post-assessment design. A baseline assessment of students, parents and teachers, based on self-report questionnaires, was to be conducted first. This was to be followed by a locally designed awareness campaign, developed from the *Awareness Manual* (Hoven *et. al* 2008) and conducted for two weeks to one month. One month after the end of the campaign, a post-assessment questionnaire of students, parents and teachers was to be administered. The *Study Procedures Manual*, developed specifically for this study, was distributed to and guided the research activities at each site (Hoven *et al.* 2004b).

Questionnaires were developed to assess the effect of the campaigns on the mental health awareness of students, parents and teachers. Each of the questionnaires, as well as the *Awareness Manual*, *Procedures Manual* (Hoven *et al.* 2004a) and the *Data Entry Manual* (Musa *et al.* 2004), were translated and back-translated for use in the eight local languages of the study: Armenian, Arabic, Azeri, Chinese, Georgian, Hebrew, Portuguese and Russian.

Prior to launching the study, staff at each site were trained in the facets of study methodology using the *Procedures Manual*. Training was assisted by Columbia University staff, either in person or via telephone-conference calls. Each site deliberated how to best conduct the pre-awareness campaign to fit their particular milieu. The child assessment was based on the self-report questionnaires, which were initially distributed to students in randomly selected classrooms in schools enrolling youth ages 10–11-years old, and students 16–17 years of age. To standardize these efforts, the procedures manual detailed the methodology for selecting a stratified sample of schools according to size and location (urban or rural), as well as providing detailed instructions for selecting classrooms in each school to capture samples for both youth age groups of interest. Instructions for random sampling included training on the use of provided tables of random numbers.

The target sample for youth was 400 per site, 200 per age group or N = 3600. Student questionnaires were to be completed during one classroom session; parent questionnaires were to be completed at the school, if possible, or sent home and brought back to school by the students. Teacher questionnaires were to be distributed and collected by study personnel. Study participants were assured that all information would be kept confidential. Institutional Review Board approvals were obtained at the study coordinating site (Columbia University) and at each of the nine country sites.

The Web was used for dissemination of information, data entry programmes and the transmission of study manuals. A Web-based email link facilitated exchange of information and questions. All data were was double entered and transmitted to the study coordinating centre (Columbia University) for analysis.

## Awareness manual

The *WPA-WHO Awareness Manual* (Hoven *et al.* 2004b) was developed for use in child mental health awareness campaigns, and was designed so that it could be adapted locally and administered by either a psychiatrist or other well-trained mental health providers. The manual was designed to inform and guide the campaigns by providing five critical elements: purpose and contextual issues for planning a campaign; mental health content areas; selection of target populations; campaign implementation methodologies, and an annotated reference of websites and other resources. The informational content explores a range of important issues, including healthy child development, mental retardation and epilepsy, as well as common childhood psychiatricdisorders, e.g. depression, anxiety, conduct disorders, PTSD, substance abuse and schizophrenia. Suicide was intentionally folded in as an area to focus on in an awareness campaign. Similarly, stigma, service use and treatment issues were also included. The awareness manual elaborates upon and stresses the need for employing local contexts appropriate for utilizing different campaign methods at the least cost. The annotated references of worldwide authoritative sources are divided into potential user groups, e.g children, parents and families; policy-makers and NGOs, and health care professionals. Recognizing the influence of racial, ethnic and cultural differences (Moscicki 1999), creativity and local resources were taken into account in fashioning site-specific campaigns, rather than proposing a fixed standard model.

## Evaluation measures

The Mental Health Awareness Questionnaire for students assessed demographics, including but not limited to, age, gender and school grade. In an effort to determine general level of impairment in the student population, as well as comparability of samples across sites, the Strengths and Difficulties Questionnaire (SDQ) (Goodman 1999), an instrument to assess behaviours, thoughts and feelings was utilized. Additional questions designed to gather information about the students' opinions concerning child mental health problems were included. These questions addressed different issues, including the students' knowledge of and attitudes about mental health. Questions also assessed the students' views about mental health treatment for children. Finally, there were a number of baseline-specific and follow-up-specific questions, including those about the child's desire for more knowledge about child mental health. The follow-up questions concerned other aspects of the campaign and its effectiveness in increasing knowledge about child mental health, and sought to ascertain whether the campaign altered attitudes, especially the students'.

The Mental Health Awareness Questionnaire for parents and teachers, except for the SDQ, paralleled the content of the student questionnaire. These questionnaires aimed to determine the knowledge and attitudes of parents and teachers about child mental health treatment issues. Baseline questions addressed parent and teacher knowledge of child mental health and their own attitudes about the recent awareness campaign. The follow-up questions were designed to assess changes from baseline responses, as well as views of the effectiveness of the campaign, and whether it played a role in increasing the respondent's knowledge of or change in attitudes about child mental health.

## Overview of study results

The nine-country study explored and tested the suitability and appropriateness of different media approaches, selected in each country by locals who best knew which of the available modalities among the many suggested in the *Awareness Manual* had the greatest possibility for effective transmission of mental health information for youth in their specific culture. Baseline assessment included N = 3574 participants: 2471 students, 607 parents, and 495 teachers. Participation at follow-up (N = 2450) included 1954 students, 260 parents, and 236 teachers.

Some general results, true for all sites:

◆ Mothers at all sites comprised from two-thirds to nearly all parent participants.

◆ Teachers as well were mostly female, ranging from over 50 per cent to 100 per cent.

◆ Pre-campaign interest in knowing more about mental health was low for all participants, the lowest being expressed by students, and only moderate interest was subscribed to by teachers and by parents.

◆ In contradistinction to pre-campaign expression of interest in mental health, post-campaign desire to know more increased at every site. For example, at one post-campaign site, 90 per cent of teachers reported post-campaign that they wanted to know more about mental health;

◆ All groups of participants claimed an increase in knowing enough about child mental health problems: students from 27 to 51 per cent; teachers from 20 to 41 per cent, and parents from 26 to 34 per cent.

◆ Probably the most convincing and heartening of results, affirming the success of the awareness campaigns, is indicated by the general post-campaign increase in reported level of comfort reported by all groups in entering into discussions of emotional problems in youth. Thus, 75 per cent of teachers felt more comfortable in discussing these problems with students, or with other school personnel, and 68 per cent reported greater comfort in discussing such student emotional problems with parents. Post-campaign, 60 per cent of parents also reported feeling more comfortable talking to their children about emotional problems, while 46 per cent felt more at ease in discussing these problems with teachers. Children themselves, in general, reported feeling more comfortable (post-campaign) in talking to others: to teachers or counsellors (59 per cent), to parents or relatives (55 per cent) and to friends (59 per cent).

In sum, the awareness campaigns seemed to have 'loosened tongues', that is, increased willingness to 'expose dark secrets' and to tell 'what must be told'.

Given the wide variation and extraordinary differences in cultures, languages, race/ethnicity, religion, population size, level of economic development, and nature of the workforce (Maris *et al.* 2000; De Leo and Evans 2004; Didiot 2004; Kleinman 2004; Lee *et al.* 2007), the fact that the nine selected countries participating in the WPA Study were able to partially or completely successfully comply with most of the very tight parameters for the conduct of the study, as well as with the rigorous data entry procedures, was an achievement per se. This is especially laudable inasmuch as the near draconian budgetary restrictions of this study pilot sorely hampered anything approaching an expensive publicity programme for bolstering 'awareness'. Six of the nine countries were able to finish both pre-campaign and post-campaign requirements, while all nine demonstrated adherence to training, learning basic field methods for epidemiological research, including sample selection procedures, interviewing techniques, data entry and data reporting, all the while conforming to all confidentiality procedures, thereby protecting the privacy of study participants.

The awareness programme has, thus, been shown to have great potential for opening communication pathways, thereby providing broader avenues of intervention (Hoven *et al.* 2008). Moreover, this simultaneous, cross-stakeholder approach (parents, teachers and students) can be effective in changing attitudes about mental health and fostering a willingness of troubled youth to speak openly with parents and teachers (and they in turn with the students) about their emotional problems, empowers each stakeholder to be appropriately responsive. Expanding knowledge and understanding of mental illness among the most universal youth stakeholders, parents, teachers as well as among the youth themselves, potentially enhances early detection by multiplying the number of eyes and ears attuned to any individual youth who may be suffering, often silently (Steele and Doey 2007). Evidence shows that awareness programmes increase mental health literacy, but that it must be strengthened with more focused suicide preventive interventions in order to help suicidal pupils (Goldney and Fisher 2008). The awareness programme is designed to be offered in addition to, and not to replace, any other interventions which have proven to be affective in reaching youth who are at known elevated risk (Burns *et al.* 2007). The programme is, thus, intended to expand the scope and reach of existing suicide prevention programmes, as well as to be a free-standing programme in places where children's mental health services are essentially non-existent.

## Discussion

These results are heartening, but do such efforts as these seem likely to help to stem the tide of youthful suicide? While recognizing that some researchers originally warned of potential problems associated with use of such education methods with children and adolescents (Shaffer *et al.* 1996), we, nonetheless, believe that campaigns such as those conducted in this pilot can be very important for suicide prevention, provided that:

1 They are based on sound, accurate information (e.g based on documents such as the *Awareness Manual*);

2 Have a simultaneous key-stakeholder (parents, teachers and youth) approach;

3 Do not over-reach, inappropriately raising expectations for formal services that may not exist;

4 Do not follow simple didactic methods, but rather engage all stakeholders; and

5 Include psychiatrically or psychologically trained individuals, at least in the design phase of the campaign.

It also seems useful to develop a sense of connectedness among stakeholders in resolving child mental health problems, so that all who are involved have an investment in positive results: higher degree of mental health, lesser amount of mental illness, and fewer suicides.

Epidemiological studies over the past several decades have identified problems of mental illness and suicide throughout the world (De Leo and Evans 2004). They demonstrate annual rise in suicide rates during the quarter century from the mid-1950s to the late 1970s, among youth (ages 15–24) (Moscicki 1999; Gould *et al.* 2003; De Leo and Evans 2004; Wasserman *et al.* 2005); where, for example, during this period in the United States, the rate more than tripled for boys, and more than doubled for girls. In the 1990s, these rates largely declined. We simply do not know what accounts for such fluctuations (Gould *et al.* 2003). Also, we are unsure as to how generalizable throughout the world such rates may be, as there is much imprecision in rates gathered from different WHO Regions (Cantor 2000; Timmermans 2005).

As noted, the WPA/WHO/IACAPAP Awareness task force successfully conducted studies of child mental health awareness in nine countries on different continents simultaneously. The goal was to test the feasibility and separate requirements of waging awareness campaigns in different cultures, using different languages, and in countries at varying levels of economic development. These efforts ultimately led to important insights relevant for conducting larger-scale child mental health awareness campaigns, which appear to have potential to augment existing youth suicide prevention efforts, especially in under-resourced environments.

Of utmost importance, however, is to be very fastidious about the correctness of information that is transmitted in awareness campaigns, to avoid untoward effects from the passing on of false facts. A brief synoptic treatment of mental disorders is clearly insufficient for making diagnoses, and doing so could wrongly identify people. Not only could those who are not at great risk come to think that they are, but also those who are at high risk might feel falsely safe, when they are not. For example, first identified cases of HIV-AIDS in the mid-1980s (Centers for Disease Control and Prevention 2001) suggested that people at risk for acquiring HIV were: gay white men, Haitians, intravenous drug abusers, and haemophiliacs. The information was 'correct' based on the first cases that had turned up; however, the CDC's publication of these findings had the unfortunate effect of inducing a false feeling of security and safety for persons not on the CDC at-risk list. The AIDS epidemic, at the time, had already been shown to involve heterosexual transmission in Africa, and soon began showing up in other populations not identified at first as being at high risk. What may have ensued is the kind of carelessness that would produce avoidable and unnecessary infections, had there been better information available.

The limited information obtained in this study certainly appears promising for bostering suicide prevention efforts. It should be noted, however, that the questions asked, about mental health–mental illness were general. No specific assessment of suicide risk was made. However, as the WPA-WHO-IAPACAP Awareness Task Force determined, withholding child mental health information is unethical, so that the challenge before us was to find a way to make such information available and useful to as many persons, especially youth, as possible, so as to contribute to their taking steps to reduce rates of suicide. We believe mental health awareness campaigns, which succeed in opening pathways of communication about these issues, can make a significant contribution to this effort. They can help to reduce stigma, shame and distress of families with mentally ill and suicidal children, and improve awareness that mental health problems are treatable and suicide is preventable. However, in-depth studies about how information is perceived by students, parents and teachers and how to motivate and ensure referral of vulnerable young persons for care and treatment, are required to further promote suicide prevention.

## Conclusions: lighting a candle is not sufficient

Finally, it would be overly optimistic to expect that such a brief exposure, as an awareness campaign without follow-up activity, can sustain a lasting effect. 'Lighting a candle' is by no means sufficient to illuminate the darkness surrounding mental illness and suicide; in fact, we feel that such a brief exposure is soon extinguished, and even worse raises false hopes of relief when it is not followed by making resources available, or at the very least, directing those who feel that there may be need for ameliorative action that there are places to consult for help. The *Awareness Manual* does introduce such sources, but even that manual, up to date at time of publication, soon requires updating. And projects aiming to change attitudes and behaviour require consistent action into the future.

What is desperately needed to realize such change is a dramatic increase of effort, extended over a long period of time. Let us give an example: In November 1981, a 31-year-old surgical resident, returning to the hospital after a brief dinner break, was accosted by two muggers who attempted to rob him. Although he was carrying only five dollars, he ran and/or offered resistance and was fatally shot. The incident occurred just outside below our own present offices at Columbia University-New York State Psychiatric Institute.

The accounts among others in *New York Times* that followed revealed that the area had long been considered unsafe, and lacking in proper lighting and police protection. There had been a number of similar incidents occurring when nurses finishing their work shifts were walking home. Nothing of consequence, however, was done until the time of this incident involving a male surgeon from a prominent medical family. The earlier incidents did not bring about any response involving increasing safety and security. However, after Dr John Chase Wood Jr's demise, sodium vapour lamps were installed all around the area; the dark shadows were no more. Security personnel were assigned to patrol duty and electronic surveillance was installed. The chances for a repeat of this kind of attack were now much more remote.

We understand, of course, that this account is only a metaphor, but we feel that in like manner, only when the mystery and dark shadows which continue to surround topics like mental illness and suicide are exposed, brought into full view, and discussed openly, will there result a sufficient call for change, enabling the provision of help for the troubled and a stronger safety net for those on the verge of suicide.

## References

Beautrais AL, Joyce PR, Mulder RT (1996). Risk factors for serious suicide attempts among youths aged 13 through 24 years. *Journal of the American Academy of Child and Adolescent Psychiatry*, **35**, 1174–1182.

Bertolote JM, Fleischmann A, De Leo D *et al.* (2003). Suicide and mental disorders: do we know enough? *British Journal of Psychiatry*, **183**, 382–383.

Brezo J, Paris J, Barker ED *et al.* (2007). Natural history of suicidal behaviors in a population-based sample of young adults. *Psychological Medicine*, **37**, 1563–1574.

Burns J, Morey C, Lagelee A *et al.* (2007). Reach out! Innovation in service delivery. *Medical Journal of Australia*, **187**, S31–S34.

Cantor CH (2000). Suicide in the western world. In K Hawton K and K van Heeringen K, eds, *The International Handbook of Suicide and Attempted Suicide*, pp. 9–28. John Wiley and Sons, Chichester.

Carpinello SE (2005). *Saving Lives in New York: Suicide Prevention and Public Health, Approaches and Special Populations*. New York Office of Mental Health, New York.

Centers for Disease Control and Prevention (2001). HIV and AIDS—United States, 1981–2000. Available at http://www.cdc.gov/mmwr/preview/mmwrhtml/mm5021a2.htm.

Coleman L (1987). *Suicide Clusters*. Faber and Faber, Boston.

Coleman L (2005). *The Copycat Effect: How The Media and Popular Culture Trigger The Mayhem in Tomorrow's Headlines*. Simon and Schuster, New York.

De Leo D and Evans R (2004). *International Suicide Rates and Prevention Strategies*. Hogrefe and Huber, Cambridge.

Didiot B (2004). *L'Etat du Monde 2005*. Boréal, Montreal.

Fisher P and Shaffer D (1984). Methods for investigating suicide in children and adolescents. In HS Sudak, AB Ford and NB Rushforth, eds, *Suicide in the Young*, pp. 139–157. John Wright, Boston.

Ford AB, Rushforth NB, Sudak HS (1984). The causes of suicide: Review and comment. In HS Sudak, AB Ford and NB Rushforth, eds, *Suicide in the Young*, pp. 159–169. John Wright, Boston.

Friend T (2003). Letter from California.: Jumpers: the fatal grandeur of the Golden Gate Bridge. *The New Yorker*.

Goldney RD and Fisher LJ (2008). Have broad-based community and professional education programs influenced mental health literacy and treatment treatment-seeking of those with major depression and suicide ideation? *Suicide and Life-Threatening Behavior*, **38**, 129–142.

Goodman R (1999). The extended version of the Strengths and Difficulties Questionnaire as a guide to child psychiatry caseness and consequent burden. *Journal of Child Psychology and Psychiatry, and Allied Disciplines*, **40**, 791–799.

Gould M, Jamieson P, Romer D (2003). Media contagion and suicide among the young. *American Behavioral Scientist*, **46**, 1269–1284.

Gould MS, Marrocco FA, Kleinman M *et al.* (2005). Evaluating iatrogenic risk of youth suicide screening programs—a randomized controlled trial. *Jama-Journal of the American Medical Association*, **293**, 1635–1643.

Gould MS, Shaffer D, Greenberg T (2003). The epidemiology of youth suicide. In RA King and A Apter, eds, *Suicide in Children and Adolescents*, pp. 1–40. Cambridge, Cambridge University Press, Cambridge..

Hawton K and Van Heeringen K (2000). *The International Handbook of Suicide and Attempted Suicide*. Wiley and Sons, Chichester.

Hoven CW, Doan T, Musa GJ, *et al.* (2008). Worldwide child and adolescent mental health begins with awareness: a preliminary assessment in nine countries. *International Journal of Psychiatry*, **20**, 261–270.

Hoven CW, Musa G, Wicks J *et al.* (2004a). *Procedures Manual: A School-based Assessment of the Effectiveness of Awareness Campaigns about Child and Adolescent Mental Health*. The Presidential World Psychiatric Association (WPA), Program on Global Child Mental Health, in collaboration with The World Health Organization (WHO) and The International Association for Child and Adolescent Psychiatry and Allied Professions (IACAPAP), Columbia University/New York State Psychiatric Institute, New York.

Hoven CW, Tyano S, Agossou TA *et al.* (2004b). *Expanding Awareness of Mental Health in Childhood and Adolescence: The Awareness Program Manual*. The Presidential World Psychiatric Association (WPA), Program on Global Child Mental Health, in collaboration with The World Health Organization (WHO) and The International Association for Child and Adolescent Psychiatry and Allied Professions (IACAPAP). Available online at: http://www.icaf.org/resources/papers/awareness_program_manual.pdf.

Katz AH (1970). *Mission of Man*, 1st ed. New York, Philosophical Library, New York.

Kleinman A (2004). Culture and depression. *New England Journal of Medicine*, **351**, 951–953.

Lee DTS, Kleinman J, Kleinman A (2007). Rethinking depression: An ethnographic study of the experiences of depression among Chinese. *Harvard Review of Psychiatry*, **15**, 1–8.

Leenaars AA (2004). *Psychotherapy with Suicidal People: A Person-centered Approach*. John Wiley and Sons Ltd, Chichester.

Mann JJ and Arango V (1999). The neurobiology of suicidal behavior. In DG Jacobs, ed., *The Harvard Medical School Guide to Suicide Assessment and Intervention*, pp. 98–114. Jossey-Bass, San Francisco.

Mann JJ, Apter A, Bertolote J *et al.* (2005). Suicide prevention strategies—a systematic review. *Journal of the American Medical Association*, **294**, 2064–2074.

Maris RW, Berman AL, Silverman MM (2000). Racial, ethnic, and cultural aspects of suicide. In RW Maris, AL Berman and MM Silverman, eds, *Comprehensive Textbook of Suicidology*, pp. 170–192. The Guilford Press, New York.

Mittendorfer-Rutz E, Rasmussen F, Wasserman D (2004). Restricted fetal growth and adverse maternal psychosocial and socioeconomic conditions as risk factors for suicidal behaviour of offspring: a cohort study. *Lancet*, **364**, 1135–1140.

Moscicki EK (1999). Epidemiology of suicide. In DG Jacobs, ed., *The Harvard Medical School Guide to Suicide Assessment and Intervention*, pp. 40–51. Jossey-Bass, San Francisco.

Musa GJ, Doan T, Hoven CW (2004). *Data Entry Manual: A School-based Assessment of the Effectiveness of Awareness Campaigns about Child and Adolescent Mental Health*. The Presidential World Psychiatric Association (WPA), Program on Global Child Mental Health, in collaboration with The World Health Organization (WHO) and The International Association for Child and Adolescent Psychiatry and Allied Professions (IACAPAP). Columbia University/New York State Psychiatric Institute, New York.

Patel V, Saraceno B, Kleinman A (2006). Beyond evidence: the moral case for international mental health. *American Journal of Psychiatry*, **163**, 1312–1315.

Pfeffer CR (2003). Assessing suicide behavior in children and adolescents. In RA King and A Apter, eds, *Suicide in Children and Adolescents*, pp. 211–226. Cambridge University Press, Cambridge.

Sartorius N and Schulze H (2005). *Reducing the Stigma of Mental Illness: A Report from a Global Programme of the World Psychiatric Association*. Cambridge University Press, Cambridge.

Shaffer D (1988). The epidemiology of teen suicide: an examination of risk factors. *Journal of Clinical Psychiatry*, **49**, 36–41.

Shaffer D, Gould MS, Fisher P *et al.* (1996). Psychiatric diagnosis in child and adolescent suicide. *Archives of General Psychiatry*, **53**, 339–348.

Shafii M, Whittinghill JR, Dolen DC *et al.* (1984). Psychological reconstruction of completed suicide in childhood and adolescence. In HS Sudak, AB Ford and NB Rushforth, eds, *Suicide in the Young*, pp. 271–294. John Wright, Boston.

Shneidman ES (2004). *Autopsy of a Suicidal Mind*. Oxford University Press, Oxford.

Steele MM and Doey T (2007). Suicidal behaviour in children and adolescents. Part 2: Treatment and prevention. *Canadian Journal of Psychiatry–Revue Canadienne de Psychiatrie*, **52**, 35S–45S.

Timmermans S (2005). Suicide determination and the professional authority of medical examiners. *American Sociological Review*, **70**, 311–333.

Wasserman D (2001). *Suicide—An Unnecessary Death*. Taylor and Francis, London.

Wasserman D, Cheng Q, Jiang GX (2005). Global suicide rates among young people aged 15–19. *World Psychiatry*, **4**, 114–120.

WHO (2007). *World Suicide Prevention Day*. http://www.who.int/mediacentre/news/statements/2007/s16/en/index.html, accessed 27 December 2007.

Wolk-Wasserman D (1986). Attempted suicide: the patient's family, social network and therapy. Doctoral dissertation, Karolinska Institute, Sweden, Stockholm.

Yang LH, Kleinman A, Link BG *et al.* (2007). Culture and stigma: adding moral experience to stigma theory. *Social Science and Medicine*, **64**, 1524–1535.

# CHAPTER 68

# Suicide prevention by education and the moulding of attitudes

David Titelman and Danuta Wasserman

## Abstract

In this chapter the challenge of influencing the attitudes to suicide prevention in key individuals or gatekeepers, such as clinicians, school personnel, social planners, and researchers in mental health and suicide prevention, is addressed. Based on experiences from several training programmes, the importance of a psychological perspective on suicidality is seen as relevant, even in population-based research and prevention. One focus in the discussion is on the distinction between having an immediate impact on conscious attitudes and the more difficult challenge of influencing less conscious, individual and cultural ambivalent attitudes to suicide prevention. In light of the universal stigma of and taboo against the topic of suicide, the ability of prevention specialists to withhold judgement and reflect on their own emotional responses to self-destructiveness is considered as an aspect of a scientific attitude. In addition, an anthropological elucidation of mental ill-health and suicide is called for as a supplement to the biopsychosocial, stress–vulnerability paradigm in suicide-preventive training programmes.

## Introduction

What is high-quality education in suicide prevention? The complexity of this question derives from its elements 'education' and 'suicide prevention', both of which continue to be universal social and scientific challenges. In a critical review of national suicide-preventive programmes, DeLeo (2002) recommended multidisciplinary education as the most relevant prevention strategy today. Mann *et al.* (2005), in a review of published prevention studies worldwide, similarly found that education was an effective strategy, particularly when directed to gatekeepers, for example, primary care physicians. One can conclude from these reviews that the severely distressed individual's susceptibility to wishing his or her own death may be counterbalanced—and suicide prevented—by better knowledge and by attitude change in gatekeepers, and that education of suicide-prone individuals as well as of caregivers, other gatekeepers, and those in power to shape society, may contribute to making suicide an 'unnecessary death' (Wasserman 2001a).

Attitudes to suicide on the one hand represent conscious ideas and self-reported behaviours, that is, phenomena that in evaluation studies might be measured on attitude scales. However, attitudes also have unconscious underpinnings, which can only be inferred retrospectively from complex narratives and from manifest action in real-life situations. An example of an unconsciously shaped attitude is the universal taboo against suicide, which does not solely denote a cultural, religious, or instinctive prohibition against killing oneself, but also a phobic attitude to approach—in deed or in thought—anything that has to do with suicide, suicide research and prevention included. Whereas the prohibitive function of the suicide taboo may protect people from taking their lives, the phobic aspect may, in interaction with other factors, contribute to promoting suicides.

A methodological challenge in population-based suicide prevention, including education, is that results reflecting the effects of a given prevention strategy are often not obtainable for statistical reasons, for example, when large enough cohorts or samples aren't available. Moreover it is often essential to supplement robust information on suicide rates, however reliably this information may reflect changes in health in a given population, with experience-near narratives and coherent theoretical descriptions of what has been achieved and how.

The Gotland study, a clinically based yet public-health oriented suicide-preventive intervention (Rutz *et al.* 1989; Rutz 1992; Rutz *et al.* 1995), which was the brainchild of the Swedish Committee for Prevention and Treatment of Depression (Eberhard *et al.* 1992), is an example of how to combine qualitative and quantitative approaches in evaluating the effects of attitude moulding; this project provides real-life illustrations of some of the questions and didactic challenges that are addressed in this chapter.

The principal intervention in this project was a training program given to all of the eighteen general practitioners working in the Swedish island of Gotland, the population of which was about 55,000 when the project was initiated in 1980. The main focus of the two days of lectures and discussions they took part in during the first year of the project was on contemporary methods of diagnosis and treatment of depression; a year later there was a follow-up day of lectures on other themes related to depression and suicidality. An immediate effect of the intervention was that the prescription rate of antidepressants increased and that suicide rates decreased from an annual average of 22 suicides per 100,000 inhabitants in 1979–1982 to 15.5 in 1983–1985.

However, in a follow-up study three years after the project period, the total suicide rate in Gotland had returned to its original, baseline level. One explanation may be that the half-life of attitude change in health-care organizations is short, and that continuous education in psychiatric practices are required to achieve sustainable results. In a subsequent commentary, Rutz and Wålinder (2000) noted that the fact that at follow-up the prescription of antidepressants remained stable at its new, higher level indicates that medication alone did not account for the intermittent reduction of suicides. The most obvious other variable that might explain the decrease of suicides during the project period was the patient–doctor relationship, which in the typical case was intensified while the project was running, or this relationship in interaction with the changed prescription practices. Either way, Rutz and Wålinder concluded, intense, empathic doctor–patient relationships contribute to reducing suicide rates among patients seen by general practitioners.

Improved doctor–patient relationships in general health care and psychiatry may be included among the salutogenic educational and attitude-related targets of individual-based prevention as well as of prevention directed towards vulnerable groups. Related goals are to advance openness to individual differences in the community at large or in social milieus other than clinics, for example, in schools, work places, and military settings, and to counteract the stigmatization of suicide attempters or other vulnerable individuals or groups.

A number of relatively recent studies (Oyama et al. 2004; Samuelsson and Åsberg 2002; Szántó et al. 2007; Valentini et al. 2004) in agreement with Rutz's work as well as with many of the studies reviewed by Mann et al. (2005), for example, Hannaford et al. (1996), Kelly (1998), Lin et al. (2001), Naismith et al. (2001), Pfaff et al. (2001), Rihmer et al. (2001), Takahashi et al. (1998), all bear out that education may have suicide-preventive effects.

## The National Swedish Prevention of Suicide and Mental Ill-Health (NASP) training programmes

Ultimately aiming at reducing suicide rates in the population, the training programmes at NASP, the Karolinska Institute, Stockholm, Sweden where both authors are active, have the objective of disseminating scientific knowledge and inspiring a science-based attitude to suicide prevention. The mental health professionals, social planners, administrators, and researchers who are students in the programmes are also regarded as suicide-preventive key persons who in turn are expected to influence the attitudes of others.

The programmes include arrangements in which students reflect on their personal values and attitudes to suicide. This emphasis, which in part derives from the clinical orientation and training of the NASP faculty and has evolved from the encounters with students from different professional and cultural backgrounds, does not exclude a parallel focus on the importance for mental health or ill-health of medical, physical, economical, and social conditions. These and other aspects, such as the availability of means for taking one's life, or cultural and social pressures, may play a role similar to that of attitudes in tipping the scale of the complex interaction of factors that in the end may either elicit or prevent a suicide.

The mixed professional background of the students is in harmony with the assumption that suicide can be fully elucidated only with a multidisciplinary approach. Although there is consensus on this view among researchers worldwide, implementing a multidisciplinary framework when teaching suicide prevention can be difficult. Not only do lecturers and seminar leaders need to be skilled in their respective subspecialties, but, in order to communicate effectively with students with heterogeneous professional backgrounds, they also need to be able to present their work in a theoretically integrated way and to place it within a framework of a complex stress–vulnerability model of mental health and ill-health. Taking into account that students will have emotionally coloured attitudes not only to suicidal patients or individuals, but also to competing theories on suicide, we face a challenge in promoting reflection and openness to the complexities of topic(s).

A particular facet of suicidal behaviours, which almost paradoxically has come to light in the research-oriented programmes rather than in the clinical ones (in which this perhaps is taken for granted), is that the real-life interface between the prevention specialist or researcher and the real or imagined beneficiary of the prevention efforts, for example, an individual member of a population cohort, is psychological. Depressive affect, anxiety, and the wish to die all belong to subjective experience, even when these phenomena are studied in terms of neurobiology, epidemiology, anthropology, or some specialized causal hypothesis in psychology. The prevention worker's attitudes to suicide prevention are affected by actual experiences, which may have been gratifying or disappointing, as well as by privately motivated and envisioned expectations, hopes, and fears about influencing—ultimately saving—suicidal individuals. Whether a clinician or a researcher, the engaged professional may empathize, neglect, outright reject, or directly or indirectly expose the vulnerable individual to mixtures of these attitudes. Clinicians usually appreciate the opportunity to address countertransference issues, i.e. their emotional response to suicidal individuals (Maltsberger and Buie 1972). It is a recurring experience that our research and master students, too, ask for seminars in which their personal values and views on suicide may be discussed.

### Suicide prevention: theory and practice

This programme is a one and-a-half-year, part-time course for physicians, nurses, social workers, and psychologists working in psychiatry, child and adolescent psychiatry, general medicine, and social services. It has been given as a specialization single-subject course at Karolinska Institutet on a regular basis since 1993 (Wasserman 1993). The first programme, which was organized as a part time, 200-hour course covering two years, but condensed into a one-and-half year, three-semester programme in 2003 (with the same number of hours), gives an orientation on neurobiological, epidemiological, social, psychological, philosophical, and historical perspectives on suicide. Lectures are given on pharmacological and psychotherapeutic treatment strategies and on prevention programmes for near-suicide patients as well as for non-clinical vulnerable groups such as refugees and immigrants, the aged, and the young.

In closed small-group seminars that run throughout the entire course, students have the opportunity to relate their newly acquired theoretical knowledge to previous habits of thought and to clinical experiences. Through role playing the students also learn to lead a psychological autopsy after a suicide or a suicide attempt. The seminars are lead by clinically experienced and psychotherapeutically trained group leaders.

In addition to attending lectures and seminars, the students in this programme carry out a suicide-preventive research and development project in their workplaces with supervision from the NASP faculty, and describe it in a written report. Examples of topics for such projects are: writing local guidelines for the care of psychiatric patients at risk for suicide, or routines for the support and follow-up of individuals hospitalized after a suicide attempt; organizing courses in suicide prevention and support of trainers and supervisors; local epidemiological or small-scale treatment studies; carrying out and evaluating psychological autopsies; writing a qualified research plan, for example, for a doctoral dissertation in suicidology or suicide prevention. Together with the reflection and dialogue in the seminar groups, the implementation of a suicide-preventive project constitutes an accommodative element of the programme, aimed at fostering integration of the material given in the lectures (Piaget 1958; Wasserman 1993).

In a doctoral dissertation, Ramberg (2003), using questionnaires, studied the impact of the programme on the students' and their workplaces (Aish *et al.* 2000; Ramberg and Wasserman 2000, 2003, 2004a, b). The respondents, all from Stockholm, were 617 psychiatric co-workers who filled out the questionnaires before, immediately after, and one-and-a-half years after the completed programme. Half of the respondents worked in training units from which personnel were sent to the programme. The other half worked in non-trained units and served as controls. The main findings were that the respondents in the training units were to a significant extent more positive about working with suicidal patients after the programme than were those working in control units. Another observation was that the wish for training was greatest among psychiatric nurses and assistant nurses, whereas physicians and psychologists either tended to believe that they were already sufficiently knowledgeable in the field, or state that they did not wish to study it. The strengthening of the psychiatric personnel's motivation and sense of security in working with suicidal patients was significant in the training units regardless of which treatments methods they believed to be the best. In a subsequent study Ramberg and Wasserman (2003, 2004a, b) found that programme graduates often encounter organizational or other difficulties that stand in the way of implementing their suicide-preventive expertise. We conclude that, although an immediate impact on the conscious attitudes of psychiatric co-workers—participating students as well as their colleagues—was documented, further studies are called for to clarify the organizational obstacles and personal inhibitions that often stand in the way of suicide-preventive initiatives in the psychiatric workplace. The role of unacknowledged ambivalent attitudes to suicide prevention should also be studied in this context.

## Love is the Best Kick

This is the name of a three-day training programme for teachers and other gatekeepers, including clinicians in child and adolescent psychiatry, who are accessible for young people for discussing important but difficult existential issues. The name of the programme is the same as that of a 46-minute documentary film, jointly produced by NASP and the Swedish film director Göran Setterberg. Four young adults are portrayed in the film. All four, two men and two women, have survived a suicide attempt during adolescence and they describe the struggle, each person in their own way, to find a new orientation and a stable identity as an adult in the years following the suicidal crisis.

The participants in this course learn to use the film to stimulate discussions with young people. Basics of adolescent psychology are included in the programme, as is the importance of creating a psychologically safe and respectful setting for the intended discussions. Participants who complete the programme receive a copy of the film, teaching materials, and a certificate authorizing them to use the film in schools, youth centres, and other appropriate settings.

The impact on young persons who watch the film and take part in a guided discussion was evaluated by Alin-Åkerman (2002). The specific focus of the evaluation was whether this experience strengthens the youngster's awareness of and ability to deal with the life challenges they are facing. Two groups of secondary school students were compared. Both groups included individuals with suicide-related problems and others without known problems. Participants in the intervention group saw the film, took part in a group discussion, and were interviewed and tested with psychological tests before and after the intervention. Those in the control group were interviewed and tested at the same intervals without having seen the film or having taken part in an organized discussion.

The young men and women in the intervention group, whether they were known to have suicide-related problems or not, appreciated the opportunity to talk about important issues about life and death in a safe context. They all underscored that there was little room for such exchanges in their everyday lives and that they would normally hesitate to burden others with their concerns, or to openly expose these thoughts to others. It was clear that the film worked a catalyst for these discussions.

As to the attitudes of school staff and mental health professionals who take part in the training programme, the encounter with the personal fates of the four young adults featured in the film usually has an immediate and rather dramatic impact. In course evaluations the participants report that they left the programme wanting to do more to help the young. However, as the empathic identification with a suicidal person individual is easily offset by a simultaneous impulse to withdraw from him or her (Titelman 1997; Wolk-Wasserman 1985, 1986), there is a great need to support those who make themselves available as partners for serious conversation and relationship-building with the young. Again, attitude 'maintenance' is a necessary supplement to mere inspiration.

*Love is the Best Kick*—the film, the course, and the study manual—works well as a tool for communicating with adolescents. The programme adds structure and motivation to those who work with the young in schools and other relevant locations and provides opportunities to discuss issues that may otherwise remain secret and drive a lonely young person to destructive acting out.

### A research course on the scientific evaluation of interventions aimed at preventing mental ill-health and suicide

This annual, one-week research course was initiated in 2000 as a mental-health module of the World Health Programme, a postgraduate scheme supported by the Karolinska International Research and Training Committee (KIRT) at the Division of International Health (IHCAR) at Karolinska Institutet. The focus of the course week is primarily on epidemiology, although there has been some variation in content. The course attracts PhD students and established researchers from all over the world, who are given the opportunity to present their own work during the course week. Some participants return year after year to what in effect has evolved as an international network of researchers in suicidology and suicide prevention.

In 2006 the course had a clinical perspective that included the evaluation of psychotherapies with suicidal patients (Hendin *et al.* 2006) and presentations of psychoanalytically informed experiential as well as group-based studies focusing on the interaction of psychological development, traumatization and biological, social, and psychological vulnerability and protective factors.

In their evaluations of the course in 2006, students reported that it was meaningful to reflect on the experiential dimensions of their research subjects when these were envisioned men or women in risk of suicide in an otherwise relatively anonymous research context. To mention one example where the added psychological dimension was rewarding, a project on the role of the media in instigating suicidal behaviour among adolescents was dramatically enriched by the opportunity for the project leader to reflect on group psychology and identification phenomena with the aid of psychoanalytic theories.

### Master programme in public health sciences with a focus on mental health promotion and suicide prevention

The master programme was first given as a one-year programme, which in addition to applying the stress–vulnerability paradigm, included an orientation in public health science as well as courses in quantitative and qualitative research methodology. Specific courses focusing on population-based suicide prevention were also included, for example, 'The environmental fraction in the causation of suicide and how it can it be controlled', 'The role of the media in facilitating or preventing suicide', and 'Clinical and nonclinical population groups vulnerable to suicide.'

The programme attracted students with academic backgrounds in medicine, psychology and sociology. Although the principal focus of the programme was on research and public health perspectives, as the programme advanced, the students' interests gravitated towards clinical and philosophical issues, foremost questions about the right to choose death, and on their own emotional responses to the topic. In line with these interests, a two-week course on ethics in research in mental health and suicide research was perceived by the students as a high point in the programme. Questions that were addressed in the ethics course were, for example: Is suicide ever acceptable? Should it always be prevented? What are our own values and fears towards suicide and towards talking openly about it? In the generally positive student evaluations of this programme one complaint recurred: it was felt to be too condensed, too intense.

A new, two-year master programme, which replaced the one-year programme in the autumn of 2007, is designed according to the principles of so-called Bologna Declaration, an agreement on synchronizing higher education in Europe, signed by forty-six countries. The two-year programme is open to international researchers, research-interested clinicians, social planners, and other qualified professionals with an interest either in the training programme in its entirety or in topics addressed in single-subject course modules within the programme.

The content of the previous master programme is extended in the two-year programme with course modules on psychophysiological stress research and on salutogenic perspectives on mental health, including cultural and anthropological aspects. The fourth term is devoted to an advanced level, 30-credit (European Credit Transfer and Accumulation System, ECTS) master thesis.

## A scientific attitude

In the context of the mentioned methodological and epistemological challenges—the complex nature of attitudes to suicide, the centrality of psychological dimensions of suicidal behaviours, the overlap between individual- and population-based approaches, and the multifactorial, biopsychosocial explanatory perspective—it is relevant to underscore a particular element of a scientific attitude: the ability to suspend judgement when faced with the complex causation and the phenomenological ambiguity of suicide-nearness and suicide. This ability complements other aspects of a scientific approach, such as separating observations from inference and otherwise safeguarding the reliability and validity of one's work. It must sometimes be upheld in the face of pressures to provide simple answers, although, in clinical situations, when the immediate task is to save a life, direct and unambiguous action is usually necessary. The following example of being pressed to take action in an extreme situation, yet able to think clearly enough to postpone acting, was given by a student in one of our programmes who unexpectedly found herself in a situation in which she was pushed not to save a life, but to promote a death:

> As an unplanned effect of his treatment, a somatically ill, elderly patient in our unit had lost consciousness and was given life-sustaining treatment. His family agreed with the head of the unit that it would be appropriate and in agreement with the patient's own wishes to discontinue his life-sustaining treatment. There was little reason [except for a sound scepticism about the objectivity of any close relative of any individual] to question that the family's assessment was made in earnest. I could not, however, make myself carry out his recommendation and instruct the staff to 'pull the plug', I just couldn't do it. After some time, the patient came to and was grateful for having been restored to life. I, too, was grateful for having had the presence to think about the fragility of the wish to live under such difficult circumstances, and about the possibility that the patient had other wishes simultaneously to wishing to die, as we had discussed in the programme. I felt strengthened by what I had learned about the

risk for drawing quick conclusions with regard to an allegedly unambiguous wish to end your life.

(Student's personal communication. Words within brackets added).

## Addressing the suicide taboo

When confronted with what is destructive in life, our inclination to oversimplification or avoidance may in part be caused by anxiety. Life's destructive sides include physical decay and mental disintegration in old age, but also the self-destructiveness seen in serious psychopathology. Is not anxiety, in fact, generally at work behind a phobic attitude to both suicide and suicide prevention? Miscalculated ideas and actions on the part of close relatives, medical staff, social workers, and psychotherapists are in any case not uncommon in interactions with suicidal individuals, particularly, perhaps, with the young, whom we simply do not wish to perceive as suicidal (Laufer 1995). As noted, in clinical work, such responses are understood as reflecting countertransference difficulties, sometimes including unconscious hate of the suicidal patient (Gabbard 2003; Kernberg 2004; Maltsberger and Buie 1972; Winnicott 1958; Wolk-Wasserman 1985, 1987).

We have emphasized that suicidality in real life is always presented as a psychological event: the conscious wish to die is consciousness, or, more specifically, a self-consciousness disorder. As such it is something distinctly human, related to, among other things, the capacity for guilt feelings. It is noteworthy in this context that Kandel (2005), whose focus is neurobiological, has pointed out that malignant self-destructiveness (of which inordinate self-punitive tendencies may be a derivative) is a response to severe stress that is specifically human, a reaction not found in other mammals. The therapist's or scientific investigator's—or the suicide-preventive gatekeeper's—emotional response to the suicidal person, which can shift between engagement and indifference and which probably always includes an element of identification (sometimes in the form of aggressive, 'projective identification'), is a similarly human reaction in the service of ridding oneself of anxiety as well as of finding a way of remaining open to the patient to be helped or to the scientific question to be explored. Whatever applies in the individual situation, the aversion against suicide merits being approached with caution and reflection; it, too, is an aspect of the human predicament and may even reflect a human potential for suicide.

In trying to strengthen the capacity of students for intellectual and emotional containment of the challenges of suicide and suicidal behaviour, the timing of didactic interventions is critical. When we have invited students to reflect on their own attitudes too early, they have sometimes responded with discomfort and an unwillingness to open up to the questions. A typical disavowing a reaction has been: 'Why this? We are here to learn science, not discuss philosophy.' When, on the other hand, we have postponed such discussions too long, we have received evaluations such as 'Great programme, but too little time to reflect on the "philosophy of suicide" and on our own attitudes'. Our overall experience is that students, struggling to understand suicide and developing their professional skills in working with suicide prevention, gradually appreciate that suicidality always has multiple meanings and causes, which, particularly in the case of a complete suicide may not be knowable, and that epistemological and practical–philosophical reflection, including disciplined self-reflection, are essential in the quest to understand these phenomena.

Educational efforts in the mental health field need to be renewed and repeated continuously. As assimilative learning needs to be supplemented by accommodative activity in cognitive development, training events of different kinds need to be followed by new in- or output—inviting students to generate knowledge *actively* is crucial—to maintain and fortify the effects of teaching programmes (Wasserman 1993). Students, further, probably need to achieve a personal identification with their teachers or mentors to carry on as influential teachers themselves.

## Conclusion

Education frequently has an impact on the conscious attitudes to suicide and its prevention, but it is difficult to gauge the effects of educational programmes on deep-seated and relatively fixed attitudes and on the students' character-grounded anxieties and defences related to the topic of suicide.

The question remains whether the influence of education is lasting and whether educational programmes affect unconscious, ambivalent attitudes to suicide prevention at all. The challenge of addressing this and other questions in suicidology and suicide prevention will hopefully fall upon researchers who combine scientific specialization with an ability to reflect on socially, culturally and individually varied perceptions of the suicidal predicament as well as of the ways in which we try to counteract it.

## References

Aish AM, Ramberg IL, Wasserman D (2000). Measuring attitudes of mental health-care staff towards suicidal patients. *Archives of Suicide Research*, **6**, 309–323.

Alin-Åkerman B (2002). How do we find and support the vulnerable students? In *Decade of Reform: Achievements, Challenges, Problems*. II, pp. 364–369. Conference on second generation reforms, IMF Headquarters, Washington, DC. Klaipedia, Klaipedia University, Lithuania.

DeLeo D (2002). Why are we not getting any closer to preventing suicide? *British Journal of Psychiatry*, **181**, 372–374.

Eberhard G, Holmberg G, von Knorring A-L et al. (1992). *Diagnostik och Behandling av Depressioner* [Diagnostics and treatment of depression]. Eskils Tryckeri AB, Sweden.

Gabbard GO (2003). Miscarriages of psychoanalytic treatments with suicidal patients. *International Journal of Psychoanalysis*, **84**, 249–261.

Hannaford PC, Thompson C, Simpson M (1996). Evaluation of an educational programme to improve the recognition of psychological illness by general practitioners. *British Journal of General Practice*, **46**, 333–337.

Hendin H, Haas AP, Maltsberger JT et al. (2006). Problems in psychotherapy with suicidal patients. *American Journal of Psychiatry*, **163**, 67–72.

Kandel ER (2005). *Psychiatry, Psychoanalysis, and the New Biology of Mind*. American Psychiatric Association, Arlington.

Kelly C (1998). The effects of depression awareness seminars on general practitioners knowledge of depressive illness. *Ulster Medical Journal*, **67**, 33–35.

Kernberg OF (2004). *Aggressivity, Narcissism, and Self-destructiveness in the Psychotherapeutic Relationship*. Yale, New Haven and London.

Laufer ME (1995). A research study into adolescent suicide. In M Laufer, ed., *The Suicidal Adolescent*, pp. 103–118. Karnac, London.

Lin EH, Simon GE, Katzelnick DJ *et al.* (2001). Does physician education on depression management improve treatment in primary care? *Journal of General Internal Medicine*, **16**, 614–619.

Maltsberger JT and Buie DH (1972). Countertransference hate in the treatment of suicidal patients. *Archives of General Psychiatry*, **30**, 625–633.

Mann A, Apter A, Bertolote J *et al.* (2005). Suicide prevention strategies: a systematic review. *Journal of American Medical Association*, **294**, 2064–2074.

Naismith SL, Hickie IB, Scott EM *et al.* (2001). Effects of mental health training and clinical audit on general practitioners' management of common mental disorders. *The Medical Journal of Australia*, **175**, 42–47.

Oyama H, Koida J, Sakashita T *et al.* (2004). Community-based prevention for suicide in elderly by depression screening and follow-up. *Community Mental Health Journal*, **40**, 249–263.

Pfaff JJ, Acres JG, McKelvey RS (2001). Training general practitioners to recognise and respond to psychological distress and suicidal ideation in young people. *The Medical Journal of Australia*, **174**, 222–226.

Piaget J (1958). *The Development of Thought: Equilibrium of Cognitive Structures*. Viking, New York.

Ramberg IL (2003). Promoting suicide prevention: an evaluation of a programme for training trainers in psychiatric clinical work. Doctoral dissertation, Department of Public Health Sciences, Karolinska Institutet, Stockholm.

Ramberg IL and Wasserman D (2000). Prevalence of reported suicidal behaviour in the general population and mental health-care staff. *Psychological Medicine*, **30**, 1189–1196.

Ramberg IL and Wasserman D (2003). The roles of knowledge and supervision in work with suicidal patients. *Nordic Journal of Psychiatry*, **57**, 365–371.

Ramberg IL and Wasserman D (2004a). Benefits of implementing an academic training of trainers program to promote knowledge and clarity in work with psychiatric suicidal patients. *Archives of Suicide Research*, **8**, 331–343.

Ramberg IL and Wasserman D (2004b). Suicide-preventive activities in psychiatric care: evaluation of an educational programme in suicide prevention. *Nordic Journal of Psychiatry*, **58**, 389–394.

Rihmer Z, Belso N, Kalmar S (2001). Antidepressants and suicide prevention in Hungary. *Acta Psychiatrica Scandinavica*, **103**, 238–239.

Rutz W (1992). Evaluation of an educational program on depressive disorders given to general practitioners in Gotland: Short- and long-term effects. Doctoral Dissertation. Linköping University, Sweden, Linköping.

Rutz W and Wålinder J (2000). Depressions behandling i primärvården – kompetens, engagemang och empati ger resultat [Treatment of depression in primary care: competence, engagement, and empathy yield results]. *Läkartidningen*, **97**, 3638–3639.

Rutz W, von Knorring J *et al.* (1995). Prevention of male suicides: lessons from Gotland study. *Lancet*, **345**, 524.

Rutz W, Wålinder J *et al.* (1989). An educational program on depressive disorders for general practitioners on Gotland: background and evaluation. *Acta Psychiatrica Scandinavica*, **79**, 19–26.

Samuelsson M and Asberg M (2002). Training program in suicide prevention for psychiatric nursing personnel enhance attitudes to attempted suicide patients. *International Journal of Nursing Studies*, **39**, 115–121.

Szantó K, Kalmar S, Hendin H *et al.* (2007). A suicide prevention program in a region with a very high suicide rate. *Archives of General Psychiatry*, **64**, 914–920.

Takahashi K, Naito H, Morita M *et al.* (1998). Suicide prevention for the elderly in Matsunoyama Town, Higashikubiki County, Niigata Prefecture: psychiatric care for elderly depression in the community [in Japanese]. *Seishin Shinkeigaku Zasshi*, **100**, 469–485.

Titelman D (1997). Survivor siblings: the case of schizophrenia. A response to 'Impact of Adolescent Suicide on Siblings and Parents' by Brent, Moritz, Bridge, Perper, and Canobbio. *Suicide and Life-Threatening Behaviour*, **27**, 323–324.

Wasserman D (1993). The role of transference and countertransference in the teaching and learning of suicidology. In U Bille-Brahe and H Schildt, eds, *Intervention and Prevention: Proceedings from the 4th European Symposium on Suicidal Behaviour*, pp. 127–129. University Press of Southern Denmark, Odense.

Wasserman D ed. (2001a). *Suicide—An Unnecessary Death*. Martin Dunitz, London.

Wasserman D (2001b). A stress–vulnerability model and the development of the suicidal process. In D Wasserman, ed., *Suicide—An Unnecessary Death*, pp. 13–28. Martin Dunitz, London.

Winnicott DW (1958). Hate in the countertransference. In DW Winnicott, ed., *Through Paediatrics to Psycho-analysis*, pp. 194–203. Tavistock, London.

Wolk-Wasserman D (1985). The intensive care unit and the suicide attempt patient. *Acta Psychiatrica Scandinavica*, **71**, 581–595.

Wolk-Wasserman D (1986). Suicidal communication of persons attempting suicide and responses of significant others. *Acta Psychiatrica Scandinavica*, **73**, 481–499.

Wolk-Wasserman D (1987). Some problems connected with the treatment of suicide attempt patients: transference and countertransference aspects. *Crisis*, **8**, 69–82.

Valentini W, Levav I Kohn R et al. (2004). An educational training programme for physicians for diagnosis and treatment of depression [in Portuguese]. *Rev Saude Publica*, **38**, 522–528.

# CHAPTER 69

# The role of mass-media in suicide prevention

Michael Westerlund, Sylvia Schaller and Armin Schmidtke

## Abstract

Although disputed, most researchers in the field of suicide and mass media agree that the studies carried out to date have substantiated the existence, under certain circumstances, of genuine suicidal 'contagion' from suicide reports in the media. The fact that many studies have demonstrated an association between media reporting of suicide and actual suicidal behaviour has also prompted the issue of various types of recommendations on how the media *should* report on the subject of suicide to avoid imitative behaviour. The purpose of this chapter is to discuss and identify the problems associated with research on suicide and the media, with a number of seminal articles published over the years serving as examples.

## Introduction

Fear of people imitating suicidal behaviour described in the media can be traced back to the publication in 1774 of Wolfgang von Goethe's epistolary novel *The Sorrows of Young Werther*. In it, the young hero, downcast because of unrequited love, takes his life by shooting himself. Under the novel's influence, many young European men apparently emulated Werther's self-destructive act. The authorities' fears of a proliferation in juvenile suicides resulted in the book being banned in Italy, Leipzig and Copenhagen. Whether the novel did indeed precipitate a suicide epidemic has never been reliably established, but the American sociologist D P Phillips (1974) coined the expression 'Werther effect' to denote a putative relationship between media accounts of suicidal acts and individuals' imitation of this behaviour.

Over the years, research has been conducted on various forms of media, such as the daily press, television, film, music, literature and the Internet, and dealt with fiction as well as authentic accounts of real cases. Almost without exception, these studies belong in the tradition that may be termed 'social psychology' or public health research on the media reports' *effects* on individuals.

Although the results are not unequivocal, research on imitation effects indicate that media coverage of suicide can precipitate suicidal behaviour in some cases. Here, the word 'precipitate' should be emphasized, since this type of research on effects does not deal with any long-term, attitude-moulding aspects of the media. Nor do the majority of studies pay any attention to *which* individuals are at higher or lower risk of being affected by the media's suicide coverage, except that some studies indicate what appears to be a higher risk for adolescents than for their elders. Littmann (1985) emphasizes that 'copycat suicides' can hardly be deemed to stem solely from media influence. In his view, the victims concerned must already be in states that make them extremely susceptible to various types of media representation. Wasserman (1984) and Stack (1987), too, have asserted that the imitation effects of the media's suicide coverage are considerably more limited than many researchers have claimed, and that they arise almost exclusively from reports on celebrities' suicidal acts. Nonetheless, most researchers in this field agree that the studies carried out to date have substantiated the existence, under certain circumstances, of genuine suicidal 'contagion' from suicide reports in the media: 'Media accounts are potentially harmful: how suicide is described in the news contributes to what behavioural scientists call "suicide contagion" or copycat suicides' (Becker *et al.* 2004, p. 112).

In this chapter, the problems associated with research on suicide and the media are discussed, with a number of seminal articles published over the years serving as examples. The selection of articles and studies conforms in major respects to extensive summaries and meta-analyses of this research field, notably those by Schmidtke and Schaller (2000), Pirkis and Blood (2001), Gould (2001) and Stack (2005). This presentation is confined to exemplifying and discussing results from studies of the daily press and television, where the absolute majority of surveys of suicide and the media conducted to date have dealt with these two media. Where television is concerned, studies of both fictional and non-fictional events are included. The chapter ends with a summary and discussion of methodological and theoretical aspects of the research. The Internet is covered in a separate chapter.

# Newspaper studies

### How is suicide presented in the daily press?

Studies dealing with the manner in which the media portray suicidal acts are relatively limited in number, and consist primarily of investigations of the daily press. It is important to note that this type of media coverage varies from one country and continent to another, partly owing to publicity rules and traditions and to legislation. How often suicidal events are reported, where in the newspaper such reports are located, how the headlines are worded and how far the repercussions of suicide are presented as positive or negative are examples of the kinds of differences that have attracted attention (Schmidtke and Schaller 2000).

In one study, which may largely be said to summarize what many previous investigations have indicated, official cause of death data were compared with reported suicides in five major Hong Kong-based dailies in the year 2000 (Au *et al.* 2004). According to the official sources, there were 902 suicides during the year and the newspapers reported on 422 of these, in a total of 978 different articles. In a third of the cases, photographs were published. In over 70 per cent of the news articles, the suicide victims were named. The method used was mentioned in the headline in more than 90 per cent of the reports on suicide cases. Description of these cases was also clearly selective: considerably more attention was paid to adolescents' suicides than to their elders', and the publications tended more often to report suicides where the persons concerned were married or unemployed. Suicides in which the cause had been associated to partner problems were over-reported, while suicides said to be caused by family-related problems were under-reported. In their summary and discussion of the results, the authors take the view that the press coverage of suicide cases is clearly sensation-oriented, stereotyped and incorrect, and that they depart entirely from, for example, the World Health Organization's (WHO) recommendations (WHO 2000) on how suicidal events should be reported. The real-life situation based on official data and the real-life situation described by the dailies often diverge, and by extension, this may result in the public being misled and having mistaken perceptions of the reasons why certain people commit suicide.

Previous studies have also pinpointed a discrepancy between media representations of suicide and official data. In the view of Fishman and Weiman (1997), news reporting of suicide is based on stereotypes, myths and sheer errors, and this is serious in view of the news media's pivotal role in societies. The authors compared the causes of suicide as presented in two Israeli dailies with official data on causes of death between 1972 and 1988. In their comparison, they refer to similarities and differences between 'mediated reality' and 'official reality'. The official data contained particulars of individuals' sex, age, nationality, marital status and, where known, cause of suicide. Of a total of 4164 official suicidal events, the newspapers reported 1885. Overall, the analysis showed that adolescents and the Arab population were over-represented in the Israeli newspapers' reports of suicidal events. References to financial straits and love problems were also over-represented in the dailies, while mental problems were under-represented as causes of suicidal events. Official data also showed that disappointments associated to love relationships were a significant cause of men's suicidal acts, but in the mediated reality of the press, this motive was treated as unimportant and, instead, presented as more of a reason for female suicides.

A number of content analyses of European daily newspapers indicate this bias, moreover, in the reporting of suicidal events (Shepard and Barraclough 1978; Gappmair 1980; Tantalo and Marchiori 1981; Kuess and Hatzinger 1986; Michel *et al.* 1995; Fekete and Schmidtke 1996). In summary, these studies show that:

- Reports on celebrities' suicidal acts are given most coverage;
- The emphasis is laid on suicides in which violent or unusual methods are used;
- A disproportionately large share of reports cover adolescent suicides;
- Underlying causes of suicidal acts are often neglected;
- Information on other options and preventive measures is usually lacking.

# Is there any relation between newspapers' presentation of suicide and actual suicidal behaviour?

For three early studies of the impact of media on individuals' suicidal behaviour, the initial assumption was that the absence of coverage in the daily press comprising suicide reports would result in a decrease in the number of actual suicides in the community (Motto 1967, 1970; Blumentahl and Bergner 1973). Suicide data from periods of press strikes and lockouts in the USA were analysed on this basis and compared with data during periods when press distribution functioned normally. None of the surveys showed any general decline in the number of suicide cases. However, the two later studies demonstrated a certain decrease, during the periods when newspapers were not published, in the number of suicides among women aged under 35.

In a 1974 study, Phillips adopted a reverse approach and investigated, instead, the suicide rate during the months when daily newspapers in the USA reported on suicidal events on their front pages. These results showed a significant rise in the number of suicides after twenty-six cases of front-page coverage, and a decrease in the number of suicides in seven cases. Two key factors that Phillips demonstrated were that the increase in suicides was correlated with the amount of publicity given to suicide cases on the front pages of newspapers, and the fact that this effect was most pronounced among younger people.

Since its publication, the Phillips study has been developed and replicated by a number of researchers. The results from these studies are, however, not entirely congruent. Unlike Phillips, Wasserman's (1984) study demonstrated no general rise in national suicide rates in the USA during the months when suicidal events were reported on the newspapers' front pages, compared with the months when there were no such reports. On the other hand, a significant increase in suicide rates was found in the months when material concerning celebrities' suicides was published on the front pages. In line with this finding, Stack (1987), too, found evidence that the only associations with elevated suicide rates that were discernible were for reports on artists' and politicians' suicides. In further analysis of the same material, however, Stack (1990a) found that suicide rates also rose, but not to the same extent, when non-celebrities' suicides were reported. Like Phillips' results, both Wasserman's and Stack's studies showed that suicide rates rise in proportion to the quantity of material published about suicide cases.

Most studies, of whether newspapers prompt imitation (or 'copycat') effects in terms of an increase in suicidal behaviour, were based on American conditions and data. This has prompted researchers to urge caution to avoid excessively far-reaching interpretations and generalizations of these results. Sucessively, surveys in other countries and continents have been carried out. Jonas (1992) compared suicide figures from the German state of Baden-Würtemberg during the period 1968–1980 with newspaper articles on famous people's suicides during the same period. The suicide figures registered daily entailed an improvement in methods compared with the previous American studies, which were based on suicide figures at an aggregate level, thereby excluding scope for reliably stating whether a suicide took place before or after the newspapers' reports on a specific suicide case. Jonas's analyses indicated a significant increase in the number of suicides during the weeks after suicide coverage in the press. Moreover, in two separate studies analysing the relation between Japanese dailies' coverage of suicides and actual suicides, the authors were able to demonstrate a significant increase in suicides during the months in which suicide reports appeared in the press (Ishii 1991; Stack 1996).

There have also been studies in which the problem area has been approached in virtually the opposite way, i.e. by identifying and starting with actual suicides rather than media coverage of suicide cases. Barraclough et al. (1977), for example, identified all the suicides taking place in Portsmouth (UK) between 1970 and 1972, and then collected articles and notices about suicide cases from the local daily from approximately the same period. They were able to work out the probability of suicides taking place in the days after newspaper coverage of suicides, and compare it with the probability of there *not* being any suicides in the days after the coverage. For men under the age of 45, the number of suicides rose significantly after newspaper coverage of suicide, but this did not apply to women or older men. A similar Canadian study, however, did not succeed in demonstrating any direct correlation between media reporting and actual suicides (Littmann 1985).

Regarding gender differences, Hassan (1995) demonstrated a significant increase in the number of suicides among men after publication in Australian dailies of articles about suicide events. This increase was not to be found among women. This gender difference was assumed to be due to the press mainly reporting men's suicidal acts, thereby boosting the risk of copycat behaviour among men in particular. Men also read these dailies to a larger extent than women.

Support has also been cited for the incidence of suicide clusters (defined as time-limited series of further suicidal acts, such as suicide attempts, by susceptible individuals) after reporting of specific suicides in the daily press. In two articles, Ashton and Donnan (1979, 1981), point to an almost epidemic increase in the number of suicides by burning in England and Wales in the year after a political suicide that was highly publicized in the press in which this method was used. Veysey et al. (1999), too, reported a rise in the number of suicides in the UK by means of glycol poisoning after an investigation of this method had been reported in one daily, *The Independent*.

## Television

### Is there any relation between TV programmes about suicide and actual suicidal behaviour?

#### General studies

One example of a general structural research approach is Lester's (1994) survey of the relationship between suicide rates for adolescents in the years 1960–1970, and American households' TV ownership during the same period. Lester did not find that fluctuations in suicide rates were related to changes in TV ownership, but he found that they were correlated with household income.

In an Australian study, senior school pupils from three randomly selected schools answered a set of questions about TV-watching habits, including the types of content they preferred to watch, and underwent a series of validated tests for depression, risk-taking behaviour, suicidal behaviour and drug use (Martin 1996). To summarize, the results showed that the pupils who stated that they had watched more than two programmes about suicide on television also, to a higher degree, subjected themselves to risks, took more drugs, watched more videos and had more personal experience of attempted suicide and depression. In a subsequent pilot study of a more qualitative nature, 12 subjects aged 17–25 who had recently had self-harming episodes were interviewed about their experience of the media and suicide, and about whether they felt that they themselves had been influenced by media accounts of suicides (Zahl and Hawton 2004). The majority stated that they had been influenced by media coverage, and four of the respondents thought that specific programmes had induced them to harm themselves.

#### Non-fictional presentations

A high proportion of the studies concerning TV programmes about suicide confirm the above-mentioned studies regarding press reporting of suicide events and actual suicides. Bollen and Phillips (1982) showed that suicide numbers rose during a ten-day period after a suicide report in a TV news programme. Phillips and Carstensen (1986) showed a significant rise in the number of teenage suicides during seven-day periods after TV news about suicides. It was notable that this occurred irrespective of whether the news concerned individuals' suicide acts or consisted of reports of a more general nature on the subject of suicide. In a further study, material relating to the state of California was analysed (Phillips and Carstensen 1988). These results, too, showed that there was a significant correlation between TV coverage of suicide and actual suicidal acts. This correlation existed for all age groups, but was particularly strong for teenagers.

Stack (1990b) investigated the assocation between TV reporting of suicide events and the actual suicidal behaviour of elderly people's suicides, and analysed them in relation to national suicide data for the 65-and-over age group in the USA. The results showed that ten suicides were committed by elderly people in months where general TV news about suicide was broadcast. When TV specifically covered suicidal acts among elderly, an average of nineteen suicides monthly were committed by elderly people.

The studies described above thus indicate that there is an association between TV coverage of suicide and actual suicides. However, there are several studies that question this relationship. These include the study by Horton and Stack (1984) analysing the relationship between news about suicide on the American national

TV and nationwide suicide figures. After controlling for other variables, such as unemployment, divorces and seasonal effects, the analysis showed that there was no correlation between the TV news about suicide and actual suicides. Kessler *et al.* (1988, 1989) repeated the study by Phillips and Carstensens (1986). The period of analysis was extended, and televised material was collected from more archives than in the original study. The method of analysis was also improved, making it possible to define the degree of exposure to news about suicide. The results were partially contradictory, but indicated no distinct imitation effect.

In a subsequent Israeli study, the starting point was analysis of the impact of a documentary broadcast in which a young girl was interviewed about her suicide plans—plans that she then put into practice, committing suicide (Shoval *et al.* 2005). National suicide data eight weeks before and four weeks after the broadcast were compared with the same periods in the previous year. The results showed no significant difference in the number of suicides or suicide attempts between the period before and the period after the broadcast. However, a significant fall was noted in the age of individuals who performed suicide attempts in the week before the documentary was broadcast, compared with the same week in the previous year. In the week before the broadcast, the forthcoming documentary was given a great deal of publicity, and this prompted the authors to conclude that repeated broadcasts of documentaries about suicide may entail elevated risks for vulnerable individuals among the viewers.

### Fictional presentations

As for studies of the impact, of fictional accounts of suicide on actual suicide numbers, Holding (1975) investigated the effects of the TV series *Befrienders*, which was broadcast by the BBC in the UK over 11 weeks in 1972. The series was about Samaritans, an organization involved in suicide prevention, and each episode concerned a severe predicament that culminated in a suicidal situation. Holding compared the number of suicides and suicide attempts in Edinburgh ten weeks before the series was broadcast, during the series and ten weeks after it with the suicide figures in the corresponding periods in the previous three years, and also with those in the year after the series was broadcast. The results did not show any influence of the series on the numbers of either suicides or suicide attempts. On the other hand, the series did result in a rise in the number of people contacting Samaritans.

Several British studies have investigated the effects of an episode of *Eastenders*, the popular soap opera, in which the character Angie attempted suicide by taking a drug overdose with alcohol. Three small-scale studies identified an increase in the number of deliberate self-poisoning cases in the week after the episode was broadcast (Ellis and Walsh 1986; Fowler 1986; Sandler *et al.* 1986). The impact of this episode was also surveyed in two somewhat more extensive studies (Platt 1987; Williams *et al.* 1987). A significant increase in the number of suicide attempts among women, albeit not specifically those in the same age group as Angie, was shown. It was also possible to discern a rise among self-poisoning cases of the method used by the Angie character.

During the 1990s, a number of studies of the possible impact of the British hospital series *Casualty* on suicidal acts among viewers were carried out. Collins (1993) noted an increase in the number of teenage girls seeking care following a *Casualty* episode, in which a 15-year-old girl overdosed with paracetamol tablets.

Waldron *et al.* (1993), too, noted a rise in the number of women seeking care; but similar increases were also discernible on other occasions, and the authors, therefore, reached the opinion that the causes were seasonal, rather than a matter of the impact of a TV series. When the same episode was broadcast again in July 1993, its possible influence in cases of deliberate self-poisoning or self-harm was examined by Simkin *et al.* (1995). The results showed that although a certain increase in absolute figures was observed, there was no statistically significant correlation between the episode broadcast and cases of deliberate self-poisoning or self-harm.

In November 1996, another episode of *Casualty* was broadcast in which, again, a character (a pilot) attempted suicide by overdosing with paracetamol tablets. Hawton *et al.* (1999) investigated the possible effects of the episode in terms of the numbers of self-poisoning cases at accident and emergency departments and psychiatric clinics in the UK. It was not possible to demonstrate any relation between deaths from paracetamol poisoning and the episode broadcast. On the other hand, a significant increase was found in the number of cases of deliberate self-poisoning over a three-week period after the episode was broadcast, and especially of cases in which individuals had overdosed with paracetamol. In contrast, Pell and Murdoch (1999) noted a decrease in the number of cases of attempted suicide by deliberate self-poisoning in Scotland after the episode concerned had been broadcast. In another article by these authors, concerning the TV series *Casualty* and its impact, they expressed the view that paracetamol overdose is such a common means of self-poisoning that it is difficult to associate with its incidence the effects of specific media reports (Veysey *et al.* 1999). The results of their own study of the effects of a *Casualty* episode, in which a character attempted suicide by glycol poisoning, which is a method less common than the use of paracetamol, showed a significant increase in such cases in the month when the episode was broadcast.

The studies described above, about fictional representations, are all based on the broadcasting of a *single* episode describing individuals' suicidal behaviour and its impact on actual suicidal acts. A study by Schmidtke and Hafner (1988) took the opportunity to analyse the persistence of possible effects over time of a six-episode German series that was broadcast twice, in 1981 and 1982. The series was about a 19-year-old male student who commits suicide by jumping in front of a train. The results showed a significant increase, after the broadcasts in both years, in the number of suicides in which the victims used the same method as the student in the TV series. This effect persisted for at least 70 days and was most evident in men aged 15–19.

A number of researchers have also indicated that TV films and series dealing with suicide do not necessarily have adverse effects alone. Holding (1975), for example, postulated that broadcasting the TV series *Befrienders* represented an increase in awareness about the suicide prevention carried out by Samaritans, the British organization (which describes itself as 'a confidential emotional support service for anyone in the UK and Ireland'). O'Connor *et al.* (1999) also argues that broadcasting the 1996 episode of *Casualty* discussed above presumably increased public knowledge of the harmful effects that may result from a high intake of paracetamol.

The studies conducted in the USA obtained contradictory results regarding the association between fictional accounts of suicide and actual suicidal behaviour. Two studies showed an increase in the number of suicide attempts among adolescents in the aftermath of films about young people's suicidal acts being shown on TV (Ostroff *et al.* 1985; Gould and Shaffer 1986). Three follow-up studies for the same purpose, however, yielded the opposite results (Phillips and Paight 1987; Gould *et al.* 1988; Berman 1988). None of the studies showed any increase in the number of completed suicides among young people in connection with TV films about adolescents' suicidal acts being shown.

Another example of contradictory results has its starting point in Phillips's (1982) study of soaps' impact on actual suicides in the USA. The results showed that the number of suicides appeared to rise immediately after a soap episode with suicide as a theme had been broadcast. When Kessler and Stipp (1984) analysed the same data again, after correcting the data they found, in contrast to Phillips, that there was no correlation between soaps dealing with suicide and actual suicidal behaviour.

## Methodological aspects

### Studies on an aggregate level

In many of the surveys carried out, it cannot be reliably demonstrated that an account of a suicidal act was actually published before the observed increase in suicide (Baron and Reiss 1985). Moreover, no study has presented any actual evidence that people who took their lives after genuinely reading and absorbing a specific account of suicide (Schmidtke and Hafner 1988). Another central criticism is that, in the majority of cases, insufficient attention had been paid to the characteristics of either the suicide model or the imitator, or the interplay between the two (Baron and Reiss 1985). In the studies where sufficient attention had nonetheless been paid to these patterns, this interplay had occurred on a general level, for example between celebrities and non-celebrities, men and women or adolescents and non-adolescents. In two controlled studies, by McDonald and Range (1990) and Higgins and Range (1996), the methodological problems described above were largely avoided in that the researchers knew that the individuals concerned had actually seen the newspaper accounts, and that this took place before they were asked about their attitudes towards suicide. In studies of this type, it is also possible to control the characteristics of the suicide model, i.e. the manner in which the suicide event was presented. However, the problem with such studies is that the dependent variable is always a matter of individuals' attitudes towards suicide, for example the probability of the individual imitating suicidal behaviour that has been described. However, these attitudes do not necessarily have anything to do with actual behaviour, i.e. how the individuals then act (Pirkis and Blood 2001). It should also be added that the results from the two above-mentioned studies contained no indication that the survey participants might consider imitating suicidal acts after these acts had been reported in newspaper articles.

Studies of non-fictional TV representations of suicide do not, on the whole, provide as much evidence as the surveys of daily newspapers' coverage for the existence of an imitation effect (Pirkis and Blood 2001). However, Gould (2001), for example, argues that although previous studies in the area displayed a certain ambiguity in their results, subsequent studies support the assumption that an imitation effect does exist. Broadly speaking, the investigations of TV news programmes may be criticised on the same grounds as the studies of dailies, i.e. they fail to demonstrate that the accounts

of suicide events have genuinely preceded the actual suicides, or that the people who committed suicide had actually seen the TV programmes (Marks 1987; Mastroianni 1987). Neither do the majority of the studies take into account the characteristics of either the viewers or the suicide models, or the interplay between them (Clark 1989). Another aspect that should be borne in mind is that the majority of these studies were carried out in the USA and are based on the same data. This raises questions about the scope for generalizing the results to apply to other contexts (Pirkis and Blood 2001).

### Interaction between the media explorer and the responder

Studies of fictional accounts of suicide on television share the same methodological problems as those referred to above. In addition, the association between the programmes and the actual suicides is, overall, weaker than that between the latter and the non-fictional programmes (Pirkis and Blood 2001). Berman's (1988) view is that if it is true that fictional presentations of suicide may result in an imitation among individuals who view them, what this presumably involves is a complex interaction between the form taken by the programmes concerned and the traits of the viewers who watch them. Research in the field has not succeeded in exploring these factors or taking them into consideration. Some relevant and important questions that should be posed in response to the findings of these studies are:

1 Is there evidence that a person who subsequently commited suicide watched the film?

2 Is there evidence that the film influenced the person to commit suicide?

3 What characteristics describe those most predisposed to imitate a suicide stimulus?

4 What characteristics of the film stimulus make it more (or less) likely to stimulate an imitative suicide?

5 What are the true magnitude and duration of any observed effect?

6 Is there evidence for any beneficial outcome of the presentation of films depicting suicide?

7 Are those suicides which follow a film presentation likely to have occurred at some later date due to some other precipitant?

Berman's view is that these issues have been left unanswered in the studies that have been implemented concerning fictional accounts of suicide and their impact on actual suicides. However, Gould (2001) is of the opinion that, although many results may be said to be contradictory, there is nonetheless extensive evidence that even fictional representations of suicide can exert an imitation effect.

As for the contradictory results—and the contradictory *interpretations* of the results—to which studies of the media's imitation effect on suicidal behaviour have given rise, Schmidtke and Schaller (2000) point to an interesting fact. In their meta-analyses, they found that researchers with a more clinical background more often reach the conclusion that the media genuinely produce a suicidal imitation effect, while researchers with a more sociological background adopt a considerably more critical attitude towards such results in their studies. Moreover, researchers whose career bases are the research departments of media organizations have hardly ever come up with any results supporting the hypothesis that media accounts of suicide can be 'contagious'. The notion of researchers' background and subject affiliation affecting the research results produced in various ways is, perhaps, an uncomfortable truth; but it is decidedly not something specific to the research field of suicide and the media. On the contrary, this is very common in most areas where researchers from disparate scientific backgrounds meet. Neither need this be seen as something exclusively negative: based on a more interdisciplinary perspective, the various interpretations and results may be seen as enriching a discussion on the content of research and its choice of methods and theoretical foundations.

## Social learning theory

Research on the media's effects on actual suicidal behaviour has also been criticised for having a weak (or vague) theoretical basis. Thus, researchers have had difficulty in clearly explaining *why* media presentations should have any effect on people's behaviour at all. In so far as studies have nonetheless been linked to some theoretical framework, the researchers have leaned mainly on *social learning theory*. Schmidtke and Schaller (2000) hold the view that, in order to study imitative effects produced by the media it is essential to understand the general theoretical assumptions on how people learn by imitating models. They also believe that it is vital to distinguish the term 'imitation effect' from 'contagious effect', the latter being a notion that is often bandied about in the context of the media and suicide:

> Contagion implies a kind of infectious disease, not allowing the 'infected' person to act and to choose for him/herself. Learning by modelling refers to the acquisition of new patterns of behaviour through the observation of the behaviour of one or more models. Therefore, imitation is not limited to learning from real-life models.

Much of the groundwork for social learning theory was done by Albert Bandura (1977a), the American psychologist. His basic thesis is that verbal transfer of information and observation of other people's acts (models) make up the basis for the acquisition of all types of human behaviour: 'By synthesizing features of different models into new amalgams, observers can achieve through modeling novel styles of thought and conduct' (Bandura 1974).

Accordingly, people are not only affected by experience of their own acts. We also regulate our own behaviour in response to observations of other people's acts and their repercussions. Witnessing others being punished, for example, for something they have done is as clear a lesson as being punished oneself. In terms of the media, the basic idea is that individuals learn from media models about which kinds of behaviour are rewarded and which are not (and are sometimes punished). Phillips (1985), for example, with social learning theory as his starting point, thinks that suicide—which is presented in the media as an acceptable, or even glamorous, solution to a particular type of problem—may serve as a model for others who have similar problems. The act of the suicide model may, with that kind of reporting, be said to have been rewarded.

## Identification with the model

One central tenet of social learning theory is that the imitator must identify with the model in some way (Bandura 1977b). In their summary, Pirkis and Blood (2001) point out that much of the research on the media and suicide has been criticised for not taking into consideration the characteristics of the imitator, the model or the interplay between them. There has been a tendency to lump all media consumers together. In the studies where factors concerning characteristics of the models and imitators have nonetheless been partially considered it has, for example, been evident that media accounts of celebrities' suicides pose a greater risk of imitation (Wasserman 1984; Stack 1990a). This may be connected with an assumption of social theory regarding vertical identification, i.e. that individuals who perceive themselves as subordinate imitate the behaviour of their perceived superiors (Tarde 1903; Pirkis and Blood 2001). Stack (1990b) also argues that the effect of media suicide reporting is intensified if the model and imitator belong to the same social category (e.g. in terms of age, sex and ethnicity): this indicates a type of horizontal identification, i.e. individuals tend to identify with those who most resemble themselves. In their summary, Schmidtke and Schaller (2000) cite several studies in which the results have indicated that media accounts of young people's suicidal acts tend mainly to prompt imitation by adolescents, while accounts of elderly people's acts mainly affect the elderly. These findings also indicate an apparent association with respect to ethnicity and imitative suicidal behaviour.

## Dose–response effect

As mentioned above, there is thus substantial evidence that nonfictional media reports on suicides exert a stronger imitative effect than fictional ones, and this is also supported in social learning theory (Pirkis and Blood 2001). In Bandura's (1977b) view, the level of reality presumably plays a key part in imitation of models: individuals do not identify as strongly with fictional characters as with real-life ones. An additional factor in social learning theory that may be worth considering in this context is the idea that there is a 'dose effect' that intensifies (or weakens) imitative behaviour. In connection with the media and suicide, this would mean that the more suicide models that are reported in the media, or the more a specific suicide model is reported, the more likely imitation becomes. This is supported by a number of studies showing that the imitation effect increases when publicity is more extensive (Phillips 1974; Wasserman 1984; Stack 1987).

# Suicide-preventive measures in the media

Regarding daily newspapers' reporting of suicide and the imitation effect, Gould writes in her review and summary of research in the area that 'the existence of suicide contagion no longer needs to be questioned' (2001, p. 200), and also that 'Overall, the evidence to date suggests that suicide contagion is a real effect. There is substantial evidence of the significant impact of nonfictional stories on subsequent suicides' (ibid., p. 216).

Pirkis and Blood (2001), in their summary of 33 studies of the daily press and suicide, arrive at a similar viewpoint and think that, although some studies have their methodological limitations, the results show that there is an association between newspaper reports of suicide and actual suicidal acts.

Stack's (2005) studies, based on non-fictional reporting of suicides, show more of an imitation effect than studies of fictional accounts. His review of 419 results from 55 studies of non-fictional media reports on suicide shows that:

1 In studies where a celebrity's suicidal act was reported, the imitative effect was 5.27 times higher than in other studies;

**2** In studies focusing on reports in which negative definitions of suicide were central, the imitative effect was 99 per cent less likely to be found;

**3** In studies based on TV programmes about suicide, the imitative effect was 79 per cent less likely than for reports in the daily press;

**4** In studies focusing on suicide among women, the imitative effect was 4.89 times higher than in other studies.

Moreover, in their review of studies in the field, Schmidtke and Schaller (2000) conclude that 'there is substantial evidence for an imitative effect'.

The fact that many studies have demonstrated an association between media reporting of suicide and actual suicidal behaviour has also prompted the issue of various types of recommendations on how the media *should* report on the subject of suicide to avoid imitative behaviour. Studies have also been carried out in which the essential purpose has been to investigate whether implementation of such recommendations has any effect on the incidence of actual suicidal acts.

Some studies have shown that suicide-preventive measures involving the media directly can influence both the manner in which suicide is reported in the media and the actual suicide rate. These studies are the surveys by Sonneck, Etzersdorfer and Nagel-Kuess of suicides in the Vienna underground and reports on the same in the daily press (Etzersdorfer *et al.* 1992; Sonneck *et al.* 1994; Etzersdorfer and Sonneck 1998). Ever since the Vienna underground opened in 1978, both suicide attempts and suicides had taken place, but from 1984 there was a relatively large increase in suicidal acts there—one that could not be linked to an extension of the underground system or an increase in the number of passengers. On the other hand, it was noted that Austrian daily newspapers reported on these suicides in a dramatic and sensational way, and this prompted the Austrian Association for Suicide Prevention, in June 1987, to launch recommendations to improve the standard of media reporting. After implementation of these recommendations, there was an appreciable change in this reporting: the dailies published brief, non-sensational announcements on inner pages, and some stopped reporting suicide. A corresponding decrease in the number of suicides and suicide attempts relating to underground trains was observed in Vienna after the implementation of recommendations.

In Switzerland, too, researchers have evaluated the results of implementing suicide-preventive recommendations in the media (Michel *et al.* 1995; Frey *et al.* 1997; Michel *et al.* 2000). In a study of how newspapers reported on suicide, a coding and rating system was developed that permitted an 'imitation-risk score' to be calculated for each type of suicide report. Of the roughly 400 publications investigated over an 8-month period, 151 articles about suicide were found. The analysis showed that nearly half (47 per cent) of the headlines for these articles could be regarded as sensational, and that inappropriate pictures were published in 20 per cent of cases. Altogether, the researchers estimated that 44 per cent of the suicide articles constituted a high imitation risk. After the recommendations on suicide prevention for the media were issued, a follow-up study was carried out. This showed that although the number of articles about suicide actually rose, they were shorter and less frequently located on the front page as before. Headlines, illustrations and the articles themselves were deemed to be less sensational and glorifying, and the overall imitation risk to which the press material could give rise was considered lower after the implementation of recommendations.

In a study from Estonia, an association was found between the style of media reporting and readers' comments (Sisask *et al.* 2005). Inappropriate reporting of suicidal acts included comments expressing over-simplified attitudes towards suicide.

In 2000, WHO issued its publication *Preventing suicide. A resource for media professionals*, which has been circulated worldwide. The summary of what the media should and should not include in their reporting on suicide was as follows:

## What to do

◆ Work closely with health authorities in presenting the facts.

◆ Refer to suicide as a completed suicide, not a successful one.

◆ Present only relevant data, on the inside pages.

◆ Highlight alternatives to suicide.

◆ Provide information on helplines and community resources.

◆ Publicize risk indicators and warning signs.

## What not to do

◆ Don't publish photographs or suicide notes.

◆ Don't report specific details of the method used.

◆ Don't give simplistic reasons.

◆ Don't glorify or sensationalize suicides.

◆ Don't use religious or cultural stereotypes.

◆ Don't apportion blame.

The American Foundation for Suicide Prevention (AFSP) has also issued recommendations for the media's reporting of suicide (http://www.afsp.org). Scientists from the Annenberg Public Policy Center were involved in both the recommendation process (Annenberg Public Policy Center *et al.* 2002) and the evaluation (Jamieson *et al.* 2003).

## Conclusion

The studies and meta-analyses of the association between accounts of suicide in the media and actual suicidal acts showed that:

◆ The more publicity a suicide receives, the more actual suicide acts take place;

◆ The imitation effect is more marked in adolescents than in adults;

◆ Similarities between the suicide model and potential suicide imitators is a major factor in the commission of suicidal acts;

◆ The risk of an imitation effect appears to be elevated if the suicide model described is a celebrity;

◆ The risk of an imitation effect also appears to be elevated if the mediated account relates to an authentic, rather than a fictional, suicide;

◆ Reports on suicide in the daily press appear to have a greater effect than those on television;

◆ Dramatic and sensationalist descriptions of suicide cases in the media entail a greater risk of imitative suicides than balanced accounts.

## References

American Foundation for Suicide Prevention (AFSP). Accessed at: http://www.afsp.org.

Annenberg Public Policy Center *et al.* (2002). Reporting on suicide: recommendations for the media. *Suicide and Life-Threatening Behaviour*, **32**, 7–12.

Ashton JR and Donnan S (1979). Suicide by burning: a current epidemic. *British Medical Journal*, **2**, 769–770.

Ashton JR and Donnan S (1981). Suicide by burning as an epidemic phenomenon: an analysis of 82 deaths and inquests in England and Wales in 1978–79. *Psychological Medicine*, **11**, 735–739.

Au JSK, Yip PSF, Chan CLW *et al.* (2004). Newspaper reporting of suicide cases in Hong Kong. *Crisis*, **25**, 161–168.

Bandura A (1974). Behaviour theory and the models of man. *American Psychologist*, **29**, 859–869.

Bandura A (1977a). *Social Learning Theory*. Prentice-Hall, Englewood Cliffs.

Bandura A (1977b). Self-efficacy: towards a unifying theory of behavioural change. *Psychological Review*, **84**, 191–215.

Baron JN and Reiss PC (1985). Same time next year: aggregate analyses of the mass media and violent behaviour. *American Sociological Review*, **50**, 347–363.

Barraclough B, Shepherd D, Jennings C (1977). Do newspaper reports of coroners' inquests incite people to commit suicide? *British Journal of Psychiatry*, **131**, 528–532.

Becker K, Mayer M, Nagenborg M *et al.* (2004). Parasuicide online: can suicide websites trigger suicidal behaviour in predisposed adolescents? *Nordic Journal of Psychiatry*, **58**, 111–114.

Berman AL (1988). Fictional depiction of suicide in televison films and imitation effects. *American Journal of Psychiatry*, **145**, 982–986.

Blumentahl S and Bergner L (1973). Suicide and newspapers: a replicated study. *American Journal of Psychiatry*, **130**, 468–471.

Bollen KA and Phillips DP (1982). Imitative suicides: a national study of the effects of television news stories. *American Sociological Review*, **47**, 802–809.

Clark DC (1989). Impact of television news reports. *Suicide Research Digest*, **3**, 1–2.

Collins S (1993). Health prevention messages may have paradoxical effect. *British Medical Journal*, **306**, 926.

Ellis SJ and Walsh S (1986). Soap may seriously damage your health. *Lancet*, **1**, 686.

Etzersdorfer E, Sonneck G, Nagel Kuess S (1992). Newspaper reports and suicide. *New England Journal of Medicine*, **327**, 502–503.

Etzersdorfer E and Sonneck G (1998). Preventing suicide by influencing mass-media reporting: the Viennese experience 1980–1996. *Archives of Suicide Research*, **4**, 67–74.

Fekete S and Schmidtke A (1996). Attitudes toward suicide in the mass media. Paper presented at the American Association of Suicidology 29th Annual Conference: Suicide—Individual, Cultural, International Perspectives, Missouri.

Fishman G and Weiman G (1997). Motives to commit suicide: statistical versus mass mediated reality. *Archives of Suicide Research*, **2**, 199–212.

Fowler BP (1986). Emotional crisis imitating television. *Lancet*, **1**, 1036–1037.

Frey C, Michel K, Valach L (1997). Suicide reporting in the Swiss print media: responsible or irresponsible? *European Journal of Public Health*, **7**, 15–19.

Gappmair B (1980). Suizidberichterstattung in der Press [Suicide reporting in the press]. Salzburg, Dissertation.

Gould MS and Shaffer D (1986). The impact of suicide in televison movies: evidence of imitation. *New England Journal of Medicine*, **315**, 690–694.

Gould MS, Shaffer D, Kleinman M (1988). The impact of suicide in television movies: replication and commentary. *Suicide and Life-Threatening Behaviour*, **18**, 90–99.

Gould MS (2001). Suicide and the media. *Annals of the New York Academy of Sciences*, **932**, 200–224.

Hassan R (1995). Effects of newspaper stories on the incidence of suicide in Australia: a research note. *Australian and New Zealand Journal of Psychiatry*, **29**, 480–483.

Hawton K, Simkin S, Deeks JJ *et al.* (1999). Effects of a drug overdose in a television drama on presentation to hospital for self poisoning: time series and questionnaire study. *British Medical Journal*, **318**, 972–977.

Higgins L and Range LM (1996). Does information that a suicide victim was psychiatrically disturbed reduce the likelihood of contagion? *Journal of Applied Social Psychology*, **26**, 781–785.

Holding TA (1975). Suicide and befrienders. *British Medical Journal*, **3**, 751–752.

Horton H and Stack S (1984). The effect of television on national suicide rates. *Journal of Social Psychology*, **123**, 141–142.

Ishii KI (1991). Measuring mutual causation: effects of suicide news on suicides in Japan. *Social Science Research*, **20**, 188–195.

Jamieson PE, Jamieson KH, Romer D (2003). The responsible reporting of suicide in print journalism. *American Behavioural Scientist*, **46**, 1643–1660.

Jonas K (1992). Modeling and suicide: a test of the Werther-effect. *British Journal of Social Psychology*, **31**, 295–306.

Kessler RC and Stipp H (1984). The impact of fictional television suicide stories on US fatalities: a replication. *American Journal of Sociology*, **90**, 151–167.

Kessler RC, Downey G, Milavsky JR *et al.* (1988). Clustering of teenage suicides after television news stories about suicides: a reconsideration. *Journal of Psychiatry*, **145**, 1379–1383.

Kessler RC, Downey G, Stipp H *et al.* (1989). Network television news stories about suicide and short-term changes in total US suicides. *Journal of Nervous and Mental Disorders*, **177**, 551–555.

Kuess S and Hatzinger R (1986). Attitudes toward suicide in the print media. *Crisis*, **7**, 118–125.

Lester D (1994). Young adult suicide and exposure to television: a comment. *Social Psychiatry and Psychiatric Epidemiology*, **29**, 110–111.

Littmann SK (1985). Suicide epidemics and newspaper reporting. *Suicide and Life-Threatening Behaviour*, **15**, 43–50.

Marks A (1987). Television and suicide; comment. *New England Journal of Medicine*, **316**, 877.

Martin G (1996). The influence of television suicide in a normal adolescent population. *Archives of Suicide Research*, **2**, 103–117.

Mastroianni GR (1987). Television and suicide: comment. *New England Journal of Medicine*, **316**, 877.

McDonald DH and Range LM (1990). Do written reports of suicide induce high-school students to believe that suicidal contagion will occur? *Journal of Applied Social Psychology*, **20**, 1093–1102.

Michel K, Frey C, Schlaepfer TE *et al.* (1995). Suicide reporting in Swiss print media: frequency, form and content of articles. *European Journal of Public Health*, **5**, 199–203.

Michel K, Frey C, Wyss K *et al.* (2000). An exercise in improving suicide reporting in print media. *Crisis*, **21**, 71–79.

Motto JA (1967). Suicide and suggestibility: the role of the press. *American Journal of Psychiatry*, **124**, 252–256.

Motto JA (1970). Newspaper influence on suicide: a controlled study. *Archives of General Psychiatry*, **23**, 143–148.

O'Connor S, Deeks JJ, Hawton K *et al.* (1999). Effects of a drug overdose in a television drama on knowledge of specific dangers of self-poisoning: population-based surveys. *British Medical Journal*, **318**, 978–979.

Ostroff RB, Behrends RW, Lee K *et al.* (1985). Adolescent suicides modelled after television movies. *American Journal of Psychiatry*, **142**, 989.

Pell J and Murdoch R (1999). A causal association cannot yet be inferred. *British Medical Journal*, **319**, 1131.

Phillips DP (1974). The influence of suggestion on suicide: Substantive and theoretical implications of the Werther effect. *American Sociological Review*, **39**, 340–354.

Phillips DP (1982). The impact of fictional television stories on US adult fatalities: new evidence on the effect of the mass media on violence. *American Journal of Sociology*, **87**, 1340–1359.

Phillips DP (1985). The Werther effect: suicide and other forms of violence are contagious. *The Sciences*, **7**, 32–39.

Phillips DP and Carstensen LL (1986). Clustering of teenage suicides after television news stories about suicide. *New England Journal of Medicine*, **315**, 685–689.

Phillips DP and Paight DJ (1987). The impact of televised movies about suicide: a replicative study. *New England Journal of Medicine*, **317**, 809–811.

Phillips DP and Carstensen LL (1988). The effect of suicide stories on various demographic groups. *Suicide and Life-Threatening Behaviour*, **18**, 100–114.

Pirkis J and Blood RW (2001). *Suicide and the Media. A Critical Review.* Commonwealth Department of Health and Aged Care, Canberra.

Platt S (1987). The aftermath of Angie's overdose: is soap (opera) damaging to your health? *British Medical Journal Clinical Research Edition*, **294**, 954–957.

Sandler DA, Conell PA, Welsh K (1986). Emotional crisis imitating television. *Lancet*, **1**, 856.

Schmidtke A and Hafner H (1988). The Werther effect after television films: new evidence for an old hypothesis. *Psychological Medicine*, **18**, 665–676.

Schmidtke A and Schaller S (2000). The role of mass media in suicide prevention. In K Hawton and K van Heeringen, eds, *The International Handbook of Suicide and Attempted Suicide*, pp. 675–697. John Wiley & Sons, Chichester:

Shepard D and Barraclough BM (1978). Suicide reporting: information or entertainment? *British Journal of Psychiatry*, **132**, 283–287.

Shoval G, Zalsman G, Polakevitch J *et al.* (2005). Effect of the broadcast of a television documentary about a teenager's suicide in Israel on suicidal behaviour and methods. *Crisis—The Journal of Crisis Intervention and Suicide Prevention*, **26**, 20–24.

Simkin S, Hawton K, Whitehead L *et al.* (1995). Media influence on parasuicide: a study of the effects of a television drama portrayal of paracetamol self-poisoning. *British Journal of Psychiatry*, **167**, 754–759.

Sisask M, Värnik A, Wasserman D (2005). Internet comments on media reporting of two adolescents' collective suicide attempt. *Archives of Suicide Research*, **9**, 87–98.

Sonneck G, Etzersdorfer E, Nagel Kuess S (1994). Imitative suicide on the Viennese subway. *Social Science and Medicine*, **38**, 453–457.

Stack S (1987). Celebrities and suicide: a taxonomy and analysis, 1948–1983. *American Sociological Review*, **52**, 401–412.

Stack S (1990a). A reanalysis of the impact of non-celebrity suicides: a research note. *Social Psychiatry and Psychiatric Epidemiology*, **25**, 269–273.

Stack S (1990b). Audience receptiveness, the media, and aged suicide, 1968–1980. *Journal of Aging Studies*, **4**, 195–209.

Stack S (1996). The effect of the media on suicide: evidence from Japan, 1955–1985. *Suicide and Life-Threatening Behaviour*, **26**, 132–142.

Stack S (2005). Suicide in the media: a quantitative review of studies based on nonfictional stories. *Suicide and Life-Threatening Behaviour*, **35**, 121–133.

Tantalo M and Marchiori C (1981). La reppresintazione de suicido della stamp quotidiana [The representation of suicide in the daily press]. *Rivista Italiana di Medicina Legale*, **3**, 405–449.

Tarde G (1903). *The Laws of Imitation.* Holt, New York.

Veysey MJ, Kamanyire R, Volans GN (1999). Antifreeze poisonings give more insight into copycat behaviour. *British Medical Journal*, **319**, 1131.

Waldron G, Walton J, Helowicz R (1993). Medical messages on television: copycat overdoses 'coincidental'. *British Medical Journal*, **306**, 1416.

Wasserman I (1984). Imitation and suicide: a re-examination of the Werther effect. *American Sociological Review*, **49**, 427–436.

Williams JMG, Lawton C, Ellis SJ *et al.* (1987). Copycat suicide attempts. *Lancet*, **2**, 102–103.

World Health Organization (2000). *Preventing Suicide: A Resource for Media Professionals.* Department of Mental Health, Social Change and Mental Health. World Health Organization, Geneva.

Zahl DL and Hawton K (2004). Media influences on suicidal behaviour: an interview study of young people. *Behavioural and Cognitive Psychotherapy*, **32**, 189–198.

# CHAPTER 70

# The role of the Internet in suicide prevention

Michael Westerlund and Danuta Wasserman

## Abstract

Among websites relating to suicide, approximately 40 per cent represent a suicide-preventive view. However, research shows that pro-suicide sites usually rank higher on search results pages, and are more frequently searched for. These pro-suicide sites and other forms of online pro-suicide communication have tried to spread a view of suicide as an acceptable solution to life's problems. They have also increased access to potent suicide methods, through the long lists they contain. They have added to persuasion and group pressure to fulfil suicide plans, glorifying those who have committed suicide, and given rise to a new form of suicide pact—'net suicides'.

This chapter also discusses the scope for statutory prohibition and regulation of pro-suicide websites, and ways in which Internet-based systems are used as suicide-preventive support.

## Introduction

The Internet is no make-believe world. It is populated by real people from diverse social and cultural backgrounds. And what happens on the Internet has repercussions on actual human beings. Parts of the Internet can, and should, be seen as virtual social environments where people meet and exchange thoughts, feelings and experiences. Just as in physical environments, there are both positive and constructive virtual social settings and those that are clearly destructive.

In one study on how a suicide event was presented in various Internet media, and of the comments from readers to which this event gave rise, inadequate reporting of the event proved to elicit comments that simplified suicide problems to a high degree (Sisask *et al.* 2005). As the authors state, we should not underestimate the role played by the Internet in shaping attitudes towards suicide among the general public.

## How much material about suicide is online and what is it about?

A search for the keyword 'suicide' in 1997, using the Inktomi/Hotbot search engine, generated 130,000 'hits' (Baume *et al.* 1997). In 1999, 50,000–100,000 results were obtained with what were then the most popular search engines (Thompson 1999). A comparison with the many millions of hits obtained from a search for the same word in 2008 may be interesting. A search on Google, for example, now yields more than 65 million hits for 'suicide'. Does this tell us that suicide must, as many people think, be regarded as a growing problem on the Internet? All it shows, in fact, is that a vast number of web pages contain the word 'suicide'. Unless we investigate the content of these pages we cannot know what they are about.

One quantitative study of how the subject of suicide is presented on the Web was based on hits for the words *självmord* (Swedish for 'suicide') and 'suicide' generated by Google (Westerlund 2008). Overall, this study shows that web pages of institutional origin (public agencies, other organizations and companies) on the subject predominate on the Internet (84 per cent) and that the content provided by these institutions concerns research and prevention, and may thus be termed 'suicide-preventive'. But besides these institutional pages, whose manner of communication is largely reminiscent of the more traditional mass media, there are private pages (16 per cent) characterized more by multiple communication, personal confessions and narratives, and an alternative, pro-suicide stance.

Notwithstanding the predominance of the institutional websites, representing a suicide-preventive attitude, the Internet has thus provided a previously non-existent opportunity to publish material and discuss, confess and seek contact on a subject that has always been strongly taboo and therefore 'belonged' to only a few voices in public discourse. This opportunity has resulted in both constructive and strongly destructive contributions. Summing up, the study indicates two parallel trends in how the subject of suicide is represented on the Net:

It extends and supplements the presentation of suicide and suicide prevention in traditional mass media.

It provides virtual social environments (both constructive and destructive) where new forms of discourse and formerly unheard voices—with no possible place in public and mass-media discourse previously—put forward alternative explanatory models on the subject of suicide.

Both the supplementary suicide-related material now found on the Web and the scope for new forms of communication about suicide can presumably help to change the way in which suicide is perceived and portrayed. Accordingly, by extension, they can also affect the views and notions about suicide that prevail in our society and culture (Westerlund 2008).

In another study based on material collected using search engines, Biddle *et al.* (2008) analysed the results obtained when they used 12 simple keywords and phrases (such as 'suicide', 'suicide methods' and 'how to kill yourself') to search for information about suicide, using the four search engines Google, Yahoo!, MSN and Ask. Since studies of online behaviour have shown that users seldom look beyond the first ten hits on the first results page (iProspect 2006, Hansen *et al.* 2003, Eysenbach and Kohler 2002), the authors confined themselves to these ten results for each search phrase on each search engine. This yielded a total of 480 results to analyse. Summarizing these findings, nearly 30 per cent of the results may be said to consist of web pages whose content was dominated by information about suicide methods, and whose messages about suicidal acts ranged from incitement or clear encouragement to non-rejection.

In contrast to the above-mentioned web pages, 121 (25 per cent) of the hits were pages focusing on suicide prevention and pages that were clearly opposed to suicidal acts (Biddle *et al.* 2008). A further 70 results (15 per cent) were pages with academic or policy-oriented content. Overall, these two categories, totalling 40 per cent of the results, may be interpreted as representing a suicide-preventive view to some degree.

Although web pages with a more suicide-preventive attitude thus predominated among the results—a finding that tallies with that of Westerlund (2008)—Biddle *et al.* (2008) nevertheless point out that pro-suicide web pages, pages containing factual information about suicide methods and chat rooms with general discussions about suicide were the results where the highest number of hits were usually found on results pages. They also found that the three websites topping the search results were clearly pro-suicide, with the well-known (notorious) *alt.suicide.holiday* (ASH) ranked first. The website ranked fourth was Wikipedia, which also has a long list of suicide methods. The study showed, furthermore, that these four top-ranking websites not only describe various suicide methods but also evaluate them.

The authors found, moreover, that the four search engines differed (Biddle *et al.* 2008). Google and Yahoo! generated the largest number of pro-suicide results while MSN generated most suicide-preventive and academic results. This indicates that it is possible to influence the presentation of search results. It should be fruitful for Internet companies providing search engines, through optimization strategies, to attempt to maximize the probability of suicidal individuals finding websites that offer help and support instead of the risk of being ushered onto websites that are dangerous to life.

In an American study designed similarly to those discussed above, the starting point was to investigate the websites that suicidal people may encounter if they use online search engines (Recupero *et al.* 2008). The search terms used were 'suicide', 'how to commit suicide', 'suicide methods' and 'how to kill yourself'. The first 30 search results for each phrase, using Google, Yahoo!, Ask, Lycos and Dogpile, were collected and analysed. After elimination of the websites that had already been found once ('repeat listings'), 373 unique URLs remained. These were classified as either 'pro-suicide', 'anti-suicide', 'suicide-neutral,' 'not a suicide site' or 'error'. As in the studies by Biddles *et al.* (2008) and Westerlund (2008), the findings showed that 'anti-suicide' websites (29.2 per cent) were more frequent in the search results than websites categorized

as 'pro-suicide' (11 per cent). However, the authors point out that although the pro-suicide websites are fewer, in quantitative terms, they are highly accessible, as are the websites containing very potent suicide methods and describing them in detail. The study also shows that much of the pro-suicide content and 'how-to' suicide information in the search results were connected with the alt.suicide.holiday or Church of Euthanasias sites alone. The authors emphasize the importance of psychiatric staff asking patients about their use of the Internet. Depressed and/or suicidal patients who use the Internet are particularly in the risk zone. Staff can also help patients to find websites with preventive content and supportive functions, so that the Internet use can exert a therapeutic effect instead of constituting a threat.

In discussing the media and suicide, many researchers stress two facts: that suicide is the most frequent cause of death among teenagers in most countries (Wasserman *et al.* 2005) and that the suicide-attempt rate is high in adolescence (Becker and Schmidt 2004). Several studies have also shown that youthful individuals are more susceptible to, and influenced by, media presentations of suicide events than adults (Phillips and Carstensen 1986, Schmidtke and Schaller 2000). The findings of two studies that specifically explored the relationship between high-frequency Internet use ('Internet addiction'), depression and suicidal ideation among adolescents showed that a significant correlation among these variables exists (Ryo *et al.* 2004, Kim *et al.* 2006). The above factors, combined with the emergence of the Internet as a key medium for young people, have aroused many researchers' fears.

A study by Hagihara *et al.* (2007) set out to investigate this very question—whether there is any association between Internet use and the incidence of actual suicides. The authors are of the view that although Internet-based communication is extremely widespread today, knowledge of how it affects suicidal behaviour is virtually non-existent. The article shows that Internet use in Japanese households rose from 0 per cent in December 1992 to 88.1 per cent in March 2005, and that in 2005 there were more than 17,000 Japanese websites containing information about suicide and suicide methods. There is also the fact that by international standards Japan has had very high suicide rates, especially since the economic recession in 1998. Parallel to the analysis of a possible association between Internet use and the incidence of suicide, associations between accounts of suicide in the daily press and actual suicides, on the one hand, and between unemployment and suicide on the other were also investigated.

Suicide figures for Japanese men and women on a monthly basis were compiled for the period 1987–2005 and subsequently analysed in a linear model. In this model, the number of articles about suicide in the daily press, households' rate of Internet use and the number of unemployed people in a particular month were the independent variables. Suicide figures in the subsequent month were the dependent variable. The results showed a significant association between articles about suicide in the daily press and the number of suicides among men and women alike (Hagihara *et al.* 2007). As for the influence of Internet use and unemployment on suicide, there was a significant association for men, but not for women. The former, in the authors' opinion, can presumably be explained by the fact that men have greater access to the Internet and use it more than women. Regarding unemployment, the authors found that previous studies, too, had shown that this factor was correlated with male, but not female, suicide rates. It should be emphasized that the results show that press articles about suicide, on the one hand, and unemployment on the other are considerably stronger indicators of the incidence of suicide than Internet use, and—as we have seen—particularly among men.

There are a number of methodological weaknesses in the investigation, as the authors themselves admit. For example, the analytical model used does not take into consideration other known risk factors that affect suicide rates (such as increased misuse of alcohol and drugs, domestic violence and poor access to mental-health care). But perhaps the gravest objection that may be raised is that the study leaves out the account of *how* the Internet has been used; it considers only the fact of its use. Thus, we do not know if the users in the study came across any online material about suicide during the time when they used the Internet, let alone whether they were influenced by such material. Globally, moreover, during the period in which Internet use has become widespread all over the world, suicide rates in many countries have declined or, at least, not risen *pari passu* with a rise in Internet use (Galtung and Hoff 2007). Hagihara *et al.* (2007) also explored whether suicide rates in Japan had risen more rapidly after the introduction of the Internet than before, but found no differences. Summing up, more studies are needed, with more precise measuring methods, to allow us to see whether Internet-based communication affects the incidence of suicide and, if so, how.

## Pro-suicide websites and pro-suicide online communication

Many researchers (such as Baume *et al.* 1997, Thompson 1999, and Biddle *et al.* 2008) have reflected on the existence of so many pro-suicide websites. They have pointed out that these sites recommend suicide as a solution to life's problems, and contain detailed descriptions of methods yielding the maximum effect, and also suicide notes, death certificates and pictures of people who committed suicide. People who try to discourage others from putting their suicide plans into effect are 'evicted' from websites of this type. Instead, suicide is advocated as a solution to individuals' problems in life, and they are advised not to seek psychiatric or other help since this is described as worse than useless. One of these pro-suicide websites, 'The Church of Euthanasia' ('Save the Planet: Kill Yourself'), has suicide as the first of its four 'pillars' or principles. It expresses the view that suicide is something intrinsically beneficial that serves the ultimate goal: saving the planet by 'a massive *voluntary* population reduction' (http://churchofeuthanasia.org/coefaq.html). The website has had the intention of launching a pro-suicide hotline to support people in their suicidal process and give them advice about methods and the like (Thompson 1999).

The pro-suicide Internet source that is presumably best known, alt.suicide.holiday or ASH, started as a Usenet newsgroup online at the end of the 1980s. Although the initial idea was to create a forum for discussing why the number of suicides increased during holiday periods, discussions rapidly came to be about the right to take one's own life and how this could 'best' be done. Nearly 20 years after its inception, ASH is still the central source of practical information about suicide, and channel of suicide communication, on the Internet. Information about methods collected by means of the many contributions and discussions has spread to numerous websites. ASH has emerged as a discussion forum about suicide as a whole, with message boards for those who are considering suicide or wish to leave suicide notes. Thompson (1999) noted that more than 900 such messages were being left monthly in 1998–99, mainly by people who were contemplating suicide or from those who had previously attempted suicide. It should also be mentioned that active discussion participants in the ASH newsgroup in 2000 opened up the possibility of chatting in real time (Internet Relay Chat, IRC) about suicide on the website alt.suicide.bus.stop (ASBS), which is close to ASH in terms of content and values.

Today, there are a large number of pro-suicide websites in several different languages on the Internet, and they often rank high on the search engines' results pages (Biddle *et al.* 2008). Many of these sites show marked similarities and also often link to one another, giving the impression of a loosely connected virtual network of pro-suicide websites whose content is shared by visitors and producers alike. The similarities among these websites consist not only in the common subject; there is also a clearly shared subcultural and countercultural standpoint, opposed to the suicide-preventive attitude and, in general, to the basic values and morality of the community at large. This is clearly reflected in both the content and the nature of these sites.

Examples of how subcultural attitudes can be constituted, in general terms, are formulated by Dick Hebdige:

> Style in subculture is, then, pregnant with significance. Its transformations go 'against nature', interrupting the process of 'normalization'. As such, they are gestures, movements towards a speech which offends the 'silent majority', which challenges the principle of unity and cohesion, which contradicts the myth of consensus.

> (*Subculture: The Meaning of Style*, 1979: 18).

The countercultural aspect is found in explicit and implicit forms in statements about suicide that are clearly diametrically opposed to the explanatory models of society as a whole. Becker and Schmidt (2004) have expressed this aspect as the existence, underlying the pro-suicide websites, of a strong 'anti-psychiatric' view. This concealed view manifests itself through the provision of information about how to take one's own life most effectively, and also through message to the effect that suicide is something the individual alone is responsible for.

The pro-suicide websites thus express an attitude that sees society and its institutions alone as a threat to the individual's self-evident rights. It may also be deduced that individuals have few or no obligations towards others and that we are all, according to this view, accountable solely to ourselves. The outcome is a low degree of solidarity. All forms of legislation, regulation, taking into custody or other institutional intervention in people's lives are considered to be evil (Westerlund 2008).

From a psychological perspective, producing the pro-suicide message can perform at least two functions (partially working together):

1 **Identity gain** Identity is forged, as we know, both exclusively (what I am not, and don't wish to be) and inclusively (what I am or want to be—where I belong). By rebelling against the values and views of the dominant culture concerning the subject of suicide, and producing alternative ones, the websites position themselves as something distinguishably 'different'. This difference assists in the construction of a special, recognizable identity.

2 **Acting-out of aggressive impulses** Notions of violence, physical self-harm, suicide and death also enable individuals to release

and act out impulses of an aggressive nature that are suppressed in our culture. This 'double whammy' can make up part of the driving force underlying production of the pro-suicide websites, replete as they are with violence and death.

## Case studies

The above-mentioned considerations may thus partially explain *why* pro-suicide websites are produced and published on the Internet. But what are their possible repercussions on visitors to these websites? What specific risks can the pro-suicide websites pose, especially for people who are already in the risk zone for suicidal acts?

A number of case studies conducted to date show that individuals have committed suicide or carried out serious suicide attempts after obtaining information about suicide methods online (Haut and Morrison 1998, Adekola *et al.* 1999, Becker *et al.* 2004a). Becker and Schmidt (2004) refer to two cases in which teenagers went online to discuss their suicide plans and find effective methods of committing suicide. These authors' writings show that they are chiefly shocked by the number of websites describing in detail, for example, the preparations and doses necessary for attaining a lethal result. Similar experience is also described by D'Hulster and Van Heeringen (2006) in an article about two serious suicide attempts that were prepared and carried out with the assistance of information obtained from the web. In the authors' view, online access to pro-suicide information can lower the threshold and exacerbate the risk of suicidal behaviour in individuals in the risk zone.

Baume *et al.* (1997) followed up three cases in which people had left messages on ASH message boards, saying that they were thinking of taking their own lives. The researchers found that these people left a series of messages that appeared to be more in the nature of diary entries of some kind about their suicidal thoughts than suicide notes as such. The messages showed how the individuals were proceeding in their suicidal process, first asking others in the discussion group which methods were best and how they should go about getting hold of the requisites. Two of the three cases, as far as the researchers could judge, resulted in completed suicides after the people concerned had obtained highly detailed information about how to perform the acts (for example, exactly how to angle a pistol in one's mouth to obtain the maximum effect) and also been encouraged by other discussion participants to fulfil their suicide plans. In one of these cases, the discussion continued afterwards with participants arguing about whether the incitement to commit suicide that had been given was appropriate. In the third case, the person did not die from the suicide attempt (carbon monoxide poisoning) but was admitted to a psychiatric clinic. After this, he urged others in the discussion forum to avoid the method he had used, but did not comment on whether he regarded himself as being helped by the psychiatric treatment he had undergone.

Summing up, Baume *et al.* (1997) pinpointed the ambivalence that many of the participants initially show in their messages in the ASH discussion forum, but also how their decision to take their own lives is strengthened under the influence of other forum members' encouragement. Ambivalence is a highly striking and prominent factor in most individuals' suicide processes (Wasserman 2001). From a therapeutic point of view, the ambivalence factor in a suicidal person is very important since it can exert a protective effect until support and treatment can be provided. In contrast, however, ambivalent and vulnerable individuals who discussed their suicidal thoughts on ASH were subjected to such massive persuasion by other discussion participants that they were unable to back out or seek help for their problems. In one of the cases, this is extremely clear: the person in question wrote 'I'm gonna do it any day now. Really. I promise!', showing that he felt obliged to proceed with the plans he had begun discussing and obtained reactions to from other participants (Baume *et al.* 1997). These plans and thoughts might possibly have been reviewed, and revised, if the circumstances had been different. The danger of websites of this type is thus what is more or less a chorus of voices in unison, inciting and urging individuals to commit suicidal acts, while voices with other solutions to life's problems are largely excluded.

Becker and Schmidt (2004), too, hold the view that since no opinions other than pro-suicide ones are tolerated at these websites their effect is to easily tip the ambivalent stance that most individuals with suicidal tendencies have regarding whether to go on living or end it all. Teenagers and other (young) adults in the risk zone are at risk of losing their doubts about and fear of suicidal acts when they are exposed to this one-sided encouragement to proceed with their suicide plans. Clear risk factors on these websites are the group pressure to commit suicide that arises and the scope offered to agree with others to commit suicide jointly. Moreover, 'chatters' or discussion participants who have previously committed suicide are glorified. This may make them attractive (ideal) models for other visitors to imitate. In the view of Becker and Schmidt (2004), the Internet thereby has a more powerful 'Werther effect' than print media, but more research is required since to date there have only been individual case studies concerning the Internet and imitation effects. Baume *et al.* (1997), too, argue that the Internet has a greater potential than other mass media to influence people in the direction of suicidal acts, mainly because of its interactive nature. Winkel *et al.* (2003) think that social learning theory can, with advantage, be used to explain why and how individuals are influenced by communicating in various online suicide forums.

## Suicide pacts on the Internet (net suicides)

In October 2004, nine people in Japan took their own lives in what was evidently a new type of suicide pact drawn up on the Internet. Suicides of this kind have since come to be termed 'net suicides' (Rajagopol 2004; Naito 2007). These incidents, which attracted a great deal of attention, were followed within two months by a further 13 deaths in four separate suicide pacts. The method used in all these suicides was carbon monoxide poisoning, using small barbecue grills to burn charcoal in small, airtight spaces. As many as 60 people a year are thought to have been dying in 'net suicides' in Japan alone, and the number is continuing to rise (Naito 2007). This phenomenon does not, however, appear to be confined to Japan. Suicide pacts entered into online have also received attention in other countries, such as South Korea, Norway and the United Kingdom (Lee 2003; Galtung and Hoff 2007; Naito 2007). Rajagopol (2004) emphasizes the difference in kind between the phenomena of suicide pacts and suicide clusters, in that the latter is characterized by a number of suicides that is limited in time and space, and later suicides have been influenced by the earlier ones. Nor, in a suicide cluster, do the individuals involved need to have been in contact with one another. The definition of a suicide pact, on the other hand, is a joint decision by two or more individuals that they will both or all commit suicide together, in a given place and at a given time. Suicide pacts used almost always to be entered into by individuals who knew one another well and had been in a close relationship—often married or cohabiting couples. In contrast, the web-related suicide pacts that have come to light so far, such as those described above, are characterized by the fact that, for example, individuals previously unknown to one another have 'met' and communicated through Internet websites and then resolved to take their own lives simultaneously. If this phenomenon becomes any more common, Rajagopol (2004) foresees a change in the epidemiological basis of suicide pacts.

Lee *et al.* (2005) are of the view that the Internet, besides 'facilitating' the drawing-up of suicide pacts, has also contributed to the spread of new suicide methods among countries and continents. In Hong Kong, for example, carbon monoxide poisoning using charcoal grills was the method chosen in 20 of the 22 suicide pacts that were publicized in 2002 and 2003. Why these charcoal grills are used to such a large extent in suicide pacts, in particular, is that this method—unlike hanging and jumping, for example—can be easily shared, and because carbon monoxide poisoning has also often been described as a relatively painless way to die. This may also result in more passive participants in a suicide pact being induced to fulfil the plan. Lee *et al.* (2005) conclude in their article that the use of charcoal grills and 'cyber suicide pacts' may be seen as examples of how globalization and the emergence of new communications technology also create new challenges to global health.

## Legislation and regulation

Case studies have thus shown how young, vulnerable individuals, in particular, are encouraged to commit suicidal acts and how detailed information about suicide methods is provided on the pro-suicide websites. These studies and the publicity given to the phenomenon of cyber suicide pacts have prompted a moral discussion about whether this kind of material and communication should be allowed at all in the public sphere. It may appear difficult to ban this communication, since suicide as such is not a criminal offence in most countries. But some writers are of the opinion that since many countries prohibit assistance in suicide, it should be possible to take legal action against these pro-suicide websites, or at least strongly question the ethical justifiability of Internet service providers (ISPs) allowing pro-suicide websites and pro-suicide communication on their web servers (Thompson 1999; Dobson 1999).

Where legislation is concerned, as mentioned above, many countries have laws that prohibit assisted suicide. However, there is an inherent problem in this issue: such legislation criminalizes assistance in an act that is not itself outlawed. Apparently what seems to be required, for the legislation to apply, is an active, quasi-physical form of assistance in a suicidal act. Were this kind of ban to be applied in an online context, it would presumably be very difficult to draw a sharp line between what is voluntary and what can be proved to constitute unauthorized assistance from another party.

Nevertheless, a few countries have taken the issue of criminalization of assisted suicide a step further. In Portugal in 1995, a regulation concerning encouragement to commit suicide was adopted.

Accordingly, a person 'who, by any means, promotes or advertises products, objects or methods designed to cause death', in such a way as to provoke or incite suicide, is liable to imprisonment for up to two years or a fine proportional to 240 days' income earned by the offender (Galtung and Hoff 2007: 111).

In January 2002 France, too, imposed a ban whereby all forms of propaganda (encouragement) of suicidal acts or dissemination of instructions about suicide methods are punishable (Galtung and Hoff 2007: 106). These countries' prohibitions could accordingly, be applied to information and communication on the Internet, but to date no such cases have been documented.

Unlike the more general bans in Portugal and France, a more specific statutory amendment, criminalizing web pages about suicide, was carried out in Australia in 2005 (and came into force in 2006). The Australian Ministry of Justice issued the following description of this amendment:

> The Criminal Code Amendment (Suicide Related Material Offences) Act 2005 makes it an offence for a person to use the internet, or another carriage service, to counsel or incite suicide or to promote or provide instruction on a particular method of committing suicide. An Internet Service Provider that knowingly hosts a suicide site may commit an offence if it aids or abets the commission of an offence (www.ag.gov.au).

The Australian prohibition is very stringent, in that it outlaws not only production and distribution of websites with method descriptions, but also receipt and possession of this type of information. Galtung and Hoff (2007) point out that since the ban is so new, there are no documented legal precedents. On the other hand, some websites were discontinued after the law came into force, and this development is to be welcomed.

Discussions about regulation and legislation are taking place in many other countries as well. In the United Kingdom, for example, discussions have been held between healthcare authorities, the Samaritans emotional support service and ISPs on what measures can be taken to combat websites that encourage people to take their own lives (Bywaters *et al.* 2006). In Denmark, a public inquiry on the issue has concluded by advising against a ban on websites that encourage or incite suicide (Danish Standing Committee on the Criminal Code 2005, Nordentoft 2006). Galtung and Hoff (2007), too, express the view in a report on an investigation of the issue from a Norwegian point of view that the disadvantages of this kind of ban presumably outweigh the advantages. In the authors' view, if suicide information were prohibited it would, in practice, be very difficult to formulate and comply with the content of such a law. Mishara and Weisstub (2007) may be said to summarize much of what are seen as the problems of legislation and regulation in the area. The matter is complex since, for example, it touches on issues concerning freedom of expression and the role of the Internet as a global communication space that is not accommodated within a single jurisdiction. The authors also think that there is, at present, insufficient scientific evidence that Internet-based information and communication have a causal effect on actual suicidal behaviour. Nor have suicide rates risen in most countries in conjunction with the Internet becoming widely available to the public.

However, most people who have studied the subject think it is very important to increase awareness of the risks that visiting pro-suicide websites may pose for people who are close to suicide. To reduce these potential risks, two measures are called for to block the most dangerous sites: ISP self-regulation and filtering of websites in homes, schools and environments where there are vulnerable young people (Coombes 2008). Galtung and Hoff (2007) cite the scope for using existing frameworks to try, in this way, to minimize the risks of suicide incitement and clearly pro-suicide websites on the Internet. One approach would, for example, be to work for an amendment in the European Convention on Cybercrime. Article 9 of the Convention, which enjoins each party to adopt 'legislative and other measures … to establish as criminal offences … producing, offering or making available, distributing or transmitting …' child pornography, could be extended to apply to pro-suicide information and communication. In the authors' opinion, the Convention could serve as a natural framework and working for such an amendment would (though difficult) be easier than starting with completely new proposals. It should be possible to argue that online communication that strongly encourages suicide, and addresses minors, can be just as harmful as child pornography.

Comparisons have also been made between encouragement of suicidal acts and 'grooming' on the Internet, i.e. establishing a trusting rapport with a minor for the purpose of sexually abusing him or her (Galtung and Hoff 2007). Sexual grooming has attracted attention globally and the UK, for example, has already introduced legal provisions to deal with it. It is comparable to incitement of suicide since, in both cases, a type of mental influence and manipulation is involved. BBC Online reported (in 2006) on the father of a boy who had killed himself in an Internet-related suicide. The father wrote: 'It is illegal to groom a child for sex, but not to kill themselves. That seems wrong. What we need is for the government to make it illegal …'

## Suicide-preventive websites and preventive online communication

As mentioned above, there is a copious supply of suicide-preventive websites on the Internet today (Biddle *et al.* 2008; Westerlund 2008). Becker and Schmidt (2004) point out that most people who spend time and communicate in these virtual environments are teenagers and young adults, i.e. the group usually said to run the highest risk of imitative or 'copycat' suicidal behaviour. On these suicide-preventive websites, people with pressing suicidal thoughts or plans are urged to seek help, and leaving suicide notes or encouraging suicide is not permitted. In the authors' opinion, chat rooms of this kind can offer individuals a chance to anonymously discuss and share their thoughts about a subject that is taboo in our culture and our society, and this may afford mitigation and relief in thoughts and feelings for some people. The links to and telephone numbers of help organizations and clinics on these websites can also make it easier for individuals in the risk zone for suicidal acts to seek help.

A number of studies have also been carried out in which the results indicate that web-based suicide communication can give suicidal individuals support and tools for dealing with their situation. An online survey in which questionnaire responses were collected at German suicide forums showed that support and confirmation from other discussion participants were valued as highly as support from friends, and higher than support from the family (Winkel *et al.* 2005). Individuals also tended to support one another to

a greater extent in the suicide forums where no discussions of suicide methods took place. The higher frequency of social support and confirmation in these forums was also correlated with the participants' valuation of reduced suicidality. A previous user study that took place over an 11-month period showed that the discussion participants on a website focusing on the subject of suicide gave one another important 'grass-roots therapy' in the form of shared experience, sympathy, acceptance and encouragement (Miller and Gergen 1998). Hostile and aggressive discussions and participants were unusual. Nevertheless, the authors did not find support for the view that the discussions resulted in any major changes in the participants. Rather, the online dialogue appeared to serve more as a form of maintenance than a means of transformation.

Although they may be insufficient, various Internet-based systems for distributing suicide-preventive information and support are currently emerging. In one article, Wang *et al.* (2005) describe an example of the kind of communication system in which communication takes place through a third party found in proximity to the person seeking help. The system also affords scope for information specially adapted for specific cases. Another, more evaluative study compared three different technologically mediated sources of psychological and emotional first aid: a telephone hotline, personal chat and an asynchronous online support group (Gilat and Shahar 2007). 'Asynchronous', in this context, means 'not occurring at the same time' or 'more independently from space or time'. Email communication, on which such a group is based, is asynchronous and thus more distanced than, for example, telephoning or chatting on the web where feedback is immediate. This may explain the difference in the results obtained. Threats of suicide proved to be much more frequent among participants in the asynchronous support group than among those who sought help and support through the other two options provided. Further research is urgently needed to find out who joins asynchronous online support groups of this type, what kind of communication takes place there and how it develops. Another example is the Israeli SAHAR (a Hebrew acronym for 'Support and Listening on the Net') project, which offers people in severe emotional distress psychological support through a website (Barak 2007). This permits anonymous communication, both synchronous and asynchronous, with knowledgeable helpers. Roughly a third of those who contact SAHAR are thought to be suicidal, and on a number of occasions the service has succeeded in helping people who have threatened to take their own lives or been, *de facto*, moving towards the commission of suicidal acts.

In three component studies whose purpose was to explore how suicidal individuals write about themselves online, it was found that suicidal people are more rigid in their views than both other groups of people in mental distress *and* individuals characterized by mental well-being (Barak and Miron 2005). Members of the suicidal group were also considerably more self-centred in their writing, expressed greater psychological pain and were more cognitively limited than individuals in the other groups. These findings tally well with those of similar investigations of suicidal writing offline, and this should, according to the authors, have a bearing on further research, psychological assessments and understanding of suicidality. A previous study, in which suicidal individuals' online writings were compared with other help-seeking individuals' writing, shows similar results (Fekete 2002).

What, then, supports the view that suicide-preventive effects can be attained through the Internet is the fact that individuals can promptly obtain emotional support and a sense of fellowship with likeminded people, whereupon they feel less socially isolated. Evidence against the view is the fact that individuals can join the virtual community without actually needing to solve their own problems or develop 'real' relationships with others. There is a risk of communication resulting in individuals merely imitating one another's problems.

## The Internet as a threat or opportunity

Some ambivalence is discernible among researchers as to whether online information and communication about suicide should be seen as an opportunity or a threat (e.g. D'Hulster and Van Heeringen 2007). Alao *et al.* (2006) formulate this issue by pointing out that the Internet, with its tremendous capacity for information and communication, can encourage suicidal behaviour by its copious supply of descriptions of potent suicide methods and pro-suicide websites where individuals with severe mental problems are advised not to seek help. There is tolerance and sometimes even advocacy of suicide as a solution to individuals' problems, and voices advising against such acts are, moreover, sometimes excluded. At the same time, in the authors' view, the Internet is a key resource for helping potentially suicidal individuals. For example, it may be used to identify people in the risk zone for suicidal acts and then communicate with them, thereby preventing such acts. If the Internet is used properly, it is a powerful communication tool that can serve to help and support suicidal individuals.

The number of Internet users is continuing to grow steadily. In Germany, for example, the number of users aged 14 and over doubled to more than 35 million in the years 2000–05. The web has increasingly developed into a communication platform for psychiatry and psychotherapy as well, and this platform can be used for the purposes of supportive information, communication and therapy (Pfeiffer-Gerschel *et al.* 2005). Hawton and Williams (2002) believe that more research is necessary to allow any certainty about whether, for example, pro-suicide websites genuinely influence individuals in the direction of suicidal behaviour, although a growing number of case studies indicate that such negative influences very much exist. Becker and colleagues (2004a, b) think that irrespective of whether the Internet is primarily a risk or an opportunity for young people who want to communicate with others about suicide, certain steps must be taken. First, it is imperative for doctors, psychotherapists and parents to be informed about the existence of these suicide websites and chat rooms. Second, issues of media use should be included in psychiatric evaluations. Third, specific guidelines on web-based communication about suicide should be drawn up as soon as possible.

Investigations of the Internet and the subject of suicide carried out to date are mostly in the nature of case studies. Although their results, as such, are extremely important, it is difficult to generalize from these case studies regarding online information and communication about suicide as a whole. The assertion that the Internet has a greater 'Werther effect' than other mass media, owing to its interactive nature, has therefore (up to now) been considered unproven. The misgivings expressed to date about the Internet and its possible influence on individuals', and especially adolescents', suicidal behaviour may also be seen in the light of the greater or lesser outbursts of media panic to which new media invariably seem to give rise. As McQuail (2005 p. 482) puts it, 'Each new popular medium has given rise to a new wave of alarm about its possible effects'.

On the one hand, the Internet generates new problems: information about suicide methods is readily available, suicide pacts are being drawn up, suicidal acts are encouraged and incited, and the proportion of imitative suicides is rising. On the other hand, the Internet has made it possible to discuss a taboo subject and obtain information about what one can do to help oneself or others with suicide problems. Thus, the question of whether the Internet primarily generates new problems or offers new remedies with respect to suicide cannot yet be answered unequivocally.

## Conclusion

Since matters relating to suicide and its underlying causes are still taboo to a high degree in our society and culture, websites on the subject have come to represent an important and controversial source of information. Suicide communication on the Internet may be said to produce new forms—or bolster previous forms—of uncertainty, risks and threats. But the scope for suicide prevention afforded by the Internet is also increasing. In human terms, the Internet has meant the partial blurring of the distinction between personal and intimate communication, on the one hand, and public communication on the other. This also has implications regarding how the subject of suicide develops and is dealt with in modern cultures and societies.

## References

Adekola A, Yolles J, Armenta W (1999). Cybersuicide: the Internet and suicide. *American Journal of Psychiatry*, **156**, 1836–1837.

Alao AO, Soderberg M, Pohl EL *et al.* (2006). Cybersuicide: review of the role of the Internet on suicide. *Cyberpsychol Behav*, **9**, 489–493.

BBC (2006). Web helped my son kill himself. 10 September, 2006.

Barak A and Miron O (2005). Writing characteristics of suicidal people on the Internet: a psychological investigation of emerging social environments. *Suicide and Life-Threatening Behaviour*, **35**, 507–524.

Barak A (2007). Emotional support and suicide prevention through the Internet: a field project. *Computers in Human Behaviour*, **23**, 971–984.

Baume PJM, Cantor C, Rolfe A (1997) Cybersuicide: the role of interactive suicide notes on the Internet. *Crises*, **18**, 73–79.

Becker K and Schmidt MH (2004). When kids seek help on-line: Internet chat rooms and suicide. *Journal of Child and Adolescent Psychiatry*, **43**, 246–247.

Becker K, Mayer M, Nagenborg M *et al.* (2004a). Parasuicide online: can suicide websites trigger suicidal behaviour in predisposed adolescents? *Nordic Journal of Psychiatry*, **58**, 111–114.

Becker K, El-Faddagh M, Schmidt MH (2004b). Cybersuicide or Werther-effect online: suicide chatrooms or forums in the World Wide Web. *Kindheit und entwicklung*, **13**, 14–25.

Biddle L, Donovan J, Hawton K *et al.* (2008). Suicide and the Internet. *British Medical Journal*, **336**, 800–802.

Brevard A, Lester D, Yang B (1990). A comparison of suicide notes written by suicide completers and suicide attempters. *Crisis*, **11**, 7–11.

Bywaters, J, Foster K, Scott J (2006). Internet sites that promote suicide. *Psychiatria Danubina*, **18**, 97.

Coombes R (2008). Safety nets—How can parents protect vulnerable children and young people from pro-suicide sites? *British Medical Journal*, **336**, 803.

D'Hulster N and Van Heeringen C (2006). Cyber-suicide: the role of the Internet in suicidal behaviour. A case study. *Tijdschr Psychiatr*, **48**, 803–807.

Dobson R (1999). Internet sites may encourage suicide. *British Medical Journal*, **319**, 337.

Eysenbach G and Kohler C (2002). How do consumers search for and appraise health information on the world wide web? Qualitative study using focus groups, usability tests, and in-depth interviews. *British Medical Journal*, **324**, 573–577.

Fekete S (2002) The Internet—a new source of data on suicide, depression and anxiety: a preliminary study. *Archives of Suicide Research*, **6**, 352–361.

Galtung A and Hoff OK (2007) *Suicide Risk and the Internet: Can the Law Give Protection?* (in Norwegian). Kolofon Forlag AS, Norway.

Gilat I and Shahar G (2007). Emotional first aid for a suicide crisis: comparison between telephonic hotline and internet. *Psychiatry*, **70**, 12–18.

Hagihara A, Tarumi K, Abe T (2007). Media suicide-reports, Internet use and the occurrence of suicides between 1987 and 2005 in Japan. *BMC Public Health*, **7**, 321.

Hansen D, Derry H, Resnick P *et al.* (2003). Adolescents searching for health information on the Internet: an observational study. *J Med Internet Res*, **5**, 25.

Haut F and Morrison A (1998). The Internet and the future of psychiatry. *Psychiatric Bulletin*, **22**, 641–642.

Hawton K and Williams K (2002). Influences of the media on suicide. *British Medical Journal*, **325**, 1374–1375.

Hebdige D (1979) *The Meaning of Style*. Methuen, London.

iProspect (2006) Search engine user behaviour. http://www.iprospect.com/premiumPDFs/WhitePaper_2006_SearchEngineUserBehaviour.pdf.

Kim K, Ryu E, Chon MY *et al.* (2006) Internet addiction in Korean adolescents and its relation to depression and suicidal ideation: a questionnaire survey. *International Journal of Nursing Studies*, 43, 185–192.

Lee D (2003). Web of despair. *Foreign Policy*, **138**, 90–91.

Lee DTS, Chan KPM, Yip PSF (2005). Charcoal burning is also popular for suicide pacts made on the Internet. *British Medical Journal*, **330**, 602.

McQuail D (2005). *Mass Communication Theory*. Sage Publications, London.

Miller JK and Gergen KJ (1998). Life on the line: the therapeutic potentials of computer-mediated conversation. *Journal of Marital & Family Therapy*, **24**, 189–202.

Mishara BL and Weisstub DN (2007) Ethical, legal and practical issues in the control and regulation of suicide promotion and assistance over the internet. *Suicide and Life-Threatening Behaviour*, **37**, 58–65.

Naito A (2007). Internet suicide in Japan: implications for child and adolescent mental health. *Clinical Child Psychology & Psychiatry*, **12**, 583–597.

Nordentoft M (2006). Criminalization of Internet pages instructing in suicide methods? *Psychiatr Danub*, **18**, 96.

Pfeiffer-Gerschel T, Seidscheck I, Niedermeier N *et al.* (2005). Suicide and Internet. *Verhaltenstherapie*, **15**, 20–26.

Phillips DP and Carstensen LL (1986). Clustering of teenage suicides after television news stories about suicide. *New England Journal of Medicine*, **315**, 685–689.

Rajagopal S (2004). Suicide pacts on the Internet. *British Medical Journal*. **329**, 1298–1299.

Recupero PR, Harms SE, Noble JM (2008). Googling suicide: surfing for suicide information on the Internet. *J Clin Psychiatry*, **13**, e1–e11.

Ryo EJ, Choi KS, Seo J *et al.* (2004). The relationship of Internet addiction, depression and suicidal ideation in adolescents. *Taehan Kanho Hakhoe Chi*, **34**, 102–110.

Schmidtke A and Schaller S (2000). The role of mass media in suicide prevention. In K Hawton and K van Heeringen, eds, *The International Handbook of Suicide and Attempted Suicide*, pp. 675–698. John Wiley & Sons, Chichester.

Sisask M, Värnik A, Wasserman D (2005). Internet comments on media reporting of two adolescents' collective suicide attempt. *Archives of Suicide Research*, **9**, 87–98.

Danish Standing Committee on the Criminal Code (2005). *Report on Criminalisation of General Calls for Suicide* (in Danish). Report No. 1462, Copenhagen.

Thompson S (1999). The Internet and its potential influence on suicide. *Psychiatric Bulletin*, **23**, 449–451.

Wang YD, Phillips-Wren G, Forgionne G (2005). E-delivery personalised healthcare information to intermediaries for suicide prevention. *International Journal of Electronic Healthcare*, **4**, 396–412.

Wasserman D ed. (2001). *Suicide—An Unnecessary Death*. Martin Dunitz, London.

Wasserman D, Cheng Q, Jiang G-X (2005). Global suicide rates among young people aged 15–19. *World Psychiatry*, **4**, 114–120.

Westerlund M (2008). Suicide and the Internet: representation, production and interaction of a problematised and taboo subject (in Swedish). Doctoral thesis, manuscript. Stockholm University, Department of Journalism, Media and Communication (JMK).

Winkel S, Groen G, Petermann F (2003). Suicidal behaviour in adolescents and young adults—benefits of suicide chat rooms on the Internet. *Zeitschrift fur klinische psychologie psychiatrie und psychotherapie*, **51**, 158–175.

Winkel S, Groen G, Petermann F (2005). Social support in suicide forums. *Praxis der Kinderpsychologie und Kinderpsychiatrie*, **54**, 714–727.

## Internet references

Australian Government Attorney-General's Department
http://www.ag.gov.au
ASBS
http://ashbusstop.org/home.html
Ask
http://www.ask.com
Church of Euthanasia
http://www.churchofeuthanasia.org
Google
http://www.google.com
Microsoft News
http://www.msn.com
Wikipedia
http://www.wikipedia.org
Yahoo!
http://www.yahoo.com
Lycos
http://www.lycos.com
Dogpile
http://www.dogpile.com

# CHAPTER 71

# Representations of suicide in cinema

## Gérard Camy

Translated from French by Camilla Wasserman

## Abstract

In this chapter, representations of suicide in fiction film from the United States, Europe and South East Asia will be presented. Cinematic representations are helpful in addressing discourses on suicide worldwide. Typically, the sufferings of the characters that consider suicide or take their lives occupy a minor part of the plot in scenarios that highlight action, cultural and social reflection, or existential interrogations. In typical Hollywood dramas, redemption, punishment, lost love and solitude are the prime reasons for suicides; often as a consequence of genuine injustice. In the European films discussed, suicides on screen often attempt to open the screenplay to comments and reflections on the various tragic circumstances that bring the protagonists to such extremities. Refusal to recognize oneself in and by society appears to be an important reason for suicide. Another recurring theme is the wish to understand the motives behind the voluntary death of a peer. Much South East Asian cinema reflects the malaise of a society, its interiorized violence, fascination with death and the distress of a youth lacking excitement.

## Suicide and cinema

In the pursuit of an audience and money, the phenomenon of suicide as the ultimate form of auto-aggression has appealed to film studios worldwide over the years. Suicide contains notorious elements of marvel, being as fascinating in its preparation and spectacular in its realization as its consequences are devastating and tragic. In the United States' the Hays Code,[1] created because of demand from the big studios in the 1930s, similarly to classification committees around the world, states that suicide should be avoided on screen (alongside abortion and sex). According to the Hays Code, suicide should be avoided and discouraged as a solution to problems in the scenario, unless it is absolutely necessary for the development of the plot; and it should never be justified or glorified. Such stipulations still exist today, for example in the text elaborated by the Canadian Film Institute to justify interdictions to those under 13. The text takes into consideration that the adolescent audience today is more and more conscious of the artificiality of cinema, and that they are 'psychologically better equipped to follow more complex films', but they also emphasize that it is important

to give depth to the characters, and to the reasons of their actions, since it is considered that adolescents are not necessarily able to face some themes without ulterior consequences. There are numerous research reports focusing on the impact of cinematographic representation, as well as images in other visual and written medias on suicidal behaviours (Michael Westerlund and colleagues discuss this topic in Chapter 69 of this book). In this chapter, however, the focus is not on the relationship between suicide rates and representations of suicide on film, rather an investigation of the representation of suicide in fiction film from the United States, Europe and South East Asia respectively. The vast majority of films depicting the suicidal process niether glorify it or present it as a solution to existential troubles. Suicide itself is rarely the subject matter of films, with some exceptions such as Virgin suicides (2000) by Sofia Coppola or Last days (2005) by Gus Van Sant, described later in this chapter. Furthermore the actual suicide is hardly ever depicted on screen: the bullet in the head of a corrupted police officer in the beginning of Cousin (1997) by Alain Corneau is one of the exceptions.

## Hollywood's melodramatic touch

In *The suicide club* (1882), Robert Louis Stevenson offers a cynical portrait of a young aristocrat who wishes to set his disenchanted pleasure-seeking friends straight by offering them the luxury of committing suicide with discretion. Stevenson intended to reason with the young and disillusioned aristocrats of his day, aesthetes who avoided seeing life as anything other than agreeable farce, and to bring them back to reality. The novel was adapted into a motion picture by David Wark Griffith in 1909; in it the director largely toned down the cynicism and focused on the devastations of suicide. This film paves the way for many films to come about suicide. Griffith himself depicts suicide as a form of redemption in his 1911 film *The sorrows of the unfaithful*.

Suicides because of love, duty or in order to avoid dishonour all correspond perfectly with the melodramatic genre; such suicides do not lack in popular history, and no less in literature or in cinema. Redemption, punishment, lost love and solitude are the prime reasons for Hollywood suicides. Behind the romanticism, drama is to be found, and in the wake of the unrestrained, despair lures. Due to a tendency to auto-censure, the act itself is nearly never depicted in most Hollywood films. An off-screen gunshot, a panorama that turns away and as a final shot, hands that can no longer hold the gun …. The plots are constructed so that the suicidal act does not have to be seen. Don Stroud's suicide in Roger Corman's film *Bloody mama* (1970) is one of the few exceptions to this rule. When Frederic March throws himself into the ocean in *A star is born* (William Wellman 1937), he has decided to die in order to not encumber his wife Janet Gaynor's life and career: thus his suicide fades in the light of her rebirth. Kirk Douglas conceives his suicide attempt in a similar fashion in the *Arrangement* (Elia Kazan 1968). He throws himself from his car in front of a tractor-trailer in a tunnel, but does not forget to lower his head at the last moment. Saved, he makes for a salutary return to life. For the young and beautiful protagonist, swept up in a life of debauchery, in *The picture of Dorian Gray* (Albert Lewin 1945), the suicide of the affectionate young Sybil is a first warning shot. The portrait of the hero that he himself has a habit of contemplating takes on a more serious expression, and the painting slowly becomes the insufferable mirror of his dignity. Dorian even hides the painting in the attic in order to not see the hideous development of his features on the canvas as he stays eternally young. In a fit of rage, he stabs the portrait, thus provoking his own death and enabling the portrait to regain its initial features. At this juncture, suicide becomes the only possibility for Dorian Gray's redemption. However, Hollywood also grants suicide as an option for criminals to escape justice, humiliation, prison and death sentences (*The parallax view*, Alan Pakula, 1974). Suicide can also be a punishment that is inflicted on a conceited person, who upon recognizing her/his faults commits suicide, like the press magnate Raymond Massey in *The fountainhead* (King Vidor, 1949). Suicide can also be the only way out of a disappointing life with solitude as sole companion, and cinematic examples are manifold: Zero Mostel in *The front* (Martin Ritt, 1976), Jane Fonda in *They shoot horses, don't they?* (Sydney Pollack, 1969), Alan Arkin as a deaf-mute in *The heart is a lonely hunter* (Robert Ellis Miller, 1968), Jack Palance in *The big knife* (Robert Aldrich, 1955), Brad Dourif in *One flew over the cuckoo's nest* (Milos Forman, 1975), Vincent d'Onofrio in *Full metal jacket* (Stanley Kubrick, 1987) and in former times Greta Garbo and Vivian Leigh in different versions of *Anna Karenina*.

Such acts of auto-destruction can also be depicted in a more indirect form: the person wishing to commit suicide arranges for someone else to eliminate them accidentally. Correspondingly, Kirk Douglas' revolver is empty when he faces Rock Hudson at the end of *The last sunset* (Robert Aldrich, 1961). Similarly, Burt Lancaster refuses to get up and remains lying down in the shadowy light of a room in the face of the murderers that are out to kill him (*The killers*, Robert Siodmak, 1946). He awaits his punishment, jaded and fed up with running away. The men enter, weapons in hand, and fire at Lancaster who hardly sits up to see who they are as he succumbs to the heavy fire. The majority of the suicides mentioned above are presented as consequences of genuine injustice, such as poor Vincent d'Onofrio in *Full metal jacket* whose obesity is the object of the humiliation he suffers. In front of the dislocated, immobile, bloody body the audience realizes the enormous waste. Numerous suicide attempts are interrupted on film; Charlie Chaplin intervenes in time to save the life of his young neighbour Claire Bloom in *Limelight* (1952). Then there is Natalie Wood who decides to attempt suicide but

forgets her initial intentions and takes a new taste to life (*Daisy Clover*, Robert Mulligan 1965). In fact, the big studios prefer scenes of desperation that turn into scenes of rebirth. In *It's a wonderful life* (Frank Capra, 1946), James Stewart cries out: 'I want to live again, please Lord let me live again!' Then there is Jose Ferrer, playing the part of Toulouse-Lautrec in John Huston's 1952 *Moulin Rouge*, who turns on the gas to kill himself, looks at one of his paintings one last time and instinctively sets out to finish it, opening a window to breathe in the fresh air of Montmartre. In fact, Hollywood also loves to treat the topic through comedy, using an optimistic approach to gain the upper hand in this situation. Bud Cort-Harold is an unrepentant suicide attempter in *Harold and Maude* (Hal Ashby, 1972). In *The end* (1978), Burt Reynolds, director and lead actor, finds out that he has an incurable disease and ravages the hospital to find a way to end his life. In *Cookie's fortune* (Robert Altman, 1998), the suicide of an eccentric widow is disguised as murder by her self-righteous niece. This dramatic situation embarks us on a humorous adventure, played in an extraordinary fashion by Glenn Close. As has been shown through these examples, suicide is found in all the big genres of Hollywood cinema. David Lynch's *Mulholland Drive* (2001) perfectly sets the scene for Hollywood suicide with a plot that rests entirely on the twofoldedness of illusion and manipulation, erasing the border between right and wrong, dream and reality. Naomi Watts' suicide adds to this ambivalence.

It is only in 1985 with *Mishima* by Paul Schrader that US cinema modifies its stance on suicide. *Mishima* tells the story of the Japanese author Yukio Mishima, until he takes his life through hara-kiri in 1970. The author, whose real name is Kimitake Hiraoka, is 45 years old when he takes his life through ritual suicide by 'seppuku' at the Ministry of Defence. Hiraoka, author of *Confessions of a mask* (1949), was fascinated with death and chose to kill himself in accordance with the Japanese tradition of ritual suicide by disembowelment. Mishima commits seppuku after an unsuccessful attempt to incite the armed forces to stage a *coup d'état* with his private army. On the morning of his death he writes: 'Life is short but I want to live in eternity.' Schrader finds his inspiration in Mishima's four novels and breaks them into a very realistic narration that is far from the melodramatic cinema described above.

In 2001, *The suicide club* was once again adapted to the screen, this time by the director Rachel Samuels. Produced by Roger Corman, the film renews the ties with the gothic film tradition, immersed in a sober and disquieting atmosphere, evoking the irony and cynicism of Stevenson's novel. Samuels explains that when she discovered Stevenson's novel she was immediately struck by the modernity and pertinence of his ideas:

> The pre-production of the film, in 1999, coincided with the beginning of the lawsuit against Doctor Kevorkian, accused of murder for having 'helped' around ten people to kill themselves. At the same point in time, shootings and other suicide pacts amongst high school students was a common feature in US media. The decadence and fin-de-siécle anomie that characterises Stevenson's novel were not far from the millenary atmosphere of 1999. Stevenson describes the modern era with all its comforts—railroads, the telegraph, elevators—where all is easy and practical, and then he asks himself: how come one can not chose one's own death with equal facility and comfort? Doctor Kevorkian's case brought the same questions to surface. These issues are at the core of the film.

http://www.pardo.ch/2000/program/105r.htm

In 2005, two directors addressed suicide (Gus Van Sant with *Last days*) and euthanasia (Clint Eastwood with *Million dollar baby*), with rare accuracy, thus opening the eyes of many others to these phenomena. Gus Van Sant staged the last days of the front man of Nirvana and idol of a generation, Kurt Cobain, before his suicide in 1994. By refusing a fine-spun reconstitution in order to better 'understand' the act or the artist, Van Sant distances himself from Hollywood's melodramatic vision, and paints a portrait of a man, a body, a silhouette that bends over progressively until it never stands up again. Van Sant offers an ethical portrait filled with affection *vis-à-vis* his subject, and the suicide is an on-screen event. Van Sant chooses to film the exterior of the house whilst Cobain, or Blake in the film, is in the studio, angry about a song made of samples by him; a scream is heard and its echo extends endlessly. Blake's body is seen behind a window and a naked ghost rises from his corpse slowly climbing a ladder. The ghost leaves the body: a representation of the climb to heaven and the liberation from the confined setting that imprisoned him. As opposed to *Last days*, *Million dollar baby* holds onto a melodramatic structure true to the Hollywood tradition described above, with themes as varied as love, relationships and friendships, but Clint Eastwood does not stop there. Maggie Fitzgerald (Hillary Swank), an unfortunate waitress persuades a cranky boxing instructor called Frankie Dunn (Clint Eastwood) to help her to become a boxing champion. Thanks to her determination, Maggie reaches the top and is about to become champion of the world. Until this point the film has no unexpected developments, but suddenly as a result of an accident during a fight, Maggie becomes paralysed; she is incapable of any kind of movement and needs artificial respiration. Despite (or because) having all of her mental capacities intact, she sees no reason to continue living. She tries to commit suicide, and finally persuades Frankie to help her to die. 'I had it all' Maggie says to Frankie, 'so don't take it away from me'. The last forty minutes of the film help us to identify with Maggies' suffering and with Frankie's tragic dilemma. Her wish to die is above all an immense cry of despair. Frankie's final decision to give her a mortal dose is also a confession of his helplessness and inability to help her to surpass her condition.

## Existential reflections of European cinema

In the long filmography of European cinema there are numerous films in which suicide occurs as an element of the scenario without being the main theme. In such films, the suicides are often inspired by real life well-known events or historical personalities like the archduke Rudolf and his mistress baroness Mary Vetsera who together committed suicide at his Mayerling hunting lodge (*Mayerling*, Terrence Young, 1969). Other examples are *Ludwig* (Luchino Visconti, 1972) or Vincent van Gogh who, suffering from a mental disorder and haunted by anxiety, shoots himself in the chest only to die a few days later (*Van Gogh*, Maurice Pialat, 1990). Likewise, the melodramatic perspective is not unique to Hollywood cinema. *Elvira Madigan* by Bo Widerberg from 1967 is an excellent example. The film tells the tragic story of a lieutenant in the Swedish army, who after having been abandoned by wife and children, deserts and flees with the famous ropewalker Elvira Madigan. By leaving his former environment, in which he had difficulties letting his ambitions as a writer blossom, the officer situates himself halfway between adolescent revolt and an adult

class-consciousness and chooses the deadlock of a total break with society. His happiness, fated to a state of unbearable isolation, crumbles with time. The stages of degradation described by Widerberg illustrate with lucidity the loss of substance of an individual when he is no longer a part of the collective. The protagonists' love slowly dies and is declared over with the gunshot and the still image of Elvira's half-closed hands holding onto a white butterfly. A second gunshot is heard off-screen alongside the flow of the river.

The suicide attempts of Michel Simon in *Boudu saved from drowning* (Jean Renoir, 1932), Djamel Debouzze's in *Angel A* (Luc Besson, 2006), Isa Miranda's in *Everybody's woman* (Max Ophuls, 1934) and Vanessa Paradis' in *The girl on the bridge* (Patrice Leconte, 1998), are all used as points of departure to a return to life for the distressed characters. The suicide attempts open the screenplay to comments and reflections on the various tragic circumstances that brought the protagonists to such extremities. In the German film *Head on* by Faith Akin (*Gegen die Wand*, 2004) two suicide attempts are depicted. Cahit is a young German of Turkish origin living a miserable life of excessive drinking and drug abuse. One night, he semi-intentionally crashes into a wall, and barely survives. At the hospital he meets a girl, Sibel, another German Turk who has tried to commit suicide. She asks Cahit to carry out a white marriage with her (one without sexual relations) to escape her family's suffocating pressure. Cahit finally agrees to take part in her plan. The two of them try to find their respective place in the new constellation. Whilst Sibel enjoys her newfound freedom, Cahit realizes that he is falling for this young woman who has brought order, happiness and hope into his life. The catastrophe is irrefutable and the two find themselves in the midst of a storm of emotions and violence.

Another recurring approach to suicide is the inquiry following the voluntary death of another person; the wish to understand the motives of such a tragic decision. In *Terminale* (Francis Girod, 1998), the happy-go-lucky life of a group of Parisian high-school students ends when one of them kills herself. Accordingly, her friends try to understand why Caroline threw herself out of the window in the middle of a philosophy lesson. At the age of 30, Anna, the female protagonist in the Dutch film *Guernsey* (Nanouk Leopold 2005), is married and a mother of three. She lives in the suburbs of a large city and she works with irrigation systems. At the time of one of her visits abroad, she discovers the corpse of one of her colleagues who has killed herself. Nobody seems to know the reasons for the suicide. Distressed, Anna realises that even those we hold close remain strangers to us. Her outlook on her family changes and she starts to question what she means to them. Similarly, in *The passenger* (Eric Caravaca, 2004), Thomas finds out about his long since forgotten brother's suicide. He identifies the body at the forensic institute in Marseille. The casket has to be repatriated to Saintes-Maries-de-la-Mer but Thomas refuses to sign the burial demand. He wants a few days to understand the reasons for his brother hanging himself and decides to go there by car. Thomas moves in to his brother's old home at the port and gets to know his old companion and his nephew Lucas, but does not tell them about his brother's suicide. In losing his brother, Thomas changes his outlook on life and learns that he never played a part in the memory of the one he wants to remember.

For the director Philippe Garrel, the suicide attempt is an intimate and autobiographic subject, introduced in both *Elle a passé tant d'heures sous les sunlights...* (1984) and *Night wind* (*Le vent de la nuit*, 1998). In the first film, there is still hope when Garrel himself hesitates in front of an open window, only to finally abandon the thought of suicide, thinking about his child and symbolically addressing himself to an entire generation: 'I don't think about suicide anymore, life is long you know, I have to continue.' However, in the second film, which is about ageing, the darkness is absolute, and the hero Serge is always ready to go, with his arm of 'delivery' constantly at hand. Hélène, an older disillusioned woman, cuts her veins in public. Refusing to recognize oneself in and by society thus appears to be an important reason for suicide. Some film-makers will however encourage further reflection giving their characters' suicides social and political significance. Agnès Varda gives a cynical humorous touch to the cliché of happiness in her film *Happiness* (*Le bonheur*) from 1965. In the film, a television personality says that happiness is found 'through submission to man'. Thérèse finds out that her husband has a mistress. Whilst the latter declares that two women mean two times the fun without hurting either one of them, Thérèse refuses this submission and kills herself. The end is perfectly immoral: the husband marries his mistress who now becomes his companion at home, at the table and in bed. All the more reckless is Robert Bresson's *Mouchette* from 1967, in which a heroine in despair confronts the cruel stupidities of adults, the suffering of her mother, the bestial desire that ends all innocence and the rage of a society that humiliates childhood. Valerian Borowczyk uses a convent for the symbolic representation of the Polish totalitarian system in *Behind convent walls* (*Intérieur d'un couvent*, 1977), based on a novel by Stendahl. The abbess wishes to impose a constrained set of rules on the sisters, but she does not succeed in getting all of them to respect her. Her stubbornness drives two sisters to madness and suicide, but the abbess finally dies as well. Borowczyk addresses a cynical response to those in rule: all systems imposed through force are doomed to vanish. Ken Loach describes men and women who struggle to keep their self-respect in a society full of social violence, crystallised in the working conditions and life of unemployment that he illustrates. In the dilapidated Glasgow of *My name is Joe* (1998), Peter Mullan is an unemployed former alcoholic who tries to save his friend Liam, a drug-addict sucked into the destructive spiral of misery, drugs, theft and low-paid jobs. One night Liam desperately seeks his friend, submerged by guilt for having double-crossed him and unable to follow his advice, he hangs himself by throwing himself out the window. The scene is tragic. Joe hangs over the lifeless body that dangles along the wall of the building whilst crying and screaming out his hatred towards an insensitive society that eliminates the weak with extraordinary brutality. Is suicide the only response to the inhuman rigidity of such a venture?

Wished for and planned death on film has often incited fervent debates. When the British filmmaker Michael Powell made *Peeping Tom* in 1960, the subject provoked a wide range of reactions. Mark Lewis (Carl Boehm), a young film-maker who is haunted by an intuitive fear, shut away in a morbid solitude, lures women to his studio and films the fear of his victims as they realise their impending death. An amazing film to some, whilst others consider it a clinical case of a pathologist, *Peeping Tom* analyses voyeurism by placing the viewer in the very uncomfortable position as film-maker, victim and camera simultaneously. Lewis is finally exposed by his neighbour and the police, and subsequently, kills himself

in a scene of great horror. Through the meticulous mise-en-scène of his own death, the viewer involuntarily assists in the making of the film. At this point of the film, Powell intelligently abandons the subjective camera, removing from Lewis the role as 'director' of his own death. The lapse between what is filmed with Lewis' camera and what Powell shows the viewer marks a distance between the protagonist and an ensuing de-dramatization. In fact, Powell refuses to show the suicide through the device installed by Lewis. The latter will not be able to see his proper death and the angle chosen by Powell is that of a spectator situated close by. The immediate consequences of the suicide are off-screen: what remains to be shown is the blood on the foot of the camera and the wall, the suffering and the spasms, the corpse, the horror and the impression of yet another dreadful waste.

Incurable illness and traumatizing accidents may be the cause of depression and reflections on life and death. In *The sea within* (Alejandro Amenábar, *Mar adentro*, 2004), Ramón (Javier Bardem) cannot move his head because of an accident in his youth. For almost thirty years he is bedridden and unhappy, his only opening to the world is the window in his room through which he can see the sea. Although family surrounds him, Ramón has but one wish: to decide over his own death and to end his life with dignity. Inspired by the true story of Ramón Sampedro, who featured regularly in the media in Spain; the film echoes back his struggle to receive the right to die with dignity. He ended his life on 12 January 1998 without accusing those who helped him. Amenabar explains that upon realizing what an admirable man Sampedro was he decided to make the film. He concentrated on the last months of his life, and the film celebrates life itself whilst addressing euthanasia and assisted suicide in a frank manner. Tackling such a delicate subject, Amenabar felt obliged to take a position:

> Assisted suicide is a delicate subject that has to be treated with care in order to not encourage people to kill themselves or others. As a director, I tried to be respectful towards handicapped and sick people. At the same time I had to respect what had happened. If I had been in Ramón's position, I would not have wanted to die, but I think that he was right in saying that his life belonged to him and that he could do what he wanted with it. This is why I think assisted suicide should be permitted.

The actor, Javier Bardem, follows the same line of reasoning:

> I think that as long as the people who are suffering are conscious, like Ramón Sampedro, and that it is not a question of an impulsive act or connected to depression, I support their choices all the way. If someone in my family in such a position would ask me, I would try to help that person, even if it would break my heart. Actually, I think that it would be as cruel to force a person with such an illness to die as it would be to force someone like Ramón to live. Everyone should be in charge of their own lives as they wish, and if someone is not capable of doing something like this on his/her own, we should have the right to help out. For me, it is the ultimate act of love.

Without ever flirting with morbid melodrama, Amenabar conveys Ramón's moral dilemmas in a poetic and humorous way, consequently opening the doors to societal debate. Through his meticulous film-making, he succeeds in incorporating all the questions that this predicament provokes. By asking his actors to improvise with the text as a starting point, thus animating the reactions they had following the interviews with the Sampedro family, Amenabar succeeds in multiplying the points of views surrounding the subject. Consequently, even if the director and protagonist take a stance for assisted suicide, the method they undertook in the making of the film prevented any clear-cut definitions or answers to the dilemma.

## The malaise of Asian cinema

Whilst Stevenson's *Suicide club* from 1882 was written with a certain sense of irony, *The complete manual of suicide* (1993) is a serious work in which the Japanese author, Wataru Tsurumi, describes in detail ten ways to commit suicide. He argues that there is no religion or law in Japan that is opposed to suicide, and that collective suicide has always been a part of Japanese culture. In explaining the increase in suicides in Japan this morbid best-seller, along with numerous websites and chat rooms, has often been criticised by public institutions as the source of, in particular, collective suicides. Suicide, along with luxury or eroticism, is taboo in the West, or in countries with a Christian tradition, but this is not the case in Japan. Japanese directors of the 1960s and 1970s like Yasuzo Masumura or Nagisa Oshima (as well as the author Yukio Mishima who orchestrated his own death), treat suicide in a manner which often mixes eroticism and suicide. Mishima made a short film called *Yukoku* in 1965, describing in detail the suicide of a soldier who feels dishonoured because he did not assist in the *coup d'état* in 1936. Malleable aestheticism erupting from ritual suicide (Mishima) and unprudish sex and flirting with death (Masumura, Oshima) were means to provoke scandals and to renounce the immobility of social classes. *Blind beast* (Masumura 1969) and *The realm of the senses* (Oshima 1976) both describe, in different ways, absolute passion; two lovers consider that the climax of love is to put an end to life together. In Japan, erotic death or sacrifice is an accepted means to settle some sort of conflict. When a situation is inextricable and harmony is disturbed, one way to bring back order is by eliminating the object of discord, which sometimes happens to be oneself. Suicide is merely one way of dying and the soul continues to live in the cycle of deaths and rebirths. However, in the light of the high number of suicides among particularly young people, Japanese directors have confronted the problem at stake by trying to provoke the public. Their approach, often influenced by 'gore',[2] sometimes appears more spectacular than it is pedagogical: *Marebito* was shot with a digital camera in a couple of days by Takashi Shimizu and is a nightmaresque scorching experience of absolute horror. Masuoka, the protagonist, a film enthusiast who films everything around him, films the suicide of an old man in the subway with an awestruck gaze. Profoundly traumatised, he withdraws, camera at hand, into the Tokyo subway in search for that ultimate fear that will propel him into insanity.

In *Jisatsu Circle* (Sono Shion, 2002) a collective suicide of fifty-four female high school students early on set the tone of the film. The metro is unable to stop because of the quantity of blood of the joint suicide. In the wake of the horror, genuine reflection on the suicides is to be found through the inquiry of a police inspector. At first, reasons for the suicides seem obscure: the harmful effects of a pop group, the Internet, Japanese society ... and then the tragedy triggers an epidemic of collective and individual suicides with no antecedent. When twenty-something high school students throw themselves off the roof of their school, the inspector changes the focus onto the moment of the group decision: What drives these adolescents to the decision to jump at the same time? As far as he is concerned someone must be pulling the strings and manipulating these premature yet unaware youths. The policeman notices the curious appeal a girl's band of 13-year-olds hold on his daughter and he digs deeper into the meaning of one of their choruses, 'Mail me'. Pursuing his inquiry he discovers an Internet site that incites adolescents to kill themselves. Sono Shion's film goes well beyond conventions, it is violent but it also denunciates the rigidity of Japanese society. He doesn't hesitate to show the foolishness of an act with such tragic and irreversible consequences. The *Jisatsu manual* (2003) by Osamu Fukutani is not as subtle as the *Jisatsu Circle*. The film can be situated at the crossroad of harmful opportunism and genuine work of a surrealist film. Fukutani's ambiguous approach, equally cautionary and condemning, does not propose any tangible moral and does not take a stand in relation to this plague of twenty-first century Japan. The hero of the film, Yu, is a young journalist, who on his boss's orders leads an inquiry on collective suicide. Through these sinister acts, Yu tries to break the mystery of suicide as a whole: what drives someone to end their life? His investigation leads him to Ricky, a young mysterious woman who in various chat rooms with suicide as focus, provides the most 'motivated' with a dvd called the 'Jisatsu Manual' (Suicide Manual). In the dvd she incites the spectators to commit suicide, introducing them to different ways of killing themselves. Yu becomes obsessed with the film, which brings about despair tainted with a sometimes baroque touch. Is he also the prey of the 'spirit of suicide'? The film offers an interesting basis of discussion about the morbid influences that may lead to suicide, but the systematic stigmatization of the video and the Internet, as well as the over-simplification of the characters, detracts from its worth. However, the nightmarish ending, in which Yu relinquishes the wish to understand for the wish to die, gives a stifling impression of an inescapable and tragic destiny. A great popular success, Yuichi Onuma made a follow-up to the *Jisatsu manual*, the tedious *The manual 2 intermediate level*.

The analysis of contemporary Japan is at its best in *Bashing* by Masahiro Kobayashi (2005). Kobayashi tells the story of the sad return of Yuko, former hostage in Iraq. The story is inspired by a real event. Her imprisonment and the publicity that came with it greatly humiliated the authorities and disgraced her family. Her father, forced to quit his work, sees no other way out than suicide. Public opinion, however, thinks that she should have died instead. As the title suggests, Yuko is harassed, showered with phone calls, insulted in the street, fired. Yuko is a foreigner in her own land. Profoundly upset by her father's suicide but refusing to follow his path, she decides to return to Iraq; a desperate yet determined reaction to the social and human rejection that she is victim of.

South Korean cinema also shows proof of a similar obsession with suicide, especially those of adolescents. *Memento mori* by Kim Tae-Yong and Min Kyu-Dong (*Yeogo goedam II*, 1999) is an excellent example. In a South-Korean secondary school for girls, Min-ah discovers the diary that two of her schoolmates write together. As she is reading the diary she experiences strange hallucinations. Later at the nurse's office, she is witness to an intimate embrace between the writers of the journal, Hyo-Shin and her girlfriend Shi-Eun. A few days later when the girls are getting ready for their annual health examination, Hyo-Shin throws herself out the window. Contrary to what one might think, Shi-Eun does not seem to be affected by her death and appears indifferent in the days that follow. From this moment on, strange phenomenon that will change Min-ah's life ensue. Hyo-Shin's suicide, the ghost that haunts the school hallways and a next to adult-free closed environment establish the scenery of the film. *The virgin suicides* and *Battle royale* (Kinju Fukusaku 2001) come to mind, but the two young directors manage to convey a personal style, primarily thanks to the disconcerting mix of genres and the fragmented and original narrative style. The captivating and effective montage helps the spectator penetrate the two inseparable girls' thoughts; whose bickering provokes quite a lot of laughter. Behind the comedic appearance drama is hidden a love story that leads to suicide.

*Memento mori*, alongside films by directors such as Park Chan-Wook and Kim Ki-Duk, as well as Kim Jee-Woon and Hong Sang-Soo, are part of a current in Korean cinema with focus on obsessions with death: a kind of death that fascinates adolescents and young adults to such an extreme that it exercises a power of destructive attraction on them. Suicide is for them an act of defiance, an enticement, an almost child-like game, a sort of performance to imitate idols such as Kurt Cobain. This cinema reflects the malaise of a society, its interiorized violence and the distress of youth lacking excitement. *Suicide designer* (Jeon Soo-Il 2003) is a brilliant yet disturbing example of such cinema. In the first shot, the camera intriguingly moves forward in a dark hallway, the silhouette of first a man, and then a woman appears. Sounds of footsteps in water and eerie drumming create an oppressive atmosphere. The camera keeps on moving forward slowly, almost in slow motion, suddenly the camera makes a quarter of a turn towards a staircase. At the top of a menacing stone monument immobile spectators wait for a performance to begin. A white sheet is lifted, stained and dripping with blood. A woman with long black hair, trembling with fear and smudged with blood is attached to a rope. A ghastly melody accompanies the scene. It is in fact nothing but a performance in which a woman simulates her own suicide. Then another evasive character appears, Sung, writer, art and jazz enthusiast with an obscure line of work: suicide designer. 'There are two ways of becoming God: by writing, or by directing people towards their death. I help people to die', he explains with unabashed cynicism. Desperate people contact him over the Internet, and he then sketches out and carries out their suicide according to their wishes. He considers his job as a work of art and provides such ambiguous motivations for his vocation as a writer's exultation, existential megalomania and lucrative business. Once again Stevenson's *Suicide club* comes to mind. Not unlike the Japanese films *Jisatsu Circle* and the *Jisatsu manual*, the red line of the scenario is an inquiry. A video-artist and his brother who is a taxi driver meet a naive young nymphomaniac and have sex with her. Stunned by her suicide, the two men independently decide to understand the causes of her suicide and find out about Sung. The ambience is grisly and dark and reality is mixed with abstruse and tragic fantasy: Is being alive nothing but a question of perception? In *Tale of cinema* by Hong Sang-Soo from 2005, the unease of Korean youth is once again portrayed through the temptation of suicide. The Thai film *Nothing to lose* (Danny Pang 2002) also depicts two young people who want to commit suicide. Somchai, a chronic gambler who has lost everything, and Gogo, a disillusioned girl, happen to attempt their respective

suicides on the same rooftop. Somchai is overtaken by his wish to live and endeavours to convince Gogo not to jump. Discovering their respective stories, they decide to use the willpower they had to kill themselves to take revenge on life and the people that made it unliveable for them. From there on, they get out on the road, much like Bonnie and Clyde or Thelma and Louise, with nothing to lose, scorning death.

To conclude, one example of Middle Eastern cinema will be mentioned, the interesting and profound film by the Iranian director Abbas Kiarostami, *A taste of cherry*. In the film, that won the Palm d'Or at Cannes in 1997, Kiarostami envisions suicide as the only option to the hellish life on earth and the stagnated future of an Iran devoured by fundamentalism. Still, the film remains unrelentingly optimistic and humanistic despite its pessimist outcome. The scenario is simple: Mr Badli drives around the surroundings of Teheran in search for a person who, in exchange for remuneration, would be willing to help him to end his life. The protagonists' motivations are never explained, but the discussions with the different characters he meets confront him over again with one essential question: Why not try to live?

## Cinematic visions of adolescent despair

Representations of adolescent suffering and suicide often appear all the more tragic and incomprehensible. Film-makers worldwide prove fascination for the theme, as it is of great concern to us all. Explanations are often sought in existing socio-economic and cultural contexts. In this fashion, Roberto Rossellini explores suicide in two of his films, *Germany year zero* (*Germania anno zero*, 1948) and *The greatest love* (*Europa'51*, 1952). An abandoned child, criminal by mistake, finds no place of reassurance and roams the street of a war-ravaged Berlin. He finds a demolished building from which he throws himself in a scene of dreadful violence. The camera does not move and observes the boy from a respectable distance. His feet move toward the emptiness, stays immobile for a second before the boy brutally lets himself fall. The camera follows his descent. A new shot fixates the little lifeless body, as lonely as before the fall. In a parallel shot, the child is seen calling for help, trying to get in touch with his mother who is too busy, trying to reconnect with the past. On screen, he does not die immediately after his fall; his mother has the time to realize how she has forsaken her own son. After her son's death, the mother's intense guilt spurs her to change direction in life to the great displeasure of her husband. With these two films, Rossellini provokes reflection on the causes of child suicides by calling to mind the responsibilities of society and the family, refusing to see the distress and existential anxiety of children facing a past too present and a worrisome future. Taking the leap to more contemporary cinema, Tom Moore, in his 1986 masterpiece, *Good night, mother* tackles the problem of adolescent suicide. Sissy Spacek informs her mother, Anne Bancroft, of her intention to kill herself with the same gun her father used to kill himself. She commits suicide despite her mother's desperate interference. At last the mother is forced to admit her daughter's right over her own soul and life. Four years later with *Dead poets' society* by Peter Weir, the director points to the responsibility of the family, and the father in particular, at the time of the son's suicide.

In recent years, *The virgin suicides* (Sofia Coppola 2000) and *Ken Park* (Larry Clark 2004) have both opened the door to interesting discussion concerning adolescent suicide. The off-screen narration told in a melancholic voice by a narrator/witness, immediately establishes Sofia Coppola's 2000 film, *The virgin suicides* as a chronic of suicide. 'Cecilia was the first one to go' the off-screen voice tells us, thus foretelling us the tragic end of the five Lisbon sisters and inscribing the events to come in an inescapable progression towards death. The Lisbon sisters live in an affluent North-American suburb at the end of the 1970s, together forming a homogenous and undifferentiated whole: transparent creatures that form one body of which the dominant trait is their blondness. Their unity is confirmed by recurring circular figures throughout the film. When the youngest sister ends her life at a party given in her honour, the mother (Kathleen Turner), paragon of virtue who suffocates her offspring through puritan education, collects her daughters around her to stop them from contemplating the horror scene. Her arms encircle and surround the adolescents who seem to be more or less compliant with her rigid rearing techniques. Whenever a member of the group drifts away from the community she is in danger. At the surprise party, Cecilia asks her strict mother if she can go to her room: the camera isolates her while she slowly climbs the staircase in a white virginal dress. Shortly thereafter she kills herself. The symbolic break of the circle represents the disintegration of the family and by extension of society. Lux, another one of the sisters, wakes up alone in the morning on the football field, abandoned by her lover after their first night of love-making; her body is white, fragile and she is untidy, lost in the enormous grass-field. The catastrophe is imminent and the process of death underway. The Lisbon sisters no longer have the strength to survive or to run away, they are let down and disgusted by their own existence over which they hold no control. They no longer want to suffer and decide to escape through suicide. They plan their death as a cinematographic scenario that will unveil their suffering to the world. *The virgin suicides* is not a suicide apologetic, but a critique of the social rigidity of an era. The collective suicide of the four remaining Lisbon sisters contributes to the resurfacing of the hypocrisy and conformism of a social class that seems to be living on borrowed time. The sisters' disappearance will forever stay with the boys of the neighbourhood and change their lives, but the tragedy does not seem to affect the community as a whole, which continues with its everyday life. The death of the young girls does not influence the egoistic and materialistic society around them as a means of possible spiritual regeneration. In response to the suicide of their daughters, the social suicide of their parents is set in motion; beginning with the dismissal of their father, a high school teacher.

Ken Park, a teenage redhead, prepares his backpack and gets ready for school. He leaves his house and goes to a skate park. He then puts his camera in front of him, turns it on, takes out a gun and shoots himself in the head. With this scene, Larry Clark opens his film, *Ken Park*, from 2004. With *Ken Park*, Larry Clark continues in the same vein as the collective suicide of the blonde heroines in Sofia Coppola's film: an extreme act that is generated by suffocating puritanism. The ghost of the adolescent follows the spectator for the rest of the film, which shows us the ravaged lives of various teenagers left to themselves in a North-American suburb. *Ken Park* depicts teenagers who grow up and who survive; at whatever costs their family or society around them have to pay. Ken Park's dazzling and violent suicide influences and pervades the collective unconscious of a group of teenagers in a dormant little town in California. The teenagers in the film try to balance their way through the transitory age of adolescence. They find transitory release of distress and show resistance through unrestrained sexuality. When a father of one of the protagonists, in an act of fury, breaks his son's skateboard and prime sign of identity, the tone is given. *Ken Park* is a narrative of adolescents broken by the depravation of their parents and sacrificed in the course of the collapse of the family.

With *Kamataki* Claude Gagnon received a handful of prices at the Festival de Montréal in 2005. In the film, the Quebecois film-maker proposes a serene look on a 'return to life'. After the death of his father and a subsequent suicide attempt, the young Ken Antoine is sent to his Japanese uncle Takuma, brother of his father. Takuma is a renowned ceramicist who makes kamataki, unvarnished pottery. The cultural and generational differences are enormous between the young, confused and disillusioned Ken from Montreal and his uncle, a wise man, famous artist and practicing Buddhist in the Japanese countryside. Ken is juxtaposed into an unknown universe, exotic yet disturbing at the same time. Beauty, ugliness, sweat, sex and his uncle trouble and bustle the still fragile young man. Without noticing, Ken discovers beauty where he least expects it and takes up contact with life again. Just like he knows how to give birth to, feed and look after the intense fire of his oven, Takuma will also know how to reignite Ken's flame.

## Conclusion

Passing from the rather conventional, often romantic, yet rarely realistic Hollywood cinema, to the intense and pessimistic imagery of suicide in a lot of European film, to the raw outlook reflecting a societal interrogation common in Asian movies, suicide on screen is above all a dramatic, painful and violent element of unforeseen or anticipated nature. A small number of films lead to genuine reflection on this tragedy that touches a great number of teenagers worldwide. Although the majority of feature films, of which a revealing yet limited selection have been introduced in this chapter, do not encourage suicide, very few sincerely examine the path that leads to the so-called passing to the act. Suicide in cinema takes an abridged form. Depression as a possible cause of suicide is scarcely in focus on screen. The sufferings of the characters who consider suicide or take their lives occupy but a minor part of the plot in scenarios that highlight action (Hollywood), cultural and social reflection (Japan and Korea), and finally an existential interrogation that borders on the too abstract (Europe). Suicide merely depicted as a heroic act or as a failure effectively trivialises the act, and may lead to teenagers concluding that ending one's life is an acceptable death. *The virgin suicides* entails serious reflection on the slow progression towards suicide that each one of the girls face, yet the film suggests suicide as the only solution to their sufferings. Behind this decision, the solitude and impossibility to confide lure and yet again become the triggering factors of suicide on screen. In no way is fiction film an instrument of therapy.

## Notes

1. The Hays Code is a code of censure for the production of films. The code was established by the US senator, Williman Hays, president of the Association of Motion Picture Producers and The Motion Picture Producers

and Distributors of America. The Hays Code was written in 1930 and put into practice as of 1934 until 1966.

2. The term 'gore' signifies 'coagulated blood' or 'abundance of blood'. In cinema the gore genre designates horror films or thrillers with bloody scenes. Gore films are found in all countries (usually Z series), but the Italian film-makers Mario Brava or Dario Argento are the forerunners of the genre.

## References

Interview with Rachel Samuels (on www.pardo.ch/2000/program/105r.htm)
Details on the production, directors, actors, plots, etc of the films discussed can be found on
http://www.imdb.com

# PART 10B

## Public Health Strategies: Early Detection and Health Promotion

# CHAPTER 72

# Early detection of mental ill-health, harmful stress and suicidal behaviours

Andrej Marušič, Brigita Jurišić, Dejan Kozel, Milan Mirjanič, Ana Petrović, Jerneja Svetičič and Maja Zorko

## Abstract

Success in early detection of harmful stress, mental ill-health, and suicidal behaviour is substantially dependent on system solutions at the macro level. Suicide prevention interventions and strategies can only be effective if cross-disciplinary knowledge and skills, at different stages of the suicidal process and on different vulnerable groups are combined. In this chapter, traditionally well-known vulnerable groups, such as people with depression and alcohol misuse, are discussed at different stages of the suicidal process, in order to increase early detection. Early recognition is also important in demographic groups that have been neglected to date in suicide prevention, such as mothers with pre-natal and post-natal mental disorders, persons with diabetes mellitus, spinal cord injury disabilities and adult childhood cancer survivors, as well as young vulnerable people for whom harmful stress can be a suicidal trigger. In regard to the implementation and process optimization of individual interventions, lessons from management and, in particular, from social marketing, can provide a key contribution.

## Public mental health: definition and history

The origin of public mental health, as a branch of public health can be traced back to the nineteenth century, when one of the major concerns facing public health doctors was the epidemics of infectious diseases in Europe, namely of cholera. Accordingly, the first role of public health became that of social reform within the field of sanitation: housing, fresh water supply, construction of sewages, etc. The obvious public mental health component of this social intervention was an indirect one, as spending money for the relief of the living conditions of the underprivileged classes simultaneously led to an improvement in mental health.

Public health has remained concerned with primary prevention of diseases ever since, either by eliminating the causes or by enhancing host resistance. Unfortunately, the majority of mental disorders have not yet proved susceptible to this approach. Measures to prevent mental disorders, such as introducing dietary intervention to eliminate pellagra, which is a nicotinic acid deficiency causing somatic symptoms and apathy, depression and dementia; the widespread use of penicillin to eliminate general paralysis of patients with syphilis, and neonatal screening programmes to detect phenylketonuria and congenital hypothyroidism, have over time become common and made an important impact. There are several other opportunities for prevention by early intervention that have not been properly exploited yet, e.g. the detection of perinatal mental disorders in mothers, follow-up and counselling of parents with mental ill-health, prevention of pathological bereavement reactions and of post-traumatic stress disorders, and finally, prevention of suicidal behaviour (Kendell 1997). Early detection and focusing on high-risk groups are two of the main domains of public health, in general, and of public mental health, in particular.

Despite efforts to achieve a conceptual turnaround in understanding mental health in the past few decades, it is evident that the present 'state of the art' of mental health has not yet been fully successful in achieving a public health perspective and/or status. In order to improve this situation, we have to answer the question 'What options should be chosen to involve and integrate mental health within public health?' Our current understanding of mental health at present tends to be perceived solely in relation to mental disorders and the prevention thereof. There is also harmful stress, an important cause of mental ill-health and, last but not least, suicidal behaviour.

If one considers all these aspects of mental health, it is obvious that public mental health should deal with subpopulations affected by mental ill-health as well as with interventions aimed at the whole population by preventing mental ill-health and promoting mental well-being. It is necessary for public health and mental health experts to replace the notion of mental health as exclusively dealing with health determinants and supplement it with health indicators of the interplay between harmful life circumstances or events, the quality of health care and health promotion. Life events and circumstances are known to have a considerable effect on our health, in general, with mental health being the most acutely responsive and sensitive reaction. For example, harmful stress is an extremely negative life event, especially in people with mental ill health or for those lacking well-functioning mental resiliency.

In the past, public mental health has not figured high on public health agendas due to the relative insusceptibility of mental disorder to prevention and the absence of mental health indicators. These, in turn, have presented an important opportunity for public mental health to develop further as it is appropriate to consider mental health both as health determinant and health indicator. Mental health indicators provide an opportunity to study mental health in the broader social context. According to the so-called concept of sociosomatics (Kleinman and Becker 1998), as opposed to psychosomatics, mind and body interactions are reframed as mind and body in social context. The direct impact of social context on bodily or illness experiences are expected: social forces shape psychophysiological processes, and patterns of symptoms are identified as local idioms of distress and cultural syndromes (Kleinman and Becker 1998). This concept is also relevant for the cross-cultural understanding of suicidal risk.

## Suicide as a public mental health problem

Presence of mental ill-health has been recognized as being of major importance to all societies and age groups, related to a loss of quality of life, it may cause human suffering, disability, increased social exclusion (mainly due to stigma) and mortality (also due to higher suicidal risk). Accordingly, mental disorders have to be detected as early as possible to improve prognosis and also to decrease mortality—mainly via prevention of suicidal risk. Moreover, as far as primary prevention is concerned, the harmful effect of stress is usually linked to negative life events, which often causes mental disorders and needs to be prevented. The latter cannot be tackled without considering the social context of the interaction between the mind and body.

An assessment of mental health indicators and determinants is a prerequisite for the successful prevention of mental disorders and promotion of mental health. This is even more obvious if we single out the major public mental health concern—suicide. About 70 per cent of deaths worldwide due to suicide occur in the age group 25–64 which, from the socio-economic point of view, are the most productive years. Suicide poses a great economic burden to society due to lost future productivity (see Chapter 49 in this book). However, this burden will differ from state to state and from continent to continent, depending on specific suicide rates in these states and age distribution of suicides in a given country. As far as Europe and North America are concerned, suicide claims substantially more life years, and more personal income, between the ages of 20–64 than either of the other two major killers, cardiovascular diseases and cancer. The average number of years of lost productivity due to suicide is twice the number of those due to cerebrovascular disease and ischaemic heart disease. In Slovenia, which has one of the highest suicide rates in the world, death from suicide is the leading cause of future lifetime income lost; the first leading cause of *valued years of potential life*

*lost* (VYPLL); the second leading cause of *working years of potential life lost* (WYPLL) with an average number of 21.7 years per person dying prematurely; the second leading cause of *premature years of potential life lost* (PYPLL) with 29.7 years per person that died prematurely, and the third leading cause of premature death, 15.9 per 100,000 inhabitants aged 0–64 (Šešok *et al.* 2004).

Public health measures for screening and early detection of vulnerable groups, especially during times of great change and potentially harmful stress (caused by loss and other life events), are more effective than measures taken in the later stages of suicidal process when suicide risk is known to be higher. Such efforts can only be achieved if mental health indicators and determinants of mental health are well-known and implemented through every day mental health policies.

## Early detection of mental ill-health: suicidality as a process

### Detection of suicide risk in earlier stages of the suicidal process: from negative thoughts to suicidal thinking

Any kind of negative thinking, among others feelings of guilt, low self-esteem, lack of confidence, a desire not to wake up in the morning, a wish to be dead, or suicidal thinking—with or without suicidal plan or intent—is frequently associated with low mood, which may occur in the context of various mental disorders, especially depression. Suicide is also more likely in those with an underlying depressive or neurotic personality or those who are emotionally labile (see Figure 72.1). The core problem in this context appears to be poor detection by primary care practitioners (Lepine *et al.* 1997), although primary care educational programmes that target recognition and treatment of depression show an increase in antidepressant prescriptions and, in some cases, a decrease in suicidal rates (Kelly 1998; Rihmer *et al.* 2001; Marušič *et al.* 2004; Szántó *et al.* 2007). Despite significant improvement in early detection and effective treatment for depression, as evidenced by several studies (Guthrie *et al.* 2001; Motto and Bostrom 2001; Cedereke *et al.* 2002; Mann *et al.* 2005), depression is frequently under-treated or unnoticed in the primary care setting (Thies-Flechtner *et al.* 1996; Brown *et al.* 2005) with the majority of people committing suicide having had contact with a primary care physician within the last month of life (Andersen *et al.* 2000, Luoma *et al.* 2002). (See also Chapter 62 in this book.)

Enhanced and systematic types of intervention are another step forward in improving detection and treatment of depression and in preventing suicidal behaviour (Mann *et al.* 2005). In fact, several studies have reported better management of depression in primary care due to more complex interventions and systematic changes that help ensure improved treatment (Katon *et al.* 1996; Pignone *et al.* 2002; Gilbody *et al.* 2003). The success of these interventions may be linked to an improved satisfaction of patients' needs and solution of their problems in relation to depression. It is suggested that better implementation of existing guidelines for treatment by qualitatively improved interventions, which are more flexible and patient-oriented, provide an improvement of delivery of solutions for patients' problems and patients' needs and result in improvement of the patients' adherence to treatment. When we think about tailoring improved interventions for management of depression in

| Mental state contributing | | Suicidal process stage | | Traits contributing |
| --- | --- | --- | --- | --- |
| | | | | |
| depression | → | negative thinking | ← | neuroticism |
| | | ▼ | | |
| | | passive suicidal thinking | | |
| | | ▼ | | |
| | | active suicidal thinking | | |
| | | ▼ | | |
| | | suicidal plan | | |
| | | ▼ | | |
| | | suicidal intent | | |
| impulsiveness | → | ▼ | ← | impulsivity |
| | | suicidal attempt | | |
| aggression | → | ▼ | ← | aggressivity |
| | | suicide | | |

**Fig. 72.1** The development of suicide behaviour from an unspecific negative thought to the attempted or the completed suicide through several stages (being influenced by various mental states and personality traits) as potential points for various public health measures to take place.

primary care settings we must be aware of the time and provision restraints within general practices. In this regard, interventions based on improved systematic collaboration between general practitioners and nurses, beside an enhanced role of the health care provider in the treatment process, is a valuable option. Multifaceted interventions that upgrade common treatment in primary care, like telephone care management with structured cognitive behavioural psychotherapy (Simon *et al.* 2004), seem feasible as they fit well within the busy primary care setting (Hunkeler *et al.* 2000).

## Detection of suicide risk at later stages of the suicidal process: from suicidal thinking to attempting suicide

Impulsive and aggressive personality traits, in persons with, for example, bipolar disorder and mental disorder related to disinhibiting psychotropic substance misuse, are also linked to the suicidal process (see Figure 72.1). Impulsivity speeds up the process, while aggression is crucial in the progression from suicidal attempt to completion. Suicidal behaviour associated with aggression is far more likely to be fatal.

Impulsivity and aggression are usually increased in a social network where the likelihood of taking disinhibiting psychotropic substances, such as alcohol or cocaine, is higher. More data is available for alcohol-related suicide risk than drug-induced suicide risk, with acute and chronic alcohol misuse having long been identified as a potential risk factor for suicidal behaviour (Wasserman and Värnik 1998; Wasserman 2001). Studies show that approximately 40 per cent of people with alcohol problems have attempted suicide, and binge drinking in adolescents is often a more accurate indicator of suicidal behaviour than depression and stressful events (Windle 2004). Alcohol increases suicidal risk through psychological distress, aggression and impulsivity, as well as through impaired cognitive function, such as decision-making and problem-solving strategies (Hufford 2001).

If alcohol-related suicidal risk is to be detected earlier we need to be aware of the main covariants of this relationship. Temporary binge drinking, suicidal threats, comorbidity with depression, loss of close friends, poor social support, living alone, unemployment and serious somatic health problems have all been identified as specific risk factors in this high vulnerability group, where the male:female ratio can be as high as 5:1 (Murphy 2000). Individuals with alcohol dependency syndrome who show more significant signs of dependency, who have an associated mental disorder as a result of alcohol dependence, are separated or divorced are at higher risk of suicidal behaviour (Preuss *et al.* 2003; Värnik *et al.* 2007). Negative self-image, loss of self-respect, loss of independence and hopelessness are all factors which speed up the suicidal process in individuals combined with harmful alcohol use (Demirbas *et al.* 2003). If we are to detect and prevent suicidal behaviour in earlier stages of the suicidal process sooner we must focus on:

◆ Prevention of harmful alcohol use and effective treatment of alcohol-related mental disorders in the population, for example in workplaces and military settings;

◆ Screening for suicidal behaviour and presence of other mental disorders in people with harmful alcohol use in all levels of the health care system and the occupational health service;

◆ Treatment of depression in individuals with harmful alcohol use;

◆ Detection of other relevant risk factors in alcohol-dependent individuals who are at greater risk for suicidal behaviour, e.g. individuals with poor social support (already divorced or getting divorced, unemployed, socially isolated etc.) and of those with poor physical health in social service offices and in religious congregations.

Suicidal depressed males with atypical (impulsive and aggressive) and clinically unrecognized depression (also relevant in the later stages of the suicidal process) may be overlooked by the medical health care system (Rutz 1999). (See also Chapter 35 in this book.) Accodingly, suicidal ideation and behaviour related to a typical depression is more difficult to prevent.

Availability of violent means of committing suicide, for instance access to firearms, plays an important role in the later stages of the suicidal process and public health legislation which restricts or prevents gun ownership is an important protective factor (see Chapter 77). Other contributing factors that may be important at this stage in the mental state of the suicidal are the presence of role models, either in the individual's social network or through portrayal by the media (see also Chapter 69).

# Early detection of suicidal behaviour by addressing the needs of highly vulnerable groups

## Chronic somatic disease as vulnerability

Success in preventing suicidal behaviour is linked to the early detection of high-risk factors. The most relevant risk factor is depression, with a prevalence of major depression in approximately 5% of the population (Lönnqvist 2000; Wasserman 2006) and 60% of suicides being associated with mood disorder, principally major depressive disorder and bipolar disorder (Mann *et al.* 2005). For an overview of suicidal behaviour in somatic diseases see Chapter 40 in this book.

People with disabilities, chronic physical illness associated with severe pain or painful treatment procedures and dire outcomes are one such group. Any chronic somatic disease is associated with an increased prevalence of mood disorders, depression and related suicidal ideation (Mayou 1997). While more than half of all cases of suicide are diagnosed with depression (Bertolote *et al.* 2003), the inability to recognize depression is more pronounced in the group with somatic diseases, and associated suicidal ideation and behaviour is more difficult to prevent.

Early detection of the risks of suicidal behaviour amongst patients with somatic diseases is essential, particularly those with comorbid depression, with a public health emphasis on the following:

♦ Sensitivity to depressive signs and symptoms should be emphasized by specialists at secondary care level (outpatients' services should consider depression as an important obstacle to a motivated and continuously followed prevention).

♦ Improved recognition and appropriate treatment of depression, at primary care level, increasing the effectiveness of preventing suicidal ideation and behaviour.

♦ Introduction of non-governmental organizations to increase mental ill-health and suicide awareness. Patients with chronic somatic illness usually participate in associations that provide information, education, assistance and other benefits. In these organizations, attention to early detection and prevention of depression and suicidal behaviour can be monitored.

## Diabetes mellitus and suicidality

Diabetes is unique in its combination of the burden of diet and exercise, coupled with invasive blood glucose monitoring and, often, multiple daily insulin injections on the individual (Harris

*et al.* 2003). Further, the chronic nature of the course of this disease makes it a high risk factor for suicide. Recent studies have estimated the prevalence of depression in individuals with diabetes may be at least twice the rate observed in the general population, negatively impacting on patients' quality of life and glycaemic control (Anderson *et al.* 2001). There is a surprising lack of studies on the suicidal behaviour of diabetics. Although 90–95 per cent of those diagnosed have non-insulin dependent diabetes mellitus (NIDDM) (Boswell *et al.* 1997), the most widely reported cases are of insulin misuse among the young with insulin-dependent diabetes mellitus (IDDM). Goldston *et al.* (1997) observed an association between suicidal thoughts and non-compliance of medical regimen amongst this group, whilst Kyvik *et al.* (1994) discovered suicide might be an underestimated cause of death among people with IDDM, and Dahlquist and Kallen (2005) reported an increased, but statistically insignificant, suicide rate. A recent study of 420 people with NIDDM and IDDM (Kozel and Maruši'c 2006) showed that more than 40% had a prevalence for depressive symptoms, with 32.8% of those showing symptoms admitting to active suicidal ideation, in marked contrast to the 8.5% with active suicidal ideation where serious depressive symptoms were absent.

## Surviving life-threatening disease: adult childhood cancer survivors

Cancer is another chronic somatic illness associated with depression, which can, understandably, lead to an increased suicidal risk. Depressive symptoms associated with cancer range from normal sadness, through acute stress response, to major depression (Massie and Holland 1990). Steps similar to those outlined for patients with diabetes mellitus should be taken at all non-governmental levels as well as at primary and secondary health care levels.

An especially interesting vulnerable group is that of childhood cancer survivors in adulthood. There is growing evidence that the experience of cancer in childhood, or adolescence, may lead to long-term physical or psychosocial consequences of illness and its treatment, due to having faced a potentially deadly illness and possibly traumatic hospitalization, feelings of helplessness and anxiety and altered contacts with social circles. Jereb (2000) reported on emotional consequences found in 79 per cent of long-term survivors, and Bürger-Lazar (1999) showed these patients have different personality characteristics compared to their peers without a history of cancer. Cancer survivors are found to be more introverted and emotionally unstable, less persistent and assertive, with lower self-esteem, having difficulty gaining independence and, as a result, often lack social support. When compared to their siblings, childhood cancer survivors report depressive symptoms around 1.6 times more frequently (Zebrack *et al.* 2002). Even though long-term survivors may be cancer-free for a number of years, many of them are faced with an increased risk of cancer recurrence (Jazbec *et al.* 2004) and physical impairments. These have been described as risk factors for both depression and suicidal behaviour at all stages—negative thoughts, passive and active suicidal thoughts, suicidal plan and intent, and attempted and completed suicide. Indeed, Recklitis *et al.* (2003) detected suicidality in 13.9 per cent of the adult survivors of childhood cancer, all of them also showing significant psychological distress associated with their dissatisfaction with physical appearance and poor physical health.

Our study, which was one of the first investigations to tackle the problem of depression and suicidality in adulthood childhood cancer survivors, showed that significant depressive symptoms are three times more frequent in cancer survivors (13 per cent) than in their controls (Svetičič et al. 2005). The symptoms were often coupled with being female, having lower education, being single or divorced, not attending association group meetings and reporting weaker sociability. The latter was also associated with suicidal thoughts and plans. Groups did not differ in frequency of suicidal features, but, interestingly, suicide-related variables were in association with having depressive symptoms only in the cancer survivors group.

We should, however, also point that other studies show a certain appreciation for life found in individuals who survived cancer, possibly as a result of having fought a battle with a potentially deadly disease in their early years, the battle that could possibly protect them from suicidal behaviour (e.g. Chesler et al. 1992; Zeltzer 1993). These studies, including our investigation (Svetičič et al. 2005) have not shown an increased risk of suicidal behaviour among adult childhood cancer survivors. Nevertheless, special attention should be paid to those with depressive disorders. Depression is approximately twice as frequent as in a population with no history of chronic childhood disease. Primary health care workers, specialists and non-governmental organizations in touch with survivors need to be aware of the increased likelihood of depressive symptoms and the associated suicidal risk in this group. Furthermore, strategies aimed at de-stigmatization of the disease, patients' integration into society and working on their often lowered self-esteem and weakened sociability should also be considered.

### Facing life-long disability due to spinal cord injury

As well as coming to terms with permanent physical disability, and all its consequences, spinal cord injury patients also need to face the additional burden placed on them by society. The permanent physically disabled are often treated differently, for example people may be especially kind to them, they speak louder, feel tense, ask too much about the illness or disability and patronise them as if they were either younger or in some way inferior (Zaviršek 2000). An individual's self view is highly influenced not only by important restrictions due to disabilities (Prout and Prout 1996), but also by the reactions of the social environment, which can affect the disabled's self-esteem. For example, due to a noticeable difference in their physical appearance, individuals with physical disabilities attract more attention than others that do not have instantly visible handicaps. Nosek and his colleagues (1996) claim that low quality of life in spinal cord injury individuals is more a consequence of barriers set by the environment than the disability itself as far as psychological and psychopathological adjustment are concerned. However, depression, sleep disturbance, suicidal thoughts and guilt can occur in 60 per cent of patients (de Carvalho et al. 1998), whereas the suicide rate can be up to ten times higher among paraplegics than their uninjured peers (Rish et al. 1997). In general, this group suffers from psychosocial maladjustment and substance abuse, which is an additional generator of vulnerability. Five years after trauma, suicide statistics for spinal cord injured patients are significantly lower, although they never drop to the same level as their uninjured peers. Our results on individuals with paraplegia, tetraplegia or amputation following a motor vehicle accident in Slovenia (Jurišič and Marušič in press) showed extremely high suicidality rates for all the groups, which correlated with low total self-esteem, presence of post-traumatic stress disorder symptoms

and, interestingly, but not surprisingly, a history of suicide in the family. Intrusive thoughts, feelings and images of the accident correlated with suicidal thinking and planning of suicide.

We can conclude that patients with spinal cord injury need good psychosocial rehabilitation, especially paying attention to patients' self-image following their medical care, in particular when they return to their own social contexts. These results also support our intent to seriously consider self-image and especially suicide risk in patients with permanent physical disabilities, something that has been rather neglected so far.

### Focusing on negative life events and harmful stress in youth

In several countries, suicide is now the second or third most frequent cause of death amongst 15–24-year-olds (Evans et al. 2004). An increased rate of suicide towards the end of adolescence indicate youths as another important vulnerability group where early detection should be of primary concern from a public health perspective. Change is an important risk factor for adolescent suicides. Adolescence brings about physical growth, maturation and development. Adolescents need to become familiar with these changes, which often cause confusion and difficulties. Low self-esteem, for example, as a negative development outcome represents a risk factor for suicide by itself and in correlation with depression (Hawton and van Heeringen 2002). Psychological autopsies of suicide show that depression is present at the time of death in most adolescents who die by suicide (Hawton and James 2005). Depression, anxiety, hopelessness and low self-esteem are important risk factors for adolescent suicide. Conduct disorders, substance abuse, impulsivity and aggressiveness as personality traits, together with a history of suicide attempt(s) and a family history of suicide in this vulnerability group were also pointed out by Zametkin et al. (2001).

Adolescent suicide can be accelerated by psychosocial stressors, such as recent loss, rejection and failure, which are a significant and very common characteristic of adolescence. The most influential environmental factors are a history of abuse, other adverse life events, school problems, problems in peer-relations and a dysfuntional family (Evans et al. 2004). The family is a predominant source of influence on the adolescent's suicidal behaviour. Family risk factors can be divided into three groups: loss of social support (death, parental separation or divorce), variability in parental functioning (affective disorders, suicidal tendencies, alcohol misuse) and physical and psychological violence. The strong influence of adverse events on adolescents may be due to a more limited capacity of younger people to cope with such stressors (Dube et al. 2001).

Many risk factors for adolescent suicide may not be identified in time, thereby making it difficult to predict and prevent suicide. Adolescents tend to appear as rather unpredictable, and although there may be warning signs, they are often uncommon and hard to identify. Depression or distress symptoms in adolescents are also different from those of the adult population. However, suicidal ideation is relatively common in the adolescent population (Zametkin et al. 2001) and simply focusing on these would help detect early suicidal risk. An Australian programme that trained primary care physicians to recognize and respond to psychological distress and suicidal ideation in young people led to an increased identification of suicidal patients (Huey et al. 2004). A substantial number of adolescents in need do not search for appropriate help, which is why more accessible clinical help and crisis services are needed. Prevention should be based on raising awareness of the problem of adolescent suicide, training gatekeepers (general practitioners, teachers etc.) to identify those at risk and providing education about community mental health resources. There is a need for better cooperation between different professions as well as the formation of concrete activities for young people, such as how to develop a positive attitude to life and to improve coping abilities and problem-solving, etc.

## Early detection and policy-making: social marketing

Success in early detection of harmful stress, mental ill-health, and suicidal behaviour is substantially dependent on systematic solutions at the macro level. Good policy-making is essential in order to select and implement cost-effective interventions that can optimize the use of usually modest or limited resources. Suicide prevention interventions and strategies can only be effective by the combination of knowledge and skills used in different disciplines at different stages of the suicidal process and on different vulnerability groups. Lessons from management and in particular from social marketing, both until now, scarcely employed approaches in suicide prevention, can provide a key contribution to the implementation and process optimization of individual interventions.

Social marketing is the application of commercial marketing technologies to the analysis, planning, execution, and evaluation of programmes designed to influence the voluntary behaviour of target audiences in order to improve their personal welfare and that of their society (Andreasen 1995). In previous decades, the social marketing approach has proven to be effective in tackling social issues like improving physical activity, tobacco use prevention, prevention of drunk driving and so on, all via the so-called marketing behavioural change (Malafarina and Loken 1993; Andreasen 1995; Kotler et al. 2002). The social marketing approach is based on the following two key points (Andreasen 1995):

1 The aim is to achieve benefit through influencing or changing behaviour;

2 The target group has a primary role in the social marketing process.

The social marketing conceptual perspective and inventory of tools, like customer orientation, audience segmentation, marketing research, strategic planning, competitive positioning and so on, could provide a valuable opportunity for suicide prevention, due to the explicit focus on tailoring evidence-based and cost-effective programmes. In fact, providing cost-effective and evidence-based interventions is an essential argument in the advocacy of preventive programmes to policy-makers in general, and suicide preventive action in particular. Hence, evaluation of interventions should be planned and incorporated in the programme outline from the outset of the strategy planning process in order to foresee possibilities and limitations of the evaluation for single interventions. From this perspective, social marketing can be considered a promising possibility, due to a broad inventory of concepts and tools that are almost unknown to the field of mental disease and suicide prevention, and that can be applied for designing and improving cost-effective and evidence-based interventions.

Based on social marketing information (Andreasen 1995; Weinreich 1999; Kotler et al. 2002) a summary of necessary steps in establishing and setting up effective suicide prevention services is proposed. 'Steps' is perhaps not the most appropriate term as the actions listed below are not necessarily performed in sequence:

♦ **Formative research**. Formative research is primary research that is carried out before a social marketing campaign (Andreasen 1995). It is conducted to analyse the issue to be tackled in a given environment and provide the basis for determining programme focus, objectives and goals. As already stated, an effective suicide prevention service should be designed and implemented based on specific environmental characteristics, such as suicidal behaviour determinants, indicators, risk factors etc. Moreover, the understanding of suicide prevention services for those who should be targeted must be enhanced. Questions like 'How accessible is the service?', 'How user friendly is the service?' and 'What are the physical and (especially) psychological barriers in using the prevention service?' must be answered.

♦ **Selection of interventions and target groups**. This step is based on the knowledge and experience gathered through formative research. Due to the need for tailoring cost-effective interventions, selection and design of clearly defined interventions aiming at clearly defined and specific target groups is essential for optimizing the resources and achieving the best outcome. Possible interventions and target groups must be analysed, compared and selected with regard to the relevant criteria outlined before the intervention starts.

♦ **Strategic planning and integration**. Strategic planning is the detailed designing and planning of mission objectives, specific tasks, responsibilities, time schedules and procedures for selected interventions. The aim of strategic planning is to improve efficacy and efficiency of selected interventions in the implementation process, since it is not just what you do that is important, but also how you do it. In this perspective, integration and optimization of planned activities with existing initiatives and infrastructure is crucial in order to achieve not just cumulative, but also synergistic effects, of combined interventions.

♦ **Pre-testing and implementation**. Pre-testing is the precursor of the implementation phase, as it is useful in detecting weaknesses and deficits of the planned actions, and as a consequence in saving money that would be spent on less effective, or ineffective, solutions. After pre-testing, the implementation phase begins. The impementation phase must be defined and managed very carefully, since even a great strategy can fail if the implementation process is inaccurate or uncoordinated.

♦ **Evaluation**. Evaluating interventions, which can be divided into process evaluation and outcome evaluation, is an essential part of setting up effective suicide prevention programmes. First, evaluation of implementation processes provides information and knowledge on how to improve or optimize selected interventions, e.g. availability and quality of the service, effectiveness of the implementation process, quality and strength of the established network etc. Secondly, the outcome evaluation can provide evidence of success for implemented interventions (e.g. impact on the prevalence of suicide attempts, impact on completed suicides), which is the basic argument for justifying the use of resources and for gathering funds for future activities.

Generic strategies for suicide prevention should be culturally sensitive and targeted to the specific understandings and attitudes of those to whom the messages are directed (Jenkins and Singh 2000). In addition to the adequate understanding of target users, services should meet their needs in order to improve user participation. This kind of perspective, which has already been used in social marketing theory and practice, was named the 'customer-centred mindset' by Andreasen (1995). In our case, the orientation is high-risk groups for suicide, thus it is from there that the establishment of cost-effective interventions should start.

## Conclusion

In many countries, suicide prevention is left to the enthusiasm of a few individuals and is, consequently, disorganized and without a proper national programme or strategy. A lack of vision is often coupled with a lack of strategy. The question 'Why?' has yet to be fully answered, while the following have often not even been asked 'Who?' 'With whom?' 'What', 'Where' and 'How?' Suicide prevention is usually based on a combination of the best possible pharmacological approach together with some psychotherapeutical appproaches, but there is a lack of communication between health and social care sectors, governmental and non-governmental organizations. Consequently, there is great need for continuity in preventive work, which requires, among other things, greater communication between sectors and disciplines dealing with the suicidal process. If we follow the suggestions of the social marketing perspective, it should depend on a country's capacity to form an effective social network with effective suicide prevention as the aim. The following aspects are necessary for suicide prevention to be truly effective:

- Suicide prevention in the community provided by the community as a whole, making it well-integrated and locally active.

- A health and social care network as dense as possible providing continuous assessment of risk and ongoing prevention.

- An optimal social care and occupational (or educational) provision, ensuring all are supported and kept outside dangerous levels of suicide risk.

Finally, the ethical question that suicide prevention should always balance: the person's right to freedom versus their right to be safe and healthy needs. This topic needs to be examined more deeply in a sophisticated scientific and ethical discussion.

## References

Andersen UA, Andersen M, Rosholm JU et al. (2000). Contacts to the health care system prior to suicide: a comprehensive analysis using registers for general and psychiatric hospital admissions, contacts to general practitioners and practicing specialists and drug prescriptions. *Acta Psychiatrica Scandinavica*, **102**, 126–136.

Anderson RJ, Freedland KE, Clouse RE et al. (2001). The prevalence of comorbid depression in adults with diabetes: a meta-analysis. *Diabetes Care*, **24**, 1069–1078.

Andreasen AR (1995). *Marketing Social Change: Changing Behaviour to Promote Health, Social Development, and the Environment*. Jossey-Bass Publishers, San Francisco.

Bertolote JM, Fleischmann A, DeLeo D et al. (2003). Suicide and mental disorders: do we know enough? *The British Journal of Psychiatry*, **183**, 82–83.

Boswell EB, Anfinson TJ, CB Nemeroff (1997). Depression associated with endocrine disorders. In MM Robertson and CLE Katona, eds, *Depression and Physical Illness*, pp. 255–270. John Wiley in Sons Ltd, Chichester.

Brown GK, Ten Have TR, Henriques GR et al. (2005). Cognitive therapy for the prevention of suicide attempts: a randomised controlled trial. *JAMA*, **294**, 563–570.

Bürger-Lazar M (1999). Psihološke značilnosti mladih odraslih, ki so v otroštvu ali mladostništvu preboleli raka. [Psychological characteristics of childhood cancer survivors]. Unpublished Master's Thesis. Faculty of Arts, Department of Psychology, Ljubljana.

Cedereke M, Monti K, A Ojehagen (2002) A telephone contact with patients in the year after a suicide attempt: does it affect treatment attendance and outcome? A randomised controlled study. *European Psychiatry*, **17**, 82–91.

Chesler MA, Weigers M, Lawther T (1997). How am I different? Perspectives of childhood cancer survivors on change and growth. In DM Green and GJ D'Angio, eds, *Late Effects of Treatment for Childhood Cancer*, pp. 78–98. Willey-Liss, New York.

Dahlquist G and Kallen B (2005). Mortality in childhood-onset type 1 diabetes: a population-based study. *Diabetes Care*, **28**, 2384–2387.

de Carvalho SAD, Andrade MJ, Tavares MA et al. (1998). Spinal cord injury and psychological response. *General Hospital Psychiatry*, **20**, 353–359.

Demirbas H, Celik S, Ilhan IO et al. (2003). An examination of suicide probability in alcoholic in-patients. *Alcohol and Alcoholism*, **38**, 67–70.

Dube SR, Anda RF, Felitti VJ et al. (2001) Childhood abuse, household dysfunction, and the risk of attempted suicide throughout the life span: findings from the adverse childhood experiences study. *JAMA*, **286**, 3089–3096.

Evans E, Hawton K, Rodham K (2004). Factors associated with suicidal phenomena in adolescents: a systematic review of population-based studies. *Clinical Psychology Review*, **24**, 957–979.

Gilbody S, Whitty P, Grimshaw J et al. (2003). Educational and organizational interventions to improve the management of depression in primary care. *JAMA*, **289**, 3145–3151.

Goldston DB, Kelley AE, Reboussin DM et al. (1997). Suicidal ideation and behaviour and noncompliance with the medical regimen among diabetic adolescents. *Journal of the American Academy of Child and Adolescent Psychiatry*, **36**, 1528–1536.

Guthrie E, Kapur N, Mackway-Jones K et al. (2001). Randomised controlled trial of brief psychological intervention after deliberate self-poisoning. *BMJ*, **323**, 135–138.

Harris T, Cook DG, Victor C et al. (2003). Predictors of depressive symptoms in older people—a survey of two general practice populations. *Age and Ageing*, **32**, 510–518.

Hawton K and James A (2005). Suicide and deliberate self-harm in young people. *British Medical Journal*, **330**, 891–894.

Hawton K and van Heeringen K (2002). *The International Handbook of Suicide and Attempted Suicide*. Wiley, London.

Huey SJ Jr, Henggeler SW, Rowland MD et al. (2004). Multisystemic therapy effects on attempted suicide by youths presenting psychiatric emergencies. *Journal of the American Academy of Child and Adolescent Psychiatry*, **43**, 183–190.

Hufford R (2001). Alcohol and suicidal behaviour. *Clinical Psychology Review*, **21**, 797–811.

Hunkeler EM, Meresman JF, Hargreaves WA et al. (2000). Efficacy of nurse telehealth care and peer support in augmenting treatment of depression in primary care. *Archives of Family Medicine*, **9**, 700–708.

Jazbec J, Ećimović P, Jereb B (2004). Second neoplasms after treatment of childhood cancer in Slovenia. *Pediatric and Blood Cancer*, **42**, 574–581.

Jenkins R and Singh B (2000). General population strategies of suicide prevention. In K Hawton and K van Heeringen, eds, *The International Handbook of Suicide and Attempted Suicide*, pp. 597–615. Wiley, London.

Jereb B (2000). Model for long-term follow-up of survivors of childhood cancer. *Medical and Pediatric Oncology*, **34**, 256–258.

Jurišić B and Marušič A (in press). Suicidal ideation and behaviour and some pyschological correlates in physically disabled motor vehicle accident survivors. *Crisis*.

Katon W, Robinson P, Von Korff M (1996). A multifaceted intervention to improve treatment of depression in primary care. *Archives of General Psychiatry*, **53**, 1026–1031.

Kelly C (1998). The effects of depression awareness seminars on general practitioners knowledge of depressive illness. *Ulster Medical Journal*, **67**, 33–35.

Kendell R (1997). How psychiatrists can contribute to the public health. *Advances in Psychiatric Treatment*, **3**, 188–196.

Kleinman A and Becker AE (1998). 'Sociosomatics': the contributions of anthropology to psychosomatic medicine. *Psychosomatic Medicine*, **60**, 389–393.

Kotler P, Roberto N, Lee N (2002). *Social Marketing: Improving the Quality of Life*, 2nd edn. SAGE Publications, London.

Kozel D and Marušič A (2006). Individuals with diabetes mellitus with and without depressive symptoms: could social network explain the comorbidity? *Psychiatrica Danubina*, **18**, 12–8.

Kyvik KO, Stenager EN, Green A et al. (1994). Suicides in men with IDDM. *Diabetes Care*, **17**, 210–212.

Lepine JP, Gastpar M, Mendlewicz J et al. (1997). Depression in the community: the first pan-European study DEPRES (Depression Research in European Society). *International Clinical Psychopharmacology*, **12**, 19–29.

Lonnqvist JK (2000). Psychiatric aspects of suicidal behaviour: depression. In K Hawton and K van Heeringen, eds, *The International Handbook of Suicide and Attempted Suicide*, pp. 107–120. Wiley, London.

Luoma JB, Martin CE, Pearson JL (2002). Contact with mental health and primary care providers before suicide: a review of the evidence. *American Journal of Psychiatry*, **159**, 909–916.

Malafarina K and B Loken (1993). Progress and limitations of social marketing: a review of empirical literature on the consumption of social ideas. *Advances in Consumer Research*, **20**, 397–404.

Mann JJ, Apter A, Bertolote J et al. (2005). Suicide prevention strategies. *JAMA*, **294**, 2064–2074.

Marušič A and Farmer A (2001). Toward a new classification of risk factors for suicide behaviour. *Crisis*, **22**, 43–46.

Marušič A, Roškar S, Dernovšek M et al. (2004). An attempt of suicide prevention: the Slovene Gotland Study. In *Program and Abstracts of the 10th European Symposium on Suicide and Suicidal Behaviour*, p. 77. ICS, Copenhagen.

Massie MJ and Holland JC (1990). Depression and the cancer patient. *Journal of Clinical Psychiatry*, **51**, 12–17.

Mayou RA (1997). Depression and types of physical disorder and treatment. In MM Robertson and CLE Katona, eds, *Depression and Physical Illness*, pp. 2–38. John Wiley, Chichester.

Motto JA and Bostrom AG (2001). A randomized controlled trial of postcrisis suicide prevention. *Psychiatric Services*, **52**, 828–833.

Murphy GE (2000). Psychiatric aspects of suicidal behaviour: substance abuse. In K Hawton and K van Heeringen, eds, *The International Handbook of Suicide and Attempted Suicide*, pp. 135–146. Wiley, London.

Nosek MA, Fuhrer MJ, Potter C (1995). Life satisfaction of people with physical disabilities: relationship to personal assistance, disability status, and handicap. *Rehabilitation Psychology*, **40**, 191–202.

Pignone MP, Gaynes BN, Rushton JL et al. (2002). Screening for depression in adults: a summary of the Evidence for the U.S. Preventive Services Task Force. *Annals of Internal Medicine*, **136**, 765–776.

Preuss UW, Schuckit MA, Smith TL et al. (2003). Predictors and correlates of suicide attempts over 5 years in 1,237 alcohol-dependent men and women. *American Journal of Psychiatry*, **160**, 56–63.

Prout HT and Prout SM (1996). Global self-concept and its relationship to stressful life conditions. In BA Bracken, ed., *Handbook of Self-concept: Developmental, Social and Clinical Considerations*, pp. 78–98. John Wiley and Sons, Inc., New York.

Recklitis C, O'Leary T, Diller L (2003). Utility of routine psychological screening in the childhood cancer survivor clinic. *Journal of Clinical Oncology*, **21**, 787–792.

Rihmer Z, Belso N, Kalmar S (2001). Antidepressants and suicide prevention in Hungary. *Acta Psychiatrica Scandinavica*, **103**, 238–239.

Rish BL, Dilustro JF, Salazar AM et al. (1997). Spinal cord injury: a 25-year morbidity and mortality study. *Military Medicine*, **162**, 141–148.

Rutz W (1999). Improvement of care for people suffering from depression: the need for comprehensive education. *International Clinical Psychopharmacology*, **14**, 27–33.

Šešok J, Roškar S, Marušič A (2004). Burden of suicide and … have we forgotten the open verdicts? *Crisis*, **25**, 47–50.

Simon GE, Ludman EJ, Tutty S et al. (2004). Telephone psychotherapy and telephone care management for primary care patients starting antidepressant treatment. *JAMA*, **292**, 935–942.

Svetičič J, Bucik V, Jereb B, Marušič A (2005). Depresivnost in samomorilno vedenje oseb, ki so v otroštvu ali mladostništvu preživele raka [Depression and suicidal behaviour in childhood cancer survivors]. (Neobjavljeno diplomsko delo [Unpublished graduate thesis]). Faculty of Arts, Department of Psychology, Ljubljana.

Szántó K, Kalmar S, Hendin H et al. (2007). A suicide prevention program in a region with a very high suicide rate. *Archives of General Psychiatry*, **64**, 914–920.

Thies-Flechtner K, Muller-Oerlinghausen B, Seibert W et al. (1996). Effect of prophylactic treatment on suicide risk in patients with major affective disorders: data from a randomized prospective trial. *Pharmacopsychiatry*, **29**, 103–107.

Värnik A, Kõlves K, Väli M et al. (2007). Do alcohol restrictions reduce suicide mortality? *Addiction*, **102**, 251–6.

Wasserman D ed (2001). *Suicide—An Unnecessary Death*. Martin Dunitz, London.

Wasserman D (2006). *Depression: The Facts*. Oxford University Press, Oxford.

Wasserman D and Värnik A (1998). Reliability of statistics on violent death and suicide in the former USSR, 1970–1990. *Acta Psychiatria Scandinavica*, **394**, 34–41.

Weinreich NK (1999). *Hands-on Social Marketing: A Step-by-Step Guide*. SAGE Publications, London.

Windle M (2004). Suicidal behaviours and alcohol use among adolescents: a developmental psychopathology perspective. *Alcoholism, Clinical and Experimental Research*, **5**, 29–37.

Zametkin AJ, Alter MR, Yemini T (2001). Suicide in teenagers: assessment, menagement and prevention, *JAMA*, **286**, 3120–3125.

Zaviršek D (2000). *Handicap as a Cultural Trauma: Historization of Images, Bodies and Everyday Practices of Affected People*. Zalozba/* cf, Ljubljana.

Zebrack BJ, Zeltzer LK, Whitton J et al. (2002). Psychological outcomes in long-term susrvivors of childhood leukemia, Hodgkin's disease and non-Hodgkin's lymphoma: a report from the Childhood Cancer Survivor Study. *Pediatrics*, **110**, 42–52.

Zeltzer LK (1993). Cancer in adolescents and young adults: psychosocial aspect, long-term survivors. *Cancer Supplement*, **71**, 3463–3468.

# CHAPTER 73

# The role of schools, colleges and universities in suicide prevention

Madelyn S Gould, Anat Brunstein Klomek and Kristen Batejan

## Abstract

The present chapter reviews school-based suicide prevention strategies. School-based suicide prevention efforts have usually been designed separately for high school and college/university students, but the underlying strategies are similar, having two general goals: case finding with accompanying referral and treatment or risk factor reduction. Promising empirically based prevention strategies include screening for at-risk youth, gatekeeper training programmes, and skills training for students. Positive results from new 'hybrid' curriculum programmes may lead to overcoming the long-standing reluctance to implement curriculum-based strategies due to deleterious effects formerly reported for suicide 'awareness' curriculum programmes. Continuing evaluation studies of all the specific programmes reviewed in this chapter are needed, particularly as they are adapted to the cultural context in which a programme is to be implemented. A remaining challenge is to overcome the obstacles that have impeded the development and implementation of suicide prevention programmes in developing countries in Asia, Africa and South America. Today there is a marked disparity in the prevalence of school-based programmes between developing and developed countries.

## Introduction

School-based prevention strategies are a significant feature of most national suicide prevention agendas (Taylor 1997; Wasserman *et al.* 2004). Seventeen out of the eighteen countries of the WHO European region that have established suicide-prevention initiatives administer suicide-prevention sessions in the schools, with schools being a much higher-focus arena than the workplace, housing areas, or within the military (WHO 2002). The popularity of school-based suicide prevention strategies reflects the convenience with which adolescents and young adults can be reached, enabling prevention programmes to be carried out in a cost-effective

manner (Shaffer and Gould 2000). A comprehensive plan for suicide prevention in schools involves a continuum of activities, including health promotion, prevention, intervention and postvention (Locke 2007). The present chapter will focus primarily on prevention efforts that target the general student population, while recognizing the critical role that school mental health services play in addressing the treatment needs of the acutely distressed or suicidal student. Policies regarding involuntary leaves of absence (for example, when a student is required to leave school for a semester after a suicide attempt), re-entry protocols and parental notification for suicidal students are also of major importance to colleges and universities in their efforts to prevent suicides on campus (Appelbaum 2006; The Jed Foundation 2006).

School-based suicide prevention efforts have usually been designed separately for high school and college/university students, with consequent documents presenting prevention models for children and youth in schools (e.g. Guo and Harstall 2002; Gould and Kramer 2001) or college and university settings (Suicide Prevention Resource Center 2004; The Jed Foundation 2006). Yet despite distinct initiatives, the underlying suicide prevention strategies are similar, having two general goals: case finding with accompanying referral and treatment or risk factor reduction (Centers for Disease Control and Prevention 1994; Gould *et al.* 2003). The case-finding strategies to be reviewed include suicide 'awareness' educational curricula, screening, and gatekeeper training. The risk reduction strategy to be reviewed is skills training. This chapter will review the empirical evidence for the effectiveness of each strategy and present recent programmes exemplifying each goal. School-based prevention efforts have also occasionally included telephone crisis services (hotlines) and means restriction in their suicide prevention armamentarium, but these will not be reviewed within the scope of this chapter, which is focusing on more prototypical school-based suicide prevention strategies. The current review is based on a comprehensive but not exhaustive review of prevention programmes and research available in English language journals and Internet resources, using PsycINFO, MedLine, and Google Scholar as the main search engines.

## Case-finding strategies

### Suicide awareness educational curricula

Most suicide awareness curriculum programmes have been implemented at the high school-level with only minimal suicide prevention curricula taught at universities (Hazell *et al.* 1999). These educational programmes seek to increase awareness of suicidal behaviour in order to facilitate self-disclosure and prepare teenagers to identify at-risk peers and take responsible action (Kalafat and Elias 1994). The underlying rationale of these programmes is that teenagers are more likely to turn to peers than adults for support in dealing with suicidal thoughts (Ross 1985; Kalafat and Elias 1994; Hazell and King 1996). While components of some programmes have focused on faculty, staff and/or parents, the core of the programmes has been the student curriculum (Kalafat *et al.* 2003). Suicide awareness curricula have typically employed a model explaining suicide as an understandable response to stress and downplayed suicide as a symptom of an underlying mental illness (Garland *et al.* 1989; Shaffer and Gould 2000); although some curriculum-based programmes have promoted the concept that suicide is directly related to mental illness, usually major depression (Ciffone 1993, 2007). The curriculum often includes a videotape of a suicidal youth presenting warning signs, such as sadness, irritability, explicit statements of suicidal intent, or giving away possessions. Promotion of help-seeking has also been a key component of the programmes. Several studies have evaluated school-based suicide awareness programmes (Shaffer *et al.* 1991; Silbert and Berry 1991; Vieland *et al.* 1991; Ciffone 1993; Kalafat and Elias 1994; Kalafat and Gagliano 1996; Portzky and van Heeringen 2006; Ciffone 2007). Improvements in knowledge (Silbert and Berry 1991; Kalafat and Elias 1994; Portzky and van Heeringen 2006) and attitudes (Ciffone 1993; Kalafat and Elias 1994; Kalafat and Gagliano 1996; Portzky and van Heeringen 2000; Ciffone 2007) have been found. Despite positive changes in knowledge, studies have reported no effects on coping styles or levels of hopelessness (Portzky and van Heeringen 2006). Furthermore, other studies have reported no benefits (Shaffer *et al.* 1990, 1991; Vieland *et al.* 1991) or detrimental effects of suicide prevention education programmes (Overholser *et al.* 1989; Shaffer *et al.* 1991). Detrimental effects have included a decrease in desirable attitudes (Shaffer *et al.* 1991); a reduction in the likelihood of recommending mental health evaluations to a suicidal friend (Kalafat and Elias 1994); more hopelessness and maladaptive coping responses among boys after exposure to the curriculum (Overholser *et al.* 1989); and negative reactions among students with a history of suicidal behaviour, including their not recommending the programmes to other students, and feeling that talking about suicide in the classroom 'makes some kids more likely to try to kill themselves' (Shaffer *et al.* 1990); yet these detrimental effects have not been found universally (Portzky and van Heeringen 2006). Other limitations of this strategy are that baseline knowledge and attitudes of students are generally sound (Shaffer *et al.* 1991; Kalafat and Elias 1994), and changes in attitudes and knowledge are not necessarily highly correlated with behavioural change (Kirby 1985;

McCormick *et al.* 1985; Portzky and van Heeringen 2006). On the other hand, psycho-educational programmes are rated by secondary school principals, superintendents, and school psychologists as more acceptable, appropriate and effective than other school-based suicide prevention strategies, such as screening programmes (Miller *et al.* 1999; Eckert *et al.* 2003; Scherff *et al.* 2005).

### Curricula programmes

Two educational curricula rated as promising by the National Registry of Evidence-Based Programs and Practices (NREPP), a federally funded programme in the US (Rodgers *et al.* 2007), are Lifelines (Kalafat *et al.* 2003) and Signs of Suicide (SOS) http://www.mentalhealthscreening.org (Aseltine and DeMartino 2004), which can be considered 'hybrid' or 'composite' programmes in light of their augmenting their curriculum with another suicide prevention strategy. Lifelines includes gatekeeper training, i.e., education for gatekeepers, such as teachers, school staff and parents, as well as curriculum for students; SOS augments its curriculum with screening of students. The Lifelines programme focuses on teaching students to seek adult help for troubled peers, and also addresses administrators, faculty, staff and parents to increase the likelihood that these gatekeepers can identify, engage and obtain help for at-risk youth (Kalafat 2003). The programme implementation initially reviews school policies and procedures with administrators, followed by presentations to faculty and parents. The student curriculum, presented by regular classroom teachers, cannot be implemented until the components with the gatekeepers are completed because the gatekeepers have to be appropriately prepared to respond to students' referrals of at-risk peers (Kalafat *et al.* 2007). There is evidence that Lifelines may increase students' expressed intent to tell an adult about an at-risk peer (Kalafat *et al.* 1993, 2007). The curricula can be implemented with fidelity by trained school personnel and sustained over a period of years (Kalafat and Ryerson 1999; Kalafat *et al.* 2007).

SOS, which was developed by the non-profit organization Screening for Mental Health, Inc., has the basic message that suicidal behaviour is directly related to mental illness and needs appropriate psychiatric treatment. SOS is a 2-day school-based intervention which includes two components. The first is an educational curriculum (via video and group discussion) in which the students learn the acronym ACT: *Acknowledging* the signs of suicide that others display; letting the other know you *Care* and want to help; and *Telling* a responsible adult. The curriculum is followed by a brief anonymous self-screening for depression and other risk factors associated with suicide. The screen is considered a self-education tool. The students evaluate their own level of risk and depending on their score on the screen the students are provided instructions about seeking treatment. An evaluation of the SOS programme, reported high satisfaction by school personnel (Aseltine 2003) and a short-term decrease in students' suicide attempts; although neither help-seeking behaviour nor suicide ideation were affected (Aseltine and DeMartino 2004). The reduced suicide attempt rate was interpreted by the evaluators as having been due in part to increased understanding of depression and suicide (Aseltine and DeMartino 2004). The extent to which the educational or screening components of the SOS programme were responsible for the changes is not known.

There was a period of declining interest in curriculum-based suicide awareness programmes in schools in the mid-1990s (Kalafat 2003) given the conflicting evidence for their efficacy (Guo and Harstall 2002); however, the Surgeon General's Call to Action to Prevent Suicide in 1999 (Surgeon General 1999) and the recent promising findings of Lifelines and SOS, as noted above, have spurred a new interest in school-based *composite* curriculum programmes in the US. Elsewhere the evidence of possible harmful effects of earlier didactic suicide awareness curricula has precluded any recommendation of curriculum programmes for school-aged youth (Beautrais *et al.* 2007).

## Screening

A prevention strategy that has received increased attention is case-finding through direct screening of individuals. Screening strategies are based on the valid premise that suicidal adolescents are under-identified, suffer from an active, often treatable, mental illness, and exhibit identifiable risk factors (Gould *et al.* 2003). Screening programmes involve self-report and individual interviews to identify youngsters at risk for suicidal behaviour (Reynolds 1991; Shaffer and Craft 1999; Thompson and Eggert 1999; Joiner *et al.* 2002). School-wide screenings, involving multi-stage assessments, have focused on depression, substance abuse problems, recent and frequent suicidal ideation, and past suicide attempts. Evidence for the clinical validity and reliability of school-based screening procedures has emerged. Use of the Suicidal Ideation Questionnaire in a midwestern high school in the US yielded a sensitivity ranging from 83–100 per cent with specificity from 49–70 per cent (Reynolds 1990). The Suicide Risk Screen's use among 581 students in seven US high schools had a sensitivity ranging from 87–100 per cent with specificity from 54–60 per cent (Thompson and Eggert 1999). Among 2004 teenagers from eight New York metropolitan area high schools, Columbia *TeenScreen* exhibited a sensitivity of approximately 88 per cent and specificity of 76 per cent (Shaffer and Craft 1999). Moreover, many high risk adolescents were previously unidentified. Recently, Columbia Suicide Screen (CSS), completed by 1729 ninth–twelfth graders, had a sensitivity and specificity of 75 per cent and 83 per cent, respectively (Shaffer *et al.* 2004). Systematic clinical evaluations using interviews such as the Suicidal Behavior Interview (Reynolds 1990) and the Diagnostic Schedule for Children (Shaffer and Craft 1999) have provided the suicidal status criteria in these studies. A recent examination of a potential shortcoming of these programmes—the concern that asking a youngster about suicidal thoughts and behaviour may trigger subsequent suicidal ideation and behaviour—found that there was no evidence of an iatrogenic effect of asking about suicide (Gould *et al.* 2005). Neither distress nor suicidality increased among the general population or high-risk students who were asked about suicidal ideation/behaviour. On the contrary, the findings suggested that asking about suicidal ideation/behaviour may have been beneficial for students with depression or past suicide attempts.

## Screening programmes

A screening programme for high school populations that has been rated as promising by NREPP is the TeenScreen (Shaffer *et al.* 2004; Rodgers *et al.* 2007; http://www.teenscreen.org) and a recent programme designed for college populations is the US College Screening Project developed by the American Foundation for Suicide Prevention (Haas *et al.* 2003). Briefly, a screening includes completion of the Columbia Health Screen (CHS) or other self-administered screening instruments. Participants who score 'positive' are interviewed by an on-site mental health professional to determine if further evaluation is necessary. Lastly, the parents of those who need further evaluation are offered assistance with obtaining an appointment in the community. Research has shown that teens at risk for suicide are identified through the screening (Shaffer *et al.* 2004) and that the screen can identify students not previously identified (Shaffer and Craft 1999). Currently, the TeenScreen programme is active in more than 400 communities throughout the US and has been implemented in Panama, South Korea, Colombia, Canada and Taiwan. Versions of the questionnaire have been translated into Spanish and Chinese (McGuire, personal communication). The flexibility of the programme and the services that are offered to sites allows the programme to be implemented around the world. The TeenScreen staff work with communities to develop screening that can accommodate their specific needs and resources. In the US, the President's New Freedom Commission on Mental Health (2003) named the TeenScreen programme as a model programme for identifying at-risk youth and linking them to intervention services. The US College Screening Project (Haas *et al.* 2003) uses a web-based service to reach students and invite them to participate in a screening questionnaire including topics of depression, suicidal behaviour and suicidal ideation (past and present), anxiety, substance abuse, and eating disorders (Haas *et al.* 2003). Students are only identified by their log-in ID and if they meet criteria for significant psychopathology requiring treatment, a clinician will contact them via email to discuss their personalized diagnosis and treatment options. Because these screenings are anonymous, counselling services cannot require or force students into treatment even if they are screened and deemed at-risk of suicide. In the pilot test, only 25 per cent of students completed the questionnaire, and six were identified and referred for treatment (Haas *et al.* 2003). While this statistic may be troubling because the yield of the programme is not impressive, the College Screening Project may fuel awareness of mental health issues among students and potentially decrease stigma surrounding receiving help or being labelled as mentally ill. Two universities in the US have been using this screening programme since 2002, but there is no evaluative study published as yet.

Although screening appears to be a promising suicide prevention strategy, a number of challenges still need to be addressed (Gould *et al.* 2003). First, suicidal risk 'waxes and wanes' over time, therefore multiple screenings may be necessary to minimize 'false negatives' (Berman and Jobes 1995). Second, school-wide student screening programmes have been rated by high school principals and other school personnel as significantly less acceptable than curriculum-based and staff in-service programmes, as noted previously; although most respondents in these studies have had either no or minimal exposure to screening programmes (Miller *et al.* 1999; Eckert *et al.* 2003; Scherff *et al.* 2005). Moreover, some community members have also voiced opposition to screening efforts, describing these efforts as a violation of the family's right to privacy (Ashford 2005) because of their misconception that the screening of their children is mandatory (Weist *et al.* 2007). Third, screenings in general school populations tend to yield large numbers of false positives (e.g. Hallfors *et al.* 2006), placing a significant burden on schools and services. Fourth, schools need to have the capacity to follow up with students identified as at-risk by a screen, and have appropriate interventions in place before any screening programme is implemented (Gutierrez *et al.* 2004; Hallfors *et al.* 2006). Finally, the ultimate success of this strategy is dependent on the effectiveness of the referral (Gutierrez *et al.* 2004). Considerable effort must be made to assist the families and adolescents in obtaining help if it is needed. Nevertheless, school-based screening is considered a promising prevention strategy to identify at-risk youth and is being increasingly recommended as part of national suicide prevention strategies (e.g. Beautrais *et al.* 2007) and as an integral component of a public health approach to early identification and intervention for behavioural health problems (President's New Freedom Commission on Mental Health 2003; World Health Organization 2001).

## Gatekeeper training

The purpose of gatekeeper training is to develop the knowledge, attitudes, and skills to identify students at risk, determine the levels of risk, and make referrals when necessary (Garland and Zigler 1993; Kalafat and Elias 1995; Gould *et al.* 2003). The programmes to train school personnel as gatekeepers are based on the premise that suicidal youth are under-identified and that we can increase identification by providing adults with knowledge about suicide. Only 9 per cent of a national random sample of US high school teachers believed they could recognize a student at risk for suicide, and while the overwhelming majority of counsellors knew the risk factors for suicide, only one in three believed they could identify a student at risk (King *et al.* 1999). Research examining the effectiveness of gatekeeper training is limited, but the findings are encouraging, with significant improvements in school personnel's knowledge, attitudes, intervention skills, preparation for coping with a crisis, referral practices (Shaffer *et al.* 1988; Garland and Zigler 1993; Tierney 1994; Mackessy-Amiti *et al.* 1996; King and Smith 2000; Wyman *et al.* 2008) and general satisfaction with the training (Nelson 1987). Consistent with the reports that in-service training programmes are more acceptable than school-wide screening programmes (Miller *et al.* 1999;, Eckert *et al.* 2003; Scherff *et al.* 2005), 46 per cent of school districts in Washington, DC have gatekeeper training programmes, while no districts employ group screening of students (Hayden and Lauer 2000).

## Gatekeeper programmes

Increasingly popular gatekeeper programmes include LivingWorks' Applied Suicide Intervention Skills Training (ASIST) (http://www.livingworks.net) and Question Persuade and Refer (QPR) (QPR Institute, http://qprinstitute.com).

ASIST is an internationally disseminated programme designed as 'suicide first-aid'. Developed in Canada, LivingWorks has coordinating centres in Australia, New Zealand and Norway. Its programmes are delivered through a network of community-based registered trainers in Canada, Australia, Norway and the United States. Smaller numbers of trainers are located in Guam, Hong Kong, Russia, and Singapore. ASIST is a two-day workshop involving highly interactive skills-training designed to enhance the 'suicide intervention competencies' of participants (Turley *et al.* 2000).

The ASIST suicide intervention model (SIM) is divided into three phases:

1 Connecting, which involves recognising and responding to warning signs (reframed as 'invitations') and asking directly about suicide;

2 Understanding, which involves identifying reasons for dying and reasons for living, and collaboratively reviewing current risk status; and

3 Assisting, which involves developing safe plans specific to the identified risks and obtaining a commitment to the safe plans by both the gatekeeper and the caller.

The ASIST programme has been field-tested in a variety of settings, including Norway (Guttormsen *et al.* 2003; Silvola *et al.* 2003) and Australia (Turley *et al.* 2000; Pearce *et al.* 2003), where pre and post differences in attitudes and knowledge have been examined. However, to date, there has been no controlled study of its effectiveness. The National Suicide Prevention Lifeline, a national network of telephone crisis services (hotlines) in the US, has recently selected ASIST as the gatekeeper training programme to be used to train the counsellors in its network, and is conducting a pilot-controlled trial of its efficacy. LivingWorks has also developed shorter programmes, such as the half-day SafeTALK training programme, to complement its longer ASIST suicide intervention training, but evaluations of SafeTALK are not yet available.

QPR targets all adults in contact with potentially suicidal youths (e.g. teachers, counsellors, coaches, cafeteria workers). The acronym QPR stands for the three steps gatekeepers are taught in order to help prevent suicide: Question, Persuade and Refer (Quinnett 1995, 2007). The programme is designed to enhance each adult gatekeeper's ability to recognize signs of youth contemplating suicide, give the adults the skills to approach and question the youth about suicide, and to refer the youth to treatment. QPR offers a variety of programmes. The basic training programme is a one- to two-hour training course. The training programme can also be done through a web-enabled, interactive CD-ROM. This one-hour online training is convenient and time effective. The QPR training has been translated to different languages including Spanish, Japanese and Korean (Quinnett, personal communication). The QPR training programme has the standard core programme, but it can be customized to cultural, social, religious, ethic and racial contexts. The programme can be individually tailored to the referral and resource information. Such customization of this training programme is critical to its international acceptance. Pre- and post-tests of QPR have shown that adults increase their knowledge as well as self-efficacy (QPR Institute, http://qprinstitute.com). The first group-based randomized trial of the QPR gatekeeper training in 32 schools on 252 school staff in the US (Wyman *et al.* 2008) has shown that training increased the school staff members' knowledge of suicide warning signs. Moreover, their awareness of intervention behaviours and ratings of their preparation and efficacy to perform a gatekeeper role in their school and their access to referral and treatment services was improved. Training developed self-perceived preparedness among teachers and support staff, as well as among counsellors and nurses. However, after training, only a small proportion of staff (14 per cent) increased their number of queries of students about suicidal thoughts. These staff tended to be those who were already communicating with students before training. Similarly, the majority of referral behaviours occurred in those school staff already in close communication with students.

## Peer gatekeeper training programmes

Peer gatekeeper training, which is a specific type of gatekeeper training programme, is an expansion of peer helper programmes. While peer *helper* programmes usually involve general helping skills training (e.g. basic training in empathy and active listening), peer *gatekeeper* training provides skill-specific training for suicide risk assessment (Stuart *et al.* 2003). The rationale underlying these peer programmes is similar to suicide awareness programmes: suicidal youth are more likely to confide in a peer than an adult (e.g. Kalafat and Elias 1994), but peer gatekeeper training programmes usually have a greater emphasis on teaching strategies that involve active engagement with a suicidal youth. The role that peers play varies considerably by programme, with some limited to listening and reporting any possible warning signs and others involving counselling responsibilities. Many peer programmes address serious mental health problems, such as drug abuse, eating disorders, and depression, with 24 per cent of programmes in Washington State involving some suicide prevention role (Lewis and Lewis 1996). Empirical evaluations of these programmes are quite limited (Lewis and Lewis 1996) and are often confined to student satisfaction measures (Morey *et al.* 1993). A recent evaluation of the Many Helping Hearts peer gatekeeper training programme was conducted by Stuart *et al.* (2003) in eight schools in Vancouver Island in British Columbia, Canada. This training programme covered active listening skills, self-care and setting limits, crisis theory, signals of suicide, suicide risk assessment, role-play scenarios involving suicidal youth, and community resources. The training involved two half day sessions, approximately 1 week apart. A total of 65 adolescents participated in the evaluation, which employed a questionnaire administered before the training, immediately after the completion of training, and 3 months following training. Significant improvements in knowledge, attitudes, and skills occurred after training and were maintained over a 3-month period of time. However, without a control group or evaluation of actual helping behaviour, only tentative support for the efficacy of training peer helpers in suicide risk assessment is provided by this study. Of particular concern with peer programmes are the potential negative side-effects, which have rarely been examined. For example, after gatekeeper training with QPR, youth (aged 11–14 years, or 15–18 years) rated themselves lower than older individuals in the likelihood that they would ask someone if they were suicidal and go with a suicidal person to get help (QPR Institute, http://qprinstitute.com). This highlights the likely unrealistic expectations of training young children or adolescents to engage a suicidal peer. To date, there is not a sufficient body of evidence documenting the efficacy or safety of peer gatekeeper programmes.

Overall, school-based gatekeeper training programmes are a promising suicide prevention strategy, but a number of caveats exist: First, recent research indicates that this intervention training should not attempt to target all adults in a school, since successful assistance of suicidal students appears to be dependent on the adult's pre-existing empathy and communication style with students (Wyman *et al.* 2008). Procedures have to be developed to identify such empathetic school personnel. Second, no *direct measures* of staff members' interactions with students have been included in the research evaluation; rather only *self-reports* of school staff members' knowledge of suicide warning signs, intervention behaviours and preparedness have been employed. These self-reported outcomes are merely preliminary indicators of gatekeeper training programmes' efficacy. Third, the research has not determined the actual extent to which suicidal students were identified and referred, whether service utilizsation increased, or whether the mental health of students improved (Wyman *et al.* 2008). Fourth, many vulnerable youth appear to be reluctant to tell adults about their distress (Gould *et al.* 2004; Wyman *et al.* 2008) limiting the potential of gatekeeper training if the programmes do not adequately address this challenge. Lastly, gatekeeper training programmes as well as other case-finding strategies require adequate referral networks, treatment resources, or other effective sources of support prior to any implementation of these programmes.

Another means to enhance the skills of potential community and school-based gatekeepers is through 'pre-employment university training of professionals' (Waring *et al.* 2000, p. 583). Programmes such as the Youth Suicide Prevention–National University Curriculum Project in Australia focus on the development of curricula for use in the professional education of physicians, nurses, secondary school teachers, and journalists (Waring *et al.* 2000). A preliminary evaluation of this curriculum in thirty Australian universities has yielded encouraging results, with increases in knowledge and improvements in attitudes. The vast majority of the university students reported that the curriculum was relevant to their careers and that it increased their interest in the issue of youth suicide. While more extensive and longer-term evaluation is needed to determine the impact of such programmes on the more distal outcomes of enhanced mental health and reduced suicide among youth, targeting professionals during their pre-employment university training appears to be a promising strategy to complement the more conventional gatekeeper programmes, which focus their efforts on on-the-job training.

## Risk-factor reduction strategies

### Skills training of students

In contrast to suicide *awareness* curriculum in schools, skills training programmes emphasize the development of problem-solving, coping, and cognitive skills, as suicidal youth have deficits in these areas (e.g. Asarnow *et al.* 1987; Cole 1989; Rotheram-Borus *et al.* 1990). It is hoped that an 'immunization' effect can be produced against suicidal feelings and behaviours. The reduction of suicide risk factors (e.g. depression, hopelessness, and drug abuse) is also a targeted outcome. Health promotion programmes have many of the same goals as skills training strategies; although health promotion programmes are usually more expansive in scope, focusing on a broader range of health-enhancement and problem-avoidance activities (Waring *et al.* 2000).

### Skills training programmes

MindMatters (Wyn *et al.* 2000) was piloted in twenty-four schools in Australia, drawn from all educational systems and each state and territory in the country. The programme was developed for secondary schools to promote mental health and has the following goals: instil an understanding of suicidal risk and mental illness; enhance resilience and interpersonal relationships (e.g. reduce bullying and harassment); cope with grief and loss; and create a positive school environment where students feel valued and safe (Wyn *et al.* 2000, http://cms.curriculum.edu.au/mindmatters/). The feasibility of exporting the Australian MindMatters to the United States was assessed through a research protocol involving discussion with and endorsement ratings by forty-two participants, including administrators, teachers, parents, and students from four US communities (Evans *et al.* 2005). Each stakeholder group indicated that they would be likely to support and implement the programme. MindMatters is implemented in the classroom and provides the trained staff with a resource kit containing material on the programme goals.

The Zuni Life Skills Development Curriculum was developed as a culturally sensitive skills training programme for the Zuni tribe who are a part of the Pueblo people of New Mexico (LaFromboise and Howard-Pitney 1994, 1995). The curriculum was developed because of the concern about its rising rate of youth suicide. There are three components incorporated into the programme: cognitive problems, addressing negative views of the self and how to build self-esteem; behavioural problems, learning to cope with self-destructive behaviour and thoughts; and finally emotional problems, focused on identifying emotions and stress (LaFromboise and Howard-Pitney 1994, 1995). This programme was rated as promising by the NREPP (Rodgers *et al.* 2007).

Another skills training programme rated as promising by NREPP is the Reconnecting Youth (RY) Prevention Research Program, a programme that includes suicide prevention in its broader focus on reducing multiple risks among potential high school dropouts (Eggert *et al.* 2001). The programme focuses on drug abuse, depression, and suicidal thoughts (Eggert *et al.* 1994, 2001), as well as building self-esteem, decision-making, coping with anger and depression, and better peer relations. RY is concerned with the at-risk youth's ability to manage stressors through improved decision making and a strong social support network (Commission on Adolescent Suicide Prevention 2005). The semester-long elective, named the Personal Growth Class, is targeted at students with poor attendance records who appear to be potential dropouts. Programmes that were adapted from RY include CARE (Care, Assess, Respond, Empower)—formerly called Counsellor's CARE (C-CARE), a brief one-on-one intervention, and CAST (Coping and Support Training), a small-group skills building intervention (Randell *et al.* 2001). CARE includes a 2-hour, one-on-one computer-assisted suicide assessment followed by a 2-hour motivational counselling and social support intervention. CAST consists of 12 55-minute group sessions administered over 6 weeks. Both programmes have been rated as 'effective' suicide prevention programmes by NREPP (Rodgers *et al.* 2007).

Several evaluation studies have shown promising results of skills training and health promotion programmes, with some evidence for reductions in completed and attempted suicides (Zenere and Lazarus 1997) and improvements in attitudes, emotions and distress coping skills (Klingman and Hochdorf 1993; Orbach and Bar-Joseph 1993).

In two evaluations of the Zuni Life Skills programme, the intervention group demonstrated a significant decrease in ideation, hopelessness, hostility, and the view of the negative self; and an improvement in students' ability to manage and cope with stress, recognize suicidal symptoms, and use appropriate resources (LaFromboise and Howard-Pitney 1995). However, self-efficacy skills

and active listening showed no intervention effect (LaFromboise and Howard-Pitney 1995).

The most systematic evaluations of skills training have been conducted by the team of researchers who have focused on programmes for students at high risk for school failure or drop-out (Eggert *et al.* 1995; Randell *et al.* 2001; Thompson *et al.* 2000, 2001, see Eggert *et al.* 2001 for a detailed review). Enhancements of protective factors, such as self-esteem and social support resources, and reductions in risk factors, such as decreased suicide behaviours and ideation as well as depression, anger, hopelessness and stress, following the 'active' interventions were consistently found, while the control 'intervention as usual' did not yield an increase of protective factors. However, intervention as usual sometimes produced significant reductions in suicide risk behaviours (Eggert *et al.* 1995; Randell *et al.* 2001). Thus, as it is not clear which aspects of the skills-training programme were responsible for risk reduction, which is also a limitation of other trials (Zenere and Lazarus 1997). Consequently, studies clarifying this are needed. Moreover, a recent evaluation by Cho and colleagues (2005) demonstrated *negative* effects of RY at a 6-month follow up with the at-risk youth. Students bonded with other at-risk youth, had a lower grade point average, and a higher level of anger. Another study, evaluating the fidelity of RY, showed that while students were satisfied with the skills they developed, unexpectedly, being exposed to the intervention programme caused increased alcohol use and anger among the students (Sanchez *et al.* 2007). Grouping at-risk youth, with similar behavioural and/or emotional problems, seems to be a potential flaw of this intervention, eliciting untoward iatrogenic effects (Cho *et al.* 2005). Interview studies investigating the reasons for the increases in alcohol use and anger among the students in the intervention programme are necessary to understand how to modify this type of intervention.

Overall, the evaluation studies of skills training programmes have yielded encouraging data; however, the deleterious effects reported among high-risk students participating in the RY programme are disconcerting. These iatrogenic effects may be specific to a particular population (e.g. students at risk for drop-out) or implementation format (e.g. small group in contrast to one-on-one interventions) but clearly additional research is needed to determine the specific elements that contributed to RY's risks in order to evaluate the extent to which other programmes may be susceptible to similar problems.

## Postvention/crisis intervention

In the process of promoting the mental health of survivors, 'postvention thus becomes prevention' (Webb 1986, p. 477). The major goals of postvention programmes are to assist survivors in the grief process, identify and refer those individuals who may be at risk following the suicide to health-care facilities, provide accurate information about suicide while attempting to minimize suicide contagion, and implement a structure for ongoing prevention efforts (Hazell 1993; Underwood and Dunne-Maxim 1997; Gould *et al.* 2003). The rationale for school-based postvention/crisis intervention is that a timely response to a suicide is likely to reduce subsequent morbidity and mortality in fellow students, including suicidality, the onset or exacerbation of psychiatric disorders (e.g. PTSD, major depressive disorder) and other symptoms related to pathological bereavement (Brent *et al.* 1993a, b, 1994).

## Postvention programmes

The value of suicide postvention is increasingly being recognized worldwide. Following the 2001 meeting of the International Association for Suicide Prevention (IASP), researchers in Italy developed the SOPRoxi postvention programme in response to a lack of postvention planning throughout Italy as a whole. This programme involves the primary elements of identifying at-risk survivors, conducting psychological screening and assessments of these individuals, and offering interventions and support in various formats. The SOPRoxi is intended for use in schools as well as in other public spheres (Scocco *et al.* 2006). For use at the high school level or younger, Underwood and Dunne-Maxim (1997) and Kerr *et al.* (2003) in the US created comprehensive postvention handbooks which offer pertinent background information, step-by-step guidelines, and appendices of helpful documents for the postvention process. Specific actions to be taken by the crisis-response team include debriefing faculty, staff and students; identifying and contacting at-risk students; sitting in on the deceased child's classes on the day following the death; and making contact with the media, parents of survivors, and the victim's family. In response to the varied levels of postvention planning reported by colleges and universities, Webb (1986) outlined a set of postvention guidelines specifically tailored to the needs of a college or university setting. Webb's response plan hinges upon the establishment of a counselling service, which is charged with the responsibility of rapidly making contact with those individuals close to the suicide victim; supporting the campus community as a whole; avoiding glamorization of the death; and returning campus events to a normal state as soon as possible (Webb 1986). Though this plan is comprehensive enough to address most suicide deaths on an academic campus, it is also important to consider exceptions. For example, Petretic-Jackson *et al.* (1996) proposed that special considerations are necessary when conducting a postvention programme after a suicide completed by a high-profile student athlete. Petretic-Jackson *et al.* (1996) draw attention to team dynamics such as rapport with the coach as a leadership figure, close family-like bonds, and resilient athletic mentality. Petretic-Jackson *et al.* suggest that these unique elements be utilized to the advantage of the postvention programme.

Despite the proliferation of postvention programmes, the existing research on their efficacy is sparse. Hazell and Lewin (1993) examined the efficacy of 90-minute group counselling sessions offered to groups of 20–30 students on the seventh day following a suicide. No differences in outcome were found between counselled subjects and matched controls. It was unclear whether this was due to inclusion criteria for postvention counselling (close friends of deceased student), the intervention itself, the duration of the distress or whether short-term effects dissipated by the assessment at eight months after the death. An encouraging, though small and methodologically limited study by Poijula *et al.* (2001), found that no new suicides took place during a four-year follow-up period in schools where an adequate intervention took place, whereas the number of suicides significantly increased after suicides with no adequate subsequent crisis intervention.

It is imperative for postvention crisis interventions to be well planned and evaluated; otherwise not only may they not help survivors, but they may potentially exacerbate problems through the induction of imitation, as a case example of a school suicide postvention programme has illustrated (Callahan 1996).

## Conclusion

According to the European Network on Suicide Prevention established by the World Health Organization (WHO) in 2000, school-based suicide prevention programmes are a preferred strategy in many countries of the WHO European region (Wasserman *et al.* 2004). A national suicide prevention strategy commenced in Australia in 1999, building upon its former national youth suicide prevention strategy, and New Zealand's national strategy developed in 2006 has youth prevention as one of several focuses. The national strategy for suicide prevention of the United States, published in 2001, includes the goal of increasing the number of evidence-based suicide prevention programmes in schools, colleges, and universities. The South-East Asia WHO Region (SEAR), is also working to increase the focus on suicide prevention in school settings.

Another important WHO initiative in Geneva resulted in a published resource for teachers and other school staff about suicide prevention in schools (WHO 2000). In light of this growing worldwide focus on suicide prevention, it is evident that schools, colleges and universities will be subject to ever-increasing prevention activities. It is imperative that these efforts employ empirically based programmes. Moreover, programmes will need to be adapted to the cultural traditions of each community. For example, the WHO's cooperative work with SEAR countries to implement school-based suicide prevention programmes has recognized the regions various traditional knowledge, and have incorporated such non-Western wisdom in problem-solving and life-skills training programmes to improve youth mental health (SEAR 2007).

No school-based strategy reviewed in this chapter is without its unique strengths and limitations, and continuing evaluation studies of all these school-based suicide prevention strategies are needed before their efficacy can be firmly established. Nevertheless, in countries with sufficient educational and mental health service infrastructures to support school-based suicide prevention strategies, several promising empirically based prevention strategies have been identified and are recommended for use now, including screening for at-risk youth, gatekeeper training programmes, and skills training for students. The positive results from new curriculum programmes may overcome the long-standing reluctance to implement any curriculum-based strategy. Registries of evidence-based programmes and practices, such as NREPP in the US (http://www.nrepp.samhsa.gov/index.htm), are a recommended mechanism by which professionals and community members engaged in suicide prevention planning can keep abreast of empirically based prevention programmes.

While suicide prevention remains a recognized challenge in developed countries, it is especially daunting in developing countries in Asia, Africa and South America, where suicide prevention remains largely ignored (Khan 2005). Many factors impede the development of successful suicide prevention programmes (see Khan 2005 for a review), and communicable diseases as well as maternal and child health take precedence over mental health, which has a very low priority (Khan 2005).

# References

Appelbaum PS (2006). 'Depressed? Get Out!' Dealing with suicidal students on college campuses. *Psychiatric Services*, **57**, 914–916.

Asarnow J, Carlson G, Guthrie D (1987). Coping strategies, self-perceptions, hopelessness, and perceived family environments in depressed and suicidal children. *Journal of Consulting and Clinical Psychology*, **55**, 361–366.

Aseltine R (2003). An evaluation of a school based suicide prevention program. *Adolescent and Family Health*, **3**, 81–88.

Aseltine RH Jr and DeMartino R (2004). An outcome evaluation of the SOS Suicide Prevention Program. *American Journal of Public Health*, **94**, 446–451.

Ashford E (2005). The fight over screening students to prevent suicide. *Education Digest: Essential Readings Condensed for Quick Review*, **71**, 52–56. http://www.eddigest.com.

Beautrais A, Fergusson D, Coggan C et al. (2007). Effective strategies for suicide prevention in New Zealand: a review of the evidence. *New Zealand Medical Journal*, **120**, 1251.

Berman AL and Jobes DA (1995). Suicide prevention in adolescents (age 12–18). *Journal of Suicide and Life Threatening Behavior*, **25**, 143–154.

Brent DA, Perper JA, Moritz GM et al. (1993a). Bereavement or depression? The impact of the loss of a friend to suicide. *Journal of the American Academy of Child and Adolescent Psychiatry*, **32**, 1189–1197.

Brent DA, Perper JA, Moritz GM et al. (1993b). Adolescent witness to a peer suicide. *Journal of the American Academy of Child and Adolescent Psychiatry*, **32**, 1184–1188.

Brent DA, Perper JA, Moritz GM et al. (1994). Major depression or uncomplicated bereavement? A follow-up of youth exposed to suicide. *Journal of the American Academy of Child and Adolescent Psychiatry*, **33**, 231–239.

Callahan J (1996). Negative effects of a school suicide postvention program—a case example. *Crisis*, **17**, 108–115.

Centers for Disease Control and Prevention (CDC) (1994). Programs for the prevention of suicide among adolescents and young adults; and suicide contagion and the reporting of suicide: recommendations from a national workshop. *Morbidity and Mortality Weekly Report*, **43**, 1–19.

Cho H, Hallfores DD, Sanchez V (2005). Evaluation of a high school peer group intervention for at-risk youth. *Journal of Abnormal Child Psychology*, **33**, 363–374.

Ciffone J (1993). Suicide prevention: a classroom presentation to adolescents. *Social Work*, **38**, 197–203.

Ciffone J (2007). Suicide prevention: an analysis and replication of a curriculum-based high school program. *Social Work*, **52**, 41–49.

Cole DA (1989). Psychopathology of adolescent suicide: hopelessness, coping beliefs, and depression. *Journal of Abnormal Psychology*, **98**, 248–255.

Commission on Adolescent Suicide Prevention (2005). Preventive interventions and treatments for suicidal youth. In DL Evans, EB Foa, RE Gur et al., eds, *Treating And Preventing Adolescent Mental Health Disorders: What We Know And What We Don't Know, A Research Agenda For Improving The Mental Health Of Our Youth*, pp. 471–486. Oxford University Press, New York.

Eckert TL, Miller DN, DuPaul GJ et al. (2003). Adolescent suicide prevention: school psychologists' acceptability of school-based programs. *School Psychology Review*, **32**, 57–76.

Eggert LL, Thompson EA, Herting JR et al. (1994). Prevention Research Program: reconnecting at-risk youth. *Issues in Mental Health and Nursing*, **15**, 107–135.

Eggert LL, Thompson EA, Herting JR et al. (1995). Reducing suicide potential among high-risk youth: tests of a school-based prevention program. *Suicide and Life-Threatening Behavior*, **25**, 276–296.

Eggert LL, Thompson EA, Herting JR et al. (2001). Reconnecting youth to prevent drug abuse, school dropout and suicidal behaviors among high-risk youth. In EF Wagner and H Waldron, eds, *Innovation in Adolescent Substance Abuse Interventions*, pp. 51–84. Elsevier Science Ltd, Oxford.

Evans SW, Mullett E, Weist MD et al. (2005). Feasibility of the *MindMatters* school mental health promotion program in American schools. *Journal of Youth and Adolescence*, **34**, 51–58.

Garland A, Shaffer D, Whittle B (1989). A national survey of school-based, adolescent suicide prevention programs. *Journal of the American Academy of Child and Adolescent Psychiatry*, **28**, 931–934.

Garland AF and Zigler E (1993). Adolescent suicide prevention: current research and social policy implications. *American Psychologist*, **48**, 169–182.

Gould MS and Kramer RA (2001). Youth suicide prevention. *Journal of Suicide and Life-Threatening Behavior*, **31**, 6–31.

Gould MS, Greenberg T, Velting D et al. (2003). Youth suicide risk and preventive interventions: a review of the past 10 years. *Journal of the American Academy of Child and Adolescent Psychiatry*, **42**, 386–405.

Gould MS, Marrocco MA, Kleinman M (2005). Evaluating iatrogenic risk of youth suicide screening programs: a randomized controlled trial. *JAMA*, **293**, 1635–1643.

Gould MS, Velting D, Kleinman M et al. (2004). Teenagers' attitudes about coping strategies and help-seeking behavior for suicidality. *Journal of the American Academy of Child and Adolescent Psychiatry*, **43**, 1124–1133.

Guo G and Harstall C (2002). *Efficacy of Suicide Prevention Programs for Children and Youth. HTA 26: Services A. Health Technology Assessment*. Alberta Heritage Foundation for Medical Research, Alberta.

Gutierrez PM, Watkins R, Collura D (2004). Suicide risk screening in an urban high school. *Journal of Suicide and Life-Threatening Behavior*, **43**, 421–428.

Guttormsen T, Høifødt TS, Silvola K et al. (2003). Applied suicide intervention skills training: an evaluation. *Tidsskr Nor Lægeforen*, **123**, 2284–2286.

Haas AP, Hendin H, Mann JJ (2003). Suicide in college students. *American Behavioral Scientist*, **46**, 1224–1240.

Hallfors D, Brodish PH, Khatapoush S et al. (2006). Feasibility of screening adolescents for suicide risk in 'real-world' high school settings. *American Journal of Public Health*, **96**, 282–287.

Hayden DC and Lauer P (2000). Prevalence of suicide programs in schools and roadblocks to implementation. *Journal of Suicide and Life Threatening Behavior*, **30**, 239–251.

Hazell P (1993). Adolescent suicide clusters: evidence, mechanisms and prevention. *Australian and New Zealand Journal of Psychiatry*, **27**, 653–665.

Hazell P and King R (1996). Arguments for and against teaching suicide prevention in schools. *Australian and New Zealand Journal of Psychiatry*, **30**, 633–642.

Hazell P and Lewin T (1993). An evaluation of postvention following adolescent suicide. *Journal of Suicide and Life-Threatening Behavior*, **23**, 101–109.

Hazell P, Hazell T, Waring T et al. (1999). A survey of suicide prevention curricula taught in Australian universities. *Australian and New Zealand Journal of Psychiatry*, **33**, 253–259.

Joiner TE, Pfaff JJ, Acres JG (2002). A brief screening tool for suicidal symptoms in adolescents and young adults in general health settings: reliability and validity data from the Australian National General Practice Youth Suicide Prevention Project. *Behavioral Research and Therapy*, **40**, 471–481.

Kalafat J (2003). School approaches of youth suicide prevention. *American Behavioral Scientist*, **46**, 1211–1123.

Kalafat J and Elias M (1994). An evaluation of a school-based suicide awareness intervention. *Journal of Suicide and Life-Threatening Behavior*, **24**, 224–233.

Kalafat J and Elias M (1995). Suicide prevention in an educational context: broad and narrow foci. *Journal of Suicide and Life-Threatening Behavior*, **25**, 123–133.

Kalafat J and Gagliano C (1996). The use of simulations to assess the impact of an adolescent suicide response curriculum. *Journal of Suicide and Life-Threatening Behavior*, **26**, 359–364.

Kalafat J and Ryerson DA (1999). The implementation and institiutionalization of a school-based youth suicide prevention program. *Journal of Primary Prevention*, **19**, 157–175.

Kalafat J, Elias M, Gara MA (1993). The relationship of bystander intervention variables to adolescents' response to suicidal peers. *Journal of Primary Prevention*, **13**, 231–244.

Kalafat J, Haley D, Lubell K *et al.* (2007). *Evaluation of Lifelines Classes: A Component of the School-community-Based Maine Youth Suicide Prevention Project. Draft Report Prepared for the National Registry of Evidence-Based Programs and Practices.* Rutgers University Graduate School of Applied and Professional Psychology, Piscataway.

Kalafat J, O'Halloran S, Underwood M (2003). *Lifelines: A School-based Youth Suicide Response Program.* Rutgers Graduate School of Applied and Professional Psychology, Piscataway.

Kerr MM, Brent DA, McKain B *et al.* (2003). *Postvention Standards Manual: A Guide for a Schools' Response in the Aftermath of a Sudden Death.* University of Pittsburgh, Services for Teens at Risk (STAR-Center), Pittsburgh.

Khan MM (2005). Suicide prevention and developing countries. *Journal of the Royal Society of Medicine*, **98**, 459–463.

King KA and Smith J (2000). Project SOAR: a training program to increase school counselors' knowledge and confidence regarding suicide prevention and intervention. *Journal of School Health*, **70**, 402–407.

King KA, Price JH, Telljohann SK *et al.* (1999). High school health teachers' perceived self-efficacy in identifying students at risk for suicide. *Journal of School Health*, **69**, 202–207.

Kirby D (1985). Sexuality education: a more realistic view of its effects. *Journal of School Health*, **55**, 421–424.

Klingman A and Hochdorf Z (1993). Coping with distress and self harm: the impact of a primary prevention program among adolescents. *Journal of Adolescent Psychiatry*, **16**, 121–140.

LaFromboise TD and Howard-Pitney B (1994). The Zuni Life Skills Development Curriculum: a collaborative approach to curriculum development. *American Indian and Alaska Native Mental Health Research: The Journal of the National Center, Monograph Series*, **4**, 98–121.

LaFromboise TD and Howard-Pitney B (1995). The Zuni Life Skills Development Curriculum: description and evaluation of a suicide prevention program. *Journal of Counseling Psychology*, **42**, 479–486.

Lewis MW and Lewis AC (1996). Peer-helping programs: helper role, supervisor training, and suicidal behavior. *Journal of Counseling and Development*, **74**, 307–313.

LivingWorks (2007). *ASIST: Applied Suicide Intervention Skills Training.* Available online at http://www.livingworks.net.

Locke J (2007). Framework for developing institutional protocols for the acutely distressed or suicidal student. Presented to the Suffolk University ADAPT Conference, Boston, 13 April.

Mackesy-Amiti ME, Fendrich M, Libby S *et al.* (1996). Assessment of knowledge gains in proactive training for postvention. *Suicide and Life-Threatening Behavior*, **26**, 161–174.

McCormick N, Folcik J, Izzo A (1985). Sex-education needs and interests of high school students in a rural New York county. *Adolescence*, **20**, 581–592.

Miller DN, Eckert TL, DuPaul GJ *et al.* (1999). Adolescent suicide prevention: acceptability of school-based programs among secondary school principals. *Journal of Suicide and Life-Threatening Behavior*, **29**, 72–85.

Morey RE, Miller CD, Rosen LA *et al.* (1993). High school peer counseling: the relationship between student satisfaction and peer counselors' style of helping. *School Counselor*, **40**, 293–300.

Nelson F (1987). Evaluation of a youth suicide prevention school program. *Adolescence*, **88**, 813–825.

NREPP, SAMHSA's National Registry of Evidence-based Programs and Practices. Available online: http://www.nrepp.samhsa.gov/index.htm.

Orbach I and Bar-Joseph H (1993). The impact of a suicide prevention program for adolescents on suicidal tendencies, hopelessness, ego identity, and coping. *Journal of Suicide and Life-Threatening Behavior*, **23**, 120–129.

Overholser JC, Hemstreet A, Spirito A *et al.* (1989). Suicide awareness programs in the schools: effect of gender and personal experience. *Journal of the American Academy of Child and Adolescent Psychiatry*, **28**, 925–930.

Pearce K, Rickwood D, Beaton S (2003). Preliminary evaluation of a university-based suicide intervention project: impact on participants. *Australian e-Journal for the Advancement of Mental Health*, **2**.

Pena JB and Caine ED (2006). Screening as an approach for adolescent suicide prevention. *Journal of Suicide and Life-Threatening Behavior*, **36**, 614–637.

Petretic-Jackson P, Pitman L, Jackson T (1996). Suicide postvention programs for university athletic programs. *Crisis Intervention*, **3**, 25–41.

Poijula S, Wahlberg KE, Dyregrov A (2001). Adolescent suicide and suicide contagion in three secondary schools. *International Journal of Emergency Mental Health*, **3**, 163–168.

Portzky G and van Heeringen K (2006). Suicide prevention in adolescents: a controlled study of the effectiveness of a school-based psycho-educational program. *Journal of Child Psychology and Psychiatry*, **47**, 910–918.

President's New Freedom Commission on Mental Health (2003). *Achieving the Promise: Transforming Mental Care in America. Final Report.* DHHS Pub. No. SMA-03–3832. US Department of Health and Human Services, Rockville.

Quinnett P (1995). *QPR: Ask a Question, Save a Life.* The QPR Institute, Spokane. Available online at http://www.qprinstitute.com.

Quinnett P (2007). *QPR Gatekeeper Training for Suicide Prevention: The Model, Rationale and Theory.* Available online at http://www.qprinstitute.com.

Randell BP, Eggert LL, Pike KC (2001). Immediate post-intervention effects of two brief youth suicide prevention interventions. *Journal of Suicide and Life-Threatening Behavior*, **31**, 41–61.

Reynolds WM (1990). Development of a semi-structured clinical interview for suicidal behaviors in adolescents. *Psychological Assessment*, **2**, 382–390.

Reynolds WM (1991). A school-based procedure for the identification of adolescents at risk for suicidal behaviors. *Family Community Health*, **14**, 64–75.

Rodgers RL, Sudak HS, Silverman MM *et al.* (2007). Evidence-based practices projects for suicide prevention. *Journal of Suicide and Life-Threatening Behavior*, **37**, 154–164.

Ross CP (1985). Teaching children the facts of life and death: suicide prevention in the schools. In ML Peck, NL Farberow, RE Litman, eds, *Youth Suicide*, pp. 147–169. Springer, New York.

Rotheram-Borus MJ, Trautman PD, Dopkins SC *et al.* (1990). Cognitive style and pleasant activities among female adolescent suicide attempters. *Journal of Consulting and Clinical Psychology*, **58**, 554–561.

Sanchez V, Steckler A, Nitirat P *et al.* (2007). Fidelity of implementation in a treatment effectiveness trial of reconnecting youth. *Health Education Research*, **22**, 95–107.

Scherff AR, Eckert TL, Miller DN (2005). Youth suicide prevention: a survey of public school superintendents's acceptability of school-based programs. *Journal of Suicide and Life-Threatening Behavior*, **35**, 154–169.

Scocco P, Frasson A, Costacurta A *et al.* (2006). SOPRoxi: a research-intervention project for suicide survivors. *Crisis*, **27**, 39–41.

SEAR (World Health Organization Regional Office for Southeast Asia) (2007). *Suicide Prevention: Emerging from Darkness—What can be Done?* Available at http://www.searo.who.int.

Shaffer D and Craft L (1999). Methods of adolescent suicide prevention. *Journal of Clinical Psychiatry*, **60**, 70–74.

Shaffer D and Gould MS (2000). Suicide prevention in schools. In K Hawton and K van Heeringen, eds, *The International Handbook of Suicide and Attempted Suicide*, pp. 645–660. John Wiley and Sons Ltd, Chichester.

Shaffer D, Garland A, Gould M *et al.* (1988). Preventing teenage suicide: a critical review. *Journal of the American Academy of Child and Adolescent Psychiatry*, **27**, 675–687.

Shaffer D, Garland A, Vieland V *et al.* (1991). The impact of curriculum-based suicide prevention program for teenagers. *Journal of the American Academy of Child and Adolescent Psychiatry*, **30**, 588–596.

Shaffer D, Scott M, Wilcox H *et al.* (2004). The Columbia Suicide Screen: validity and reliability of a screen for youth suicide and depression. *Journal of the American Academy of Child and Adolescent Psychiatry*, **43**, 71–79.

Shaffer D, Vieland V, Garland A *et al.* (1990). Adolescent suicide attempters. Response to suicide-prevention programs. *JAMA*, **264**, 3151–3155.

Silbert KL and Berry GL (1991). Psychological effects of a suicide prevention unit on adolescents' levels of stress, anxiety and hopelessness: implications for counselling psychologists. *Counselling Psychology Quarterly*, **4**, 45–58.

Silvola K, Høifødt TS, Guttormsen T *et al.* (2003). Applied suicide intervention skills training. *Tidsskr Nor Lægeforen*, **123**, 2281–3.

Stuart C, Waalen JK, Haelstromm E (2003). Many helping hearts: an evaluation of peer gatekeeper training in suicide risk assessment. *Death Studies*, **27**, 321–333.

Suicide Prevention Resource Center (2004). *Promoting Mental Health and Preventing Suicide in College and University Settings*. Suicide Prevention Resource Center, Newton.

Taylor SJ, Kingdom D, Jenkins R (1997). How are nations trying to prevent suicide? An analysis of national suicide prevention strategies. *Acta Psychiatrica Scandinavica*, **95**, 457–463.

The Jed Foundation (2006). *Framework for Developing Institutional Protocols for the Acutely Distressed or Suicidal College Student*. The Jed Foundation, New York.

The Surgeon General (1999). *The Surgeon General's Call to Action to Prevent Suicide*. Available online at http://www.surgeongeneral.gov/library/calltoaction.

Thompson EA and Eggert LL (1999). Using the suicide risk screen to identify suicidal adolescents among potential high school dropouts. *Journal of the American Academy of Child and Adolescent Psychiatry*, **38**, 1506–1514.

Thompson EA, Eggert LL, Herting JR (2000). Mediating effects of an indicated prevention program for reducing youth depression and suicide risk behaviors. *Journal of Suicide and Life-Threatening Behavior*, **30**, 252–271.

Thompson EA, Eggert LL, Randell BP *et al.* (2001). Evaluation of indicated suicide risk prevention approaches for potential high school dropouts. *American Journal of Public Health*, **91**, 742–752.

Tierney RJ (1994). Suicide intervention training evaluation: a preliminary report. *Crisis*, **15**, 69–76.

Turley B, Pullen L, Thomas I *et al.* (2000). *Living Works Applied Suicide Intervention Skills Training (ASIST): A Competency-Based Evaluation*. Lifeline Australia Inc., Melbourne.

Underwood MM and Dunne-Maxim K (1997). Managing sudden traumatic loss in the schools. University of Medicine and Dentistry of New Jersey. *New Jersey Adolescent Suicide Prevention Project*, 1–134.

Vieland V, Whittle B, Garland A *et al.* (1991). The impact of curriculum-based suicide prevention programs for teenagers: an 18-month follow-up. *Journal of the American Academy of Child and Adolescent Psychiatry*, **30**, 811–815.

Waring T, Hazell T, Hazell P *et al.* (2000). Youth mental health promotion in the Hunter region. *Australian and New Zealand Journal of Psychiatry*, **34**, 579–585.

Wasserman D, Mittendorfer-Rutz E, Rutz W *et al.* (2004). *Suicide Prevention in Europe: The WHO European Monitoring Survey on National Suicide Prevention Programmes and Strategies*. NASP, Stockholm.

Webb NB (1986). Before and after suicide: a preventive outreach program for colleges. *Suicide and Life-Threatening Behavior*, **16**, 469–480.

Weist M, Rubin M, Moore E *et al.* (2007). Mental health screening in schools. *Journal of School Health*, **77**, 53–58.

World Health Organization (2001). *The World Health Report 2001. Mental Health: New Understanding, New Hope*. Available at http://www.who.int/whr/en.

World Health Organization (2002). Suicide Prevention in Europe: The WHO European Monitoring Survey on National Suicide Prevention Programmes and Strategies. Available at http://www.euro.who.int/document/e77922.pdf.

World Health Organization Department of Mental Health (2000). *Preventing Suicide: A Resource for Teachers and other School Staff*. Available at http://www.who.int/mental_health/media/en/62.pdf.

Wyman PA, Brown CH, Inman J *et al.* (2008). Randomized trial of a gatekeeper training program for suicide prevention: impact on school staff after one year. *Journal of Consulting and Clinical Psychology*, **76**, 104–115.

Wyn J, Cahill H, Holdsworth R *et al.* (2000). MindMatters, a whole-school approach promoting mental health and well-being. *Australian and New Zealand Journal of Psychiatry*, **34**, 594–601.

Zenere FJ and Lazarus PJ (1997). The decline of youth suicidal behavior in an urban, multicultural public school system following the introduction of a suicide prevention and intervention program. *Journal of Suicide and Life-Threatening Behavior*, **27**, 387–403.

# Public Health Strategies: Controlling the Access to Means of Suicide

# CHAPTER 74

# Protecting bridges and high buildings in suicide prevention

Annette Beautrais and Sheree Gibb

## Abstract

Suicide by jumping is a relatively uncommon method of suicide in most countries. However, in some places where there is accessible high-rise housing, jumping accounts for a significant proportion of suicides. While, internationally, most suicides by jumping occur from residential housing units, preventive efforts have tended to focus on a relatively small number of sites (often bridges) which have acquired notoriety as sites for suicide. A small number of studies suggest that the installation of safety barriers at these sites is an effective approach to reducing suicides by jumping. The extent to which lessons and principles from these examples may be applied to other jumping sites has yet to be fully explored.

## Introduction

Evidence leads to three major generalizations about the relationships between the accessibility of a specific method of suicide and suicidal behaviour:

1   As a general rule, restricting access to a specific method will result in reduced rates of mortality and morbidity by that method.

2   However, if the method that is restricted is substituted by another method, reductions in method-specific rates of suicide may not translate to reductions in overall rates of morbidity and mortality.

3   It should be noted that even in cases where substitution may eventuate, method restriction may still be justifiable. If it becomes apparent that some specific feature of the social or physical environment facilitates or encourages suicidal behaviour, it may be argued that it is ethical to remove access to that feature even though there is risk of substitution.

Because of the complex relationships between access to methods and suicidal behaviours, it is important that policies aimed at methods reduction are subject to thorough monitoring and evaluation.

The potential reduction of suicide rates by restricting access to means of suicide is addressed in a large body of research (Cantor *et al.* 1996; Beautrais 2000; Daigle 2005). In this chapter the focus will be one method of suicide: jumping from bridges and high buildings. The prevalence of suicide by jumping, characteristics of those who die by jumping, features of bridges and high buildings

which may encourage suicidal people to jump, and evidence for various approaches to prevent suicide by jumping is described.

## Epidemiology

There are marked national and international differences in rates of suicide by jumping. In part, jumping appears to be more common in some countries, city states or cities in which there are a large number of accessible high-rise buildings. For example, suicide by jumping accounts for approximately 60 per cent of suicides in Singapore (Ung 2003), 45 per cent in Hong Kong (The Hong Kong Jockey Club Centre for Suicide Research and Prevention 2005), 30 per cent in New York City (Fischer *et al.* 1993), but only 7 per cent in Switzerland (Reisch and Michel 2005), 6 per cent in Norway (Statistics Norway 1982) and Australia (Australian Bureau of Statistics 2001), 5 per cent in England and Wales (Gunnell and Nowers 1997), 4 per cent in Sweden (Statistics 2002), and less than 2 per cent in New Zealand (Ministry of Health 2006). There is little research that has explored reasons for jumping being more common in some cities, but less so in others with equal volume and accessibility to high-rise buildings. In addition to availability, the factors that may contribute to preferences for a particular method in a population include culturally determined views and attitudes to accepted methods of suicide, the role of media influences in shaping population attitudes about methods of suicide, the perceived lethality of various methods and the personal acceptability of the method (Clarke and Lester 1989). There is need for more research about the reasons for choice of jumping as a method of suicide.

Because of the high lethality of the method, there are sound reasons to try to prevent suicides by jumping in those countries in which it is a common method of suicide, and even in countries in which suicides by jumping are relatively uncommon. The tendency of clustering of such suicides to specific sites that consequently gain notoriety as suicide sites justifies preventive interventions.

## Characteristics of those who die by suicide by jumping

Some studies have suggested that individuals who choose jumping as a method of suicide tend to be younger, male and more often to have psychotic disorders than those who choose other methods

(Cantor *et al.* 1989; Ku *et al.* 2000; Beautrais 2001; Lindqvist *et al.* 2004). However, other studies have not found such differences (Prevost *et al.* 1996; Gunnell *et al.* 1997). For example, in Australia, 38 per cent of a series of suicides from a bridge in Adelaide, 45 per cent from a series of deaths from Brisbane bridges and 27 per cent from a series of deaths from a Melbourne bridge had psychotic illnesses (Pounder 1985; Cantor *et al.* 1989, Coman *et al.* 2000). In contrast, suicides from the Clifton Suspension Bridge in Bristol included only 10 per cent with psychosis, and suicides from Beachy Head in the United Kingdom included 9 per cent with psychosis, while deaths from the Jacques Cartier Bridge in Montreal included only 13 per cent with psychosis (Nowers and Gunnell 1996; Prevost *et al.* 1996; Surtees 1982). The inconsistency in findings from studies of jumping might be explained by such factors as the small numbers of suicides in some of these descriptive studies (for example, thirty-two suicides in the Adelaide series described above), the proximity of some jumping sites to psychiatric hospitals—the psychiatric hospital was only metres from the bridge in Auckland, New Zealand, for example (Beautrais 2001), the notoriety of the site in question, and the frequency of suicide by jumping in the countries of study. Nevertheless, in some countries where suicide by jumping is common, reports suggest one quarter of those who chose jumping had psychotic symptoms at the time of their attempt (Ku *et al.* 2000).

Suicide is often an impulsive act and it has been shown that most people who survive suicide attempts do not go on to die by suicide (Owens *et al.* 2002). Studies of people who attempted suicide by jumping but were restrained (Seiden 1978) or survived (Rosen 1975) found that most did not ultimately die by suicide. Researchers who studied individuals who made both fatal and non-fatal suicide attempts by jumping in Hong Kong found that half were described as impulsive by their psychiatrists (Ku *et al.* 2000). These findings suggest that restricting access to sites for jumping may delay or avert some fraction of impulsive suicide attempts and suicides.

## Features of sites chosen for suicide by jumping

Sites for suicide attempts by jumping include bridges and viaducts, high-rise public, residential and institutional buildings (including hotels, psychiatric hospitals and multi-storey car parks), and cliffs and terraces. In countries in which suicide by jumping is a common method of suicide most people attempt suicide from their home, from relatives' homes, or from nearby familiar places (Ku *et al.* 2000). However, an issue of particular concern is that specific sites or structures may acquire reputations, symbolic significance or iconic status as places for suicide (Beautrais 2001). Often these sites may be in public places, in attractive locations and may be aesthetically pleasing structures in themselves. These features appear to influence the appeal of the site for suicide. Sites which become notorious as places for suicide by jumping have emerged both in countries where suicide by jumping is common and in those in which it is rare. For example, in Hong Kong, where suicide by jumping accounts for almost half of all suicides, the new Tsing Ma Bridge has quickly acquired a reputation for suicide (see http://www.info.gov.hk/gia/general/2003121/15/1015173. htm for more detail). In New Zealand, where jumping accounts for <2 per cent of all suicides, Grafton Bridge had a long-standing national reputation as a suicide site (Beautrais 2001). Sites which

acquire iconic reputations for suicide are sometimes referred to as 'hotspots' (Reisch and Michel 2005). All significant suicide hotspots, internationally, are, in fact, jumping sites (Aitken *et al.* 2006). For example, the Golden Gate Bridge in San Francisco is the most popular public suicide site in the world, with an average of almost 20 suicides per year (Gunnell *et al.* 2005). It is interesting to note that sites may acquire reputations for suicide in spite of relatively small numbers of suicides from these sites. For example, Grafton Bridge in Auckland had a local reputation as a site for suicide despite having only one suicide per year (Beautrais 2001). Similarly small numbers were associated with other iconic sites—the Bern Muenster Terrace with four deaths per year (Reisch and Michel 2005), and the Bristol Suspension Bridge with an average of eight suicides each year (Bennewith *et al.* 2007). While there is no clear account of the mechanisms by which such sites acquire iconic status as places for suicide, it seems likely that this process would involve the development of local history, traditions and myths.

The public nature of sites that become notorious for suicide by jumping may lead to the witnessing of suicides by the public or that members of the public may be placed at risk. For these reasons, suicides from such sites tend to attract media coverage which, in turn, tends to promote and perpetuate the notoriety and appeal of the site. There is some evidence that people tend to make their choice of suicide methods based upon their perceptions of what they understand to be certain to achieve death: quick, readily available methods with a low risk of disfigurement (Lester 1988). Jumping fulfils some of these conditions. On the other hand, the symbolism and romanticism associated with an iconic or symbolic suicide site appear to play a decisive additional role for those who chose to jump from such sites (Seiden and Spence 1983–84).

## Preventive approaches

There are a series of approaches to preventing suicide by jumping. Installing barriers or safety nets to restrict access to specific sites is one preventive approach. A limited number of studies have evaluated the impact of installing barriers or safety nets at sites which acquire notoriety for suicide by jumping. These studies suggest that barriers significantly reduce suicides by jumping at the site and in the surrounding area. It is less clear, however, whether such restrictions reduce overall rates of suicide.

Examples of this approach include the installation of barriers on the Clifton Suspension Bridge in Bristol, England which halved the number of deaths from 8 to 4 per year, with no evidence of an increase in suicide at other sites in the area, and no overall change in the rate of suicide in the surrounding region (Bennewith *et al.* 2007). The installation of a safety net at the Bern Muenster Terrace in Switzerland eliminated suicides from the site, again with no evidence of substitution of another site (Reisch and Michel 2005). The *removal* of safety barriers at Grafton Bridge in Auckland, New Zealand, led to a fivefold increase in suicides from the site (Beautrais 2001) and their reinstallation eliminated suicides with no apparent substitution of other sites (Beautrais *et al.* submitted).

Similar reductions in suicides from sites to which access has been restricted, usually by the installation of barriers but sometimes by prohibiting access to the structure, have been reported (but not formally evaluated) for the Empire State Building, the Ellington Bridge in Washington DC, the Eiffel Tower, the Jacques

Cartier Bridge in Montreal, the Bloor Street Viaduct in Toronto, the Bosphoros Bridge in Istanbul and the Sydney Harbour Bridge (Aitken *et al.* 2006). Barriers may be effective in reducing suicides at these sites by averting impulsive attempts, by preventing access to sites which have symbolic significance for suicide (for which other less attractive sites are not substituted), or by forcing attempters to substitute less lethal methods. Arguments for installing barriers to prevent jumping are strengthened by observations that suicide rates by jumping increased in Singapore as the number of high-rise housing buildings increased (Lester 1994), and decreased after the Kobe earthquake in Japan, perhaps, in part, because the earthquake destroyed many high-rise buildings (Shioiri *et al.* 1999). Barriers at jumping sites may take various forms but evidence suggests they need to be 155cm or higher to prevent suicides and must be built in such a way that they do not offer a foothold for potential jumpers (Berman 1990; Reisch *et al.* 2006).

A second preventive approach that is used at known sites for suicide by jumping is to erect signs providing contact details of telephone help lines for suicidal individuals. In some cases telephones are provided from which individuals can make direct calls to helplines. This approach is underwritten by the expectation that many people planning to jump will be ambivalent about wanting to die and, if provided with ready access to a helpline, will use it. There are limited formal evaluations of this intervention and some concerns that such signs may risk promoting the idea of suicide to whose who had not previously contemplated it (Glatt 1987).

A further approach involves using surveillance and patrols at popular sites. Examples of this approach include closed circuit surveillance cameras, and site patrols by police, dedicated suicide patrol officers or unpaid volunteers. For example, the Golden Gate Bridge has security cameras and has been patrolled by a team of dedicated suicide prevention officers since 1996 (Reed 1996). However, there have been no formal evaluations of such measures and in many places in which they have been implemented, suicides have apparently not declined. There are concerns that these measures may be ineffective because patrols cannot monitor all parts of a structure (for example, a long bridge) at one time, even with the assistance of security cameras.

## Control of media reporting

As noted above, suicides from iconic public sites often lead to extensive media coverage. While these incidents may be newsworthy the reports may inadvertently promote the site for suicide, endorse the symbolic status of the site and risk imitative suicide attempts (Pirkis and Blood 2001; Yip *et al.* 2006). For these reasons an additional approach to reducing suicides by jumping involves muted media reporting of such incidents, and of preventive measures implemented at specific sites, since reports of these may also advertise the site as a place for suicide (King and Frost 2005). Evidence for the effectiveness of this approach is provided by the reduction in suicides by jumping in front of trains in the Viennese subway following the adoption of muted media reporting practices about these incidents (Etzersdorfer and Sonneck 1998). While it may be difficult to establish the extent to which prudent media reporting may lead to reductions in suicides, there may be opportunities to make 'naturalistic' evaluations at specific sites. Findings from some studies suggest that opportunities for media reporting are reduced when barriers reduce suicides at specific sites, with

this reduction in reporting being associated with fewer suicides by jumping from all sites in the local area (Gunnell *et al.* 2005).

## Prudent planning of buildings

A further approach involves collaboration with local or national building industries including architects, town planners and construction companies, to encourage the incorporation of safety features (such as barriers, safety glass in rooftops, enclosed stairwells, restricted access to rooftops and balconies, restricted window apertures) into designs of new buildings. Such efforts should particularly concern residential housing and institutions such as hospitals, prisons and juvenile detention centres. There appear to be no evaluations of such approaches. In addition, it would appear to be prudent for hospitals to move existing psychiatric inpatient facilities, or in the planning of new ones, and position them on lower floors of buildings from which patients are not able to jump to their deaths.

## Monitoring trends in suicide mortality

A useful adjunct to the practical measures outlined above includes the development of systems to monitor overall trends in suicide mortality with particular responsibility for identifying jumping sites which emerge as common sites for suicide, and implementing appropriate measures to minimize suicides from these sites.

## Discussion

In countries in which jumping accounts for a significant proportion of all suicides there is clear justification for implementing measures to reduce suicides by this method. Even in places where jumping plays only a small part of the overall suicide rates, it is justifiable to attempt to reduce these suicides. As discussed above, a range of preventive approaches exist. Thus far, however, the best evidence for the effectiveness of any approach comes from a small number of evaluations of the impact of installation (or *removal*) of safety barriers at sites which have become popular as places from which to die by suicide by jumping. The principles and lessons learned from these examples may be applicable to other jumping sites such as high-rise residential housing units and car park buildings.

Although barriers at jumping sites can help to reduce suicides, efforts to install barriers are frequently met with resistance. Often, the public view is that erecting barriers will decrease the aesthetic appeal of a site, or that suicide is inevitable in suicidal individuals and therefore barriers will be ineffective. In a study of public attitudes to suicide by jumping, Miller (2006) asked 2770 people to estimate how many people attempting to jump from the Golden Gate Bridge would have eventually died by suicide if they had been prevented from jumping off the bridge. More than a third of respondents replied that all would eventually die by suicide, and a further 40 per cent replied that 'most' would eventually die by suicide. As noted above, this perception is not supported by the research evidence. Another common reason for not installing barriers is cost. While advocates for suicide prevention argue that a socially responsible society would invest in measures to prevent a relatively small number of suicides by vulnerable members, opponents argue that the costs and lack of benefit for most of the society's members do not warrant the expense. A further reason advanced for not installing barriers is that other sites or methods would inevitably be substituted. There is no strong evidence to support this argument. First, suicide by jumping is a highly lethal method—if substitution occurs it is likely to be towards a less lethal method. Second, recent studies suggest that installing barriers at a popular site may, in fact, reduce suicides at other local sites, presumably because of the reduced media coverage of suicides at the notorious site (Bennewith *et al.* 2007). Third, people who survived suicide attempts by jumping from the Golden Gate and Oakland Bay Bridges in San Francisco said they would not have used any other method if the bridge had not been available (Rosen 1975).

Paradoxically, it seems that the best evidence for reducing suicides by jumping comes from a small number of studies in countries in which suicide by jumping is relatively uncommon. Studies of interventions to reduce suicides by jumping in countries where jumping accounts for a significant fraction of all suicides are lacking. There is a clear need for more investment in implementing and evaluating a range of preventive measures in these countries and, indeed, wherever suicides by jumping are a significant problem.

## Conclusion

There is increasing evidence that suicide by jumping can be prevented at specific sites by the installation of appropriate safety barriers and that, in some cases, this measure may decrease suicides by jumping in the surrounding area. This evidence suggests that installing barriers is the current 'best practice' and socially responsible approach to reducing suicides by jumping. However, there is a need to explore the extent to which the principles learned from these examples can be applied to a range of preventive approaches to reduce method-specific mortality and morbidity, and overall rates of mortality and morbidity.

## References

Aitken P, Owens C, Lloyd-Tomlins S *et al.* (2006) *Guidance on Action to be Taken at Suicide Hotspots.* http://www.csip-plus.org.uk/RowanDocs/SuicideHotspots.pdf. [cited 5 April 2007]. Devon Partnership NHS, Peninsula Medical School, Care Services Improvement Partnership, Mental Health in England.

Australian Bureau of Statistics (2001) *Briefing Paper Suicides 2001.* Australian Bureau of Statistics, Canberra.

Beautrais AL (2001). Effectiveness of barriers at suicide jumping sites: a case study. *Australian and New Zealand Journal of Psychiatry,* **35,** 557–562.

Beautrais AL (2000) *Restricting Access to Means of Suicide in New Zealand. A Report Prepared for the Ministry of Health on Methods of Suicide in New Zealand 1997–1996.* Ministry of Health, Wellington.

Beautrias AL, Gibb SJ, Fergusson DM *et al.* (submitted) Removing bridge barriers stimulates suicides: an unfortunate natural experiment.

Bennewith O, Nowers M, Gunnell D (2007). Effect of barriers on the Clifton suspension bridge, England, on local patterns of suicide: implications for prevention. *British Journal of Psychiatry,* **190,** 266–267.

Berman AL (1990). Suicide prevention in public places. In AL Berman, ed., *Suicide Prevention: Case Consultations,* pp. 3–24. New York, Springer.

Cantor C, Turrell G, Baume P (1996) *Access to Means of Suicide by Young Australians: A Background Report.* Australian Institute for Suicide Research and Prevention, Carina, Queensland.

Cantor CH, Hill MA, McLachlan EK (1989). Suicide and related behaviour from river bridges: a clinical perspective. *British Medical Journal,* **155,** 829–835.

Clarke RV and Lester D (1989). *Suicide: Closing the Exits.* Springer Verlag, New York.

Coman M, Meyer AD, Cameron PA (2000). Jumping from the Westgate Bridge, Melbourne. *Medical Journal of Australia,* **172,** 67–69.

Daigle MS (2005). Suicide prevention through means restriction: assessing the risk of substitution. A critical review and synthesis. *Accident Analysis and Prevention,* **37,** 625–632.

Etzersdorfer E and Sonneck G (1998). Preventing suicide by influencing mass-media reporting. The Viennese experience 1980–1996. *Archives of Suicide Research,* **4,** 67–74.

Fischer EP, Comstock GW, Monk MA *et al.* (1993). Characteristics of completed suicides: implications of differencs among methods. *Suicide and Life-Threatening Behaviour,* **23,** 91–100.

Glatt KM (1987). Suicide prevention at a suicide site. *Suicide and Life-Threatening Behaviour,* **17,** 299–309.

Gunnell D and Nowers M (1997). Suicide by jumping. *Acta Psychiatrica Scandinavica,* **96,** 1–6.

Gunnell D, Nowers M, Bennewith O (2005). Suicide by jumping: Is prevention possible? *Suicidologi,* **10,** 15–17.

King E and Frost N (2005). The New Forest Suicide Prevention Initiative (NFSPI). *Crisis,* **26,** 25–33.

Ku KH, Nguyen DGH, Ng YK (2000). Suicide attempts by jumping from height. *Hong Kong Journal of Psychiatry,* **10,** 21–26.

Lester D (1988). Why do people choose particular methods for suicide? *Activitas Nervosa Superior (Praha),* **30,** 312–314.

Lester D (1994). Suicide by jumping in Singapore as a function of high-rise apartment availability. *Perceptual and Motor Skills,* **79,** 74.

Lindqvist P, Jonsson A, Anders Hedelin A *et al.* (2004). Are suicides by jumping off bridges preventable? An analysis of 50 cases from Sweden. *Accident Analysis and Prevention,* **36,** 691–694.

Miller M, Azrael D, Hemenway D (2006). Belief in the inevitability of suicide: results from a national survey. *Suicide and Life-Threatening Behaviour,* **36,** 1–11.

Ministry of Health (2006) *New Zealand Suicide Trends. Mortality 1921–2003 Hospitalisations for Intentional Self-harm 1978–2004.* Ministry of Health, Wellington.

Nowers M and Gunnell D (1996). Suicide from the Clifton Suspension Bridge in England. *Journal of Epidemiology and Community Health,* **50,** 30–32.

Owens D, Horrocks J, House A (2002). Fatal and non-fatal repetition of self-harm. Systematic review. *British Journal of Psychiatry,* **181,** 193–199.

Pirkis J and Blood RW (2001). Suicide and the media. Part I: Reportage in nonfictional media. *Crisis: Journal of CrisisIntervention and Suicide,* **22,** 146–154.

Prevost C, Julien M, Brown BP (1996). Suicides associated with the Jacques Cartier Bridge, Montreal, Quebec 1988–1993: descriptive analysis and intervention proposal. *Canadian Journal of Public Health,* **87,** 377–380.

Reed S (1996). Patrols help reduce Golden Gate suicide rate. http://www.csip-plus.org.uk/RowanDocs/SuicideHotspots.pdf [cited 5 April 2007]. *US News,* 5 April 2007.

Reisch T and Michel K (2005). Securing a suicide hot spot: effects of a safety net at the Bern Muenster Terrace. *Suicide and Life-Threatening Behaviour,* **35,** 460–467.

Reisch T, Schuster U, Michel K (2006). Suicide prevention on bridges in Switzerland. Poster presented at the 11th Symposium on Suicide and Suicidal Behaviour, Portoroz, Slovenia, 9–12 September 2006

Rosen DH (1975). Suicide survivors. A follow-up study of persons who survived jumping from the Golden Gate and San Francisco-Oakland Bay Bridges. *The Western Journal of Medicine,* **122,** 289–294.

Seiden RH (1978). Where are they now? A follow-up study of suicide attempters from the Golden Gate Bridge. *Suicide and Life-Threatening Behaviour*, **8**, 203–216.

Seiden RH and Spence M (1983–84). A tale of two bridges: comparative suicide incidence on the Golden Gate and San Francisco–Oakland Bay Bridges. *Omega—Journal of Death and Dying*, **14**, 201–209.

Shioiri T, Nishimura A, Nushida H *et al.* (1999). The Kobe earthquake and reduced suicide rate in Japanese males. *Archives of General Psychiatry*, **56**, 282–283.

Statistics Sweden (2002) *Statistical Yearbook of Sweden. Official Statistics of Sweden*. Statistics Sweden, Stockholm.

Statistics Norway (1982). http://www.ssb.no/english/subjects/03/01/10/dodsarsak_en/tab-2004–02–27–09-en.html [accessed 2 February 2005] Surtees SJ.

Surtees SJ (1982). Suicide and accidental death at Beachy Head. *British Medical Journal*, **284**, 321–324.

The Hong Kong Jockey Club Centre for Suicide Research and Prevention (2005) *Prevention of Suicide is Everybody's Business*. The Hong Kong Jockey Club: Centre for Suicide Research and Prevention, Hong Kong.

Ung EK (2003). Youth suicide and parasuicide in Singapore. *Annals of the Academy of Medicine*, **32**, 12–18.

Yip PSF, Fu KW, Yang KCT *et al.* (2006). The effects of a celebrity suicide on suicide rates in Hong Kong. *Journal of Affective Disorders*, **93**, 245–52.

# CHAPTER 75

# Prevention of suicide by jumping

## Experiences from Taipei City (Taiwan), Hong Kong and Singapore

Ying-Yeh Chen and Paul Yip

## Abstract

Nearly 80 per cent of the population of Hong Kong and Singapore live in high-rise buildings. High-rise buildings provide an opportunity for committing suicide by jumping, and elevated rates of suicide by this method are observed in the above-mentioned cities. An analysis of the suicides in Singapore, Hong Kong and Taipei can increase understanding and improve possibilities for prevention.

## Introduction

In Taiwan, jumping suicide rates vary greatly across different levels of urbanization; the more urbanized cities/counties, with greater density of high-rise buildings, were found to have as much as a fourfold increase in incidence rate compared to the less urbanized districts (Lin and Lu 2006). In Taipei City, the largest metropolitan area in Taiwan, with a population of 2,600,000 (Department of Budget Accounting and Statistics, 2004), there are about 35 per cent of households living on the sixth floor or higher. Taipei City is one of the cities in Taiwan with high rates for jumping suicide (Lu and Chen 2006). The overall suicide rate in Taipei City was 17.3 per 100,000 population in 2006, which was lower than the national average 19.3 per 1,000,000 population. However, the average proportion of suicide by jumping in Taipei City was about 20 per cent, which was much greater than in Taiwan as a whole (8 per cent), and was the largest among all the cities in Taiwan (Lu and Chen 2006).

In Hong Kong and Singapore, nearly 80 per cent of the population lives in high-rise buildings, which provide a very accessible method for people committing suicide by jumping. Suicide by jumping is the most common method of suicide in Hong Kong and Singapore, 50 per cent and 74 per cent in 2005 respectively. In Singapore, a very significant change of method of suicides was observed during the rapid transition to urbanization in Singapore. The proportion of jumping among suicide deaths in Singapore has increased from 18 per cent in 1960–1964 to 74 per cent in 2000–2004. It has replaced hanging as the leading method of suicide since the early 1980s. In Hong Kong, jumping has replaced hanging as the most common method of suicide since 1980s as more high-rise buildings were built. The easy accessibility to potential jumping sites was an important contributing factor to the increase in jumping suicide rates in Hong Kong, Singapore and Taipei City.

## Where do they jump?

Data analysed by the Center for Suicide Research and Prevention in Hong Kong (2005) suggests that home residence is the most common place to jump: about 80 per cent of jumping suicides. However, suicide 'hotspots' in the community do exist. There have been about ten suicide deaths from jumping from the Tsing-Ma Bridge in Hong Kong since its opening in 1997.

A study conducted by Chen et al. (2008) analysed jumping suicides committed between 2002–2005 in Taipei, and had shown that private residential buildings comprised the highest proportion (67 per cent) of all jumping suicides, followed by business office buildings (13 per cent), hospitals (8 per cent) and shopping malls (5 per cent). However, hospitals and shopping malls were actually the two sites with the highest estimated risk. The number of jumping suicide per 1000 sites were 307 per 1000 hospitals, and 275 per 1000 shopping malls, compared to 0.7 per 1000 residential buildings (Chen and Lu 2008). The relative risks of jumping suicide in hospitals and shopping malls are much higher than other structures in Taipei, indicating that hotspots do exist in places where patterns of suicidal jumps mostly occur from high-rise residences. Restricting suicide from these two types of sites could prevent 13 per cent of suicide by jumping.

## Characteristics of individuals who commit suicide by jumping

Studies examining jumping suicide from high-rise residences usually found that the rates were higher among elderly people (Copeland 1989; Abrams et al. 2005; Lu and Chen 2006) and younger adults. For the older age group, a jump from their own residence is accessible, and is comparatively easier to accomplish than hanging, especially for those living in high-rise buildings. For younger adults, some show very impulsive behaviour, particularly with a relationship break-up or other problems.

Several studies have indicated that the gender distribution of those who jumped from residential buildings resemble general suicide victims (Fischer *et al.* 1993; Yip 1997). In Taipei, however, jumping suicide rates were equal in men and women (Lu and Chen 2006; Chen and Lu 2008), which is different from the gender profiling of jumping suicide in other countries. This indicates that jumping suicide is a relatively preferred method of suicide among women in Taipei, as the male:female suicide gender ratio in Taipei is about 2:1 (Kuo *et al.* 2006; Lin and Lu 2008). Differences in method availability and cultural acceptability may drive higher jumping suicide rates among women in Taipei City.

## Safety measures

Method availability relates to direct physical access to, familiarity with, and the technical skills and planning required to use the method. The factor of accessibility is a more dominant factor, especially among older adults with serious illness, since this restricts the use of other methods.

It is reasonable to expect that the unavailability of certain methods may reduce the number of people attempting suicide, or at least provide an opportunity to intervene as the person seeks another method. Although there is no formal report in Taipei, increasing the height of walls in the upper floor parking lots of a shopping mall has decreased number of cases that jumped from the site (Figure 75.1). Similarly, Times Square, one of the busiest shopping centres in Hong Kong, contains a courtyard-style building, in which there were a few incidences of suicide by jumping from higher floors into the centre court during 2002–2003. As a result, the height of the transparent partitions the upper floors was raised. After the additional safety measures were implemented there were no more suicides by jumping, and the aesthetics of the mall were largely retained.

Sensational reporting of suicide from specific places can lead to a copycat effect, as seen in three cases of jumping from Times Square in Hong Kong, in which the victims were very similar in their profile: young adults with mental illness.

The suicides from the Tsing Ma bridge in Hong Kong were also different from the general suicide population. A careful reporting on suicides from suicide hotspots, for example, avoiding mention of the specific location, would reduce the copycat effect. It seems that this is not practical in news reporting. However, if we were aware of the possibility of excess risk in copycat suicides, it would certainly be an option worth exploring for the sake of protecting the vulnerable individuals in society. Media reporting of suicide from the parking lot of the shopping mall could create an impression that it is a good and potential place for jumping suicide.

## Conclusion

The prevention of suicide by jumping can be achieved by building higher walls or fences at jump-sites, and decreasing media coverage

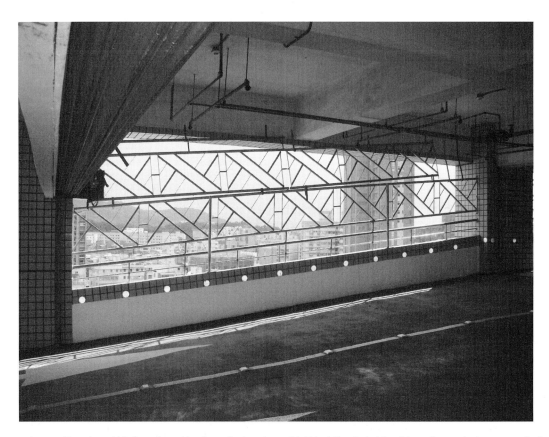

**Fig. 75.1** After several cases of jumping suicide from the parking floor of a shopping mall in Taipei City, the height of the wall was raised to prevent further jumps.

of such suicides. These strategies may be especially effective for communities with a large number of high-rise buildings.

## References

Abrams RC, Marzuk PM, Tardiff K *et al.* (2005). Preference for fall from height as a method of suicide by elderly residents of New York City. *American Journal of Public Health*, **95**, 1000–1002.

Chen YY, Gunnell D, and Lu TH (2009). A descriptive epidemiological study of sites of suicide jumps in Taipei, Taiwan. *Injury Prevention*, **15.**

Copeland AR (1989). Suicide by jumping from buildings. *American Journal of Forensic and Medical Pathology*, **10**, 295–298.

Department of Budget Accounting and Statistics. The statistical abstract of Taipei City. Taipei: Taipei City Government, Republic of China 2004.

Fischer EP, Comstock GW, Monk MA *et al.* (1993). Characteristics of completed suicides: implications of differences among methods. *Suicide and Life-Threatening Behaviour*, **23**, 91–100.

Kuo CJ, Chen YY, Chiu CH *et al.* (2006). Comparison of demographic characteristics between suicide completers and suicide attempt in Taipei City. *Taipei City Medical Journal*, **3**, 992–999.

Lin JJ and Lu TH (2006). Association between the accessibility to lethal methods and method-specific suicide rates: an ecological study in Taiwan. *Journal of Clinical Psychiatry*, **67**, 1074–1079.

Lin JJ and Lu TH (2008). Suicide mortality trends by sex, age and method in Taiwan, 1971–2005. *BMC Public Health*, **8**, 6.

Yip PS (1997). Suicides in Hong Kong, 1981–1994. *Social Psychiatry and Psychiatric Epidemiology*, **32**, 243–250.

# CHAPTER 76

# Restriction of access to drugs and medications in suicide prevention

Antoon Leenaars, David Lester,
Gaspar Baquedano, Chris Cantor,
John F Connolly, Emilio Ovuga,
Silvia Pelaez Remigio and
Lakshmi Vijayakumar

## Abstract

Suicide by prescription drugs and medications is a very common method of suicide in many countries. In 1972, Oliver and Hetzel first called attention to the adverse effects of easy availability of medications in Australia; they also reported that restriction of drugs and medications decreased the rate of suicides. Results for different countries support these observations; yet there is a lack of impact on clinical practice. Experiences from some countries are presented, which suggests, despite great variation around the world, that the way physicians and other mental health professionals act needs to be more congruent with existing evidence-based knowledge. Of course, even if medication is associated to risk, it can be asked if restriction makes a difference. The sparse research suggests that restriction of access to drugs and medications reduces the suicide rate. Governments and the WHO could be involved more; for example, to promote educational programmes, and to define standards and agreements among pharmaceutical companies, national health services, medical associations, and the population in general. Much more research and clinical action are needed.

## Introduction

Restriction of drugs and medications is consistent with a report on suicide prevention of the World Health Organization (WHO). After careful analysis of all measures by an international team of researchers, headed by Bertolote (1993), a series of tactics to prevent suicide that had support in the scientific literature were proposed. The team provided some basic steps for the prevention of suicide, among them controlling the environment: e.g. gun possession control, detoxification of domestic gas, detoxification of car emissions, and control of toxic substance availability.

## Early research from Australia

Controlling the environment is not foreign to practising clinicians worldwide (Leenaars 2005). Restriction of access to drugs or control of medications—or toxic substance—availability is common practice. In 1972, Oliver and Hetzel first called attention to the adverse effects of easy availability of medication in Australia. They examined the mortality data for the period of 1955 to 1970 in Australia; a period of significant increase in suicide, and the increase of availability of sedative agents. They found that the increase of suicide with prescription drugs wholly accounted for the increase in the suicide rate, although it was difficult to establish definitively that sedatives and, in particular, barbiturates were the cause. These substances were, however, overwhelmingly implicated. Concern mounted, not only about the deaths, but also about abuse and other mismanagements.

To test this hypothesis further, they studied a 1967 law that restricted the allowable quantity of sedatives, controlled the strength of barbiturates, and allowed for no repeats of the prescriptions. Data showed that after the law was introduced, there was not only a decline in usage, but also a decrease in suicides, as well as in undetermined causes of deaths. Thus it was concluded that the falling rates of suicide in Australia were genuine, and furthermore, the data showed that there were no substitutions with other means of suicide. They concluded that a causal relationship underlies the association observed between the ready availability of potentially lethal quantities of therapeutic substances and death by self-injury from this cause. Suicide by other means had been largely unchanged; thus, the data showed no substitution with other drugs or other methods. Finally, they concluded that a proportion of deaths, due to drug ingestion, would not have occurred had the means not been so readily available.

Oliver and Hetzel suggested measures to diminish the ready availability of medications by individual wrapping of pills, and the restriction of usage by better education of all concerned.

## Research from different continents

There are further studies on the five continents to support Oliver and Hetzel's observation. An array of current studies, as well as some observations from the continents and implications worldwide, is presented.

In the United States from 1960 to 1974, Lester (1990a) found that the suicide rate using barbiturates was associated with the annual sales of barbiturates, and with the accidental death rate from barbiturates. Lester (1990b) found that in the US from 1950 to 1984, the accidental death rate from prescription drugs, specifically from barbiturates, was positively associated with the suicide rates from these methods. Lester and Abe (1990) replicated this result for all medicaments in Japan. Thus these countries show the same result as noted in Australia.

Gunnell et al. (1997) found that British sales of paracetamol, and the rate of attempting suicide with paracetamol in the Oxford area, were positively associated for 1976–1993. The same was found also for France as a whole. The attempted and completed suicide rates by paracetamol were positively associated in both Britain and France over time. In France, however, paracetamol is sold in smaller amounts (package limit in the UK was 12 grams, where in France it was 8 grams), and the attempted suicide rate using paracetamol was lower in France than in Britain (Gunnell et al. 1997).

In Sweden, Isacsson and colleagues (1995) found that suicide rates were higher for antipsychotics and anxiolytics, and lower for analgesics. Analysis of the data indicated that the number of suicides by each medication, and the number of prescriptions, was strongly positively associated. Furthermore, in Sweden, Carlsten et al. (1996) found that the suicide rate using barbiturates declined as the sales of barbiturates declined rapidly from 1977–1992, and the same parallel was found for analgesics and for neuroleptics/antidepressants. Sundquist et al. (1996) found that, in southern Sweden, the greater the sales of tranquillizers and hypnotics/sedatives in the municipalities, the higher the suicide rate; however, this pattern was not evident for antidepressants or neuroleptics. Of course, correlations imply associations and not necessarily causality; other factors, such as mental health conditions in the region, may also have accounted for the results.

Japan offers an interesting test of Oliver and Hetzel's finding. In Japan, prior to 1961, barbiturates were available over the counter without a prescription. From February 1961, the Pharmacy Act S.49 required prescriptions both for barbiturates and meprobamate. Lester and Abe (1989) examined the use of sedatives for suicide prior to and after the implementation of the Act. The suicide rate using sedatives and hypnotics peaked at 7.05 per 1,000,000 per year in 1958. Thereafter, the suicide rate by sedatives and hypnotics declined consistently. When the Pharmacy Act was implemented in 1961, the suicide rate using sedatives and hypnotics was already declining; however, the decline did increase a little after the implementation of the Act. Furthermore, the suicide rate by all other methods was examined for the same time period: it began declining even earlier, after 1955 in fact, and continued to decline until 1965. There was thus no increase in other methods after the Act, and no evidence that people switched methods for suicide once prescriptions were required for sedatives and hypnotics.

In the United Kingdom (UK), both Brewer and Farmer (1985) and Forster and Frost (1985) noted that completed and attempted suicide by overdoses paralleled the prescription rate for hypnotics, tranquillizers and other psychotropic drugs. Forster and Frost estimated that 1000 fewer prescriptions resulted in 3.8 fewer attempted suicides. Similar associations have been noted in Scotland (McMurray et al. 1987) and Australia (Buckley et al. 1995). Thus, data from the different continents support the practice of the restriction of access to lethal medications.

## Impact on clinical practice

Controlling the availability of medication may be the most viable strategy to prevent suicide. Yet despite the recommendations of the WHO, and the research indicating the importance of education of the suicidal person and their families on the importance of having medication locked up or under control when a person is suicidal (Leenaars 2005), there continues to be a lack of impact on clinical practice globally. Wislar and colleagues research (1998), for example, exemplifies this absence. They conducted a chart review in an emergency department of a hospital of youths receiving mental health evaluation, with 40 per cent being suicide-related events. Suicide-related events were defined as behaviour involving self-directed injuries, e.g. cutting, jumping, or thoughts about self-injury or death. Chart reviews provided no evidence that means restriction education was provided to the young patients and/or their parents. Wisler et al.'s study, including other similar experiences, calls for greater attention by physicians and other mental health professionals to controlling the environment in the treatment of suicidal patients. Oliver and Hetzel stated the same, but also called for other strategies, such as surveillance and restricting the prescribed amount and/or dosage.

Over 30 years ago, Oliver and Hetzel noted that the implications of their findings were obvious. The more recent studies support the 'obvious'; yet there is a lack of application. Even in countries such as the US and Canada, where medication can be obtained only by prescription, there is, as Wislar and colleagues (1998) showed, a *lack of application, both in policies and in the individual clinical practice.* Physicians and other mental health professionals' knowledge and attitudes need to be reshaped.

## Experiences from some countries

In order to obtain information on the present topic from a geographically broader area, the first author asked some people on each continent to reflect on the issues at hand (Gaspar Baquedano, Mexico; Chris Cantor, Australia; John Connolly, Ireland; Emilio Ovuga, Uganda; Silvia Palaez Remigio, Uruguay, and Lakshmi Vijayakumar, India). They were asked specifically, once they read the research to date, to reflect on the role of the physician, and on the way medications are obtained by prescription or over the counter.

Countries like Australia, Canada, Ireland, and the US require prescriptions, but in Mexico, medications without prescriptions are easily accessible in pharmacies. Physicians in Mexico are also prone to hand out large quantities of medication to patients. This, as in other regions, is a reflection of the belief by the government, and the people themselves, that if you have medications then the health system is adequate. In much of Latin America, the situation is the same. In Uruguay, for example, only medical doctors can prescribe medication. However, if a person wants to buy a drug, they can buy it without a prescription, but at higher prices. Psychotropic drugs cannot be obtained without a physician's prescription. There are restrictions in place regarding the sale of such drugs as neuroleptics, benzodiazapines and antidepressants. People are encouraged to visit the doctor and, as a result, can buy medication at cheaper prices. If a person wants other non-psychotropic drugs (many lethal), they are always available. Of course people can stockpile money to obtain the drugs, even if they are poor, just as they can stockpile available drugs.

Availability of lethal means increases the environmental fraction of the suicide risk (WHO 2006). It is, furthermore, easy to conclude, as elsewhere, that poverty dictates availability—not legislation—if there is any. In other countries, the state is even worse. In India, for example, drugs can be easily obtained in drug stores. Even though there is legislation, the majority of psychotropic medications are available without physician's prescription. This situation is repeated in much of Asia. Africa is no different; Uganda, for example, lacks legislation to control drugs. Therefore, even before one introduces means restriction, the very control of availability needs to be managed. Physicians and health professionals need to strongly support public health action; and in countries where there is a lack of knowledge about suicide risks (e.g. a lack of sufficient labelling of potential lethality by pharmaceutical companies), in many regions and legislation, these should be implemented immediately.

The problems that affect availability of medications are, furthermore, complicated by violence (WHO 2002). In countries such as Uganda, owing to poverty and breakdown of essential drug regulatory mechanisms, following years of conflict and war, medications of all types are readily available, ranging from analgesics and antibiotics through psychotropics to pesticides. Where there is a lack of central regulatory mechanisms, in addition to large populations of rodents and insects, the role of physicians in controlling the amounts of permitted medications that they can prescribe is not sufficient, as people in Uganda often ingest large quantities of pesticides or swallow quartz cells from wrist watches, or a cocktail of analgesics, antibiotics and anti-malarial drugs in a bid to end their lives. Control of harmful medications will require multifaceted approach targeting, not only health providers and members of the general public, but also special groups including government officials, traders, farmers, insecticide producers, veterinarians, pharmacy specialists, owners of pharmacies, and drug companies.

## Prevention approaches

Of course, the control of availability of medications and drugs, which can be used as a mean of suicide, is not sufficient. The control of medication involves not only a duty to restrict access to what are dangerous and lethal products when misused, but also to prescribe appropriately, rationally and adequately for mental illnesses. Physicians play a great and decisive role here. The prescribing of large quantities, as seen in Mexico, is lethal. One should prescribe according to risk; this will mean greater education for physicians. For example, Chris Cantor from Australia tells of a patient who was prescribed the sleeping tablet chloral hydrate. The GP had been concerned that benzodiazapines might be used for a suicide attempt, so chloral hydrate was prescribed instead. The physician had been attending to risk issues but prescribed the worst possible sleeping tablet. Each of the authors could report such individual cases. Information to physicians and health professionals is obviously incomplete, even in Australia, Europe, North America, Africa, Asia, and South America. Wislar et al.'s study (1998) further shows that patients and their families need to be educated, by encouraging them to dispose of excess unused tablets. This is especially important with patients who do not comply with treatment regimes. This leads to stockpiling of large amounts of unused medications that are readily accessible as a means of suicide, as well as posing a danger to others, particularly children, the elderly, and animals. This is, as noted, further complicated by the practice of prescribing large dosages in countries such as, for example, Mexico. This problem must be addressed as a matter of urgency. There is, for example, in Dublin, Ireland, a scheme that was introduced for the proper disposal of unused medication. The initiative involved not only physicians and pharmacists, but also the patients and their families. Public information on the dangers of medication, measures to control availability and dispose of medication is necessary worldwide.

A basic question from a public health perspective is: Does research support the positive effect of the implementation of strategies to control availability of drugs? The research cited indicated that the availability of medication is associated to risk. Thus, it can be asked, does restriction of access to drugs and medications reduce the risk? The research shows that this approach, indeed, has an influence on decreasing suicide rates; however, more studies are needed.

Melander et al. (1991) compared data in two towns in Sweden from 1978. One of the towns (Malmö) had instituted prescription surveillance, and an information campaign about medication use, after it was found that the city had the highest suicide rate and prescription rate for anxiolytic–hypnotic drugs (AHD) in the country. The campaign resulted in a 25 per cent decrease in suicide, a 12 per cent decrease in AHD prescriptions, and a 40 per cent decrease in AHD abuse. In the other comparable city (Gothenberg), where no such campaign was carried out, the suicide rates were found to increase during the following seven years. These observations suggest that restricting prescriptions can decrease AHD abuse and suicide.

Reducing the size of packs of paracetamol in the UK in 1998 resulted in a 31 per cent reduction in cases of self-poisoning with paracetamol in Birmingham (Hughes et al. 2003). In a recent review of studies Morgan and Majeed (2004) concluded that admissions to liver units, admissions for liver transplants and emergency room admissions for paracetamol poisoning had declined in the UK after the packaging restrictions in 1998.

## Conclusion

Despite the clear evidence, since the work of Oliver and Hetzel 1972, restriction of easily available drugs and medication does not appear to be implemented on most continents. The facts are unequivocal. Oliver and Hetzel called for control of the availability of means for suicide. The way of obtaining prescriptions needs to be regulated; physicians and other mental health professionals can play a major role here, not only in education, but also in means restriction. The problem is, however, more complex; the references to the continents shows this. More can be done.

Governments and agencies need to be aware of these issues in order to promote international cooperation, establishing educational campaigns, and international agreements among pharmaceutical companies, national health services, and medical associations. Within the context of cultural sensitivities, international standards need to be developed. The WHO could be involved in defining standards, establish campaigns and international agreements among pharmaceutical companies, national health services, medical associations and populations in general. The implications of the research, as Oliver and Hetzel noted in 1972, are obvious: more practical applications are needed.

## References

Bertolote J (1993). *Guidelines for the Primary Prevention of Mental, Neurological, and Psychosocial Disorders: Suicide.* World Health Organization, Geneva.

Brewer C and Farmer R (1985). Self-poisoning in 1984. *British Medical Journal,* **290,** 391.

Buckley NA, Whyte IM, Dawson AH *et al.* (1995). Correlations between prescriptions and drugs taken in self-poisoning. Implications for prescribers and drug regulation. *Medical Journal of Australia,* **162,** 194–197.

Carlsten A, Allebeck P, Brandt L (1996). Are suicide rates in Sweden associated with changes in the prescribing of medications? *Acta Psychiatrica Scandinavica,* **94,** 94–100.

Forster D and Frost C (1985). Medicinal self-poisoning and prescription frequency. *Acta Psychiatrica Scandinavica,* **71,** 567–574.

Gunnell D, Hawton K, Murray V *et al.* (1997). Use of paracetamol for suicide and non-fatal poisoning in the UK and France. *Journal of Epidemiology & Community Health,* **51,** 175–179.

Hughes B, Durran A, Langford NJ *et al.* (2003). Paracetamol poisoning. *Journal of Clinical Pharmacy & Therapeutics,* **28,** 307–310.

Isacsson G, Wasserman D, Bergman U (1995). Self-poisonings with antidepressants and other psychotropics in an urban area of Sweden. *Annals of Clinical Psychiatry,* **7,** 113–118.

Leenaars A (2005). Effective public health strategies in suicide prevention are possible: a selective review of recent studies. *Clinical Neuropsychiatry,* **2,** 21–31.

Lester D (1990a). The use of prescribed medications for suicide. *International Journal of Risk & Safety in Medicine,* **1,** 279–281.

Lester D (1990b). Accidental death rates and suicide. *Activitas Nervosa Superior,* **32,** 130–131.

Lester D and Abe K (1989). The effect of controls on sedatives and hypnotics and their use for suicide. *Clinical Toxicology,* **27,** 299–303.

Lester D and Abe K (1990). The availability of lethal methods for suicide and the suicide rate. *Stress Medicine,* **6,** 275–276.

McMurray JJ, Northridge DB, Abernethy VA *et al.* (1987). Trends in analgesic self-poisoning in West-Fife, 1971–1985. *The Quarterly Journal of Medicine,* **65,** 835–843.

Melander A, Henricson K, Stenberg P *et al.* (1991). Anxiolytic–hypnotic drug: relationship between prescribing, abuse and suicide. *European Journal of Clinical Pharmacology,* **41,** 525–529.

Morgan O and Majeed A (2004). Restricting paracetamol in the United Kingdom to reduce poisoning. *Journal of Public Health,* 8 December, e-publication.

Oliver R and Hetzel B (1972). Rise and fall of suicide rates in Australia: relation to sedative availability. *The Medical Journal of Australia,* **2,** 919–923.

Sundquist J, Ekedahl A, Johansson S (1996). Sales of tranquillizers, hypnotics/sedatives and antidepressants and their relationship with underprivileged area scores and mortality and suicide rates. *European Journal of Clinical Pharmacology,* **51,** 105–109.

Wislar J, Grossman J, Kruesi J *et al.* (1998). Youth suicide-related visits in an emergency department serving rural counties: implications for means restriction. *Archives of Suicide Research,* **4,** 75–87.

World Health Organization (2002). *World Report on Health and Violence.* World Health Organization, Geneva.

World Health Organization (2006). *Preventing Disease through Healthy Environments.* World Health Organization, Geneva.

# CHAPTER 77

# Gun availability and control in suicide prevention

Antoon Leenaars

## Abstract

Although countries differ in the most frequent methods of suicide, firearms are a preferred method in some countries. It is a method with high case fatality. Individual (case–control) studies and population studies show that restriction of firearms reduces suicide. This is especially evident in the young. Further, population studies show that gun control, such as strict licensing and restricted availability of firearms, is effective. Individual and population studies also found that one must especially control the availability of firearms to people with mental disorders. Canada's Criminal Law Amendment Act of 1977 (Bill C-51) illustrates the effect of legislating means restriction when one controls for confounding social and economic factors. The young show the most significant decrease in suicide rates, not substituting guns with other methods of suicide. Studies on firearms and suicide across the globe support the studies from Canada. Yet, there are researchers who espouse the opposite and the debate has been polemic. More research is needed to strengthen the conclusion on the positive effects of gun control laws worldwide.

## Introduction

One public health approach to suicide prevention is restricting the means of suicide: today there is prevailing consensus that this method can be effective (Stengel 1964; Kreitman 1976; Leenaars *et al.* 2000; World Health Organization 2002, 2006). Erwin Stengel (1964) was one of the first in the twentieth century to propose a public health approach as a means to decrease the incidence of suicide, noting, for example, that the detoxification of domestic gas (from coal gas with high carbon monoxide content to natural gas) might have reduced the suicide rates in nations where the switch had taken place. Subsequent research on the detoxification of domestic gas in England supported Stengel's proposal (Kreitman 1976). A comprehensive review of the research around the globe supports the approach more generally, often called controlling the environment (Leenaars *et al.* 2000). After careful analysis of all measures by an international team of researchers, headed by Bertolote (1993), a series of tactics to prevent suicide that had support in the empirical literature were proposed. Among the tactics were gun possession control, detoxification of domestic gas, detoxification of car emissions

and control of toxic substance availability. Gun control legislation is often cited as the prototypical example of public health intervention to prevent suicide (Bertolote 1993; Leenaars *et al.* 1998; WHO 2006). Gun control is, for example, an excellent example because guns are a lethal method and easy availability can obviously facilitate death. One would predict that availability would increase suicide and that stricter gun laws would reduce the suicide rate. There are ample laws, for example, in Australia, Canada, New Zealand and the United States to allow for scientific investigation. In this chapter, a review is performed of the research on the association of the availability of the guns and suicide, and on the effect of gun control legislation or laws on suicide.

In a public health perspective, one can study the association between firearms and suicide at an individual and population level, sometimes called the ecological level. Each level has its limitations and benefits. The individual (case–control) empirical studies problem is finding reasonable controls and allowing for generalizations, often from small groups to larger groups in society. The population studies problem includes the 'ecological fallacy' when drawing conclusions about individuals from groups (aggregate) data. Each approach has its weaknesses and its strengths.

## Ecological studies on gun availability and suicide

Availability of guns is difficult to measure; oftentimes only indirect findings are available, e.g. the accidental death rate by firearms and the percentage of firearms used for crimes such as murder (Lester 2000). There are, however, a few studies on actual firearm ownership, such as measured by gun licences. In the United States, measures of actual firearm ownership are available in nine regions (but not for all states). Markush and Bertolucci (1984) found that in the US the actual ownership was positively associated with suicides by shooting and the total suicide rate. Lester (1988a) replicated that ownership was positively associated with the firearm suicide rate. Lester (1988b) found that ownership of firearms in Australia was positively associated with suicide by shooting; Carrington and Moyer (1994a) reported that firearm suicide was associated with ownership in Canada; and Etzersdorfer, Kapusta and Sonneck (2006) concluded that the same was valid in Austria.

Killias (1993) and Lester (1996) both found a positive association between the percentage of households with guns and suicide by shooting in twelve nations. A longitudinal analysis of firearm availability in an array of countries—US, Switzerland, Finland, France, Canada, Sweden, Australia, the Netherlands, England and Wales, Scotland, Norway, Spain and New Zealand—support the association; the study confirms the same patterns and associations of households owning firearms and suicide (Ajdacic-Gross et al. 2006). The international data, further, showed that the proportion of firearm suicides decreased simultaneously with the decrease in the proportion of homes owning guns. Consequently, the following question surfaced among public health professionals: would restriction of the means reduce suicides and violence in general (Leenaars 2006, 2007)?

## Individual level studies on guns and suicide

The case–control studies indicate that a gun in the home is significantly associated with a higher risk of suicide, especially among the young (Miller and Hemenwey 1999). Kellerman et al. (1992), in a frequently cited study, found that people who died by suicide were more likely to have a gun in the home. They studied all cases of suicide that occurred in the home during thirty-two months in two urban areas, Shelby County, Tennessee and King County, Washington. They controlled for sex, race, age range and confounding variables such as failure to graduate from high school, living alone, consumption of alcohol, current medication, and hospitalization. After controlling for the confounders, the presence of a gun was highly significant. The risk was higher when the gun was a handgun, loaded and kept in unlocked storage. Cummings et al. (1997) overcame the common problem of informational bias in case–control studies on suicide. They studied the actual handguns present in the home by analysing whether the purchase of a gun from a licensed dealer was associated with the suicides of 353 people using any method to kill themselves during the period 1980–1992. They controlled for social factors (confounders) such as income and education, and showed that the person who died by suicide was more likely to have had a gun and to have purchased a gun as compared to matched controls.

Not only studies across age groups, but also the study by David Brent on adolescents have shown similar results. Brent et al. (1988), in a pilot study, noted that a small group of adolescents who died by suicide (N = 27), compared to a psychiatric control group, had more often had firearms available in the home. In a larger-scale study (N = 47), Brent et al. (1991) showed that the presence and accessibility of firearms in the home of adolescents committing suicides were significant factors in the deaths. Guns were twice as likely to be in the home; the more guns, the greater the risk. Handguns did not differ from long guns with respect to risk. Alcohol was associated; the people who died by suicide with guns were more frequently intoxicated. A third case–control study (Brent et al. 1993), with a larger sample (N = 67), replicated the finding: the association between suicide and guns in the home is significant. Even if one controls for mental health disturbance (psychopathology), there is a particularly high risk. Subsequent case–control studies replicated the finding (Beautrais et al. 1996; Bailey et al. 1997). Brent et al. (1993) showed statistically that one can generalize the results of the individual cases to the community

as a whole, not just for adolescents, but for the whole population (Miller and Hemenway 1999; Lester 2000). However, from a public health perspective, the individual case studies must be supplemented by population studies.

The research at the individual level showed that the association of guns and suicide is not simplistic. Psychopathology and drug/alcohol abuse, especially alcohol, are associated in the equation (Miller and Hemenway 1999). If a suicidal person, for example, has a mental disorder, the risk of the gun in that home greatly increases the risk for suicide.

## Gun control laws and suicide in Canada

Although countries differ in the most frequent method of suicide, firearms are a preferred method in a number of countries. This is true in Canada, for example. Gun control, by strict licencing and restricted availability of firearms, is often cited as the prototypical example of public health intervention to prevent suicide (Bertolote 1993; Leenaars et al. 1998).

An opportunity to study the preventive effects of legislative means restriction, e.g. gun control laws, on suicide is provided by Canada's Criminal Law Amendment Act of 1977 (Bill C-51), enforced since 1978. This Act required an acquisition certification for all firearms, restricted the availability of some types of firearms to certain types of individuals, set up procedures for handling and storing firearms, required permits for those selling firearms, and increased the sentences for firearm offences. Early commentators on the impact of this Act (Mundt 1990), reported little impact of the Act on firearm suicide in Canada, but presented only simple charts with no statistical analysis of the trends. Lester and Leenaars (1993, 1994) reported a comprehensive study on the preventive effects on suicide the Act had demonstrated in Canada. The results suggested that strict firearm control laws might well have been associated with changes in suicide rates due to the reduced use of firearms for suicide, and no overall switching from firearms to other methods for suicide. Lester and Leenaars' results suggest that Bill C-51 in Canada appeared to have had a significant positive impact, namely, lowering the rate of suicide by guns.

Subsequently, Leenaars and Lester (1997a) examined whether the restriction of firearms in Bill C-51 in Canada had a preventive impact for those of all ages or only for some ages. The results showed that the percentage of suicides using firearms decreased only for those aged 15–64, while it increased for those aged 65+. Thus, the general conclusion seems to be that the impact of making the gun control laws stricter in Canada on suicide was not apparent in those over the age of 65, but significantly so in the young. Shneidman and Farberow (1957) had already shown that the suicidal elderly have a stronger intent to die than younger adults. They are less ambivalent and there is a chronic course (Leenaars 2004). Younger suicides are generally more situationally disturbed and impulsive (Leenaars 2004). Perhaps the younger individual may be sufficiently delayed by increased difficulty in obtaining the preferred method for suicide so that the suicidal pain has passed by the time he or she has succeeded in obtaining the means for suicide. This argues for the waiting period hypothesis. Considering the elderly, the result is consistent with other research (Lester 1992) suggesting that education programmes, crisis intervention services and telephone crisis centres are less effective with the elderly than with young adults. Thus, much more thought must be given and research undertaken to devising tactics for preventing suicide in the elderly (Richman 1993).

## Gender effects

There is evidence that men and women may respond differently to restricted access to lethal methods for suicide. A study by Leenaars and Lester (1996) was designed, therefore, to explore whether the 1977 gun control law in Canada had different effects on men and women in their use of guns for suicide. The results indicated that the passage of C-51 seemed to have had a greater preventive impact on suicide as well as on homicide in women than in men, possibly because more men switched suicide method. This phenomenon is called displacement. Carrington (1999) subsequently suggested that significant downward changes in death rates for suicide for both men and women occurred, with no evidence for switching method in both sexes. Recent re-evaluations found that the intervention had an impact on both men and women, probably because more men use firearms, but some men, indeed, showed displacement to other methods when committing suicide (Leenaars et al. 2003). Thus, public health approaches, such as gun control, may have limits in their preventive effects. The decrease of suicides among women is in agreement with other findings showing that suicidal women respond better to clinical intervention programmes, educational endeavours, use of telephone crisis centres, and receiving care for psychiatric disturbances (Lester 1995). Thus, it makes sense that this would be true with tactics of environmental control, but research to explain the phenomenon and for developing gender-specific interventions is lacking.

## Social factors

In a review of gun control studies, Stack (1998) pointed out that gun control studies rarely take into account other societal factors (confounders) which may influence the suicide rate—factors such as divorce, unemployment and the age structure of the population. A study by Leenaars and colleagues (2003) examined whether social changes might have had an impact on suicide rates from guns. Birth, marriage and divorce rates as measures of domestic integration—a social variable which Durkheim (1897) argued was critical in determining suicide rates—the unemployment rate (Platt 1984), median family income and the percentage of the males aged 15–24 years as a percentage of the total male population (a group with one of Canada's highest suicide rates) were studied. The results showed that the passage of Bill C-51 in Canada in 1977, introducing stricter gun control, appears to have been followed by a significant reduction in the suicide rate by firearms, even after controlling for some social variables. Thus, it appears that even if one controls for social variables, gun control succeeds in preventing suicides. There may, of course, have been social changes other than those considered that might be responsible for changes in the suicide rates, and the use of a different set of indicators such as alcohol and drug consumption the percentage of foreign-born, social class and education levels should be studied in the future, if and when the necessary data become available.

However, some researchers have disputed the conclusion that gun restriction has prevented suicide in Canada and elsewhere (Rich et al. 1990; Sloan et al. 1990; Kassirer 1991). Rich et al. (1990) reported, using a small sample, that stricter gun-control laws in Toronto were followed by decrease in suicide using guns, but at the same time an increase of suicide using other methods, like subway jumping, was observed. However, Carrington and Moyer (1994b) replicated the positive findings for gun control in Ontario. They also showed that most of Canada's provinces had either stable or decreasing rates of firearm suicides, following C-51 (Carrington and Moyer 1994a). Results on related phenomena of homicide (Leenaars and Lester 2001) and accidental deaths (Leenaars and Lester 1997b) hold equal promise.

There have been two subsequent laws in Canada, Bill C-17 and C-68. Bill C-17 in 1991 tightened the screening provisions for firearm acquisition (FAC). A more complete search of an applicant's personal and criminal records and 28-day waiting periods were required. Bridges (2004), following Leenaars and Lester's design, examined the impact of the bill and showed a significant decrease after passage of Bill C-17 in the rate of suicides involving firearms and the percentage of suicides using firearms. Bill C-68 was more an attempt at people control than gun control. It required people to register all shotguns and rifles. It was to be implemented in 1999, then 2001, then in 2003, and so on. The bill has encountered mounting problems and has yet to be enacted. The bill itself, unlike C-17, for example, is controversial in Canada and has met with significant opposition: the current government, in fact, introduced a bill on June 19, 2006 to rescind the bill. To date, the bill is still in limbo.

Farmers, hunters, indigenous people and many other people in Canada, as elsewhere around the world, have been against such registration of guns. They view this act as a control of common rights. Environmental controls, at least within public health, are known to be more effective than people controls. Simply stated, not all controls are accepted. This debate is not unusual about gun control worldwide (Leenaars 2006).

## Gun control laws in other countries

Beautrais, Fergusson and Horwood (2006) examined the impact of more restrictive firearm legislation (Amendment to the Arms Act 1992) in New Zealand on suicides involving firearms. The amendment restricted accessibility, required confidentiality checks of two references, and introduced more strict storage and safety requests. After the legislation, it was shown that firearm-related suicide decreased dramatically, especially in youth. Thus, the New Zealand study not only replicated the Canadian findings, but also supported the finding that the tactic was especially useful with young people, a high-risk group for suicide globally (Wasserman et al. 2005).

In the last twenty years or so, the positive effects of gun control laws have also been studied in the United States and Australia; these studies too support the research of Leenaars and Lester, the most comprehensive studies to date on any continent (Lester 2000). For example, in the US, Ludwig and Cook (2000) examined the association of guns and suicide with the implementation of the Brady Handgun Violence Protection Act and noted a decrease of suicide by firearms in older adults (age >55); when there was no reduction in suicide by all methods. The authors attributed this to interim waiting periods for firearms acquisition in the Brady Law, which has since been dropped in the permanent law. Maxwell and colleagues (1984), Medoff and Magaddino (1983) and Sommers (1984) have also reported that the restrictions in the selling and purchasing of guns played the most significant role in reduced suicide rates. These restrictions were especially important in the control of buying of guns by people with mental health disorders (psychopathology). A waiting period was also important (Medoff and Magaddino 1983). The various studies also offered some data on the fact that these impacts were true even if one controls for some social factors. The number of factors that were studied, however, were few. This warrants caution in over-generalizing, something Leenaars and his colleagues (2003) attempted to rectify. Thus, it is of note that waiting periods, like restriction of sale to some people such as those with mental disorders (psychopathology), may be important. Further studies need to explore what is effective not only at an individual level, but also at national and international levels. The science of controlling the environment for the means is at that stage now. Probably regional differences will emerge. For example, the US is known to be well above the average among industrialized nations in firearm violence (Hahn *et al.* 2003).

In Australia, after a 1996 firearm massacre in Tasmania in which thirty-five people died, the Australian government undertook gun law reforms. Legislation restricted the sale of semi-automatic shotguns and rifles to civilians. Gun registration was legislated and the prohibition of private sales was implemented. Chapman *et al.* (2006), using official statistics, showed that after the law there was an accelerated decline in firearm deaths, especially suicides. This Australian example once more showed that removing lethal means in the environment could be associated with a sudden and ongoing reduction in suicides and related phenomena of homicide and accidental deaths. This finding is consistent at both the individual and population levels of analysis.

Kleck (1991), Britt *et al.* (1996) and Kleck (1997) argued that gun control fails to reduce the rate of suicide and violence in general. Hemenway (1999) pointed out problems in Kleck's analysis. Also, Leenaars *et al.* (2003) addressed Kleck's arguments about statistics and designs at a population level, by using interrupted time series analyses and controls for possible confounders, and showed that the associations between the availability of guns and suicide hold. Cummings *et al.* (1997) showed the same at an individual level. The discussion, of course, will continue (Leenaars 2006).

## The applicability of gun control worldwide

The tactic of controlling the environment is more complex than gun control, although it is a prototypical example. Referring to gun control as a means for suicide prevention in Canada and in the US probably makes sense, because it is those countries' main method of suicide. It is a highly lethal method. However, in other countries, guns are not a frequent means. For example, in Cuba, firearms are the least frequent means for committing suicide in the nation: hanging is the most common for men and immolation the most frequent for women. The main suicide method in Lithuania is also hanging. This is true in Australia. In China and India, the common methods are poisoning by insecticides or pesticides and hanging. Hanging and drowning are the most popular in Ireland. Hanging is the most common method in Thailand, but the use of firearms is increasing. Firearm suicides have increased in Russia. The same are true in Columbia (WHO 2002). Hanging and the use of firearms are the main methods in South Africa. There is great variation in means of committing suicide and, although gun control may make little sense in some regions of the five continents, the tactic of controlling the environment may well have increasing applicability, as suggested in the WHO report (Bertolote 1993), and as studies on different continents show (Leenaars *et al.* 2002).

## Conclusion

There are numerous studies on the impact of guns on suicide, such as firearm ownership, availability of guns, guns in the home and firearm storage, and gun control legislation (see Lester 2000; Leenaars 2007; Miller and Hemenway 1999 for reviews). Studies on the availability of guns show that if present, the rate of use for the means of suicide increases. Ownership shows the same pattern. Individual-level studies show that the more guns in the home, the more suicides, especially among the young. Population-level studies show the same patterns and associations. There are consistencies (commonalities) in the empirical studies, both individual and ecological. Most of the empirical studies, together with gun control law studies across the globe, show that availability of a potentially dangerous means affects the rate of use of the means for death (WHO 2006). Firearms are a method with high case fatalities, not only for suicide, but also for homicide.

## References

Adjacic-Gross V, Killias M, Hepp U *et al.* (2006). Changing times: a longitudinal analysis of international firearm suicide data. *American Journal of Public Health*, **96**, 1752–1755.

Bailey J, Kellerman A, Somes G *et al.* (1997). Risk factors for violent death of women in the home. *Archives of Internal Medicine*, **157**, 777–782.

Beautrais A, Fergusson D, Horwood L (2006). Firearms legislation and reduction in firearms-related suicide deaths in New Zealand. *Australian and New Zealand Journal of Psychiatry*, **40**, 253–259.

Beautrais A, Joyce P, Mulder R (1996). Access to firearms and the risk of suicide. *Australian and New Zealand Journal of Psychiatry* **30**, 741–748.

Bertolote J (1993). *Guidelines for the Primary Prevention of Mental, Neurological and Psychosocial Disorders: Suicide*. World Health Organization, Geneva.

Brent D, Perper J, Allman C *et al.* (1991). The presence and accessibility of firearms in the homes of adolescent suicides. *Journal of the American Medial Association*, **266**, 2989–2995.

Brent D, Perper J, Goldstein G *et al.* (1988). Risk factors for adolescent suicide. A comparison of adolescent suicide victims with suicidal inpatients. *Archives of General Psychiatry*, **45**, 581–588.

Brent D, Perper J, Moritz G *et al.* (1993). Firearms and adolescent suicide. *American Journal of Diseases of Children*, **147**, 1066–1071.

Bridges F (2004). Gun control law (Bill C-17), suicide, and homicide in Canada. *Psychological Reports*, **94**, 819–826.

Britt C, Bondua D, Kleck G (1996). A reassessment of the DC gun law: some cautionary notes on the use of interrupted time series designs for policy impact-assessment. *Law and Society Review*, **30**, 361–380.

Carrington P (1999). Gender, gun control, suicide and homicide in Canada. *Archives of Suicide Research*, **5**, 71–75.

Carrington P and Moyer S (1994a). Gun availability and suicide in Canada. *Studies on Crime and Crime Prevention*, **3**, 168–178.

Carrington P and Moyer S (1994b). Gun control and suicide in Ontario. *American Journal of Psychiatry*, **151**, 606–608.

Chapman S, Alpers P, Aglo K *et al.* (2006). Australia's 1996 gun law reforms: faster falls in firearm deaths, firearm suicides, and a decade with mass shootings. *Injury Prevention*, **12**, 365–372.

Cummings P, Koepsell T, Grossman D *et al.* (1997). The association between the purchase of a handgun and homicide and suicide. *American Journal of Public Health*, **87**, 974–978.

Durkheim E (1897). *Le Suicide*. Felix Alcan, Paris.

Etzersdorfer E, Kapusta N, Sonneck G (2006). Suicide by shooting is correlated to rate of gun licenses in Austrian counties. *Wiener Klinische Wochenschrift*, **118**, 464–468.

Hahn R, Bilukha O, Crosby A *et al.* (2003). First reports evaluating the effectiveness of strategies for preventing violence: firearms laws. *Morbidity and Mortality Weekly Report*, **2**, 11–20.

Hemenway D (1999). Risk and benefits of gun ownership. Letter. *Journal of the American Medical Association*, **282**, 135–136.

Kassirer J (1991). Firearms and the killing threshold. *New England Journal of Medicine*, **325**, 1647–1650.

Kellerman A, Rivara F, Somes G *et al.* (1992). Suicide in the home in relation to gun ownership. *New England Journal of Medicine*, **327**, 467–472.

Killias M (1993). International correlations between gun ownership and rates of homicide and suicide. *Canadian Medical Association Journal*, **148**, 1721–1725.

Kleck G (1991). *Point Blank*. Aldine de Gruyter, New York.

Kleck G (1997). *Targeting Guns: Firearms and their Control*. Aldine de Gruyter, New York.

Kreitman N (1976). The coal gas story. *British Journal of Preventive and Social Medicine*, **30**, 86–93.

Leenaars A (2004). *Psychotherapy with Suicidal People*. John Wiley and Sons, Chichester.

Leenaars A (2006). Suicide by shooting and gun ownership (licenses) in Austria: would gun restriction help? *Wiener Klinische Wochenschrift*, **118**, 439–441.

Leenaars A (2007). Gun-control legislation and the impact on suicide. *Crisis*, **28**, 50–57.

Leenaars A and Lester D (1996). Gender and the impact of gun control on suicide and homicide. *Archives of Suicide Research*, **2**, 223–234.

Leenaars A and Lester D (1997a). The impact of gun control on suicide and homicide across the life span. *Canadian Journal of Behavioural Science*, **29**, 1–6.

Leenaars A and Lester D (1997b). The effects of gun control on the accidental death rate from firearms in Canada. *Journal of Safety Research*, **28**, 119–122.

Leenaars A and Lester D (2001). The impact of gun control (Bill C-51) on homicide. *Journal of Criminal Justice*, **29**, 287–294.

Leenaars A, Cantor C, Connolly J *et al.* (2000). Controlling the environment to prevent suicide: international perspectives. *Canadian Journal of Psychiatry*, **45**, 639–644.

Leenaars A, De Leo D, Goldney R *et al.* (eds) (1998). The prevention of suicide: controlling the environment. *Archives of Suicide Research*, **4**, 1–107.

Leenaars L, Moksony F, Lester D *et al.* (2003). The impact of gun control (Bill C-51) on suicide in Canada. *Death Studies*, **27**, 103–124.

Lester D (1988a). Gun control, gun ownership and suicide prevention. *Suicide and Life-Threatening Behaviour*, **18**, 176–180.

Lester D (1988b). Restricting the availability of guns as a strategy for suicide prevention. *Biology and Society*, **5**, 127–129.

Lester D (1992). *Why People Kill Themselves*, 3rd edn. Charles C. Thomas, Springfield.

Lester D (1995). Preventing suicide in women and men. *Crisis*, **16**, 79–84.

Lester D (1996). Gun ownership and rates of homicide and suicide. *European Journal of Psychiatry*, **10**, 83–85.

Lester D (2000). *Why People Kill Themselves: A 2000 Summary of Research on Suicide*. Charles C. Thomas, Springfield.

Lester D and Leenaars A (1993). Suicide rates in Canada before and after tightening firearm control laws. *Psychological Reports*, **72**, 787–790.

Lester D and Leenaars A (1994). Gun control and rates of firearm violence in Canada and the United States. *Canadian Journal of Criminology*, **36**, 463–464.

Ludwig J and Cook P (2000). Homicide and suicide rates associated with implementation of the Brady Handgun Violence Protection Act. *Journal of the American Medical Association*, **284**, 585–591.

Markush R and Bertolucci A (1984). Firearms and suicide in the United States. *American Journal of Public Health*, **74**, 123–127.

Maxwell S, Stolensky D, Goodman N *et al.* (1984). Suicide by firearms. *New England Journal of Medicine*, **310**, 46–49.

Medoff M and Magaddino J (1983). Suicides and firearm control laws. *Evaluation Review*, **7**, 357–372.

Miller M and Hemenway D (1999). The relationship between firearms and suicide: a review of the literature. *Aggression and Violent Behaviour*, **4**, 59–75.

Mundt D (1990). Gun control and rates of firearm violence in Canada and the United States. *Canadian Journal of Criminology*, **32**, 137–154.

Platt S (1984). Unemployment and suicidal behaviour. *Social Science and Medicine*, **19**, 93–115.

Rich C, Young J, Fowler R *et al.* (1990). Guns and suicide. *American Journal of Psychiatry*, **147**, 342–346.

Richman J (1993). *Preventing Elderly Suicide*. Springer, New York.

Shneidman E and Farberow N (eds) (1957). *Clues to Suicide*. McGraw-Hill, New York.

Sloan J, Rivera F, Reay D *et al.* (1990). Firearm regulation and rates of suicide: a comparison of two metropolitan areas. *New England Journal of Medicine*, **322**, 369–373.

Sommers, P (1984). The effect of gun control laws on suicide rates. *Atlantic Economic Journal*, **12**, 67–69.

Stack S (1998). Research on controlling suicide: methodological issues. *Archives of Suicide Research*, **4**, 95–99.

Stengel E (1964). *Suicide and Attempted Suicide*. Penguin, Baltimore.

Wasserman D, Cheng Q, Jiang GX (2005). Global suicide rates among young people aged 15–19. *World Psychiatry*, **4**, 114–120.

World Health Organization (2002). *World Report on Violence and Health*. World Health Organization, Geneva.

World Health Organization (2006). *Preventing Disease Through Healthy Environments*. World Health Organization, Geneva.

# CHAPTER 78

# Restrictions of access to pesticides in suicide prevention

Michael R Phillips and David Gunnell

## Abstract

Intentional pesticide ingestion is one of the most common methods of suicide, accounting for up to one-third of all suicides worldwide. The importance of intentional ingestion of pesticides was initially recognized in Asia and the Western Pacific but it is becoming evident that it is also a significant problem in Africa and, to some extent, in Latin America. Pesticides are employed in about 300,000 suicides annually—primarily in the rural areas of low-and middle-income countries (LAMIC)—so limiting access to these lethal agents could, theoretically, substantially reduce the global burden of mortality due to suicide. Organophosphate pesticides are responsible for a large proportion of pesticide self-poisonings and the majority of deaths.

## Introduction

Intentional pesticide ingestion is thought to account for over a third of the global burden of suicide (Gunnell et al. 2007a). The differential availability of pesticides in rural versus urban communities, differences in the type and method of use of pesticides, and the high case fatality after intentional pesticide ingestion compared to other methods of self-poisoning are important determinants of cross-national and cross-regional differences in the rates and demographic characteristics of suicide (Eddleston 2000; Gunnell and Eddleston 2003; Buckley et al. 2004; London et al. 2005; Bertolote et al. 2006; Gunnell et al. 2007a). In almost all countries self-poisoning is the most common form of self-harm (WHO 2006) but—with the exception of pesticides and a few other toxins—fatality from self-poisoning is much lower than with most other forms of suicidal behaviour (hanging, jumping, firearm, drowning etc.) so the proportion of all suicidal acts that are fatal is low, usually less than 1 in 20. But in countries, regions and population cohorts where a high proportion of self-poisoning is by pesticide ingestion, the relatively high case-fatality of this method—varying from under 8 per cent for chlorpyrifos to over 70 per cent with paraquat and aluminium phosphide (Fitzgerald et al. 1978; Chugh et al. 1991; Eddleston et al. 2005)—increases the overlap between low-intent non-fatal suicidal behaviour and high-intent fatal suicidal behaviour. This results in higher case fatality and a higher proportion of suicide deaths in females, who more often engage in low-intent suicidal behaviour by self-poisoning than males.

## Characteristics of those who die by pesticide ingestion

Suicidal behaviour is the outcome of the interaction of a wide variety of individual-, family- and community-level risk factors. The relative importance of these risk factors varies for each separate suicidal act; but the likelihood that particular risk factors are relevant in a specific case is influenced by their background prevalence in the community and population group of which the individual is a member. The higher rates of suicide in locations where large numbers of community members have easy access to pesticides suggests—but does not prove—that pesticide availability (like handgun availability) is a risk factor for suicide. The presumed mechanism is that readily available pesticides are commonly used in impulsive, low-intent suicidal acts that (unlike self-poisoning with medication) result in death because of the toxicity of the agents and the low technical level of available treatment services.

Research shows that many intentional pesticide ingestions are impulsive acts following acute interpersonal crises in persons who do not have underlying mental disorders (Eddleston and Phillips 2004; Conner et al. 2005; Konradsen et al. 2006; Alex et al. 2007), though these individuals may be more impulsive than other community members. The pesticides are typically chosen on the basis of availability without consideration of their perceived lethality (Eddleston et al. 2006). Thus, in most LAMIC that have large agricultural populations, patterns of pesticide use are a more important determinant of suicide rates than the prevalence and treatment rates for mental disorders. For example, the relatively high rates of suicide in Sri Lanka and China do not appear to be due to higher levels of mental illness or higher rates of self-harm, but rather to the higher lethality of self-harm acts (Eddleston and Gunnell 2006; Eddleston et al. 2006).

Another possible component of the public health impact of pesticides is that long-term, low-level exposure to organophosphate pesticides in those who frequently handle pesticides and in members of rural households that store pesticides may directly increase the risk of suicide and/or impulsiveness (London et al. 2005). Case–control research and cross-sectional studies have shown a relationship between chronic exposure to pesticides and depression, anxiety, suicide and overall mortality (Parron et al. 1996; Stallones and Beseler 2002; London et al. 2003; van Wijngaarden 2003;

London *et al.* 2005). There is, moreover, a plausible biological pathway involving an imbalance in cholinergic pathways (implicated in depressive disorders) and inhibition of cholinesterase that could explain the relationship between pesticide exposure and suicide (Gunn 1976; Smith 1996). However, this area is still controversial (Goetz *et al.* 1994; Colosio *et al.* 2003; London *et al.* 2005) so more research is needed before definitive conclusions can be drawn.

## Economic burden

Treatment of intentional pesticide ingestion places a heavy drain on the economic and medical resources of poor rural communities (Eddleston 2000; Srinivas Rao *et al.* 2005). The 1990 report on pesticides by the World Health Organization and United Nations Environment Programme (WHO and UNEP 1990) estimated two million hospitalizations from pesticide poisoning worldwide each year and a 2007 analysis estimates 230,000–400,000 global deaths from intentional pesticide ingestion annually (Gunnell *et al.* 2007a). Most of these hospitalizations and deaths occur in the rural areas of LAMIC where pesticide use is most prevalent. Intentional pesticide ingestion is typically more medically serious than occupational exposure (which is usually transcutaneous or respiratory) (Eddleston 2000) so it is more likely to require emergency resuscitation and the prolonged use of intensive care beds. The management of pesticide poisoning is complex and different pesticides require different approaches (Buckley *et al.* 2004; Eddleston *et al.* 2005), so well-trained personnel who have access to appropriate drugs and equipment are essential. Such resources are often not available in the rural areas of LAMIC, so many who ingest pesticides die despite emergency resuscitation by local medical personnel (WHO and UNEP 1990; Phillips *et al.* 2002).

## Awareness

Until recently the vast majority of published research on the prevalence, methods, causes and prevention of suicide focused on the situation in developed countries where pesticides are a relatively uncommon cause of death, so it is not surprising that the role of pesticides received so little attention from suicidologists. This failure to recognize the magnitude of the problem is compounded by the international agencies and pesticide producers interested in pesticide safety who usually avoid the issue of self-poisoning because of its political sensitivity. For example, most official documents from the Intergovernmental Forum on Chemical Safety (IFCS) focus almost exclusively on occupational and accidental pesticide poisoning even though the majority of hospitalizations and deaths are from intentional self-poisoning (Konradsen *et al.* 2005).

More recently, increased awareness of the magnitude of the problem of suicide by intentional ingestion of pesticides has lead to a flurry of research and the initiation of the WHO Pesticides and Health Initiative in 2004 (WHO 2004), a collaborative effort of the WHO Department of Mental Health and Substance Abuse, the WHO Department of Injuries and Violence Prevention and the WHO Programme on the Promotion of Chemical Safety. The field is still in the preliminary, descriptive stages, but systematic assessments of different methods of restricting pesticide availability (Konradsen *et al.* 2007b) and of medically managing intentional pesticide poisoning (Pawar KS *et al.* 2006) are currently underway.

## How could restricting access to pesticides decrease suicides?

Strategies to reduce suicides by restricting access to commonly used methods are best focused on those methods associated with high case-fatality. Three potential mechanisms could explain how restricting access to lethal means such as pesticides can prevent suicides. In cases of impulsive suicidal behaviour where the intent to die is not strong, increasing the difficulty of obtaining the means for suicide may give individuals greater opportunity to think through their options and reduce the likelihood that they will follow through with the suicidal act (Daigle 2005). Where the intent to die is stronger but the suicidal behaviour is impulsive, postponing the act by making it harder to obtain the necessary means will afford a greater opportunity for other preventive interventions to take place, though this is unlikely to be helpful in those LAMIC settings in which there are no other preventive services available. Finally, irrespective of impulsivity or intent, reducing the lethality of the available means will result in lower case-fatality rates.

Assuming all other factors are held constant, restricting access to a commonly used lethal means of suicide can have four possible outcomes:

1   A permanent reduction in both fatal and non-fatal suicidal behaviour;

2   A permanent reduction in fatal suicidal behaviour with a corresponding increase in non-fatal suicidal behaviour as individuals use less lethal means;

3   A temporary reduction in fatal suicidal behaviour with a gradual return to pre-restriction fatality rates as individuals start using alternative, equally fatal means (i.e. 'substitution');

4   An increase in fatal suicidal behaviour as individuals replace the restricted means with an even more lethal alternative.

Case fatality varies widely by type of pesticide (Eddleston 2000; Eddleston *et al.* 2005). Consequently, in nations or communities with a large agricultural workforce as patterns of pesticide use change over time the balance between fatal and non-fatal suicidal behaviours will change and—given the predominance of young people and females among attempted suicides—the gender ratio and age distribution among completed suicides will also change. Increased use and availability of more toxic pesticides would lead to higher rates of completed suicide, particularly in women and young people. Alternatively, limiting the use and/or access to the most lethal pesticides, reducing the lethality of available pesticides, and improving the rates of successful resuscitation following pesticide ingestion would decrease the rates and case-fatality of self-poisoning and—assuming limited substitution of pesticides for equally or more lethal methods of self-harm—result in a lower rate of completed suicide, particularly in women and young people. Confirmation of this relationship comes from agricultural-intensive countries where rapid changes in the pattern of pesticide use were associated with dramatic changes in the rates and demographic characteristics of suicides; as seen when paraquat was introduced in Western Samoa (Bowles 1995) and when WHO

Class I pesticides were banned in Sri Lanka (Roberts *et al*. 2003; Gunnell *et al*. 2007b).

Several mediating factors will influence the impact on suicide rates of different approaches to pesticide restriction.

1 The case-fatality of the restricted pesticide(s);

2 The degree to which the programme is adopted by the target community;

3 The potential degree of substitution by alternative methods and the relative lethality of the alternative methods (Daigle 2005);

4 The proportion of all suicides that are impulsive and low intent (Conner *et al*. 2005);

5 Access to crisis services and other forms of mental health care; and

6 Access to medical resuscitation services that can effectively manage poisoning by pesticide ingestion.

## What methods are available for restricting access to pesticides?

A number of factors confound efforts to restrict access to pesticides in rural communities of LAMIC. First, governments are often reluctant or unable to implement and monitor the pesticide management policies they adopt. Second, influential agrochemical companies resist any approaches that decrease the use of their products. Third, in some countries unregulated black market production and sale of the most toxic pesticides circumvent government regulations. Fourth, rural communities have limited resources to develop, test and promulgate pesticide restriction programmes. Fifth, farmers are often reluctant to adopt practices that decrease their ready access to the agricultural chemicals they consider necessary to their economic survival. Lastly, there may be substitution of restricted pesticides by other pesticides or by alternative, more lethal, methods of self-harm. The following approaches to limiting access to pesticides have been proposed:

♦ **Ban the most toxic pesticides**. Several international policy instruments address the problem of access to lethal pesticides (Konradsen *et al*. 2003), but LAMIC encounter substantial difficulty in implementing these international conventions (London and Bailie 2001; Alex *et al*. 2007; Konradsen *et al*. 2007b). Many LAMIC do not live up to the standards of the international Code of Conduct on the Distribution and Use of Pesticides (FAO 2002); this Code does not directly address the issue of self-harm but, if followed, would prohibit the use of WHO Class I pesticides in most developing countries and, thus, probably result in decreased case-fatality following intentional pesticide ingestion (Konradsen *et al*. 2003). Even if LAMIC do adopt the international guidelines, they need to undertake ongoing surveillance to ensure that restriction of one method doesn't lead to the substitution of an equally lethal method and to provide the information needed to change the guidelines in response to rapidly changing patterns of pesticide use. For example, following the gradual restriction of WHO Class I organophosphates in Sri Lanka from 1984 through 1995 there was substitution with endosulfan—a Class II organocholine pesticide—that proved just as toxic as many of the banned substances (Roberts *et al*. 2003). Appreciation of this effect led

Sri Lanka's Registrar of Pesticides to ban endosulfan and there is evidence that the cumulative impact of Sri Lanka's policy of banning the most toxic pesticides has resulted in a reduction in suicides (Gunnell *et al*. 2007b).

♦ **Promote secure storage in homes, fields or a centralized community location**. This method of restricting access is supported by the agrochemical industry because, unlike other pesticide restriction strategies, it does not result in decreased sales of their products. The method has recently been adopted in small test sites in China, India and Sri Lanka (WHO 2006). Locked boxes for storage of pesticides are installed in homes, in fields or at a central point in the local village. The keys for the boxes are held by a trusted family member or a respected community figure (Vijayakumar *et al*. 2005); in some locations the husband and wife hold separate keys so they both must be present to open the lockbox. Given the cost involved in constructing the boxes and the inconvenience of using the boxes, external funding is often necessary to manufacture the boxes and ongoing public education efforts are needed to ensure that end-users actually employ the installed boxes. There is also a concern that highlighting the location of storage and potential lethality of pesticides could result in an increase in their use in acts of self-harm (Konradsen *et al*. 2007b), so detailed qualitative and quantitative research will be needed before the potential benefits and risks of this approach can be determined. Preliminary results of an ongoing evaluative study in Sri Lanka (Konradsen *et al*. 2007a, b) indicate that seven months after installing lockable pesticide storage boxes on houses in a rural area there was a substantial decrease in the access to pesticides in the 172 households with the boxes; but provision of the boxes resulted in many farmers storing their pesticides at home rather than in their fields—potentially increasing ease of access to the pesticides if the boxes were left unlocked, as occurred in 27 of the 172 households at the 7-month evaluation.

♦ **Establish a minimum pesticide list**. A huge range of pesticides in a variety of formulations are available, making it difficult for end users and government agencies to make informed decisions about the relative cost–benefit of different products. Developing minimum (or essential) pesticide lists would, like essential drug lists, help bring clarity to the bewildering array of choices available. Such lists would decrease pesticide use to a minimum, exclude the more toxic compounds and require a thorough assessment of the efficacy, safety and cost of new products before inclusion on the list (Eddelston *et al*. 2002).

♦ **Promote Integrated Pest Management (IPM) programmes**. These programmes restrict use of pesticides that are highly toxic and pesticides to which pests have proven resistant, they encourage less frequent application of pesticides, and they promote the use of alternative physical and biological control methods. Taken together these steps usually lead to a drastic reduction in the overall use of pesticides and, thus, decreased availability of pesticides in farmers' households (Kenmore 2002; Konradsen *et al*. 2003).

♦ **Apply a tax to pesticides that increases with pesticide lethality**. This approach would decrease, but not eliminate, the availability of the most toxic pesticides. An alternative method of achieving the same goal would be to subsidize the less lethal pesticides (Gunnell and Eddleston 2003).

- **Limit usage of pesticides in each village or community to a small number of licensed individuals who would apply pesticides for all community members**. This would get the pesticides out of community members' homes and ensure that only a few community members regularly handled pesticides. There would, however, be substantial difficulty in establishing a separate licencing procedure, funding and monitoring the activities of the licenced individuals, and, most importantly, getting community acceptance for the programme.

- **Training pesticide retailers to recognize potentially suicidal individuals**. As part of the licensing of pesticide retailers they might be required to undergo regular training in the recognition of those at risk of impulsive self-harm. For example they might ask screening questions of their would-be customers about their reason for requesting a particular product, their experience in previous use of the product and the crops for which it will be used. They might be advised not to sell their products to very young people.

- **Limit sale of pesticides to single-use amounts**. This would ensure that no residual pesticides were left in the home or field. An alternative method of achieving the same objective would be to develop mechanisms for ensuring that unused pesticides are returned to the vendor immediately after application (Gunnell and Eddleston 2003).

## Conclusion

The importance of pesticide self-poisoning on the global burden of suicide has been recognized for over twenty years (Jeyaratnam 1985; WHO and UNEP 1990) but suicidologists—most of whom work in developed countries where pesticide ingestion is uncommon—have only recently become interested in the problem. Research in the area is still in its preliminary, descriptive stages.

Given that about one-third of all suicides worldwide are by pesticide ingestion, restricting access to pesticides should be a key component of the global effort to reduce suicides. Attempts to restrict access by encouraging governments of LAMIC to adopt international guidelines have had limited effect, largely because no real attempt has been made to adjust the guidelines to the resource structure and rapidly changing agricultural practices of each country or, more importantly, to understand and address the attitudes and incentives of key stakeholders in the target communities.

In the absence of effective regulation, several countries rely heavily on the agrochemical industry to promote safe use (Konradsen et al. 2003). Training about safe usage by agrochemical firms often results in increased knowledge but does not necessarily result in changed behaviour (Ellis 1998; Atkins and Lesinger 2000). Moreover, this training often leads to increased market penetration of the products (the goal of the industry) and, thus, an increase in the availability of pesticides. Approaches to limiting access by improving local storage and management of pesticides—the preferred approach to restricting access of the agrochemical industry—have only recently been attempted, their long-term benefit (or harm) remain to be proven.

Despite these limitations, there has been a dramatic increase in awareness about the public health importance of intentional pesticide ingestion, partly stimulated by the WHO Pesticides and Health Initiative. In this environment there is reason to hope that some LAMIC—particularly the economically strong LAMIC such as China and India—will mobilize the political will needed to implement international guidelines and, possibly, conduct targeted research in this area.

To ensure that this temporary increase in attention on the problem of intentional pesticide ingestion results in a long-term benefit, organizations and individuals concerned with suicide prevention must ensure that adopted pesticide restriction programmes are not stand-alone programmes. Rather, such programmes should be incorporated into comprehensive regional or national suicide prevention plans that aim to address the underlying causes of self-harm behaviours (Mann et al. 2005).

## References

Alex R, Prasad J, Kuruvilla A et al. (2007). Self-poisoning with pesticides in India. *British Journal of Psychiatry*, **190**, 274–275.

Atkins J and Lesinger K (eds) (2000) *Safe and Effective Use of Crop Protection Products in Developing Countries*. CABI Publishing, London.

Bertolote J, Fleischmann A, Eddleston M et al. (2006). Deaths from pesticide poisoning: a global response. *British Journal of Psychiatry*, **189**, 201–203.

Bowles J (1995). Suicide in Western Samoa: an example of a suicide prevention program in a developing country. In R Diekstra, ed., *Preventive Strategies on Suicide*, pp. 173–206, Brill, Leiden.

Buckley N, Karalliedde L, Dawson A et al. (2004). Where is the evidence for treatments used in pesticide poisoning? Is clinical toxicology fiddling while the developing world burns? *Journal of Toxicology: Clinical Toxicology*, **42**, 113–116.

Chugh S, Dushyant F, Ram S et al. (1991). Incidence & outcome of aluminium phosphide poisoning in a hospital study. *Indian Journal of Medical Research*, **94**, 232–235.

Colosio C, Tiramani M, Maroni M (2003). Neurobehavioural effects of pesticides: state of the art. *Neurotoxicology*, **24**, 577–591.

Conner K, Phillips M, Meldrum S et al. (2005). Low-planned suicides in China. *Psychological Medicine*, **35**, 1197–1204.

Daigle M (2005). Suicide prevention through means restriction: Assessing the risk of substitution: a critical review and synthesis. *Accident Analysis and Prevention*, **37**, 625–632.

Eddelston M, Karalliedde I, Buckley N et al. (2002). Pesticide poisoning in the developing world—a minimum pesticides list. *Lancet*, **360**, 1163–1167.

Eddleston M (2000). Patterns and problems of deliberate self-poisoning in the developing world. *Quarterly Journal of Medicine*, **93**, 715–731.

Eddleston M and Gunnell D (2006). Why suicide rates are high in China. *Science*, **311**, 1711–1713.

Eddleston M and Phillips M (2004). Self poisoning with pesticides. *BMJ*, **328**, 42–44.

Eddleston M, Eyer P, Worek F et al. (2005). Differences between organophosphorus insecticides in human self-poisoning: a prospective cohort study. *Lancet*, **366**, 1452–1459.

Eddleston M, Karunaratne A, Weerakoon M et al. (2006). Choice of poison for intentional self-poisoning in rural Sri Lanka. *Clinical Toxicology*, **44**, 283–286.

Ellis W (1998). Private–public sector co-operation to improve pesticide safety standards in developing countries. *Medicina del Lavoro*, **89**, 112–122.

FAO (2002). *International Code of Conduct on Distribution and Use of Pesticides*. Food and Agricultural Organization, Rome.

Fitzgerald G, Barniville G, Flanagan M et al. (1978). The changing pattern of paraquat poisoning: an epidemiologic study. *Irish Medical Journal*, **71**, 103–108.

Goetz C, Bolla K, Rogers S (1994). Neurologic health outcomes and Agent Orange: Institute of Medicine report. *Neurology*, **44**, 801–809.

Gunn D (1976). Alternatives to chemical pesticides. In D Gunn and J Stevens, eds, *Pesticides and Human Welfare*, pp. 241–255, Oxford University Press, Oxford.

Gunnell D and Eddleston M (2003). Suicide by intentional ingestion of pesticides: a continuing tragedy in developing countries. *International Journal of Epidemiology*, **32**, 909–203.

Gunnell D, Eddleston M, Phillips MR *et al.* (2007a). Worldwide patterns of fatal pesticide self-poisoning. *BMC Public Health*, **7**, 357.

Gunnell D, Fernando R, Hewagama M *et al.* (2007b). The impact of pesticide regulations on suicide in Sri Lanka. *International Journal of Epidemiology*, doi:10.1093/ije/dym164.

Jeyaratnam J (1985). Health problems of pesticide usage in the Third World. *British Journal of Industrial Medicine*, **42**, 505–506.

Kenmore P (2002). Integrated pest management. *International Journal of Occupational and Environmental Health*, **8**, 173–174.

Konradsen F, Dawson A, Eddleston M, Gunnell D (2007a). Pesticide self-poisoning: thinking outside the box. *Lancet*, **369**, 169–170.

Konradsen F, Pieris R, Weerasinghe M *et al.* (2007b). Community uptake of safe storage boxes to reduce self-poisoning from pesticides in rural Sri Lanka. *BMC Public Health*, **7**, 13–15.

Konradsen F, van de Hoek W, Cole D *et al.* (2003). Reducing acute poisoning in developing countries—options for restricting the availability of pesticides. *Toxicology*, **192**, 249–261.

Konradsen F, van der Hoek W, Gunnell D *et al.* (2005). Missing deaths from pesticide self-poisoning at the IFCS Forum IV. *Bulletin of the World Health Organization*, **83**, 157–158.

Konradsen F, van der Hoek W, Peiris P (2006). Reaching for the bottle of pesticide—a cry for help. Self-inflicted poisonings in Sri Lanka. *Social Science and Medicine*, **62**, 1710–1719.

London L and Bailie R (2001). Challenges for improving surveillance for pesticide poisoning: policy implications for developing countries. *International Journal of Epidemiology*, **30**, 564–570.

London L, Flisher A, Wesseling C *et al.* H (2003). Neuropsychiatric evaluation in subjects chronically exposed to organophosphate pesticides. *Toxicological Sciences*, **72**, 267–271.

London L, Flisher A, Wesseling C *et al.* (2005). Suicide and exposure to organophosphate insecticides: cause or effect? *American Journal of Industrial Medicine*, **47**, 308–321.

Mann J, Apter A, Bertolote J *et al.* (2005). Suicide prevention strategies: a systematic review. *JAMA*, **294**, 2064–2074.

Parron T, Hernandez A, Villanueva E (1996). Increased risk of suicide with exposure to pesticides in an intensive agricultural area: a 12-year retrospective study. *Forensic Science International*, **79**, 53–63.

Pawar KS, Bhoite RR, Pillay CP *et al.* (2006). Continuous pralidoxime infusion versus repeated bolus injection to treat organophosphorus pesticide poisoning: a randomised controlled trial. *Lancet*, **368**, 2136–2141.

Phillips M, Yang G, Zhang Y *et al.* (2002). Risk factor for suicide in China: a national case–control psychological autopsy study. *Lancet*, **360**, 1728–1736.

Roberts D, Karunarathna A, Buckley N *et al.* (2003). Influence of pesticide regulation on acute poisoning deaths in Sri Lanka. *Bulletin of the World Health Organization*, **81**, 789–798.

Smith C (1996). *Elements of Molecular Neurobiology*. Wiley, New York.

Srinivas Rao C, Venkateswarlu V, Surender T *et al.* (2005). Pesticide poisoning in south India: opportunities for prevention and improved medical management. *Tropical Medicine and International Health*, **10**, 581–588.

Stallones L and Beseler C (2002). Pesticide poisoning and depressive symptoms among farm residents. *Annals of Epidemiology*, **12**, 389–394.

van Wijngaarden E (2003). Mortality of mental disorders in relation to potential pesticide exposure. *Journal of Occupational Environmental Medicine*, **45**, 564–568.

Vijayakumar L, Pirkis J, Whiteford H (2005). Suicide in developing countries (3): Prevention initiatives. *Crisis*, **26**, 120–124.

WHO (2004). *The Impact of Pesticides on Health: Preventing Intentional and Unintentional Deaths from Pesticide Poisoning*. World Health Organization, Geneva.

WHO (2006). *Safer Access to Pesticides: Community Interventions*. World Health Organization, Geneva.

WHO and UNEP (1990). *Public Health Impact of Pesticides used in Agriculture*. World Health Organization and United Nations Environment Programme, Geneva.

# CHAPTER 79

# Prevention of metropolitan and railway suicide

Karl-Heinz Ladwig, Esther Ruf,
Jens Baumert and Natalia Erazo

## Abstract

Railway suicides account for a minority of <10 per cent of all suicides, although they are considered a major public health issue because of their tremendous consequences on functioning of the transportation system and their deteriorating impact on the mental health of staff and bystanders. Railway suicide is a particularly violent method, and case fatality is 90 per cent of all attempts. However, case fatality in metro systems of >60 per cent are rare. More men than women choose the track as a means of suicide with a trend towards a balanced distribution in metro systems. Victims are predominately young with a median age stratum in the range of 25–34 years. For men, a prevalence peak in April and a low in December has been observed. The weekly distribution shows a peak at the beginning of the week and a low on weekends. Railway suicide behaviour patterns include jumping, lying and wandering, some individuals present deviant behaviour prodromal to the attempt. Attractiveness of the method derives from high levels of opportunity and low levels of self-perceived costs.

Prevention may rely on a package of different structural and communicative tools. Inhibiting access to the track, by providing barriers at places of advanced risk and surveillance systems, are among structural means. Inhibiting media coverage and education of gatekeepers to increase awareness and skilfulness in contact with potentially vulnerable subjects on station platforms are among communicative tools. Railway suicide prevention is a realistic option: however, enhancement of research in this field is urgently needed.

## Introduction

The first steam engine—critical to the invention of the modern railroad and trains—dates back to the very beginning of the nineteenth century. In 1825, *Locomotion No.1* was the first steam locomotive engine for railways that carried both goods and passengers on regular schedules in England. The success of this and other early local railway experiences influenced the development of railways elsewhere in Britain and abroad, leading to a first trunk line, opening in 1837, which connected the rapidly industrializing towns in England (for details see Evans and Gough 2003).

The Victorian railway rapidly acquired a double-edged perception in the view of the public: as 'a vast, dramatic, and highly visible expression of technology triumphant' but with the railway accident 'as a uniquely sensational and public demonstration of the price which that triumph demanded—violence, destruction, terror and trauma' (Harrington 2003, p. 203). In validation of Emile Durkheim's prediction stating that 'the more the land is covered in railroads, the more general becomes the habit of seeking death by throwing one's self under a train' (cited by Clarke 1994, p. 401), the development of the railroad network apparently reached a critical density in a short time to become a suicide mean: the first railway suicide to be officially recorded in the reports of the British Registrar General was a male subject in the year 1852 (Clarke 1994). More than 10 years later, in 1864, the first female suicide was recorded but female incidences in that year mounted quickly to five cases.

Since then, the railroad system, including metropolitan railways built under the ground in large cities, has become one of the most prominent transportation means in industrialized and emerging countries, carrying millions of passengers every day. Among critical incidences with involvement of damage to persons, suicide acts on the track nowadays hold the most prominent position (Rådbo et al. 2005). Each railway suicide is an individual tragedy, but is often also a cause of trauma amongst train drivers, employees, emergency personal and bystanders who witness the event or deal with the aftermath of the incident, including removing the body. The British Rail Safety and Standards Board estimates the total cost of suicides (trackside and at stations) to the industry in 2003 was more than £61 000 per suicide and accounted for several million pounds per year. This includes delay to trains, lost working time as a result of trauma suffered by staff and the equivalent value of trauma as a minor injury (Samaritans 2008).

## Definition and epidemiology

### Definition

Suicides on railway or subway tracks are classified in the mortality recording in accordance with the tenth revision of the *International Classification of Diseases* (ICD-10) category as 'intentional self-harm by jumping or lying in front of a moving object' (code X81). In principle, there are no basic differences in terms of suicidal behaviour between railway systems that serve as urban underground transportation (metro) and those who provide long-distance transportation, especially if the suicide attempt is accomplished within the railway station or along the platform. Nevertheless, several specific aspects have to be taken into consideration, which will be addressed in the following.

### Case fatality

Railway suicide is considered as a particularly serious 'hard' suicide method, which does not allow ambivalent behaviour, and no control over the effects of the attempt is available once the suicidal act is initiated. In contrast to less violent suicide methods (e.g. self-poisoning), it is largely impossible to solicit help after initiating a suicide attempt on the track (Veress and Szabo 1980; Deisenhammer et al. 1997; Erazo et al. 2005).

However, epidemiological reports from different European countries elucidate a stable proportion of survivors on the overground railway track in the range between 6–13 per cent (Veress and Szabo 1980; Lindekilde and Wang 1985; Schmidtke 1994; Deisenhammer et al. 1997; Kerkhof 2003; Erazo et al. 2005). The case fatality of urban metro suicides is even lower. In the international comparison study of O'Donnell and Farmer (1992), case fatality rates of metro suicides greater than 60 per cent were rare. Case fatality in London was 55 per cent (O'Donnell and Farmer 1994) while in the Munich subway study, the overall case fatality rate reached 66 per cent (Ladwig and Baumert 2004). Survivors generally sustain severe injury, such as major head injuries or amputation of upper and lower extremities (Maclean et al. 2006; Guth et al. 2006). An evanescent minority receives little, if any, injury irrespective of the mode of the railway system (Guggenheim and Weisman 1972).

## Prevalence and trends

### Prevalence (railway)

Epidemiological evidence concerning railway prevalence from populations in Europe and elsewhere are scarce. No data on this topic from the USA have been published so far. Limited and mostly outdated data from Hungary in the 1960s (Veress and Szabo 1980) pointed to a proportion of 2.7 per cent of all suicides, 3.1 per cent in Denmark (Lindekilde and Wang 1985), and 2.5 per cent in Brisbane, Australia (Emmerson and Cantor 1993). Schmidtke (1994) analysed 6090 cases of railway suicides in Germany in the study period of 1976–1984, revealing a proportion of 5.7 per cent in males and 4.2 per cent in females of all suicides. In Austria, Deisenhammer et al. (1997) analysed data from 552 cases in the years 1990–1994, and found a proportion of 5.7 per cent of all suicides. Van Houwelingen and Beersma (2001) analysing the study period of 1980 to 1994 reported an excess annual ratio of 10–14 per cent of railway-to-all-suicides for The Netherlands. Baumert et al. (2006) registered 8653 fatal railway suicide attempts over a 10-year observation period on the German railway net, which accounted for an average of 7.0 per cent of all suicides in the German population. This proportion, reflecting an average of three fatal railway suicide attempts per day, underscores that railway suicides are of major public concern. Around 80 per cent of 80–100 fatalities occurring on the Swedish railroad each year are considered suicides, which

account for about 5 per cent of all suicides in Sweden (Rådbo et al. 2005).

### Prevalence (metro)

International comparisons of prevalence figures of metro suicides are compromised by major differences in track length and number of passengers using the transportation system. Ladwig and Baumert (2004) assessed incidence of subway suicides relative to total mortality in 1999 (0.8 per cent) and its relative proportion to all suicides (4.1 per cent). In general, rates within cities appear to be independent of national rates of all suicide methods (Ranayake et al. 2007).

### Trends

The British SOVRN Project (Abbott et al. 2003) observed a steady increase of suicide numbers from 1996–1997 (153 cases) to 2000–2001 (203 cases) on the British East Coast Main Line (ECML) connecting London with Scotland. During the 1990s, suicide deaths in Japan on just one rail network, operated by the East Japan Railway Company, increased from 81 per year at the start of the decade to 212 in 1999 (Fernandes 2003). Based on the grounds of 10-year representative central critical incidence registry (1991–2000) of all person accidents for the German railway system, Baumert et al. (2006) revealed an average annual percentage change of +1.8 (95 per cent CI 0.1 to 3.4) for subjects younger than 65 years. Contrary to a substantial decrease of all suicides over the same observation period, these findings translate into an approximately 20 per cent increase of railway suicides among this age group within this timeframe. In contrast, the incidence of fatal railway suicide attempts for subjects aged >65 years exhibited a favourable decrease, on average by –6.2 per cent per year. As for underground railways, O'Donnell and Farmer (1994) found an increase in mean annual numbers from 36.1 (1940–1949) to 94.1 (1980–1989). Ladwig and Baumert (2004) determined a stable incidence of subway suicides in Munich over a 20-year observation period, again despite a pronounced decline in total suicide mortality in the Munich population.

## Patients' characteristics

### Sex ratio

In the general population, substantially more men than women commit suicides with a male:female ratio of 3.2:1 within European countries (Schmidtke 1997). Erazo et al. (2004b) analysed 4003 fatal railway suicides over a 6-year period (1997–2002) and revealed a male:female ratio of 2.70:1 (p >0.0001), which was almost identical with the sex ratio of railway suicides revealed by Schmidtke (1994) more than a decade before. The excess railway suicide risk of males was also confirmed in the SOVRN Project (Abbott et al. 2003). Apparently, these figures mirror to some extent the general sex distribution of fatal suicides in Western societies. However, in contrast to these findings, the sex ratio of suicide victims in subway systems differs considerably. Here, Ladwig and Baumert (2004) observed a near to equal sex distribution, which is supported by findings from O'Donnell and Farmer (1992, 1994) and Sonneck et al. (1994). Interestingly, when analysing sex differences in fatal railway suicides (after stratifying by open track and station area), it appears that the striking male preponderance of railway suicides decreases from 1:2.85 to 1:2.46 (Erazo et al. 2005).

## Age distribution

Elderly people are known to have the highest suicide risk (Conwell and Brent 1995). In contrast, O'Donnell and Farmer (1992) in their multinational approach and Sonneck *et al.* (1994) in their analysis of the Vienna subway system, report that the majority of metro suicides were committed by 20–29-year-olds. Furthermore, O'Donnell and Farmer (1994) identified a peak age group in the London study of 25–34 years, which was exactly the case in the Munich study (Ladwig and Baumert 2004). In the SOVRN Project (Abbott *et al.* 2003), suicide deaths in overground railway suicides peaked within the age band of 31–40 years; still, however, leaving over one quarter in the age stratum of >50 years.

## Mental illness

Evidence from retrospective psychological autopsy studies confirmed a substantial degree of psychiatric morbidity in these patients. Mishara (1999) reanalysed patient records from 129 subjects, who committed suicide in the Montreal metro, and found 73 per cent had received inpatient psychiatric treatment (e.g. major depression, schizophrenia) at the time of death. The majority of the SOVRN patients suffered from signs of mental disorders, where many of these were present for over a year and some for more than a decade (Abbott *et al.* 2003, p. 51). Recently, van Houwelingen and Kerkhof (2008) revealed in a study of 57 train suicides in The Netherlands that 53 per cent received psychiatric care at the time of suicide, with 49 per cent of them being inpatients. Compared to general suicides, functional non-affective psychoses were over-represented. However, loneliness and sudden ending of an intimate relationship are also possible triggers (O'Donnell *et al.* 1996).

# Behavioural patterns and personal characteristics

## Time patterns

Seasonality is often seen in violent methods of deliberate self-harm (Maes *et al.* 1993; Hakko *et al.* 1998), especially in males (Meares *et al.* 1981; Micciolo *et al.* 1991), and was confirmed by railway track suicides revealing a prevalence peak in April and September followed by a low in December for men (Schmidtke *et al.* 1994; Deisenhammer *et al.* 1997; Erazo *et al.* 2004b). Concerning the weekly distribution, studies indicate a peak at the beginning of the week and a low on weekends (Angermeyer and Massing 1995; Schmidtke *et al.* 1994; Deisenhammer *et al.* 1997; van Houwelingen and Beersma 2001; Erazo *et al.* 2004b). Apparently for subjects at risk the beginning of the working week triggers feeling of personal failure and isolation.

As for circadian patterns, it is generally believed that suicides by all means are largely restricted to daytime (Barraclough 1976). In an analysis of 4003 railway suicide cases, Erazo *et al.* (2004b) looked two-dimensionally at clock time and time of the year, and found that peaks of the summer half year compared to those in the winter half year were clearly shifting to earlier and later clock times, respectively, corresponding to time of sunrise and sunset. In the male subgroup, a pronounced late evening peak after sunset was observed, whereas the female subgroup was characterized by a single morning peak and no evening peak. These findings support previous analyses of sex-specific interaction patterns of season and clock time of excess railway suicide risk (Schmidtke *et al.* 1994; van Houwelingen and Beersma 2001).

## Behavioural patterns

Guggenheim and Weisman (1972) were the first to describe four distinct patterns of suicidal behaviour on railway tracks. People who manifest these behaviours were termed jumpers, liers, touchers and wanderers. Accordingly, jumpers are those who leap or tumble directly in front of an oncoming train in the presence of passengers and other bystanders. Liers, seldom observed entering the pit, lie down across the tracks, generally in a prone position, and await the approach of a train or for the train to start. Decapitation, in the latter cases, is not a rare event. Touchers get into contact with the electrical sources by being killed through electrocution from a high-volt electrical conductor. Wanderers walk along the pit and are hit by the collision with the train in a walking position. Subway drivers often experience suicides by wanderers as particularly traumatogenic, because they may be exposed to a 'final' look from the suicidal person. Analysing suicide data for the German Railway Suicide Project, we additionally identified some rare cases of 'chaired suicides' (one incidence with wheelchair bound persons, several incidences with couples). In one case, a young mother had committed suicide on the track with two infants in her arms.

## Deviant behaviour

Relevant indicators of suicidal intent may be removal of shoes (O'Donnell *et al.* 1996), sudden dropping of belongings as the train approaches, possession of items that ordinarily would be left home (e.g. framed family pictures), erratic behaviour, possibly with indications of alcohol/drug intoxication, or conversely over-deliberate moves, faces hidden, avoidance of eye contact (Clarke and Poyner 1994; Gaylord and Lester 1994). Interestingly, in China, departing from ordinary dress to clothing in traditional ethic fashion alerts subway staff (Gaylord and Lester 1994).

## Method choice

Key factors presumed to influence railway track method choice remain largely speculative. It is also most likely that the different behavioural patterns (jumpers, liers, etc.) bear different choice-structuring properties. Intuitively, suicide death on the open track, accomplished by wanderers or liers and not witnessed by the public, point to a more thoughtful and hopeless 'accounting balance' consideration than is the case with a public death in the metro system with numerous bystanders. Accordingly, Guggenheim and Weisman (1972) learnt from jumper survivors to be well aware of the public nature of their attempt. They reported feeling '*full of hate for everyone*' and wanting '*to punish the whole world*'.

Mishara (2007) interviewed Metro suicide attempters in a hospital emergency room and revealed as omnipresent belief that suicide on the track results in a certain and painless death. According to the SOVRN project, railway suiciders choose places near their vicinity—the 'proximity factor'. The choice-structuring concept presented by Carke and Lester (1989) underscores, first of all, the complexity of the cognitive progression from ideation to action (Cantor and Baume 1998) and, by applying the concept on railway suicides, the fatal attractiveness of the method. As illustrated in Table 79.1, opportunities are high—no knowledge and skills are required to reliably produce the desired result—costs may in some cases be even of benefit (inconvenience to others), and among other issues, misperception (certainty of death) may be widespread.

**Table 79.1** Choice-structuring properties of metro and railway suicides (modified Clarke and Lester 1988)

| Opportunities | Railway suicide characteristics | Perceived as |
|---|---|---|
| Availability | Unrestricted access (not everywhere) | High |
| Familiarity with the method | Imitation learning (proximity factor) | To a certain degree |
| Technical skills | Not necessary | |
| Planning | Often spontaneous, impulsive | Not needed |
| **Costs** | | |
| Pain | Presumably not | Painful, but quick |
| Courage | High | Low, because *being killed* |
| Consequences of failure | Amputation of extremities, head injuries etc. | Perceived as unlikely |
| Messiness/disfigurement after death | High | Not considered as important |
| Danger | High | |
| Inconvenience to others | Substantial traumatization | Attractive to a subpopulation |
| **Other issues** | | |
| Certainty of death | Failure in up to 40% of cases | Perceived as high |
| Time taken to die while conscious | No data available | Perceived as immediately dead |
| Scope for second thoughts | No ambiguity possible | Not intended |

# Prevention strategies

Current knowledge of predictors of suicidal behaviour is largely unable to anticipate concrete individual acting (Mann *et al.* 2005). Nevertheless, primary and secondary suicide prevention for railway and metro systems is possible (O'Donnell *et al.* 1994; Mishara 2007), even though it should rely on the synergistic effect of a package of different structural and communicational means, each of which has a very limited individual influence.

## Structural means

Undoubtedly, '*closing the access*' by inhibiting access to the track is by far the most effective method to prevent track-related suicide behaviour. However, extensive track length (e.g. currently more than 36,000 km in Germany) impedes complete fencing-in, and makes this approach financially untenable as is the case with installing secure barriers with automatic doors in metro systems (Mishara 2007). However, the French TGF (Train à Grande Vitesse) fast track railway system is hermetically sealed, thus successfully inhibiting suicides (personal communication).

A realistic alternative is to provide barriers at places of advanced risk—hotspots. Erazo *et al.* (2004a) identified clusters of increased suicide prevalence analysing 5731 railway suicides in Germany over a 5-year observation period. Of these, >75 per cent were in the proximity of psychiatric hospitals. It is most likely that specific

approaches in these risk areas are more feasible and may substantially contribute to suicide prevention. However, with the passage of time new hotspots emerge, and a special task force and surveillance is needed as a continuous effort. More awareness is warranted when planning psychiatric hospitals in the proximity of railway lines. Planning and development of psychiatric facilities at a distance within a circle of about 2–3 miles from a railway line should be prevented by law. Visibility of railway tracks from psychiatric facilities should be strictly inhibited.

Further structural means refer to the installation of mirrors, flash lights, warning signals and television surveillance systems, mainly for platforms on railway and metro stations. Success in the east Japanese metro system, however, was not convincing (personal communication 2005). The same holds true for tools to mitigate the collision with the body (e.g. airbags, baskets) on the train. Drainage pits in metro systems, however, may be successful in decreasing mortality, due to a gap of space below the track, which prevents an attempter from making bodily contact with the train (Clarke and Poyner 1994; Coats and Walter 1999; Ratnayake *et al.* 2007).

## Communicative means

### Media effects

Railway and metro suicides have often led to extensive media coverage in the past. Media effects on suicides have been convincingly evaluated in the pioneering work of Schmidke and Häffner (1988), which showed that a fictional television drama of the intentional death of a male student on the railway track led to a substantial increased in the subsequent incidences of railway suicides for male subjects in the same age group. Etzersdorfer and Sonnek (1998) showed by their experience in Vienna that it is possible to prevent imitative suicides by influencing mass media to limit reports and depictions of railway and metro suicides as much as possible.

### Announcements

Automatically transmitted announcements in trains, and on station platforms along trunk lines, may reach tens of thousands of passengers simultaneously. Thus, railway companies are advised to design announcement protocols that inform passengers and bystanders about a critical incident leading to a breakdown of railway traffic but avoid promotion and further implementation of railway suicide into the subconscious of the passengers (e.g., the German Railway Company now uses the wording 'due to a medical rescue operation underway' as standard operation procedure).

### Poster campaigns

Poster campaigns addressing help for high-risk subjects may, under defined circumstances, be a prevention option: to avoid counter-productive promotion of suicidal ideation and fantasies dealing with the railway as a concrete suicide mean, nationwide poster campaigns in railway stations targeted at persons with increased suicidal risk should focus solely on addressing concrete help (telephone hotline, Samaritans) for those who feel hopeless and desperate. Under no circumstances should the campaign address concrete suicide means and it should also avoid mentioning any understanding of the motives of suicidal plans.

### Hotspot education

Once a psychiatric facility has been 'infected' by imitation behaviour with a high degree of virulence (Hazell 1993), going back to normal

**Table 79.2** Gatekeeper functions for employers and other personal working in the proximity of railroad station platforms

| |
|---|
| Being familiar with and alert for particular vulnerable time windows of excess risk for railway suicides |
| Increasing awareness of deviant behaviour |
| Encouraging staff members to use initative in case of being confronted with at-risk subjects |
| Educating basic skills on how to approach at-risk subjects properly |

is unethical, and specific approaches to avoid in-hospital psychiatric suicides are warranted (Vogel *et al.* 2001).

### Gatekeepers

Taking the German railway company as an example for a transportation system typical in highly developed countries, one will come across several tens of thousands of employers who are working on a daily schedule in the proximity of station platforms. Additionally, some thousands of persons are engaged as police force in this particular setting, as are Samaritans and railway chaplains. All these specialists may serve as 'organizational gatekeepers whose contact with potentially vulnerable populations provides an opportunity to identify at-risk individuals and direct them to appropriate assessment and treatment' (Mann *et al.* 2005, p. 2067). Advanced vocational training in these subjects should include basic knowledge and skills in approaching persons at risk (see Table 79.2). Awareness programmes for railway staff members have led to successful primary interventions (for example in the Montreal metro system) resulting in a substantial number of people being intercepted' before a possible suicide attempt (Mishara 1999).

## Conclusion: situation on the five continents

Suicides on the track of metro and railway systems are perceived as serious public health issues around the world. This has been proven in particular for metro suicides, including analyses from the Far East (Hong Kong, Tokio), Middle- (Mexico City) and South America (Caracas) and the USA (San Francisco) (see O'Donnell and Farmer 1992; Ratnayake *et al.* 2007). Nevertheless, data on prevalence, case fatality and patient characteristics remain scarce, especially for railway suicides (Mishara 2007). At present, most epidemiological findings are available from European countries (Austria, England, Germany, Sweden, The Netherlands). However, findings from India (Chowdhury *et al.* 2000) elucidate that railway suicides are also a reality in developing countries. Surprisingly, to date, no reports on railway suicides are available from Australia (except one report by Emmerson and Cantor 1993), USA, or Middle- and South America—although indirect evidence and anecdotal reports prove that railway track suicides occur in the USA (Guth *et al.* 2006) and in Brazil (Fernandes 2003).

## References

Abbott R, Young S, Grant G *et al.* (2003). *Railway Suicide: An Investigation of Individual and Organisational Consequences. A report of the SOVRN (Suicides and Open Verdicts on the Railway Network) Project*. Doncaster and South Humber Healthcare NHS Trust, Doncaster.

Angermeyer MC and Massing W (1985). The monthly and weekly distribution of suicide. *Social Science and Medicine*, **21**, 433–441.

Barraclough BM (1976). Time of day chosen for suicide. *Psychological Medicine*, **6**, 303–305.

Baumert J, Erazo N, Ladwig KH (2006). Ten-year incidence and time trends of railway suicides in Germany from 1991 to 2000. *European Journal of Public Health*, **16**, 173–8.

Cantor H and Baume PJM (1998). Access to methods of suicide: what impact? *Australian and New Zealand Journal of Psychiatry*, **32**, 8–14.

Carke RV and Lester D (1989). *Suicide: Closing the Exits*. Springer, New York.

Chowdhury AN, Dutta S, Chowdhury S (2000). Eco-psychiatry: suicidal behaviour at Calcutta metro rail: a prospective study. *International Medical Journal*, **7**, 27–32.

Clarke M (1994). Railway suicide in England and Wales, 1850 – 1949. *Social Science and Medicine*, **38**, 401–407.

Clarke RV and Poyner B (1994). Preventing suicide on the London underground. *Social Science and Medicine*, **8**, 443–446.

Coats TJ and Walter DP (1999). Effect of station design on death in the London underground: observational study. *British Medical Journal*, **319**, 957.

Conwell Y and Brent D (1995). Suicide and aging, I: patterns of psychiatric diagnosis. *International Psychogeriatrics*, **7**, 149–164.

Deisenhammer EA, Kemmler G, De Col C *et al.* (1997). [Railroad suicides and attempted suicides in Austria 1990–1994. Extending the hypothesis mass media transmission of suicidal behavior]. *Nervenarzt*, **68**, 67–73.

Emmerson B and Cantor C (1993). Train suicides in Brisbane, Australia, 980–1986. *Crisis*, **14**, 90–94.

Erazo N, Baumert J, Ladwig KH (2004a). [Regional and local clusters of railway suicides.] *Nervenarzt*, **75**, 1099–1106.

Erazo N, Baumert J, Ladwig KH (2004b). Sex-specific time patterns of suicidal acts on the German railway system. An analysis of 4003 cases. *Journal of Affective Disorders*, **83**, 1–9.

Erazo N, Baumert J, Ladwig KH (2005). Factors associated with failed and completed railway suicides. *Journal of Affective Disorders*, **88**, 137–143.

Etzersdorfer E and Sonnek G (1998). Preventing suicide by influencing mass-media reporting: the Viennese experience 1980–1996. *Archives of Suicide Research*, **4**, 67–84.

Evans AKB and JV Gough (eds) (2003). *The Impact of the Railway on Society in Britain. Essays in Honour of Jack Simmons*. Ashgate, Aldershot.

Fernandes J (2003). Suicide on the tracks. Journal of International Transport Workers' *Federation*, **11**.

Gaylord MS and Lester D (1994). Suicide in the Hong Kong subway. *Social Science and Medicine*, **38**, 427–430.

Guggenheim FG and Weisman AD (1972). Suicide in the subway. Publicly witnessed attempts of 50 cases. *Journal of Nervous and Mental Disease*, **155**, 404–409.

Guth AA, O'Neill A, Pachter HL *et al.* (2006). Public health lessons learned from analysis of New York City subway injuries. *American Journal of Public Health*, **96**, 631–633.

Hakko H, Räsänen P, Tiihonen J (1998). Secular trends in the rates and seasonality of violent and non-violent suicide occurrences in Finland during 1980–95. *Journal of Affective Disorders*, **50**, 49–54.

Harrington R (2003). On the tracks of trauma: railway spine reconsidered. *Social History of Medicine*, **16**, 209–223.

Hazell P (1993) Adolescent suicide clusters: evidence, mechanisms and prevention. *The Australian and New Zealand Journal of Psychiatry*, **27**, 653–665.

Kerkhof A (2003). Railway suicides: who is responsible? *Crisis*, **24**, 47.

Ladwig KH and Baumert J (2004). Patterns of suicidal behaviour in a metro subway system. A study of 306 cases injured by the Munich subway, 1980–1999. *European Journal of Public Health*, **14**, 291–5.

Lindekilde K and Wang AG (1985). Train suicide in the county of Fyn 1979–82. *Acta* Psychiatrica Scandinavica, **72**, 150–154.

Maclean AA, O'Neill AM, Pachter HL *et al.* (2006). Devastating consequences of subway accidents: traumatic amputations. *American Journal of Surgery*, **72**, 74–76.

Maes M, Cosyns P, Meltzer HY *et al.* (1993). Seasonality in violent suicide but not in non-violent suicide or homicide. *American Journal of Psychiatry Association*, **150**, 1380–1385.

Mann JJ, Apter A, Bertolote J *et al.* (2005). Suicide prevention strategies: a systematic review. *Journal of American Medical Association*, **294**, 2064–2074.

Meares R, Mendelsohn FAO, Milgrom-Friedman J (1981). A sex difference in the seasonal variation of suicide rate: a single cycle for men, two cycles for women. *British Journal of Psychiatry*, **138**, 321–325.

Micciolo R, Williams T, Zimmermann-Tansella CH *et al.* (1991). Geographical and Urban rural variation in the seasonality of suicide: some further evidence. *Journal of Affective Disorders*, **21**, 39–43.

Mishara BL (1999). Suicide in the Montreal subway system: characteristics of the victims, antecedents, and implications for prevention. *Canadian Journal of Psychiatry*, **44**, 690–9.

Mishara BL (2007). Railway and metro suicides. Understanding the problem and prevention potential. *Crisis*, **28**, 36–43.

O'Donnell I and Farmer RDT (1992). Suicidal acts on metro systems: an international perspective. *Acta Psychiatrica Scandinavica*, **86**, 60–63.

O'Donnell I and Farmer RDT (1994). The epidemiology of suicide on the London Underground. *Social Science and Medicine*, **38**, 409–418.

O'Donnell I, Farmer R, Catalan J (1996). Explaining suicide: the views of survivors of serious suicide attempts. *British Journal of Psychiatry*, **168**, 780–786.

O'Donnell I, Farmer R, Tranah T (1994). Introduction. *Social Science and Medicine*, **38**, 399–400.

Rådbo H, Svedung I, Andersson R (2005). Suicides and other fatalities from train-person collisions on Swedish railroads: a descriptive epidemiologic analysis as a basis for systems oriented prevention. *Journal of Safety Research*, **36**, 423–428.

Ratnayake R, Links PS, Eynan R (2007). Suicidal behaviour on subway systems: a review of the epidemiology. *Journal of Urban Health*, **84**, 766–781.

Samaritans (2008). http://www.samaritans.org/your_emotional_health/ publications/reducing_suicide_railways.aspx.

Schmidtke A (1994). Suicidal behaviour on railways in the FRG. *Social Science and Medicine*, **38**, 419–426.

Schmidke A (1997). Perspective. Suicide in Europe. *Suicide and Life-Threatening Behavior*, **27**, 127–136.

Schmidtke A and Häfner H (1988). The Werther effect after television films: new evidence for an old hypothesis. *Psychological Medicine*, **18**, 665–676.

Sonneck G, Etzersdorfer E, Nagel-Kuess S (1994). Imitative suicide on the Viennese subway. Social Science and Medicine, **38**, 453–457.

Van Houwelingen CA and Beersma DG (2001). Seasonal changes in 24-h patterns of suicide rates: a study on train suicides in the Netherlands. *Journal of Affective Disorders*, **66**, 215–213.

Van Houwelingen CA and Kerkhof AJ (2008). Mental healthcare status and psychiatric diagnoses of train suicides. *Journal of Affective Disorders*, **107**, 281–284.

Veress L and Szabó T (1980). Die Besonderheiten der am Eisenbahnkörper verübten Selbstmorde [The particularities of suicides committed on the railway track]. *Suizidprophylaxe*, **7**, 401–426.

Vogel R, Wolfersdorf M, Wurst FM (2001). [How and to what extent is suicide postvention part of the routine of health care professionals in psychiatric hospitals after inpatient suicide?] *Psychiatrische Praxis*, **28**, 323–325.

# CHAPTER 80

# Prevention of suicide due to charcoal burning

Paul Yip

## Abstract

A new method for suicide, charcoal-burning poisoning, was initiated in Hong Kong in 1998, and has replaced hanging as the second most commonly used method of suicide in the last five years. It has also spread to other regions, for example, Taiwan and Japan. Furthermore, the use of charcoal-burning suicide has drawn a new cohort of individuals into the suicide population. The profiles of the charcoal-burning poisoning death are different from the non-charcoal-burning deaths: there are more males, less psychiatric illness and more financial problems among these cases. Restricting access to charcoal has been proposed to reduce the number of charcoal-burning deaths. The idea is not to completely remove it from the market, but rather to set up barriers to obtaining the suicide means. This means that there is a wider window of opportunity for intervention.

## Introduction

Since 1998, Hong Kong has experienced a new method of suicide: charcoal-burning poisoning suicide. Usually this is done indoors, generally in a small sealed room by inhaling the fumes of carbon monoxide generated by charcoal burning—about 80 per cent of charcoal-burning deaths occur at home. This method accounted for 2.0 per cent of suicide deaths in 1998, rising to 26.4 per cent in 2003 (see Figure 80.1; Yip and Lee 2007). It has replaced hanging as the second most frequently used suicide method in Hong Kong. Furthermore, charcoal burning suicide is not a local phenomenon restricted to Hong Kong. One of the first charcoal-burning suicide victims occurred in Taiwan in 1999, and the individual stated explicitly in his suicide note that he had learned this method from reading a Hong Kong newspaper on the Internet. Since then, the number of suicide deaths resulting from charcoal burning ranked first in Taipei City in 2005, and on a territory-wide level in 2006. At the same time, Taiwan has experienced an historically high suicide rate—20.0 per 100.000 in 2006—which is more than three times the rate during 1993 (6.3 per 100,000). The increase is mainly attributable to the suicide death from charcoal-burning poisoning. Suicide deaths by other means have not increased at similar rates.

Yip and Lee (2007) and Kuo *et al.* (2008) revealed that the socio-demographic and clinical characteristics of charcoal-burning suicide victims are distinct from those of other cases. The charcoal-burning

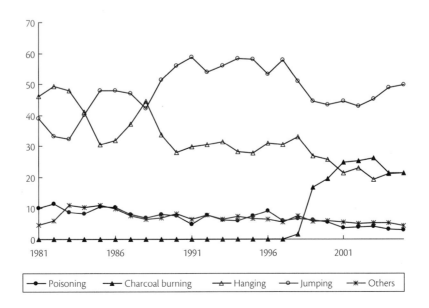

**Fig. 80.1** The proportion of suicide methods in Hong Kong, 1981–2005.

— Poisoning    — Charcoal burning    — Hanging    — Jumping    — Others

suicide victims are predominately aged 25–54, mostly men, unmarried and had relatively less history of substance abuse or other mental disorders. They were more likely to have financial troubles (see also Lee *et al.* 2002; Chan *et al.* 2005; Liu *et al.* 2007). Macau, the formerly Portuguese colony located 70 kilometres south-west of Hong Kong, has also reported twelve deaths by charcoal burning, out of the sixty suicide deaths in 2000 (*Macau Daily* 2000). Japan too reported a significant increase in suicide deaths due to charcoal burning, from less than 1 per cent to about 7 per cent (Takahashi 2008).

Charcoal burning has also commonly been used in suicide pacts in Hong Kong and Taiwan. In 2002 and 2003, 20 of 22 suicide pacts (91 per cent) used charcoal burning (Lee *et al.* 2005). Previous studies have shown that the methods of suicide used by suicide pacts are generally less violent, and the most common means is poisoning by fumes (Rajagopal 2004). Several perceived characteristics of charcoal burning make it attractive in suicide pacts. Charcoal burning is often portrayed as painless and effective, and hence, passive partners in suicide pacts could be more easily enticed into the act. It is non-disfiguring and is often perceived as a romantic and easy form of death. The messiness and pain associated with gunshots, jumping, hanging or drug poisoning are likely to discourage the submissive participants in a pact. Furthermore, unlike other methods of suicide, such as jumping from heights and hanging, it can easily be shared.

## Suicide prevention effort: some restrictions in charcoal sales

Charcoal is readily available in local markets, supermarkets and convenience stores in Hong Kong. However, it is not an essential and daily household item. It is mainly used for recreational activities (outdoor barbecue especially in Hong Kong) or religious ritual practice (especially in Taiwan for worshipping ancestors). Restriction of the easy access to charcoal is one of the possible prevention methods, and it is also a method that is consistent with international standards of best practice for suicide prevention. Indeed, restricting access to the methods of self-inflicted death has received very strong support both from the World Health Organization (WHO 2001; Hendin *et al.* 2008) and the International Association for Suicide Prevention (Mishara 2006). One suggestion is to remove the charcoal from open shelves, thus, making it necessary for the customer to ask a shop assistant to obtain charcoal for purchase. Such a restriction could be useful. The idea is not to completely remove it from the market, but to set up barriers to obtain the suicide means. This means that there is a wider window of opportunity for intervention.

In Hong Kong, we have launched a pilot study among all supermarkets and convenience stores in one district. A restriction of charcoal sales has been imposed by removing it from the open shelves of stores in this district. Preliminary results have suggested that this simple restriction has reduced charcoal-burning suicides, as opposed to a comparable district which does not use this measure. Nor is there any obvious substitution for other methods. This is not a question of no access; rather this is a proposal *to slow access* for those who would seek charcoal at a time of heightened distress.

Research evidence has also shown that restricting access to a specific method of suicide can often lead to fewer deaths. One classic example was a change in the nature of cooking gas in the United Kingdom (Kreitman 1976): a more recent effort involved a change in the packaging of paracetamol in UK, which led to a decrease in deaths from paracetamol poisoning by 21 per cent (Hawton 2002). Also, building barriers on a bridge in New Zealand (Beautrais 2001) (similar to a previously successful effort in Canada), gun safety training in the US (Hemenway *et al.* 1995), and restricting the sales of specific lethal pesticides in mainland China have been suggested as methods for suicide prevention (Pearson *et al.* 2002; Yip *et al.* 2008).

It is particularly important to understand that, based on our monitoring of Hong Kong's suicides, the use of charcoal burning has not been a substitute for other methods (Yip and Lee 2007). The extent to which a society is prepared to impose relatively minor restrictions on all members (which might cause some inconvenience), in order to protect a minority of people who are mentally ill or severely distressed is a reflection of that society's compassion and kindness to its vulnerable fellow citizens.

## Conclusion

Suicide is a very complex phenomenon that requires multilayered interventions. Education in life skills, providing and improving services for persons who suffer from medically significant depression, and aiding individuals and families at times of turmoil or distress are all important steps that must be taken. Nevertheless, restricting means is one proven method that has been shown to be cost-effective and relatively simple to implement when it is supported by the community. Thus, we strongly advocate the development of a concerted, sustained and collective approach to suicide prevention that uses, among others things, strategies to control means of suicide (e.g. charcoal sales) as one of its important tools.

## References

Beautrais A (2001). Effectiveness of barriers at suicide jumping sites: a case study. *Australian and New Zealand Journal of Psychiatry*, **35**, 557–562.

Chan K, Yip P, Au J, Lee D (2005). Charcoal-burning suicide in post-transition Hong Kong. *British Journal of Psychiatry*, **186**, 67–73.

Hawton K (2002). United Kingdom legislation on pack sizes of analgesics: background, rationale, and effects on suicide and deliberate self-harm. *Suicide and Life-Threatening Behavior*, **32**, 223–229.

Hemenway D, Solnick SJ, Azrael DR (1995). Firearm training and storage. *Journal of the American Medical Association*, **273**, 1733–1734.

Hendin H, Phillips MR, Vijayakumar L *et al.* (2008). Suicide and Suicide Prevention in Asia. World Health Organization, Geneva.

Kreitman N (1976). The coal gas story. United Kingdom suicide rates, 1960–71. *British Journal of Preventive and Social Medicine*, **30**, 86–93.

Kuo CJ, Conwell Y, Yu Q *et al.* (2008). Suicide by charcoal burning in Taiwan: implications for means substitution by a case-linkage study. *Social Psychiatry and Social Epidemiology*, **43**, 286–290.

Lee D, Chan K, Lee S *et al.* (2002). Burning charcoal: a novel and contagious method of suicide in Asia. *Archives of General Psychiatry*, **59**, 293–294.

Lee D, Chan K, Yip P (2005). Charcoal burning is also popular for suicide pacts made on the internet. *British Medical Journal*, **330**, 602.

Liu K, Beautrais A, Caine E *et al.* (2007). Charcoal burning suicides in Hong Kong and urban Taiwan—an illustration of the impact of a novel method of suicide on overall regional rates. *Journal of Epidemiology and Community Health*, **61**, 248–253.

*Macau Daily* (2000). Charcoal burning suicide killed 12 people this year. 23 November.

Mishara B (2006). *Report on the 2nd International Workshop on Secure Access to Pesticides, in conjunction with the IASP Asia-Pacific Regional Conference on Suicide Prevention*. IASP, Singapore.

Pearson V, Philips MR, He F *et al.* (2002). Attempted suicide among young rural women in the People's Republic of China: possibilities for prevention. *Suicide and Life-Threatening Behavior*, **32**, 359–369.

Rajagopal S (2004). Suicide pacts and the Internet. *British Medical Journal*, **329**, 1298–1299.

Takahashi Y (2008). Japan. In P Yip, ed., *Suicide in Asia: Causes and Prevention*, pp. 7–18. The University of Hong Kong Press, Hong Kong.

WHO (2001). *World Health Report 2001*. World Health Organization, Geneva.

Yip P and Lee DTS (2007). Charcoal burning suicides and strategies for prevention *Crisis*, **28**(suppl. 1), 21–27.

Yip P, Liu K, Law CK (2008). Years of life lost from suicide in China. *Crisis*, **29**, 131–136.

# CHAPTER 81

# Restriction of alcohol consumption in suicide prevention

Danuta Wasserman and Gergö Hadlaczky

## Abstract

Alcohol consumption is related to suicide rates on an aggregate level. Given that a causal relationship is also supported by both natural experiments and studies on an individual level, restricting access to alcohol can arguably prevent suicides. Sensitivity of suicide rates to changes in alcohol consumption varies from one region to another, depending on cultural drinking habits. Identifying the key characteristics of cultures where changes in alcohol consumption most affect suicide rates may help in deciding where alcohol restriction policies may be effective in reducing suicide.

## Introduction

Determining whether a death by alcohol overdose is due to suicide or an accident may be difficult, even in a situation where the deceased had a history of suicide ideation or attempts. Deaths due to acute intoxication are automatically classified as 'unintentional poisoning by alcohol' (Michalodimitrakis et al. 1997). While suicides can be identified by the existence of suicide notes, the incidence of note-leaving is only some 15–30 per cent of suicides overall (O'Donnell et al. 1993; Shioiri et al. 2005). The difficulty of identifying cases in which alcohol is used to commit suicide impedes the study and prevention of such cases.

However, alcohol also plays a part in cases where the method of suicide is not alcohol per se, but the suicide is nevertheless alcohol-related. Post-mortem investigations have revealed alcohol in the blood of 45 per cent of Swedish (Ferrada-Noli et al. 1996), 36–40 per cent of Finnish (Öhberg et al. 1996; Pirkola et al. 2003), 35–48 per cent (depending on the time period) of Estonian (Värnik et al. 2007), 28–29 per cent of American (Mendelson and Rich 1993; Garlow 2002) and 20 per cent of Dutch (Hansen et al. 1995) suicide victims.

Psychological autopsies of suicide victims showed evidence of diagnosable alcoholism in 40 per cent of the Finnish and Northern Irish cases (Henriksson et al. 1993; Foster et al. 1997), 39 per cent of cases in Sri Lanka (Abeyasinghe and Gunnell 2008) and 33 per cent in Hungary (Zonda 2006). By comparison, in the general population in Europe and the USA, lifetime prevalence is approximately 20 per cent for alcohol dependence in males and 8 per cent for females (Prytz 1998; Wasserman 2001).

While alcohol abuse or dependence is itself a psychiatric diagnosis, it is also closely related to other mental illnesses. Of patients with affective disorders, including depression and bipolar disorders, 20–30 per cent have a comorbid alcohol disorder (Wasserman 2006). This is also true of approximately 33 per cent of those with schizophrenia and 30 per cent with lifetime panic disorders (Frye and Salloum 2006). Having more than one disorder of any kind appears to increase the probability of suicidal behaviour, partly because it is more difficult to diagnose and therefore treat comorbid disorders and partly because of the burden these diseases represent. Of those who die by suicide, 44–72 per cent have more than one diagnosable mental disorder, one of which is often alcohol-related (Henriksson et al. 1993; Lonnqvist et al. 1995; Seguin et al. 2006).

Since alcohol is used as a means of committing suicide, and alcohol abuse and dependence also appear to be related to suicidal behaviour (Beautrais et al. 1996), removing alcohol may arguably result in a lower number of suicides. This prevention approach is similar to other strategies aimed at restricting means of suicide. Thus, the purpose of this chapter is to discuss this strategy and how it may help in reducing all types of alcohol-related suicides, not just those caused by alcohol poisoning.

## Effect of change in alcohol consumption on suicide rates

A number of studies have shown that a change in the alcohol consumption of the inhabitants of a particular area is positively related to suicide rates in that area (Skog and Elekes 1993; Skog et al. 1995; Wasserman et al. 1998; Ramstedt 2001a; Razvodovsky 2007). In other words, when consumption rises or falls, suicide rates follow suit. However, sensitivity of suicide rates to changes in alcohol consumption varies from one area to another (Lester 1993; Norström 1995; Razvodovsky 2007). Measured with such statistical techniques as time-series analysis, this information can be useful for planning suicide-prevention strategies based on alcohol reduction and estimating the extent of a decrease in suicide that may be expected when alcohol consumption falls, i.e. the prospects of the prevention succeeding.

In Sweden, for example, it has been calculated that a one-litre decrease in per capita alcohol consumption would result in a 13 per cent decline in suicide (Norström 1995). The same fall in alcohol consumption would bring about a decline in suicide of approximately 5 per cent in Hungary (Skog and Elekes 1993), 4 per cent in the USA and Canada (Caces and Harford 1998; Ramstedt 2005), 3 per cent in France (Norström 1995) and Portugal (Skog et al. 1995) and no significant decrease at all in Switzerland (Gmel et al. 1998).

These differences in the effect of alcohol on suicide may possibly be explained by cultural differences in drinking habits, which may be categorized in terms of 'wet' and 'dry' drinking cultures, depending on levels of alcohol consumption and intoxication-oriented drinking (Ramstedt 2001a). Examples of dry alcohol cultures in Europe are Nordic countries like Norway, Finland and Sweden, where mean annual consumption between 1951 and 1995 was relatively low at 4.1, 6.4, and 6.5 litres per capita respectively. These dry alcohol cultures are characterized by high levels of intoxication-oriented drinking (especially on weekends). Southern countries like Italy, Portugal and France, on the other hand, are examples of wet alcohol countries, with relatively high alcohol consumption (15.6, 15.9 and 21.6 litres for the same years as above) and low intoxication-oriented drinking. The UK, Denmark and Germany, with medium levels of consumption (7.5, 9.3 and 11.4 litres respectively), may serve as examples of intermediate countries between wet and dry cultures (Ramstedt 2001a).

Heavy drinking may be less tolerated in cultures with low alcohol consumption, and may therefore be more likely to lead to severed social networks and consequently suicide (Norström 1995). Moreover, individual-level studies have shown that alcohol intoxication can often lead to impulsive and aggressive behaviour (Sher 2006), where the former may turn suicidal ideation into a suicide attempt and the latter may turn an attempt into completed suicide by influencing the choice of method. In fact, Oei et al. (2006) showed that suicide victims with alcohol in their blood were more likely to die by violent means, such as gunshot or strangulation, than those without alcohol in their blood.

Given the above considerations, the effect of alcohol consumption on suicide rates may be greater in dry countries characterized by low consumption and high intoxication-oriented drinking than in wet countries characterized by high alcohol consumption and low intoxication-oriented drinking. In testing this hypothesis, Ramstedt (2001a) compared fourteen western European countries grouped into one of either 'wet', 'medium' or 'dry' alcohol-consumption categories. As expected, suicide rates were found to be more sensitive to changes in alcohol consumption in the dry drinking cultures than in the medium and wet ones. However, no difference was found between the latter two groups (medium and wet). The greatest alcohol-associated change in suicide rates was found in the 15–34 age groups, for both genders, followed by the 35–49 age group for males and the female 70+ age group in the dry countries (Finland, Norway and Sweden).

It has been pointed out that while the wet/dry theory may explain differences in the sensitivity of suicide rates to changes in alcohol consumption in European countries, it fails to do so in countries like Russia, other former Soviet republics and Eastern European countries. Owing to their high alcohol consumption, these countries appear to have a wet alcohol culture; nevertheless, their suicide rates appear to be highly sensitive to changes in alcohol consumption, like the dry alcohol cultures of northern Europe

(Pridemore 2006). Possibly even more important than the level of alcohol consumption is the frequency of intoxication, as well as the type of beverage used for intoxication. A number of studies have shown that consumption of spirits (such as vodka, rum, whisky and gin) alone was significantly related to suicide (Gruenewald et al. 1995; Norström and Rossow 1999; Ramstedt 2005). In line with the above notion that intoxication transforms near-suicidal behaviour into completed suicide, it makes sense that the consumption of beverages with the highest potency for intoxication should have the greatest impact on suicide. Razvodovsky (2007) used the fatal alcohol-poisoning rate—possibly an even better proxy for intoxication-oriented drinking—as a suicide predictor in a time series analysis in Belarus, and found further support for this relationship.

Studies by Wasserman et al. (1994) and Värnik et al. (1998a, b) of an anti-alcohol campaign initiated in 1985 by Gorbachev in the former Soviet Union, as a part of 'perestroika' (restructuring), provided good opportunities to shed light on how suicide rates correlate with restrictions in alcohol consumption in the population. Alcohol prices were raised substantially during the strict reform and sales were limited. Suicide rates fell sharply during the period 1984–1988, with a 32 per cent decline occurring among men and 19 per cent among women. Alcohol played a part, estimated as attributable fractions, in approximately 50 per cent of the men's and 27 per cent of the women's suicides in the former USSR as a whole during this period (Wasserman et al. 1994, 1998). Furthermore, the decline was strongly correlated with alcohol consumption for both sexes, but especially for men in the workforce aged 25–54. This age group is similar to that of people found to be most responsive in terms of suicide to changes in alcohol consumption in the study of 14 European countries by Ramstedt (2001a).

Another natural experiment took place in Denmark between 1917 and 1918, when alcohol prices were raised to boost state revenue in order to combat the economic shortages caused by the First World War. In this study, too, the data suggested a decrease in suicide rates associated with reduced drinking in the population (Skog 1993). Such studies are of importance for suicide-preventive efforts because it is only in such quasi-experimental conditions that the cause of the change in alcohol consumption, such as the price increase, is known. This makes it possible to rule out, to some extent, the idea that the relationship between alcohol consumption and suicide is spurious, i.e. caused by a third underlying variable. The problem is that not even such studies can entirely rule out this possibility. Amongst the number of changes that occurred in the former Soviet Union during perestroika, as well as those in Denmark, changes in alcohol consumption were probably not the only factor that may have affected suicide rates.

However, individual-level studies in Denmark and Estonia (a former Soviet republic) support the causal connection between alcohol consumption and suicide. In Denmark, it was shown that the above-mentioned rise in alcohol prices was followed by a fall in suicide rates, but only among alcoholics (Skog 1991, 1993). Värnik et al. (2007) analysed blood alcohol concentration (BAC) in suicide victims in Estonia before, during and after the alcohol restrictions initiated by Gorbachev during perestroika. Each suicide case was assigned to either a 'no-alcohol' group or to one of three 'alcohol-positive' groups, according to BAC levels. The low alcohol-positive group comprised suicide cases where BACs were found to be between 0.5 per mille (‰) and 1.49‰; the intermediate group had BACs of 1.5–2.49‰ and the high group consisted of all cases with BAC levels above 2.5‰. During the alcohol restriction period, male suicides decreased by 11 per cent, 42 per cent, and 61 per cent in the low, intermediate and high alcohol groups respectively, and corresponding decreases were found in female suicides: 13 per cent, 43 per cent and 71 per cent. The number of no-alcohol suicides remained more or less stable during the same period of alcohol restrictions (with a small increase of 4 per cent for men and decrease of 1 per cent for women). After perestroika, when the alcohol restrictions were abolished, suicides increased among men (by 23 per cent for the low, 26 per cent for the intermediate and 50 per cent for the high alcohol groups). The number of suicides where no alcohol was observed in the blood remained relatively constant during this period (with a 4 per cent decrease for men and a 9 per cent increase for women) as well. This study shows a clear pattern in the decrease of alcohol-related suicides during the period of alcohol restriction and an increase in alcohol-related suicides after its abolition. Further, the lack of change in the non-alcohol group over the whole study period suggests a cause and effect relationship between alcohol and suicide.

## Other effects of alcohol on society

Restrictions on alcohol may also have beneficial effects other than a decrease in suicide. An increase in alcohol consumption is associated with rises in all-cause mortality (Norström 2001), overall accident mortality (Skog 2001), liver cirrhosis mortality (Ramstedt 2001b) and homicide (Rossow 2001) in fourteen European countries studied. Counties in Alabama (USA) with alcohol prohibition also had lower rates of homicide than counties where sales were allowed (Joubert 1994). Further, in Russia it was shown that the large fluctuations in overall mortality rates between 1984 and 1994 were most probably due to changes in alcohol consumption. Strongly alcohol-associated variation in deaths due to homicide, violence, accidents and suicide were observed during this period (Leon *et al.* 1997). In the city of Izhesk, Russia, almost 50 per cent of premature male all-cause deaths were related to hazardous drinking. This may be generalized to a large number of cities in Russia (Leon *et al.* 2007).

## Regional measures to reduce alcohol consumption

The WHO Expert Committee on Problems Related to Alcohol Consumption recommends eight strategies to reduce alcohol consumption in a region (WHO 2007). Those listed below are of interest for suicide prevention:

♦ *Government regulation of sales.* Given the positive correlation between the number of outlets and alcohol consumption, it is important to regulate the number of outlets and alcohol sales at retail level. Licensing can be used to regulate private operators, by enabling the government to give, suspend or withdraw the licences of private operators seeking to sell alcohol.

♦ *Alcohol prices and taxes.* Regulation of prices and taxes is an effective method of reducing alcohol consumption. This seems to apply particularly to young people: it can be used to reduce the proportion of heavy drinkers and the amount of binge drinking, as well as delaying intentions to start drinking.

The age group shown to be most sensitive to this strategy across fourteen European countries was 15–34 years (Ramstedt 2001a).

♦ *Bans.* Examples are a minimum age for alcohol purchase and bans on drinking on streets and public places or in specific circumstances.

♦ *Restrictions on alcohol marketing.* Exposure to alcohol advertising has significant effects on the drinking habits of young people, in particular.

♦ *Education.* People can be educated about alcohol-related harm in many different ways, such as mass-media campaigns, use of the Internet, labelling of alcoholic beverage containers with relevant messages, family initiatives, etc. Young people can be reached in classroom settings but unfortunately, owing to lack of attractiveness and sustainability, educational campaigns do not appear to be as effective as other methods of reducing alcohol consumption.

## Conclusions

Aggregate-level and individual-level studies have shown that reductions in overall national or regional alcohol consumption are likely to lead to a decrease in national and regional suicide rates respectively. Sensitivity of suicide rates to change in alcohol consumption seems, however, to depend substantially on cultural factors. High frequency and intensity of alcohol intoxication, as well as high availability and consumption of spirits, in particular, appear to be key components of the type of drinking culture in which suicide rates are most sensitive to changes in alcohol consumption.

It is important to remember that, to a high degree, the effectiveness of the methods of reducing alcohol consumption described above depends on how well they are enforced and how well counterproductive activity, such as bootlegging and home brewing, is controlled. Further, since alcohol is associated with a vast number of harmful effects besides suicide and mental ill-health, such as liver cirrhosis, vehicle accidents and violent crimes, the synergic effects of reducing alcohol consumption should be considered in policy creation.

## References

Abeyasinghe R and Gunnell D (2008). Psychological autopsy study of suicide in three rural and semi-rural districts of Sri Lanka. *Social Psychiatry and Psychiatric Epidemiology*, **43**, 280–285.

Beautrais AL, Joyce PR, Mulder RT *et al.* (1996). Prevalence and comorbidity of mental disorders in persons making serious suicide attempts: a case–control study. *American Journal of Psychiatry*, **153**, 1009–1014.

Caces F and Harford T (1998). Time series analysis of alcohol consumption and suicide mortality in the United States, 1934–1987. *Journal on Studies of Alcohol*, **59**, 455–461.

Ferrada-Noli M, Ormstad K, Asberg M (1996). Pathoanatomic findings and blood alcohol analysis at autopsy (BAC) in forensic diagnoses of undetermined suicide. A cross-cultural study. *Forensic Science International*, **78**, 157–163.

Foster T, Gillespie K, McClelland R (1997). Mental disorders and suicide in Northern Ireland. *British Journal of Psychiatry*, **170**, 447–452.

Frye MA and Salloum IM (2006). Bipolar disorder and comorbid alcoholism: prevalence rate and treatment considerations. *Bipolar Disorder*, **8**, 677–685.

Garlow SJ (2002). Age, gender, and ethnicity differences in patterns of cocaine and ethanol use preceding suicide. *American Journal of Psychiatry*, **159**, 615–619.

Gmel G, Rehm J, Ghazinouri A (1998). Alcohol and suicide in Switzerland—an aggregate-level analysis. *Drug and Alcohol Review*, **17**, 27–37.

Gruenewald PJ, Ponicki WR, Mitchell PR (1995). Suicide rates and alcohol consumption in the United States, 1970–89. *Addiction*, **90**, 1063–1075.

Hansen AC, Kristensen IB, Dragsholt C et al. (1995). Alcohol, drugs and narcotics in suicides in the Aarhus police district (in Danish). *Ugeskr Laeger*, **157**, 1524–1527.

Henriksson MM, Aro HM, Marttunen MJ et al. (1993). Mental disorders and comorbidity in suicide. *American Journal of Psychiatry*, **150**, 935–940.

Joubert CE (1994). 'Wet' or 'dry' county status and its correlates with suicide, homicide, and illegitimacy. *Psychological Reports*, **74**, 296.

Leon DA, Chenet L, Shkolnikov VM et al. (1997). Huge variation in Russian mortality rates 1984–94: artefact, alcohol, or what? *Lancet*, **350**, 383–388.

Leon DA, Saburova L, Tomkins S et al. (2007). Hazardous alcohol drinking and premature mortality in Russia: a population based case–control study. *Lancet*, **369**, 2001–2009.

Lester D (1993). Alcohol use and abuse, suicide and homicide. *Psychological Reports*, **73**, 346.

Lonnqvist JK, Henriksson MM, Isometsa ET et al. (1995). Mental disorders and suicide prevention. *Psychiatry and Clinical Neuroscience*, **49**, S111–116.

Mendelson WB and Rich CL (1993). Sedatives and suicide: the San Diego study. *Acta Psychiatrica Scandinavica*, **88**, 337–341.

Michalodimitrakis MN, La Grange R et al. (1997). Suicide by alcohol overdose. *Journal of Clinical and Forensic Medicine*, **4**, 91–94.

Norström T (1995). Alcohol and suicide: a comparative analysis of France and Sweden. *Addiction*, **90**, 1463–1469.

Norström T (2001). Per capita alcohol consumption and all-cause mortality in 14 European countries. *Addiction*, **96**, S113–1128.

Norström T and Rossow I (1999). Beverage specific effects on suicide. *Nordic Studies on Alcohol and Drugs*, **16**, 109–108.

O'Donnell I, Farmer R, Catalan J (1993). Suicide notes. *British Journal of Psychiatry*, **163**, 45–48.

Oei TP, Foong T, Casey LM (2006). Number and type of substances in alcohol and drug-related completed suicides in an Australian sample. *Crisis*, **27**, 72–76.

Öhberg A, Vuori E, Ojanpera I et al. (1996). Alcohol and drugs in suicides. *British Journal of Psychiatry*, **169**, 75–80.

Pirkola S, Isometsa E, Lonnqvist J (2003). Do means matter? Differences in characteristics of Finnish suicide completers using different methods. *Journal of Nervous and Mental Disease*, **191**, 745–750.

Pridemore WA (2006). Heavy drinking and suicide in Russia. *Social Forces*, **85**, 413–430.

Prytz H (1998). Alkoholismens epidemiologi [The epidemiology of alcoholism]. In Nordén A, ed., *Alkohol som sjukdomsorsak [Alcohol as a cause of illness]*, pp. 64–70. Stockholm, Nordstedts Förlag.

Ramstedt M (2001a). Alcohol and suicide in 14 European countries. *Addiction*, **96**, S59–75.

Ramstedt M (2001b). Per capita alcohol consumption and liver cirrhosis mortality in 14 European countries. *Addiction*, **96**, S19–33.

Ramstedt M (2005). Alcohol and suicide at the population level–the Canadian experience. *Drug and Alcohol Review*, **24**, 203–208.

Razvodovsky YE (2007). Suicide and alcohol poisoning in Belarus between 1970 and 2005. *Adicciones*, **19**, 297–303.

Rossow I (2001). Alcohol and homicide: a cross-cultural comparison of the relationship in 14 European countries. *Addiction*, **96**, S77–92.

Seguin M, Lesage A, Chawky N et al. (2006). Suicide cases in New Brunswick from April 2002 to May 2003: the importance of better recognizing substance and mood disorder comorbidity. *Canadian Journal of Psychiatry*, **51**, 581–586.

Sher L (2006). Alcohol consumption and suicide. *Quarterly Journal of Medicine*, **99**, 57–61.

Shioiri T, Nishimura A, Akazawa K et al. (2005). Incidence of note-leaving remains constant despite increasing suicide rates. *Psychiatry and Clinical Neurosciences*, **59**, 226–228.

Skog OJ (1991). Alcohol and suicide: Durkheim revisited. *Acta Sociologica*, 193–206.

Skog OJ (1993). Alcohol and suicide in Denmark 1911–24—experiences from a 'natural experiment'. *Addiction*, **88**, 1189–1193.

Skog OJ (2001). Alcohol consumption and mortality rates from traffic accidents, accidental falls, and other accidents in 14 European countries. *Addiction*, **96**, S49–58.

Skog OJ and Elekes Z (1993). Alcohol and the 1950–90 Hungarian suicide trend—is there a causal connection? *Acta Sociologica*, **36**, 33–46.

Skog OJ, Teixeira Z, Barrias J et al. (1995). Alcohol and suicide—the Portuguese experience. *Addiction*, **90**, 1053–1061.

Värnik A, Kolves K, Vali M et al. (2007). Do alcohol restrictions reduce suicide mortality? *Addiction*, **102**, 251–256.

Värnik A, Wasserman D, Dankowicz M et al. (1998a). Age-specific suicide rates in the Slavic and Baltic regions of the former USSR during perestroika, in comparison with 22 European countries. *Acta Psychiatrica Scandinavica Supplementum*, **394**, 20–25.

Värnik A, Wasserman D, Dankowicz M et al. (1998b). Marked decrease in suicide among men and women in the former USSR during perestroika. *Acta Psychiatrica Scandinavica Supplementum*, **394**, 13–19.

Wasserman D (2001). Alcoholism, other psychoactive substance misuse and suicide. In Wasserman D, ed., *Suicide—An Unnecessary Death*, pp. 49–57. Martin Dunitz, London.

Wasserman D (2006). *Depression: The Facts*. Oxford University Press, Oxford.

Wasserman D, Varnik A, Eklund G (1994). Male suicides and alcohol consumption in the former USSR. *Acta Psychiatrica Scandinavica*, **89**, 306–313.

Wasserman D, Varnik A, Eklund G (1998). Female suicides and alcohol consumption during perestroika in the former USSR. *Acta Psychiatrica Scandinavica Supplementum*, **394**, 26–33.

WHO (2007). *Expert Committee on Problems Related to Alcohol Consumption*. World Health Organization, Geneva.

Zonda T (2006). One hundred cases of suicide in Budapest: a case-controlled psychological autopsy study. *Crisis*, **27**, 125–129.

# PART 11

# Survivors of Suicide Loss

# CHAPTER 82

# Why suicide loss is different for the survivors

Edward J Dunne and Karen Dunne-Maxim

## Abstract

People who are bereaved by suicide are confronted with a number of unique circumstances which hold the potential for complicating or even completely derailing their recovery process. First, they must work through the considerable stigma, which still surrounds this type of death. This chapter examines some of the historical and contemporary manifestations of societal reactions to death by suicide as a way of establishing a background for understanding the aspects of suicide bereavement, which distinguish it from other types of bereavement. These reactions are described based on the authors' work with more than 2000 survivors over the past 25 years. Not all survivors experience all of these reactions, and the intensity of the reactions will differ for each individual and even over time for the same individual. Yet, their common appearance in many survivors warrants special attention to them as a way of understanding the grieving process of those bereaved by suicide. Particular attention is paid to the tasks of the treating clinician when intervention is initiated. They are directed specifically at stigma reduction as a means of avoiding complicated mourning as well as familial discord. The chapter also draws attention to the special needs of young children who survive a loved one's suicide.

## Introduction

Sudden and traumatic deaths throw the survivors into a severe psychological crisis. Not having anticipated the loss, they must begin the task of imagining their future lives without their loved one at the same time that they are actually living without them. The many difficult aspects of grieving under these circumstances pose some of the greatest challenges to the bereaved, and expose them to an increased likelihood of complicated and even morbid grief outcomes. If the death is by suicide, the possibility of pathological outcomes is increased. This phenomenon has been studied by Rando (1993). Sakinofsky (2007), in a review of treatment interventions for the people bereaved by suicide, cited numerous investigations, which found clear differences in the length, intensity of grief as well as an increase of depressive sequelae for these survivors when contrasted with the more typically bereaved (Brent *et al.* 1993; Brent *et al.* 1995; Seguin 1995; Brent *et al.* 1996; Bailley *et al.* 1999; Cerel *et al.* 1999; Harwood *et al.* 2002; Cvinar 2005). Several first person accounts, for instance, those by Bolton (1984),

Fine (1999), and Alexander (1998) support and give substance to these more empirical accounts. This literature suggests a variety of emotional and behavioural reactions, which are unique to suicide, summarized by Sakinofsky as hiding the actual cause of the death from others, obsession with the motivation of the suicide victim, and viewing the suicide as an act of aggression directed against them as an act of retribution. Our work with survivors has led us to the appreciation that not all survivors experience each of these reactions, and that the intensity with which they are experienced will vary. Unquestionably, the single most important factor which complicates suicide bereavement is the stigma associated with this type of death. Whether real or imagined, reacting to stigma serves to place an additional layer of burden on the bereaved and becomes intertwined with the other emotional reactions of grief.

## Suicide and stigma

In his extensive review of suicide, Colt (1991) asserts that negative reactions to suicide can be traced as far back as primitive cultures, which denied traditional burial because they believed that the spirit of the departed would haunt the village. Neither the Greeks nor the Romans were indifferent to suicide and began the practice of punishing the families following an unsanctioned suicide. Early Christian teaching opposed suicide and associated it with eternal damnation. The Jewish faith began prohibiting funeral rites following a suicide at around the same time. In the Middle Ages, civil authority was invoked to prevent suicide. Colt, for instance, reported the example of a medieval widow who was required to pay damages to the Crown after her husband took his own life. Various states, in the New World, enacted laws prohibiting the burial of suicides within traditional cemeteries, while the Catholic church prohibited funeral rites to suicide victims until the Second Vatican Council in 1962. By depriving the surviving family of the customary funerary rituals, these societies and institutions were practicing a crude form of suicide prevention. However, these practices provided an early incentive to surviving families to hide or deny the actual cause of death, thus, creating the stigma which surrounds this type of death. It is the additional burden of stigma which drives the grieving process of many surviving families. Even in the absence of specific social opprobrium around survivors, stigma may be internalized and blame self-imposed.

# What does suicide grief look like?

Although it is not possible to predict with accuracy for any given individual their response to a loss to suicide, several distinct themes seem to characterize the grieving of most people in this situation. The following list summarizes our observations over several years of working with survivors.

## Shock and denial

With the possible exception of families who have lived through multiple serious suicide attempts by a loved one, the most likely initial response to a completed suicide is shock and denial. This stems both from the unexpectedness of the death as well as the desire to avoid the stigma attached to it. As the survivors gradually accommodate the facts of the death, many move through a phase of acceptance of the death, but not the cause. Some refuse, at first, to label the death a suicide even when the facts are quite unambiguous. This denial may continue for days or months, and runs the risk of becoming a permanent part of the survivor's narrative about their lost relative. This places them at risk for subsequent trauma when others hold an opposing point of view. Such an extreme reaction is increasingly rare as societal opinions about suicide have evolved, however, the more ambiguous the details of the death—i.e. no suicide note, overdosing on substances of abuse, unexplained accidents—the more likely the survivor will persist in attributing the death to some other cause, and therefore the greater likelihood of subsequent trauma when the cause finally becomes more certain. It is not unknown for people within the same family to hold different beliefs about the cause of the death, thereby complicating the grief of all. Whole societies can fall victim to this if the suspected suicide is well-known and admired (i.e. Marilyn Monroe). In these instances, this form of denial can persist for years.

## Search for the why

People are often troubled by the ambiguity surrounding a suicide and may find themselves obsessively involved in searching for an explanation. Completed suicides are, of course, very complex events and it is unlikely that any single fact will suffice as an explanation (lost job, divorce, etc.). Nevertheless, many survivors experience repeated distress when each of their early explanations is undone by subsequent information and a new explanation has to be found. Some survivors find this uncertainty intolerable and will latch onto an overly simplistic explanation (i.e. 'she drove him to do it'), which requires them to deny more nuanced explanations. In many cases, however, the 'why' is not actually knowable, and the survivor continues the search until settling for the possibility that they may never know the complete story. This searching for the 'why' is unique to suicide deaths, and has been found in some individuals as many as 20 years after their loss.

## Blaming

In their search for an explanation, survivors frequently blame others whom they perceive has having failed to keep their loved one from harm. This most typically is directed towards caregivers who were directly responsible for the safety of the victim (therapists, hospitals, physicians, etc.), but can include other family members, employers, school systems, or even song lyricists. Blaming can result in protracted conflict within a family as different members hold different people responsible. Blaming is reinforced by the larger community, which frequently holds family members responsible and communicates this through a variety of ways (direct accusations, innuendo, etc.). A most powerful source of blame is the media, which tries to fix responsibility in order to provide an easy explanation for a complicated event. For example, a United States newspaper article on the simultaneous suicides of four teenagers was headlined 'Four unloved kids take their lives'. Feeling blamed results in social withdrawal and isolation on the part of the survivors, which further complicates grief.

## Guilt

It is very difficult for survivors of a suicide to avoid examining their own behaviour before the death. Frequently, they discover actions (or inaction), which they believe caused or at least contributed to the suicide. They often exaggerate their role in the outcome, overlooking more probable causes such as an underlying mental illness. This leads to obsessive thoughts about how they might have behaved differently, frequently associated with magical thinking characterized by such phrases as 'if only I had …' or 'if only she …'. This can prolong the period before the death is fully accepted and can lead to delayed resolution of grief.

## Anger

Anger directed towards the deceased is a unique feature of deaths by suicide. Survivors may find their grief complicated by intense feelings of abandonment or resentment about being placed in this situation. This interferes with the expression of the feelings of loss, which are more typical of bereavement. Survivors may find themselves oscillating between these conflicting emotions and may need a great deal of time to eventually reconcile them.

## Anxiety

People who lose a loved one to suicide frequently find themselves worrying about the possibility that someone else, or even themselves, may choose to end their own life. This specific fear is not typical of 'natural' deaths, but may occur when the loss is through homicide or infectious disease. Anxiety among survivors may lead them to behaviours which interfere with recovery, such as over-protectiveness and hypervigilance of other family members or excessive worry about their own impulse control. In more severe instances, the anxiety is generalized, leading to a state of chronic apprehension about possible loss.

## Relief

People who survive the death of a loved one, who had suffered from a chronic physical illness, may experience some sense of relief when the ill person dies because the burden of caring for them is lifted. Usually, however, these survivors anticipate the death and are preparing themselves for it. Although they may be conflicted about feeling relief, they are usually able to justify it on the basis of the relief from suffering the deceased has achieved. People who share their lives with chronically mentally ill relatives, however, do not usually anticipate death, yet may experience relief when they find that they no longer have to worry about the deceased (particularly if they had been previously suicidal). This sense of relief is disconcerting, however, since it suggests that they are actually glad about the death. It is unusual for them to justify this on the basis of the relief the victim achieves. This conflict results in the additional burden of excessive guilt about one's own feelings.

These grief patterns usually come unanticipated by survivors, who then may be at a loss in dealing with them. Although world culture is replete with depictions of grieving, it is only rarely that one is exposed to examples of people mourning the loss of a loved one to suicide. Lacking specific information about this particular loss, the survivor questions the legitimacy, not only of their own reactions, but also of those close to them who are also grieving. In the presence of stigma, this questioning can lead to anxiety, anger, and conflict with precisely the people who would otherwise be a source of support—other family members. For this reason, we advocate for early intervention based on the family psychoeducation model (Dunne 1992), in which the family receives education about suicide and suicide grief. In this model, the family is helped to normalize their reactions and is steered away from thoughts and behaviours which may complicate the grief. Our experience has taught us that the best outcomes happen when the intervention is early, specific, and non-blaming. The tasks for a clinician making such a post-vention effort are detailed in the following paragraph. Our experience also teaches us that the majority of survivors are remarkably resilient. Most can avoid long-term negative outcomes with the proper intervention, many without any intervention at all. Some survivors, however, may need extra help at this time, and it is wise to normalize the utilization of support groups as well as the mental health system.

## Task of the post-vention clinician

Recommendations are based on the assumption of an early, preferably within the first week, contact with the family. Modifications will be needed if the family is contacted later.

1 Help the family make decisions about funeral arrangements, which are in keeping with usual family traditions around mourning.

2 Educate family about the high correlation between suicide and major mental illnesses, emphasizing the biological underpinnings of these illnesses (depression, schizophrenia, bipolar disorder, especially).

3 Encourage the family to accept and share with others the actual cause of the death.

4 Educate the family about typical psychological reactions to suicide as a means of normalizing them and depriving them of some of their potential for negative outcomes.

5 Acknowledge the family's heightened sense of anxiety and contract for safety and consideration among family members.

6 Help the family respect the individual grieving styles of its members. Remind them that all people grieve differently and at different paces.

7 Connect the family to other sources of support through local survivor support groups, literature, and the Internet.

8 If the young children are involved, help the family plan and rehearse what and how they will be told about the death.

## The special case of children as survivors

Children who survive the suicide of someone close to them have very specific needs which need to be attended to. Their grief reactions may be quite different from that of their parents, and clinicians must help the family negotiate this, while respecting each other's unique process. A most common public misconception is that it is not wise to tell children the truth when a death in the family is a suicide. Instead, children are frequently told that the cause of death was an accident or some physical illness such as a heart attack. This is most frequently an outgrowth of the belief that children will somehow be protected from the stigma related to suicide if they do not know the truth. Sometimes people are motivated by the fear that knowledge that a loved one died by suicide might encourage children to consider suicide in the future. Countless clinical examples from adults who were misinformed about the true cause of a family member's death underscore the potential for difficulty in this approach. These 'unknowing' survivors frequently report being on guard and suspicious about the family 'secret'. Most often, they learn the truth in inappropriate circumstances and without support (i.e. in schoolyards, through newspaper accounts, etc.). An additional complication is that once they learn the true nature of the death they have to go through an additional grieving process, even if the loss occurred years earlier. Thus, telling children the facts in a straightforward way, being mindful of their capacity to understand death in general based on their developmental stage, is a crucial first intervention. This should be done in a supportive atmosphere and the clinician can be present to help the caregiver relay the facts if necessary. One explanation given to younger children describes the suicide as a 'brain attack' or a sickness which came over the brain and made their thinking unclear. Older children can better understand mental illness as a cause whose roots are biological and affect brain chemistry.

Understandably, children will grow through this loss as a function of the strength of their adult caregivers. Thus, providing the family with education and support can contribute greatly to a healthy outcome in surviving children. This underscores the value of an initial psychoeducational intervention as mentioned above. It is here that the adults can be taught the appropriate language for describing the death to children. A list of interventions that can be helpful for child survivors is presented below.

## Intervention for children who suffer a loss through suicide

1 Encourage their age-appropriate participation in rituals associated with honouring the deceased. Children have similar needs as adults to do something concrete in the midst of grieving.

2 Encourage discussion about the life of the deceased rather than focusing on the manner in which they died.

3 Emphasize to caregivers the importance of maintaining a normal routine for children as best as possible. Keeping familiar surroundings, activities and relationships will greatly help to lessen their anxiety.

4 Facilitate their expression of feelings. Normalize them as something all are going through. Even validate that anger is appropriate.

5 Be aware that children may experience an exaggerated sense of responsibility ('if only I had done my school work my father would not have died') and help them to put this into proper perspective.

6  Anticipate that they may have academic setbacks. Grieving, confusion and the uncertainty can affect performance. Work out strategies with teachers to help them with this.

7  Expect complaints about somatic illnesses (headaches, stomach aches, etc.). Help them to verbalize their feelings during this time. Explore the possibility of school phobias related to stigma avoidance being expressed in this manner.

8  Provide them with opportunities to meet with other children who have experienced a loss. This can be accomplished through groups or individual arrangements.

9  Expose them to the stories of other children going through the grieving process.

## Factors affecting stigma surrounding a death by suicide

In the past 30 years, especially in the United States, but elsewhere as well, as reported by Andriessen (2004, 2007) and Jobes and colleagues (2000), knowledge about and attitudes towards suicide have undergone a substantial shift towards greater understanding and empathy. Self-help groups dealing specifically with survivors of a loved one's suicide began to surface in the early 1980s, not only in the United States, but in Europe too (Grad 2006). Members from these groups were subsequently responsible for the increase in awareness of suicidologists for the need to study survivor issues. In turn, suicidologists began investigating survivor families and became open to hearing their particular stories as they attempted to quantify the impact of losing someone to suicide. This greater willingness to listen to survivors prompted a number of celebrities to talk about their own experiences with suicide in their own families. The celebrities' candour about a previously taboo subject helped change the attitudes of the general public regarding suicide. In addition, the American Foundation for Suicide Prevention and the American Association of Suicidology, as well as the International Association for Suicide Prevention, the professional organizations dealing with suicide all expanded their focus to include divisions specifically dedicated to understanding and helping survivors. They aligned with them in lobbying governments to fund research on survivors and to provide resources for them. This culminated in a national strategy for suicide prevention proposed by the US Surgeon General (2001), which addressed the issue of suicide survivors. Currently, there are over 500 survivors of suicide support groups in the United State and the rest of the world. This has led to an increase in sophistication in general about suicide and, particularly, its close correlation with mental illness, and as stigma around mental illness has declined over the past three decades, so too has the stigma associated with suicide.

Despite these gains, most mental health professional graduate programmes and medical schools do not include survivor issues as part of their curriculum. Ironically, however, it is this group of professionals who are most likely to be among the first responders when a suicide occurs in a family. Unfortunately, this lack of training leaves the clinician woefully inexperienced at a critical juncture.

## Conclusion

The unique circumstances surrounding a death by suicide require both specialized knowledge and skills on the part of the clinicians who work with the survivors.

In addition to advocating for including survivor issues as part of training curriculum for new clinicians, there is a pressing need to find opportunities to educate those clinicians who are currently in practice. Countless clinical examples of their naivete in working with this population reinforces this problem. Taking into account the genetic factors inherent in mental illness, as well as the efffect of 'modelling', underscores the fact that appropiate postvention with these families is a significant step toward prevention. When one considers that, worldwide, there are 877,000–1 million or more suicides annually, the number of individuals affected by this traumatic loss is staggering. Thus, in the vast array of suicide prevention efforts, educating those who provide clinical services to the survivors looms as one of the most important.

## References

Alexander V (1998). *In the Wake of Suicide: Stories of the People Left Behind*. Jossey-Bass, New York.

Andriessen K (2004). Suicide survivor activities, an international perspective. *Suicidologi*, **9**(2), 26–31.

Andriessen K (2007). A gathering at the seaside: the first international postvention seminar. *Surviving Suicide*, **19**, 3–10.

Bailley SE, Kral MJ, Dunham K (1999). Survivors of suicide do grieve differently: empirical support for a common sense proposition. *Suicide and Life-Threatening Behaviour*, **29**, 256–271.

Brent DA, Moritz G, Bridge J et al. (1996). Long-term impact of exposure to suicide: a three-year controlled follow-up. *Journal of the American Academy of Child and Adolescent Psychiatry*, **35**, 646–653.

Brent DA, Perper J, Moritz G et al. (1993). Adolescent witnesses to a peer suicide. *Journal of the American Academy of Child and Adolescent Psychiatry*, **32**, 1184–1188.

Brent DA, Perper J, Moritz G et al. (1995). Posttraumatic stress disorder in peers of adolescent suicide victims: predisposisng factors and phenomenology. *Journal of the American Academy of Child and Adolescent Psychiatry*, **34**, 209–215.

Bolton I (1984). *My Son ... My Son ... A Guide to Healing after Death, Loss, or Suicide*. Bolton Press, Atlanta.

Cerel J, Fristad MA, Weller EB et al. (1999). Suicide-bereaved children and adolescents: a controlled longitudinal examination. *Journal of the American Academy of Child and Adolescent Psychiatry*, **38**, 672–679.

Colt GH (1991). *The Enigma of Suicide*. Summit Books, New York.

Cvinar JG (2005). Do suicide survivors suffer social stigma: a review of the literature. *Perspectives in Psychiatric Care*, **41**, 14–21.

Dunne EJ (1992). Psychoeducational strategies for survivors of suicide. *Crisis*, **13**, 35–40.

Fine C (1999). *No Time to Say Goodbye*. Random House, New York.

Grad O (2006). How can we help survivors in a clinical practice? *Psychiatria Danubia*, **18**, 1–27.

Harwood D, Hawton K, Hope T et al. (2002). The grief experiences and need of bereaved relatives and friends of older people dying through suicide: a descriptive and case control study. *Journal of Affective Disorders*, **72**, 189–194.

Jobes DA, Luoma JB, Hustead LA et al. (2000). In the wake of suicide: survivorship and postvention. In RW Maris, AL Berman, MM Silverman, eds, *Comprehensive Testbook of Suicidology*, pp. 536–561. Guilford, New York.

Rando TA (1993). *Treatment of Complicated Mourning*. Research Press, Champaign.

Sakinovsky I (2007). The aftermath of suicide: managing survivors' bereavement. *Canadian Journal of Psychiatry*, **52**, 129–136.

Seguin M (1995). Parental bereavement after suicide and accident: a comparative study. *Suicide and Life-Threatening Behaviour*, **25**, 489–494.

# CHAPTER 83

# Therapists as survivors of suicide loss

Onja T Grad

## Abstract

When a patient in an inpatient or outpatient setting—whether in therapy or after ending it—commits suicide, this act provokes a lot of distressful feelings in their therapist. Besides very personal reactions of shock, grief and regret, therapists often feel guilt, failure and incompetence connected to their professional performance. They are afraid of being blamed by their colleagues and/or of legal litigation from the family of the deceased. If they work in an institution they fear how the management will react to this event. Therapists need help and support, preferably in a form of standardized procedure, which is also presented in this chapter.

## Introduction

> The emotions were far too numerous to be documented here, but the one that stands out in my mind is the pervasive feeling I had of being alone. I was going to be standing on my own, a virtual child in the very adult world of psychology.
> Spiegelman and Werth (2005, p. 38)

> How can you be strong and meet the community needs when you want to disappear into some dark hole and weep a river of tears?
> Fleming (1997, p. 133)

If a patient who is, or used to be, in any kind of therapy commits suicide, the event makes his/her therapist a suicide survivor. Even though suicide is characterized as being both an occupational and predictable hazard (Chemtob *et al.* 1989; Valente 2003), it has nevertheless proven to be an ordeal for the therapists (Kleespies *et al.* 1990), what's more, quite damaging (Farberow 2001; Dexter-Mazza and Freeman 2003), and with a tremendous and long-lasting effect on every caregiver. Litman, in one of the first articles on the topic (1965), believes that a client's suicide represents a crisis for the therapist, both professionally and personally. He claims that the professional role serves the caregiver as a defensive and reparative function to help overcome the pain which they feel as a human being. The longer therapists practice their clinical work, the more likely it is that they will experience this anxiety-provoking event; studies show that 97 per cent of clinicians fear a client's suicide (Pope and Tabachnik 1993). The numbers of caregivers who confirm having survived their patient's suicide vary according to studies, from 22 per cent (Dexter-Mazza and Freeman 2003) to 47 or 50 per cent (Cryan *et al.* 1995; Hendin *et al.* 2000), to as much as 68 per cent (Alexander *et al.* 2000). It is even more disturbing if a patient's suicide happens in the formative years of a trainee, whether they be a future psychiatrist, clinical psychologist, psychiatric registered nurse, or other health professional. Some authors found that patient suicide happens to one-third of residents (Ellis *et al.* 1998), while others claimed up to 61 per cent (Pilkinton and Etkin 2003), representing a large number of future professionals only just starting their working career.

Every suicide has a profound effect on the immediate environment. Not only family and friends, but many others who were in personal or professional contact with the suicidal person, can be seriously affected. Therapists, consultants, supervisors, nurses, social workers, family physicians, and many other caregivers involved will most likely be disturbed, frightened and influenced by the patient's fatal decision. If a patient dies of a cardiovascular or some other malignant disease, the death is both expected and accepted, and the various caregivers see little or no personal involvement in it. Suicide, though often strongly connected to the outcome of certain diseases (such as depression), can easily be interpreted as the therapist's unfinished business and responsibility. In comparison to other deaths, suicide is perceived as an unnatural and avoidable death, one which the therapist was closely connected to and should have been able to prevent. This is a standpoint strongly held by the family, society and, especially, by therapists themselves. Litman (1965) refers to this as a 'taboo area of psychology', which is probably the crucial reason why the topic was almost untouched for so many years. While suicide has been studied since the beginning of humankind, only within the past 50 years has attention been turned towards bereaved relatives of a family in which a suicide has occurred. Therapists as suicide survivors were neglected to an even greater extent throughout the development of suicidological research, even though the majority of patients who commit suicide had been in some kind of therapy (Gitlin 1999; Valente 2003).

Why so much avoidance to explore the subject? Brown (1987a, b) mentions four possible explanations:

1 Too great a burden of taking care of patients on the trainees, which might be jeopardized if the problems were revealed;

**2** Fear on the part of staff leaders that this disclosure might affect the morale of their team;

**3** The trainees themselves feel that the patient's suicide was partly their failure or even fault and are therefore reluctant to talk about it;

**4** There is a general difficulty of accepting any death of a patient, and especially so if it was self- inflicted.

The first written statement about the therapist's own reactions to a patient's suicide was by Freud, who articulated the suppressed feelings after the event had occurred to him (Litman 1965). For a long time afterwards there were few personal reflections from therapists and almost no studies on the topic. There are many reasons for this: suicide provokes strong feelings of failure in therapists and their supervisors or consultants; there is a fear of reactions from the patient's family, including legal litigation; and there is a belief among therapists and within their environment that they will be able to deal with the problem themselves (Grad and Michel 2005). However, therapists are neither prepared for, nor immune to, the disruptive impact of suicide on their professional belief system and on their professional standing (Brown 1987b; Dewar *et al.* 2000; Valente 2003).

## Therapist's reactions after a patient's suicide

'There is a terrible sense of failure at having let down those who have put their trust in you' (Alexander *et al.* 2000, p. 1572). When a patient commits suicide, the therapist can be notified about the disastrous event in many different, sometimes disturbing ways: some receive the news from the family of the patient, some are informed first thing when coming to work, some come across the obituary, and some only find out about the suicide when the patient does not show up for the therapy session. Regardless of how the information is received, it first provokes shock and disbelief in the therapist, just as it does in anyone close to the deceased suicidal person (Chemtob *et al.* 1988a; Kleespies 1993; Grad 1996; Hendin *et al.* 2000, 2004).

In most of the studies, therapists reported that they had experienced various emotional reactions on a very personal level. Their most frequently experienced feelings were: grief, feelings of betrayal and anger towards the patient, guilt, fear of blame, embarrassment, self-doubt, inadequacy, shame (Michel 1997; Grad *et al.* 1997; Grad and Zavasnik 1998; Hendin *et al.* 2000; Grad and Michel 2005), anger towards the patient or the consultant (Chemtob *et al.* 1989), denial and avoidance, fear of being accused of negligence (Yousaf *et al.* 2002), fears of litigation and retribution from the psychiatric community (Gitlin 1999), and, especially in younger therapists who were still in training, anxiety (Kleespies 1993). All these reactions were connected to many factors regarding therapy and the bond between the therapist and the patient, such as: how long and how closely the therapist had worked with the patient; the therapist's degree of professional commitment (Litman 1965); how much anger and hostility was involved in the relationship (Jones 1987); the level of predictability of suicide; the method and location of suicide; the emotional involvement with the patient (Valente 1994); the therapist's countertransference with the patient; the setting in which they were working with the patient (private or institutional); whether the therapist

was the only one responsible for the patient or whether the patient's treatment was the responsibility of a team; whether the therapist was at the beginning of their career or an experienced one; whether the therapist had constant supervision for that specific therapy or not (Grad 1996). It is also very important whether the therapist, their consultant and the whole team have an explanation for the patient's suicide. Motto (1979), in one of the pioneering articles on the topic, stresses two issues: first, the importance of the therapist's own current life cycle (they can be faced with thier own mortality for the first time, or once again after some time), and second, the therapist's theoretical, philosophical and clinical backgrounds at the time of a patient's suicide. It is equally important to know that the therapist's personality (Hendin *et al.* 2004), his\her therapist's personalites own previously experienced losses and his\her therapist's personalites age and gender (Grad *et al.* 1997) play a significant role in determining his\her therapist's personalites feelings and reactions 'after'.

Similar emotional reactions of a therapist after a patient's suicide were reported in most of the studies and thus seem to be quite expected and universal. On the affective level the most frequent and painful feelings therapists experienced were guilt, sadness and incompetence (Kolodny *et al.* 1979; Jones 1987; Grad *et al.* 1997; Hendin *et al.* 2000; Valente 2003; Hendin *et al.* 2004), which were closely connected to the cognitive feelings of fear of blame, litigation and loss of professional standing (Chemtob *et al.* 1988b). Both grief and guilt reflected the close relationship with the patient, but also the fear that the relatives (feeling guilty as well) would sue the therapist or the institution. This generalized fear may provoke unfavourable and unhelpful reactions from the administrative staff, additionally burdening the therapist.

Many studies proved that experiencing the suicide of a patient is more difficult when the therapist is still in training (Ellis and Dickey 1998; Yousaf *et al.* 2002; Dexter-Mazza and Freeman 2003; Ruskin *et al.* 2004). It is true that the trainee has limited legal responsibilities, but otherwise they function as a competent and fully responsible therapist who treats the patient on their own. The trainee's emotional reactions are similar to those described by the more experienced therapists, only more severe and with long-lasting effects. Trainees are not adequately prepared for such an event happening to them and they are not warned of the impact it might have on them (Pilkinton and Etkin 2003). They are poorly prepared to deal with suicidal patients. Furthermore, there is a substantial difference between informational or knowledge competence with regard to risk factors and the demographics of suicide and the actual ability to effectively manage or treat the suicidal patients (Dexter-Mazza and Freeman 2003). As trainees are not yet permanently and closely intertwined into a clinical team, with which they work at the time of suicide, they can feel less support from the colleagues when the tragic event occurs. It has been proved that the impact of a patient's suicide was more severe for those trainees who perceived less social integration in their professional network (Ruskin *et al.* 2004).

There were some differences found between male and female therapists (Grad and Michel 1994; Grad *et al.* 1997) when experiencing a patient's suicide. While female respondents (75 per cent) predominantly preferred to vent their feelings, their male colleagues helped themselves either by going on with work as usual (30 per cent) or talking about their feelings (30 per cent). As most leading positions in mental health in Western settings are held by men, it is possible that they prefer the working routine to stay unchanged after suicide in their environment occurs. Which then implicitly influences the people, men and women, working underneath them, having to deal with the situation in a similar fashion.

Experiencing and surviving a patient's suicide entails, along with many negative outcomes, some beneficial ones as well (Courtenay and Stephens 2001). One beneficial (or formative) outcome has been described by therapists as learning from the experience to develop more thorough and comprehensive risk assessment skills in the formative years. One of the studies (Hendin *et al.* 2004) has found that the less distressed therapists had a greater capacity to view their misfortunes as learning opportunities rather than as occasions for self-reproach. Negative outcomes were many: the therapists felt isolated, disillusioned, and vulnerable, they were lacking confidence and/or they became afraid of clinical contact.

Most of the described feelings and behaviour patterns were obtained from the respondents inside the psychiatric and psychological field; however, the reactions described by the general practitioners, who had treated suicidal patients were very similar. Compared to psychotherapists, family doctors did not differ in feelings of grief; they also became more cautious with other patients after experiencing a patient's suicide, and they spoke less with colleagues and friends about the event than did psychotherapists. They also differed significantly in other ways: they reported feeling a lesser amount of guilt, they used the supervisor's help less frequently, and they had more difficulties in revealing their feelings after the event to their colleagues (though this is probably indicative of the attitudes and culture in both groups) (Grad and Zavasnik 1998).

## Helpful and unhelpful procedures

Whenever the suicide of a patient occurs, therapists are in need of post-traumatic debriefing and various other procedures, some self-chosen and some prescribed. The procedure should give the therapist the space and time they need for support, understanding and a forum for expressing and accepting their different feelings.

### Helpful procedures

Brown (1987a) proposes a few steps: any therapist working with suicidal patients should have been prepared in advance for the possibility of experiencing a completed suicide of one of their patients. Afterwards, it is necessary to share the responsibility, talk about one's own feelings and fears, perform the psychological autopsy and agree on the procedure concerning the relatives.

Basically there are three different needs to be fulfilled after a patient's suicide (Ellis and Dickey 1998): administrative needs that monitor the occurrence of adverse patient events in order to improve quality; educational needs that take care of the level of suicide-related training (Midence *et al.* 1996) and provide supervision to each trainee; and emotional needs that support any therapist in distress after the trauma of patient suicide.

It seems that while administrative and possibly also educational needs are often fulfilled, the emotional needs can become a problem both from the side of the institution and that of the therapist. This might be the reason why there are many different suggestions in the literature on how to organize help. All the respondents in the different studies agreed that therapists should have had a chance to express themselves afterwards and that any support was helpful

and appreciated (Courtenay and Stephens 2001). However, the proposed procedures about how to achieve this varied. Some authors claimed that even the participation in the study and the interview helped the participants to further process their feelings (Kleespies *et al.* 1993). Most respondents in the range of studies mentioned that talking to family and friends, to the close team of colleagues, individual colleagues and to consultants or supervisors was most helpful (Chemtob *et al.* 1989; Grad *et al.* 1997; Grad and Zavasnik 1998; Alexander *et al.* 2000; Valente 2003). This can be done in special supervisor–therapist meetings or group meetings, where the therapist can tell their story about the patient; alternatively, it can be done by writing a narrative—whichever suits them best (Valente 2003). Some authors propose 'away days' (Walmsley 2003). Reviews of the case or psychological autopsies can be helpful if they are geared towards learning rather than blaming (Alexander *et al.* 2000). At the same time, however, other authors think that institutional responses and case reviews are rarely helpful (Hendin *et al.* 2000). One message that is clearly useful is that therapists' fantasies of having ultimate control over patient's lives should be limited (Gitlin 1999).

### Unhelpful procedures

When suicide occurs in any institution, it provokes many fears, not only among clinicians, but among the management as well. This often results in some legal, disciplinary proceedings, which may add to, rather than diminish, the already existing distress of the medical staff and the therapist. We are living in a 'blame culture' (Alexander *et al.* 2000), where scapegoating and witch hunting are not rare even in academic circles. If psychological autopsies add to self-doubts and distress of the therapist (Goldstein and Buongiorno 1984) and evolve in public shaming, they seem to be counterproductive. In this respect, publicity in the media—especially sensationalist reporting—is additionally distressing for the therapist (Alexander *et al.* 2000).

Some authors found that outside counsellors, who have been drafted in to assist, are considered unhelpful (Courtenay and Stephens 2001); others, meanwhile, have proposed that an independent institution come in to help in the case of a patient's suicide (Hendin *et al.* 2000). In light of these contradictory statements, it is obvious that planning any help in advance that would be universally useful is a difficult, if not impossible, job. Perhaps it is wiser to prepare a framework of procedures and then listen to the survivor's needs or the needs of the team that experienced the patient's suicide to fill the framework with their contents.

## A proposed protocol

Proposing any particular protocol that would be useful for every therapist and every team of different caregivers would be a daring act. The therapist's bereavement after a patient has committed suicide is too individual and too personal to fit into a framework of rigid procedures.

In consideration of the above, every protocol should nevertheless include:

1  Compulsory part:
   ♦ Organize a meeting for everybody who dealt with the patient to gather and talk—either about the patient, the treatment or the therapist themself;

- Appoint a supervisor (insider, outsider) to lead the debriefing, and to decontaminate the atmosphere of blame and self-blame;
- Appoint a consultant (one person or a board of specialists in the field) to listen to the patient's history and treatment (go through the chart), and try to find a common understanding of the suicidal act;
- Take the required legal and administrative actions;
- Give clear instructions concerning contact with patient's relatives, about the funeral, how to inform and help other patients (if necessary), etc.

2 Offered, but self-chosen part:

- Offer the therapist time and a setting to acknowledge, express and understand their own feelings;
- Offer the therapist the chance to be counselled (or supervised) by a colleague or a consultant;
- Allow the therapist time off work or off specific responsibilities if the therapist expresses this wish;
- Facilitate bereavement and normalize this behaviour;
- Limit the therapist's fantasies of having ultimate control over patient's lives (Gitlin 1999), every suicide is a decision made by the patient themself;
- Offer counselling if long-term effects appear—insecurity, quicker hospitalization of suicidal patients, not accepting suicidal patients in treatment, burnout syndrome, and even change of career.

Both parts are equally important, but deciding how to combine them is a matter for each individual therapist and institution (Grad 2005). Indeed, when a therapist (similarly to the bereaved relative) works through the feelings and thoughts after the loss of a patient, he may gain in wisdom and experience on how to treat well but also how to accept different consequences better.

## Conclusion

Experiencing a patient's suicide is a rite of passage for each therapist: 'to survive it is testimony to one's hardiness, endurance, and being a real physician' (Gitlin 1999, p. 1630).

It is necessary to think about 'before and after'. Rule number one is to offer good training programmes for the trainees in psychiatry, psychology and nursing that prepare future clinicians for the real work with a suicidal patient. If they do experience a patient's suicide (and they probably will, as this is an inevitable occupational hazard of working with selected suicidal population), every institution should prepare a flexible postvention protocol to support and serve the individual needs of the therapist and diminish their feelings of being socially isolated from their colleagues. The best solution would be to achieve a balance between prescribed, compulsory, formal procedures, which will serve administrative and educational needs of the therapist and the institution, and the self-chosen, more informal ones that offer the therapists the most appropriate and convenient form to accept this difficult experience in their professional life.

## References

Alexander DA, Klein S, Gray NM *et al.* (2000). Suicide by patients: questionnaire study of its effect on consultant psychiatrists. *British Medical Journal*, **320**, 1571–1574.

Brown HN (1987a). The impact of suicide on therapists in training. *Comprehensive Psychiatry*, **28**, 101–112.

Brown HN (1987b). Patient suicide during residency training: Incidence, implications and program response. *Journal of Psychiatric Education*, **11**, 201–216.

Chemtob CM, Hamada RS, Bauer G *et al.* (1988a). Patients' suicides: frequency and impact on psychiatrists. *American Journal of Psychiatry*, **145**, 224–228.

Chemtob CM, Hamada RS, Bauer G *et al.* (1988b). Patient suicide: frequency and impact on psychologists. *Professional Psychology Research and Practice*, **19**, 416–420.

Chemtob CM, Bauer G, Hamada RS *et al.* (1989). Patient suicide: occupational hazard for psychologists and psychiatrists. *Professional Psychology Research and Practice*, **20**, 294–300.

Courtenay KP and Stephens JP (2001). The experience of patient suicide among trainees in psychiatry. *Psychiatric Bulletin*, **25**, 51–52.

Cryan EMJ, Kelly P, McCaffrey B (1995). The experience of patient suicide among trainees in psychiatry. *Psyhiatric Bulletin*, **19**, 4–7.

Dexter-Mazza ET and Freeman KA (2003). Graduate training and the treatment of suicidal clients: the student's perspective. *Suicide and Life-Threatening Behaviour*, **33**, 211–218.

Dewar I, Eagles J, Klein S *et al.* (2000). Psychiatric trainees' experiences of, and reactions to, patient suicide. *Psychiatric Bulletin*, **24**, 20–23.

Ellis TE and Dickey TO (1998). Procedures surrounding the suicide of a trainee's patient: a national survey of psychology internships and psychiatry residency programs. *Professional Psychology Research and Practice*, **29**, 492–497.

Ellis TE, Dickey TO, Jones EC (1998). Patient suicide in psychiatry residency programs: a national survey of training and postvention practices. *Academic Psychiatry*, **22**, 181– 89.

Farberow NL (2001). The therapist-clinician as survivor. In OT Grad, ed., *Suicide Risk and Protective Factors in the New Millennium*, pp. 11–21. Cankarjev dom, Ljubljana.

Fleming G (1997). The isolated medical proactitioner. *Crisis*, **18**, 132–133.

Gitlin MJ (1999). A psychiatrist's reaction to a patient's suicide. *American Journal of Psychiatry*, **156**, 1630–1634.

Goldstein LS and Buongiorno PA (1984). Psychotherapists as suicide survivors. *American Journal of Psychotherapy*, **38**, 392–398.

Grad OT (1996). Suicide—how to survive as a survivor. *Crisis*, **17**, 136–142.

Grad OT (2005). Suicide of a patient: what do we need? *Book of Abstracts, XXIII: World Congress of International Association of Suicide Prevention*, p. 40. Durban, South Africa.

Grad OT and Michel K (1994). Losing a patient by suicide: a male–female perspective. *Fourth International Conference on Grief and Bereavement in Contemporary Society*, p. 136. Swedish National Association for Mental Health, Stockholm.

Grad OT and Michel K (2005). Therapists as client suicide survivors. In K Weiner, ed., *Therapeutic and Legal Issues for Therapists who have Survived a Client Suicide*, pp. 71–81. The Haworth Press, Binghamton.

Grad OT, Zavasnik A, Groleger U (1997). Suicide of a patient: gender differences in bereavement reactions of therapists. *Suicide and Life-Threatening Behaviour*, **27**, 379–386.

Grad OT and Zavasnik A (1998). The caregivers' reactions after suicide of a patient. In RJ Kosky, HS Eshkevari, RD Goldney *et al.*, eds, *Suicide Prevention—The Global Context*, pp. 287–291. Plenum Press, New York.

Hendin H, Lipschitz A, Maltsberger JT *et al.* (2000). Therapists' reactions to patients' suicides. *American Journal of Psychiatry*, **157**, 2022–2027.

Hendin H, Pollinger Hass A, Maltsberger JT *et al.* (2004). Factors contributing to therapist's distress after the suicide of a patient. *American Journal of Psychiatry*, **161**, 1442–1446.

Jones FA (1987). Therapists as survivors of client suicide. In EJ Dunne, JL McIntosh and K Dunne-Maxim, eds, *Suicide and its Aftermath*, pp. 126–141. Norton, New York.

Kleespies PM, Smith R, Becker BR (1990). Psychology interns as patient suicide survivors: incidence, impact and recovery. *Professional Psychology Research and Practice*, **21**, 257–263.

Kleespies PM (1993). The stress of patient suicidal behaviour: implications for interns and training programs in psychology. *Professional Psychology Research and Practice*, **24**, 477–482.

Kolodny S, Binder RL, Bronstein AA *et al.* (1979). The working through of patients' suicides by four therapists. *Suicide and Life-Threatening Behaviour*, **9**, 33–46.

Litman RE (1965). When patients commit suicide. *American Journal of Psychiatry*, **19**, 570–576.

Michel K (1997). After suicide: who counsels the therapist? *Crisis*, **18**, 128–130.

Midence K (1996). The effects of patient suicide on nursing staff. *Journal of Clinical Nursing*, **5**, 115–120.

Motto JA (1979). The impact of patient suicide on the therapist's feelings. *Weekly Psychiatry Update Series*, **3**, 7.

Pilkinton P and Etkin M (2003). Encountering suicide: the experience of psychiatric residents. *Academic Psychiatry*, **27**, 93–99.

Pope K and Tabachnik B (1993). Therapists' anger, hate, fear and sexual feelings: national survey of therapist responses, client characteristics, critical events, formal complaints, and training. *Professional Psychology Research and Practice*, **24**, 142–153.

Ruskin R, Sakinofsky I, Bagby RM *et al.* (2004). Impact of patient suicide on psychiatrists and psychiatric trainees. *Academic Psychiatry*, **28**, 104–110.

Spiegelman JS and Werth JL (2005). Don't forget about me: the experiences of therapists-in-training after a client has attempted or died by suicide. *Women & Therapy*, **28**, 35–57.

Valente SM (1994). Psychotherapists reactions to the suicide of a patient. *American Journal of Orthopsychiatry*, **64**, 614–621.

Valente SM (2003). Aftermath of a patient's suicide: a case study. *Perspectives in Psychiatric Care*, **39**, 17–22.

Walmsley P (2003). The patient suicide and its effect on staff. *Nursing Management*, **10**, 1–3.

Yousaf F, Hawthorne M, Sedgwick P (2002). Impact of patient suicide on psychiatric trainees. *Psychiatric Bulletin*, **26**, 53–55.

# CHAPTER 84

# How to help survivors of suicide loss

Franz Baro, Arlette J Ngoubene-Atioky, Jan Toye and Marc Vande Gucht

## Abstract

Survivors, i.e. relatives and friends of persons who have died by suicide, experience a plethora of emotional and societal difficulties. Due to the complicated nature of grieving in the aftermath of a suicide, emotional and social support to survivors can only ameliorate the life functioning of this population. The present chapter outlines therapeutic resources that will be beneficial to this unique group. Therapeutic groups, and many other group-related activities, have been established to assist survivors of suicide. Descriptive information with regards to these groups and how to create them is provided. The chapter ends with recommendations on additional resources and services for survivors of suicide.

## Introduction

Complicated grieving is defined as the emotional state of an individual who suffers from a loss due to crisis-related circumstances (e.g. depression, anxiety, cancer, etc.). Suicide is among contextual factors that clearly undermine the grieving process. Survivors of suicide suffer from a series of emotional sequelae following the traumatic, and sometimes rapid, death of their loved ones. Survivors of suicide are at risk for depression, suicidal ideation, anxiety, and negative existential values (Mitchell *et al.* 2005; Zisook and Kendler 2007 ; Sveen and Walby 2008).

In addition to common bereavement symptoms such as confusion, sadness, guilt, and anger, survivors of suicide may have recurrent rumination of a plausible avoidance of the suicidal act. They may also blame themselves for the suicidal act, and believe the cause of, or lead the deceased to commit suicide. Some survivors of suicide may perceive the suicide as a tangible expression of rejection from the deceased (Sveen and Walby 2008). If the deceased is a family member (e.g. a child), the homeostasis of the family is likely to be disrupted. Anguish may be experienced, especially if the deceased was the primary caregiver or the principal source of familial income (Hopmeyer and Werk 1994). Feelings of shame over societal stigma of suicide may also be present (Ellenbogen and Gratton 2001). These feelings of shame may be accentuated by the survivor's age and/or cultural affiliation. Children and adolescent survivors of suicide are more likely to take responsibility for the suicide than adult survivors of suicide. Children and adolescent survivors of suicide are also more at risk for major depressive disorder, post-traumatic stress disorder, and impaired social adjustment (Sethi and Barghava 2003). Moreover, in certain religions, such as Catholicism, suicide may be perceived as a sin, which may bring shame and desolation to survivors. Ultimately, the cultural identity of the family determines the intensity and evolution of the grieving process, as well as the emanation and severity of the aforementioned bereavement symptoms (Stack 1998).

Due to the sudden and traumatic nature of suicide, emotional assistance becomes fundamental to survivors. This chapter provides an overview of best practice for psychological and emotional assistance for survivors of suicide, with a strong emphasis on group-related assistance. We will first delineate common psychological and emotional assistance that is currently available to this population, followed by practical resources considered to be of the utmost benefit to them.

## Therapeutic services

Literature differentiates emotional support provided to survivors of suicide into two categories: individual and group support. Groups are facilitated by professionals, peers, or experienced individuals (Parkes 1972). The individual is conceptualized as belonging to a spherical social environment and emotional assistance follows a systematic theoretical orientation (Raphael 1983). The individual is placed at the centre of this social sphere, and is influenced by immediate and remote contextual factors. Due to the crisis-related circumstance of the loss, survivors are, therefore, in need of immediate and remote members of their social realms in order to cope and move beyond their grief (Bronfenbrenner 1977; De Clerq and Dubois 2001). Provision of support from one's social sphere is empowering.

Feminist and humanistic ideas of empowerment, and unconditional positive regard, have also been therapeutic orientations employed with survivors of suicide (World Health Organization 2000). The ultimate goal is to provide a community-based environment in which survivors will gain support, disclose their emotional burden, and finally, be able to live a well-functioning life.

The cultural identity of the survivor determines the type of resources that will be employed to recover their loss (Andriessen 2004).

## Individual therapy

Professional support mostly consists of individual or group therapy, which is facilitated by an accredited mental health professional, e.g. psychologist, psychiatrist, social worker, or licensed therapist/ counsellor. Individual therapy for adults usually serves as a transition to group therapy, especially for survivors not ready for group interactions. Individual therapy may provide survivors with some needed additional one-on-one support; support that they may seek due to the deleterious consequences that suicide may have on an entire family. Individual therapy becomes a place to re-evaluate and disclose issues outside of the familial realm, a place where the survivors may feel more comfortable disclosing particular issues. Individual therapy may be appropriate for survivors of suicide whose pre-existing mental health condition was worsened by the complicated grief. Individual therapy is also generally warranted for individuals who do not feel comfortable participating in group interactions.

Special consideration should be given to the young population, whose developmental stage determines the emerging bereavement symptoms, as well as the appropriateness of services provided. Some children may be too young to openly express their emotional reaction, or to comprehend the nature and circumstances of suicide. The therapeutic intervention does not lie in how to hide the suicidal act from the child, but rather how suicide is explained and appropriately processed (Cain 2002). Due to the societal stigma of suicide, parents or loved ones may be inclined to conceal the cause of death from the child (Sveen and Walby 2008). Although controversy exists with regard to this matter, it is usually recommended that the child be informed of the circumstance of the death; however, providing specific details regarding the suicidal act should be avoided. Some studies reveal the benefit of informing children of the suicidal act rather than hiding it (Cain and Fast 1966; Cain 2002). It is believed that significant harm is done when the child is not allowed to properly grieve the death of a loved one. Grieving is, indeed, a significant part of living; the sudden death of loved ones ascertains some psycho-education, which implies the education of survivors of suicide on practical ways to cope with their grief, life, suicide, and the grieving process. The use of simple culturally appropriate terms rather than psychological or adult jargon to explain the suicide of a parent or a loved one is essential (Cain 2002). Therapy also focuses on allowing the child to reconstruct themself, through drawing or telling small stories. Narrative or play therapy is, therefore, strongly recommended for these groups that are still unable to appropriately describe their emotional state. Child survivors of suicide would also be reassured that most of the practical needs fulfilled by the deceased will be met and provided by close loved ones (Cain 2002). Suicide prevention is also critical for this population, as it serves to halt the perpetuation of a suicidal act within a social circle. Research does indicate a higher prevalence of mental health disorders in survivors who are relatives or close loved ones of the deceased by suicide (Sveen and Walby 2008).

## Group therapy

Although individual therapy can be beneficial, it has mostly been in conjunction with group therapy, as it is perceived to be critical for survivors to go back to a seemingly normal lifestyle. The term *therapeutic group* applies to a set of individuals, whose:

> broad purpose [is to increase] people's knowledge of themselves and others, assisting people to clarify the changes they most want to make in their own life, and giving people some of the tools necessary to make these desired changes.
>
> Corey and Corey (1987)

Due to potential derogatory perceptions of the word *therapy*, and its sometimes non-applicability worldwide, other terms such as group discussions, group narratives, group coping, or spiritual groups may be more culturally appropriate. Nonetheless, all these terms are synonymous with therapeutic group, as these groups all serve to support and assist the survivors of suicide.

In a study by Hopmeyer and Werk (1994), adult participants who attended self-help or peer support-type of bereavement groups reported an overall satisfaction with regards to the support they received. Although minimal studies exist on the benefit of child survivors support groups, the few studies that have examined these groups denote a decrease in anxiety and depressive symptoms among participants (Pfeiffer *et al.* 2002; Mitchell *et al.* 2007). Social isolation and loneliness are quite common among survivors of suicide (Moore 1995). Group therapy allows for a gradual transition, because of the pseudo-societal reality formed within group sessions.

Therapeutic groups rely on interpersonal relationships to address and overcome grief. Most groups follow Yalom's (1995) theory on group therapy. Yalom ascertained that groups provided a safe pseudo-reality environment where survivors of suicide were able to disclose complex emotions, receive, and reciprocate positive and empowering feedback. Yalom recommended an average of 6–10 members in the 2-hour time period of each group interaction. Groups are either structured (with a predetermined agenda for each session) or unstructured, which implies that members are in charge of the themes of each group session. They may be open, allowing inclusion of additional group members at any given time, or closed, with a set number of group members from beginning to end. All groups are facilitated by one or two experienced mediators. The facilitator does not lead or moderate group discussions; the facilitator's role is to intervene and participate in extreme situations. Maintenance of confidentiality, civility, and all the predetermined rules of the group is upheld by the facilitator. The facilitator also holds experiential and practical knowledge with regards to suicide and survivors' experiences. Yalom denoted the facilitator's role in providing some practical and educational information to group members; however, group interaction was believed to be the primary source of healing.

Certain groups, however, hold a strong psycho-educational focus, while others only incorporate group interaction and self-disclosures. The overall nature and atmosphere of the group is mostly determined by the group facilitator and the group members. Different types of groups may therefore emerge: most groups that are believed beneficial to survivors of suicide are self-help/peer-related groups (Moore 1995). These groups are facilitated by either an experienced survivor of suicide, or a professional with experience in complicated grief. Groups may be psycho-educational, which implies educating survivors of suicide on practical ways to cope with their grief, or peer-related, where survivors manage the agenda and the overall evolution of the group.

Mitchell *et al.* (2003) offers a comprehensive description of the application of narrative theory in a therapeutic group for survivors of suicide: narrative therapeutic groups mostly consist of the use of life stories as therapeutic tools for healing. Rituals and any other culturally appropriate ways of grieving may apply in peer support group. Peer support may be appropriate for survivors of a collective suicide. France is currently seeing the emergence of collective (group) suicide within its youth (France Television 2008). Survivors of a same collective suicide may reunite and help each other cope with their collective loss. Constantino *et al.* (2001) examined the effectiveness of post-vention groups for widowed survivors of suicide: group members reported a significant decrease in depression, psychological distress, and grief. A significant improvement in social adjustment was also observed. Hence, in peer-related groups, the nature, duration, and specific tasks of the group will be moderated by group members, whose expertise and knowledge in a particular culture will be critical to the positive therapeutic process and outcome of the group.

## Practical resources

The World Health Organization (2000) reports that traditional self-help groups are predominant in English-speaking countries; and other non-traditional therapeutic resources may be available to survivors originating from non-English speaking areas. Andriessen (2004) reports a prevalence of services in north-western and mid-European regions, countries such as Belgium, France, Ireland, Norway, Sweden, and the UK have the largest number of services available to survivors of suicide. In countries where limited resources are available, it becomes critical to provide a model of how to set up self-help groups that would be beneficial to regional survivors of suicide. Literature denotes several critical factors to consider when any individual, organization, or network is interested in establishing a support group for survivors of suicide (Moore 1995; WHO 2000; Andriessen 2004):

- *Knowledge of survivors of suicide and personal health*: what is your experience and knowledge on this topic? How aware are you of the community resources available to survivors of suicide? Do you have good conflict resolution skills? Do you have previous experience in leading a group? Do you consider yourself emotionally capable of creating such group? It is recommended that the facilitator seeks supervision prior to the creation of the group to ensure readiness and capacity to venture in group facilitation.

- *Primary goal and duration of the group*: determine your target population: family, widowed, or women survivors of suicide. Is it a transition group or a group that will accompany each member through all stages of grief? Is there a predetermined termination of the group: weeks, months, years?

- *Structure of the group*: is it a closed or an open group? Is it a structured or unstructured group? Is it a psycho-educational or disclosure-focused group? What would be the length of time of the group meetings? How frequently will group members meet?

- *Preliminary procedure*: how are members recruited? Are there any specific screening procedures to select and admit members into the group? What are the pre-existing rules or code of ethics that you believe need to be respected by each group member before the beginning of the group sessions?

- *Cultural underlying factors that may influence group dynamics and group process*: what is the cultural background of group members? If members originate from the same community, what cultural factors are critical to consider in situation of complicated grief? What cultural factors will influence the name of the group, the group process and its outcome? What culturally appropriate interventions will it be critical to implement in group sessions?

- *Location of group meetings*: consideration of confidentiality and each member's comfort will need to be taken. Would the group sessions occur in an office, in a park, or in a house?

- *The nature and personality of group members*: group discussion will demand the participation and appreciation of civility, respect, and non-destructive manners. Are group members aware of their rights, privileges, and role in the group? Are group members prepared and advised with regards to the structure and evolution of therapeutic groups? Are group members functioning enough to participate in group discussion (no severe pre-existing mental health condition or limited social skills)?

Further resources and recommendations on how to establish a group for survivors of suicide is available in the 2000 Report on survivors of suicide from the WHO Department of Mental Health (WHO 2000).

## Network Resources

The establishment of support groups throughout a particular geographical location increases the likelihood of the establishment of national and international network for survivors of suicide. International networks can only benefit survivors, as the sharing of valuable resources will further impact survivors' functioning. The International Network for Survivors of Suicide was founded in 2000, and many other national networks have also been established (Andriessen 2004). The World Health Organization (WHO) founded the WHO International Network for Suicide Prevention and Research, which seeks to increase awareness and prevention of suicide. Survivors of suicide, group facilitator, and local organization's enrolment and participation in these national and international networks will allow for a systematic provision of services to this community.

With the advance of technology, many forums and online networks have emerged to support survivors of suicide. These provide a cybernetic environment, where survivors receive practical advice, and are able to disclose and receive support anonymously. Some forums or networks are created specifically for a particular group of survivors of suicide (parents or widows, survivors of suicide). Although these boards can be beneficial, due to their online characteristics, caution must be taken to maintain confidentiality of users, as well as to ensure the active participation of users in real-life social activities. It is recommended that survivors of suicide visit official national networks, which have been established in Belgium, Germany, and many other European countries: a directory of available national services and additional reliable resources are available for survivors of suicide (Andriessen 2004). *Go for Happiness* is an example of social network available for Belgian survivors of suicide; it is a non-profit organization founded by survivors of suicide for the prevention of depression and suicide in young people.

Go for Happiness provides survivors of suicide an opportunity to volunteer and to advocate socially for the prevention of suicide, and works on the creation of a European platform in this field. Further resources for survivors of suicide include the circulation of several national newsletters published in France, Germany, and the UK; these newsletters can provide survivors and mental health professionals additional references and resources on survivors of suicide (Andriessen 2004).

## Conclusions

Due to the difficult contextual factors of suicide, survivors are in need of fundamental resources that will help them grieve, heal, and function. Group-related resources and support are believed essential to this population. The aforementioned resources are, therefore, basic services that have been shown to be beneficial to survivors of suicide. Caution must, however, be taken with regards to the applicability of some resources cross-nationally. It is therefore recommended to establish group support or network nationwide in order to ensure a better shaping of resources for survivors of suicide.

### References

Andriessen K (2004). Suicide survivor activities, an international perspective. *Suicidologi*, **9**, 26–31.

Bronfenbrenner U (1977). *The Ecology of Human Development*. Harvard University Press, Cambridge.

Cain AC (2002). Children of suicide: the telling and the knowing. *Psychiatry*, **65**, 124–136.

Cain AC and Fast I (1966). Children's disturbed reactions to parent suicide. *American Journal of Orthopsychiatry*, **36**, 873–880.

Constantino RE, Sekula L, Rubinstein EN (2001). Group intervention for widowed survivors of suicide. *Suicide and Life-Threatening Behaviour*, **31**, 428–441.

Corey MS and Corey G (1987). *Groups: Process and Practice*, p. 9. Brooks/Cole, Pacific Grove.

DeClerq M and Dubois V (2001). Crisis intervention model in the French-speaking countries. *Crisis*, **22**, 32–38.

Ellenbogen S and Gratton F (2001). Do they suffer more? Reflections on research comparing suicide survivors to other survivors. *Suicide and Life-Threatening Behaviour*, **3**, 83–90.

France Television (2008). *Tentative de suicide collectif via internet*. http://nord-pas-de-calais-picardie.france3.fr/info/43302794-fr.php

Go for Happiness (Ga voor Geluk) Foundation and NGO, Zwartschaapstraat 24, 1755 Gooik, Belgium. http://www.gavoorgeluk.be

Hopmeyer E and Werk A (1994). A comparative study of family bereavement groups. *Death Studies*, **18**, 243–256.

Mitchell AM, Gale DD, Garand L *et al.* (2003). The use of narrative data to inform the psychotherapeutic group process with suicide survivors. *Issues in Mental Health Nursing*, **24**, 91–106.

Mitchell AM, Wesner S, Garand L *et al.* (2007). A support group intervention for children bereaved by parental suicide. *Journal of Child and Adolescent Psychiatric Nursing*, **20**, 3–13.

Mitchell AQ, Kim Y, Prigerson HG *et al.* (2005). Complicated grief and suicidal ideation in adult survivors of suicide. *Suicide and Life-Threatening Behaviour*, **35**, 498–506.

Moore MM (1995). Counseling survivors of suicide: implications for group postvention. *The Journal for Specialists in Group Work*, **20**, 40–47.

Parkes M (1972). *Bereavement Studies of Grief in Adult Life*. Tavistock Press, London.

Pfeiffer C, Martins P, Mann J *et al.* (2002). Group interventions for children bereaved by the suicide of a relative. *Journal of the American Academy of Child and Adolescent Psychiatry*, **41**, 505–513.

Raphael B (1983). *The Anatomy of Bereavement*. Basic Books Inc., New York.

Sethi S and Bhargava S (2003). Child and adolescent survivors of suicide. *The Journal of Crisis Intervention and Suicide Prevention*, **24**, 4–6.

Stack S (1998). Gender, marriage, and suicide acceptability: a comparative analysis. *Sex Roles*, **38**, 501–520.

Sveen CA and Walby FA (2008). Suicide survivors' mental health and grief reactions: a systematic review of controlled studies. *Suicide and Life-Threatening Behaviour*, **38**, 13–29.

World Health Organization Department of Mental Health (2000). *Preventing Suicide: How to Start a Survivor's Group*. http://www.who.int/mental_health/media/en/61.pdf

Yalom ID (1995). *The Theory and Practice of Group Psychotherapy*. Basic Books, New York.

Zisook S and Kendler KS (2007). Is bereavement-related depression different than non-bereavement-related depression? *Psychological Medicine*, **37**, 779–794.

# Young People and Suicide

# CHAPTER 85

# Suicide on all the continents in the young

Alan Apter, Cendrine Bursztein, José M Bertolote, Alexandra Fleischmann and Danuta Wasserman

## Abstract

This chapter reviews the epidemiology of suicidal behaviours in young people in selected countries on the five continents. The chapter indicates that suicide is a global public health problem, and an issue of major concern in developing countries as much as it is in the well-studied developed parts of the world. Patterns of suicidal behaviours in the various continents have some similarities and some differences in aspects such as male:female ratio, cultural and societal risk factors and relative rates in different age groups. For example, in North America, Australia and New Zealand all indigenous populations show the same pattern of high suicidality. Also, after a long period of increasing rates among males in the West, there is now a significant drop in rates of young male suicides. In contrast to the other continents, Asia shows a unique pattern of higher suicide rates in young women compared to young men. Furthermore, a high use of self-poisoning with pesticides can be found in this part of the world.

## Introduction

Most of the research on suicidal behaviour among the young focuses on developed countries; these include European countries, the United States of America, Canada, Japan, New Zealand and Australia. Much less is known about the other parts of the world regarding epidemiology of suicidal behaviours, specific risk factors and special characteristics or methods of suicide.

Out of the 193 WHO Member States, only a hundred have available information on suicide in the age groups 5–14 and 15–24, by males and females. No countries provide anywhere near comprehensive data on non-fatal suicidal behaviours (see http://www.who.int/mental_health/prevention/suicide/country_reports/en/index.html).

Data on suicide rates from developing countries often simply do not exist (Wasserman et al. 2005). When available, figures on suicide are underestimated and are not reliable due to underreporting result of inefficient civil registration systems. There are also variations in coroners', doctors', and hospital practices when issuing death certificates. Additionally, there are differences in the extent to which family and friends may try to conceal the cause of death due to social stigma, religious sanctions, and legal and economic issues associated with suicide (Vijayakumar et al. 2005).

Few studies have compared suicidal behaviours cross-culturally in young people from diverse parts of the world. Data that do exist from developing countries point to clear differences between patterns of suicide in these countries when compared to developed countries. Various authors have suggested that these observed differences may be related to a variety of factors including population increases (Zhang 1998), cultural, religious, and legal attitudes toward suicide (Sartorius 1995; Kelleher et al. 1998; Ruzicka 1998), major political changes (Sartorius 1995), health service factors (Sartorius 1995), the role of acute stressors, personality traits (Phillips et al. 2002a) and socio-economic factors (Sartorius 1995).

In addition, there have not been as many psychological autopsy studies for the young, which allow a better understanding of the relationships between suicide and mental disorders, as there have been for adults. A review of the existing literature on young people points toward mood, substance-related, and disruptive behaviour disorders as being the disorders most frequently associated with completed suicides. However, as expected, most studies came from Western countries (Fleischmann et al. 2005).

Hence, the present chapter attempts to provide a preliminary review of the epidemiology of suicidal behaviours in young people in different countries, based on the World Health Organization (WHO) data and a literature review of electronic database (PUBMED). Information from the WHO database is regularly updated and was last accessed for this chapter during March 2008. Readers of this chapter can check on the WHO website for further update of the data (http://www.who.int/mental_health/prevention/suicide/country_reports/en/index.html).

For the reasons given above, the data on global suicide statistics in youth presented are unfortunately incomplete. Additionally, a great deal of data on suicide has not been collected systematically in various parts of the world. Thus, there is a lack of accurate figures concerning the spread of the problem of suicidal behaviours in youth in most developing countries in Africa, South and Central America, and Asia.

## Central and South America

In general, the suicide rates in this part of the world are quite low (see Table 85.1). Yet apart from some research conducted in

**Table 85.1** Youth suicide rates in selected countries by age and sex*

| Country | Year | Age 5–14 years | | | Age 15–24 years | | |
|---|---|---|---|---|---|---|---|
| | | M | F | All | M | F | All |
| Sri Lanka | 1991 | 3.0 | 2.0 | 2.5 | 59.0 | 42.0 | 71.5 |
| Russia | 2004 | 3.6 | 1.0 | 2.3 | 47.4 | 8.2 | 28.1 |
| Lithuania | 2004 | 2.7 | 0.5 | 1.6 | 42.9 | 7.4 | 25.5 |
| Finland | 2004 | 1.2 | 0.8 | 0.8 | 33.1 | 9.7 | 21.7 |
| New Zealand | 2000 | 1.0 | 0.3 | 0.7 | 30.4 | 5.7 | 18.2 |
| Latvia | 2004 | 1.6 | 0.0 | 0.8 | 21.9 | 4.0 | 13.1 |
| Poland | 2004 | 1.1 | 0.4 | 0.8 | 20.6 | 2.7 | 11.8 |
| Ireland | 2005 | 0.7 | 0.4 | 0.5 | 20.4 | 3.2 | 11.9 |
| Norway | 2004 | 0.0 | 1.0 | 0.5 | 20.3 | 7.3 | 14.0 |
| Argentina | 2003 | 1.1 | 0.7 | 0.9 | 19.2 | 5.5 | 12.4 |
| Canada | 2002 | 0.9 | 0.9 | 0.9 | 17.5 | 5.2 | 11.5 |
| Australia | 2003 | 0.5 | 0.5 | 0.5 | 17.4 | 3.6 | 10.7 |
| Chile | 2003 | 1.4 | 0.3 | 0.8 | 17.3 | 4.0 | 10.8 |
| Japan | 2004 | 0.4 | 0.4 | 0.4 | 16.9 | 8.4 | 12.8 |
| United States | 2002 | 0.9 | 0.3 | 0.6 | 16.5 | 2.9 | 9.9 |
| Austria | 2005 | 0.6 | 0.2 | 0.4 | 15.7 | 3.6 | 9.8 |
| Czech Republic | 2004 | 0.9 | 0.6 | 0.7 | 15.5 | 2.1 | 9.0 |
| China (Hong Kong SAR) | 2004 | 0.5 | 0.8 | 0.9 | 15.4 | 9.0 | 12.2 |
| Sweden | 2002 | 0.7 | 0.5 | 0.6 | 14.6 | 4.5 | 9.7 |
| Switzerland | 2004 | 0.2 | 0.0 | 0.1 | 14.5 | 4.9 | 9.8 |
| Hungary | 2003 | 1.4 | 0.0 | 0.7 | 14.4 | 3.4 | 9.0 |
| Thailand | 2002 | 0.6 | 0.5 | 0.6 | 13.8 | 3.8 | 8.9 |
| Ecuador | 2004 | 2.1 | 2.2 | 2.1 | 13.0 | 10.3 | 11.7 |
| France | 2003 | 0.7 | 0.2 | 0.4 | 12.5 | 3.7 | 8.1 |
| Singapore | 2003 | 0.8 | 0.8 | 0.8 | 12.2 | 8.9 | 10.5 |
| Republic of Korea | 2004 | 0.6 | 0.7 | 0.6 | 11.3 | 8.0 | 9.7 |
| Mauritius | 2004 | 0.0 | 0.0 | 0.0 | 11.2 | 5.2 | 8.2 |
| Israel | 2003 | 0.5 | 0.0 | 0.2 | 10.9 | 0.9 | 6.0 |
| Germany | 2004 | 0.4 | 0.2 | 0.3 | 10.5 | 2.7 | 6.7 |
| Mexico | 2003 | 0.8 | 0.5 | 0.7 | 10.1 | 2.8 | 6.4 |
| United Kingdom | 2004 | 0.1 | 0.0 | 0.1 | 8.0 | 2.3 | 5.2 |
| China (mainland, selected rural areas) | 1999 | 1.3 | 1.0 | 1.2 | 8.0 | 12.9 | 10.4 |
| Netherlands | 2004 | 0.7 | 0.2 | 0.5 | 7.3 | 2.6 | 5.0 |
| Brazil | 2004 | 0.3 | 0.3 | 0.3 | 6.9 | 2.4 | 4.6 |
| Italy | 2002 | 0.2 | 0.2 | 0.2 | 6.5 | 1.5 | 4.1 |
| Spain | 2004 | 0.5 | 0.1 | 0.3 | 6.4 | 2.1 | 4.3 |
| Portugal | 2003 | 0.0 | 0.0 | 0.0 | 5.6 | 1.6 | 3.7 |
| China (mainland, selected rural and urban areas) | 1999 | 0.9 | 0.8 | 0.8 | 5.4 | 8.6 | 6.9 |
| Greece | 2004 | 0.4 | 0.0 | 0.2 | 3.0 | 0.3 | 1.7 |
| China (mainland, selected urban areas) | 1999 | 0.5 | 0.4 | 0.4 | 3.0 | 4.1 | 3.5 |
| Philippines | 1993 | 0.0 | 0.0 | 0.0 | 2.7 | 2.7 | 2.7 |
| Peru | 2000 | 0.1 | 0.1 | 0.1 | 1.7 | 1.9 | 1.8 |
| Egypt | 1987 | 0.0 | 0.0 | 0.0 | 0.0 | 0.0 | 0.0 |

* Rank-ordered by 15–24 male suicide rates.

Source: World Health Organization (2008). Regularly updated by the WHO and last accessed 16 March 2008: http://www.who.int/mental_health/prevention/suicide/country_reports/en/index.html.

Mexico (published mostly in Spanish) and Brazil, data on suicidal behaviours in Central and South American countries are sparse, unreliable and out of date.

Data from Mexico points to important variations between states: the states with the highest suicide mortality were Campeche and Tabasco (9.68 and 8.47 per 100,000, respectively), and the lowest rates were seen in Chiapas and the state of Mexico (1.03 and 1.99 per 100,000, respectively). Over a decade, the greatest increase by age group was seen in women 11–19 years old (from 0.8 per 100,000 in 1990 to 2.27 per 100,000 in 2001). The largest increase in men also occurred among the 11–19 age group (from 2.6 per 100,000 in 1990 to 4.5 per 100,000 in 2001). There were changes in suicide methods, with hanging now being the method most frequently used by both men and women of all ages (Puentes-Rosas *et al.* 2004).

In Chile, a clear rise in the suicide rates in both males and females can clearly be seen when comparing data from 1995 and 2003: In 1995, the rates were 6.5 per 100,000, 11.3 for males and 1.7 for females. In 2003, a total rate of 10.4 per 100,000 was reported, 17.8 for males and 3.1 for females (WHO 2008). It is not clear if this significant increase is due to better reporting, or to a true increase in suicide in the Chilean population; moreover, specific trends of suicide in youth remain unclear.

Suicide in Brazil shows a total rate of 4.0 per 100,000 in the 15–24 age group, 6.0 for males and 2.0 for females (Mello-Santos *et al.* 2005).

Although suicide rates among young people are still relatively low, the increase has become a reason for great concern. Mello-Santos *et al.* (2005) show an alarming increase in suicide rates (1900 per cent) in the 15–24 male age group between 1980–2000 in Brazil. As portrayed in another study, in urban areas of Brazil, suicide is the sixth most frequent cause of death among young people, having increased by 42.8 per cent from 1979 to 1998 (De Souza *et al.* 2002). In a 20-year period, the suicide rate in this age range increased ten-fold, from 0.4 to 4.0. The greatest increase was seen among males, in whom it increased approximately 20 times (0.3 to 6.0). The increase in suicide among females aged 15–24 was approximately 4 times (from 0.5 to 2.0) (Mello-Santos *et al.* 2005).

A series of studies conducted in selected areas in Brazil show that the vast majority of young suicide victims had only primary schooling. However, in the last year, reports showed that there was a proportional drop in this group, with a rise in the proportion of young people with more schooling (De Souza *et al.* 2002).

Regarding gender in the general population, Brazilian studies confirm the tendency for a higher suicide rate among Brazilian males than among Brazilian females, at a ratio of 3:1 and in agreement with international studies (Krug *et al.* 1998; Bertolote and Fleischmann 2002). The average age of individuals committing suicide in Brazil has been decreasing in recent years, which is in keeping with the global tendency (Mello-Santos *et al.* 2005).

## North America and Europe

Mortality data from the WHO show that suicide rates of youth in Europe vary. There are very high rates in the Russian Federation and former Soviet states, along with Finland and Ireland (see Table 85.1). These countries have rates of youth suicide two to three times higher than the United States and Canada. On the other hand, countries in the Mediterranean region including Italy, Greece, Spain, Portugal, France and Israel show low youth suicide rates (see Table 85.1).

Israeli Arab children and adolescents display a lower incidence, compared to Jews: during 1996–2000, in the 15–24 age group the suicide rate was of 7.2 per 100,000 in Arab males and 0.9 in females, compared to a rate of 11.8 in Jewish males and 2 in females (Haklai *et al.* 2005). Although an increase has been observed over the past decade in Arab adolescents, the rates are still much lower than for the Jewish population (Morad *et al.* 2005).

In the United States, rates of attempted and completed suicide are especially high among young Native Americans (Wallace *et al.* 1996; Borowsky *et al.* 1999; Anderson *et al.* 2002), a pattern observed among indigenous peoples worldwide (Cantor and Neulinger 2000; Beautrais 2001; Boothroyd *et al.* 2001). Berlin (1987) found that tribes with the highest suicide rates had higher rates of alcoholism, incarceration, unemployment, and lack of retention of traditional Native American culture (Bridge *et al.* 2006).

Whites traditionally have had higher suicide rates than non-whites in the United States, but the gap has been narrowing due to an increase in youth suicide among African-American males (Shaffer *et al.* 1994; Joe and Kaplan 2002; Centers for Disease Control and Prevention 2005). Assimilation and loss of traditional protective factors may also partially explain the class gradient in suicide among young African-Americans, with risk increasing with higher social class (Gould *et al.* 1996). Hispanic youth in the USA are not disproportionately represented among suicide completers (Demetriades *et al.* 1998), but still show higher rates of suicidal ideation and attempted suicide (Grunbaum *et al.* 2004).

The three leading methods of suicide among youth in the United States are firearms, hanging, and poisoning, respectively, whereas in most other Western countries hanging and vehicular exhaust predominate, followed by firearms and poisoning (Cantor and Neulinger 2000; Beautrais 2001; Centers for Disease Control and Prevention 2005). With limitations on availability of firearms, the United States and Australia have seen a decline in the use of firearms, and partially, substitution of other methods such as hanging and vehicle exhaust (Beautrais 2001; Centers for Disease Control and Prevention 2004; Bridge *et al.* 2005). Suicide by jumping is a relatively uncommon method of suicide in most countries (Gunnell and Nowers 1997), although jumping from a height is the primary method of choice for suicide completers in China (Hong Kong Special Administrative Region), (Hau 1993).

The US has seen a recent drop in suicide rates in adolescent males—a drop that is mirrored in other Western countries. The reasons for this are controversial, but may be related to the increased use of SSRI medications in the population. Indeed, after the FDA recently issued a black box warning regarding the dangers of SSRIs, the most recent figures in the US showed resurgence (Gibbons *et al.* 2007).

## Africa

The literature from the various Arab countries is sparse, although, rates are probably quite low because Islam prohibits taking one's own life (see Part 1 in this book). Rates of suicide attempts in hospitalized populations have no significant associations with religiousness among Arabs (Okasha 2004). For example, the crude rate of suicide attempts in Cairo was found to be 38.5 per 100,000. There was a high percentage in the 15–44 age group, with no major difference between the genders. There is reason to believe that, as in many other places, suicide mortality is underestimated. A crude estimate of suicide in Egypt would be about 3.5 per 100,000 (Okasha and Lotaief 1979). A study in 1981–1982 showed that the majority of suicide attempters were young women belonging to large, overcrowded families. They showed a higher tendency to be single, literate and unemployed than the corresponding age group in the general population. Drug overdose was the method most commonly used. The majority made their attempt at home when there was somebody nearby, and 31 per cent had made previous 'non-serious' attempts. Dysthymic adjustment, affective and personality disorders were the most common diagnoses encountered (Okasha *et al.* 1986).

More recent suicide statistics from South Africa show that 9 per cent of all teenage deaths are due to suicide. Also, one in every twelve adolescents has attempted suicide at least once. In terms of choice of method, hanging was the most common method (36.2 per cent), followed by shooting (35 per cent), poisoning (9.8 per cent), gassing (6.5 per cent) and burning (4.1 per cent). A serious comorbid factor of concern is that 5 per cent of suicide victims had positive levels of blood alcohol (Schlebusch *et al.* 2003).

It was also shown that 43.3 per cent of suicides were committed by blacks, 38.4 per cent by whites, 15.9 per cent were coloured, and 2 per cent Asians. Nearly one-quarter of black patients studied by Schlebusch *et al.* (2003) were youths 18 years and younger. This reflects a change from earlier South African research (Forster and Keens, 1988), which concluded that suicidal behaviour among black South Africans was rare, due to close family ties and cultural taboos against suicide (Cheetham 1988). Schlebusch points to various factors to explain the increase in suicidal behaviour in post-apartheid South Africa, which has become less isolated. These factors include the HIV-AIDS epidemic; high crime and violence rates; high stress levels; high unemployment levels; the impact of socio-economic and related forces in South Africa; societal factors such as social disintegration; and uncertainty regarding personal future (including increasing competitiveness in education and career advancement).

Another study by Flisher *et al.* (2004) reports a significant increase in youth suicide between 1968 and 1990 in South Africa, especially marked in the male population. At this point, the mechanisms involved in the rise of youth suicide remain purely speculative, but risk factors may include drug and alcohol abuse, an increase in family dissolution (Maris 1985, 1981), and the changing roles of men and women in society (McClure 1994).

Conclusions should be regarded with caution as the last data year in this study was 1990. Flisher *et al.* (2004) point to the interesting finding that similar patterns of rise in youth suicide, particularly affecting young white males, can be found between the South African population with populations in Europe and the USA, and attention to trends in these countries may be helpful in the prediction of future trends in youth suicide in South Africa.

## Asia

There are not many papers on suicidal behaviour of young people in the Asian region. In all the South East Asia Region (SEARO) countries, an increase in the number of suicides has been noticed in urban areas, suggesting that it maybe linked to urbanization, industrialization, migration and changing socio-economic patterns. One striking aspect of the suicide rates in the SEARO is a higher suicide rate in young women than young men, which is found in southern India and also observed in China and Singapore (Vijayakumar *et al.* 2005).

A study of the methods of suicide reveals that across SEARO countries, self-poisoning with a variety of substances ranging from pesticides to commonly available household products is the commonest method, ranging from 70 per cent in Sri-Lanka to 60 per cent in rural China, 23 per cent in Thailand, 47 per cent in Indonesia and 37 per cent in India (Gunnell and Eddleston 2003). Hanging is the other frequently adopted method. A comparison with the West indicates that gunshot injuries are not common in SEARO.

A study on suicidal behaviour among young people in Singapore (Ho Kong Wai *et al.* 1999) found that females were more at risk of suicidal behaviour than males. Suicidal behaviour was rare in the population below 13 years of age. There were significant differences in prevalence among the three main ethnic groups living in the country: young Singaporeans of Indian origin appear to be more at risk compared with their Malaysian and Chinese counterparts. This has also been observed in neighbouring Malaysia (Chia and Tsoi 1972).

Many theories have been proposed to explain this difference. Malays being entirely Muslim have traditionally low suicide rates as Islam views suicide as an absolute taboo. Conversely, Hindu attitudes towards suicide have traditionally been fairly tolerant (Ho Kong Wai *et al.* 1999) (see also Part 1, Chapter 4 in this book).

Latest available information on suicide rates in India dates from 2002 and points to a total of 10.5 per 100,000 in the total population, 12.8 for males and 8.0 for females (WHO 2008).

Different rates of suicide have been reported in India with a clear gradient increasing from north to south. Though detailed urban/rural comparisons are not available, in India, nearly 50–60 per cent of suicides still occur in rural areas. This variation may not reflect the exact picture of urban/rural differences due to differential reporting in rural versus urban areas. Many factors, such as societal and family pressures, limited access to health care, education and employment determinants, may play a role in these variations (Wun Jung and Tanvir 2004).

In Vellore, southern India, it was noted that the rates of suicides are several times higher than those reported anywhere in the world, especially in young women. Moreover, the leading cause of death in the 10–19 age group was suicide. The average suicide rate for young women aged 15–19 was 152 per 100,000, and for young men 69 per 100,000. Hence, the suicide rate for young women aged 15–19 was 70 times higher than the 2.1 per 100,000 in 1998 in the UK. The most common methods of suicide were hanging (44 per cent), poisoning with insecticide (40 per cent), self-immolation (9 per cent), and drowning (7 per cent). All the self-immolation was by girls (Aaron *et al.* 2004).

A recent study in this particular area showed (Aaron *et al.* 2004) a suicide rate ten times higher than the national average. It can not be excluded that the reported rates of suicide in other parts of India are low, because identification of suicides is difficult owing to inefficient registration systems, non-reporting of deaths, variable standards in certifying death, and the legal and social consequences of suicide. Various factors that contributed to adolescent suicide in Vellore area included acute stressors similar to those found in other studies: family conflicts, domestic violence, academic failures, unfulfilled romantic ideals, and mental illness. As mentioned earlier, in rural areas, the easy availability of pesticides in the homes of most families makes poisoning the preferred method of deliberate self-harm. The limited access to a well-equipped health facility where pesticide poisoning can be managed resulted in high rates of mortality (Aaron *et al.* 2004; Eddleston *et al.* 2006).

Additionally, it seems that the influence of the deeply rooted religious belief of Hindus and Buddhists in rebirth and karma (i.e. not regarding death as the final step) and self-sacrifice cannot be overlooked as a potential contributing factor to the high suicide rates in the country. Self-immolation, exclusively used by adolescent girls, might be indicative of such cultural and religious factors (Wun Jung and Tanvir 2004).

Latest available information on suicide rates in Sri-Lanka in the 15–24 age group dates from 1991, and points to an alarmingly high rate of 59 per 100,000 for males and 42 for females (WHO 2008).

A study carried out in the 1980s in the north of Sri Lanka (Ganeswaran *et al.* 1984) reveals that the 15–34 age group is most threatened by suicide. It is equally important to note that the suicide rate among the female rural population has been on the increase (Bolz 2002).

Suicide rates in Sri Lanka (40 per 100,000) greatly exceed those of the United Kingdom (7.4/100,000), United States (12/100,000), and Germany (15.8/100,000) (Eddleston *et al.* 1998). A leading method of committing suicide in Sri Lanka is ingestion of pesticides, which are readily available in rural farming households. Suicide attempts tend to be fatal, especially in the rural areas where rescue facilities are seldom available (Jeyaratnam 1990; Eddleston *et al.* 2002, 2006). Further reasons for high mortality rates include the toxic nature of the substances involved, lack of antidotes, distances between hospitals and patients, and overburdened medical staff (Desapriya *et al.* 2004).

A report from Sri Lanka (Bolz 2002) described possible reasons for the high suicide rates: conflicts between collectivism and individualism, rigid hierarchical structure, repressive education, and conflict between native and foreign culture, which is now easily accessible through cinema and television (Wun Jung and Tanvir 2004).

As is the case for many developing countries, China does not have a complete registration system. The official mortality data provided to WHO are based on 10 per cent of the population only. Rates of suicide in China vary widely across the country: according to selected rural or urban areas, ranges from 3.4–3.5 to 10.4 in the 15–24 age group, with 3–8 per 100,000 for males and 4.1–12.9 for female: suicide rates in China (Hong Kong SAR) thus point to a total of 11.0 in the 15–24 age group, 13.1 per 100,000 for males and 8.9 for females (WHO 2008).

Suicides in China are estimated to account for 19 per cent of all suicide deaths worldwide, with young females in the 15–24 age group particularly vulnerable. Despite this, there is a lack of information on the prevalence and predictors of depression and suicide ideation in Chinese adolescents (Hesketh *et al.* 2002).

Certain patterns of suicide that characterize Western countries are reversed in China. For example, the suicide rate in youths in rural areas in China is three times greater than the urban rates (Phillips and Yang 2004); in the younger age groups, they occur among women rather than men. The high suicide rate in young Chinese women contrasts with the high rate of attempted suicide in young women in the West (Cooper and Sartorius 1996). Like in many other places, national rates for attempted suicide are unknown in China.

In the attempt to explain the high Chinese rate in young women and in rural areas, it is implied that the sociocultural factors, acute stress and the readily availability of pesticides are more important than the psychiatric factors (Phillips *et al.* 2002b), which are regarded as the major influence in the West (Cooper and Sartorius 1996). Studies do show that the prevalence of depression is relatively low by international standards—perhaps less than 0.76 per 1000, which is as much as 100 times less than in North America (Lee and Kleinman 1997).

However, Phillips *et al.* (2007) state that the potential insensitivity to depression of translated diagnostic instruments makes it difficult to assess the relationship of depressive symptoms to suicide in non-Western cultures. Hence, adding culture-appropriate probes about depressive symptoms to standardized diagnostic instruments identifies many Chinese subjects with unrecognized depression.

China's data may suggest several points about gender inequality: the relatively low status of women in a society that is still patriarchal, the deeply frustrating constraints on their opportunities, and the cruelty displayed toward them. Many of the suicide attempts among these young girls might be calls for help that unintentionally become fatal because of the limited medical care available (Ji *et al.* 2001).

In all Asian countries, a key factor in suicide prevention is increased control of poisonous pesticides, which has been shown, in the case of Sri Lanka, to drastically reduce suicide rates (Gunnell *et al.* 2007).

## Australia and the Western Pacific

While the overall suicide rate has remained relatively stable in Australia, and is comparatively favourable in an international context, a different picture emerges when trends for specific age groups are examined with rates rising dramatically among younger people. Latest available information on suicide rates in Australia dates from 2003 and shows a total rate of 10.7 per 100,000 suicides in the 15–24 age group, 17.4 for males and 3.6 for females (WHO 2008). In 2003, suicide accounted for 19.9 per cent of total male deaths and 13.1 per cent of total female deaths registered in the 15–19 age group, and for 26.1 per cent of total male deaths and 11.6 per cent of total female deaths registered in the 20–24 age group (Australian Bureau of Statistics 2005).

Rates for males aged 15–24 have more than tripled over the past 40 years. Youth suicide is second only to motor vehicle traffic accidents as a cause of death in young Australians (Australian Bureau of Statistics 1997). Comparable rates for females, however, have shown no significant changes (Cantor *et al.* 1999), and suicide rates among older adult populations have generally declined across Australia over a similar period, though the decline has been erratic and patterns have varied between states (Cantor *et al.* 1999).

La Vecchia *et al.* (1994) also found that overall suicide trends of Australia and New Zealand followed those of North America. This suggests that ongoing North American trends may be relevant to Australian developments.

Rural areas often demonstrate greater suicide rates. Suicide rates in young males in the 15–24 age group were higher than overall male rates in all areas, especially in rural and remote areas. Suicide rates for young females suggested the same pattern as for males, but due to small numbers, these conclusions were unreliable. Rural migration, unemployment, abuse of alcohol, medical service utilization, socio-economic status and resource deprivation are possible risk factors requiring examination (Cantor and Neulinger 2000).

Significantly higher firearm suicide rates have been found in rural areas for both genders. In metropolitan and provincial areas, males were found to use carbon monoxide poisoning (vehicle exhaust gas) and drugs or poisons, and females to use drugs or poisons, significantly more than rural areas (Cantor and Slater 1997).

It is believed that the actual Aboriginal rate of suicide may be as much as two to three times higher than figures indicate. Collecting accurate information on Aboriginal suicide is difficult due to remote communities, unsystematic recording procedures, and because Aboriginal people define their aboriginality by identification, the Aboriginal culture (Cantor and Neulinger, 2000). The past decade has seen suicide become a significant contributor to premature Aboriginal mortality. Today, Aboriginal suicide rates in children and adolescents are possibly two to three times that of non-Aboriginal Australians (Elliott-Farrelly 2004).

Suicide rates in New Zealand show a very high rate of 30.4 per 100,000 for males aged 15–24 (see Table 85.1). Rates of male youth suicide began to increase in the 1970s, and then showed an abrupt increase over the period from the mid-1980s to the mid-1990s. However, in the years 1995–1999, the male youth suicide rate in New Zealand declined. In addition, there has been a steady increase in the rate of female youth suicide. In 1985, females accounted for 20 per cent of youth suicides (age 15–24), and in 1999, 31 per cent of youth suicides were female (Beautrais 2003).

For both young males and females, data suggest that young Maori males and females are approximately one-and-a-half times more likely to die by suicide than non-Maori young people (Beautrais 2003).

In 2000, the rate of suicide for Maori youth was 25.7 per 100,000, compared with the non-Maori rate of 16.2 per 100,000; the rates for young Maori males were 43.5 per 100,000, and the rate of suicide for young Maori females was 7.4 per 100,000 (New Zealand Ministry of Health 2002).

In New Zealand, the commonly used methods of suicide vary with gender. For young males, the most frequently used methods are hanging, vehicle exhaust gas, and firearms. Over the last two decades, there have been substantial increases in the use of both hanging and vehicle exhaust gas, and a decline in the use of firearms. In females, the most commonly used methods of suicide are hanging, vehicle exhaust gas and self-poisoning. There have been major changes in female methods of suicide, which changed from self-poisoning as the leading method in 1980 and has declined over the years (with self-poisoning accounting for 8 per cent of female suicide deaths in 1999), to increases in the use of hanging and vehicle exhaust gas. The use of hanging increased fivefold from 1980 to 1999, with hanging accounting for the majority (almost 85 per cent) of all female suicide deaths in 1999. These figures show that, for both genders, hanging has become increasingly common, in both male and female youth suicides (Beautrais 2003).

Japan has one of the highest overall suicide rates of industrialized countries. It has been rising throughout the 1990s—a decade of economic stagnation, failing businesses and growing levels of unemployment in the country. Suicide victims are mostly young people. Among those in the 15–24 age group, it is the second leading cause of death. The general suicide rate per 100,000 in Japan increased from 1995 to 2000 from 17.2 in 1995 to 24.1 in 2000 (Desapriya and Iwase 2003).

The cases of Internet suicide, which are popular in Japan, have highlighted a disturbing trend toward younger people taking their lives. Among school and college students, the 54 per cent increase in 2003, as compared to the previous year, was alarming, and was observed mostly among elementary and middle school students.

Some point to a profound and growing alienation among young people who are under enormous pressure to succeed at school and university and to find and keep a job. Over the past decade, competition for the top schools and universities has become increasingly intense, and unemployment among young people has risen sharply. These pressures are compounded by a culture in which relationships, even within the family, continue to be rather formal. As a result, young people often feel isolated and unable to discuss their personal problems.

Summing up, global suicide rates have been fluctuating over recent decades, decreasing in developed countries such as the USA, countries in the European Union, and Japan, and increasing in Eastern Europe, especially in Russia and countries of the former Soviet Union, Brazil, Sri Lanka, and China (Wasserman *et al.* 2005). What appears to be common in the countries that have increasing suicide rates is the turmoil following the rapid changes in the economic system. One striking aspect of the suicide rates in some Asian countries, such as in southern India, China and Singapore, is the higher suicide rate in young women than young men (Wun Jung and Tanvir 2004).

## Conclusion

This chapter indicates that suicide, in general, and especially in young people, is a global public health problem and an issue of major concern in developing countries as much as it is in the well-studied developed parts of the world. It is clear that in many developing countries on all continents, suicide rates are high by international standards. Patterns of suicidal behaviours in the various continents differ in some aspects (e.g. male:female ratio in Asia compared to other continents, cultural and societal risk factors), but are similar in others (e.g. increasing relative rates of youth suicide over the last decades on all continents). This essential information should be used when developing preventive measures in varying cultures.

The lack of appropriate epidemiological data in many parts of the world—especially in South America, North Africa and vast parts of Asia—needs to be addressed urgently as a first step in allowing appropriate preventive efforts to be developed, based on the specific characteristics of risk factors and epidemiology.

## References

Aaron R, Joseph A, Abraham S *et al.* (2004). Suicides in young people in rural southern India. *Lancet*, **363**, 1117–1118.

Anderson PL, Tiro JA, Price AW *et al.* (2002). Additive impact of childhood emotional, physical, and sexual abuse on suicide attempts among low-income African-American women. *Suicide and Life-Threatening Behavior*, **32**, 131–138.

Australian Bureau of Statistics (1997). *Causes of Death, Australia*. ABS Catalogue no. 3303.0. Australian Bureau of Statistics, Canberra.

Australian Bureau of Statistics (2005). *Suicides: Recent Trends.* ABS Xatalogue no. 3309.0.55.001. Australian Bureau of Statistics, Canberra.

Beautrais A (2001). Child and young adolescent suicide in New Zealand. *Australian and New Zealand Journal of Psychiatry,* **35,** 647–653.

Beautrais A (2003). Suicide in New Zealand I: time trends and epidemiology. *Journal of the New Zealand Medical Association,* **116,** 1175.

Berlin IN (1987). Suicide among American Indian adolescents: an overview. *Suicide and Life-Threatening Behavior,* **17,** 218–232.

Bertolote JM and Fleishmann A (2002). A global perspective in the epidemiology of suicide. *Suicidologi,* **7,** 6–7.

Bertolote JM and Fleishmann A (2002). Suicide and psychiatric diagnosis: a world perspective. *World Psychiatry,* **1,** 181–185.

Bolz W (2002). Psychological analysis of the Sri Lankan conflict culture with special reference to the high suicide rate. *Crisis,* **23,** 167–170.

Boothroyd LJ, Kirmayer LJ, Spreng S *et al.* (2001). Completed suicides among the Inuit of northern Quebec, 1982–1996: a case–control study. *Canadian Medical Association Journal,* **165,** 749–755.

Borowsky IW, Resnick MD, Ireland M *et al.* (1999). Suicide attempts among American Indian and Alaska Native youth: risk and protective factors. *Arch Pediatr Adolesc Med,* **153,** 573–580.

Bridge JA, Barbe RP, Brent DA (2005). Recent trends in suicide among U.S. adolescent males, 1992–2001. *Psychiatr Serv,* **56,** 522.

Bridge JA, Goldstein TR, Brent DA (2006). Adolescent suicide and suicidal behavior. *Journal of Child Psychology and Psychiatry,* **47,** 372–394.

Cantor C and Neulinger K (2000). The epidemiology of suicide and attempted suicide among young Australians. *Australian and New Zealand Journal of Psychiatry,* **34,** 370–387.

Cantor C and Slater PJ (1997). A regional profile of suicide in Queensland. *Australian and New Zealand Journal of Public Health,* **21,** 181–186.

Cantor C, Neulinger K, De Leo D (1999). Australian suicide trends 1964–1997: youth and beyond? *Medical Journal of Australia,* **171,** 137–141.

Centers for Disease Control and Prevention (2004). Methods of suicide among persons aged 10–19 years—United States, 1992–2001. *Morbidity and Mortality Weekly Report,* **53,** 471–474.

Centers for Disease Control and Prevention (CDC) (2005). Homicide and suicide rates—national violent death reporting system, six states, 2003. *Morbidity and Mortality Weekly Report,* **54,** 377–380.

Cheetham RWS (1988). Suicide: cross-cultural aspects. In L Schlebusch, ed., *Suicidal Behaviour,* pp. 129–132. University of Natal, Durban.

Chia BH and Tsoi WF (1972). Suicide in Singapore. *Singapore Medical Journal,* **13,** 91–97.

Cooper JE and Sartorius N (1996). *Mental Disorders in China: Results of the National Epidemiological Survey in 12 Areas.* Gaskell, London.

De Souza ED, de Souza MC, Malaquias JV (2002). Suicide among young people in selected Brazilian State capitals. *Cad Saúde Pública, Rio de Janeiro,* **18,** 673–683.

Demetriades D, Murray J, Sinz B *et al.* (1998). Epidemiology of major trauma and trauma deaths in Los Angeles County. *Journal of the American College of Surgeons,* **187,** 373–383.

Desapriya EBR and Iwase N (2003). New trends in suicide in Japan. *Injury Prevention,* **9,** 284.

Desapriya EBR, Joshi P, Han G *et al.* (2004). Demographic risk factors in pesticide-related suicides in Sri Lanka. *Injury Prevention,* **10,** 125.

Eddleston M, Karalliedde L, Buckley N *et al.* (2006). Patterns of hospital transfer for self-poisoned patients in rural Sri Lanka: implications for estimating the incidence of self-poisoning in the developing world. *Bulletin of the World Health Organization,* **84,** 276–282.

Eddleston M, Shriff MHR and Hawton K (1998). Deliberate self-harm in Sri Lanka and overlooked tragedy in developing world. *BMJ,* **317,** 133–135.

Elliott-Farrelly T (2004). Australian Aboriginal suicide: the need for an Aboriginal suicidology? *Australian e-Journal for the Advancement of Mental Health,* **3,** 3, http://www.auseinet.com/journal/vol3iss3/elliottfarrelly.

Fleischmann A, Bertolote JM, Belfer M *et al.* (2005). Completed suicide and psychiatric diagnoses in young people: a critical examination of the evidence. *American Journal of Orthopsychiatry,* **75,** 676–683.

Flisher AJ, Liang H, Laubscher R *et al.* (2004). Suicide trends in South Africa, 1968–90. *Scandinavian Journal of Public Health,* **32,** 411–418.

Forster HW and Keen AW (1988). Black attitudes in suicide. In L Schlebusch, ed., *Suicidal Behavior, Proceedings of the First Southern African Conference on Suicidology.* pp. 98–105. Department of Medically Applied Psychology, University of Natal, Durban.

Ganeswaran T, Subramaniam S, Mahadevan K (1984). Suicide in a northern town of Sri Lanka. *Acta Psychiatrica Scandinavica,* **69,** 420–425.

Gibbons RD, Brown CH, Hur K *et al.* (2007). Early evidence on the effects of regulators' suicidality warnings on SSRI prescriptions and suicide in children and adolescents. *American Journal of Psychiatry,* **164,** 1356–1363.

Gould MS, Fisher P, Parides M *et al.* (1996). Psychosocial risk factors of child and adolescent completed suicide. *Archives of General Psychiatry,* **53,** 1155–1162.

Grunbaum JA, Kann L, Kinchen S *et al.* (2005).Youth risk behavior surveillance—United States, 2003. *Morbidity and Mortality Weekly Report,* **54,** 608.

Gunnell D and Eddleston M (2003). Suicide by intentional ingestion of pesticides: a continuing tragedy in developing countries. *International Journal of Epidemiology,* **32,** 902–909.

Gunnell D and Nowers M (1997). Suicide by jumping. *Acta Psychiatrica Scandinavica,* **96,** 1–6.

Gunnell D, Fernando R, Hewagama M *et al.* (2007). The impact of pesticide regulation on suicide in Sri Lanka. *International Journal of Epidemiology,* **36,** 1235–1242.

Haklai Z, Aburbeh M, Stein N (2005). *Suicidality in Israel.* Ministry of Health, Health Information and Computer Services, Jerusalem.

Hau KT (1993). Suicide in Hong Kong 1971–1990: age trend, sex ratio, and method of suicide. *Social Psychiatry and Psychiatric Epidemiology,* **28,** 23–27.

Hesketh T, Ding QJ, Jenkins R (2002). Suicide ideation in Chinese adolescents. *Social Psychiatry and Psychiatric Epidemiology,* **37,** 230–235.

Ho Kong Wai B, Hong C, Heok KE (1999). Suicidal behavior among young people in Singapore. *General Hospital Psychiatry,* **21,** 128–133.

Jeyaratnam T (1990). Acute pesticide poisoning: a major global health problem. *World Health Statistics Quarterly,* **43,** 139–144.

Ji J, Kleinman J, Becker AE (2001). Suicide in contemporary China: a review of China's distinctive suicide demographics in their sociocultural context. *Harvard Review of Psychiatry,* **9,** 1–12.

Joe S and Kaplan MS (2002). Firearm-related suicide among young African-American males. *Psychiatric Services,* **53,** 332–334.

Kelleher MJ, Chambers D, Corcoran P *et al.* (1998). Religious sanctions and rates of suicide worldwide. *Crisis,* **19,** 78–86.

Krug EG, Powell KE, Dahlberg LL (1998). Firearm-related deaths in the United States and 35 other high- and upper-middle-income countries. *International Journal of Epidemiology,* **27,** 214–221.

La Vecchia C, Lucchini F, Levi F (1994). Worldwide trends in suicide mortality, 1955–89. *Acta Psychiatrica Scandinavica,* **90,** 53–64.

Lee S and Kleinman A (1997). Mental illness and social change in China. *Harvard Review of Psychiatry,* **5,** 43–46.

Maris R (1981). *Pathways to Suicide: A Survey of Self-destructive Behaviours.* Johns Hopkins University Press, Baltimore.

Maris R (1985). The adolescent suicide problem. *Suicide and Life-Threatening Behavior,* **15,** 91–109.

Mc Clure GMG (1994). Suicide in children and adolescents in England and Wales 1960–1990. *British Journal of Psychiatry,* **165,** 510–514.

Mello-Santos C, Bertolote JM, Wang YP (2005). Epidemiology of suicide in Brazil (1980–2000): characterization of age and gender rates of suicide. *Revista Brasileira de Psiquiatria*, **27**, 131–134.

Morad M, Merrick E, Schwarz A *et al.* (2005). A review of suicide behavior among Arab adolescents. *Scientific World Journal*, **26**, 674–679.

New Zealand Ministry of Health (2002). *Youth Suicide Facts, Provisional 2000 Statistics (15–24-year-olds)*. Ministry of Health, Wellington.

Okasha A (2004). Focus on psychiatry in Egypt. *British Journal of Psychiatry*, **18**, 266–272.

Okasha A and Lotaief F (1979). Attempted suicide: an Egyptian investigation. *Acta Psychiatrica Scandinavica*, **60**, 69–75.

Okasha A, Lotaief F and El Mahallawy N (1986). Descriptive study of attempted suicide in Cairo. *Egyptian Journal of Psychiatry*, **9**, 53–90.

Phillips MR and Yang G (2004). Suicide and attempted suicide—China, 1990–2002. *Morbidity and Mortality Weekly Report*, **53**, 481.

Phillips MR, Li X, Zhang Y (2002a). Suicide rates in China, 1995–99. *Lancet*, **359**, 835–840.

Phillips MR, Shen Q, Liu X *et al.* (2007). Assessing depressive symptoms in persons who die of suicide in mainland China. *Journal of Affective Disorders*, **98**, 73–82.

Phillips MR, Yang G, Zhang Y *et al.* (2002b). Risk factors for suicide in China: a national case–control psychological autopsy study. *Lancet*, **360**, 1728–1736.

Puentes-Rosas E, Lopez-Nieto L, Martinez-Monroy T (2004). Mortality from suicides: Mexico, 1990–2001. *Revista Panamericana de Salud Publica*, **16**, 102–109.

Ruzicka SA (1998). Pain beliefs. What do elders believe? *Journal of Holistic Nursing*, **16**, 369–382.

Sartorius N (1995). Recent changes in suicide rates in selected eastern European and other European countries. *International Psychogeriatrics*, **7**, 301–308.

Schlebusch L, Naseema BM, Vawda N, Bosch B. (2003) Suicidal behavior in black South Africans. *Crisis*, **24**, 24–28.

Shaffer D, Gould M, Hicks RC (1994). Worsening suicide rate in black teenagers. *American Journal of Psychiatry*, **151**, 1810–1812.

Vijayakumar L, Nagaraj K, Pirkis J *et al.* (2005). Suicide in developing countries (1): frequency, distribution, and association with socioeconomic indicators. *Crisis*, **26**, 104–111.

Wallace JD, Calhoun AD, Powell KE *et al.* (1996). *Homicide and suicide among Native Americans, 1979–1992*. Centers for Disease Control and Prevention, National Center for Injury Prevention and Control. Violence Surveillance Series, No. 2, Atlanta.

Wasserman D, Cheng Q, Jiang GX (2005). Global suicide rates among young people aged 15–19. *World Psychiatry*, **4**, 114–120.

World Health Organization (2008). *Figures and Facts About Suicide*. Updated country charts at http://www.who.int/mental_health/prevention/suicide/country_reports/en/index.html, last accessed 16 March 2008.

Wun Jung K and Tanvir S (2004). Trends and dynamics of youth suicides in developing countries. *The Lancet*, **363**, 1090.

Zhang J (1998). Suicide in the world: toward a population increase theory of suicide. *Death Studies*, **22**, 525–539.

# CHAPTER 86

# Suicidal behaviour in children and adolescents in different clinical settings

Anat Brunstein Klomek, Orit Krispin and Alan Apter

## Abstract

This chapter reviews the various clinical settings in which suicidal behaviours occur among children and adolescents. The chapter focuses on primary care settings (family or paediatric practices), emergency rooms, intensive care units, mental health outpatient departments and inpatient units. The authors discuss the need for early screening of suicidality and its risk factors, management of these high-risk children and adolescents and the different clinical interventions that are available. These interventions include psychosocial and medication treatments that have varying rates of success and still need more studies. In all clinical settings a multidisciplinary approach to treatment is recommended. The importance of risk assessment and continuity of care are highlighted.

## Introduction

Suicidal behaviours among children and adolescents occur in different clinical settings and contexts. These include primary care settings (family or paediatric practices), emergency rooms (ER), and intensive care units (ICU), both in general and psychiatric hospitals, mental health outpatient departments (OPD) and inpatient units.

Although there are several treatment methods targeting suicidal behaviour in adolescents, no treatment has been proven effective enough to permit its definition as the treatment of choice for suicidal teens. The different approaches to reducing suicidal behaviour include psychotherapy, psychosocial and medication treatments that have varying rates of success. Those treatments are described in this part of the book by Spirito in Chapter 92, Brent in Chapter 91 and Malone in Chapter 93.

## Primary care settings

Paediatricians are important gatekeepers in suicide prevention. Frequently, suicidal youth seek general medical care in the month preceding suicidal acts (Pfaff et al. 1999). These routine examinations are crucial for the early screening, management and referral of high-risk youth. Gatekeeper training is designed for the early identification of individuals at risk for suicide, facilitating timely referrals to mental health services (Pfaff et al. 2001). Mental health screening should be an essential part of the routine medical examination in primary practice. The screening should include questions regarding the signs and symptoms of childhood internalizing and externalizing disorders. Paediatric providers should be proactive and systematic in assessing suicide. Assessments must include direct inquiries about suicidal ideation and behaviour (Pfaff et al. 2001). Although depression is relatively common in paediatric settings, it often goes unnoticed. Therefore, improving physicians' recognition of depression and suicide risk will facilitate timely referrals for early treatment before complications arise.

Untreated internalizing disorders among children and adolescents tend to become chronic conditions with considerable morbidity. There are currently evidenced-based treatments for uncomplicated depression and anxiety for children and adolescents. These include cognitive behavioural therapy (CBT) (Brent et al. 1997; Compton et al. 2004) and interpersonal psychotherapy (IPT-A) (Mufson et al. 1999, 2004). In addition, pharmacotherapy with selective serotonin reuptake inhibitors (SSRIs) can be very useful for both disorders (The Research Unit on Pediatric Psychopharmacology Anxiety Study Group 2001; March et al. 2004). When untreated, many of these children and adolescents will become highly predisposed to suicidal behaviour and completed suicide.

Externalizing disorders are also a risk factor for suicidality (Brent et al. 1993; Renaud et al. 1999). These include a myriad of problems related to conduct disorders, attention deficit disorders and psychosexual disorders. Paediatricians and specialists in adolescent medicine should be trained in diagnosing sexual and physical abuse, as well as the early stages of drug and alcohol abuse. Moreover, they should learn to detect the physical signs of self-injury (e.g., cutting) and disordered eating. For youth, these disorders are often the harbingers of a spectrum of high-risk behaviours that include suicide.

### Emergency room management

Young people are commonly seen in the ER following suicidal behaviour. ER and other crisis staff should be trained in communicating with suicidal teens to optimize diagnosis and treatment. Staff members should be able to establish rapport with the suicidal individual and their family, and should be educated about the importance of treatment. There are no randomized controlled trials to determine whether hospitalizing high-risk suicide attempters saves lives. Clinicians, however, should be prepared to admit suicide attempters who express a persistent wish to die or who have a clearly abnormal mental state. Regardless of the apparent mildness of the patient's suicidal behaviour, the clinician must obtain information from a third party. Discharge can be considered only when the patient's mental state and suicidality have been stabilized and a reasonable degree of safety is assured. The clinician should assure that adequate supervision and support will be available for the patient (Brent 1997; American Academy of Child and Adolescent Psychiatry 2001).

The use of firearms is the most common method for adolescents who complete suicide (Gould *et al.* 2003). Ingestion of medication is the most common method for adolescents who attempt suicide (CDC 1995). Availability and presence of firearms and lethal medication at home must be determined during assessment, and parents must be explicitly told to remove firearms and lethal medication (Brent *et al.* 1991). It is also valuable for the clinician to warn adolescents and their parents about the dangerous disinhibiting effects of alcohol and other drugs.

Increased risk of suicide potential in a child or adolescent includes a previous attempt, an intent to attempt, a lethal plan, precautions against being rescued, accessibility of lethal means (especially guns) and probability of alcohol use (Shaffer *et al.* 1996; Gould *et al.* 1998). Additional features of high-risk clinical scenarios in a child or adolescent include suicide pacts with peers, desire to join a deceased friend or relative, inadequate parental supervision and support, and inability of the child or adolescent to agree to an explicit verbal or written no-suicide contract with the clinician. The value of 'no-suicide contracts', in which the child or adolescent agrees not to engage in self-harming behaviour and to tell an adult if they are having suicidal urges, is unknown (Reid 1998). The child or adolescent might not be in a mental state to accept or understand the contract. Even after a contract has been signed by the teen, the family and clinician should maintain their vigilance (Apter 2001).

Before discharge from the ER, an appointment should be scheduled for the child or adolescent to be seen for a thorough evaluation and a follow-up plan. If this is not possible, a telephone contact with a parent or other caretaker should be scheduled. If the clinical staff has not been contacted by the parent/caretaker within a reasonable period of time, they should initiate contact. The clinician treating the suicidal child or adolescent during the days following an attempt should have experience managing suicidal crises, be available to the patient and family (e.g., initiate and receive phone calls beyond therapeutic hours), and have support available for him or herself. A referral to a specific therapist and continued contact with the child and family until a therapeutic alliance is established increases the likelihood that the patient will continue treatment.

## Intensive care units

Few studies have examined serious suicide attempts in adolescents. The most well-known study is the Canterbury (New Zealand) Suicide Project (Beautrais *et al.* 1996), which is a case–control study of 200 suicide cases, 302 medically serious suicide attempts and 1028 randomly selected control subjects. Participants were aged 13–24 with a mean age of 19.4. The gender ratio was consistent among all groups. Nearly equal numbers of males and females made serious suicide attempts. Twice as many females used overdose than males, who used CO poisoning and hanging. Low income and residential mobility were highly associated with a serious attempt. Serious attempt was also associated with childhood sexual abuse, low parental care and poor parental relationship. There was also an elevated risk for mood disorder, substance abuse and conduct disorder. In addition, legal problems and difficulties with interpersonal relationships, work and finances made a significant contribution to risk of a serious suicide attempt (Beautrais, 1998). Although no gender differences were revealed regarding the seriousness of the suicide attempt, differences were depicted between suicide attempters who were admitted to ICU compared with those who were not.

Subjects with more severe suicide attempts were characterized with lower levels of self-disclosure. Self-disclosure is comparatively more limited in males. Impaired ability of self-disclosure was found to be associated with loneliness, psychiatric illness, anxiety and aggression, which are associated with suicidal behaviours (Apter and Ofek 2001). Thus limited ability of self-disclosure may indicate the necessity of psychological intervention that focuses on intimate interpersonal relationships and the ability to share feelings with others.

## Child and adolescent mental health outpatient departments

Mental health OPDs usually encounter youth with past suicide attempts and/or current suicidal ideation. Thus the OPD is responsible for the management of suicidality. Despite the magnitude of the problem and the volume of youth suicide research, there is no specific treatment that has been proven effective for suicidal behaviour among adolescents in outpatient settings.

Research indicates that the two most prominent risk factors for both completed suicide and suicidal behaviour in adolescents are past suicide attempt and a diagnosis of a depressive disorder, each independently contributing at least a 10–30-fold increased risk for completed suicide (Gould *et al.* 1996; Shaffer *et al.* 1996).

Although the evidenced-based literature is scarce, most OPDs provide a multidimensional treatment approach involving clinical (psychological and pharmacological) interventions, common sense and supportive therapy. This approach has proven sufficient in most cases and is recommended.

## Adolescent inpatient units and residential treatment programmes

Suicidal behaviours are among the major reasons for admission to an adolescent inpatient unit in different parts of the world (Cohen *et al.* 1997). The prevalence of suicidal behaviour among inpatients is high (Robbins and Alessi 1985). Adolescent inpatients usually have a history of repeated suicide attempts and subsequent psychiatric hospitalization (Pfeffer *et al.* 1988; Cohen *et al.* 1997).

Studies have indicated that mortality rates among males are excessively higher than among females (e.g. Gould *et al.* 1998). As mentioned above, affective disorders (especially depression), schizophrenia, eating disorders (anorexia nervosa and bulimia nervosa) and borderline personality disorder are all associated with significant increased risk for suicidal behaviour (e.g. Shaffer *et al.* 1996; Gould *et al.* 1998). Serious psychiatric disorders in adolescence that require hospitalization compound suicidal risk, especially if accompanied by other risk factors for suicide and another diagnosed psychiatric disorder. In our own clinical practice we have identified four comorbid constellations that may be highly related to suicide in adolescent populations, requiring vigorous psychiatric intervention:

1 The combination of schizophrenia, depression and substance abuse;

2 Substance abuse, conduct disorder and depression;

3 Affective disorder, eating disorder and anxiety disorders;

4 Affective disorder, personality disorder cluster A in DSM terminology and dissociative disorders (Apter 2001).

A multidisciplinary approach to treatment is recommended for suicidal patients. This includes formalized suicide assessment (done conjointly by medical and nursing staff), accurate psychiatric and medical diagnosis, psychotherapeutic and/or pharmacotherapy treatment, flexible and skilled observation policy, inpatient groups focusing on risk factors and triggers of suicidal behaviour, and a referral to continuing treatment once the patient is discharged. Prevention of suicidal behaviours in adolescent inpatients mostly involves treatment of the underlying psychiatric illness and the provision of sufficient after care following discharge. Lack of continuity of care places patients at an elevated risk for additional suicide attempts (Hulten and Wasserman 1998). When referring a suicidal patient, it is critical to highlight the strategies and skills acquired by the patient and identify those that are lacking.

## Conclusion

Two prominent risk factors for both completed suicide and suicidal behaviour in adolescents are previous suicide attempts and a diagnosis of a depressive episode. Adolescents with different degrees of suicidal risk and severity are referred and/or admitted to various clinical settings. Research has yet to clearly identify the treatment of choice for suicidal patients. Regardless, clinical interventions should be based on a thorough suicide-risk assessment. Treatment strategies should be multidimensional, targeting suicidal behaviour as well as the underlying psychiatric illness and/or other personality and environmental risk factors. Given that adolescents are referred from one clinical setting to another, continuity of care (e.g. recommendation for after care, a concrete referral and a telephone follow-up) must be one of mental health practitioners' major concerns. Lack of continuity of care places patients at an elevated risk for additional suicide attempts.

## References

American Academy of Child and Adolescent Psychiatry (2001). Practice parameters for the assessment and treatment of children and adolescents with suicidal behavior. *Journal of American Academy of Child and Adolescent Psychiatry*, **40** (suppl), 24–51.

Apter A (2001). Adolescent suicide and attempted suicide. In D Wasserman, ed., *Suicide—An Unnecessary Death*, pp. 78–98. Martin Dunitz, London.

Apter A and Ofek H (2001). Personality constellations and suicidal behavior. In K van Heeringen, ed., *Understanding Suicidal Behavior: The Suicidal Process Approach to Research, Treatment and Prevention*, pp. 94–120. Wiley, New York.

Beautrais AL (1998). Risk factors for serious suicide attempts among young people: a case–control study. In RJ Kosky, HS Eshkevari *et al.* eds, *Suicide Prevention: The Global Context*, pp. 167–181. Plenum Press, New York.

Beautrais AL, Joyce PR, Mulder RT (1996). Risk factors for serious suicide attempts among youths aged 13 through 24 years. *Journal of the American Academy of Child and Adolescent Psychiatry*, **35**, 1174–1182.

Brent DA (1997). The aftercare of adolescents with deliberate self-harm. *Journal of Child Psychology and Psychiatry and Allied Disciplines*, **38**, 277–286.

Brent DA, Holder D, Kolko D *et al.* (1997). A clinical psychotherapy trial for adolescent depression comparing cognitive, family, and supportive therapy. *Archives of General Psychiatry*, **54**, 877–885.

Brent DA, Perper JA, Allman CJ *et al.* (1991). The presence and accessibility of firearms in the homes of adolescent suicides: a case–control study. *Journal of the American Medical Association*, **266**, 2989–2995.

Brent DA, Perper JA, Moritz G *et al.* (1993). Psychiatric risk factors for adolescent suicide: a case–control study. *Journal of the American Academy of Child and Adolescent Psychiatry*, **35**, 521–29.

CDC (Center for Disease Control) (1995). Suicide among children, adolescents and young adults. *Morbidity and Mortality Weekly Report*, **44**, 289–291.

Cohen Y, Spirito A, Apter A *et al.* (1997). A cross-cultural comparison of behavior disturbance and suicidal behavior among psychiatrically hospitalized adolescents in Isreal and in the United States. *Child Psychiatry and Human Development*, **28**, 89–102.

Compton SN, March JS, Brent D *et al.* (2004). Cognitive-behavioral psychotherapy for anxiety and depressive disorders in children and adolescents: an evidence-based medicine review. *Journal of the American Academy of Child and Adolescent Psychiatry*, **43**, 930–959.

Gould MS, Fisher P, Parides M *et al.* (1996). Psychosocial risk factors of child and adolescent completed suicide. *Archives of General Psychiatry*, **53**, 1155–1162.

Gould MS, King R, Greenwald S *et al.* (1998). Psychopathology associated with suicidal ideation and attempts among children and adolescents. *Journal of the American Academy of Child and Adolescent Psychiatry*, **37**, 915–923.

Gould MS, Shaffer D, Greenberg T (2003). The epidemiology of youth suicide. In RA King and A Apter, *Suicide in Children and Adolescents*, pp. 1–41. Cambridge University Press, Cambridge.

Hulten A and Wasserman D (1998). Lack of continuity—a problem in the care of young suicides. *Acta Psychiatrica Scandinavica*, **97**, 326–333.

March J, Silva S, Petrycki S *et al.* (2004). Treatment for Adolescents With Depression Study (TADS) Team. Fluoxetine, cognitive-behavioral therapy, and their combination for adolescents with depression: Treatment for Adolescents With Depression Study (TADS) randomized controlled trial. *Journal of American Medical Association*, **292**, 807–820.

Mufson L, Dorta KP, Moreau D *et al.* (2004). *Interpersonal Psychotherapy for Depressed Adolescents*. Guilford Press, New York.

Mufson L, Weissman MM, Moreau D *et al.* (1999). Efficacy of interpersonal psychotherapy for depressed adolescents. *Archives of General Psychiatry*, **56**, 573–579.

Pfaff JJ, Acres JG, Wilson M (1999). The role of general practitioners in para-suicide: a Western Australia perspective. *Archives of Suicide Research*, **5**, 207–214.

Pfaff JJ, Acres JG, McKelvey RS (2001). Training general practitioners to recognize and respond to psychological distress and suicidal ideation in young people. *The Medical Journal of Australia*, **174**, 222–226.

Pfeffer CR, Newcorn J, Kaplan G *et al.* (1988). Suicidal behavior in adolescent psychiatric inpatients. *Journal of the American Academy of Child and Adolescent Psychiatry*, **27**, 357–361.

Reid WH (1998). Promises, promises: don't rely on patients no suicide/ no violence 'contracts'. *Journal of Practical Psychiatry and Behavioral Health*, **4**, 316–318.

Renaud J, Brent D, Birmaher B *et al.* (1999). Suicide in adolescents with disruptive disorders. *Journal of the American Academy of Child and Adolescent Psychiatry*, **38**, 846–851.

Robbins DR and Alessi NE (1985). Depressive symptoms and suicidal behavior in adolescents. *American Journal of Pschiatry*, **142**, 588–592.

Shaffer D, Gould MS, Fisher P *et al.* (1996). Psychiatric diagnosis in child and adolescent suicide. *Archives of General Psychiatry*, **53**, 339–348.

The Research Unit on Pediatric Psychopharmacology Anxiety Study Group (2001). Fluvoxamine for the treatment of anxiety disorders in children and adolescents. *New England Journal of Medicine*, **344**, 1279–1285.

# CHAPTER 87

# Psychopathology and risk factors for suicide in the young
## Theoretical and empirical

Israel Orbach and Maya Iohan-Barak

## Abstract

In the first section risk factors along the categories of pathology, emotional states, personality traits, cognitive deficits, deficits in self-regulation, stressors and facilitators and inhibitors of suicidal behaviour are classified. The second section consists of a presentation of several theoretical perspectives of self-destructive behaviour in adolescents. The third section provides a review of theoretical and empirical models that try to track the interactions between the various risk factors leading to suicidal behaviour. The last section focuses on different pathways, based on different major dynamics, showing that there is more than one way to approach suicidal behaviour in adolescents.

Many risk factors have been implicated in suicidal behaviour. In order to gain some clarity in this web of multiple risk factors, a meaningful organization of the existing data is needed. In this chapter we will rely on Orbach's (1997) taxonomy of risk factors in order to facilitate in the organization of data related to suicidal behaviour in adolescents.

## Psychopathology and risk factors

Research on suicidal adolescents suggests that psychopathology is very common within this population. Post-mortem studies show that more than 90 per cent of the adolescents who commit suicide have at least one major psychiatric disorder: this is especially prominent among older adolescents who commit suicide (Gould et al. 2003). Furthermore, a leading cause for hospitalization among adolescents is suicidal behaviour. Follow-up studies on former adolescent patients show that 7.1 per cent of the inpatient males committed suicide within a 6-year follow-up (Pelkonen et al. 1996).

When considering the bearing of psychiatric illness on adolescent suicidal behaviour, two mediating variables must be accounted for: gender and comorbidity. Male and female adolescents were found to be affected differently by the different risk factors (Andrews and Lewinsohn 1992). This gender-based differentiation was recently demonstrated by Fennig et al. (2005), who found that while antisocial behaviour and depression are predicting factors for male attempters, types of defence mechanism and destructiveness are predictive for female attempters. Comorbidity is another mediating variable when assessing suicide risk in adolescents with psychiatric disorders. Beautrais et al. (1996) suggest that the likelihood for suicide by a person who suffers from one psychiatric disorder is 17.4 compared to the odds for a person with no psychiatric diagnosis. The probability for a person who suffers from two diagnoses of psychiatric disorder is 89.7. However, Houston (2004) found no such effect.

Psychiatric disorders and comorbidities are very common in adolescent suicide attempters and are described by Apter et al. in Chapter 85.

## Emotional states

### Depressed mood

Depressed mood can appear with or without a diagnosis of major depression. Depressed mood in and of itself is one of the most critical risk factors for suicidal behaviours among young adults. Wetzler et al. (1996) examined severe attempters, non-severe attempters, suicide ideators, and non-suicidal adolescents. They found that depressed mood is fundamentally associated with all forms of suicidality. Similarly, Spirito et al. (2003) found that the baseline for depressed mood was the most strongly related factor to future suicidal ideation and attempts. An additional study found that when depressed mood is controlled for, other factors may become non-significant (Wichstrom and Rossow 2002).

### Hopelessness

While a strong association has been established between hopelessness and suicide in adults (Beck et al. 1985), such an association is less clear-cut in adolescents. Multiple studies report a strong association between hopelessness and suicidal behaviour in adolescents (Horesh et al. 2003; Thompson et al. 2005), yet a recent study of Turkish adolescents found that hopelessness did not predict suicide risk within their sample (Sayar and Bozkir 2004). This seeming contradiction can be resolved considering the recent findings of Eposito et al. (2003), indicating that hopelessness may be more critical for multiple suicide attempters than for single suicide attempters. There is also some lack of clarity regarding the role of hopelessness in male versus female suicide attempters. One study found that hopelessness added significantly to the prediction of suicide risk scores in female juvenile detainees but did not add to the prediction of suicide risk scores in males (Sanislow *et al.* 2003). In a study of victims of sexual abuse who were suicidal, hopelessness was more strongly related to suicidal behaviour in male victims of sexual abuse, while depressive symptoms were more critical in the case of suicidal behaviour in female victims (Bergen *et al.* 2003). Some studies found that hopelessness increases suicide risk in youngsters who internalize anger but not in those who externalize anger, and that hopelessness plays a more significant role for older adolescents than for younger ones (Barbe *et al.* 2005). Other studies, such as that of Goldston *et al.* (2001), report that when depression is controlled for hopelessness it is no longer associated to suicidality.

### Anxiety

Excessive anxiety, especially trait anxiety, is an emotional characteristic of suicidal adolescents (Fennig *et al.* 2005). De Wilde *et al.* (1993) found that both hospitalized and non-hospitalized adolescent attempters experienced significantly more state and trait anxiety compared to non-attempters. Later, Goldston *et al.* (1999) distinguished trait anxiety, and not state anxiety, as associated with suicidal behaviour in adolescents.

### Anger, hostility and irritability

Suicidal adolescents seem to experience more anger, more hostility, and more irritability than their non-suicidal counterparts (Penn *et al.* 2003). With regard to anger, some studies show that internalized anger is more critical to suicidal behaviour than externalized anger (Cautin *et al.* 2001). Other studies point to externalized anger as the more critical of the two types as far as suicidal behaviour is concerned (Zlotnick *et al.* 2004).

### Shame, guilt, and loneliness

Feelings that are related to interpersonal relationships were also found to be associated with adolescent suicidal behaviour. Savarimuthu (2002) analysed audio-taped suicide notes of suicidal adolescents, following the path of expressed social emotions moment by moment. The investigators established that shame can be a devastating experience to the self, possibly leading to suicidal behaviour (see also Loraas 1997). Guilt feelings were found to be characteristic of suicidal young adults (Haliburn 2000). Suicidal youngsters experience far more inappropriate guilt than non-suicidal youngsters (Catalina-Zamora and Mardomingo-Sanz 2000). Suicidal adolescents also express a strong sense of loneliness (Batigun 2005). Guertin *et al.* (2001) found that sense of loneliness increases the odds of self-mutilation among suicidal adolescents almost sixfold.

### Mental pain

Shneidman (1993) introduced the concept of unbearable mental pain, or as he terms it 'psychache', (Orbach *et al.* 2003) as the immediate reason for suicidal behaviour. Shneidman's concept, psychache, refers to a generalized emotional state that is different from any specific negative emotion. In recent studies, mental pain appears as a distinguished characteristic of the emotional state of suicidal adolescents (Orbach and Iohan 2005). Evren

and colleagues (2001) found that 66.7 per cent of a given suicidal sample self-reported the reason underlying their suicidal attempt was 'to get away from boredom and pain' (Haliburn 2000).

### Emotional instability

Some suicidal adolescents are characterized by no specific emotional state of anxiety, anger, or hopelessness, but rather by rapid shifts in temperament. Such rapid shifts are related to difficulties in emotional regulation, and were found to be implicated in suicidal behaviour by some researchers (e.g. Miller *et al.* 2000)

## Personality traits

Personality traits in and of themselves do not cause suicide. The same trait can be adaptive or non-adaptive depending on the situational demands. However, when some traits interact with other risk factors it may increase the risk of suicide by intensifying the suicidal crisis.

### Impulsivity, aggression and negativism

Impulsivity, aggression, and the tendency to act out in the face of frustration and interpersonal conflict are some of the most frequent personality traits found in suicidal adolescents (Fennig *et al.* 2005; Horesh *et al.* 2003). Eliason (2001) has found that impulsivity was the best discriminator between attempters and non-attempters and that among young impulsive individuals there is a very short span time between the suicidal thought and the attempt, thus exhibiting a difficulty controlling anger. Suicidal adolescents are often described as negativistic and as rejecting outside help for their emotional problems (Deane *et al.* 2001; Orbach 1997).

### Ambitiousness and perfectionism

Other personality characteristics of suicidal adolescents are ambitiousness and perfectionism. An ambitious youngster who finds it difficult to compromise between high aspirations and the limitations of reality may choose to escape reality by taking their own life. Such a youngster may perceive compromise or failure as less bearable than death. Perfectionism is particularly critical in the development of hopelessness, although this is attenuated after controlling for depressive cognition (Donaldson *et al.* 2000). Yet socially prescribed perfectionism was found to be a primary factor in predicting the wish to die for suicide attempts among adolescents (Boerges *et al.* 1998).

### Low self esteem

Further, low self-esteem and a negative self-concept are significantly related to adolescent suicidal behaviour (Martin *et al.* 2005). By looking for adolescents with low self-esteem, researchers were able to distinguish young suicide ideators from suicide attempters (Merwin and Ellis 2004).

### Identify confusion

Finally, identity confusion, a lack of self-cohesiveness and self-integration, low self-complexity, lack of differentiation between self and parents, and discrepancies between actual self, normative self, and the ideal self, represent structural aspects of personality that are related to adolescent suicidal behaviour. These structural aspects of personality hamper the ability to regulate and cope, thereby increasing self-negativity and suicidal risk (Orbach *et al.* 1998; Brunstein-Klomek *et al.* 2005).

## Deficits

### Self-regulation

Self-regulation is conceptualized as the ability to control a range of internal systems that include affect regulation, modulation of anger, inhibition of self-destructive behaviour, minimization of negative ruminations, and self-soothing. It has been repeatedly found that suicidal youngsters encounter difficulties in regulation of negative emotions, negative cognitions, and impulsive behaviours (e.g. Esposito *et al.* 2003; Zlotnick *et al.* 1997). Negative attributional style is another self-regulation deficit that influences suicidal behaviour. Negative attributional style includes attributing positive outcomes to external forces of change and negative outcomes to the self (Schwartz *et al.* 2000; Rotheram-Borus 1988), negative self-appraisal, and negative appraisal of one's own degree of controllability of stressful events.

Fritsch and colleagues (2000) found that suicidal adolescents, as compared to non-suicidal adolescents, use more forceful and less conforming regulation strategies. Piquet and Wagner (2003) have categorized the cognitive and regulative patterns of suicidal youngsters into two systems and subsequently into four subtypes of coping strategies:

1  Approach-effortful (e.g. seeking advice and support);

2  Avoidance-effortful (e.g. 'band-aid' solution);

3  Approach-automatic (e.g. blaming others); and

4  Avoidance-automatic (e.g. alcohol and drug abuse, self-destructive thoughts).

It was found that, relative to the comparison group, the adolescent suicide attempters made fewer approach-effortful responses and less avoidance-effortful coping responses, both considered the more adaptive coping strategies of the four.

### Cognitive deficits

Problem-solving deficits are a distinct cognitive characteristic of suicidal youngsters, expressed in their tendency to produce more problematic alternatives and fewer effective alternatives in interpersonal problem-solving tasks. Metacognitively, suicidal adolescents exhibit more pessimistic appraisal of their ability to solve problems. In addition, their problem-solving abilities are compromised by their inability to produce specific autobiographic memories (see review by Specker and Hawton 2005). Suicidal adolescents are also inclined to focus on problematic aspects of a stressful situation, yet at the same time they resort more to wishful thinking strategies when confronted with a problem (Goldston *et al.* 2001). In problem situations, suicidal adolescents prefer drastic solutions and dependence on others (Orbach *et al.* 1990). A history of repetitive failures seems to condition suicidal youngsters to perceive problems as inherently unsolvable (Orbach *et al.* 1999) and as out of their control (Wilson *et al.* 1995). Suicidal youth also have a cognitive style of an automatic production of negative thoughts (Nock and Kazdin 2002). Events and situations are automatically evaluated negatively (Kienhorst *et al.* 1992). Negative attributions are assigned to oneself, others, and to the future (Rudd 2000).

## Stressors

A variety of life events have been found to be related to suicidal behaviour, including bereavement, breakdown of close relationships, interpersonal conflicts, financial difficulties, legal setbacks, or disciplinary problems (Fergusson *et al.* 2000). Different life events have a different impact at different ages. Pertaining to interpersonal conflicts, parent–child conflicts constitute a greater risk factor for early adolescence, whereas romantic difficulties constitute a greater suicide risk factor during later adolescence (Groholt *et al.* 1998).

Beyond the general pool of life events, certain specific life events have consistently been found to influence the presence of suicidal behaviour in young adults. Sexual abuse and physical abuse, for example, were found strongly associated with suicidal behaviour. Sexual abuse is statistically predictive of suicidal behaviour even after controlling for depression, hopelessness, and family dysfunction. Girls who report distress about their experience of sexual abuse have a threefold increased risk of suicidal thoughts and plans compared to non-abused girls. Similarly, male adolescents who are highly distressed about their experience of sexual abuse have a tenfold increased risk for suicide attempts compared to non-abused adolescent males. However, the relationship between sexual abuse and attempted suicide also varies along gender lines: sexually abused males face a significantly higher risk of suicide (55 per cent) than sexually abused adolescent females (29 per cent) (Martin *et al.* 2004). Similar findings were found with regard to physical abuse (Johnson *et al.* 2001).

Interpersonal stressors within the family context have also been implicated in youth suicidal behaviour. These stressors include conflicts, rejections, harsh demands and expectations, faulty communication, 'scapegoating', family dysfunction, negative attachment, and lowered parental responsiveness (Cetin 2001; Orbach 1989; Wagner *et al.* 2003). However, there is some evidence that family effects might be mediated by the adolescent's psychopathology (Wagner *et al.* 2003).

Failure, especially academic failure, also constitutes a critical life stressor associated to suicidal behaviour among youngsters. Poor academic performance (compared to above average) is associated with a fivefold increased likelihood of a suicide attempt and has long-term predictive value of suicidality (Richardson *et al.* 2005).

Losses that are early, recent, or multiple are empirically associated with suicidal behaviour. Losses can take on the form of death, separation, or parental divorce (Liu and Tein 2005). In a recent study, Orbach and Iohan (2007) studied experiences of loss among psychiatric suicide attempters, non-attempters, and controls. The types of losses studied included the loss of a close person (e.g. parent), material loss (e.g. loss of a job), mental loss (e.g. loss of faith), and physical losses (e.g. loss of good health). Compared to the non-attempters and the control group, the suicidal group reported more mental loss, physical losses, and loss of a close person. The number of losses was found to be significantly related to suicidal behaviour. The relationship between type of loss and number of loss and suicidal behaviour were sustained even after controlling for depression.

Liu and Tein (2005) found that an accumulation of such negative life events, regardless of the type of event, is a critical factor in suicidal behaviour. They report that 4–6 events have an odds ratio of 1.40; 7–9 events have an odds ratio of 2.02, and 9 and up events have an odds ratio of 3.73 (see also Roberts *et al.* 1998).

# Facilitators and inhibitors of suicidal behaviour

Facilitators and inhibitors (protective) factors can increase or decrease the probability of acting out suicidal impulses. These factors are not considered direct causes for suicide, rather they determine whether the suicidal person will act on the already existing suicidal tendencies, ideation, or wishes.

## Facilitators

### Attitudes toward death and toward ones body

Attraction to death and distorted beliefs about death, e.g. perceiving death as an improved state of life (Orbach 1994), bodily dissociation (numbness, detachment, high sensation threshold) and negative attitudes towards the body (Orbach *et al.* 1997, 2006) have been identified as facilitators of suicidal behaviour. In accordance with these findings, attraction to death and bodily dissociation make it easier for the suicidal youngster to choose death and to carry out an aggressive act against their own body.

### Vicarious exposure to sucide

Other facilitators include exposure to the suicidal acts of others, specifically when the possibility of vicariousness is more tangible. One obvious example is being made aware of the suicide of a friend (Stack 1996) or of a close relative (Gallo and Pfeffer 2003). However, a less apparent, yet no less potent form of vicarious exposure to suicide can occur through media reports of a suicidal act committed by an individual. The magnitude of suicides committed as a result of media facilitation increases in proportion to the amount, duration, and prominence of media coverage on suicide (Pirkis and Blood 2001). Suicide coverage may increase suicidal behaviour in several ways. Repeated exposure of a given suicidal act may promote identification with the attempter as well as with the method of attempt (Schmidtke and Schaller 2000; Pirkis and Blood 2001). Repetitive reporting of suicidal acts may also portray suicide as normative behaviour (Schmidtke and Schaller 2000). Furthermore, presenting suicide as a feature story has been hypothesized to promote the idealization of suicide and to engender the wish to receive attention (Orbach 1997).

### Availability of means

Availability of means is an important facilitator of suicidal behaviour, especially among impulsive suicides (Hawton *et al.* 2001). The presence of firearms within the home is a critical risk factor for suicide in adolescents (Brent *et al.* 1988; Grossman *et al.* 2005).

### Social norms

Moreover, social norms in and of themselves can facilitate suicide. In Domino and Takahashi's (1991) taxonomy study, Japanese medical students scored higher than their American counterparts on the Right to Die Scale. Differences in the scores were found related to suicide rates in the two countries.

## Inhibitors

Social support can serve as strong protective factors against suicide. Peer and family support were found to reduce various risk behaviours in youngsters who were sexually abused (Perkins and Jones 2004). Similarly, a sense of connectedness to parents or peer groups, as well as a sense of belonging to a positive school climate, was found to be strong protective factor against emotional distress and suicidal behaviour (Perkins and Jones 2004). Extra-curricular activities such as engaging in sports also contribute to suicide prevention in adolescents (Perkins and Jones 2004; Tomori and Zalar 2000).

Family cohesion in the form of mutual involvement, shared interests, and emotional support is another protective factor. This was found to be true in a longitudinal study of middle school students (Mckeown *et al.* 1998). One way that family cohesion can serve as a protective factor is that it seems to imbue its members with a sense of responsibility to family, as well as to close ones in general (Kyle 2004). Family cohesion was also found to mitigate suicidal behaviour, depression, and general life stress (Rubenstein *et al.* 1998).

A sense of self-cohesion and a strong sense of identity have been found to protect against suicidal behaviour, especially under stressful conditions. Katzir (2005) evaluated the sense of self-cohesion and identity in Israeli 18-year-olds prior to enlisting in the army, and did a follow-up on them throughout their military service. He found that young soldiers who had a strong sense of self-cohesion and identity were more resilient and less suicidal even under very stressful conditions compared to their counterparts.

The concept of religiosity as a protective factor was first introduced by Durkheim (1897, 1951). The protective value of religion lies in that it offers cohesiveness and integration (Durkheim 1897, 1951), social support and sense of belongingness (Pescosolido and Georgianna 1989), commitment to a few core life-saving beliefs (Stack 1992), rules and customs (Greening and Stoppelbein 2002) and moral obligations (Kyle 2004). Subsequently, Greening and Stoppelbein (2002) studied intrinsic and extrinsic religiosity and orthodoxy and their respective relationships to suicidality, depression, and hopelessness among a very large population of white Christian adolescents in the United States. In this study, orthodoxy emerged as a strong protective factor against suicidality (see also Hilton *et al.* 2000; Gould *et al.* 2003).

# Theoretical perspectives on suicidal behaviour in adolescents

## The stress–diathesis–hopelessness hypothesis

One of the most widely accepted theories regarding the relationship between problem-solving deficits and suicidal behaviour is the stress–diathesis–hopelessness hypothesis (SDH) developed by Schotte and Clum (1987). According to Schotte and Clum, individuals with difficulties in divergent thinking are unable to develop efficient solutions while under stress. As a result of their inability to conceive of a rational solution, their efforts are often reduced to purely psychological reactions of helplessness and hopelessness, leading individuals to view suicide as the only solution. Several authors have recently suggested elaborating the SDH hypothesis so that it considers not only the leverage of the cognitive deficits in problem-solving, but also the equally important role of the under-evaluation of one's own ability to problem-solving. Dixon *et al.* (1994) Rudd *et al.* (1994), and Yang and Clum (1996) have found that the under-evaluation of one's own ability to solve problems, rather than one's actual ability or performance, is a critical factor in the SDH process. This is also consistent with assertions that even highly intelligent individuals, who have the cognitive abilities to create solutions, may encounter problem-solving difficulties due to their lack of confidence (Shure 1997).

## Family dynamics as an explanation for suicidal behaviour in adolescents

Clinical observers of suicidal youngsters (Sabbath 1969) report that these youngsters have often experienced strong rejections by their parents from very early on in life. Sabbath gives examples of commonplace phrases employed by the parents of suicidal adolescents, conveying ruthless messages implying that the adolescent would be better of dead. One mother, for example, was in the habit of telling her 15-year-old daughter to 'drop dead.' Another example is of a father who would often convey tell his daughter: 'If you've got one rotten apple in the barrel you've got to get rid of it' (Orbach 1988).

Orbach (1986, 1988, 1989) suggests that suicidal tendencies in youth are directly linked to family situations and demands that pressure the child or adolescent to solve irresolvable problems. Some typical irresolvable problems are so because of the very nature of the problem (e.g., to excel beyond one's capability), a family problem that is disguised as a problem of the child (e.g. one parent exacerbating the child's problem and using it as leverage to keep the other parent within the family unit), limiting alternatives for solutions, and creating a new problem whenever the old one is resolved. In a recent empirical test of this theory, four experiential elements of facing irresolvable problems have emerged: feeling that the demands are unattainable (realistically so); a sense of an inextricable commitment to parental happiness; a sense that the youngster is required to behave in a problematic way; and giving up individuality for the sake of the parents (Orbach et al. 1999).

Richman (1978) found that suicidal adolescents were often the product of a family characterized by symbiosis without empathy. Symbiosis without empathy is a forced strangling bond without any expression of love and warmth. The parents demand total loyalty, yet are distant and estranged. As a result of these paradoxical conditions, the symbiotic family develops a massive generalized identity, with little distinction among the different members, and each family member is often ironically left with a feeling of isolation and loss of self. Another result of the family's extreme drive for unity is that intimate relationships outside the home become a complete taboo. Ultimately, the youngster is forced to choose between a complete break with the outside world or a complete separation from the family. Therefore, when adolescents from a symbiotic family experience failure outside the family unit, suicide often becomes a symbolic route for reunification and total fusion with there family. Thus, suicide in such youngsters is both an escape from, as well as a reunion with, the family.

## The propensity for suicidal behaviour: a biological predisposition for suicide

This theory suggests that there is a basic difference between suicidal and non-suicidal individuals in terms of an early propensity for suicidal behaviour. One version of this theory was suggested by Mann et al. (1999), and it was expanded by Wasserman (2001). According to the propensity theory, the suicidal propensity (stress–diathesis) is rooted in genetic, biological, and biochemical deficits (e.g. genetic inheritance, low serotonin activity). This propensity, which can be intensified by early and prolonged stress (e.g. mental illness, long-standing relationship problems) creates a readiness to respond to life difficulties with hopelessness, suicidal ideation, and with the planning of suicide. The suicidal propensity also involves a tendency to act out impulsively and aggressively. The propensity becomes active when it interacts with self-regulation deficits and current stressful life triggers such as acute psychiatric illness, loss, and separation or narcissistic injury.

### Self-reported reasons for suicidal behaviour

Boergers et al. (1998) studied male and female adolescents in a general hospital emergency room in terms of their self-reported reasons for their suicide attempt. The most frequently reported reason given for the suicide attempt was that they simply wanted to die, followed by the desire to be relieved from a terrible state of mind, to escape from an impossible situation, and to make people understand how desperate they feel. The rest of the reasons provided were of a more manipulative nature (e.g. to influence someone, to find out whether someone loved you). These findings were also confirmed by Haliburn (2000).

## Theoretical and empirical models of suicidal behaviour

In order to understand the relationships and interactions between the many factors involved in suicidal behaviour of adolescents in a more coherent way, several theoretical models have been introduced (Orbach 2001; Beautrais 2003; Rudd 2000; Sandin et al. 1998; Yang and Clum 1996). The various risk factors can be categorized into several main categories. The following categorization is suggested in this review: biological factors, morbidity factors, background factors (e.g. age, gender), stressors and triggers, mediating and moderating factors such as cognitive deficits, emotional deficits (e.g. depressive mood), personality aspects (e.g. impulsivity), and facilitators and inhibitors (protective factors).

Different models may use different systems of categorization. For example in some models depression is conceptualized as a mediating factor (Thompson et al. 2005) while in others, depression is conceived of as a more independent morbidity factor (Wasserman 2001). Some of the factors can appear in more than one category. For example, in Beautrais' (2003) model, life stress can appear first as an independent factor and later as a mediating factor. While some theoretical models make use of many of the factors found to be involved in suicidal behaviour, others make use of very few. Most of the theoretical models suggested emphasize interactional rather than linear models. The general trend of interaction that emerges within the various models is described as a flow from biological factors to morbidity factors, background factors, mediating factors, moderators, and finally facilitators and inhibitors.

Below, three examples of empirical examinations of theoretical models of suicidal behaviour in adolescents are described. Lewinsohn et al. (1996) examined the contribution of several independent variables on suicidal behaviour in adolescents (thoughts about death, death wishes, suicidal ideation, suicide planning, less serious suicide attempts, more serious suicide attempts, multiple suicide attempts). The independent variables included psychopathology (depression, anxiety, disruptive behaviour, and substance abuse), physical illness (number of sick days, number of doctors visits, physical symptoms), background/personal history factors (parental divorce/separation, death of a parent, teenage mother, moving away from home, suicide attempt by friend, death of a relative, poor social support, conflict with parents, everyday problems), interpersonal problems (involvement in arguments or fights, break-up with a friend, emotional over-dependency, and emotional estrangement); mediating variables (negative cognitions attribution style, self-esteem and coping skills). Lewinsohn *et al.* (1996) found that each factor (psychopathology, physical illness, environment and interpersonal) constituted a distinguished pathway to suicide with the first three showing a direct influence on suicidal behaviour. At the same time, however, all four categories were also found to have an indirect contribution mediated by the faulty cognitions.

Orbach and Iohan (2005) found a different configuration of interaction. They studied personality characteristics (negative emotional regulation, tolerance for mental pain, gender, dependency, perfectionism, and self-criticism), environmental stress (perceived stress, number of various types of loss), negative experiential aspects (mental pain), and depressive symptoms. Personality variables such as negative emotional regulation, self-criticism and perfectionism had a direct impact on suicidal behaviour (ideation, tendencies, and attempts). These variables, as well as a tendency for dependence, were found to have an additional indirect impact as well, mediated first by perceived pressure and number of losses and then by mental pain and depressive symptoms. In contrast to Lewinsohn's *et al.* (1996) model, Orbach and Iohan's model separated between personality aspects (e.g. perfectionism) and more subjective aspects (e.g. mental pain). However, similar to the Lewinsohn *et al.* (1996) model, multiple interactions were found among the independent and mediating factors.

Rather than following the interactional flow of different factors, Roberts *et al.* (1998) examined the accumulative impact of different contributing factors. Among other factors, they studied lifetime suicide attempts, age, gender, socio-economic status, depression, loneliness, life stress, fatalism, pessimism, and self-esteem. They computed the odd ratios of each variable for suicidal behaviour and found depression, lifetime suicide attempts, and life stress to have the highest odds ratios respectively. They also found that the odd ratios for having one of the 6 factors examined was 3.48, and for 6 factors the odd ratios increased to 67. Other empirical models have discovered different factor structures and interactions for male and female adolescents (Lewinsohn *et al.* 2001).

## Pathways to suicide

Achenbach (1991) has distinguished between externalizing pathologies and internalizing pathologies in youth. Externalizing pathologies include such symptoms as delinquent behaviour, aggressive behaviour, impulsivity, oppositional behaviour, and hyperactivity. Internalizing pathologies include withdrawal, somatic complaints, anxiety, depression, inhibition, and being self-demanding. These two types of pathologies can be linked to different pathways of suicidal behaviour in adolescents independent of negative life events. Similar findings were reported by Vermerien *et al.* (2002).

Orbach (1997) has also distinguished between different pathways to suicide in general, positing three clusters of suicidal behaviour. The depressive perfectionist cluster (the internalizing cluster) is hypothesized to be mediated by severe negative emotions. The aggressive impulsive cluster (externalizing cluster) is hypothesized

to be mediated by deficits in impulse control. The disintegrating cluster characterized by panic, severe anxiety and psychiatric pathology is hypothesized to be mediated by a severe loss of control.

As Wagner and Hustead (2002) perceive it, the pathways to youth suicidal behaviour are paved upon child–family relationships. One such pathway is the child-driven pathway wherein the suicidal behaviour is primarily enabled by the child's problems. This pathway is characterized by children who develop insecure or disrupted attachments towards the parents despite their parents' supportiveness and competence. Furthermore, the child's relationship with, and treatment of, their parents is distinctively negative and aggressive. This pathway involved children with high psychopathology to parents with low psychopathology. The child has a short history of suicidal behaviour, yet their suicide attempts are highly lethal and driven by an attempt to escape pain and do not implicate the family. The second pathway is the parent-driven pathway wherein the child's suicidal behaviour is primarily enabled by the parents. This pathway involves parents who are poorly competent, and who are insecure in their attachment to the suicidal child. Their treatment of and relationship with the suicidal child is marked by aggression and negativity. In this pathway the parents are highly psychopathological and the child is low in psychopathology. The child has a long history of suicidal behaviour, yet their attempts are low in lethality. The attempts are described as interpersonal and communication-based, and the family is implicated in precipitating the attempt. The third pathway posited by Wagner and Hustead is the reciprocal pathway characterized by poor parental competence and support, high parental and child psychopathology, mutual parent and child insecure attachments, long history of suicidal behaviour and parent and child mutual perceptions of negative–aggressive relationships. This pathway usually results in lower lethality of attempts that are described as interpersonal messages and as being precipitated by the family. The authors report finding strong empirical supports for the first and third pathways and somewhat weaker support for the second pathway.

From a different perspective, Blatt (1995) posits personality develops as a consequence of a complex interaction between two fundamental lines: (a) the development of the capacity to establish mature and satisfying interpersonal relationships and (b) the development of a realistic, positive, and integrated self-definition and identity. An overemphasized interpersonal relatedness may lead to an anaclitic (or dependent) depression, whereas overemphasized individuality and self-definition may result in self-critical (or introjective) depression. Anaclitic depression involves a deep longing to be loved and cared for. The overly individualized person is characterized by self-criticism, feelings of inferiority, and guilt. Each of these imbalances were found to be related to suicidal behaviour in different ways (see also Brunstien-Klomek *et al.* 2005; Fehon *et al.* 2000; Orbach and Iohn 2005). Both anaclitic depression and introjective depression were found to be implicated in suicidal behaviour.

Applying a cognitive approach, Dieserud *et al.* (2001) offer a two-path model of suicide attempt for all ages that is somewhat parallel to Blatt's two pathway model. The first pathway begins with low self-esteem, loneliness, and separation or divorce, advancing to depression, then hopelessness, suicide ideation, and finally a suicide attempt. The second pathway begins with low self-esteem and a low sense of self-efficacy, followed by negative self-appraisal of one's own problem-solving capacity, and poor interpersonal problem-solving skills, finally leading to suicide. This model emphasizes the importance of addressing both depression and hopelessness, as well as problem-solving deficits when working with suicide attempters.

## Conclusion

There is an abundance of information on suicidal behaviour in general and on adolescent suicidal behaviour in particular. Unfortunately, the natural conclusion—that we have a good understanding and knowledge of this tragic phenomenon—is not fully accurate. One reason for this counterintuitive reality is that empirical findings have been transmitted through various and non-concurring theories and terminologies. It is our belief that the first step to furthering our knowledge of suicide is to promote a coherent organization of the data for the sake of advancing conceptual clarity. Further, the present review shows that there that there is more than one pathway or one dynamic of suicidal behaviour. It is evident that these should be taken in consideration when prevention programmes are planned. One size does not fit all and different prevention programmes should be tailored for each dynamic or pathway. Such efforts can help us to better define our future goals in the study of suicide and eventually lead to an improved effort in the prevention of suicidal behaviour in adolescents.

## References

Achenbach TM (1991). *Manual for the Youth Self-Report and 1991 Profile.* University of Vermont, Department of Psychiatry, Burlington.

Andrews JA and Lewinsohn PM (1992). Suicidal attempts among older adolescents: prevalence and co-occurrence with psychiatric disorders. *Journal of the American Academy of Child and Adolescent Psychiatry*, **31**, 655–662.

Barbe RP, Williamson DE, Bridge JA *et al.* (2005). Clinical differences between suicidal and nonsuicidal depressed children and adolescents. *Journal of Clinical Psychiatry*, **66**, 492–498.

Batigun AD (2005). Suicide probability: an assessment terms of reasons for living, hopelessness and loneliness. [Intihar Olasiligi: Yasami Surdurme Nedenleri, Umutsuzluk ve Yalnizlik Acisindan Bir Inceleme.] *Turk Psikiyatri Dergisi*, **16**, 29–39.

Beautrais AL (2003). Life course factors. *The American Behavioral Scientist*, **46**, 1137–1156.

Beautrais AL, Joyce PR, Mulder RT *et al.* (1996). Prevalence and comorbidity of mental disorders in persons making serious suicide attempts: a case–control study. *American Journal of Psychiatry*, **153**, 1009–1014.

Beck AT, Steer RA, Kovacs M *et al.* (1985). Hopelessness and eventual suicide: a 10-year prospective study of patients hospitalized with suicidal ideation. *American Journal of Psychiatry*, **142**, 559–563.

Bergen HA, Martin G, Richardson AS *et al.* (2003). Sexual abuse and suicidal behavior: a model constructed from a large community sample of adolescents. *Journal of the American Academy of Child and Adolescent Psychiatry*, **42**, 1301–1309.

Blatt SJ (1995). The destructiveness of perfectionism: implications for the treatment of depression. *American Psychologist*, **50**, 1003–1020.

Boergers J, Spirito A, Donaldson D (1998). Reasons for adolescent suicide attempts: associations with psychological functioning. *Journal of the American Academy of Child and Adolescent Psychiatry*, **37**, 1287–1293.

Brent DA, Perper JA, Goldstien CE *et al.* (1988). Risk factors for adolescent suicide: a comparison of adolescent suicide victims with suicidal inpatients. *Archives of General Psychiatry*, **45**, 581–588.

Brunstein-Klomek A, Orbach I, Meged S *et al.* (2005). Self complexity of suicidal adolescents. *International Journal of Adolescent Medicine and Health*, **17**, 267–273.

Catalina-Zamora ML and Mardomingo-Sanz MJ (1997). Psychiatric pathology associated to suicidal attempts. [Patalogia psiquiatrica asociada en los intentos de suicidio.] *Revista de Psiquiatria Infanto Juvenil*, **1**, 17–20.

Cautin RL, Overholser JC, Goetz P (2001). Assessment of mode of anger expression in adolescent psychiatric inpatients. *Adolescence*, **36**, 163–170.

Cetin FC (2001). Suicide attempts and self-image among Turkish adolescents. *Journal of Youth and Adolescence*, **30**, 641–651.

De Wilde EJ, Kienhorst IC, Diekstra RF *et al.* (1993). The specificity of psychological characteristics of adolescent suicide attempters. *Journal of the American Academy of Child and Adolescent Psychiatry*, **32**, 51–59.

Deane FP, Wilson CJ, Ciarrochi J (2001). Suicidal ideation and help-negation: not just hopelessness or prior help. *Journal of Clinical Psychology*, **57**, 901–914.

Dieserud G, Roysamb E, Ekeberg O *et al.* (2001). Toward an integrative model of suicide attempt: a cognitive psychological approach. *Suicide and Life-Threatening Behavior*, **31**, 153–168.

Dixon WA, Heppner PP, Rudd MD (1994). Problem-solving appraisal, hopelessness, and suicide ideation: evidence for a mediational model. *Journal of Counseling Psychology*, **41**, 91–98.

Domino G and Takahashi Y (1991). Attitudes toward suicide in Japanese and American medical students. *Suicide and Life-Threatening Behavior*, **21**, 345–359.

Donaldson D, Spirito A, Farnett E (2000). The role of perfectionism and depressive cognitions in understanding the hopelessness experienced by adolescent suicide attempters. *Child Psychiatry and Human Development*, **31**, 99–111.

Durkheim E (1897). *Le suicide*. Felix Alcan, Paris.

Durkheim E (1951). *Suicide*. Free Press, New York.

Eliason RV (2001). The roles of cognitive rigidity and impulsivity in adolescent suicide attempts. *Dissertation Abstracts International: Section B: The Sciences and Engineering*, **62**, 1075.

Esposito C, Spirito A, Boergers J *et al.* (2003). Affective, behavioral, and cognitive functioning in adolescents with multiple suicide attempts. *Suicide and Life-Threatening Behavior*, **33**, 389–399.

Evren C, Ogel K, Tamar D *et al.* (2001). The characteristics of inhalant users. [Ucucu madde kullanicilarinin ozellikleri.] *Bagimlik Dergisi*, **2**, 57–60.

Fehon DC, Grilo CM, Martino S (2000). A comparison of dependent and self-critically depressed hospitalized adolescents. *Journal of Youth and Adolescence*, **29**, 93–106.

Fennig S, Geva K, Zalsman G *et al.* (2005). Effect of gender on suicide attempters versus nonattempters in an adolescent inpatient unit. *Comprehensive Psychiatry*, **46**, 90–97.

Fergusson DM, Woodward LJ, Horwood LJ (2000). Risk factors and life processes associated with the onset of suicidal behaviour during adolescence and early adulthood. *Psychological Medicine*, **30**, 23–39.

Fritsch S, Donaldson D, Spirito A *et al.* (2000). Personality characteristics of adolescent suicide attempters. *Child Psychiatry and Human Development*, **30**, 219–235.

Gallo CL and Pfeffer CR (2003). Children and adolescents bereaved by a suicidal death: implications for psychosocial outcomes and interventions. In RAE King and AE Apter, eds, *Suicide in Children and Adolescents*, pp. 294–312. Cambridge University Press, New York.

Goldston DB, Daniel SS, Reboussin BA *et al.* (2001). Cognitive risk factors and suicide attempts among formerly hospitalized adolescents: a prospective naturalistic study. *Journal of the American Academy of Child and Adolescent Psychiatry*, **40**, 91–99.

Goldston DB, Sergent-Daniel S, Reboussin DM *et al.* (1999). Suicide attempts among formerly hospitalized adolescents: a prospective naturalistic study of risk during the first 5 years after discharge. *Journal of the American Academy of Child and Adolescent Psychiatry*, **38**, 660–671.

Gould MS, Greenberg T, Velting DM *et al.* D (2003). Youth suicide risk and preventive interventions: a review of the past 10 years. *Journal of the American Academy of Child and Adolescent Psychiatry*, **42**, 386–405.

Greening L and Stoppelbein L (2002). Religiosity, attributional style, and social support as psychosocial buffers for African American and White adolescents' perceived risk for suicide. *Suicide and Life-Threatening Behavior*, **32**, 404–417.

Groholt B, Ekeberg O, Wichstrom L *et al.* (1998). Suicide among children and younger and older adolescents in Norway: a comparative study. *Journal of the American Academy of Child and Adolescent Psychiatry*, **37**, 473–481.

Grossman DC, Mueller BA, Riedy C *et al.* (2005). Gun storage practices and risk of youth suicide and unintentional firearm injuries. *Journal of the American Medical Association*, **293**, 707–714.

Guertin T, Lloyd-Richardson E, Spirito A *et al.* (2001). Self-mutilative behavior in adolescents who attempt suicide by overdose. *Journal of the American Academy of Child and Adolescent Psychiatry*, **40**, 1062–1069.

Haliburn J (2000). Reasons for adolescent suicide attempts. *Journal of the American Academy of Child and Adolescent Psychiatry*, **39**, 13–14.

Hawton K, Townsend E, Deeks J *et al.* (2001). Effects of legislation restricting pack sizes of paracetamol and salicylate on self poisoning in the United Kingdom: before and after study. *British Medical Journal*, **322**, 1203–1207.

Hilton SC, Fellingham GW, Lyon JL (2000). Suicide rates and religious commitment in young adult males in Utah. *American Journal of Epidemiology*, **155**, 413–419.

Horesh N, Orbach I, Gothelf D *et al.* (2003). Comparision of the suicidal behavior of adolescent inpatients with borderline personality disorder and major depression. *Journal of Nervous and Mental Disease*, **191**, 582–588.

Houston JL (2004). Impact of comorbidity on self-reported suicidal ideation and future suicidal behavior in an adolescent residential care sample. *Dissertation Abstracts International: Section B: The Sciences and Engineering*, **64**, 3526.

Johnson JG, Cohen P, Kasen S *et al.* (2001). Association of maladaptive parental behavior with psychiatric disorder among parents and their offspring. *Archives of General Psychiatry*, **58**, 453–460.

Katzir Y (2005). The relations between ego identity formation and suicide tendencies within soldiers in their first months of their military training. Dissertation thesis. Department of Education, Bar-Ilan University, Ramat-Gan.

Kienhorst C, de Wilde EJ, Diekstra RF *et al.* (1992). Differences between adolescent suicide attempters and depressed adolescents. *Acta Psychiatrica Scandinavia*, **85**, 222–228.

Kyle JA (2004). Familial and social support as protective factors in African Americans at risk for suicide. *Dissertation Abstracts International: Section B: The Sciences and Engineering*, **65**, 2004–2099.

Lewinsohn PM, Rohde P, Seeley JR (1996). Adolescent suicidal ideation and attempts: prevalence, risk factors, and clinical implications. *Clinical Psychology: Science and Practice*, **3**, 25–46.

Lewinsohn PM, Rohde P, Seeley JR *et al.* (2001). Gender differences in suicide attempts from adolescence to young adulthood. *Journal of the American Academy of Child and Adolescent Psychiatry*, **40**, 427–434.

Liu X and Tein JY (2005). Life events, psychopathology, and suicidal behavior in Chinese adolescents. *Journal of Affective Disorders*, **86**, 195–203.

Loraas JA (1997). Shame, symptom-expression, and destructive behavior in adolescent depression. *Dissertation Abstracts International: Section B: The Sciences and Engineering*, **58**, 2687.

Mann JJ, Waternaux C, Haas GL *et al.* (1999). Toward a clinical model of suicidal behavior in psychiatric patients. *American Journal of Psychiatry*, **156**, 181–189.

Martin G, Bergman HA, Richardson AS *et al.* (2004). Sexual abuse and suicidality: gender differences in a large community sample of adolescents. *Child Abuse and Neglect*, **28**, 491–503.

Martin G, Richardson AS, Bergen HA *et al.* (2005). Perceived academic performance, self-esteem and locus of control as indicators of need for assessment of adolescent suicide risk: implications for teachers. *Journal of Adolescence*, **28**, 75–87.

McKeown RE, Garrison CZ, Cuffe SP *et al.* (1998). Incidence and predictors of suicidal behaviors in a longitudinal sample of young adolescents. *Journal of the American Academy of Child and Adolescent Psychiatry*, **37**, 612–619.

Merwin RM and Ellis JB (2004). Children's reasons for living, self-esteem, and violence. *Archives of Suicide Research*, **8**, 251–261.

Miller AL, Wyman SE, Huppert JD *et al.* (2000). Analysis of behavioral skills utilized by suicidal adolescents receiving dialectical behavior therapy. *Cognitive and Behavioral Practice*, **7**, 183–187.

Nock MK and Kazdin AE (2002). Parent-directed physical aggression by clinic-referred youths. *Journal of Clinical Child and Adolescent Psychology*, **31**, 193–205.

Orbach I (1986). The 'insolvable problem' as a determinant in the dynamics of suicidal behavior in children. *American Journal of Psychotherapy*, **40**, 511–520.

Orbach I (1988). *The 'Insolvable Problem' in the Dynamics of Suicidal Behavior in Children*. Jason Aronson Inc., Lanham.

Orbach I (1989). Familial and intrapsychic splits in suicidal adolescents. *American Journal of Psychotherapy*, **43**, 356–367.

Orbach I (1994). Dissociation, physical pain, and suicide: a hypothesis. *Suicide and Life-Threatening Behavior*, **24**, 68–79.

Orbach I (1997). A taxonomy of factors related to suicidal behavior. *Clinical Psychology: Science and Practice*, **4**, 208–224.

Orbach I (2001). Therapeutic empathy with the suicidal wish: principles of therapy with suicidal Individuals. *American Journal of Psychotherapy*, **55**, 166–184.

Orbach I and Iohan M. (2005). Distress and regulation in female suicide attempters. Unpublished Manuscript. Department of Psychology, Bar-Ilan University.

Orbach I and Iohan M (2007).Stress, distress, emotional regulation and suicide attempts in female adolescents. In R Tatarelli, M Pompili and P Giradi, eds, *Suicide in Psychiatric Disorders*, pp. 295–314. Nova Science Publishers, New York

Orbach I, Bar-Joseph H, Dror N (1990). Styles of problem-solving in suicidal individuals. *Suicide and Life-Threatening Behavior*, **20**, 56–64.

Orbach I, Gilboa-Schechtman E, Sheffer A *et al.* (2006). Negative bodily self in suicide attempters. *Suicide and Life Threatening Behavior*, **36**, 136–153.

Orbach I, Mikulincer M, Blumenson R *et al.* D (1999). The subjective experience of problem irresolvability and suicidal behavior: dynamics and measurement. *Suicide and Life-Threatening Behavior*, **29**, 150–164.

Orbach I, Mikulincer M, Gilboa-Schechtman E *et al.* (2003). Mental pain and its relationship to suicidality and life meaning. *Suicide and Life-Threatening Behavior*, **33**, 231–241.

Orbach I, Mikulincer M, King R *et al.* (1997). Threshold for tolerance of physical pain in suicidal and nonsuicidal adolescents. *Journal of Consulting and Clinical Psychology*, **65**, 646–652.

Orbach I, Mikulincer M, Stein D *et al.* (1998). Self-representation of suicidal adolescents. *Journal of Abnormal Psychology*, **107**, 434–439.

Pelkonen M, Marttunen M, Pulkkien E *et al.* (1996). Excess mortality among former adolescent male outpatients. *Acta Psychiatrica Scandinavia*, **94**, 60–66.

Penn JV, Esposito CL, Schaeffer LE *et al.* (2003). Suicide attempts and self-mutilative behavior in a juvenile correctional facility. *Journal of the American Academy of Child and Adolescent Psychiatry*, **42**, 762–769.

Perkins DF and Jones KR (2004). Risk behaviors and resiliency within physically abused adolescents. *Child Abuse and Neglect*, **28**, 547–563.

Pescosolido BA and Georgianna S (1989). Durkheim, suicide, and religion: toward a network theory of suicide. *American Sociological Review*, **54**, 33–48.

Piquet ML and Wagner BM (2003). Coping responses of adolescent suicide attempters and their relation to suicidal ideation across a 2-year follow-up: a preliminary study. *Suicide and Life-Threatening Behavior*, **33**, 288–301.

Pirkis J and Blood RW (2001). Suicide and the media: (1) Reportage in nonfictional media. *Crisis*, **22**, 146–154.

Rubenstein JL, Halyon A, Kasten L *et al.* (1998). Suicidal behavior in adolescents: stress and protection in different family contexts. *American Journal of Ortthopsychiatry*, **68**, 274–284.

Richardson AS, Bergen HA, Martin G *et al.* (2005). Perceived academic performance as an indicator of risk of attempted suicide in young adolescents. *Archives of Suicide Research*, **9**, 163–176.

Richman J (1978). Symbiosis, empathy, suicidal behavior, and the family. *Suicide and Life-Threatening Behavior*, **8**, 139–149.

Roberts RE, Roberts CR, Chen RY (1998). Suicidal thinking among adolescents with a history of attempted suicide. *Journal of the American Academy of Child and Adolescent Psychiatry*, **37**, 1294–1300.

Rotheram-Borus MJ (1988). Hopelessness, depression, and suicidal intent among adolescent suicide attempters. *Journal of the American Academy of Child and Adolescent Psychiatry*, **27**, 700–704.

Rudd MD, Rajab MH, Dahm PF (1994). Problem-solving appraisal in suicide ideators and attempters. *American Journal of Orthopsychiatry*, **64**, 136–149.

Rudd MD (2000). The suicidal mode: a cognitive-behavioral model of suicidality. *Suicide and Life-Threatening Behavior*, **30**, 18–33.

Sabbath JC (1969). The suicidal adolescent: the expendable child. *Journal of the American Academy of Child Psychiatry*, **8**, 272–285.

Sandin B, Chorot P, Santed MA *et al.* (1998). Negative life events and adolescent suicidal behavior: a critical analysis from the stress process perspective. *Journal of Adolescence*, **21**, 415–426.

Sanislow CA, Grilo CM, Fehon DC *et al.* (2003). Correlates of suicide risk in juvenile detainees and adolescent inpatients. *Journal of the American Academy of Child and Adolescent Psychiatry*, **42**, 234–240.

Savarimuthu A (2002). Commitment to living: a microanalytic study of the emotion of shame and the perceived erosion of social bonds in two cases of adolescent suicide. *Dissertation Abstracts International Section A: Humanities and Social Sciences*, **62**, 7927.

Sayar K and Bozkir F (2004). Predictors of suicide intent and lethality in a sample of adolescent suicide attempters. [Intihar Girisiminde Bulunan Ergenlerde Intihar Niyeti ve Olumculugun Belirleyicileri.] *Yeni Symposium: Psikiyatri, Noroloji ve Davranis Bilimleri Dergisi*, **42**, 28–36.

Schotte DE and Clum GA (1987). Problem-solving skills in suicidal psychiatric patients. *Journal of Consulting and Clinical Psychology*, **55**, 49–54.

Schmidtke A and Schaller S (2000). The role of mass media in suicide prevention. In K Hawton and K van Heeringen, eds, *The International Handbook of Suicide and Attempted Suicide*, pp. 675–697. John Wiley and Sons Ltd, Chichester.

Schwartz JAJ, Kaslow NJ, Seely J *et al.* (2000). Psychological, cognitive, and interpersonal correlates of attributional change in adolescents. *Journal of Clinical Child Psychology*, **29**, 188–198.

Shneidman ES (1993). Commentary: suicide as psychache. *Journal of Nervous and Mental Disease*, **181**, 145–147.

Shure MB (1997). Interpersonal cognitive problem solving: primary prevention of early high risk behaviors in preschool and primary years.

In GW Albee *et al.*, eds, *Primary Prevention Works: Issues in Childrens' and Families' Lives*, pp. 167–188. Sage, Thousand Oaks.

Specker AEM and Hawton K (2005). Social problem solving in adolescents with suicidal behavior: a systematic review. *Suicide and Life-Threatening Behavior*, **35**, 365–387.

Spirito A, Valeri S, Boergers J *et al.* (2003). Predictors of continued suicidal behavior in adolescents following a suicide attempt. *Journal of Clinical Child and Adolescent Psychology*, **32**, 284–289.

Stack S (1992). Religiosity, depression, and suicide. In JFE Schumaker, ed., *Religion and Mental Health*, pp. 87–97. Oxford University Press, New York.

Stack S (1996). The effect of the media on suicide: evidence from Japan, 1955–1985. *Suicide and Life-Threatening Behavior*, **26**, 132–142.

Thompson EA, Mazza JJ, Herting JR *et al.* (2005). The mediating roles of anxiety, depression, and hopelessness on adolescent suicidal behaviors. *Suicide and Life-Threatening Behavior*, **35**, 14–34.

Tomori M and Zalar B (2000). Sport and physical activity as possible protective factors in relation to adolescent suicide attempts. *International Journal of Sport Psychology*, **31**, 405–413.

Vermeiren R, Ruchkin V, Leckman PE *et al.* (2002). *Exposure to Violence and Suicide Risk in Adolescents: A Community Study*. Springer, Germany.

Wagner BM and Hustead L (2002). Family profiles of adolescent suicide attempters. Paper presented at the annual meeting of the American Association of Suicidology, Bethesda.

Wagner BM, Silverman MA, Martin CE (2003). Family factors in youth suicidal behaviors. *American Behavioral Scientist*, **46**, 1171–1191.

Wasserman D (2001). A stress–vulnerability model and the development of the suicidal process. In D Wasserman, ed., *Suicide: An Unnecessary Death*, pp. 13–27. Martin Dunitz, London.

Wetzler S, Asnis GM, Hyman RB *et al.* (1996). Characteristics of suicidality among adolescents. *Suicide and Life-Threatening Behavior*, **26**, 37–45.

Wichstrom L and Rossow I (2002). Explaining the gender differences in self-reported suicide attempts: a nationally representative study of Norwegian adolescents. *Suicide and Life-Threatening Behavior*, **32**, 101–116.

Wilson KG, Stelzer J, Bergman JN *et al.* (1995). Problem solving, stress, and coping in adolescent suicide attempts. *Suicide and Life-Threatening Behavior*, **25**, 241–252.

Yang B and Clum GA (1996). Effects of early negative life experiences on cognitive functioning and risk for suicide: a review. *Clinical Psychology Review*, **16**, 177–195.

Zlotnick C, Donaldson D, Spirito A *et al.* (1997). Affect regulation and suicide attempts in adolescent inpatients. *Journal of the American Academy of Child and Adolescent Psychiatry*, **36**, 793–798.

Zlotnick C, Wolfsdorf BA, Johnson B *et al.* (2004). Impaired self-regulation and suicidal behavior among adolescent and young adult psychiatric inpatients. *Archives of Suicide Research*, **7**, 149–157.

# CHAPTER 88

# Psychodynamic and family aspects of youth suicide

Robert A King

## Abstract

The psychodynamic approach to suicide examines the meaning and origins of suicidal behaviour in terms of the vicissitudes of feelings, motives, self-concept, and interpersonal relationships. Negative or poorly differentiated self-concept; maladaptive defensive or attachment style; and isolative, avoidant, or self-critical personality traits appear to be important risk factors for suicidality in youth.

Across diverse national contexts, adolescent suicidality is associated with family factors such as parental psychopathology, negative life events, family discord, negative parent–child relationship (including abuse and neglect), and low perceived family support. Further research is needed to understand the intervening variables linking such family factors to suicide, including delineating the relative contributions of shared genetic risk (e.g. for psychopathology or maladaptive traits) versus the negative developmental impact of adverse family environment.

The developmental challenges of adolescence increase the vulnerability to suicidal ideation and behaviour. How specific national or cultural contexts mitigate or exacerbate these factors remains an important area for further study.

## Introduction

### The psychodynamic approach

Psychodynamic theorizing about youth suicide had its origins in efforts to understand the perceived epidemic of student suicides in Germany and Austria in the years before the First World War. Themes which emerged from the Vienna Psychoanalytic Society's 1910 symposium (Friedman 1967) on the topic were the role of guilt, aggression turned against the self, and thwarted love. Sadger emphasized the importance of libidinal or attachment elements: 'the only person who puts an end to his life is one who has been compelled to give up all hope of love.' In contrast, Stekel emphasized the aggressive and self-punitive aspects of suicide: 'No one kills himself who has never wanted to kill another, or at least wished the death of another' (Friedman 1967, p. 97). This perspective was later elaborated in Menninger's (1938) dictum that suicide was rooted in the threefold wish to kill, the wish to be killed, and the wish to die, and summarized in Shneidman's (1980) pithy

aphorism that suicide is murder in the 180th degree. It was Freud (1917), however, who combined the aggressive, libidinal, and object relations perspectives in his notion that, in melancholia, the attack on the self is driven by the threatened loss of an intensely needed, but ambivalently loved object (or internalized other), who is felt to be potentially hateful, critical, or rejecting of the subject.

Following these early leads, the contemporary psychodynamic approach to suicide complements the biological, sociological, and nosological approaches by examining the meaning of suicidal behaviour in terms of feelings, motives, interpersonal relationships, and their conflicts (King 2003). For example, in looking at the immediate experiential antecedents of suicidal action, we may ask, what are the unbearable affects from which suicide appears to offer a means of escape (Baumeister 1990)? What are the developmental experiences that predispose to experiencing the self as the intolerable origin or locus of this pain? What kinds of internal or external events trigger suicidal feelings and behaviour, and what is their significance in the broader context of the suicidal youngster's life? The psychodynamic approach is also a developmental one that attempts to understand the origins of the vulnerability to suicide and depression in the related developmental trajectories of the capacity for self-care and comfort, the ability to reach out for and sustain protective affiliations, and the regulation of self-esteem (King and Apter 1996). As a corollary, the psychodynamic approach is also concerned with how different coping, defensive, and attachment styles influence the vulnerability to suicide via the quality of affect regulation and internal object relations. Since the matrix of these capacities are believed to lie in the child's early experiences of being cared for, comforted, and cherished, the psychodynamic approach is interested in how different family contexts may serve to increase or buffer the developing youngster's potential suicidal risk. Finally, the psychodynamic perspective seeks clues as to how, in a given culture, the challenges of specific developmental epochs, such as adolescence, may confer a particular vulnerability to suicidal behaviour (Tabachnik 1981).

### The international context

Reliable cross-national or cross-cultural data on the psychosocial variables associated with youthful suicidal behaviours are sparse (Evans *et al.* 2004; Colucci and Martin 2007b); most studies are limited to comparisons of rates, gender ratios, or method (Kelleher and Chambers 2003; Gould *et al.* 2003b; Bridge *et al.* 2006; Colucci and Martin 2007a). UNICEF (2007) reports, such as the recent comprehensive score-card of child and adolescent well-being in economically advanced nations, provide a rich overview of socio-economic indicators, family structure, and self-reported measures of family and peer relations, risk and health behaviours, and personal well-being; these data, however, have not systematically been brought into relationship with those on national rates of attempted or completed youth suicide. Table 88.1 shows the most recent (WHO 2007) youth suicide data for selected countries, together with their rank-order on the UNICEF summary dimensions

**Table 88.1** Youth suicide rates and measures by age of well-being in selected countries[a]

| Country | Year | 5–14 years | 15–24 years | Rank order | |
|---|---|---|---|---|---|
| | | All | All | Subjective well-being | Family and peer relationships |
| Russia | 2004 | 2.3 | 28.1 | | |
| Lithuania | 2004 | 1.6 | 25.5 | | |
| Finland | 2004 | 0.8 | 21.7 | 11 | 17 |
| New Zealand | 2000 | 0.7 | 18.2 | | |
| Iceland | 2004 | 0.0 | 16.2 | | |
| Norway | 2004 | 0.5 | 14.0 | 8 | 10 |
| Latvia | 2004 | 0.8 | 13.1 | | |
| Japan | 2004 | 0.4 | 12.8 | | |
| Argentina | 2003 | 0.9 | 12.4 | | |
| Belgium | 1997 | 0.5 | 12.4 | 16 | 5 |
| China (Hong Kong SAR) | 2004 | 0.6 | 12.2 | | |
| Ireland | 2005 | 0.5 | 11.9 | 5 | 7 |
| Poland | 2004 | 0.8 | 11.8 | 19 | 14 |
| Austria | 2005 | 0.4 | 11.8 | 9.8 | 16 |
| Canada | 2002 | 0.9 | 11.5 | 15 | 18 |
| Australia | 2003 | 0.5 | 10.7 | | |
| Singapore | 2003 | 0.8 | 10.5 | | |
| United States | 2002 | 0.6 | 9.9 | | 20 |
| Switzerland | 2004 | 0.1 | 9.8 | 6 | 4 |
| Sweden | 2002 | 0.6 | 9.7 | 7 | 15 |
| Hungary | 2003 | 0.7 | 9.0 | 13 | 6 |
| Czech Republic | 2004 | 0.7 | 9.0 | 17 | 19 |
| France | 2003 | 0.4 | 8.1 | 9 | 13 |
| Denmark | 2001 | 0.3 | 7.5 | 12 | 9 |
| China (mainland, selected areas) | 1999 | 0.8 | 6.9 | 10 | 1 |
| Germany | 2004 | 0.3 | 6.7 | | |
| Mexico | 2003 | 0.7 | 6.4 | | |
| Israel | 2003 | 0.2 | 6.0 | 18 | 12 |
| United Kingdom | 2004 | 0.1 | 5.2 | 20 | 21 |
| Netherlands | 2004 | 0.5 | 5.0 | 1 | 3 |
| Spain | 2004 | 0.3 | 4.3 | 2 | 8 |
| Italy | 2002 | 0.2 | 4.1 | | |
| Portugal | 2003 | 0.0 | 3.7 | 14 | 2 |
| Greece | 2004 | 0.2 | 1.7 | 3 | 11 |

From: *World Health Organization: Country Suicide Reports*, (http://www.who.int/mental_health/prevention/suicide/country_reports/en/index.html) accessed 11/30/07

UNICEF: *Child poverty in perspective: An overview of child well-being in rich countries*. Innocenti Report Card 7 Florence, UNICEF Innocenti Research Centre, 2007.

a; in descending order of suicide rates for 15–24 y.o.

of subjective well-being and family and peer relationships. The World Values Survey (Inglehart *et al.* 1998) also provides a source of age-graded data from different countries on variables such as life and home satisfaction, happiness, trust in family, etc.

Work by Offer and colleagues (Offer *et al.* 1988) provide extensive comparative data on multiple facets of adolescents' self-image around the world.

# Individual psychodynamic factors: self-concept, object relations, personality factors, intense affect states

## Self-concept

Although self-esteem or self-concept is sometimes discussed in suicide research (Fergusson and Lynskey 1995; Overholser *et al.* 1995) as though it were a unitary concept, it is important to go beyond global measures of self-worth. The work of Harter distinguishes different facets of adolescent self-concept, with those aspects salient to peers (perceived appearance, peer likeability, and athletic competence) and those salient to parents (scholastic competence and behavioural conduct) exercising an impact on depression, hopelessness, and suicidality via independent paths (Harter *et al.* 1992). Examining the self-representations of suicidal Israeli adolescents, Orbach and colleagues found suicidal adolescents showed a less complexly differentiated and integrated organization of self-attributes, and an increased discrepancy between perceived actual and desired self, suggesting a vulnerability to 'uneven processing of positive and negative information, confusion, and [over]simplicity' (Orbach *et al.* 1998, p. 435). In addition, suicidal adolescents evidenced not only an increased number of negative self-descriptions and negative descriptions of parents, but also a self-perception of being less differentiated from their parents with respect to these negative traits (negative symbiosis) (Klomek *et al.* 2007).

Distorted object relations parallel suicidal adolescents' maladaptive defensive styles. Overuse of displacement is connected with increased risk for suicidal and aggressive behaviours, while sublimation is probably a protective factor. A study (Apter *et al.* 1997) of suicidal Israeli adolescents found a preponderance of immature ego defences (including the use of displacement), which appeared to amplify aggression, with the maladaptive overuse of introjection, displacement, and repression resulting in increased aggression and negative affects directed against the self.

## Attachment

Bowlby and colleagues' (Thompson 2006) work on attachment styles has provided a fruitful model for linking early infant experiences of caretaking and later enduring styles of interaction or response to interpersonal loss or frustration that may confer vulnerability to depression and suicidality. Although the relative role of experience and constitutional factors in shaping maladaptive attachment styles remains uncertain, attachment style is an important determinant, even in later childhood and adolescence, of the quality of perceived stress, support, and closeness with others (Blatt 1995; Shahar *et al.* 2003; Collins and Steinberg 2006). A study by Adam *et al.* (1996) of the attachment status of suicidal adolescents compared to non-suicidal psychiatric controls, found that suicidal adolescents are more likely to show 'unresolved'

or 'preoccupied' attachment styles, which might be coloured by these adolescents' acute state. In contrast, a longitudinal study of offspring of depressed parents did not find that early childhood attachment status predicted suicide status in adolescence (Klimes-Dougan *et al.* 1999).

## Personality traits and defensive styles

Impulsive aggression (i.e. impulsively reacting to provocation or frustration with hostility or aggression) is a major risk factor for adolescent suicidality independent of diagnosis and appears to play a role in the familial transmission of suicidal behaviour (King *et al.* 2003; Bridge *et al.* 2006; Melhem *et al.* 2007), at least in part independent of depression. Personality traits including neuroticism (a temperamental propensity for negative affects such as embarrassment, guilt, fear, anger), introversion, and avoidant traits (Brent *et al.* 1994) have also been associated with adolescent suicide in settings diverse as North America (Hewitt *et al.* 1997; Enns *et al.* 2003), New Zealand (Beautrais *et al.* 1999), Scandinavia (Nordstrom *et al.* 1995), Turkey and Iran (Irfani 1978).

Blatt and colleagues (1995)have distinguished two personality subtypes conferring vulnerability to depression: the *dependent* and the *self-critical*, each associated with distinctive attachment styles and characteristic preoccupations and forms of dysphoria. Individuals with dependent subtype have insecure–ambivalent attachment styles and a propensity for struggles with attachment figures, over-value dependent relationships, and are vulnerable to feeling helpless or abandoned in the face of perceived loss. In contrast, individuals with strong self-critical traits tend to be anxiously preoccupied with issues of achievement, perfectionism, and self-worth, to de-emphasize the importance of intimate relationships, and to react to perceived failure with feelings of guilt, humiliation and perceived loss of control.

A growing body of research has examined the role of these factors in suicidality in both adults and adolescents, with some suggestion that dependent individuals are more prone to depression triggered by rejections and losses, while self-critical individuals are more likely to become depressed in response to perceived achievement failures (King 2003). In addition, self-critical adolescents experience more negative interpersonal and achievement-related life events and fewer positive ones (Shahar *et al.* 2003). In some, but not all (Shaffer *et al.* 1996), studies, high self-criticism (Enns *et al.* 2003) and perfectionism (Boergers *et al.* 1998), have been found to be associated with suicidal behaviour and ideation in adolescents, over and above the variance explained by hopelessness (Hewitt *et al.* 1997) and depressive cognitions (Donaldson *et al.* 2000), but with variable findings as to the contribution of these traits independent of psychiatric diagnosis (Gould *et al.* 1998). Other studies have noted a high level of discrepancy between the perceived actual self and ideal selves of suicidal adolescents (Orbach *et al.* 1998).

Self-critical and perfectionistic traits may be a particularly important risk factor for certain self-demanding, high-achieving youngsters (King 2003), as evidenced by completed suicides in elite Israeli adolescent conscripts (Apter *et al.* 1993; King *et al.* 2007) and Oxford university students (Hawton *et al.* 1995), especially those who show who are perfectionistically anxious (Shaffer 1974; Allan *et al.* 1998) or appear to value achievement at the expense of social relatedness (King *et al.* 2007).

## Escape from unbearable affects

Suicidal behaviour and ideation usually occur in the context of a desperate attempt to escape from a seemingly intolerable affective state—what Shneidman (1998) refers to as 'psychache' or psychic pain and Williams (2001) as 'entrapment'—feelings such as rage, isolation or abandonment, or severe anxiety (Hendin 1991; Hendin *et al.* 2007). Other unbearable affects associated with suicidality are often, but not necessarily, linked to depression; these include intense hopelessness, helplessness, humiliation, self-criticism (Flamenbaum and Holden 2007) or self-hatred or, less often in adolescence, fear of fragmentation, profound anhedonia (Nock and Kazdin 2002), or a sense of inner deadness.

A study of British adolescent self-poisoners (Hawton *et al.* 1982) found that the commonest affect states preceding the suicide attempt were anger, loneliness, feeling unwanted, or worry about the future, while two-thirds of US adolescent ideators or attempters seen in an emergency ward reported intense anger, hopelessness, or depression (Beautrais *et al.* 1997; Negron *et al.* 1997). Although overwhelming, these intense feelings are often difficult for some adolescents to process or describe; thus, among New Zealand (Beautrais *et al.* 1997), British (White 1974), and Dutch (Kienhorst *et al.* 1995) adolescent attempters, from one-third to over half were unable to describe a precipitant or give an explanation or motive for their act. It is unclear whether this inability to articulate feelings or interpersonal situations is an acute deficit related to a state of intense affective arousal and/or a more persistent deficit in the capacity to differentiate feeling states or use verbal mediators in the service of social problem-solving (Rourke *et al.* 1989; Brent 1997; Evans *et al.* 2005a; Speckens and Hawton 2005; McAuliffe *et al.* 2006).

The crises that precipitate youthful suicidal behaviour are most often commonplace events that cannot be viewed simply as extraordinary external factors. Rather, their significance lies in the dangerous reverberations they evoke in potentially vulnerable youngsters. In addition to amplifying the impact of such upsets, the psychopathological factors associated with adolescent suicidality, in many cases, also increase the likelihood of such crises occurring in a youngster's life.

These risk factors all increase the probability of conflicts and upsets with peers, romantic partners, parents, and other authority figures. At the same time, these same factors are likely to amplify the youth's adverse reactions to upsetting events, increasing what Shneidman (1985, 1986) has termed *perturbation* in the form of agitation and pressure to take precipitous action. The frequency and impact of such precipitants may vary with diagnosis or other risk factor, with legal/disciplinary crises especially common in youngsters with disruptive diagnoses and substance abuse (Gould *et al.* 2003a), and interpersonal separations serving more often as a precipitant in adolescents with weakened parental support (Marttunen *et al.* 1993).

## Family factors

Around the world, family factors, operating via a range of mechanisms, play an important role child and adolescent suicidal behaviour (Wagner *et al.* 2003; Gould *et al.* 2003a; Evans *et al.* 2004; Flouri 2005; Bridge *et al.* 2006; Colucci and Martin 2007b).

Many studies (Gould *et al.* 2003a; Flouri 2005; Bridge *et al.* 2006), including those in the US (Brent *et al.* 1996, 2003; Brent and Mann 2006), New Zealand (Fergusson *et al.* 2000), and elsewhere have found family psychopathology, especially a history of parental depression, core anxiety, substance abuse, antisocial personality disorder and or suicidal behaviour, to be an important risk factor for prepubertal and adolescent suicide attempts and completion. As with other aspects of family environment, the extent to which reflects the negative impact on the child of an adverse family environment and parenting behaviours vs shared genetic risk factors for psychiatric disorder or maladaptive traits cannot be determined in most studies. Indeed, gene X environment studies suggest that stressful early life experiences (e.g. abuse) may have an especially negative impact on children with certain genotypic vulnerabilities (Rutter *et al.* 2006). For a discussion of genetic factors, see Chapters 26 and 27 in this book.

A history of suicidal behaviour in family members is associated with youth suicide behaviour in a wide range of countries and ethnic groups, including Alaskan Native and American Indian (Blum *et al.* 1992), Swiss (Buddeberg *et al.* 1996), Dutch, Slovenian (Tomori *et al.* 2001), German (Lieb *et al.* 2005), and Swedish and Turkish adolescents (Eskin 1995). A prospective study of a German community sample (Lieb *et al.* 2005) found that a suicide attempt by a mother was associated with a several-fold increase in risk of suicide ideation or attempt in the adolescent offspring. A history of depression and sexual abuse in parents is an especially potent risk factor for suicidality in offspring, especially those with mood disorder and impulsive aggression (Melhem *et al.* 2007).

Both in the months preceding a suicidal episode or over their entire life time, negative life events, especially those that involve disruption of emotional ties with significant others, increase the risk of child and adolescent suicidal behaviour (Cohen-Sandler *et al.* 1982; Beautrais *et al.* 1996; King *et al.* 2001), in some studies even after controlling for psychiatric diagnosis (Gould *et al.* 1996). Frequent separations and disruptions of important family relationships might be speculated to be a marker for parental psychopathology and/or to predispose youngsters to an insecure or anxious attachment style and propensity to depression and to interfere with the development of self-regulatory capacities (King 2003).

In population-based studies, findings are mixed as to the whether parental divorce, non-intact home, or single-parent status are risk factors for youth suicidal behaviour (Beautrais 2000; Evans *et al.* 2004; Bridge *et al.* 2006), especially after adjusting for parental psychopathology. A study of 34 nations found a significant correlation between national rates of divorce and suicide rates in 15–24-year-olds (especially males) (Johnson *et al.* 2000); an analysis of 54 nations found suicide rates in 15–24-year-olds was significantly positively correlated with national divorce rates and negatively correlated with reported 'home satisfaction' (as measured in the World Values Survey) (Wu and Bond 2006). Although national divorce rates and reported home satisfaction were modestly correlated, it is unclear whether other unmeasured socio-economic variables might influence this apparent relationship. Foster care or living apart from both parents appear to increase suicidal risk in adolescents according to studies from New Zealand (Beautrais *et al.* 1996), Switzerland (Gex *et al.* 1998), France (Chastany) and Finland (Kaltiala *et al.* 1999).

Various forms of family discord (e.g., high conflict or low cohesion) and negative parent–child relationships, e.g., low parental involvement and warmth, poor parent child communication, harsh discipline, are associated with youthful suicidal behaviour (Wagner *et al.* 2003; Flouri 2005).

Family discord has been found to be associated with increased risk of suicidal behaviour in US (Reinherz *et al.* 1995), Hong Kong (Stewart *et al.* 1999), Native American (Borowsky *et al.* 1999), Icelandic (Bjarnason and Thorlindsson 1994), Swiss (Gex *et al.* 1998), Dutch, Slovenian (Tomori *et al.* 2001), and New Zealand (Fergusson and Lynskey 1995; Beautrais *et al.* 1996) youth. However, the direction of causality between family conflict and adolescent suicidal behaviour is difficult to determine from this literature (Trautman and Shaffer 1984; Tomori *et al.* 2001), because of the predominance of cross-sectional over longitudinal study designs, and, with few exceptions, a reliance on adolescent self-reports, rather than observational (Williams and Lyons 1976) or parental reports (Fergusson and Lynskey 1995; Klimes-Dougan *et al.* 1999; Wagner *et al.* 2000).

Low perceived parental care or support is a risk factor for adolescent suicidality in many studies, (Dubow *et al.* 1989; Marttunen *et al.* 1993; Groholt *et al.* 1997; McKeown *et al.* 1998; West *et al.* 1999; Evans *et al.* 2004; Flouri 2005), even after controlling for various forms of family adversity (Beautrais *et al.* 1996) and interpersonal and school problems (Simons and Murphy 1985). It has been proposed that low perceived parental care may interfere with youngster's developing the ability to see their body and self as worth caring for and protecting, as opposed to a source of distress (Khantzian and Mack 1983; King and Apter 1996; Orbach *et al.* 2001; King 2003; Orbach 2003).

Low parental involvement (Flouri 2005), emotional responsiveness (Fergusson and Lynskey 1995), or expressiveness and greater negative expressed emotion (Wedig and Nock 2007) and perceived parental rejection or lack of warmth (Garber *et al.* 1998; Ruchkin *et al.* 2003) are all associated with increased risk of adolescent suicidality.

In contrast, good family relationships, including perceived high family cohesion, parent–child connectedness, high parental academic expectations and supervision, and time spent together may have a protective effect in reducing suicidal behaviour (Rubenstein *et al.* 1989; Borowsky *et al.* 2001; King *et al.* 2001; Evans *et al.* 2004; Kidd *et al.* 2006).

Family systems theory has proposed that family-wide difficulties and conflicts in communication, problem-solving, and relationship styles can predispose adolescents to suicidal behaviour (Richman 1986; Wagner 1997). For example, Orbach and colleagues (Orbach *et al.* 1999) have proposed that suicidal behaviour may represent an attempt to coerce change in what is perceived as an intolerable family situation. Wagner (1997) proposes a nuanced nosology of family influences on offsprings' suicidality that distinguishes between 'child-driven', 'reciprocal', and 'parent-driven' family profiles. In the child-driven case, the suicidal behaviour is not primarily interpersonally motivated or communicative, but rather driven by severity of the child's psychopathology, despite the relatively competent, supportive parenting. At the other extreme, in parent-driven cases, parental psychopathology, deficient problem-solving and communication skills, and lack of perceived parental support evoke self-destructive behaviour in the child in an attempt to retaliate or coerce concern. In the intermediate reciprocal type, the child's suicidal behaviour results from an interaction of child vulnerabilities and family dysfunction.

## Physical and sexual abuse

Physical and sexual abuse are among the most harmful forms of adverse early experience associated with subsequent suicidal behaviour (Evans *et al.* 2005b), as documented in Swiss (Buddeberg *et al.* 1996; Gex *et al.* 1998), New Zealand (Fergusson *et al.* 1996), French (Choquet *et al.* 1997), and Native and other American adolescents (Blum *et al.* 1992; Borowsky *et al.* 1999). Whether the effects of abuse are direct ones, mediated by factors such as depression or other maladaptive traits, or shared genetic vulnerabilities with the abusing parent is unclear (Melhem *et al.* 2007). As noted earlier, children with certain genotypes may be particularly sensitive to the deleterious impact of abuse (Rutter *et al.* 2006)

## Mediating mechanisms of early adverse experiences

The mechanisms by which early adverse experiences are linked to subsequent suicidality are complex and difficult to disentangle. Using a structural equations approach to analyse cross-sectionally collected data, one study (Yang and Clum 2000) found maladaptive psychological traits in the child played an important mediating role in the association between early negative life events (such as maltreatment, family instability, and poor general family environment) and later suicidal ideation. The impact of early negative life events on later suicidality was largely accounted for by the former's effects on impaired psychological functioning (self-esteem, external locus of control, hopelessness, and problem-solving deficits). One longitudinal study found that the link between late adolescent suicide attempts and early childhood maltreatment and maladaptive parenting was mediated by an elevated risk for interpersonal difficulties in middle adolescence (Johnson *et al.* 2002), while another longitudinal study found the relationship between early physical abuse and adolescent suicidality largely unmediated, save for the exception of adolescent internalizing disorders (Salzinger *et al.* 2007).

## Adolescence as a period of vulnerability

Adolescence is a time of tremendous developmental shifts that may leave youngsters especially vulnerable to suicidal ideation and behaviour, as evidenced by the marked rise of suicidal behaviours and completed suicide with the onset of adolescence (Tabachnik 1981; King *et al.* 2003; King 2007; WHO 2007). Among the developmental factors conferring risk are:

1 Efforts to become more independent from parents, with a resulting increase in parent–child conflicts;

2 Increased risk-taking behaviours and impulsivity, reflecting in part neurobiological shifts and immaturities; and

3 A shift in primary attachment and reliance from parental figures to peers.

The social ecological model (Kidd *et al.* 2006) emphasizes the importance of reciprocal relationships between contextual factors (family, peers, school, culture) and individual factors (e.g. hopelessness, depression) in shaping adolescents' vulnerability to suicidal behaviour and ideation. A full exploration of this model lies beyond the scope of this chapter, but it is important to note that perceived parental support, peer relationships, and connectedness to school appear to act both independently and in tandem to confer or mitigate risk of adolescent suicidality. Perceived lack of connection to family, peer, or school all render adolescents more vulnerable to suicidal behaviour and ideation.

The recent UNICEF Innocenti Report Card (UNICEF 2007) provides data for 27 economically advanced countries on the percentage of 15-year-olds endorsing specific negative, anomic feelings ('I feel like an outsider or left out of things', 'I feel awkward and out of place', and 'I feel lonely.') In all but 11 or the 27 countries, no more than 5–10 per cent of youngsters endorsed these feelings. However, endorsement rates greater than 10 per cent were found in Belgium, Canada, Denmark, France, Germany, Iceland, Japan, New Zealand, Portugal, Switzerland and the Russian Federation. Strikingly, 18 per cent of Japanese youngsters endorsed 'I feel awkward and out of place' and 30 per cent endorsed 'I feel lonely.' These results can be viewed in the context of the corresponding national youth suicide rates shown in Table 88.1.

## Identity

The concept of identity, as defined by Erikson (1963), links notions of internal coherence and persistence over time with 'self representations that serve to define the individual in a variety of social contexts' (Abend 1995). As such, identity depends not only on the developmental coherence of the self, but also its congruence with the social roles and opportunities that given culture offers a youngster. Although much empirical developmental research has shifted away from global notions of identity to focus on more specific self-concepts (Steinberg and Morris 2001), identity remains a key psychoanalytic concept for understanding youth suicide, especially in the context of indigenous groups and other cultures undergoing rapid change, with attendant weakening of traditional social structures and practices (Larson and Wilson 2004; Beautrais and Fergusson 2006; Lester 2006).

The utility of the concept is illustrated by an ambitious empirical study of cultural mainstream and Aboriginal (First Nations) youth in which the authors (Chandler and Proulx 2006) elaborated a normative theory of adolescent identity development and applied it to understanding the wide differences in youth suicide rates across different First Nation communities in British Columbia. The authors discerned two distinctive identity strategies—the Essentialist and the Narrative/Relational—that were employed by different adolescents to conceptualize their own and others' personal continuity over time.

The Essentialist strategy seeks 'grounds for sameness in some specific feature or aspect of the self ranging from the concrete, i.e. name, physical features through the abstract that is imagined to have endured despite acknowledged change in other quarters' (Chandler and Proulx 2006, p. 131). In contrast, the relational/narrative strategy concentrates on the 'functional relations or narrative connections between admittedly different moments or time-slices in one's unfolding identity … the existence of some storied form or "narrative glue" that link up aspects of the self over time', tying together earlier and later ways of being' (Chandler and Proulx 2006, p. 131). Both modes permit development and elaboration over time of self accounts that have room for both sameness and change and most youngsters, as they moved through adolescence, passed through a series of different transitions in their schemas for maintaining the continuity of their identity.

Among community adolescents, over 80 per cent of aboriginal youth saw their own and others' personal continuity in relational or narrative terms; in contrast, 80 per cent of culturally mainstream, i.e. non-aboriginal, youth saw personal persistence from an essentialist perspective. These divergent findings emphasize that adolescents in different cultures define their identities in different ways, with aboriginal youth in this case seeing their life trajectories in a more socially embedded fashion.

Next, in a blind comparison of the interview protocols for a sample of suicidal and non-suicidal hospitalized adolescent psychiatric inpatients, as well as a group of non-hospitalized controls, 85 per cent of the actively suicidal youngsters lacked any coherent strategies for a sense of self-continuity.

The authors next explored the hypothesis that the incidence of youth suicide in various First Nations communities would vary inversely with an index of 'cultural continuity' measuring the extent to which the group had preserved ties to their cultural past and exercised local control over self-governance and health, education, policing, and cultural resources. Although aboriginal youth have on average a 5–7 times higher suicide rate than the British Columbia youth population as a whole, 90 per cent of the aboriginal youth suicides occur in only 15 per cent of the 200-plus bands. Those bands with the highest levels of cultural continuity had few if any youth suicides, while those with the lowest index of protective cultural continuity had youth suicide rates more than 100 times the national average. (Further study is of course needed to clarify the role of potential intervening variables such as socio-economic status, educational and economic opportunity, family status, rates of substance abuse, etc.)

## Conclusion

A review of the psychodynamic and family factors associated with youth suicide suggests many potential openings for prevention and treatment. The prominence of parental psychopathology, family discord, and abuse as risk factors for adolescent suicidality underlines the preventive importance of including a focus on family and parent–child work in treating parents with affective or substance abuse disorders, especially those with personal histories of abuse (Melhem *et al.* 2007). In addition to family-focused interventions (Harrington *et al.* 1998) to reduce or mitigate family conflict, maladaptive communication styles, negative life events, and perceived lack of support, individual psychotherapeutic interventions for the adolescent patient are usually also indicated to address low self-esteem, hopelessness, and deficits in problem-solving and affect regulation (as well as specific psychiatric disorders, if present). Psychodynamically oriented psychotherapy provides one potential avenue for clarifying and rectifying distortions in self-concept and object relations, improving affect tolerance and social problem-solving skills, and fostering healthy ongoing development. Much empirical research is needed, however, to clarify the relative merits of different therapeutic approaches for specific subtypes of adolescent suicidality (Apter and King 2006).

### References

Abend SM (1995). Identity. In B Moore and B Fine, eds, *Psychoanalysis: The Major Concepts*, pp. 471–474. Yale University Press, New Haven.

Adam KS, Sheldon-Keller A, West M (1996). Attachment organization and history of suicidal behavior in clinical adolescents. *Journal of Consulting and Clinical Psychology*, **64**, 264–272.

Allan WD, Kashani JH, Dahlmeier JM *et al.* (1998). Anxious suicidality: a new subtype of childhood suicide ideation? *Suicide and Life-Threatening Behavior*, **28**, 251–260.

Apter A and King RA (2006). Management of the depressed, suicidal child or adolescent. *Child and Adolescent Psychiatric Clinics of North America*, **15**, 999–1013.

Apter A, Bleich A, King RA *et al.* (1993). Death without warning? A clinical postmortem study of suicide in 43 Israeli adolescent males. *Archives of General Psychiatry*, **50**, 138–142.

Apter A, Gothelf D, Offer R *et al.* (1997). Suicidal adolescents and ego defense mechanisms. *Journal of the American Academy of Child and Adolescent Psychiatry*, **36**, 1520–1527.

Baumeister RF (1990). Suicide as escape from self. *Psychological Review*, **97**, 90–113.

Beautrais AL (2000). Risk factors for suicide and attempted suicide among young people. [Review]. *Australian and New Zealand Journal of Psychiatry*, **34**, 420–436.

Beautrais AL and Fergusson DM (2006). Indigenous suicide in New Zealand. *Archives of Suicide Research*, **10**, 159–168.

Beautrais AL, Joyce PR, Mulder RT (1996). Risk factors for serious suicide attempts among youths aged 13 through 24 years. *Journal of the American Academy of Child and Adolescent Psychiatry*, **35**, 1174–1182.

Beautrais AL, Joyce PR, Mulder RT (1997). Precipitating factors and life events in serious suicide attempts among youths aged 13 through 24 years. *Journal of the American Academy of Child and Adolescent Psychiatry*, **36**, 1543–1551.

Beautrais AL, Joyce PR, Mulder RT (1999). Personality traits and cognitive styles as risk factors for serious suicide attempts among young people. *Suicide and Life-Threatening Behavior*, **29**, 37–47.

Bjarnason T and Thorlindsson T (1994). Manifest predictors of past suicide attempts in a population of Icelandic adolescents. *Suicide and Life-Threatening Behavior*, **24**, 350–358.

Blatt SJ (1995). The destructiveness of perfectionism. Implications for the treatment of depression. *American Psychologist*, **50**, 1003–1020.

Blum RW, Harmon B, Harris L *et al.* (1992) American Indian–Alaska native youth health. *The Journal of the American Medical Association*, **267**, 1637–1644.

Boergers J, Spirito A, Donaldson D (1998). Reasons for adolescent suicide attempts: associations with psychological functioning. *Journal of the American Academy of Child and Adolescent Psychiatry*, **37**, 1287–1293.

Borowsky IW, Ireland M, Resnick MD (2001). Adolescent suicide attempts: risks and protectors. *Pediatrics*, **107**, 485–493.

Borowsky IW, Resnick MD, Ireland M *et al.* (1999). Suicide attempts among American Indian and Alaska native youth. *Archives of Pediatrics and Adolescent Medicine*, **153**, 573–580.

Brent DA (1997). The aftercare of adolescents with deliberate self-harm [Review]. *Journal of Child Psychology and Psychiatry and Allied Disciplines*, **38**, 277–286.

Brent DA, Bridge J, Johnson BA *et al.* (1996). Suicidal behavior runs in families. A controlled family study of adolescent suicide victims. *Archives of General Psychiatry*, **53**, 1145–52.

Brent DA, Johnson BA, Perper J *et al.* (1994). Personality disorder, personality traits, impulsive violence, and completed suicide in adolescents. *Journal of the American Academy of Child and Adolescent Psychiatry*, **33**, 1080–1086.

Brent DA and Mann JJ (2006). Familial pathways to suicidal behavior— understanding and preventing suicide among adolescents. *The New England Journal of Medicine*, **355**, 2719–2721.

Brent DA, Oquendo M, Birmaher B *et al.* (2003). Peripubertal suicide attempts in offspring of suicide attempters with siblings concordant for suicidal behavior. *American Journal of Psychiatry*, **160**, 1486–1493.

Bridge JA, Goldstein TR, Brent DA (2006). Adolescent suicide and suicidal behavior. [Review]. *Journal of Child Psychology and Psychiatry*, **47**, 372–394.

Buddeberg C, Buddeberg FB, Gnamm G *et al.* (1996). Suicidal in Swiss students: an 18-month follow-up survey. *Crisis: Journal of Crisis Intervention and Suicide*, **17**, 78–86.

Chandler M and Proulx T (2006). Changing selves in changing worlds: youth suicide on the fault-lines of colliding cultures. *Archives of Suicide Research*, **10**, 125–140.

Choquet M, Darves-Bornoz JM, Ledoux S *et al.* (1997). Self-reported health and behavioral problems among adolescent victims of rape in France: results of a cross-sectional survey. *Child Abuse and Neglect*, **21**, 823–832.

Cohen-Sandler R, Berman AL, King RA (1982). Life stress and symptomatology: determinants of suicidal behavior in children. *Journal of the American Academy of Child and Adolescent Psychiatry*, **21**, 178–186.

Collins WA and Steinberg L (2006). Adolescent development in interpersonal context. In W Damon and RM Lerner, series eds, and N Eisenberg, vol. ed., *Handbook of Child Psychology, vol 3: Social, Emotional, and Personality Development*, pp. 1003–1067. John Wiley and Sons, Hoboken.

Colucci E and Martin G (2007a). Ethnocultural aspects of suicide in young people: a systematic literature review part 1: rates and methods of youth suicide. *Suicide and Life-Threatening Behavior*, **37**, 197–221.

Colucci E and Martin G (2007b). Ethnocultural aspects of suicide in young people: a systematic literature review part 2: risk factors, precipitating agents, and attitudes toward suicide. *Suicide and Life-Threatening Behavior*, **37**, 222–237.

Donaldson D, Spirito A, Farnett E (2000). The role of perfectionism and depressive cognitions in understanding the hopelessness experienced by adolescent suicide attempters. *Child Psychiatry and Human Development*, **31**, 99–111.

Dubow EF, Kausch DF, Blum MC *et al.* (1989). Correlates of suicidal ideation and attempts in a community sample of junior high and high school students. *Journal of Clinical Child Psychology*, **18**, 158–166.

Enns MW, Cox BJ, Inayatulla M (2003). Personality predictors of outcome for adolescents hospitalized for suicidal ideation. *Journal of the American Academy of Child and Adolescent Psychiatry*, **42**, 720–727.

Erikson EH (1963). *Childhood and SOCIETY*. Norton, New York.

Eskin M (1995). Suicidal behavior as related to social support and assertiveness among Swedish and Turkish high school students: a cross-cultural investigation. *Journal of Clinical Psychology*, **51**, 158–172.

Evans E, Hawton K, Rodham K (2004). Factors associated with suicidal phenomena in adolescents: a systematic review of population-based studies. [Review]. *Clinical Psychology Review*, **24**, 957–979.

Evans E, Hawton K, Rodham K (2005a). In what ways are adolescents who engage in self-harm or experience thoughts of self-harm different in terms of help-seeking, communication and coping strategies? *Journal of Adolescence*, **28**, 573–587.

Evans E, Hawton K, Rodham K (2005b). Suicidal phenomena and abuse in adolescents: a review of epidemiological studies. *Child Abuse and Neglect*, **29**(1), 45–58.

Fergusson DM, Horwood LJ, Lynskey MT (1996). Childhood sexual abuse and psychiatric disorder in young adulthood: II. Psychiatric outcomes of childhood sexual abuse. *Journal of the American Academy of Child and Adolescent Psychiatry*, **35**, 1365–1374.

Fergusson DM and Lynskey MT (1995). Childhood circumstances, adolescent adjustment, and suicide attempts in a New Zealand birth cohort. *Journal of the American Academy of Child and Adolescent Psychiatry*, **34**, 612–622.

Fergusson DM, Woodward LJ, Horwood LJ (2000). Risk factors and life processes associated with the onset of suicidal behaviour during adolescence and early adulthood. *Psychological Medicine*, **30**, 23–39.

Flamenbaum R and Holden RR (2007). Psychache as a mediator in the relationship between perfectionism and suicidality. *Journal of Counseling Psychology*, **54**, 51–61.

Flouri E (2005). Psychological and sociological aspects of parenting and their relation to suicidal behavior. *Archives of Suicide Research*, **9**, 373–383.

Freud S (1917). Mourning and melancholia. In *The Standard Edition of the Complete Psychological Works of Sigmund Freud*, vol 14, pp. 289–300. Vintage, London.

Friedman P (1967). On suicide: with particular reference to suicide among young students. In P Friedman, ed., *Discussions of the Vienna psychoanalytic society—1910*. International Universities Press, New York.

Garber J, Little S, Hilsman R *et al.* (1998). Family predictors of suicidal symptoms in young adolescents. *Journal of Adolescence*, **21**, 445–457.

Gex CR, Narring F, Ferron C *et al.*A (1998). Suicide attempts among adolescents in Switzerland: prevalence, associated factors and comorbidity. *Acta Psychiatrica Scandinavica*, **98**, 28–33.

Gould MS, Fisher P, Parides M *et al.* (1996). Psychosocial risk factors of child and adolescent completed suicide. *Archives of General Psychiatry*, **53**, 1155–1162.

Gould MS, Greenberg T, Velting DM *et al.* (2003a). Youth suicide risk and preventive interventions: a review of the past 10 years. [Review]. *Journal of the American Academy of Child and Adolescent Psychiatry*, **42**, 386–405.

Gould MS, King R, Greenwald S *et al.* (1998). Psychopathology associated with suicidal ideation and attempts among children and adolescents. *Journal of the American Academy of Child and Adolescent Psychiatry*, **37**(9), 915–923.

Gould MS, Shaffer D, Greenberg T (2003b). The epidemiology of youth suicide. In RA King and A Apter, eds, *Suicide in Children and Adolescents*, pp. 1–41. Cambridge University Press, Cambridge.

Groholt B, Ekeberg O, Wichstrom L *et al.* (1997). Youth suicide in Norway, 1990–1992: a comparison between children and adolescents completing suicide and age- and gender-matched controls. *Suicide and Life-Threatening Behavior*, **27**, 250–263.

Harrington RC, Kerfoot M, Dyer E *et al.* (1998). Randomized trial of a home-based family intervention for children who have deliberately poisoned themselves. *Journal of the American Academy of Child and Adolescent Psychiatry*, **37**, 512–518.

Harter S, Marold DB, Whitesell NR (1992). Model of psychosocial risk factors leading to suicidal ideation in young adolescents. *Development and Psychopathology*, **4**, 167–188.

Hawton K, Cole D, O'Grady J *et al.* (1982). Motivational aspects of deliberate self-poisoning in adolescents. *British Journal of Psychiatry*, **141**, 286–291.

Hawton K, Simkin S, Fagg J *et al.* (1995). Suicide in Oxford university students, 1976–1990. *British Journal of Psychiatry*, **16**, 44–50.

Hendin H (1991). Psychodynamics of suicide, with particular reference to the young. *American Journal of Psychiatry*, **148**, 1150–1158.

Hendin H, Maltsberger JT, Szanto K (2007). The role of intense affective states in signaling a suicide crisis. *Journal of Nervous and Mental Disease*, **195**, 363–368.

Hewitt PL, Newton J, Flett GL *et al.* (1997). Perfectionism and suicide ideation in adolescent psychiatric patients. *Journal of Abnormal Child Psychology*, **25**, 95–101.

Inglehart R, Basanez M, Moreno A (1998). *Human Values and Beliefs: A Cross-cultural Sourcebook*. University of Michigan Press, Ann Arbor.

Irfani S (1978). Personality correlates of suicidal tendency among Iranian and Turkish students. *Journal of Psychology*, **99**, 151–153.

Johnson JG, Cohen P, Gould MS *et al.* (2002). Childhood adversities, interpersonal difficulties, and risk for suicide attempts during late adolescence and early adulthood. *Archives of General Psychiatry*, **59**, 741–749.

Johnson GR, Krug EG, Potter LB (2000). Suicide among adolescents and young adults: a cross-national comparison of 34 countries. *Suicide and Life-Threatening Behavior*, **30**, 74–82.

Kaltiala HR, Rimpela M, Marttunen M *et al.* (1999). Bullying, depression, and suicidal ideation in Finnish adolescents: school survey. *British Medical Journal*, **319**, 348–351.

Kelleher MJ and Chambers D (2003). Cross-cultural variation in child and adolescent suicide. In RA King and A Apter, eds, *Suicide in Children and Adolescents*, pp. 170–197. Cambridge University Press, Cambridge.

Khantzian EJ and Mack JE (1983). Self-preservation and the care of the self. *Psychoanalytic Study of the Child*, **38**, 209–232.

King RA (2003). Psychodynamic approaches to youth suicide. In RA King and A Apter, eds, *Suicide in Children and Adolescents*, pp. 150–169. Cambridge University Press, Cambridge.

King RA (2007). Adolescence. In A Martin and FR Volkmar, eds, *Lewis' Child and Adolescent Psychiatry: A Comprehensive Textbook*, pp. 279–291. Lippincott Williams and Wilkins, Philadelphia.

King RA and Apter A (1996). Psychoanalytic perspectives on adolescent suicide. *Psychoanalytic Study of the Child*, **51**, 491–511.

King RA, Apter A, Zohar A (2007). Towards a typology of adolescent suicide. In L Mayes and M Target, eds, *Developmental Science and Psychoanalysis: Integration and Innovation*, pp 315–327. Karnac Books, London.

King RA, Ruchkin VV, Schwab-Stone M (2003). Suicide and the 'continuum of adolescent self-destructiveness': is there a connection? In RA King and A Apter, eds, *Suicide in Children and Adolescents*, pp. 41–62. Cambridge University Press, Cambridge.

King RA, Schwab-Stone M, Flisher AJ *et al.* (2001). Psychosocial and risk behavior correlates of youth suicide attempts and suicidal ideation. *Journal of the American Academy of Child and Adolescent Psychiatry*, **40**, 837–846.

Kidd S, Henrich CC, Brookmeyer KA *et al.* (2006). The social context of adolescent suicide attempts: interactive effects of parent, peer, and school social relations. *Suicide and Life-Threatening Behavior*, **36**, 386–395.

Kienhorst IC, De Wilde EJ, Diekstra RF *et al.* (1995). Adolescents' image of their suicide attempt. *Journal of the American Academy of Child and Adolescent Psychiatry*, **34**, 623–628.

Klimes-Dougan B, Free K, Ronsaville D *et al.* (1999). Suicidal ideation and attempts: a longitudinal investigation of children of depressed and well mothers. *Journal of the American Academy of Child and Adolescent Psychiatry*, **38**, 651–659.

Klomek AB, Zalsman G, Apter A *et al.* (2007). Self-object differentiation in suicidal adolescents. *Comprehensive Psychiatry*, **48**, 8–13.

Larson R and Wilson S (2004). Adolescence across place and time: globalization and the changing pathways to adulthood. In RM Lerner and L Steinberg, *Handbook of Adolescent Psychology*, 2nd edn, pp. 299–330. John Wiley and Sons, Hoboken.

Lieb R, Bronisch T, Höfler M *et al.* (2005). Maternal suicidality and risk of suicidality in offspring: findings from a community study. *The American Journal of Psychiatry*, **162**, 1665–1671.

Lester D (2006). Suicide among indigenous peoples: a cross-cultural perspective. *Archives of Suicide Research*, **10**, 117–124.

Marttunen MJ, Aro HM, Lonnqvist JK (1993). Precipitant stressors in adolescent suicide. *Journal of the American Academy of Child and Adolescent Psychiatry*, **32**, 1178–1183.

McAuliffe C, Corcoran P, Keeley HS *et al.* (2006). Problem-solving ability and repetition of deliberate self-harm: a multicentre study. *Psychological Medicine*, **36**, 45–55.

McKeown R E, Garrison CZ, Cuffe SP *et al.* (1998). Incidence and predictors of suicidal behaviors in a longitudinal sample of young adolescents. *Journal of the American Academy of Child and Adolescent Psychiatry*, **37**, 612–619.

Melhem NM, Brent DA, Ziegler M *et al.* (2007). Familial pathways to early-onset suicidal behavior: familial and individual antecedents of suicidal behavior. *American Journal of Psychiatry*, **164**, 1364–1370.

Menninger K (1938). *Man Against Himself*. Harcourt Brace, New York.

Negron R, Piacentini J, Graae F *et al.* (1997). Microanalysis of adolescent suicide attempters and ideators during the acute suicidal episode. *Journal of the American Academy of Child and Adolescent Psychiatry*, **36**, 1512–1519.

Nock MK and Kazdin AE (2002). Examination of affective, cognitive, and behavioral factors and suicide-related outcomes in children and young adolescents. *Journal of Clinical Child and Adolescent Psychology*, **31**, 48–58.

Nordstrom P, Shalling D, Asberg M (1995). Temperamental vulnerability in attempted suicide. *Acta Psychiatrica Scandinavica*, **92**, 155–160.

Offer D, Ostrov E, Howard KI *et al.* (1988). *The Teenage World: Adolescents' Self-image in Ten Countries.* Plenum Medical, New York.

Orbach I (2003). Suicide and the suicidal body. 2002 Dublin Award Address. *Suicide and Life-Threatening Behavior*, **33**, 1–8.

Orbach I, Mikulincer M, Blumenson R *et al.* (1999). The subjective experience of problem irresolvability and suicidal behavior: dynamics and measurement. *Suicide and Life-Threatening Behavior*, **29**, 150–164.

Orbach I, Mikulincer M, Stein D *et al.* (1998). Self-representation of suicidal adolescents. *Journal of Abnormal Psychology*, **107**, 435–439.

Orbach I, Stein D, Shan-Sela M *et al.* (2001). Body attitudes and body experiences in suicidal adolescents. *Suicide and Life-Threatening Behavior*, **31**, 237–249.

Overholser JC, Adams DM, Lehnert KL *et al.* (1995). Self-esteem deficits and suicidal tendencies among adolescents. *Journal of the American Academy of Child and Adolescent Psychiatry*, **34**, 919–928.

Reinherz HZ, Giaconia RM, Silverman AB *et al.* (1995). Early psychosocial risks for adolescent suicidal ideation and attempts. *Journal of the American Academy of Child and Adolescent Psychiatry*, **34**, 599–611.

Richman J (1986). *Family Therapy for Suicidal People.* Springer, New York.

Rourke BP, Young GC, Leenaars AA (1989). A childhood learning disability that predisposes those afflicted to adolescent and adult depression and suicide risk. *Journal of Learning Disabilities*, **22**, 169–174.

Rubenstein JL, Heeren T, Housman D *et al.* (1989). Suicidal in 'normal' adolescents: risk and protective factors. *American Journal of Orthopsychiatry*, **59**, 59–71.

Ruchkin VV, Schwab-Stone M, Koposov RA *et al.* (2003). Suicidal ideation and attempts in juvenile delinquents. *Journal of Child Psychology and Psychiatry*, **44**, 1058–1066.

Rutter M, Moffitt TE, Caspi A (2006). Gene–environment interplay and psychopathology: multiple varieties but real effects. *Journal of Child Psychology and Psychiatry*, **47**, 226–261.

Salzinger S, Rosario M, Feldman RS *et al.* (2007). Adolescent suicidal behavior: associations with preadolescent physical abuse and selected risk and protective factors. *Journal of the American Academy of Child and Adolescent Psychiatry*, **46**, 859–866.

Shaffer D (1974). Suicide in childhood and early adolescence. *Journal of Child Psychology and Psychiatry*, **15**, 275–291.

Shaffer D, Gould MS, Fisher P *et al.* (1996). Psychiatric diagnosis in child and adolescent suicide. *Archives of General Psychiatry*, **53**, 339–348.

Shahar G, Henrich CC, Blatt SJ *et al.* (2003). Interpersonal relatedness, self-definition, and their motivational orientation during adolescence: a theoretical and empirical integration. *Developmental Psychology*, **39**, 470–483.

Shneidman ES (1980). Suicide. In ES Shneidman, ed., *Death: Current Perspectives,* pp. 416–434. Mayfield Publishing, Palo Alto.

Shneidman ES (1985) *Definition of Suicide.* Wiley, New York.

Shneidman ES (1998). *The Suicidal Mind.* Oxford University Press, New York.

Simons RL and Murphy PI (1985). Sex differences in the causes of adolescent suicide ideation. *Journal of Youth and Adolescence*, **14**, 423–434.

Speckens AE and Hawton K (2005). Social problem solving in adolescents with suicidal behavior: a systematic review. *Suicide and Life-Threatening Behavior*, **35**, 365–387.

Steinberg L and Morris AS (2001). Adolescent development. *Annual Review of Psychology*, **52**, 83–110.

Stewart SM, Lam TH, Betson C *et al.* (1999). Suicide ideation and its relationship to depressed mood in a community sample of adolescents in Hong Kong. *Suicide and Life-Threatening Behavior*, **29**, 227–240.

Tabachnik N (1981). The interlocking psychologies of suicide and adolescence. *Adolescent Psychiatry*, **9**, 399–410.

Thompson RA (2006). The development of the person: social understanding, relationships, conscience, self. In W Damon and RM Lerner, series ed., and N Eisenberg, vol. ed., *Handbook of Child Psychology, vol 3: Social, Emotional, and Personality Development*, pp. 24–98. John Wiley and Sons, Hoboken.

Tomori M, Kienhorst C, de Wilde E *et al.* (2001). Suicidal behaviour and family factors among Dutch and Slovenian high school students: a comparison. *Acta Psychiatrica Scandinavica*, **104**, 198–203.

Trautman PD and Shaffer D (1984). Treatment of child and adolescent suicide attempters. In HS Sudak, AB Ford and N Rushforth, eds, *Suicide in the Young*, pp. 307–323. John Wright, Boston.

UNICEF (2007). *Child Poverty in Perspective: An Overview of Child Well-being in Rich Countries.* UNICEF Innocenti Research Centre. Innocenti Report Card 7, Florence.

Wagner BM (1997). Family risk factors in child and adolescent suicidal behavior. *Psychological Bulletin*, **121**, 246–298.

Wagner BM, Aiken C, Mullaley PM *et al.* (2000). Parents' reactions to adolescents' suicide attempts. *Journal of the American Academy of Child and Adolescent Psychiatry*, **39**, 429–436.

Wagner BM, Silverman MAC, Martin CE (2003). Family factors in youth suicidal behaviors. *American Behavioral Scientist*, **46**, 1171–1191.

Wedig MM and Nock MK (2007). Parental expressed emotion and adolescent self-injury. *Journal of the American Academy of Child and Adolescent Psychiatry*, **46**, 1171–1178.

West ML, Spreng SW, Rose SM *et al.* (1999). Relationship between attachment, felt security, and history of suicidal behaviours in clinical adolescents. *Canadian Journal of Psychiatry*, **44**, 578–582.

White HC (1974). Self-poisoning in adolescents. *British Journal of Psychiatry*, **124**, 24–35.

Williams M (2001). *Suicide and Attempted Suicide.* Penguin Books, London.

Williams C and Lyons CM (1976). Family interaction and adolescent suicidal behavior: a preliminary investigation. *Australian and New Zealand Journal of Psychiatry*, **10**, 243–252.

World Health Organization (2007). *Country Suicide Reports.* Retrieved on 30 November 2007 from http://www.who.int/mental_health/prevention/suicide/country_reports/en/index.html.

Wu WCH and Bond M (2006). National differences in predictors of suicide among young and elderly citizens: linking societal predictors to psychological factors. *Archives of Suicide Research*, **10**, 45–60.

Yang B and Clum GA (2000). Childhood stress leads to later suicidality via its effect on cognitive functioning. *Suicide and Life-Threatening Behavior*, **30**, 183–198.

# CHAPTER 89

# Psychiatric disorders in suicide and suicide attempters

Alan Apter, Orit Krispin and Cendrine Bursztein

## Abstract

This chapter reviews common psychiatric disorders and conditions which appear to be major risk factors for all types of suicidality, both non-fatal and fatal, among children and adolescents. These psychiatric conditions include personality disorders, conduct disorder, affective disorder, bipolar disorder, anxiety disorder, obsessive–compulsive disorder, schizophrenia, substance abuse, and eating disorders. Each psychiatric condition is described and discussed in terms of its unique features that are associated with suicide behaviours and its risk for suicide behaviour.

## Introduction

It appears that almost any diagnosable psychiatric disorder may increase the risk for suicide.

Psychiatric illnesses in adolescence are especially dangerous when they occur in conjunction with other risk factors for suicide (see Chapters 38 and 39 in Part 6 of the book) and when more than one illness is present (comorbidity). This chapter will deal with the common psychiatric disorders found in clinical practice that are associated with suicidal behaviour. Different treatments of suicidal young people are described in detail in Chapters 91, 92 and 93 in this part (Part 12) of the book.

## Personality disorders

### Borderline personality disorder

Borderline personality disorder (BPD) is traditionally associated with non-fatal suicide attempts but there is increasing evidence that fatal suicide is also common in these patients. Intentional self-damaging acts and suicide attempts are the 'behavioural specialty' of these patients (Gunderson 1984). Although 'affective instability' is said to be one of the critical symptoms of this disorder, many seem to have a chronic underlying depression and most of the adolescent BPD patients who require psychiatric help meet criteria for an affective disorder, usually major depression. In addition, many suffer from chronically stable depression, hopelessness, worthlessness, guilt and helplessness.

Another group of suicide related symptoms are those associated with anger. Many of these patients are very angry and even violent; others are fearful of losing control of their anger and are unable to express their aggressive feelings. Other frequent comorbid conditions that increase the likelihood of suicide are conduct disorder, bulimia and substance abuse. An additional comorbid condition of considerable interest is dissociative disorder and the common origin of this combination often seems to appear after incest or continuous non-injurious (in the physical sense) sexual abuse. Some authors report even seeing multiple personality disorder developing in these patients (Pope *et al.* 2006), although our group has never seen such a case.

About 9 per cent of patients with BPD eventually kill themselves (Stone 1989). In a series of BPD inpatients followed for 10–23 years after discharge, patients exhibiting all eight DSM III criteria for BPD at the index admission had a suicide rate of 36 per cent, compared to a suicide rate of 7 per cent in people who had 5–7 of the criteria. Patients with BPD also have high repetition rates of suicidal behaviour (Brodsky *et al.* 1997). Individuals with BPD who show impulsive and aggressive characteristics combined with over-sensitivity to minor life events are at risk for suicidal behaviour. This sensitivity often leads to angry and anxious reactions with secondary depression. These subjects tend to have suffered childhood physical and sexual abuse and use defenses such as regression, splitting, dissociation and displacement. There is often a history of alcohol or substance abuse and there appears to be a connection to an underlying disturbance of serotonin metabolism which is genetic in origin (Apter and Ofek 2001).

### Narcissistic perfectionist personality disorder

Our own experience with this personality constellation and suicide has been based on psychological autopsies of young soldiers doing their military service in the Israel Defence Force (Apter *et al.* 1993a) Many of these suicides seemed to be very different from the patients seen in the adolescent unit or in the emergency room and in fact, the vast majority had never been in contact with a mental health professional. However, once alerted to this maladaptive personality style, there seemed to be resemblances to the life patterns of some of our adolescent patients, especially those with more serious suicide attempts.

Psychological post-mortem studies of soldiers in the Israeli Defence Force (IDF) have shown some features that differ from similar studies conducted in Europe and the USA (Apter *et al.* 1993a; King and Apter 1996). Strong narcissistic and perfectionist patterns were a feature of the lives of about a quarter of the suicides, while 40 per cent showed schizoid and avoidant traits in their personalities. The IDF is for many Israeli youths a chance to prove their worth—much like a prestigious college or university career for European or American students. For many the military is a second chance to redeem earlier shortcomings or to confirm a sense of a competent identity.

These high self-expectations and hopes may also have made it difficult for these young men to acknowledge or bear even marginal difficulties or personal limitations that emerged during their subsequent active duty: any shortcoming was seen by them as devastating.

These features were often complicated by strong isolative traits, which seemed to be common to many of the suicide victims. In most cases these seemed to be lifelong personality patterns which were not related to stress or periods of depression. Their parents, teachers and friends remembered them as being 'very isolated' children. Their superior officers often termed them as being 'very private' people.

This combination of traits had several very dangerous consequences. Many of these young people seemed to have felt an overwhelming need to make a good impression on their pre-induction assessments, which are made on all Israeli teenagers at the age of 16. A good score in these assessments gives the opportunity to be assigned to a prestigious battle unit—a highly valued attainment in the eyes of Israeli society.

This is exemplified by another finding that is unusual in most studies of suicide. These subjects had much higher physical fitness ratings than the average Israeli soldier, probably reflecting their minimizing of non-specific and subjective physical symptoms, such as backache and flat feet and/or intensive training to reach high levels of fitness before conscription. Once these young men encountered perceived difficulty, they felt shame related to their unrealistically high standards, which was combined in many cases with an isolative style that prevented them from turning to peers, officers or clinicians for help or support.

> As a result, even minor setbacks (to the external observer) could rapidly spiral into disaster as burgeoning anxious preoccupation, depressive rumination and withdrawal further interfered with the recruit's ability to perform at the high levels he demanded of himself or to reach out to others, triggering a vicious cycle of isolative decompensation, with suicide as the only way out.
>
> King and Apter (1996, p.112)

Those recruits who used achievement as a kind of pseudo-mastery to substitute for a lack of real interpersonal closeness seemed especially vulnerable to this kind of catastrophic decompensation.

Some basic rules and values are essential in treating the borderline suicidal adolescent. Probably most crucial is a stable therapeutic framework with consistent and reliable care. Next, behaviour and feelings are used as the principal mode of communication. The therapist is active and uses high-energy confrontation and care (so-called therapeutic pressing). The central message is always 'doing something with the patient, not something to the patient'. This way patients feel somewhat in control, which might keep them in treatment. Reflecting their splitting mechanism, these patients alternatively feel inferior and omnipotent, angry at others and self-destructive, sensitive to rejection but usually provoking it.

Flexibility in approach, but firmness in basic values, with creativity and readiness to step away from the rules to get out of frustrating 'no way out' situations, is essential. Many of these patients cannot tolerate feeling better, as this means that the therapist is successful. These and similar frustrative situations cause countertransference problems, with a potential loss of professional objectivity; constant supervision and a support network are therefore necessary.

At least initially, the therapy is supplemented by as much structuring of the patient's life as needed. This may range from directing behaviours, to day-hospital programmes, to hospitalization. Complications often require additional structuring such as phone calls or extra sessions. Structuring, advice, and logic are not expected to generate personality change, only to temporarily improve behaviour control.

Patients who are dysphoric and highly sensitive to social approval (i.e. who are high in reward dependence and harm avoidance) are most likely to improve on selective serotonin reuptake inhibitors (SSRIs). In contrast, those who are highly fearful but not socially dependent are most likely to improve on noradrenergic uptake inhibitors such as desipramine (norpramine). Children with attention-deficit/hyperactivity disorder (who are high in novelty-seeking) are efficiently treated with drugs that increase dopamine release and inhibit its reuptake, such as methylphenidate.

## Conduct disorder

Aggressive impulsive behaviour is a major risk factor for suicidal behaviour in adolescence. A major concern is the high rate of suicidal behaviours among juvenile delinquents, especially in those who are incarcerated in remand homes or in prisons. Unfortunately, in many countries reform schools often do not have the facilities for adequate mental health treatment, while psychiatric units cannot cope with the violence and aggression displayed by these youths. Many of the risk factors for suicide are also risk factors for conduct disorder. These include broken homes, physical and sexual abuse as children, personal and familial alcoholism and substance abuse, unemployment and poverty and access to firearms.

In addition, mood disorders are often present in children who have some degree of irritability and aggressive behaviour. It may be quite difficult to make the differential diagnosis between major depressive disorder, bipolar disorder and conduct disorder. There is also a substantial comorbidity between conduct disorders and affective disorders in adolescence. Again, many factors predisposing to depression also predispose to conduct disorder including family conflict, negative life events, level of affiliation with delinquent peers and parental involvement.

Examining the Center's for Disease Control and Prevention (CDC) Youth Risk Behaviour Survey (YRBS) data for 3054 Massachusetts high school students, Woods *et al.* (1997) found lifetime suicide attempts were significantly associated with physical fights in the past year, regular tobacco use, lack of seatbelt use, gun carrying, substance use before last sexual activity, and lifetime drug use. An analysis of the national cross-sectional survey data on 11,631 high school students found significant and substantial correlations between suicide attempts and gun carrying, multiple sexual partners, condom non-use, fighting resulting in injury, driving while intoxicated, and cocaine use (Sosin *et al.* 1995). Orpinas *et al.* (1995) examined the YRBS data for 2075 Texas high school students and found that weapon-carrying and fighting resulting in injury were associated with suicidal ideation, as well as with alcohol use, number of sexual partners, and low academic performance.

Adolescent suicide attempters are also at ongoing risk for injury and death from motor vehicle accidents, substance abuse, homicide, etc. Prospective studies demonstrate a shared set of social, developmental, and psychopathological risk factors predicting completed or attempted suicide and unintentional injury or death (Fergusson & Lynskey 1995; Neeleman *et al.* 1998).

Risk factors and prognostic implications associated with adolescent suicidal behaviour differ with gender. In their psychological autopsy study of adolescent suicides, Shaffer *et al.* (1996) found that for boys, completed suicide was associated with major depression, substance abuse, and/or antisocial behaviour; in contrast, for girls, major depression and antisocial behaviour, but not substance abuse were associated with increased risk of suicide completion.

Dryfoos (1990) has summarized the extensive overlap in both the prevalence and risk factors for delinquency, substance use, teen pregnancy, and school failure, including the frequent commonalities of poverty, low resistance to deviant peers, insufficient bonding and communication with parens, and insufficient, harsh or inconsistent parental discipline or monitoring.

In conclusion, it seems as if there may be a type of suicidal behaviour characterized by low fatality suicidality related to a wide variety of other kinds of impulsive behaviours, as seen in adolescents with conduct disorders. The psychology of this form of suicidality is related to defects in impulse control similar to those seen in the borderline personality organization as described by Kernberg (1975) and may be related to defects in serotonin metabolism.

The very violent, suicidal and drug abusing adolescent usually requires some form of institution—if possible manned both by social services and mental health personnel. Interventions usually include working with families and schools and often with the police, especially where community policing is available. These young people often do not respond to traditional mental health approaches. However, when they are suicidal there is often quite extensive psychiatric comorbidity which should be treated. Theoretically, anti-aggressive medication ('serenics') should be useful for both internally and externally directed aggression but in practice this is usually not the case. Some clinicians favour the use of mood-stabilizing medications such as carbemazepine and sodium valproate.

There is significant agreement on criteria for hospitalization of patients with conduct disorder (CD) (Lock and Strauss 1994), but level of care decision-making continues to be complex and unsupported by empirical data. The psychiatric professional should choose the least restrictive level of intervention that fulfils both the short- and long-term needs of the patient. Imminent risk to self or others, such as suicidal, self-injurious, homicidal, or aggressive behaviour, or imminent deterioration in medical status, remain clear indications for the need for hospitalization (American Academy of Child and Adolescent Psychiatry 1996, 1990).

## Depression

Major depressive disorder is reported to be the most common mood disorder. It may manifest as a single episode or as recurrent episodes. The course may be somewhat protracted—up to 2 years or longer—in those with the single-episode form. Whereas the prognosis for recovery from an acute episode is good for most patients with major depressive disorder, three out of four patients experience recurrences throughout life, with varying degrees of residual symptoms between episodes. Bipolar disorders consist of at least one hypomanic, manic, or mixed episode. Mixed episodes represent a simultaneous mixture of depressive and manic or hypomanic manifestations. Although a minority of patients experience only manic episodes, most bipolar disorder patients experience episodes of both polarity (Wasserman 2006).

Among teenagers, both attempted and completed suicide is, in the great majority of cases, preceded by depressive symptoms. Depressed young people who attempt suicide often come from broken families and have had one or more relatives who have committed or attempted suicide. They have also, relatively often, run away from home and thus been brought up without favourable role models. Physical and mental abuse, as well as sexual assault, is also more common in this group. Young people who have attempted suicide often have ongoing problems at school and also difficulties in achieving workable relationships with their peers, compared with young people who are depressed and have not attempted suicide. Abuse of alcohol and drugs, impulsive behaviour and asocial behaviour are additional risk factors for attempted and completed suicide among depressed young people. Owing to the high incidence of depression among young people who have attempted suicide, it is important to make a diagnosis and provide adequate treatment at an early stage. Studies show that depressive disturbances are more common among children and young people than has previously been believed. Unfortunately, many young people with depression are not identified, partly because their depressive symptoms are often atypical and partly because adults do not readily recognize depressive symptoms in the young, owing to their wish to see their children as happy and healthy.

Major depression is most easily diagnosed when it appears acutely in a previously healthy child and in these cases the symptoms closely resemble those seen in adults. In many children, however, the onset is insidious and the child may show many other difficulties such as attention deficit disorder or separation anxiety disorder before becoming depressed.

Mood disorders tend to be chronic when they start at an early age and the children come from families where there is a high incidence of mood disorders and alcohol abuse.

In some cases the depressed adolescent may also be psychotic and have hallucinations and delusions which are usually mood congruent. When the psychotic themes are related to suicide, such as in command hallucinations or delusions of guilt, the risk for suicide is very high.

Although antidepressant medications are widely used in the treatment of depression and suicidality, the effect of medication treatment on suicidal behaviour remains unclear. Although the evidenced-based literature is gloomy, most outpatient departments provide a multidimensional treatment approach involving clinical (psychological and pharmacological) interventions, common sense and supportive therapy. This approach has proven sufficient in most cases.

Electroconvulsive therapy may also be indicated in suicidal psychotic depression in adolescence.

## Bipolar disorder

Bipolar disorder was once thought to occur only rarely in youth. However, approximately 20 per cent of all bipolar patients have their first episode during adolescence, with a peak age of onset between 15 and 19 years of age. Developmental variations in presentation, symptomatic overlap with other disorders, and lack of clinician awareness have all led to under-diagnosis or misdiagnosis in children and adolescents. Therefore, clinicians need to be aware of some of the unique clinical characteristics associated with the early-onset form. Similarly, it is important to recognize the various phases and patterns of episodes associated with bipolar disorder. Youth may first present with either manic or depressive episodes. Twenty to thirty per cent of youth with major depression go on to have manic episodes (Weller *et al.* 2002).

Adolescents with bipolar disorder are at increased risk for completed suicide. Twenty percent of adolescents with bipolar disorder made at least one medically significant suicide attempt (Weller *et al.* 2002). Lithium has been found to effectively reduce suicide rates during long-term treatment of patients with bipolar disorders (Baldessarini *et al.* 2002). Data on the efficacy of anticonvulsant mood stabilizers in reducing suicide risk are sparse (Yerevanian *et al.* 2003).

## Anxiety disorders

Anxiety has been identified as an important risk factor for suicidal behaviour in adults. A follow-up study of patients with major affective disorder (Fawcett *et al.* 1990) found that anxiety symptoms were strongly related to completed suicide within one year of assessment. There have also been studies that indicate that anxiety disorders are associated with an increased risk of suicidal behaviour (Allgulander and Lavori 1991; Mannuzza *et al.* 1992; Massion *et al.* 1993). Studies with adolescents have shown mixed results. Taylor and Stansfeld (1984) found that when compared to psychiatric outpatients, suicide attempters exhibited higher levels of anxiety (38 per cent vs 22 per cent); however, the difference was not significant. Another study (Kosky *et al.* 1986) reported that depressed suicidal ideators (of whom 39 per cent had attempted suicide) manifested high levels of anxiety (76.4 per cent), but these levels were not significantly different from those of depressed non-suicidal adolescents. Andrews and Lewinsohn (1992) found in a large community sample of adolescents a significant association between anxiety disorders and suicide attempts in males, but not in females. Most research on anxiety as a risk factor for suicidal behaviour has focused on the measurement of state anxiety. This may not be a fruitful method if state anxiety is significantly reduced following a suicide attempt. Ideally, risk factors used for predictive purposes should be stable (Hawton 1987). As such, research on the relationship between anxiety and suicidal behaviour might benefit from focusing on the measurement of anxiety as a trait rather than as a state. In fact, Apter and his colleagues (Apter *et al.* 1990, 1993b) found that adult psychiatric inpatient suicide attempters had significantly higher levels of trait anxiety than inpatient non-attempters, whereas state anxiety did not discriminate between the two groups. Moreover, trait anxiety was highly associated with a self-report scale of suicide risk. Another study (Oei *et al.* 1990) found that adult depressed patients with suicidal ideation had significantly higher levels of state and trait anxiety than depressed patients with no suicidal ideation. A study of Dutch adolescents (De Wilde *et al.* 1993) found that suicide attempters (half of them psychiatric patients and half high school students) exhibited significantly higher levels of state and trait anxiety than non-depressed non-attempters (high school students).

There are no studies on treatment of suicidal behaviour in anxiety disorders and the treatment should be based on the same considerations as those for depressive disorders, with CBT probably being the most efficacious psychotherapeutic method for the basic anxiety disorder.

## Obsessive–compulsive disorder

Obsessive–compulsive disorder (OCD) is a well-described disorder in childhood and adolescence occurring in about 3 per cent of 16-year-olds (Apter *et al.* 1997). Although effective methods of treatment are available, a substantial minority of patients do not respond to therapy and have a relatively poor prognosis. A minority will require psychiatric hospitalization (Jenike 1990). The factors contributing to treatment failure include: comorbidity with personality disorders, tic disorders, conduct disorders and oppositional disorders, dysfunctional families and the presence of depression and suicidal behaviour (Foa 1979; March and Mulle 1998). OCD is a common comorbid condition with affective disorder. About 10 per cent of unipolar depressive individuals and 21 per cent of those suffering of bipolar disorders, show comorbid OCD (Chen and Dilsaver 1995). Perugi *et al.* (1997) found 15.7 per cent of subjects with OCD have episodes of a bipolar disorder. It appears that depression is also common among adolescents with OCD (Valleni-Basile *et al.* 1994) and that depression in combination with OCD may lead to an increased risk for suicidal behaviour (Valleni-Basile *et al.* 1994; Chen and Dilsaver 1995). Non-fatal suicidal behaviour occurs in about 15 per cent of individuals suffering from OCD (Angst 1993; Hollander *et al.* 1996), principally in those showing comorbidity with antisocial behaviour or borderline personality disorder.

Adolescent inpatients with OCD show high levels of depression, suicidality, anxiety, impulsivity, violence and aggression. The fact that all the hospitalized adolescents, irrespective of their diagnosis, showed similar high scores on the BDI tend to support the notion that these depressive symptoms are non-specific and represent a reaction to illness and hospitalization.

Although the OCD adolescents resemble their inpatient counterparts on almost all the psychopathological dimensions, they do seem to differ in regards to their suicidal behaviour. This difference is however complex and not easy to explain.

First, although on a scale of suicidality ranging from no suicidality through ideation threats, gestures and attempts, the OCD inpatients are equal to the non-OCD patients, they are significantly less likely to have made an actual attempt. Second and most striking is the relationship between depression and suicidal behaviour. In the patient controls there is an expected strong correlation between levels of depression and suicidal behaviour. In the OCD group there is in fact a non-significant trend in the *opposite* direction. Similarly the relationship between both trait and state anxiety and suicidal behaviour is highly significant in the patient controls but weak and non-significant in the OCD inpatients. The same findings apply to aggression, anger and violence. The findings for the non-OCD inpatients are in accord with what is generally reported in the literature (Apter *et al.* 1993b, 1995). The findings for the OCD patients seem to indicate that the correlates of suicidal behaviour in these adolescents are different. In fact, the only significant correlate with suicidal behaviour in the OCD subjects is the presence of antisocial behaviour (Apter *et al.* 2003).

Classic psychoanalytic theory predicted that the individual suffering from OCD would be protected from both depression and suicide. This appears to be incorrect as far as depression is concerned, but may be true with regard to suicidal behaviour. The mechanism that 'protects' the OCD patients from suicidal behaviour is unclear. It may be related to the 'harm avoidance' described by Nelson *et al.* (1996) or to some more specific defense or other mechanism.

There are no studies on suicidal behaviour in OCD and the treatment should be based on the same considerations as those for depressive disorders, with CBT probably being the most efficacious psychotherapeutic method for the basic OCD.

## Schizophrenia

Schizophrenia is a common psychiatric disorder of adolescence (hence the term dementia praecox). Because schizophrenia is a serious disorder with ominous prognosis and social stigma, some clinicians are hesitant to make this diagnosis, even when there is sufficient evidence to do so. This potentially denies the child and family access to appropriate treatment, knowledge about the disorder, and specialized support services.

The differentiation between schizophrenia, psychotic depression or mania and schizoaffective disorder is not always easy in adolescence and many conceptual and nosological issues remain to be decided. The patient must then be followed longitudinally, with periodic diagnostic reassessments, to ensure accuracy. Patients and families should be educated about these diagnostic issues.

The depression in schizophrenia may be related to the fact that the young person feels that they are falling apart and becoming mentally ill and there is indeed evidence that suicidality and depression in these patients is related to good premorbid function, better insight, higher intelligence and preservation of cognitive function. Post-psychotic depression, and depressive states due to neuroleptic medications may also have a role to play in this dangerous condition.

Many schizophrenic patients are depressed and suicidal especially when they are young and have not been ill for a long time.

At least two-thirds of the suicides seen in persons with schizophrenia are related to depression, and only a small minority to the psychotic symptoms such as command hallucinations. The suicide is often shortly after discharge and thus may be related to lack of social support.

Finally, many adolescents with schizophrenia also abuse drugs and alcohol, thus increasing their risk for suicide. Sometimes the abuse is an attempt at self-medication. Anti-cholinergic medications given for the relief of extra-pyramidal symptoms (EPS) often give some adolescent patients a high to which they become addicted and those patients may simulate EPS in order to obtain these drugs. Child and adolescent onset of schizophrenia are often preceded by difficulties of attention and learning for which stimulant medications are given. Again, in the context of a developing schizophrenic condition there is a potential for abuse and drug-induced depression.

Recently Schwartz *et al.* (2006) found that depression can occur in some but not all adolescent patients with schizophrenia in the weeks following an acute psychotic episode. This depression can be quite severe and is associated with suicidal risk and actual suicidal behaviours. The schizophrenia-related depression in general shares some common features with the depression seen in major depressive episode (MDE) although in most cases it appears to be quantitatively less severe. In general, it seems that depression in schizophrenia can be distinguished from negative symptoms of schizophrenia. Finally, it appears that depression, hopelessness, and suicidality in schizophrenia are strongly related to the degree of insight and may be related to youth's sense that they are developing a mental illness. In fact, there is evidence that suicidality and depression in these patients is related to good premorbid function, better insight, higher intelligence and preservation of cognitive functions (De Hert and Peuskins 2000). Paradoxically, it is the patients with better insight and thus probably with better prognosis who are more likely to be depressed and suicidal (Schwartz *et al.* 2006). Post-psychotic depression and neuroleptic medications may also have a role in this dangerous condition. Suicide among this population often occurs shortly after discharge, and thus may be related to lack of social support. About 10–15 per cent of patients suffering from schizophrenia eventually commit suicide.

## Alcohol and drug abuse

Adolescents with Psychoactive Substance Abuse Disorder (PSUD), especially males, are more likely to commit suicide with guns than are adolescents without PSUD. Adolescent suicide also seems to be related to more chronic PSUD in subjects who have not sought treatment.

For any age group, acute intoxication often precedes suicide attempts. Intoxication for the purpose of self-medication of anxiety and despondency, which often follows a crisis, may trigger suicide in an adolescent who feels shame, humiliation or frustration. It has been suggested that adolescents may use psychoactive substances to bolster their courage to carry out the suicide attempt or suicide. Intoxication may also lead to impaired judgement and decreased inhibition and thus may facilitate suicidal behaviour.

This topic of adolescent suicide and drug abuse has been extensively reviewed by Kaminer (1996). Many studies have reported an elevated suicide-risk ratio for adults diagnosed with PSUD (Kaminer 1996).

Although there has not been extensive research on this subject in adolescence it is well-known that conduct disorders and mood disorders are frequently comorbid with both substance abuse and suicidal behaviour.

The relationship between suicide, aggression and alcoholism may be especially relevant to people with type 2 alcoholism. These people are characterized by high novelty-seeking, low harm avoidance, and low reward dependence, and there alcoholism has an early onset and is characterized by a rapid course, severe psychiatric symptoms, fighting, arrests, poor prognosis and multiple suicide attempts. Surveys have found that suicidal thoughts were experienced by more than 25 per cent of college students aged 16–19 (Kaminer 1996). This supports a general non-specificity for adolescent suicidal thoughts. However, students with PSUD had more frequent and more severe suicidal thoughts than average, and also were more likely to have a prolonged desire to be dead. PSUD was also found to be associated with more severe medical seriousness of actual suicide attempts.

Studies of completed suicide in adolescents have shown that in Scandinavia, Canada and the USA, PSUD is more common among victims than in the general adolescent population. There is some evidence that alcohol and cocaine may be especially dangerous with regard to suicide, but this is yet to be validated (Kaminer 1996).

Impulsive rather than planned suicides by adolescents have been reported in large numbers. Many adolescents manifest suicidal behaviour after an acute crisis such as perceived rejection or interpersonal conflict, an acute disciplinary act, sexual assault, or immediate loss. Intoxication for the purpose of self-medication, which often follows a crisis, may trigger suicide in an adolescent who feels shame, humiliation or frustration.

## Eating disorders

There has also been recent recognition of the very definite increased risk for suicide in girls with eating disorders (Apter *et al.* 1995). The relationship between anorexia nervosa (AN) and depression is well documented. However, the suicide potential of these adolescents has been neglected in the literature, perhaps because these youngsters use denial to a large extent and because it was felt that starvation was a suicidal equivalent, obviating the need for a direct self-attack in these patients. Recently, however, it has been pointed out that suicide is not rare in AN and suicidal behaviour may be an important indication of poor prognosis for AN. Patton (1988) followed up 460 patients with eating disorders and found that the increased standard mortality rate in anorectic patients was mostly due to suicide, with death occurring up to 8 years after the initial assessment. These findings were similar to those of the Copenhagen Anorexia Follow-up study. Projective testing of anorectic patients also shows a preponderance of suicidal indicators (Gordon *et al.* 1984). Standard mortality ratio for death and suicide were 9/6 and 58.1, respectively (Herzog *et al.* 1994).

One can speculate on this association between depression, suicide and eating disorders. It is possible that for many girls weight loss is a form of self-medication for depression since in fact many healthy women feel much better when they lose weight. These good feelings are related in many ways to social approval, but may also result from the release of endorphins from damaged muscle tissue or from vomiting. In some cases we have seen depression resulting from weight gain as if the patient was suffering from withdrawal symptoms from her addiction to thinness. However, weight loss may of itself induce quite severe depression and suicidal ideation, even in volunteers and in normal dieters. Another very dangerous form of depression occurs in treatment-resistant cases where the constant battle against gaining weight on the one hand, and the constant social pressure to gain weight on the other becomes an intolerable burden. The diary of Ellen West, a famous anorectic patient who eventually killed herself, contained the following passages:

> The most horrible thing about my life is that it is filled with continuous fear. Fear of eating but also fear of hunger and fear of fear itself. Only death can liberate me from this dread.

> Since I am doing everything from the point of view of whether it makes me thin or fat, all things lose their real value. It has fallen over me like a beast and I am helpless against it.

Adolescents with bulimia nervosa are also highly prone to suicidal behaviours as part of an impulsive and unstable life style. Many show self-mutilation and cutting but often they also make serious suicide attempts which sometimes end in suicide. In our own series of former bulimic adolescent inpatients about 3.5 per cent died from suicide in a 15-year-long follow-up. This was about 300 times higher than the risk for other former female adolescent psychiatric inpatients. Recently, the term multi-impulsive bulimia has been coined to describe the increasingly more common association between bulimia, borderline or unstable personality disorder, substance abuse, depression and conduct disorder. Most patients with this comorbid constellation of disorders are women showing high risk for replication of suicide attempts and for fatal suicide.

Eating disorder patients who are suicidal should probably be hospitalized in most cases since the risk for completed suicide is great. Most will refuse treatment and legal commitment may be necessary. Many of these patients, however, are extremely resistant to therapy. In the chronic resistant patient the mainstays of usual treatment such as family therapy or cognitive behavioural therapy may be ineffectual. In the suicidal multi-impulsive bulimic individual there may be a place for dialectic behaviour therapy (DBT) (Linehan 1993). In anorectic patients weight gain and refeeding are essential and in many individuals this will restore mood and alleviate suicidal pain. In others, weight gain can cause tremendous disappointment and this may be an incentive for suicide.

Although there was an initial enthusiasm for the SSRI treatment of bulimia, recent results have been disappointing and in the suicidal patient with extensive psychiatric comorbidity these medications are usually not effective, although most clinicians usually give them a try. Antidepressant medications are usually unhelpful in the underweight depressed, suicidal anorectic, but they are of use in preventing relapse after weight gain has been restored. Our own experience (uncontrolled without any evidence base) is that long-term open-ended supportive therapy is usually the best way to keep these patients alive in the long run, and where a therapeutic relationship is achieved suicide can be obviated although the eating disorder usually persists to a greater or lesser degree.

## Conclusions

Suicidal behaviour appears in many if not all psychiatric conditions of adolescence. Brent *et al.* (1993) found the following odds ratios (OR) for adolescent (completed) suicide risk factors: major depression (OR = 27); bipolar disorder (OR = 9); psychoactive substance use disorder (OR = 8.5) and conduct disorder (OR = 6).

It appears that suicidality cuts across nosological boundaries and thus may be regarded as an independent psychopathological dimension. This is supported by the work of Van Praag (1997) who found that biological markers for suicide were far more robust than biological markers for DSM-related nosological entities. In addition it may be that any serious debilitating mental illness leads to demoralization and hopelessness with resulting mental pain (Orbach *et al.* 2003). In any event, psychiatric illness remains the most well-defined risk factor for adolescent suicide and suicidality should be assessed in every young person suffering from a serious mental illness.

## References

Allgulander C and Lavori PW (1991). Excess mortality among 3302 patients with 'pure' anxiety neurosis. *Archives of General Psychiatry*, **48**, 599–602.

American Academy of Child and Adolescent Psychiatry (1990). *Documentation of Medical Necessity of Child and Adolescent Psychiatric Treatment: Guidelines for Use in Managed Care, Third-party Coverage, and Peer Review.*

American Academy of Child and Adolescent Psychiatry (1996). *Level of Care Placement Criteria for Psychiatric Illness.*

Andrews JA and Lewinsohn PM (1992). Suicidal attempts among older adolescents: prevalence and co-occurrence with psychiatric disorders. *Journal of the American Academy of Child and Adolescent Psychiatry*, **31**, 655–662.

Angst J (1993). Comorbidity of anxiety, phobia, compulsion and depression. *International Clinical Psychopharmacology*, **8**, 21–25.

Apter A and Ofek H (2001). Personality constellations and suicidal behaviour. In K Van Heeringen, ed., *Understanding Suicidal Behaviour: The Suicidal Process Approach to Research, Treatment, and Prevention*, pp. 94–119. Wiley, Chichester.

Apter A, Bleich A, King R *et al.* (1993a). Death without warning? A clinical postmortem study of 43 Israeli male suicides. *Archives of General Psychiatry*, **50**, 138–142.

Apter A, Gothelf D, Orbach I *et al.* (1995). Correlation of suicidal and violent behaviour in different diagnostic categories in hospitalized adolescent patients. *Journal of the American Academy of Child and Adolescent Psychiatry*, **34**, 912–918.

Apter A, Horesh N, Gothelf D *et al.* (2003). Depression and suicidal behaviour in adolescent inpatients with obsessive compulsive disorder. *Journal of Affective Disorders*, **75**, 181–189.

Apter A, Offer R, Gothelf D *et al.* (1997). Defense mechanisms in suicidal adolescents. *Journal of the American Academy of Child and Adolescent Psychiatry*, **36**, 1520–1527.

Apter A, Plutchik R, Van Praag HM (1993b). Anxiety, impulsivity and depressed mood in relation to suicide and violent behaviour. *Acta Psychiatrica Scandinavica*, **87**, 1–5.

Apter A, Van Praag HM, Sevy S *et al.* (1990). Interrelationships among anxiety, aggression, impulsiveness and mood: a serotonergically linked cluster? *Psychiatric Research*, **32**, 191–199.

Baldessarini RJ, Tondo L, Hennen J *et al.* (2002). Is Lithium still worth using? An update of selected recent research. *Harvard Review of Psychiatry*, **10**, 59–75.

Brent DA, Perper JA, Moritz G *et al.* (1993). Psychiatric risk factors for adolescent suicide: a case-control study. *Journal of the American Academy of Child and Adolescent Psychiatry*, **32**, 521–529.

Brodsky BS, Malone KM, Ellis SP *et al.* (1997). Characteristics of borderline personality disorder associated with suicidal behaviour. *American Journal of Psychiatry*, **154**, 1715–1719.

Chen YW and Dilsaver SC (1995). Comorbidity for obsessive-compulsive disorder in bipolar and unipolar disorders. *Psychiatry Research*, **59**, 57–64.

De Hert M and Peuskins J (2000). Psychiatric aspects of suicidal behaviour: Schizophrenia. In K Hawton and K van Heeringen, eds, *The International Handbook of Suicide and Attempted Suicide*, pp. 121–134. Wiley, Chichester.

De Wilde EJ, Kienhorst IC, Diekstra RF *et al.* (1993). The specificity of psychological characteristics of adolescent suicide attempters. *Journal of the American Academy of Child and Adolescent Psychiatry*, **32**, 51–59.

Dryfoos J (1990). A review of interventions to prevent pregnancy. *Advances in Adolescent Mental Health*, **4**, 121–35.

Fawcett J, Scheftner WA, Fogg L *et al.* (1990). Time-related predictors of suicide in major affective disorder. *American Journal of Psychiatry*, **147**, 1189–1194.

Fergusson DM and Lynskey MT (1995). Suicide attempts and suicidal ideation in a birth cohort of 16-year-old New Zealanders. *Journal of the American Academy of Child and Adolescent Psychiatry*, **4**, 1308–1317.

Foa EB (1979). Failures in treating obsessive–compulsives. *Behaviour Research and Therapy*, **17**, 169–176.

Gordon DP, Halmi KA, Ippolito PM (1984). A comparison of the psychological evaluation of adolescents with anorexia nervosa and of adolescents with conduct disorders. *Journal of Adolescence*, **7**, 245–266.

Gunderson JG (1984). *Borderline Personality Disorder*. American Psychiatric Association, Washington, DC.

Hawton K (1987). Assessment of suicide risk. *British Journal of Psychiatry*, **150**, 145–153.

Herzog DB, Greenwood DN, Dorer DJ *et al.* (1994). Mortality in eating disorders: a descriptive study. *International Journal of Eating Disorders*, **28**, 20–26.

Hollander E, Greenwald S, Neville D *et al.* (1996). Uncomplicated and comorbid obsessive–compulsive disorder in an epidemiologic sample. *Depression and Anxiety*, **4**, 111–119.

Jenike MA (1990). Approaches to the patient with treatment-refractory obsessive compulsive disorder. *Journal of Clinical Psychiatry*, **51**(Suppl), 15–21.

Kaminer Y (1996). Adolescent substance abuse and suicidal behaviour. *Child and Adolescent Psychiatric Clinicsof North America*, **5**, 45–58.

Kernberg OF (1975). *Borderline Conditions and Pathological Narcissism*. Jason Aronson, New York.

King RA and Apter A (1996). Psychoanalytic perspectives on adolescent suicide. *Psychoanalytic Study of the Child*, **51**, 491–505.

Kosky R, Silburn S, Zubrick S (1986). Symptomatic depression and suicidal ideation. A comparative study with 628 children. *Journal of Nervous and Mental Disease*, **174**, 523–528.

Linehan MM (1993). *Cognitive-Behavioural Treatment of Borderline Personality Disorder*. Guilford Press, New York.

Lock J and Strauss GD (1994). Psychiatric hospitalization of adolescents for conduct disorder. *Hospital and Community Psychiatry*, **45**, 925–928.

Mannuzza S, Fyer AJ, Endicott J *et al.* (1992). An extension of the acquaintanceship procedure in family studies of mental disorder. *Journal of Psychiatric Research*, **26**, 45–57.

March JS and Mulle K (1998). *OCD in Children and Adolescents: A Cognitive-behaviour Treatment Manual*. Guilford, New York.

Massion AO, Warshaw MG, Keller MB (1993). Quality of life and psychiatric morbidity in panic disorder and generalized anxiety disorder. *American Journal of Psychiatry*, **150**, 600–607.

Neeleman J, Wessely S, Wadsworth M (1998). Predictors of suicide, accidental death, and premature natural death in a general-population birth cohort. *Lancet*, **351**, 93–97.

Nelson EC, Cloninger CR, Przybec TR *et al.* (1996). Platelet serotonergic markers and Tridimensional Personality Questionnaire measures in a clinical sample. *Biological Psychiatry*, **40**, 271–278.

Oei TI, Verhoeven WM, Westenberg HG, Zwart FM, van Ree JM (1990). Anhedonia, suicide ideation and dexamethasone nonsuppression in depressed patients. *J Psychiatr Research*, **24**, 25–35.

Orbach I, Mikulincer M, Gilboa-Schechtman E *et al.* (2003). Mental pain and its relationship to suicidality and life meaning. *Suicide and Life-Threatening Behaviour*, **33**, 231–241.

Orpinas PK, Basen-Engquist K, Grunbaum JA *et al.* (1995). The co-morbidity of violence-related behaviours with health-risk behaviours in a population of high school students. *Journal of Adolescent Health*, **16**, 216–225.

Patton GC (1988). Mortality in eating disorders. *Psychological Medicine*, **18**, 947–951.

Perugi G, Akiskal HS, Pfanner C *et al.* (1997). The clinical impact of bipolar and unipolar affective comorbidity on obsessive–compulsive disorder. *Journal of Affective Disorders*, **46**, 15–23.

Pope HG, Barry S, Bodkin A *et al.* (2006). Tracking scientific interest in the dissociative disorders: a study of scientific publication output 1984–2003. *Psychotherapy and Psychosomatics*, **75**, 19–24.

Schwartz O, Zalsman G, Apter A (2006). Depression, suicidal behaviour and insight in adolescents with schizophrenia. *European Journal of Child and Adolescent Psychiatry*, **15**, 352–359.

Shaffer D, Gould MS, Fisher P *et al.* (1996). Psychiatric diagnosis in child and adolescent suicide. *Archives of General Psychiatry*, **53**, 339–348.

Sosin DM, Koepsell TD, Rivara FP *et al.* (1995). Fighting as a marker for multiple problem behaviours in adolescents. *Journal of Adolescent Health*, **16**, 209–215.

Stone M (1989). The course of borderline personality disorder. In RE Hales and AJ Frances, eds, *Review of Psychiatry*, pp. 103–122, American Psychiatric Press, Washington, DC.

Taylor EA and Stansfeld SA (1984). Children who poison themselves. I. A clinical comparison with psychiatric controls. *British Journal of Psychiatry*, **145**, 127–132.

Valleni-Basile LA, Garrison CZ, Jackson KL *et al.* (1994). Frequency of obsessive–compulsive disorder in a community sample of young adolescents. *Journal of the American Academy of Child and Adolescent Psychiatry*, **33**, 782–791.

Van Praag HM and Honig A (eds) (1997). *Depression: Neurobiological, Psychopathological and Therapeutic Advances.* Wiley, Chichester.

Wasserman (2006). *Depression. The Facts.* Oxford University Press, New York.

Weller EB, Weller RA, Sanchez LE (2002). Bipolar disorder in children and adolescents. In M Lewis, ed., *Child and Adolescent Psychiatry: A Comprehensive Textbook,* pp.1117–1121. Lippicott Williams & Wilkins, Philadelphia.

Woods ER, Lin YG, Middleman A *et al.* (1997). The asociations of suicide attempts in adolescents. *Pediatrics*, **99**, 791–796.

Yerevanian BI, Koek RJ, Mintz J (2003). Lithium, anticonvulsants and suicidal behaviour in bipolar disorder. *Journal of Affective Disorders*, **73**, 223–228.

# CHAPTER 90

# The link between physical disabilities and suicidality in children and adolescents

## Gil Zalsman and Gal Shoval

## Abstract

The existence of physical disorders and disabilities has been associated with suicidal behaviour among adults. Though relatively less often studied in children and adolescents, a growing body of evidence supports a similar link in this population as well. This chapter describes recent studies on suicidality among young patients with diabetes mellitus, bronchial asthma, human immunodeficiency virus (HIV), epilepsy, multiple sclerosis, traumatic brain injuries and physical injuries. Suggested models addressing biological, psychological and social aspects relevant to the possible pathophysiological mechanisms linking physical disorders and disabilities to suicidal behaviour in the paediatric age group are also discussed.

## Introduction

Extensive research during the past three decades has elucidated various biological, psychological and social risk factors for suicidal behaviour, such as gender, age, previous suicide attempt, substance abuse, presence of psychiatric disorders and a family history of suicide. Another intriguing risk factor that was established is the presence of a physical disorder. The existence of physical diseases or disabilities has shown repeatedly to be associated with suicidal behaviour among adult populations and, particularly, in the elderly. This significant association persisted even after adjusting for depression and substance use (Druss and Pincus 2000). Cancer, stroke, AIDS, multiple sclerosis, systemic lupus erythematosis, migraine and Parkinson's disease were found, in many large-scale studies, to elevate the risk for suicide ideation, suicide attempt as well as completed suicide (Fox *et al.* 1982; Breslau 1992; Massie *et al.* 1994; Jorm *et al.* 1995; Stenager *et al.* 1998). In the European Parasuicide Study Interview Schedule (EPSIS) survey that included 1269 patients who attempted suicide (aged 15 and older), 50 per cent were suffering from physical disorders at the time of the parasuicide, and more than a fifth rated their physical illness as a major factor precipitating the attempt (De Leo *et al.* 1999). Despite the abundant literature in adults, this issue was relatively less studied in child and adolescent populations (Lewinsohn *et al.* 1995; Ikeda *et al.* 2001).

One can assume that physical disability or disorder will serve as a negative life event and enhance the stress to the developing brain. Some recent evidence has demonstrated that the interaction between psychosocial stress and genetic vulnerability, such as having the short allele 5HTTLPR, may lead to both depression and suicidality (Caspi *et al.* 2003; Eley *et al.* 2004; Kaufman *et al.* 2004; Zalsman *et al.* 2006). The physical disorder itself may have a biological impact on the developing brain.

In a prospective controlled study of 1507 randomly selected high school students, poor physical health was found to be a specific risk factor for the development of major depressive disorder, which may lead to suicidal behaviour (Lewinsohn *et al.* 1995). In a prospective register-based study of Danish children in the 14–27 age group, physical handicap was among several risk factors for attempted suicide (Christoffersen *et al.* 2003). The existence of several physical disorders was connected with an odd ratio (OR) of 1.9.

A smaller-scale population-based, case–control study in Houston, Texas included 153 subjects aged 13–34 years, admitted to hospital emergency rooms following nearly lethal suicide attempts (Ikeda *et al.* 2001). They were compared to 513 controls. Case patients reported significantly more serious medical conditions (OR = 3.23, 95 per cent CI = 2.12–4.91). This finding also persisted when controlling for age, race, alcoholism, depression and hopelessness, with and OR in males of 4.76 (95 per cent CI = 1.87–12.17), while it was only 1.6 (95 per cent CI = 0.62–4.17) in females.

## Diabetes mellitus

Insulin-dependent diabetes mellitus (IDDM) is a serious illness that requires daily treatment, including a restrictive diet and self-injection of insulin. Its onset is typically in the second decade of life, and may lead to psychiatric consequences. In a sample of ninety-one adolescents with IDDM, the rate of suicide ideation was measured to be higher than the general population, and seems to be associated with serious, potentially life-threatening non-compliance with the medical regimen required (Goldston *et al.* 1997). It should be noted, however, that there was no significant elevation in suicide attempts among the study population. This was consistent with a previous longitudinal study of diabetic children, performed by the same group, indicating increased suicidal ideation among the cohort, associated with later medication non-compliance (Goldston *et al.* 1994).

## Bronchial asthma

Bronchial asthma is another prevalent (6–12 per cent) and chronic medical condition affecting the pediatric population. A recent study aimed at determining the association between asthma and suicide ideation among youth in the general population (Goodwin and Marusic 2004). Analysing data from the Methodological Epidemiology of Children and Adolescents (MECA) study, a large (N = 1285), multi-centre, cross-sectional designed study, suicidal ideation was more frequently reported among youth with bronchial asthma compared to healthy subjects (OR = 3.25, 95 per cent CI = 1.04–10.1). The association between asthma and suicidal ideation persisted after controlling for sociodemographic characteristics and comorbid mental disorders. This finding strengthens previous similar findings regarding the relationship between asthma and suicidality among the young (Druss and Pincus 2000; Goodwin *et al.* 2003). To the best of our knowledge, no study showed an association between asthma and suicide attempts in the children and adolescent population, although this connection has been demonstrated in adults (Levitan 1983).

## Human immunodeficiency virus

One of the significant epidemiological shifts of the HIV pandemia, in the past decade, was an increase in the rates of HIV infection among teenagers (Donenberg and Pao 2005). However, research findings regarding the impact of acquired immunodeficiency syndrome (AIDS) among the young are inconclusive. While most data indicate that affected populations suffer from increased rates of psychiatric disorders (45 per cent), including depression, anxiety, aggression and a substantial decrease in all areas of functioning (Rotheram-Borus *et al.* 2001), some studies have failed to replicate these findings (Lee and Rotheram-Borus 2002), leaving room for further research on the psychiatric aspects of this prevalent chronic disease.

## Epilepsy

Epilepsy is one of the most common neurological disorders affecting children and adolescents. Patients with convulsive disorders were found to have an increased risk for suicide in both the adult and paediatric group (Brent *et al.* 1990). Rates may be as high as twelve times than those in the general population (Jones *et al.* 2003). This association may be explained by the markedly increased rates of psychiatric comorbidity reported among patients with epilepsy, particularly the temporal lobe type. Axis I disorders range from 19–62 per cent (Fiordelli *et al.* 1993; Manchanda *et al.* 1996) in this population, with a predominance of mood disorders, reported to be as prevalent as 42–63 per cent (Silberman *et al.* 1994; Altshuler *et al.* 1999). Other common psychiatric disorders that may possibly increase suicidality are schizophrenia, substance abuse and cluster B personality disorders. Despite these elevated rates, recently, major depressive disorder has been found to be under-diagnosed and under-treated in a cohort of epileptic children aged 5–16 years (Plioplys 2003). This issue was also reviewed by others (Baker 2006) as a matter of public health concern. An interesting, related finding, comes from a recent population-based case–control study, which demonstrated that a history of either major depression or attempted suicide was independently associated with increased risk for seizure, thus suggesting that a more complex pathophysiological mechanism underlies the connection between epilepsy, depression and suicidality (Hesdorffer *et al.* 2006).

## Multiple sclerosis

Multiple sclerosis (MS) is a neurodegenerative disorder affecting primarily young women. Suicide prevalence among patients with MS was found to be approximately twice that of the general population (Stenager *et al.* 1992), accounting for 15 per cent of all patient deaths (Sadovnick *et al.* 1991). It should be noted that completed suicide in MS patients was shown to be associated with diagnosis of the disorder prior to age 30 (Stenager *et al.* 1992). This underlines the importance of monitoring these young patients in order to prevent suicide. Additional reinforcement for the importance of monitoring comes from the report on prevalent common suicide intent among MS patients (Feinstein 2002; Fredrikson *et al.* 2003).

## Traumatic brain injury

Depending on its extent and locus and on the emotional response to it, traumatic brain injury may cause different levels of psychiatric symptomatology. Major depressive disorder, suicidal ideation and suicide attempts have been reported following local and diffuse brain injuries (Fedoroff *et al.* 1992; Ownsworth and Oei 1998; Mann *et al.* 1999). Since data is scarce even for adults, let alone for children and adolescents, the findings should be received with appropriate caution. One study reported 85 suicides among a cohort of 6498 war veterans with brain injury (Achte and Anttinen 1963). In a Danish population registry study, incidence of suicide increased considerably in patients having brain concussion (three old as compared to the general population), cranial fracture (2.7-fold increase) and traumatic intracranial hemorrhage (4.1-fold increase) (Teasdale and Engberg 2001). Increased suicidality in patients with brain injury may be a result of the same risk factors as those in persons with suicidal behaviour, namely being of male gender, impulsive and a substance abuser. Such persons are more prone for traumatic injuries. Further studies focusing on traumatic cerebral injuries in the young are required to elucidate possible mechanisms linking brain injury and suicidal behaviour. For example: a dysfunction of the frontal lobe, which is essential in affective regulation, behaviour and decision-making.

## Physical injuries

Physical injuries are the single largest cause of morbidity among US children. While the annual figure of injured children is estimated to be approximately 16 million, the extent of psychiatric sequelae are still unknown (Stoddard and Saxe 2001) and are relatively understudied. The most established psychiatric disorder, following physical injuries, is post-traumatic stress disorder (PTSD), which may be severely incapacitating and central in the development of suicidality. However, PTSD is beyond the scope of this chapter, as it is discussed elsewhere in this volume. Other mental disorders that have a high probability of appearing, following a child's physical injury, are mood and anxiety disorders (Stoddard and Saxe 2001). Staff training, patient and parent education and careful psychiatric monitoring of the paediatric patients diagnosed with physical injuries are needed in order to prevent mental complications that may affect the prognosis. These measures are important also in rehabilitation. Further study is needed to shed more light on suicidality among these patients.

It is of note that physical injuries are no longer exclusively considered as 'accidents'. There are several established risk factors for a child to be injured, such as the presence of attention-deficit hyperactivity disorder (ADHD), conduct disorders or substance use (Pulkkinen 1995; Spirito *et al.* 1997; Leibson *et al.* 2001). These findings are important in developing prevention programmes to decrease physical injuries among the young, and thus prevent comorbid psychiatric morbidity, including suicide.

## Suggested models

Few models have been suggested over the years to explain the relationship between physical disorders and disabilities and suicidal behaviour in the paediatric age group. These models are mainly based on the assumption that psychological traits and states may mediate between physical disorders and suicidal behaviour. However, the literature lacks a biological model that attempts to link the effect of physical disease to a vulnerable brain. Recently, a great body of evidence has demonstrated that the neurobiology of suicidal behaviour in children and adolescents exists (Mann 2003; Zalsman and Mann 2005; Zalsman *et al.* 2006).

The four-stage model developed by Baumeister suggests an explanation to this critical psychological process that leads from having a physical disability to developing suicidal ideation and later to attempting suicide (Baumeister 1990). In stage I, the patient becomes acutely aware of his disorder and perceives it as a personal failure. In stage II, the 'failure' is attributed to self, thus, making it unacceptable. It is then that 'cognitive deconstruction' appears, resulting in emotional decline (stage III). Later, in stage IV, irrationality and disinhibition develop in a manner that may produce suicidal thoughts and behaviour. An elaboration of the Baumeister model was later suggested by Reich based on the results of the Life Events and Aging Project (LEAP) (Reich *et al.* 1996). The purpose of this controlled prospective study was to assess the

effects of recent physical disability and recent bereavement on the mental health of adults (Reich *et al.* 1989). It showed that health downturns led to a later increase in psychological distress. The Reich model suggests that health decline is the initiating condition causing both a decline in self-esteem and an increase in fatalism (Figure 90.1).

Each of these may lead to confused thinking and feelings of helplessness that, consequently, lead to suicidal ideation. It is noteworthy that the risk for suicidal ideation as a direct consequence of health decline was moderate, while the impact of health decline on self-esteem and helplessness, as mediators, was significant (p <0.001). According to this and many other models, feeling helpless may lead to suicidal ideation (Beck *et al.* 1985). Nonetheless, a direct association between health decline and suicidality was also found (p <0.05) (Reich *et al.* 1989).

These two models have significant weaknesses in the context of this chapter. First, they were contemplated on the basis of data derived from adult studies. Therefore, they may be less valid and probably only partially relevant to children and adolescents. However, we chose to describe them as we have failed to find a comprehensive integrative model linking physical disabilities and suicidality in youth populations. Full integrative adaptation of any of these models to children and adolescents requires further study on the effect on psychological variables caused by physical disorders and, therefore, is beyond the scope of this chapter. Such adaptation to youth populations should take into account the developmental perspective of children and adolescents in the context of them coping with their health downturns. Self-esteem is a prominent issue during adolescence and may, therefore, cause more vulnerability to injury in that developmental period. The same may be true, albeit to a lesser extent, for fatalism. Cognitive development is still ongoing in prepubertal children, and therefore they may be more susceptible to thought confusion and distortions that could enhance suicidal behaviour.

A second weakness of the Baumeister and Reich models lies in the absence of the social aspects, which play a central role in children's and adolescents' psychopathology. Comparing oneself to peers is very common for children and is an integral part of their

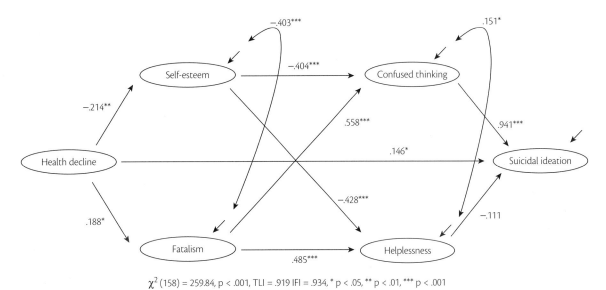

$\chi^2$ (158) = 259.84, p < .001, TLI = .919 IFI = .934, * p < .05, ** p < .01, *** p < .001

**Fig. 90.1** Graphical presentation of the full structural equation model with standardized path coefficient. From Reich *et al.* (1996) with permission.

maturation process. But contrary to the adult population, in the youth population physical disorders are less prevalent and, therefore, may lead more frequently to a narcissistic insult and inappropriate feelings of guilt, injustice or helplessness. Children and adolescents are often more impulsive and, therefore, may react dramatically to these feelings by displaying suicidal behaviour.

Finally, a future model for the relationship between physical disorders and suicidality should include the concept of unipolar mood disorder. Depression is more prevalent in children (1–2.5 per cent) and adolescents (6–8 per cent) than previously thought and is known to strongly increase suicidality. To date, the proportion of major depressive disorder among youth with physical disorders who attempt suicide is yet unknown. However, as hopelessness, low self-esteem and cognitive confusion are key features in depression, we estimate this figure to be quite high. Elucidating these data necessitates further study. Depression is a treatable and reversible psychiatric disorder. Its early detection in the prone/high-risk population of physically disabled children and adolescents may prove highly beneficial in the prevention of both additional mental distresses of the child as well as suicidal behaviour.

## Conclusion

Children and adolescents with physical ailments are a high-risk population for psychiatric disorders, in particular depression, and therefore require closer monitoring to ensure early detection and treatment that may prevent suicidality.

In summary, future studies should concentrate on deepening our knowledge of the various biological, social and psychological risk factors for suicidality among children and adolescents (Shoval *et al.* 2005, 2006). An integrative and comprehensive developmental model is yet to be formulated in order to better determine the exact role of physical disabilities on the different neuropsychological developmental axes and their consequent psychiatric sequelae.

## References

Achte KA and Anttinen EE (1963). [Suicides in brain damaged veterans of the wars in Finland]. *Fortschr Neurol Psychiatr Grenzgeb*, **31**, 645–667.

Altshuler L, Rausch R, Delrahim S *et al.* (1999). Temporal lobe epilepsy, temporal lobectomy, and major depression. *Journal of Neuropsychiatry and Clinical Neuroscience*, **11**, 436–443.

Baker GA (2006). Depression and suicide in adolescents with epilepsy. *Neurology*, **66**, S5–12.

Baumeister RF (1990). Suicide as escape from self. *Psychological Review*, **97**, 90–113.

Beck AT, Steer RA, Kovacs M *et al.* (1985). Hopelessness and eventual suicide: a 10-year prospective study of patients hospitalized with suicidal ideation. *American Journal of Psychiatry*, **142**, 559–563.

Brent DA, Kolko DJ, Allan MJ *et al.* (1990). Suicidality in affectively disordered adolescent inpatients. *Journal of the American Academy of Child and Adolescent Psychiatry*, **29**, 586–593.

Breslau N (1992). Migraine, suicidal ideation, and suicide attempts. *Neurology*, **42**, 392–395.

Caspi A, Sugden K, Moffitt TE *et al.* (2003). Influence of life stress on depression: moderation by a polymorphism in the 5-HTT gene. *Science*, **301**, 386–389.

Christoffersen MN, Poulsen HD, Nielsen A (2003). Attempted suicide among young people: risk factors in a prospective register-based study of Danish children born in 1966. *Acta Psychiatrica Scandinavica*, **108**, 350–358.

De Leo D, Scocco P, Marietta P *et al.* (1999). Physical illness and parasuicide: evidence from the European Parasuicide Study Interview Schedule (EPSIS/WHO-EURO). *International Journal of Psychiatry in Medicine*, **29**, 149–163.

Donenberg GR and Pao M (2005). Youths and HIV/AIDS: psychiatry's role in a changing epidemic. *Journal of the American Academy of Child and Adolescent Psychiatry*, **44**, 728–747.

Druss B and Pincus H (2000). Suicidal ideation and suicide attempts in general medical illnesses. *Archives of Internal Medicine*, **160**, 1522–1526.

Eley TC, Sugden K, Corsico A *et al.* (2004). Gene–environment interaction analysis of serotonin system markers with adolescent depression. *Molecular Psychiatry*, **9**, 908–915.

Fedoroff JP, Starkstein SE, Forrester AW *et al.* (1992). Depression in patients with acute traumatic brain injury. *American Journal of Psychiatry*, **149**, 918–923.

Feinstein A (2002). An examination of suicidal intent in patients with multiple sclerosis. *Neurology*, **59**, 674–678.

Fiordelli E, Beghi E, Bogliun G *et al.* V (1993). Epilepsy and psychiatric disturbance. A cross-sectional study. *British Journal of Psychiatry*, **163**, 446–450.

Fox BH, Stanek EJ III, Boyd SC *et al.* (1982). Suicide rates among cancer patients in Connecticut. *Journal of Chronic Diseases*, **35**, 89–100.

Fredrikson S, Cheng Q, Jiang GX *et al.* (2003). Elevated suicide risk among patients with multiple sclerosis in Sweden. *Neuroepidemiology*, **22**, 146–152.

Goldston DB, Kelley AE, Reboussin DM *et al.* (1997). Suicidal ideation and behaviour and noncompliance with the medical regimen among diabetic adolescents. *Journal of the American Academy of Child and Adolescent Psychiatry*, **36**, 1528–1536.

Goldston DB, Kovacs M, Ho VY *et al.* (1994). Suicidal ideation and suicide attempts among youth with insulin-dependent diabetes mellitus. *Journal of the American Academy of Child and Adolescent Psychiatry*, **33**, 240–246.

Goodwin RD, Kroenke K, Hoven CW *et al.* (2003). Major depression, physical illness, and suicidal ideation in primary care. *Psychosomatic Medicine*, **65**, 501–505.

Goodwin RD and Marusic A (2004). Asthma and suicidal ideation among youth in the community. *Crisis*, **25**, 99–102.

Hesdorffer DC, Hauser WA, Olafsson E *et al.* (2006). Depression and suicide attempt as risk factors for incident unprovoked seizures. *Annals of Neurology*, **59**, 35–41.

Ikeda RM, Kresnow MJ, Mercy JA *et al.* (2001). Medical conditions and nearly lethal suicide attempts. *Suicide and Life-Threatening Behavoir*, **32**, 60–67.

Jones JE, Hermann BP, Barry JJ *et al.* (2003). Rates and risk factors for suicide, suicidal ideation, and suicide attempts in chronic epilepsy. *Epilepsy and Behaviour*, **4**(Suppl 3), S31–S38.

Jorm AF, Henderson AS, Scott R *et al.* (1995). Factors associated with the wish to die in elderly people. *Age Ageing*, **24**, 389–392.

Kaufman J, Yang BZ, Douglas-Palumberi H *et al.* (2004). Social supports and serotonin transporter gene moderate depression in maltreated children. *Proceedings of the National Academy of Sciences of the USA*, **101**, 17316–17321.

Lee MB and Rotheram-Borus MJ (2002). Parents' disclosure of HIV to their children. *AIDS*, **16**, 2201–2207.

Leibson CL, Katusic SK, Barbaresi WJ *et al.* (2001). Use and costs of medical care for children and adolescents with and without attention-deficit/hyperactivity disorder. *JAMA*, **285**, 60–66.

Levitan H (1983). Suicidal trends in patients with asthma and hypertension. A chart study. *Psychotherapy and Psychosomatics*, **39**, 165–170.

Lewinsohn PM, Gotlib IH, Seeley JR (1995). Adolescent psychopathology: IV. Specificity of psychosocial risk factors for depression and substance abuse in older adolescents. *Journal of the American Academy of Child and Adolescent Psychiatry*, **34**, 1221–1229.

Manchanda R, Schaefer B, McLachlan RS *et al.* (1996). Psychiatric disorders in candidates for surgery for epilepsy. *Journal of Neurology, Neurosurgery and Psychiatry*, **61**, 82–89.

Mann JJ (2003). Neurobiology of suicidal behaviour. *Nature Reviews: Neuroscience*, **4**, 819–828.

Mann JJ, Waternaux C, Haas GL *et al.* (1999). Toward a clinical model of suicidal behaviour in psychiatric patients. *American Journal of Psychiatry*, **156**, 181–189.

Massie MJ, Gagnon P, Holland JC (1994). Depression and suicide in patients with cancer. *Journal of Pain Symptom Management*, **9**, 325–340.

Ownsworth TL and Oei TP (1998). Depression after traumatic brain injury: conceptualization and treatment considerations. *Brain Injury*, **12**, 735–751.

Plioplys S (2003). Depression in children and adolescents with epilepsy. *Epilepsy and Behaviour*, **4**(Suppl 3), S39–S45.

Pulkkinen L (1995). Behavioural precursors to accidents and resulting physical impairment. *Child Development*, **66**, 1660–1679.

Reich JW, Newsom JT, Zautra AJ (1996). Health downturns and predictors of suicidal ideation: an application of the Baumeister model. *Suicide and Life-Threatening Behaviour*, **26**, 282–291.

Reich JW, Zautra AJ, Guarnaccia CA (1989). Effects of disability and bereavement on the mental health and recovery of older adults. *Psychology and Aging*, **4**, 57–65.

Rotheram-Borus MJ, Lee MB, Gwadz M *et al.* (2001). An intervention for parents with AIDS and their adolescent children. *American Journal of Public Health*, **91**, 1294–1302.

Sadovnick AD, Eisen K, Ebers GC *et al.* (1991). Cause of death in patients attending multiple sclerosis clinics. *Neurology*, **41**, 1193–1196.

Shoval G, Zalsman G, Polakevitch J *et al.* (2005). Effect of the broadcast of a television documentary about a teenager's suicide in Israel on suicidal behaviour and methods. *Crisis*, **26**, 20–24.

Shoval G, Zalsman G, Sher L *et al.* (2006). Clinical characteristics of inpatient adolescents with severe obsessive–compulsive disorder. *Depression and Anxiety*, **23**, 62–70.

Silberman EK, Sussman N, Skillings G *et al.* (1994). Aura phenomena and psychopathology: a pilot investigation. *Epilepsia*, **35**, 778–784.

Spirito A, Rasile DA, Vinnick LA *et al.* (1997). Relationship between substance use and self-reported injuries among adolescents. *Journal of Adolescent Health*, **21**, 221–224.

Stenager EN, Madsen C, Stenager E *et al.* (1998). Suicide in patients with stroke: epidemiological study. *BMJ*, **316**, 1206.

Stenager EN, Stenager E, Koch-Henriksen N *et al.* (1992). Suicide and multiple sclerosis: an epidemiological investigation. *Journal of Neurology, Neurosurgery and Psychiatry*, **55**, 542–545.

Stoddard FJ and Saxe G (2001). Ten-year research review of physical injuries. *Journal of the American Academy of Child and Adolescent Psychiatry*, **40**, 1128–1145.

Teasdale TW and Engberg AW (2001). Suicide after traumatic brain injury: a population study. *Journal of Neurology, Neurosurgery and Psychiatry*, **71**, 436–440.

Zalsman G, Huang Y, Oquendo MA *et al.* (2006). A triallelic serotonin transporter gene promoter polymorphism (5-HTTLPR), stressful life events and severity of depression. *(In press)*.

Zalsman G and Mann JJ (2005). The neurobiology of suicide in adolescents. An emerging field of research. *International Journal of Adolescent Medicine and Health*, **17**, 195–196.

# CHAPTER 91

# Effective treatments for suicidal youth

## Pharmacological and psychosocial approaches

David Brent

## Abstract

There are few empirically tested treatments for suicidal adolescents. In this chapter, the relationship between adolescent depression and suicidal behaviour is reviewed, as well as the risk factors for suicidal behaviour in depressed adolescents. The impact of psychosocial and pharmacotherapeutic interventions on depression and on suicidal outcomes is reviewed, including recent reports that SSRIs may be associated with an increase in spontaneously reported suicidal adverse events. We then review the few empirically tested psychosocial interventions for the treatment of suicide-attempting adolescents, including treatments that target family interactions, cognitions, social and emotion regulation skills, and the social ecology (either social network or school) of the suicidal adolescent. Studies have also examined the impact of different aspects of clinical management, such as the development of a safety plan, providing open access to an inpatient unit, and augmenting usual care with occasional postcards from clinical staff. The possible impact of lithium, divalproex, neuroleptics, and SSRIs in the reduction of impulsive aggression and suicidal risk is also discussed. Recommendations for further research are advanced.

## Introduction

This chapter reviews proven and promising treatments for suicidal youth, beginning with the management of depression, the single most common psychiatric disorder accompanying suicidal behaviour in children and adolescents. Subsequently, the interventions that are known to target suicidal behaviour are reviewed. On the basis of this review, recommendations about best practice for the treatment of suicidal youth and for further research are delineated.

## Depression

### Depression and suicide

Depression is the single most important psychiatric risk factor for child and adolescent suicidality. Over 80 per cent of adolescent suicide attempters, and 60 per cent of adolescent suicide completers have at least one major mood disorder (Brent *et al.* 1993;

Kerfoot *et al.* 1996; Lewinsohn *et al.* 1996; Shaffer *et al.* 1996; Gould *et al.* 1998; Bridge *et al.* 2006). Since depression conveys a 10–50-fold increased risk for suicidal behaviour, it follows that improved identification and treatment of depression should be an important element in the reduction of suicidal risk. The risk for suicidal behaviour in depressed children and adolescents is particularly elevated in those whose depression is characterized by early onset, greater severity, and chronicity. Comorbid conditions, particularly substance abuse, conduct disorder, impulsive aggressive personality traits, as well a history of abuse, parent–child discord and criminality and a family history of suicidal behaviour, also contribute to an increased risk for suicidal behaviour (Lewinsohn *et al.* 1996; Brent 1997; Fergusson and Woodward 2002; Brent and Mann 2005). Because suicidality in depression is the product of the interaction between depression and personal family and social contextual factors, prevention of suicidal behaviour in depressed, suicidal individuals may require both treatment of depression as well as interventions that target these associated contextual factors.

### Treatments for depression

Both antidepressants and specific types of psychotherapy (cognitive behaviour therapy and interpersonal therapy) have been shown to be efficacious in the treatment of adolescent depression (Lewinsohn *et al.* 1990; Wood *et al.* 1996; Brent *et al.* 1997; Clarke *et al.* 1999; Mufson *et al.* 1999; March *et al.* 2004; Mufson *et al.* 2004). In Chapter 92 individual psychotherapy techniques are described. Less is known about the direct impact of these treatments for depression on suicidal ideation and behaviour, because suicidal subjects are frequently excluded from clinical trials, and suicidality is often not assessed or reported as an outcome.

### Does treatment of depression reduce the risk for suicidality?

In one study, cognitive behaviour therapy (CBT) was found to be superior to both family and supportive therapies for the treatment of adolescent depression, yet all three treatments produced comparable reductions in suicidality (Brent *et al.* 1997) in patients with current or lifetime suicidality (attempt or ideation with a plan). CBT was markedly superior to supportive therapy for the treatment of depression (Barbe *et al.* 2004). Interpersonal therapy (IPT) was found to be superior to clinical management for adolescent depression, but there was no differential impact on suicidal ideation or attempts (Mufson *et al.* 1999). In the multi-site Treatment of Adolescent Depression Study (TADS) in which fluoxetine, cognitive behaviour therapy (CBT), and the combination were compared to each other and to placebo, both fluoxetine and the combination of medication and CBT produced substantial improvements in depression relative to placebo (and to CBT alone), but only the combination treatment produced a more robust reduction in suicidal ideation compared to placebo (March *et al.* 2004). In the TADS trial, fluoxetine was associated with more suicidal events than placebo, and over the 9-month continuation and follow-up, participants who stayed in their original treatment showed a lower rate of suicidal events in the combined treatment versus fluoxetine alone (Emslie *et al.* 2006; The TADS Team 2007). However, two other large clinical trials with participants with greater severity of depression, longer duration, or higher levels of intake suicidal ideation did not find a protective effect for the combination of CBT plus medication against the occurrence of suicidal events (Goodyer *et al.* 2007; Brent *et al.* 2008).

One quality improvement study based in primary care compared the provision of specialty mental health care on-site (CBT, medication or both) versus usual care for adolescent depression (Asarnow *et al.* 2005). The quality improvement condition showed a greater reduction in depression, as well as a near-significant trend towards a reduction in the incidence of clinically significant suicidality.

### Predictors of poor response to treatment of depression

Many of the predictors of poor response to either SSRIs or cognitive therapy are also associated with suicidal behaviour: chronicity, severity, comorbidity, high hopelessness, family discord, history of abuse, and parental depression (Clarke *et al.* 1992; Brent *et al.* 1998, Emslie *et al.* 1998, Lewinsohn *et al.* 1996, 1998; Rohde *et al.* 2001; Barbe *et al.* 2004). The TADS trial confirmed several of these observations, but found one result that was in the opposite direction of several of these studies: greater cognitive distortion was associated with a larger effect size for the combined treatment, and also CBT worked best in participants that came from homes with higher incomes (Curry *et al.* 2006). Interventions that address these co-occurring difficulties may improve treatment outcomes for depression and may also provide relief of suicidality. Pharmacogenetic studies hold promise for personalizing treatment. The more functional allele of the serotonin transporter promoter gene (long allele) has been shown to predict better response of depressed children and adolescents to citalopram (Kronenberg *et al.* 2007).

### SSRIs and suicidality

A meta-analysis including over 4300 child and adolescent subjects treated with antidepressants found that new-onset or worsening suicidality occurred about 1.8 times more often in the drug condition than in placebo, with an average of 4 per cent of those on medication developing suicidality versus 2 per cent on placebo. A later re-analysis of all paediatric clinical trials using second-generation antidepressants that included newer studies and used random- rather than fixed-effects assumptions in estimating risk differences found only a 0.9 per cent risk difference in the rate of

suicidal events between antidepressant and placebo overall, and within the depressed subsample (Bridge *et al.* 2007). In contrast to the FDA report, this meta-analysis compared benefit to risk, and found that over 11 times more individuals were likely to benefit from an antidepressant for the treatment of depression than were likely to experience a suicidal event, which many would consider a favourable risk-to-benefit ratio. The risk to benefit ratio was also more favourable for adolescents versus children, except for trials of fluoxetine, in which the effects were similar. Effect size was inversely proportional, and the placebo response rate was positively correlated with the number of sites, suggesting that studies with a large number of sites may not screen out potential placebo responders and therefore may be underestimating the true effect of antidepressants on paediatric depression (Bridge *et al.* 2007). This is important because it means that the ratio of those who benefit from the drug versus those who become suicidal may underestimate the benefit to those with at least moderately severe depression.

The mechanism by which antidepressants may increase the risk for suicidal behaviour is not known, but possible explanations include increased irritability and hostility, akathisia, disinhibition, withdrawal symptoms induced by non-compliance, or development of a mixed state in those with a bipolar diathesis. The latter condition is much more likely to be induced by SSRI treatment in younger versus older patients (Martin *et al.* 2004). Data from both psychotherapy and pharmacotherapy trials show that self-reported ideation at intake is the single best predictor of a suicidal event in the clinical trial (Apter *et al.* 2006; March *et al.* 2006).

As a result of the concern raised about antidepressants and suicidality, the FDA is now requiring that clinical trials use a standard classification of suicidal events, the Columbia Classification Algorithm of Suicide Assessment (C-CASA), which has demonstrated reliability and validity (Posner *et al.* 2007). Consequently, using this system, the US Food and Drug Administration (2003) found an increase in risk for suicidal events in patients taking antiepileptic drugs versus placebo (0.43 per cent versus 0.22 per cent; http://www.fda.gov/CDER/drug/infopage/antiepileptics/default.htm). There is also a strong push for rapid publication and access to data from industry-funded studies, which traditionally have shown a strong publication bias towards publication of positive results.

The detection of a small but palpable signal for suicidality associated with SSRI treatment must be placed in a larger public health perspective. The adolescent suicide rate in the United States and in many developing countries has been declining for over a decade, a period that coincides with the introduction of SSRIs (Brent 2004). Although pharmacoepidemiology studies are correlative and evaluate group rather than individual effects, they do show a relationship between an increase in SSRI prescriptions and sales and a decline in the overall and adolescent suicide rate (Olfson *et al.* 2003; Gibbons *et al.* 2005; Ludwig and Marcotte 2005). Subsequent to the FDA warning about antidepressants, there has been a decline in the number of prescriptions of SSRIs for youth without any concomitant increase in referrals for psychotherapy, and a decline in the rate of diagnosis of adolescent depression in the United States (Libby *et al.* 2007). This decline in SSRI prescriptions has also been noted in the Netherlands and in the United Kingdom. In the United States and the Netherlands, the decline in the use of antidepressants was associated with an increase in the adolescent suicide rate in the year following the FDA announcement

(Gibbons *et al.* 2007). In contrast, the suicide rate in adolescent males and females continued to decline, and the rate of admissions for suicide attempts continued to increase, even after a dramatic decrease in the rate of SSRI prescriptions (Wheeler *et al.* 2008). Nevertheless, even a finding of *no* relationship between SSRI prescriptions and either suicide or suicide attempt rates supports the view that SSRIs do not significantly increase the risk for suicidal behaviour.

## Psychosocial interventions to target risk and protective factors for suicidal behaviour

### Psychoeducation and cognitive behavioural family therapy

Rotheram-Borus *et al.* (1996) compared a six-session family CBT plus a one-session family psychoeducation session delivered in the emergency room to family CBT alone for a largely Dominican, female adolescent sample of 140 suicide attempters (Rotheram-Borus *et al.* 1996). The psychoeducation intervention increased compliance with the intervention, so that the study compares family CBT plus psychoeducation to a lower dose of family CBT (5.7 versus 4.7 sessions attended). The educational intervention trained emergency room staff to be more supportive and less negative towards adolescent suicide attempters and their families and provided a videotape for families to explain emergency room procedures and the rationale for continued treatment. Also, the family received one emergency family therapy session to develop a coping plan for potential suicide-inducing situations and provided liaison to the outpatient staff to insure continuity of care. The family cognitive behavioural therapy was a six-session programme that focused on developing positive family problem-solving, communication, and mutual reinforcement.

At the end of treatment, the enhanced CBT group showed lower adolescent suicidal ideation and lower maternal depressive and general symptomatology, greater maternally reported family cohesion, and more positive attitudes towards treatment (Rotheram-Borus *et al.* 1996). At 18-month follow-up, the rates of attempts and of significant suicidal ideation were not different between the two groups although there was a non-significant trend for a lower re-attempt rate in the experimental group (8.7 versus 14.6 per cent) (Rotheram-Borus *et al.* 2000). The enhanced intervention had the greatest impact on maternal emotional distress and family cohesion in families of more symptomatic adolescent attempters. Due to the design, one cannot tell to what extent these findings are attributable to the emergency room intervention itself or its impact on adherence.

### Home-based family therapy

Harrington and colleagues compared a 5-session home-based family intervention plus routine care to routine care alone for 162 adolescent who made suicide attempts by overdose in a randomized clinical trial (Harrington *et al.* 1998). The experimental intervention targeted family conflict, parental distress, adolescent suicidality, and hopelessness.

While satisfaction and compliance were higher in the home-based family treatment, the experimental intervention was no better than routine care overall for reducing ideation or re-attempt.

However, among the non-depressed subgroup, the home-based treatment reduced suicidal ideation more so than did treatment as usual. The family intervention did not produce any significant changes in family climate relative to routine care, contrary to the intent of the treatment. However, there were fewer out-of-home placements in the family treatment (Byford *et al.* 1999).

### Developmental group therapy

A study compared a group therapy, termed developmental group therapy, plus usual care to usual care alone for sixty-three adolescents who had engaged in at least two episodes of deliberate self-harm within the past year. The experimental treatment focused on family conflict, problem-solving, interpersonal relationships, anger management, school problems, depression and hopelessness.

On average, participants had engaged in four prior episodes of self-harm, around half had experienced definite or probable sexual or physical abuse, and most came from socio-economically disadvantaged backgrounds. The experimental treatment consisted of a median of 8 group sessions, and a median of 2.5 individual sessions by the same therapists. Routine care was used much less often by those who were assigned to the group treatment compared to those who had routine care alone (median number of sessions 1 versus 4) and antidepressants were prescribed for a minority of participants in both treatments.

The experimental treatment, compared to routine care showed a reduction in episodes of self-harm (RR = 0.6) and a much lower rate of having two or more episodes (RR = 0.16). The time to first repetition was also longer in the experimental arm (11.9 versus 7 weeks). School attendance was improved in those subjects assigned to the experimental treatment, and the rate of behavioural disorder was lower as well (RR = 0.3). There was no differential treatment effect on depression, suicidal ideation, or global outcome.

### Skills-based therapy

A study compared a skills-based therapy (SBT) that consisted of training in problem-solving and emotion regulation versus supportive relationship therapy (SRT) for thirty-nine adolescent suicide attempters randomly in a randomized clinical trial. Treatment in both groups consisted of 6 individual sessions, and one adjunct session for over the first 3 months, followed by 3-monthly maintenance sessions. At the therapist's discretion, up to two additional family and two additional individual sessions were also available. About half of subjects had a history of two or more attempts, more than two disorders, and comorbid marijuana abuse. The randomization was balanced, except that a higher proportion of those assigned to supportive treatment had a disruptive behaviour disorder.

Both groups showed similar improvements in depression and ideation, with a trend towards better problem-solving in the SBT group. Subjects showed a non-significant trend for a higher rate of re-attempts in SBT group versus SRT at 3 months (4/15 versus 1/16) and 6 months (4/15 and 2/16). The majority of subjects in both treatments were in the non-clinical range on the Suicide Ideation Questionnaire by the end of treatment and upon 3- and 6-month follow-up. The dropout rate was higher in the experimental treatment (6/19 versus 2/19). Although the sample is too small for any definitive conclusions, this study suggests that SRT might be at least as efficacious as the experimental treatment.

## Multisystemic therapy

Multisystemic therapy (MST), a flexible, family-based treatment that involves case-management and admixtures of individual and family treatment was compared to psychiatric hospitalization and usual care in 156 youths presenting to the emergency room with suicidal ideation, suicide attempt, homicidal ideation, psychosis, or other threat of harm to self or others (Huey *et al.* 2004). MST empowers families to communicate with, monitor, and discipline their children effectively, help promote prosocial activities for children and helps children disengage from antisocial peers. In the context of suicidality, MST focuses on helping parents to identify, contain, monitor, and diminish suicidal risk. Intervention typically lasts 3 to 6 months, but is intensive, with up to daily contact, delivered in the patient and family's natural ecology—often the home and the school. A large proportion of the MST group also were hospitalized (44 per cent) and this was not accounted for in the analyses, making the results difficult to interpret. At intake, according the suicide attempt item from the Youth Risk Behaviour Survey, 31 per cent of those assigned to MST had attempted suicide versus only 19 per cent of those who were hospitalized. At post-treatment and 1-year follow-up, the rates of re-attempt in MST were 14 per cent and 4 per cent versus 9 per cent and 4 per cent, respectively, which was reported as significantly different in the paper, although no treatment-by-time interactions were reported. There were no treatment effects for suicidal ideation, depression, internalizing symptoms, or hopelessness. Parental-rated control increased in MST relative to the hospitalization group at the end of treatment, but these effects did not persist upon 1-year follow-up.

## Youth-nominated support teams (YST-1)

A study evaluated the efficacy of augmenting the connection between suicidal adolescents and individuals in their social network whom the suicidal adolescent identified as being significant and supportive. This intervention, termed Youth-Nominated Support Team (YST-1) provides psychoeducation to individuals nominated by suicidal adolescents, and facilitates weekly contact between those nominated individuals and the suicidal adolescents. Therapists encourage support people to facilitate activities with the suicidal individual in the service of overall treatment goals. A group of 289 psychiatrically hospitalized adolescents who were admitted for significant suicidal ideation or an attempt were randomized to YST-1 plus usual care or usual care alone. Subjects in both conditions as part of routine care received psychotherapy and nearly all received some psychotropic medication. Attrition was greater in the experimental intervention (24.2 versus 12.9 per cent) because of unwillingness or inability for some adolescents to involve at least two supportive individuals. This also resulted in a low (35 per cent) acceptance rate into randomization. Adolescents in the YST-1 condition most commonly nominated parents, non-parental relatives, non-adult relatives, peers, or teachers.

Suicidal ideation declined in both groups, but among girls, the YST-1 group showed a greater decline in suicidal ideation in completer analyses, although no differences were found in the proportion who had suicidal ideation at a level below clinical cut-offs. No difference was found for the 6-month rate of suicide attempts. In both intent-to-treat and in completer analyses, girls experienced greater improvement in mood-related functioning in the YST-1 condition. The effect sizes for ideation and mood-related function reported in girls were in the small-to-moderate range.

## School-based prevention

To enhance protective factors against suicide, a school-based intervention, consisting of a one-semester 'Personal Growth Class' to enhance attendance, self-esteem, sense of personal control, and association with a prosocial peer group was implemented in two of four high schools (Eggert *et al.* 1994). The intervention groups showed greater improvement in drug-related problems, self-esteem, grade-point average, and involvement with prosocial peers. A subsequent study compared this intervention plus a screen for suicidality conducted by an interviewer to a more intensive version of this class (two semesters) and to screening alone (Eggert *et al.* 1995). In all three intervention groups, suicidal youth were assigned to a case manager at the school. Surprisingly, the brief assessment intervention was as efficacious as the more extended intervention in reduction of suicidal ideation and associated risk factors, with one exception—the Personal Growth Class resulted in greater improvements in self-rated personal control. The results of this study suggest that a brief screening and contact with a case manager may be an effective and sufficient intervention in schools to reduce suicidal risk, although this awaits replication in comparison to a control intervention.

Another proposed prevention approach is on-site screening of youth for depression and suicidality, using the Columbia Suicide Screen (Shaffer *et al.* 2004). This self-report questionnaire showed a sensitivity 0.75 and specificity of 0.83 against a structured interview, with a positive predictive value of 16 per cent. The TeenScreen appears to identify at-risk youth who are not already recognized by school professionals: of adolescents identified as thinking of suicide, having attempted suicide, or being depressed, 74 per cent, 50 per cent, and 69 per cent of these youth were previously unrecognized by school personnel (Shaffer and Craft 1999). There has been no published evaluation of the TeenScreen on referral or outcome. However, there do not appear to be iatrogenic effects of screening youth for suicidal ideation (Gould *et al.* 2005). See also Chapter 68 in this book.

The Signs of Suicide (SOS) programme combines self-screening and an educational intervention (video and discussion) designed to improve high school students' efficacy in recognizing suicidal behaviour and depression and in seeking help. In five high schools, a total of 2100 students were randomly assigned to the intervention or a control condition; all students were surveyed 3 months after the intervention with regard to attitudes and knowledge about depression and suicide, help-seeking, and rate of self-reported suicide attempts. In the intervention condition, students were screened using the Columbia Depression Scale, a brief scale derived from the Diagnostic Interview Schedule for Children (Aseltine and DeMartino 2004). If they scored 16 or higher, they were instructed to seek help immediately. Upon 3-month follow-up, students were provided with a list of sources for clinical care. Students in the intervention group were 40 per cent less likely to have made a suicide attempt (3.6 versus 5.4 per cent). showed greater knowledge about depression and suicide, and more adaptive attitudes towards these problems, but without significant changes in help-seeking behaviour. The program effects on suicide attempts may have been mediated through improvements in student knowledge and attitudes.

## Development of a plan for coping with suicidal urges

A one-session combination assessment and intervention using contracting and teaching simple emotion regulation techniques for youth staying in runaway shelters judged to be a high suicidal risk was evaluated using a quasi-experimental design (Rotheram-Borus and Bradley 1991). In youth judged to be at high suicidal risk by a standard assessment, youth were asked to engage in five behavioural tasks:

1  Share three positive compliments about themself;

2  Identify three people from whom to seek support;

3  Identify various emotional states using a scalar measure known as a 'Feeling Thermometer,' and identifying situations that would elicit suicidal behaviour (see a description of the procedure in Chapter 92);

4  Develop a concrete plan for coping with these suicide-eliciting situations; and

5  Agree to a written no-suicide contract for a brief (usually less than or equal to two weeks) period.

In a pre-post evaluation, the number of attempts in shelters in the three months prior to implementation was 9, as compared to two attempts in the 18 months after the programme was implemented.

## Dialectic behaviour therapy

Dialectic behaviour therapy (DBT), a treatment that focuses on the development of emotional regulation, distress tolerance, and interpersonal social skills, has been shown in personality disordered adults to reduce recurrent suicidal and self-harm behaviour (Linehan et al. 1991, 1993, van den Bosch et al. 2002; Bohus et al. 2004). DBT has been modified for use for suicidal adolescents, by shortening the treatment from 1 year to 12 weeks, reducing the total number of skills taught, incorporating family members into treatment, and offering an optional 12-week patient consultation group (Miller et al. 1997). Their modification of DBT emphasizes the following skills: mindfulness, emotion regulation, distress tolerance, and interpersonal effectiveness (Miller et al. 2007). Identity problems, impulsivity, emotional instability, and interpersonal problems were targeted by cultivating mindfulness, distress tolerance, emotion regulation, and interpersonal effectiveness. An open pilot study of 27 14–19-year-old suicidal adolescents showed improvements in all target areas and a trend towards a lower rate of suicidal behaviour on follow-up (Miller et al. 2000).

Rathus and Miller (2002) then conducted a quasi-experimental study in which 111 suicidal adolescents with borderline personality disorder features received either DBT (N = 29) or treatment as usual (TAU) (N = 82). the latter of which consisted of twice-weekly supportive-psychodynamic therapy plus weekly family therapy (Rathus and Miller 2002). At intake, the DBT group had more previous attempts, was more depressed, and had had more previous hospitalizations. Although not statistically significant, fewer subjects made suicide attempts in the DBT condition (3.4 versus 8.6 per cent). fewer subjects were hospitalized, and the completion rates for treatment were higher in the DBT group. Within-treatment examination of the impact of DBT showed significant reductions in suicidal ideation, general symptomalogy,

and borderline symptoms. However, changes in symptomatology were not compared to the TAU group. This study supports further work in the application of DBT to the treatment of suicidal adolescents.

In a subsequent study, sixty-two adolescents with suicidal ideation or attempt were admitted to one of two psychiatric units, one of which offered inpatient DBT (Katz et al. 2004). Although subjects were not randomly assigned, admission was based on bed availability rather than any clinical indicators. Subjects were evaluated at intake, discharge, and 1 year later. The DBT condition involved ten daily DBT skills training sessions, and twice-weekly individual treatment, delivered over two weeks. Routine care consisted of a daily psychodynamic therapy group, individual psychodynamic therapy at least once a week, and a psychodynamic milieu. Both groups received pharmacotherapy and were discharged to community mental health clinics.

Both groups showed similar substantial reduction in self-reported depression, suicidal ideation, and hopelessness. There were also no differences in re-attempts, re-hospitalization or adherence to outpatient treatment. Fewer incident reports were generated on the DBT unit. This study, as the authors note, is limited by lack of randomization, blind ratings, formal fidelity checks for DBT, and relatively small sample size. While the findings do show that DBT can be delivered on an inpatient unit, results in high retention and satisfaction, and produces a reduction in targeted symptoms, this pilot study does *not* provide support to the hypothesis that DBT is superior to standard inpatient care.

## Cognitive behaviour therapy

Brown and colleagues (2005) have developed a cognitive behaviour model for adult suicide attempters that focuses almost entirely on cognitions that are associated with suicidal behaviour, which in turn is derived from a careful chain analysis of the attempt (Brown et al. 2005). Important components of the treatment include active case-management, development and monitoring of a safety plan, development of a hope kit and other coping strategies for suicidal crises. Treatment targets included improved problem-solving with increased adaptive use of social support, and improved compliance with medical, psychiatric, and substance abuse treatment. A group of 120 adult suicide attempts with high rates of depression and substance abuse were randomized to either CBT plus routine care or case management plus routine care. CBT-treated subjects were half as likely to re-attempt as those in the enhanced usual care group over the 18 month follow-up (24.1 versus 41.6 per cent) and showed great improvements on self-reported depression and hopelessness on follow-up. This approach has been adapted for adolescent suicide attempters and is now being pilot tested in five sites in a project funded by the National Institutes of Mental Health.

## Post-hospital written contact

For a description of different techniques used in different individual therapies, see Chapter 92. One of the standard interventions for individuals judged to be at high risk for suicide is psychiatric hospitalization. The risk of suicide and re-attempt is extremely high after discharge from the hospital (Kjelsberg et al. 1994). One study has found that written contact after discharge from the hospital was associated with a lower risk for suicide in adults at high suicide risk who were non-compliant with outpatient treatment (Motto and Bostrom 2001). A replication of this intervention, 'Postcards from the Edge,' was conducted on adolescent and young adult self-poisoners who were medically hospitalized (Carter *et al.* 2005). A total of 772 aged 16 and older subjects were randomized to receiving 8 postcards over 12 months plus treatment as usual versus treatment as usual alone. There were 192 episodes of self-poisoning in the control condition versus 101 events in the experimental intervention group (RR = 0.55). Patients randomized to the experimental arm used 110 fewer hospital bed-days. However, the proportion of those who re-attempted was not different between groups. This intervention appears to be an inexpensive method for reducing repetition of hospital-treated suicide attempts. However, the proportion of subjects who reattempted was not different between the experiment and control groups (15.1 versus 17.3 per cent).

## Open access to hospital

Cotgrove and colleagues conducted a randomized trial of post-hospital care of adolescent suicide attempters (Cotgrove *et al.* 1995). Subjects (N = 105) were randomized to either immediate, unquestioned readmission to hospital plus usual care, or usual care alone, and followed up one year later. Of those with open access, 6 per cent reattempted suicide versus 12 per cent of those in usual care, which, while lower, was not statistically significant. A post-hoc analysis seemed to indicate that open access was protective only for those at low or moderate risk for suicide re-attempt. Of those given open access, 11 per cent requested hospitalization.

# Pharmacological interventions

There have been no pharmacological trials that target adolescent suicidal behaviour, and very few in adults. We review studies in those agents that show efficacy in targeting impulsive aggression and/or suicidal behaviour.

## Lithium

Lithium has not been evaluated for suicidal behaviour in a double-blind controlled trial in either children or adults, although one is now ongoing in adults (Lauterbach *et al.* 2005). Naturalistic studies comparing those treated with lithium compared to those on either no treatment or alternative mood stabilizers (carbamazepine, divalproex) find a protective effect against suicide (Rifkin *et al.* 1997; Baldessarini and Tondo 2003; Goodwin *et al.* 2003). In a population-based sample of 20,638 members of a health plan aged 14 and older with a diagnosis of bipolar disorder and at least one filled prescription of lithium, divalproex, or carbamazepine, the rates of suicide attempts and completions were compared. After adjustment for age, sex, comorbid medical and psychiatric conditions, the risk of death by suicide was increased 2.7-fold, and the risk for attempted suicide resulting in hospitalization was increased 1.7-fold (Goodwin *et al.* 2003). In a similar type of study, 12,662 Medicaid patients with bipolar disorder were compared with respect to risk for suicide and attempted suicide as a function of their prescribed medication (Collins and McFarland 2008). The risks for attempted suicide were 2.7 times higher in those using divalproex, and 1.6 times higher for those using gabapentin than in those using lithium. Similarly, the risk compared to those on lithium for completed suicide was 1.5 times higher in those

on divalproex (not significant) and 2.6 times higher in those on gabapentin.

A similar analysis found that lithium was protective against suicide for patients with recurrent unipolar depression (Guzzetta *et al.* 2007). In 329 depressed patients, the risk for suicide and suicide attempts was compared while on (1149 person-years) and off (1285 person-years) lithium. The risk for completed and attempted suicide were 8.7 and 6.8 times higher, respectively, in patients during periods of non-exposure to lithium.

While the results of these studies are of interest, because patients are not randomly assigned to their medications, the results are difficult to interpret. However, a meta-analysis of clinical trials with lithium in mood disorder patients provides a compelling case for reduction of suicide risk associated with the use of lithium. In 32 trials, 1389 patients were randomized to lithium and 2069 were assigned to other compounds or placebo. Those who received other compounds were four times more likely to die by suicide than those who received lithium, and five times more likely to either die by suicide or make a suicide attempt (Cipriani *et al.* 2005).

Lithium has been used to target aggression in children and adolescents without mood disorder (Campbell *et al.* 1984; Malone *et al.* 2000). Most, but not all, find a positive effect in the reduction of aggression. These results support further exploration of the role of lithium in the management of suicidal behaviour.

## Divalproex

Two studies have found efficacy for divalproex in the management of impulsive aggression, mood lability, and behavioural symptoms in child, adolescent, and adult samples (Donovan *et al.* 2000; Hollander *et al.* 2003; Steiner *et al.* 2003). Divalproex has not been experimentally evaluated for management of suicidal behaviour. However, in naturalistic studies, lithium appeared to be superior to divalproex in preventing suicidal behaviour in bipolar adults (Goodwin *et al.* 2003; Collins and McFarland 2008).

## Neuroleptics

Three experimental studies in adults support the use of neuroleptics in the treatment of suicidal outcome in adults. One large study of schizophrenics who were judged at high suicidal risk because of suicide attempt or current suicide ideation, clozapine was found to be superior to olanzapine in reducing suicidal behaviour over a 24-month period (Meltzer *et al.* 2003). Consistent with these results, an open trial of clozapine in adolescent schizophrenic patients showed a reduction in aggressive behaviour (Kranzler *et al.* 2005). In a national sample of adult schizophrenic patients who had been hospitalized for a suicide attempt, both antipsychotic use and combined antipsychotic and antidepressant use was associated with a lower mortality due to suicide (Haukka *et al.* 2008). The combination of olanzapine/fluoxetine (OFC) was compared to lamotregine (LMG) for the treatment of bipolar depression in a 7-week trial (Brown *et al.* 2006). Patients assigned to OFC showed greater global improvement, reduction in depression, and a lower incidence of suicidal and self-injurious behaviour (0.5 versus 3.4 per cent, p <0.04). Another, unpublished study found an injectable neuroleptic to be superior to placebo in preventing recurrent suicidal behaviour in adults with a history of repeated attempts (Montgomery *et al.* 1979). While the use of neuroleptics for the management of youthful suicidal behaviour has not been evaluated, atypical neuroleptics have been shown to be efficacious in managing aggressive behaviour (Findling *et al.* 2000; Schur *et al.* 2003). The most significant drawback of this approach is the problem of significant weight gain found even in the short-term use of these medications.

## SSRIs

Fluoxetine has been shown to diminish both impulsive aggression in personality disordered patients, and the intensity and frequency of 'anger attacks' in patients with depression (Fava *et al.* 1993, 1996; Coccaro and Kavoussi 1997). However, SSRIs do not appear to prevent recurrent suicidal behaviour in adults without mood disorder (Montgomery *et al.* 1994; Verkes *et al.* 1998). No studies have evaluated the impact of fluoxetine on impulsive aggression in paediatric samples, nor has this domain been assessed as an outcome in paediatric clinical trials involving fluoxetine or other SSRIs.

## Summary

Efficacious treatments have been demonstrated for depression among youth, but it has not been conclusively demonstrated that either antidepressants or psychotherapy reduce suicidal ideation or risk for suicidal behaviour in depressed adolescents compared to control treatments. This may be in part due to exclusion of the most suicidal individuals from clinical trials, lack of careful assessment of suicidal indicators in most trials, and inadequate sample size to detect effects. In one clinical trial, the combination of CBT and medication was the only treatment superior to placebo in reducing suicidal ideation. Epidemiological evidence seems to suggest that there is a relationship between increased use of SSRIs and a decline in the adolescent suicide rate and conversely between a decline in SSRI use and an increase in adolescent suicide. While there is some evidence to support a relatively rare but palpable increase in suicidality with the treatment of SSRIs, many more youth appear to benefit from, than are harmed by, antidepressants.

Subsequent clinical trials in patients with mood disorder and other conditions at high risk for suicide should consider including suicidal subjects, improving the assessment of intake suicidal risk factors (ideation, past attempt, impulsive aggression, hopelessness) and the effect of interventions on these risk factors and on suicidal ideation and behaviour. In a recent clinical trial with treatment-resistant depressed adolescents, almost 60 per cent of participants showed clinically significant suicidal ideation upon entry, supporting the feasibility of the recruitment, management, and protection of suicidal participants in a clinical trial (Brent *et al.* 2008). This would permit a more accurate estimate of the impact of treatment on suicidal risk. Future work should also focus on the identification of predictors of treatment response and adverse events in those treated with SSRIs.

Treatment studies of adolescent suicide attempters are few, often with small samples and modest effects. The most promising results to date have been those of which found a reduction in recurrent deliberate self-harm in a pilot study of a brief intervention. On the basis of the results in adult studies, treatment trials to evaluate the efficacy of DBT and CBT for the treatment of suicidal adolescents should be developed. The role of simple after care interventions like 'Postcards from the Edge' should also be pursued (Carter *et al.* 2005).

There are several pharmacological agents with promise to reduce suicidal risk and precursors therefore, such as impulsive aggression, namely, lithium, divalproex, and atypical neuroleptics. Because each of these medications has several side-effects that make them less than desirable for adolescents (e.g., weight gain), studies should first be conducted on those for whom other reasonable psychosocial interventions have failed and where the patient has engaged in recurrent suicidal behaviour.

While there is a great deal known about the risk factors for suicidal behaviour, and the precursors thereof, there has been relatively little attempt to prevent the development of suicidal behaviour in at-risk youth. Given the association of core protective factors and low risk for suicidal behaviour, the role of interventions to strengthen protective factors to prevent onset of suicidality and other health risk behaviours should be assessed in the context of both universal and indicated prevention (Resnick *et al.* 1997; Borowsky *et al.* 2001).

## Conclusion

Despite suicide being the leading and most severe complication of psychiatric disorder, there are a paucity of studies that target individuals at high suicidal risk. Investigators have avoided these populations because of the difficulty in engaging such subjects in treatment and because of concerns of a suicide occurring in a clinical trial. On the other hand, systematic exclusion of high-risk subjects from clinical investigation truncated our knowledge about how to best treat these patients. Therefore, ethical guidelines and safeguards should be developed that allow for these studies that include suicidal individuals; in order to improve treatment for these vulnerable people.

## References

Apter A, Lipschitz A, Fong R *et al.* (2006). Evaluation of suicidal thoughts and behaviours in children and adolescents taking paroxetine. *Journal of Child and Adolescent Psychopharmacology*, **16**, 77–90.

Asarnow JR, Jaycox LH, Duan N *et al.* (2005). Effectiveness of a quality improvement intervention for adolescent depression in primary care clinics a randomized controlled trial. *Journal of the American Medical Association*, **293**, 311–319.

Aseltine RH and DeMartino R (2004). An outcome evaluation of the SOS suicide prevention program. *American Journal of Public Health*, **94**, 446–451.

Baldessarini RJ and Tondo L (2003). Suicide risk and treatments for patients with bipolar disorder. *Journal of the American Medical Association*, **290**, 1517–1518.

Barbe RP, Bridge J, Birmaher B *et al.* (2004). Suicidality and its relationship to treatment outcome in depressed adolescents. *Suicide and Life-Threatening Behaviour*, **34**, 44–55.

Bohus M, Haaf B, Simms T *et al.* (2004). Effectiveness of inpatient dialectical behavioural therapy for borderline personality disorder: A controlled trial. *Behaviour Research and Therapy*, **42**, 487–499.

Borowsky IW, Ireland M, Resnick MD (2001). Adolescent suicide attempts: risks and protectors. *Pediatrics*, **107**, 485–493.

Brent DA (1997). Practitioner review: the aftercare of adolescents with deliberate self-harm. *Journal of Child Psychology and Psychiatry* **38**, 277–286.

Brent DA (2004). Antidepressants and pediatric depression: the risk of doing nothing. *New England Journal of Medicine*, **351**, 1598–1601.

Brent DA and Mann JJ (2005). Family genetic studies of suicide and suicidal behaviour. *American Journal of Medical Genetics*, **133C**, 13–24.

Brent DA, Perper JA, Moritz G *et al.* (1993). Psychiatric risk factors of adolescent suicide: a case control study. *Journal of the American Academy of Child and Adolescent Psychiatry*, **32**, 521–529.

Brent DA, Holder D, Kolko D *et al.* (1997). A clinical psychotherapy trial for adolescent depression comparing cognitive, family, and supportive treatments. *Archives of General Psychiatry*, **54**, 877–885.

Brent DA, Kolko D, Birmaher B *et al.* (1998). Predictors of treatment efficacy in a clinical trial of three psychosocial treatments for adolescent depression. *Journal of the American Academy of Child and Adolescent Psychiatry*, **37**, 906–914.

Brent DA, Emslie GJ, Clarke GN *et al.* (2008). Switching to venlafaxine or another SSRI with or without cognitive behavioural therapy for adolescents with SSRI-resistant depression: the TORDIA randomized control trial. *JAMA*, **299**, 901–913.

Bridge J, Barbe RP, Birmaher B *et al.* (2006). Emergent suicidality in a clinical psychotherapy trial for adolescent depression. *American Journal of Psychiatry*, **162**, 2173–2175.

Bridge J, Iyengar S, Salary CB *et al.* (2007). Clinical response and risk for reported suicidal ideation and suicide attempts in pediatric antidepressant treatment: a meta-analysis of randomized controlled trials. *JAMA*, **297**, 1683–1696.

Bridge JA, Salary CR, Birmaher B *et al.* (2005). The risks and benefits of antidepressant treatment for youth depression. *Annals of Medicine*, **37**, 404–412.

Bridge JA, Goldstein TR, Brent DA (2006). Adolescent suicide and suicidal behaviour. *Journal of Child Psychology and Psychiatry* **47**, 372–394.

Brown EB, McElroy SL, Keck Jr PE *et al.* (2006). A 7-week, randomized, double-blind trial of olanzapine/fluoxetine combination verus lamotrigine in the treatment of bipolar 1 depression. *Journal of Clinical Psychiatry*, **67**, 1025–1033.

Brown GK, Have TT, Henriques GR *et al.* (2005). Cognitive therapy for the prevention of suicide attempts. *Journal of the American Medical Association*, **294**, 563–570.

Byford S, Harrington R, Torgerson D *et al.* (1999). Cost-effectiveness analysis of a home-based social work intervention for children and adolescents who have deliberately poisoned themselves. *British Journal of Psychiatry*, **174**, 56–62.

Campbell M, Small AM, Green WH *et al.* (1984). Behavioural efficacy of haloperidol and lithium carbonate: a comparison in hospitalized aggressive children with conduct disorder. *Archives of General Psychiatry*, **41**, 650–656.

Carter GL, Clover K, Whyte IM *et al.* (2005). Postcards from the edge project: randomised controlled trial of an intervention using postcards to reduce repetition of hospital-treated deliberate self-poisoning. *BMJ*, doi:10.1136/bmj.38579.455266.E0.

Cipriani A, Pretty H, Hawton K *et al.* (2005). Lithium in the prevention of suicidal behaviour and all-cause mortality in patients with mood disorders: a systematic review of randomized trials. *American Journal of Psychiatry*, **162**, 1805–1819.

Clarke G, Hops H, Lewinsohn PM *et al.* (1992). Cognitive-behavioural group treatment of adolescent depression: prediction of outcome. *Behavioural Therapy*, **23**, 341–354.

Clarke GN, Lewinsohn PM, Rohde P *et al.* (1999). Cognitive-behavioural group treatment of adolescent depression: efficacy of acute group treatment and booster sessions. *Journal of the American Academy of Child and Adolescent Psychiatry*, **38**, 272–279.

Coccaro EF and Kavoussi RJ (1997). Fluoxetine and impulsive aggressive behaviour in personality-disordered subjects. *Archives of General Psychiatry*, **54**, 1081–1088.

Collins JC and McFarland BH (2008). Divalproex, lithium and suicide among Medicaid patients with bipolar disorder. *Journal of Affective Disorders* **107**, 23–28.

Cotgrove A, Zirinsky L, Black D *et al.* (1995). Secondary prevention of attempted suicide in adolescence. *Journal of Adolescence* **18**, 569–577.

Curry J, Rohde P, Simons S *et al.* (2006). Predictors and moderators of acute outcome in the Treatment for Adolescents with Depression Study (TADS). *Journal of the American Academy of Child and Adolescent Psychiatry*, **45**, 1427–1439.

Donovan SJ, Stewart JW, Nunes EV *et al.* (2000). Divalproex treatment for youth with explosive temper and mood lability: a double-blind, placebo-controlled crossover design. *American Journal of Psychiatry*, **157**, 818–820.

Eggert LL, Thompson EA, Herting JR *et al.* (1995). Reducing suicide potential among high-risk youth: tests of a school-based prevention program. *Suicide and Life-Threatening Behaviour*, **25**, 276–296.

Eggert LL, Thompson EA, Herting JR *et al.* (1994). Preventing adolescent drug abuse and high school dropout through an intensive school-based social network development program. *American Journal of Health Promotion*, **8**, 202–215.

Emslie G, Kratochvil C, Vitiello B *et al.* (2006). Treatment for Adolescents with Depression Study (TADS): safety results. *Journal of the American Academy of Child and Adolescent Psychiatry*, **45**, 1440–1455.

Emslie GJ, Rush AJ, Weinberg WA *et al.* (1998). Fluoxetine in child and adolescent depression: acute and maintenance treatment. *Depression and Anxiety*, **7**, 32–39.

Fava M, Rosenbaum JF, Pava JA *et al.* (1993). Anger attacks in unipolar depression, Part 1: clinical correlates and response to fluoxetine treatment. *American Journal of Psychiatry*, **150**, 1158–1163.

Fava M, Alpert J, Nierenberg AA *et al.* (1996). Fluoxtine treatment of anger attacks: a replication study. *Annals of Clinical Psychiatry*, **8**, 7–10.

Fergusson DM and Woodward LJ (2002). Mental health, educational, and social role outcomes of adolescents with depression. *Archives of General Psychiatry*, **59**, 225–231.

Findling RL, McNamara NK, Branicky LA *et al.* (2000). A double-blind pilot study of risperidone in the treatment of conduct disorder. *Journal of the American Academy of Child and Adolescent Psychiatry*, **4**, 509–516.

Gibbons RD, Brown CH, Hur K *et al.* (2007). Early evidence on the effects of regulators' suicidality warnings on SSRI prescriptions and suicide in children and adolescents. *American Journal of Psychiatry*, **164**, 1356–1363.

Gibbons RD, Hur K, Bhaumik DK *et al.* (2005). The relationship between antidepressant medication use and rate of suicide. *Archives of General Psychiatry*, **62**, 165–172.

Goodwin FK, Fireman B, Simon GE *et al.* (2003). Suicide risk in bipolar disorder during treatment with lithium and divalproex. *JAMA*, **290**, 1467–1473.

Goodyer I, Dubicka B, Wilkinson P *et al.* (2007). Selective serotonin reuptake inhibitors (SSRIs) and routine specialist care with and without cognitive behaviour therapy in adolescents with major depression: randomised controlled trial. *BMJ*, **335**, 106–107.

Gould MS, King R, Greenwald S *et al.* (1998). Psychopathology associated with suicidal ideation and attempts among children and adolescents. *Journal of the American Academy of Child and Adolescent Psychiatry*, **37**, 915–923.

Gould MS, Marrocco FA, Kleinman M *et al.* (2005). Evaluating iatrogenic risk of youth suicide screening programs: a randomized controlled trial. *Journal of the American Medical Association*, **293**, 1635–1643.

Guzzetta F, Tondo L, Centorrino F *et al.* (2007). Lithium treatment reduces suicide risk in recurrent major depressive disorder. *Journal of Clinical Psychiatry*, **68**, 380–383.

Harrington R, Kerfoot M, Dyer E *et al.* (1998). Randomized trial of a home-based family intervention for children who have deliberately poisoned themselves. *Journal of the American Academy of Child and Adolescent Psychiatry*, **37**, 512–518.

Haukka J, Tiihonen J, Harkanen T *et al.* (2008). Association between medication and risk of suicide, attempted suicide and death in nationwide cohort of suicidal patients with schizophrenia. *Pharmacoepidemiology and Drug Safety*, epub ahead of print.

Hollander E, Tracy KA, Swann AC *et al.* (2003). Divalproex in the treatment of impulsive aggression: efficacy in Cluster B personality disorders. *Neuropsychopharmacology*, **28**, 1186–1197.

Huey SJ, Henggeler SW, Rowland MD *et al.* (2004). Multisystemic therapy effects on attempted suicide by youths presenting psychiatric emergencies. *Journal of the American Academy of Child and Adolescent Psychiatry*, **43**, 183–190.

Katz LY, Cox BJ, Gunasekara S *et al.* (2004). Feasibility of dialectical behaviour therapy for suicidal adolescent inpatients. *Journal of the American Academy of Child and Adolescent Psychiatry*, **43**, 276–282.

Kerfoot M, Dyer E, Harrington V *et al.* (1996). Correlates and short-term course of self-poisoning in adolescents. *British Journal of Psychiatry*, **168**, 38–42.

Kjelsberg E, Neegaard E, Dahl AA (1994). Suicide in adolescent psychiatric inpatients: incidence and predictive factors. *Acta Psychiatrica Scandinavica*, **89**, 235–241.

Kranzler H, Roofeh D, Gerbino-Rosen G *et al.* (2005). Clozapine: its impact on aggressive behaviour among children and adolescents with schizophrenia. *Journal of the American Academy of Child and Adolescent Psychiatry*, **44**, 55–63.

Kronenberg S, Apter A, Brent D *et al.* (2007). Serotonin transporter polymorphism (5-HTTLPR) and citalopram effectiveness and side effects in childen with depression and/or anxiety disorders. *Journal of Child and Adolescent Psychopharmacology*, **17**, 741–750.

Lauterbach E, Ahrens B, Felber W *et al.* (2005). Suicide prevention by lithium (SUPLI)—challenges of a multi-center prospective study. *Archives of Suicide Research*, **9**, 27–34.

Lewinsohn PM, Clarke GN, Hops H *et al.* (1990). Cognitive-behavioural treatment for depressed adolescents. *Behaviour Therapy*, **21**, 385–401.

Lewinsohn PM, Rohde P, Seeley JR (1996). Adolescent suicidal ideation and attempts: prevalence, risk factors, and clinical implications. *Clinical Psychology Science and Practice*, **3**, 25–46.

Lewinsohn PM, Rohde P, Seeley JR (1998). Major depressive disorder in older adolescents: prevalence, risk factors, and clinical implications. *Clinical Psychology Review*, **18**, 765–794.

Libby A, Brent DA, Morrato EH *et al.* (2007). Decline in treatment of pediatric depression after FDA advisory on risk of suicidality with SSRIs. *American Journal of Psychiatry*, **164**, 884–891.

Linehan MM, Armstrong HE, Suarez A *et al.* (1991). Cognitive-behavioural treatment of chronically parasuicidal borderline patients. *Archives of General Psychiatry*, **48**, 1060–1064.

Linehan MM, Heard HL, Armstrong HE (1993). Naturalistic follow-up of a behavioural treatment for chronically parasuicidal borderline patients. *Archives of General Psychiatry*, **50**, 971–974.

Ludwig J and Marcotte DE (2005). Anti-depressants, suicide, and drug regulation. *Journal of Policy Analysis and Management*, **24**, 249–272.

Malone R, Delaney MA, Luebbert JF *et al.* (2000). A double-blind placebo-controlled study of lithium in hospitalized aggressive children and adolescents with conduct disorder. *Archives of General Psychiatry*, **57**, 649–654.

March JS, Silva S, Petrycki S *et al.* (2004). Fluoxetine, cognitive-behavioural therapy, and their combination for adolescents with depression. Treatment for Adolescent Depression Study (TADS) randomized controlled trial. *Journal of the American Medical Association*, **292**, 807–820.

March J, Silva S, Vitiello B and the TADS Team (2006). The Treatment for Adolescents with Depression Study (TADS): methods and message at twelve weeks. *Journal of the American Academy of Child and Adolescent Psychiatry*, **45**, 1393–1403.

Martin A, Young C, Leckman JF *et al.* (2004). Age effects on antidepressant-induced manic conversion. *Archives of Pediatrics and Adolescent Medicine*, **158**, 773–780.

Meltzer HY, Alphs L, Green AI *et al.* (2003). Clozapine treatment for suicidality in schizophrenia: International Suicide Prevention Trial (InterSePT). *Archives of General Psychiatry*, **60**, 82–91.

Miller AL, Rathus JH, Linehan MM *et al.* E (1997). Dialectical behaviour therapy adapted for suicidal adolescents. *Journal of Practical Psychiatry and Behavioural Health*, **3**, 86.

Miller AL, Wyman SE, Huppert JD *et al.* (2000). Analysis of behavioural skills utilized by suicidal adolescents receiving dialectical behaviour therapy. *Cognitive and Behavioural Practice*, **7**, 183–187.

Miller AL, Rathus JH, Linehan MM (2007). *Dialectical Behaviour Therapy with Suicidal Adolescents*. The Guilford Press, New York.

Montgomery DB, Roberts A, Green M *et al.* (1994). Lack of efficacy of fluoxetine in recurrent brief depression and suicidal attempts. *European Archives of Psychiatry and Clinical Neuroscience*, **244**, 211–215.

Montgomery SA, Montgomery DB, Javanthi-Rani S *et al.* (1979). Maintenance therapy in repeat suicidal behaviour: A placebo controlled trial. In *Proceedings of the 10th intervention*, pp. 227–229. International Congress for Suicide Prevention and Crisis Intervention, Ottawa, Ontario.

Motto JA and Bostrom AG (2001). A randomized controlled trial of postcrisis suicide prevention. *Psychiatric Services*, **52**, 828–833.

Mufson L, Weissman MM, Moreau D *et al.* (1999). Efficacy of interpersonal psychotherapy for depressed adolescents. *Archives of General Psychiatry*, **56**, 573–579.

Mufson L, Dorta KP, Wickramaratne P *et al.* (2004). A randomized effectiveness trial of interpersonal psychotherapy for depressed adolescents. *Archives of General Psychiatry*, **61**, 577–584.

Olfson M, Shaffer D, Marcus SC *et al.* (2003). Relationship between antidepressant medication treatment and suicide in adolescents. *Archives of General Psychiatry*, **60**, 978–982.

Posner K, Oquendo M, Stanley B *et al.* (2007). Columbia Classification Algorithm of Suicide Assessment (C-CASA): Classification of suicidal events in the FDA's pediatric suicidal risk analysis of antidepressants. *American Journal of Psychiatry*, **164**, 1035–1043.

Rathus JH and Miller AL (2002). Dialectical behaviour therapy adapted for suicidal adolescents. *Suicide and Life-Threatening Behaviour*, **32**, 146–157.

Resnick MD, Bearman PS, Blum RW *et al.* (1997). Protecting adolescents from harm: findings from the National Longitudinal Study on Adolescent Health. *JAMA*, **278**, 823–832.

Rifkin A, Karajgi B, Dicker R *et al.* (1997). Lithium treatment of conduct disorders in adolescents. *American Journal of Psychiatry*, **154**, 554–555.

Rohde P, Clarke GN, Lewinsohn PM *et al.* (2001). Impact of comorbidity on a cognitive-behavioural group treatment for adolescent depression. *Journal of the American Academy of Child and Adolescent Psychiatry*, **40**, 795–802.

Rotheram-Borus MJ and Bradley J (1991). Triage model for suicidal runaways. *American Journal of Orthopsychiatry*, **61**, 122–127.

Rotheram-Borus MJ, Piacentini J, van Rossem R *et al.* (1996). Enhancing treatment adherence with a specialized emergency room program for adolescent suicide attempters. *Journal of the American Academy of Child and Adolescent Psychiatry*, **35**, 654–663.

Rotheram-Borus MJ, Piacentini J, Cantwell C *et al.* (2000). The 18-month impact of an emergency room intervention for adolescent female suicide attempters. *Journal of Consulting and Clinical Psychology* **68**, 1081–1093.

Schur SB, Sikich L, Findling RL *et al.* (2003). Treatment recommendations for the use of antipsychotics for aggressive youth (TRAAY). Part I. A review. *Journal of the American Academy of Child and Adolescent Psychiatry*, **42**, 132–1440.

Shaffer D and Craft L (1999). Methods of adolescent suicide prevention. *Journal of Clinical Psychiatry*, **60**(S2), 70–74.

Shaffer D, Gould MS, Fisher P *et al.* (1996). Psychiatric diagnosis in child and adolescent suicide. *Archives of General Psychiatry*, **53**, 339–348.

Shaffer D, Scott M, Wilcox H *et al.* (2004). The Columbia SuicideScreen: validity and reliability of a screen for youth suicide and depression.

*Journal of the American Academy of Child and Adolescent Psychiatry*, **43**, 71–79.

Steiner H, Petersen ML, Saxena K *et al.* (2003). Divalproex sodium for the treatment of conduct disorder: a randomized controlled colincal trial. *Journal of Clinical Psychiatry*, **64**, 1183–1191.

The TADS Team (2007). The Treatment for Adolescents with Depression Study (TADS): long-term effectiveness and safety outcomes. *Archives of General Psychiatry*, **64**, 1132–1144.

US Food and Drug Administration (2003). *FDA Public Health Advisory: Reports of Suicidality in Pediatric Patients being Treated with Antidepressant Medications for Major Depressive Disorder (MDD).* http://www.fda.gov/bbs/topics/answers/2003/ans01256.html.

van den Bosch LM, Verheul R, Schippers GM *et al.* (2002). Dialectical behaviour therapy of borderline patients with and without substance use problems: implementation and long-term effects. *Addictive Behaviours*, **27**, 911–923.

Verkes RJ, Van der Mast RC, Hengeveld MW *et al.* (1998). Reduction by paroxetine of suicidal behaviour in patients with repeated suicide attempts but not major depression. *American Journal of Psychiatry*, **155**, 543–547.

Wheeler BW, Gunnell D, Metcalfe C *et al.* (2008). The population impact on incidence of suicide and non-fatal self harm of regulatory action against the use of selective serotonin reuptake inhibitors in under 18s in the United Kingdom: ecological study. *BMJ*, **336**, 542–545.

Wood A, Harrington R, Moore A (1996). Controlled trial of a brief cognitive-behavioural intervention in adolescent patients with depressive disorders. *Journal of Child Psychology and Psychiatry* **37**, 737–746.

# CHAPTER 92

# Individual therapy techniques with suicidal adolescents

Anthony Spirito and Christianne Esposito-Smythers

## Abstract

This chapter provides a brief summary of the literature on individual therapy with suicidal adolescents. The primary focus is on the treatment of adolescents who have attempted suicide. Therapy techniques specific to cognitive, emotional/affective, interpersonal, and intrapsychic factors are reviewed. Techniques from cognitive behavioural therapy, dialectical behaviour therapy, psychodynamic psychotherapy, and interpersonal psychotherapy are described. An approach to psychoeducation regarding suicidality is also presented.

## Introduction

Suicidality is typically addressed in the context of the treatment of adolescent depression. However, effective treatment of the underlying condition, such as depression, does not necessarily result in a reduction in suicidality. Therefore, treatment specifically addressing suicidality is important. However, the treatment outcome literature on psychotherapy with suicidal adolescents is very limited. Consequently, there is little empirical data to support the efficacy of using the individual therapy techniques described in this chapter. Nonetheless, clinicians seek guidance on how to best treat this high-risk group.

Individual therapy is used by the majority of clinicians treating suicidal adolescents (Spirito *et al.* 2002a) and thus individual therapy techniques are of most interest to therapists. In this chapter, individual therapy techniques for treating adolescents who have attempted suicide are presented. The techniques were chosen based on the current treatment outcome literature (See Donaldson *et al.* 2003 for review), treatment protocols being tested in clinical trials, and the clinical literature.

To our knowledge, our group has published the only study of community psychotherapy for adolescent suicide attempters (Spirito *et al.* 2002a). Adolescents who had attempted suicide were interviewed 3 months following their attempt. Adolescents attended from 0 to 22 outpatient psychotherapy sessions (including home-based services) with 7.0 being the mean number attended. In this sample, 8 per cent of the participants did not attend any therapy sessions after their suicide attempt, 21 per cent attended 1–3 sessions, 31 per cent attended 4–7 sessions, 27 per cent attended 8–12 sessions, and 13 per cent attended 13 or more sessions.

Thirty-four per cent received individual therapy, and 66 per cent of the adolescents received a combination of individual and family sessions. The therapists reported that 58 per cent of the adolescents who entered treatment dropped out of therapy prematurely. The use of supportive therapy techniques was reported by approximately 75 per cent of the sample. Regarding dynamic psychotherapy methods, more than half of the adolescents reported that their therapist 'sometimes or frequently' made connections between emotional reactions and childhood experiences or emotional reactions and relationship problems. Cognitive therapy methods were taught 'sometimes or frequently' for approximately one half of the sample, and approximately one-third of the sample reported that they 'sometimes or frequently' learned behavioural techniques such as relaxation in their sessions.

In the pages that follow, we start by presenting a psychoeducation plan that can be used with suicidal adolescents and their families. This plan includes strategies to engage these adolescents and their families in treatment. The bulk of the chapter presents technique specific to the domains of functioning most commonly found to be problematic among suicidal adolescents: cognitive, affective, and interpersonal. Techniques to address intrapsychic factors are also described. However, the emphasis is on more directive techniques, especially those to address cognitive distortion and affect regulation, because of the importance of being proactive in the treatment of suicidal adolescents.

## Outcome literature on individual therapy with adolescent suicide attempters

Please also see Brent on effective treatment for suicidal youth (Chapter 91). Only two empirical studies of individual psychosocial treatments for adolescents who attempt suicide have been published, both of which were conducted in the United States. Rathus and Miller (2002) adapted Linehan's (1993) dialectical behaviour therapy (DBT) for use with suicidal adolescents. The focus of DBT is to improve distress tolerance, emotional regulation and interpersonal effectiveness. Using a quasi-experimental design, they compared treatment efficacy of DBT to treatment-as-usual (TAU) for suicidal adolescents (one-third were attempters) with borderline features. Adolescents in both groups attended approximately 24 sessions over 3 months. The DBT group, which had more severe baseline symptomatology than the TAU group, had fewer psychiatric hospitalizations and higher rates of treatment completion than the TAU group. No differences in repeat suicide attempts were found. About 40 per cent of adolescents re-attempted over the course of treatment.

Donaldson *et al.* (2005) conducted the only randomized trial to date of individual therapy. In this trial, CBT was compared to a problem-oriented supportive therapy designed to mimic standard care with adolescent suicide attempters. Both treatments were delivered in an individual format with conjoint parent–adolescent sessions. Adolescents were randomized to either 10 sessions of CBT (N = 18) or the problem-oriented supportive treatment. Seven different therapists provided both treatments to control for therapist effects. The groups were equivalent across baseline variables as well as percentage placed on medication during the study. More than half of the sample had made multiple suicide attempts. Participants in both conditions reported significant reductions in suicidal ideation and depression at 3-month follow-up but there were no between-groups differences. At 6 months, both groups retained improvement over baseline, however levels of suicide ideation and depression were slightly higher than at 3-month follow-up. Approximately one-quarter of the entire sample did not improve at follow-up with respect to suicidal ideation and approximately one-third with respect to depressed mood. Similarly, approximately 20 per cent of the patients in both conditions of the clinical trial dropped out of treatment against medical advice

## Conclusions

Empirical studies of individual therapy with adolescent suicide attempters have been conducted only in the United States to date. These studies have tested the efficacy of DBT and CBT. There have not been enough studies conducted to indicate whether these particular therapies are more efficacious than any other type of individual therapy. It is also unclear whether these therapies will be effective in community care or in other cultures.

Community therapists typically develop their own eclectic approach to therapy, do not typically have as much training and supervision in a particular therapy, and have limited time to learn new treatments. In contrast, in clinical trials, a consistent therapeutic orientation is taught and employed. It may be that a consistent therapeutic orientation across sessions, regardless of its actual content, may lead to greater improvement in symptoms (Kolko *et al.* 2000). The therapists in the Donaldson *et al.* study (2005) received weekly supervision throughout the study to ensure adherence to the protocol, a factor that has been suggested in successful treatment of other difficult-to-treat populations (Linehan 1993).

Our clinical and research programme emphasizes CBT techniques because they are action-oriented and can be used in a directive fashion, which we believe is important when working with suicidal adolescents. Consequently, in the pages that follow we describe CBT techniques in more detail than other therapeutic approaches. We believe that CBT techniques may be easier to apply in outpatient care than either family therapy or psychodynamic therapy, which tend to involve more extensive therapist training

and supervision as well as a longer treatment commitment from families. Ease of implementation of these techniques will affect both research and adoption of these techniques by clinicians, particularly in countries with fewer opportunities for training.

## Psychoeducation

Psychoeducation should include facts related to adolescent suicidal behaviour such as:

◆ The highest risk period for a repeat suicide attempt is within three months of the first attempt;

◆ More girls attempt suicide than boys but more boys complete suicide than girls;

◆ Risk factors for suicide include depression, hopelessness, a prior attempt and substance abuse, access to firearms; and

◆ Adolescents who attempt suicide often threaten to do so before the attempt.

Warning signs of depression are also useful to outline. Clinicians should educate family members about the adolescent's suicidal behaviour and instruct parents to increase their level of supervision, take all suicidal statements seriously, and restrict access to potentially lethal means, including both prescription and non-prescription medication, firearms or other weapons, toxic household chemicals, and motor vehicles (Pfeffer 1990; Freeman and Reinecke 1993).

It is also important to stress with the adolescent and family the importance of attending therapy sessions. This approach is most common in the Americas, Australia, and some European countries. It is useful to focus on the initial engagement in therapy using four basic strategies:

1  Education about the specifics of treatment;

2  An attendance contract;

3  Identification of potential treatment barriers; and

4  Problem-solving to address the barriers identified (Spirito *et al.* 2002b).

During the initial engagement in therapy, the therapist can share how treatment visits will be organized (with whom does the therapist meet, how long, content), the expected number of treatment sessions, and how visits will be scheduled. In discussing expectations for treatment, ask the adolescent what they think about coming to counselling, what they think happens in counseling, and how many visits they believe that it will take to get better. The therapist should also discuss factors that may impede adolescent treatment compliance (e.g., stigma, concerns that the therapist will side with parents against teen, parents might get upset if teen discusses family problems, etc.) and address these obstacles so they do not get in the way of attending counselling regularly.

## Cognitive factors

Rudd (2000) has outlined the fundamental assumptions of cognitive therapy for suicidal persons. First, suicidality is assumed to stem from a maladaptive suicidal belief system regarding one's self, the environment, and the future. Second, the suicidal belief system interacts with psychological/biological systems. Third, hopelessness, which consists of three core belief categories—unlovability, helplessness, and poor distress tolerance—is a central characteristic of the belief system. Fourth, cognitive vulnerabilities (faulty cognitive constructions) predispose individuals to suicidality, but these vulnerabilities may be different based on underlying psychiatric disorders. Fifth, the suicidal belief system exists at the person's core unconscious (metacognitive) and conscious (automatic) levels. The conscious level is most amenable to change.

Once suicidal behaviour occurs, it may sensitize the adolescent to future suicide-related thoughts and behaviour (Beck 1996). Beck conceptualizes these thoughts and behaviours as orienting schema. Suicidal behaviour makes the suicidal schema more easily accessible and easily triggered in future stressful situations. Once the taboo against suicide has been broken, it becomes easier to view suicide as a viable solution to life's problems. Thus, the importance of effective treatment for adolescents following a suicide attempt cannot be underestimated.

## Cognitive therapy

Cognitive therapy is highly structured and can address the cognitive distortions that are common among suicidal adolescents. Of the treatment approaches that address suicidal behaviour directly, cognitive therapy is most frequently advocated in the Americas, Australia and commonly in Europe. Pfeffer (1990) notes that a cognitive orientation in psychotherapy is useful in the management of impulsive behaviours and confronting biased perceptions of life stress, both of which are common in adolescents who attempt suicide. Below we describe a general approach to cognitive restructuring followed by a number of cognitive techniques specifically useful for suicidal persons (Freeman and Reinecke 1993). We then describe a problem-solving method that can be used to improve cognitive flexibility and decrease 'all or nothing' thinking.

## Cognitive restructuring

Suicidal adolescents also typically exhibit cognitive distortion. The *ABCDE* method, a modified version of rational emotive therapy (McClung 2000), can be useful in addressing cognitive distortions. This method is introduced as a skill that helps adolescents deal with negative beliefs or thoughts that they may experience when problems arise. The experience of negative thoughts in and of themselves is normalized for the adolescent but it is noted that they become problematic when they occur too frequently.

Each letter of the ABCDE method stands for a different step of thought changing. A stands for Activating Event. The first step in changing negative thought is to identify the activating event associated with the negative thoughts. Activating events can be positive or negative. In teaching the ABCDE method, the letter C (Consequences) is described next and the adolescent is taught to identify Consequences or feelings related to the Activating Event. Next, the adolescent is taught that the B of the ABCDE method stands for Beliefs, and that it is one's beliefs that lead one to feel badly.

Sample dialogue might be: Many people believe that negative Activating Events cause us to feel badly. For example, people believe that failing a test *causes* you to feel depressed. But that is not true. It is what occurs between the negative Activating Event and our feelings that cause us to feel bad. These things are called Beliefs and they occur between steps 1 and 3. These beliefs are typically negative and occur so quickly that we don't even know that we have them. Many of these beliefs are irrational or untrue.

The adolescent is then taught that, in order to feel better, they must argue against these beliefs or dispute them. Disputing is the fourth step, and perhaps the most important step, of thought changing. Most people don't dispute their negative beliefs and are left feeling very upset, and that is when they make unsafe decisions, such as hurting themselves.

When teaching the adolescent to dispute, we ask the adolescent to begin by asking themself two simple questions in regard to beliefs surrounding a negative activating event: (1) Is this belief true? And if it is true, (2) Is this belief helpful? If the answer is 'no' to either of these questions, then disputing is employed. The adolescent is then asked to develop an evidence for belief/evidence against belief list. Other useful questions include: What would your friend say if he/she heard this belief?; Does this belief help get you what you want?; Does this belief help you feel the way you want?; Does this belief help you avoid conflicts?; Is there another explanation for why the event occurred?

The last step begins with an E and stands for Effect. Effecting something is described as changing it. Adolescents are taught that they may not be able to change the fact that a negative activating event happened, but they can change negative beliefs and feelings surrounding the event.

## Other cognitive techniques

### Re-attribution

The therapist tries to help the adolescent change the self-statement, 'It's all my fault' to a new statement in which responsibility is attributed appropriately, perhaps to friends or parents, chance factors, or negative mood states. The therapist may initially support the adolescent's view that it is their fault but then suggests it might be worthwhile to look more closely at what the adolescent contributes to the situation and what other people contribute.

### Decatastrophizing

In this approach, the therapist helps the adolescent decide whether they are overestimating the catastrophic nature of the precipitating event. The therapist asks the adolescent, 'What would be the worst thing that will arise if _____ occurs?' 'If _____ does occur, how will it affect your life in 3 months? 6 months?' 'What is the most likely thing to happen here?' 'How will you handle it?'

### Pros and cons

The adolescent is asked to list advantages and disadvantages of different options. For example, therapist and client may examine the pros and cons of ending a romantic relationship. It can be useful to create a list of pros and cons because most adolescent suicide attempters view the world in black and white terms and don't typically view issues from both sides.

### Examination of options and alternatives

The therapist agrees with the adolescent that suicide is an option but helps the adolescent generate other options. Shneidman (1985) describes the use of this technique with a suicidal young adult who is pregnant. After agreeing that suicide is an option to her dilemma, Shneidman had the patient write a list of alternatives without regard to their feasibility, e.g., have an abortion, put the child up for adoption, raise the child on her own, etc. Then he had the young woman rank order the options from the least onerous to most onerous. Although she commented negatively on the options, this procedure helped her to see that there were other options besides suicide and she no longer ranked suicide as first or second choices.

### Scaling the severity of an event

The therapist asks the adolescent to scale the suicidal precipitant or anticipated future stressful events (on a scale from 0 to 100). Scaling the severity of an event provides a way for adolescents to view situations along a continuum rather than in a dichotomous fashion.

### Questioning of evidence

The therapist helps the adolescent question the evidence that is used to support a negative view. Socratic questions can be useful during this aspect of therapy (Overholser 1993). This technique is based on findings that suicide attempters often selectively attend to a particular set of evidence which confirms their negative interpretation.

### Reasons to live

At the end of the session, the therapist works with the adolescent to create a personal 'reasons to live' list and a coping card. The adolescent is asked to generate at least five reasons to live (e.g., to have a family of my own, to go to college) and write them on a worksheet. For the coping card, the adolescent generates a list of strategies that they can use in coping with difficult situations and phone numbers of persons to contact in an emergency. The adolescent is asked to keep the 'reasons to live' list and coping card readily available.

### Problem-solving

Deficits in problem-solving have been noted in adolescent suicide attempters. The 'SOLVE' system (Donaldson *et al.* 2003) described below covers the basic steps in problem-solving and has been implemented with adolescent suicide attempters (Donaldson *et al.* 2005). Each letter in the word SOLVE stands for a different step of the problem-solving process. S stands for Select a Problem. The second step is O or Options. After identifying the problem, the adolescent makes a list of all of the possible options—not just the ones they think would work. The bigger the list, the better the chance the adolescent has of coming up with a solution.

Often, the adolescent will have initial difficulties generating options. The therapist may need to model the skills in order to help the adolescent learn these new behaviours. Some adolescents will only generate options that they perceive to be workable solutions. The therapist can prompt the adolescent to generate a minimum of at least two strategies that they think would work as well as two strategies they think might not work very well. It is useful if the clinician illustrates a suicide attempt as a failure in problem-solving using the SOLVE system. That is, adolescents who attempt suicide often don't think that they have any options to solve their problem(s), other than to hurt themselves.

The next step in the problem-solving process is L or Likely outcomes. The adolescent takes the list of options and decides what might happen if they tried each of these options. The adolescent rates them in terms of whether selecting the option would make things better or worse. Sample therapist dialogue might be: 'Now you need to weigh each option and decide whether you think it would or would not be a helpful option. Let's take the first option you listed. Do you think this is something that would or would not help in that situation?' Then, the adolescent narrows the list down to one option and picks the Very Best One to do. Finally, the adolescent Evaluates whether or not the problem still exists. If it does, the adolescent goes back to Options, weighs the options, and picks the next Very Best One to try. The adolescent keeps doing this until the problem is solved. After problem-solving skills are successfully taught, the problem that precipitated the suicide attempt can be addressed using the same system.

### Emotional factors

Affect regulation techniques, i.e. training adolescents to recognize stimuli that provoke negative emotions and learning to reduce physiological arousal via self-talk and relaxation, are also commonly used with suicidal adolescents. These techniques can be introduced as follows: '*One thing you have told (or shown) us is that you often feel (e.g., angry, emotionally out of control). This is something that happens to a lot of the teenagers we work with who have hurt themselves. As we talked about earlier, when a negative activating event occurs, it triggers negative or untrue beliefs. These beliefs then cause negative feelings such as anger or sadness. In addition to negative feelings, these negative beliefs can also cause our body to start feeling out of control. You might experience muscle tightness, a faster heart rate, sweating, or shortness of breath and not even realize it. The more your body feels out of control, the harder it is to do problem-solving or dispute negative beliefs.*' Affect regulation strategies are most commonly used in the Americas. Below, we provide an overview of dialectical behaviour therapy, a therapy designed to specifically target affect disregulation, followed by a description of other affect regulation techniques that have been used to treat suicidal adolescents.

## Dialectical behaviour therapy

Dialectical behaviour therapy (DBT) includes a set of affect regulation techniques commonly used in the Americas and sometimes in Europe. Emotional dysregulation is the primary focus of DBT. In DBT, four sets of skills are targeted to address emotional dysregulation (Miller 1999):

1  Mindfulness skills to help alleviate confusion about oneself;

2  Emotional regulation skills to address emotional instability;

3  Distress-tolerance skills to target impulsivity; and

4  Interpersonal-effectiveness skills to address interpersonal problems.

Mindfulness skills are techniques designed to help adolescents make more balanced decisions. By helping the adolescent take the time to focus on emotions, the ultimate goal is to teach greater awareness and develop control over emotions. In emotion regulation training, adolescents are taught to identify and label emotions, reduce emotional vulnerability, increase positive experiences, and counteract negative emotion by acting the opposite of the distressing emotion.

Distress-tolerance skills include teaching adolescents to distract themselves from emotional pain, to self-soothe, and to generate pros and cons of tolerating versus not tolerating distress. Acceptance skills are designed to help the adolescent accept the fact that life involves pain but that they can learn the skills necessary to cope with distress. Interpersonal effectiveness skills are designed to help the adolescent manage interpersonal conflict more effectively.

### Chain analysis

When adolescents report instances of hurting themselves during the course of treatment, a functional analysis of this behaviour is often useful. A functional analysis adapted from Linehan's (1993) dialectical behaviour therapy with adults combines the use of problem-solving, cognitive restructuring, and other affect regulation techniques. This exercise is called a chain analysis because it takes a number of links or a chain of related behaviour, thoughts, feelings, and body sensations to lead to suicide attempt. The chain analysis helps the adolescent determine what triggered their suicide attempt and each of the negative links that followed.

First, the adolescent is asked questions regarding medication adherence, eating patterns, sleeping patterns, exercise, the use of alcohol or drugs, and other behaviours that are specific to the adolescent, such as isolating oneself when upset. These behaviours serve as vulnerability factors and if present may be included in the chain analysis. The therapist then asks the adolescent to begin the chain analysis with a behaviour that occurred earlier in the day that served as the initial trigger for a negative mood, not the actual suicide attempt, followed by the related thoughts, feelings, and body sensation. Several additional links are then completed in the same fashion up to the point of the suicide attempt.

Upon completion of all of the links, the therapist asks the adolescent to identify the 'weak links' in the chain by identifying the negative behaviours and thoughts associated with any negative body sensations and feelings. Next, the adolescent is asked to identify and record alternative adaptive thoughts and behaviours or 'strong links' that could be used to replace the 'weak links'. For example, 'disputing' and 'relaxation' are skills that an adolescent could use to replace a weak link.

The adolescent is asked to examine what the need was that they were trying to meet by engaging in dangerous behaviour and how they can get that need met in an adaptive manner in the future. Plans that can be used to address the harm the behaviour has caused and prevent future suicidal episodes are also developed.

## Other affect regulation techniques

### Feelings thermometer

One approach to affect regulation training is to show the adolescent a series of feelings cards and ask them to choose the card that best describes how they were feeling when they attempted suicide. Next, the therapist presents the adolescent with a list of general symptoms ('body talk') associated with negative affect (e.g., tension, fast heartbeat, sweating, yelling, slamming doors) and asks the adolescent to identify those associated with the feeling they experienced at the time of the attempt. The therapist notes that these body talk symptoms do not occur all at once but successively, like a set of dominos. The adolescent is then introduced to the concept of a 'feelings thermometer' (Rotheram-Borus et al. 1994). The bottom of the thermometer has a rating of '1' and stands for 'calm and cool' and the top is '10' and stands for 'extremely upset'. The adolescent is then asked to fill in lines by each rating on the

thermometer with body talk symptoms identified earlier as well as any associated negative beliefs. Next, the adolescent is asked to indicate their personal danger zone on the thermometer or the point where their body spirals so far out-of-control that they are at risk for unsafe or suicidal behaviour. Finally, the adolescent is asked to create a 'stay cool' plan to use when he/she begins to notice early 'body talk' and negative beliefs to prevent them from reaching the point of 'extreme upset' and unsafe behaviour.

### Anger management

The Match and Firecracker paradigm (Feindler and Ecton 1986) provides a means of describing the sequence of events that result in emotional dysregulation, especially anger. This concept can be introduced as follows: *A problem acts as the match that lights the fuse of the firecracker. Your mind is the fuse, and your body is the firecracker. The longer you let the problem last, the longer the fuse burns or your mind has negative thoughts and feelings, the more likely you are to feel really mad. You can put the fuse out quickly by doing things to control your negative thoughts and body symptoms.*

Feindler and Ecton (1986) developed a system of cognitive mediation techniques and anger arousal reduction methods that can be helpful in treating suicide attempters. Steps include identifying the anger trigger, altering the thoughts which led to the angry feelings, using self-statements to guide them through angry provocations, and relaxation techniques to modulate physiologic arousal. Problem-solving training, modelling, and behavioural rehearsal are used to help in applying the newly taught skills in anger-provoking situations. The ultimate goal is for adolescents to repeat calming statements to themselves during interpersonal conflicts and use relaxation techniques to minimize affective arousal.

## Interpersonal factors

### Psychodynamic psychotherapy

Psychodynamic psychotherapy addresses interpersonal factors underlying the suicidal behaviour. The therapeutic alliance and transference form the core of the therapy, especially in the beginning and middle phases of psychodynamic psychotherapy (Pfeffer 1986). Jobes (1995) has summarized key principles in psychodynamic therapy with suicidal adolescents. Suicidal adolescents often replicate earlier disturbed relationships with parents through the transference. The skilful psychodynamic therapist works through the transference to establish a good object relationship experience for the adolescent. Therapists demonstrate that they can tolerate the patient's negative, painful affect as well as the adolescent's conflicts around separation, helplessness, and dependency. The therapist's major role in the transference is to be the 'good' parent whose expectations match the adolescent's level of emotional maturity (Jobes 1995). The attention and concern of the therapist has therapeutic value as a corrective emotional experience.

### Interpersonal psychotherapy

Interpersonal Psychotherapy for Depressed Adolescents (IPT-A) is a brief treatment for depression that specifically addresses interpersonal issues as they relate to a depressive episode (Mufson et al. 1999). Although not specifically designed to address suicidality, IPT-A is naturally applicable to the suicidal feelings expressed by an adolescent in the context of discussing their depressed mood. IPT-A addresses interpersonal issues that arise with parents (separation, authority) and peers, as well as experiences with death. The techniques used to explore interpersonal conflict include exploratory questioning, encouragement of affect, clarification of conflicts, communication analysis, and role playing (Mufson *et al.* 2004).

### Intrapsychic factors

In psychodynamic psychotherapy certain intrapsychic themes common to adolescents who attempt suicide are typically addressed. Below, we review four techniques to address death fantasies, splitting, distress tolerance, and lack of self-care.

### Confronting death fantasies

Adolescents who attempt suicide view death as a viable alternative to life. This perception may be exacerbated if the adolescent has experienced the loss of an important person in their life. The therapist attempts to increase the adolescent's anxiety about death by confronting the adolescent's fantasy that death is preferable to life. Interventions may include emphasizing the finality of death and the impact of death on significant others (Fremouw *et al.* 1990).

### Splitting between positive and negative selves

Adolescent suicide attempters often have a poor self-image and view themselves very negatively. As the therapist works to keep the adolescent's view of themself positive, the opportunity exists to split the positive and negative images of the self. The goal is to help the adolescent see that the negative self associated with suicidality doesn't need to dominate the adolescent's life and that there is a part of the adolescent that wants to live. The therapist forms an alliance with this positive self (Orbach 1988).

### Self-soothing

Adolescent suicide attempters typically have limited ability to tolerate psychological pain and to self-soothe (King and Apter 1996). Helping adolescents develop external sources of support is an interim measure. The therapist typically addresses these difficulties by identifying conflicts related to attachment which in turn affect the adolescent's ability to care for themself.

### Lack of self-care

The depression experienced by adolescent suicide attempters has been associated with difficulties in self-care (King and Apter 1996). In the course of treatment, the therapist works with the adolescent to help them see that they deserve to care for themself and to explore ways to do so.

### Future research

Future research needs to consider several challenges pertinent to treatment of suicidal adolescents. First, adolescents who attempt suicide vary greatly in terms of treatment attendance. Follow-up studies of these adolescents have typically found poor adherence with outpatient treatment (Boergers and Spirito 2003). The transportability of research findings will be compromised if adolescents in community care or in certain countries are unwilling to attend a sufficient number of sessions to implement the protocol. Specific steps to encourage families to come to counselling regularly and complete the full treatment programme have been tested by Spirito *et al.* (2002b).

Second, suicidal behaviour rarely occurs in the absence of psychopathology (Shaffer *et al.* 1996). Further, adolescent suicide attempters possess great diagnostic heterogeneity. Comorbid psychiatric disorders further increase risk for suicidality. For example, rates of suicide attempts in depressed adolescents increase when they are diagnosed with a comorbid anxiety, disruptive behaviour (oppositional defiant or conduct disorder), and/or substance use disorder (Brent *et al.* 1993; Shaffer *et al.* 1996). Thus, treatment of suicidal behaviour must by necessity address the symptomatology associated with the accompanying psychiatric disorder(s).

Third, there exists evidence for at least two distinct types of suicide attempters: impulsive suicide attempters with predominant externalizing symptoms and non-impulsive suicide attempters with predominant internalizing symptoms. Relative to impulsive attempters, non-impulsive attempters have been found to have higher levels of depression and hopelessness, and a trend toward greater suicidal ideation (Brown *et al.* 1991). Further, anger turned inward has been found to be associated with hopelessness in the non-impulsive group. Thus, treatment protocols must be flexible enough to address these different presentations.

Fourth, the treatment outcome literature on adolescent suicide attempters is small, both because of the difficulties inherent in treating this population and investigator concerns about liability in clinical trials with such high-risk patients (Pearson *et al.* 2001). Adolescents with a history of suicidal behaviour have a high likelihood of continued suicidality during a research protocol, which often results in patients being removed from clinical trials. Under such conditions, a substantial percentage of suicidal adolescents may never complete treatment trials, making it difficult to accrue knowledge.

Fifth, even if therapy has been successful, adolescent suicide attempters remain vulnerable to a sudden resurgence of suicidal feelings (Beck 1996). It is important for the therapist to forewarn the adolescent and parents of the potential for resurgence of suicidality. Identifying subclinical levels of sadness or pessimism that can be managed before they reach crisis proportions, via individual efforts or booster sessions, is a priority. Therefore, research protocols may need to include both scheduled and as-needed booster sessions over a 4–6-month period which complicates the research design and follow-up.

Finally, when enrolled in trials immediately following a suicide attempt, many of these adolescents will be on one or more medications. Consequently, it is difficult to test the effectiveness of psychotherapeutic or psychosocial treatments alone. Thus, combined psychotherapeutic or psychosocial/psychopharmacologic treatments, with a standard algorithm guiding medication use, may be the research designs best suited to address the clinical and ethical realities of studying such a high-risk population.

### References

Beck AT (1996). Beyond belief: a theory of modes, personality, and psychopathology. In P Salkovskis, ed., *Frontiers of Cognitive Therapy*, pp. 1–25. Guilford Press, New York.

Berman A and Jobes D (1991). *Adolescent Suicide: Assessment and Intervention*. American Psychological Association, Washington.

Boergers J and Spirito A (2003). The outcome of suicide attempts among adolescents. In A Spirito and J Overholser, eds, *Evaluating and Treating Adolescent Suicide Attempters: From Research to Practice*, pp. 261–276. Academic Press, San Diego.

Brent D, Kolko DJ, Wartella ME *et al.* (1993). Adolescent psychiatric inpatients' risk of suicide attempt at 6-month follow-up. *Journal of the American Academy of Child and Adolescent Psychiatry*, **32**, 95–105.

Brown LK, Overholser J, Spirito A *et al.* (1991). The correlates of planning in adolescent suicide attempts. *Journal of the American Academy of Child and Adolescent Psychiatry*, **30**, 95–99.

Donaldson D, Spirito A, Esposito-Smythers C (2005). Treatment for adolescents following a suicide attempt: results of a pilot trial. *Journal of the American Academy of Child and Adolescent Psychiatry*, **44**, 113–120.

Donaldson D, Spirito A, Overholser J (2003). Treatment of adolescent suicide attempters. In A Spirito and J Overholser, eds, *Evaluating and Treating Adolescent Suicide Attempters: From Research to Practice*, pp. 295–321. Academic Press, San Diego.

Feindler E and Ecton R (1986). *Adolescent Anger Control: Cognitive-behavioral Techniques*. Pergamon Press, New York.

Freeman A and Reinecke M (1993). *Cognitive Therapy for Suicidal Behavior*. Springer Publishing Company, New York.

Fremouw W, dePerczel M, Ellis T (1990). *Suicide Risk: Assessment and Response Guidelines*. Pergamon Press, New York.

Jobes D (1995). Psychodynamic treatment of adolescent suicide attempters. In J Zimmerman and G Asmis, eds, *Treatment Approaches with Suicidal Adolescents*, pp. 137–154. John Wiley & Sons, New York.

King R and Apter A (1996). Psychoanalytic perspectives on adolescent suicide. *Psychoanalytic Study of the Child*, **51**, 491–511.

Kolko D, Brent D, Baugher M *et al.* (2000). Cognitive and family therapies for adolescent depression: treatment specificity, mediation and moderation. *Journal of Consulting and Clinical Psychology*, **68**, 603–614.

Linehan M (1993). *Cognitive Behavior Therapy of Borderline Personality Disorder*. Guilford, New York.

McClung T (2000). *Rational Emotive Therapy Adapted for Adolescent Psychiatric Inpatients*. Unpublished manual, West Virginia University School of Medicine.

Miller A (1999). Dialectical behavior therapy: a new treatment approach for suicidal adolescents. *American Journal of Psychotherapy*, **53**, 413–417.

Mufson L, Weissman MM, Moreau D *et al.* (1999). Efficacy of interpersonal psychotherapy for depressed adolescents. *Archives of General Psychiatry*, **56**, 573–579.

Mufson L, Dorta KP, Moreau D *et al.*(2004). *Interpersonal Psychotherapy for Depressed Adolescents*. Guilford, New York.

Orbach I (1988). *Children who Don't Want to Live*. Jossey-Bass, San Francisco.

Overholser JC (1993). Elements of the Socratic method: I. systematic questioning. *Psychotherapy*, **30**, 67–74.

Pearson J, Stanley B, King C *et al.* (2001). Intervention research with persons at high risk for suicidality: safety and ethical considerations. *Journal of Clinical Psychiatry*, **62**, 17–26.

Pfeffer CR (1986). *The Suicidal Child*. Guilford, New York.

Pfeffer CR (1990). Clinical perspectives on treatment of suicidal behavior among children and adolescents. *Psychiatric Annals*, **20**, 143–150.

Rathus J and Miller A (2002). Dialectical behavior therapy adapted for suicidal adolescents. *Suicide and Life-Threatening Behavior*, **32**, 146–157.

Rotheram-Borus MJ, Piacentini J, Miller S *et al.* (1994). Brief cognitive-behavioral treatment for adolescent suicide attempters and their families. *Journal of the American Academy of Child and Adolescent Psychiatry*, **33**, 508–517.

Rudd MD (2000). The suicidal mode: a cognitive-behavioral model of suicidality. *Suicide and Life-Threatening Behavior*, **30**, 18–33.

Shneidman E (1985). *Definition of Suicide*. John Wiley & Sons, New York.

Shaffer D, Gould MS, Fisher P *et al.* (1996). Psychiatric diagnoses in child and adolescent suicide. *Archives of General Psychiatry*, **53**, 339–348.

Spirito A, Stanton C, Donaldson D *et al.* (2002a). Treatment-as-usual for adolescent suicide attempters: implications for choice of comparison groups in psychotherapy research. *Journal of Clinical Child and Adolescent Psychology*, **31**, 41–47.

Spirito A, Boergers J, Donaldson D *et al.* (2002b). An intervention trial to improve adherence to community treatment by adolescents after a suicide attempt. *Journal of the American Academy of Child and Adolescent Psychiatry,* **41**, 435–442.

# CHAPTER 93

# Innovative psychosocial rehabilitation of suicidal young people

Kevin Malone and Su Yin Yap

## Abstract

This chapter examines current service provision and research in the area of youth suicide from the perspective of psychosocial rehabilitation. We examine culturally tailored programmes for suicide prevention and emphasize that adopting a community-based and culturally tailored approach is crucial in meeting the needs of suicidal young people. Gaps in the research into youth suicide are highlighted, including psychosis and substance misuse. Using these two examples, we attempt to show how the research has neglected key areas pertaining to youth suicide.

The second part of the chapter looks at service provision for suicidal young people. Gaps in the services are highlighted, namely the need to consult young people in service provision. We examine some promising areas of research that may be incorporated into tailoring services for suicidal young people. The use of Internet therapy is briefly examined and proposed as a means of tailoring services to young people by adopting their preferred technologies of communication.

We conclude by summarizing key recommendations for future research and service provision for suicidal young people.

## What is psychosocial rehabilitation?

There is a growing movement within the field of mental health towards the recovery model and psychosocial rehabilitation.

Psychosocial rehabilitation has been defined as a range of social, educational, occupational, behavioural, and cognitive interventions that aim to restore the patient's ability to function in the community (Sheth 2005). Psychosocial rehabilitation includes services aimed at long-term recovery, integration into the community, and maximization of self-sufficiency, as distinguished from the symptom-stabilization function of acute care (Barton 1999). The term psychosocial rehabilitation, in its broadest sense, covers the domains of skills training, peer support, vocational services, and community resource development (Barton 1999). The term *recovery model* is often used interchangeably with *psychosocial rehabilitation*, though rehabilitation denotes more of a focus on housing and employment.

With reference to youth suicide, it is apparent that, worldwide, the response to supporting suicidal young people falls short of this multifaceted concept of psychosocial rehabilitation.

## Who are 'young people'?

The issue of the definition of a young person is a crucial one. How we define a young person is central to shaping the mental health profession's response to youth suicide. For the purposes of this chapter, a young person is defined as 14–24 years of age. This age range encompasses three models of care: child services who are responsible for the 0–16-year-olds, the more uncommon adolescent services who provide for 16–18-year-olds, in some parts of the US and Europe, and finally, the adult services who provide care to the over 18s.

These arbitrary age segregations, while clear-cut and tidy from an administration and organisational point of view, do not serve the needs of the young people. Services specifically geared for adolescents are rare.

The Irish College of Psychiatrists (2005) have called for the establishment of a community-based dedicated psychiatric service for adolescents with the emphasis on treatment at home or in day hospitals. There is no cohesive approach to providing seamless care for young people of different ages. In addition, the models lying behind these services are very different in their approach.

The child services model of care centres on psychotherapy and family therapy, and tends toward a family systems approach. Although the global incidence of suicide by 0–15-year-olds is rare at 0.4 per 100,000, the rate has more than doubled since 1960 (Australian Institute for Suicide Research and Prevention 2003).

This trend is true for both males and females. In an Irish context, the suicide rate of 0–15-year-olds increased by 3900 per cent between 1960 and 1999. The Scandinavian countries also show a huge increase in suicides for this age group, with Norway and Finland showing a 570 per cent and 177 per cent increase respectively (Australian Institute for Suicide Research and Prevention 2003).

The adolescent model is broader in its approach, adopting a biopsychosocial model. However, internationally there is a dearth of such services aimed specifically at adolescents.

At the age of 18, young people are forced into the one size fits all adult model, a model that shows very little flexibility in tailoring care to suicidal young people. The suicidal young person, at a vulnerable point in their life, a time when they most need to feel understood, finds themselves in an adult psychiatric service, surrounded by people possibly generations older than themselves, to whom they may feel unable to relate.

Thus, it is clear that there is a gulf between child and adult mental health services' response to suicide. Service providers' creation of arbitrary age boundaries is not conducive to providing a tailored response to suicidal young people and does not provide consistency or continuity of care. Rather than sticking rigidly to age boundaries, there is a clear need for collaborations between teams in the fields of child, adolescent, and adult mental health to best meet the needs of young people. Such a dialogue across the age domains needs to address all components of psychosocial rehabilitation: skills training, peer support, vocational services, and community resource development.

## Research on psychosocial rehabilitation: what's out there?

Suicide preventative efforts worldwide can be divided in to three domains: biological intervention, psychotherapy, and social and educational. Despite the amount of literature and research into the area of youth suicide, there is a paucity of research into the psychosocial rehabilitation of suicidal young people (Hawton et al. 1998; Burns and Patton 2000; Miller and Glinski 2000).

As Comtois and Linehan (2006) argue, a central problem in addressing youth suicide is this dearth of research trials either developing new treatments or evaluating the standard of care treatments.

Most of the studies on psychosocial treatments for suicidal individuals have been carried out with predominantly adult populations (Shaffer et al. 1988; Hawton et al. 1998, 2002). Hawton et al. (1998, 2002) reviewed all randomized controlled trials targeting suicide attempters. Of the twenty-three studies, only two explicitly obtained an adolescent sample (Cotgrove et al. 1995; Harrington et al. 1998). There are dangers in generalizing results from an adult population to an adolescent population. With reference to cognitive behavioural therapy carried out with adult participants, Zametkin et al. (2001) note, it cannot be assumed that results of such studies apply also to adolescents, given the critical role of family factors in adolescent life and the possibility that developmentally, young people might be incapable of using certain cognitive behavioural approaches.

Of the relatively few studies that have been carried out on an adolescent population, evidence is far from conclusive. Greenhill and Waslick (1997) reported that no treatment programme had reduced the subsequent attempts in adolescent suicide attempters.

## Culture and suicide: culturally specific research on psychosocial rehabilitation

Across the five continents, the bulk of the research into psychosocial rehabilitation of suicidal young people has been carried out in the US.

### American Indians

Within the continent of America, there is great disparity in youth suicide rates. Suicide is currently the second leading cause of death for 15–24-year-old American Indians and Alaska Natives (AI/AN). One community that has experienced a significantly high rate of suicide are the Zuni Pueblo reservation in Arizona (LaFramboise and Howard-Pitney 1995).

LaFramboise and Howard-Pitney (1995) evaluated a culturally tailored intervention programme—the Zuni Life Skills Development Curriculum. In 1987, Zuni leaders initiated the development of a suicide prevention programme with a life-skills focus, using a model of social cognitive development. This focus on life skills is a departure from most school-based suicide intervention programmes in the US, which are based on education, developing crisis intervention techniques, and referring at-risk students. Compared to the non-intervention control group, the programme was effective in reducing some of the risk factors (e.g. hopelessness) and increasing some of the protective factors (e.g. problem-solving, stress and anger management), associated with suicide. This study provides encouraging results for a life-skills approach and a culturally tailored approach to school-based suicide intervention programmes.

Further support for culturally tailored interventions comes from May et al.'s (2005) evaluation of a community-wide suicide prevention programme in an American Indian Tribal Nation. Tribal leaders, health care providers, elders, youths, and clients all participated in the design and implementation of this intervention. As a result of more than fifty interactive community workgroups, suicide itself was not identified as one of the most important problems. The underlying issues that may lead to suicide—alcoholism, child abuse, domestic violence, and unemployment—were highlighted. As a result of these findings, the programme adopted an integrated, multidimensional approach to Adolescent Suicide Prevention. The programme began in 1990 and targeted youths aged 11–18 years. While the number of deaths by suicide remained at one to two per year between 1988–2002, the annual mean number of total self-destructive acts dropped by 61.1 per cent during the same years of the programme.

These two programmes conducted with an American Indian population are multimodal in their approach, with an emphasis on community input and involvement, life-skills building, and peer support. They are, thus, closer to the model of psychosocial rehabilitation than many other intervention programmes.

### Canada

Aboriginal males aged 15–19 have the highest suicide rate of any group in Canada. The White Stone Organization, based in Calgary, runs suicide prevention and education workshops tailored specifically to Aboriginal youth across Canada. More critically, the programme then trains these youth to conduct such presentations for peers in their own home communities. Youth leaders that have experienced suicide, family violence, and substance abuse in their own lives are credible educators and facilitators with their peers. The desire for peer leaders has been expressed by young people in the Irish Reaching Out study (Bolger et al. 2004). Interventions such as the White Stone Programme urgently need to be evaluated and rigorously tested to fully investigate their efficacy.

This culture-specific programme aims to disentangle the complex reasons behind the high rates of suicide among Aboriginal youth. The programme addresses culturally specific factors that affect suicidal youth, e.g. loss of culture and language, discrimination outside the reserve.

The 2003 Health Canada report *Preventing Youth Suicide in First Nations* stresses the need for the community-driven approaches. These community-driven approaches seek solutions from within and are best placed to investigate subcultures of suicide, and respond in a tailored fashion. It is imperative that researchers and service providers worldwide adopt a similar approach, and tackle the problem of youth suicide from a specific and tailored perspective.

## Psychosis and suicide: Australia's response

Of the few studies investigating the effect of psychosocial interventions in suicide prevention, none have involved patients with psychotic disorders despite this group being at particularly high risk of suicide (Power *et al.* 2003). As yet, there are no reports of any of these therapies being adapted for patients with psychotic disorders.

Early intervention in first episode psychosis with young people has been shown to reduce the risk of suicide in this high-risk population (Power *et al.* 2003). Between 1997 and 1999, the Australian government funded the EPPIC (Early Psychosis Prevention and Intervention Centre) with their Lifespan programme: an early intervention programme for young people (aged 15–29) presenting with first episode psychosis. Services include an early detection and crisis assessment team, an acute inpatient unit, an outpatient group programme, assertive follow-up teams and an intensive outreach mobile support team. This intervention was based on the biopsychosocial model incorporating low dose medication, cognitive-oriented individual therapy, and family and group therapies. Power *et al.*'s (2003) randomized controlled trials (RCT) of the Lifespan programme showed benefits on indirect measure of suicidality for the treatment group. It is clear that further studies involving populations with psychosis are urgently needed to address the high risk of suicide in this population.

## Substance misuse

Alcohol and substance abuse play a significant part in youth suicide. Indeed, comorbidity is the rule rather than the exception among adolescents (Volkmar and Woolston 1997).

Further research is needed to build up a comprehensive picture of the extent of the role substance abuse plays, but various studies show alcohol and substance abuse in 38–54 per cent of suicides of adolescents and young adults (Miller and Glinksi 2000).

Depressed young people with comorbid alcohol/substance abuse, conduct problems, and/or borderline personality disorder (BPD) represent a particularly high-risk profile for suicidal behaviour and completed suicide among teenagers (Brent *et al.* 1993).

Despite these research findings, the area of dual diagnosis and youth suicide has been neglected by researchers. Traditionally, research has excluded dually diagnosed patients in an attempt to attain a homogenous population sample. This exclusion provides an inaccurate profile of suicidal young people, fails to acknowledge their problems, and further hinders research into this high-risk group.

In order to address the needs of young people at risk of suicide, it an imperative for us to design treatment programmes for young people with a dual diagnosis of mental health problems and substance misuse problems, from the point of view of prevention and rehabilitation. An active substance abuse problem will make a diagnosis of a mental illness more difficult, as well as the treatment of that disorder. Dually diagnosed young people present a variety of individual, social, fiscal and political challenges to effective psychosocial rehabilitation programmes. Dually diagnosed patients require not only treatment for their mental illness, but concomitant treatment for substance abuse symptomatology as well.

# Where are we going wrong? Gaps in the research

## Consulting young people: Reaching Out study

Although there are valuable lessons to be learned from the reviewed studies, they still fall short of psychosocial rehabilitation as defined by Sheth (2005) or Barton (1999). Studies tend to look at symptom stabilization, for example measuring hopelessness, suicidal ideation, and depressive symptoms, instead of focusing on the holistic and multimodal model of psychosocial rehabilitation.

In addition, very few studies have consulted young people about how services might best be tailored and delivered to meet the specific needs of young people. In the world of commerce, the first step a company developing a product would undertake would be a needs assessment, followed by consumer consultation with feedback. The model of psychiatric and psychosocial rehabilitation care has been prescriptive for the most part, relying on the 'leave it to the professionals' adage. In treating suicidal young people, this feedback loop has been largely missing from research and treatment programmes, and instead study results and treatment programmes consistently report poor compliance.

An Irish study aimed at addressing this knowledge deficit, spoke to 14–20-year-olds in suicidal crisis admitted to the AandE department (Bolger *et al.* 2004). This study blended both quantitative and qualitative methods to examine the psychological functioning of the young people, self-reported reasons for self-harm, their view of their current psychological functioning and personal relationships, reported repetition of self-harm and their views of what type of services would be useful for young people with suicidal ideation or behaviour.

The young people stressed the importance of having someone to talk to at a time of crisis. When this person could not be a family member or friend, they emphasized the importance of an informal, 24-hour, accessible service, staffed by people with experience of mental health disorders, including alcohol and drug problems. A number of the young people mentioned the inclusion in such services of young people who have self-harmed in the past. Bolger *et al.* (2004) recommend that service providers and clinicians need to listen to the patients to best meet their needs.

## Services for suicidal young people

As a previous suicide attempt is the strongest predictor of future suicide (e.g. Shafii *et al.* 1985), the question of how best to rehabilitate suicidal young people is of utmost importance. Shaffer *et al.* (1996) report that approximately one-third of teenagers who die by suicide have made a previous suicide attempt.

### Follow-up care for suicide attempters

The majority of suicidal young people admitted to hospital after a suicide attempt do not receive follow-up care due to a lack of available resources, lack of suitable tailored treatment programmes in place, and poor adherence rates.

Bolger *et al.* (2004) highlighted the discrepancies in treatment offered to young people who present to Acccident and Emergency (AandE) departments after a suicide attempt. In 34 per cent of cases, the young person either did not see a psychiatrist or their notes were left incomplete, so it was unclear as to whether the patient had been seen by a psychiatrist. The large number of patients in this study who did not see a psychiatrist is unacceptably high. This finding raises questions about the consistency of care offered to young people who attempt suicide. It is imperative that a very high standard of care is provided to young people presenting with self-harming or suicidal behaviours as these presentations to AandE may offer a 'one-off' opportunity for therapeutic intervention.

A British study by Kapur *et al.* (2002) found that adults who had self-poisoned and received no psychosocial assessment were more likely to poison themselves again. This highlights the imperative for a psychosocial assessment after suicide attempts, as there is an indication that the assessment has therapeutic benefits. In light of this finding, Bolger *et al.* (2004) recommend that a psychosocial assessment be carried out for *all* young people who present at AandE after a suicide attempt or deliberate self-harm.

Studies show that adolescent suicide attempters have poor compliance to treatment recommendations (Shaffer *et al.* 1988) with reported adherence rates for non-hospitalized adolescents of between 20–30 per cent (Burns and Patton 2000). The issue of poor retention rates needs to be teased apart and addressed.

### First-time completers

In the case of young people who die by suicide at their first attempt, many of these suicidal young people never come to the attention of the medical profession. A British study by Vassilas and Morgan (1997) reported that only 22 per cent of males under the age of 35 years who die by suicide, and 57 per cent of females come into contact with the health services in the four weeks before death.

It is clear that first, early detection is crucial, we need to find ways of reaching out to our young people in distress, and try to equip them with the coping skills to deal with their problems. Secondly, once suicidal young people come to the attention of the health services, effective psychosocial rehabilitation programmes need to be implemented.

## Providing a tailored service for suicidal young people

### Mobile phone technology

Therapists need to tune in to how young people use modern technology as a means of communicating. Rather than seeing this technology as a barrier for therapy, it might be valuable to explore how this technology can be used to augment connectivity with the therapist as a means of developing and sustaining the therapeutic alliance. Linehan used this effectively in her DBT programme (Linehan 1995), where patients would contact their therapists by pager if they felt suicidal and the therapist would make telephone contact with them (if they made a suicide attempt the pager was not an option and the patient would have to go to the emergency room [ER]). In St Vincent's University Hospital in Ireland, mobile phone technology has been employed with patients in several ways.

First as simple dialogue for day-to-day management questions that may arise. Patients also log their next appointment into their telephone calendar for reminder, which has improved attendance at sessions. Finally, some patients have found it useful to insert a daily reminder to take their medication, and to include a brief catch phrase from the therapy session that will reinforce their engagement with therapy and encourage them on bad days. For example, one patient who had recovered from a depressive episode, which was complicated by alcohol consumption inserted a daily reminder in his phone as follows 'no jar 2day, L100'—the 'no jar' was a catch-phrase reminder from the patient not to have any alcohol (one day at a time), whereas the L100 referred to his dose of antidepressant he was taking at the time (lustral 100). These clinical anecdotes of using a technology known to young people should be explored further in properly designed clinical trials to see if it improves treatment outcome.

Services and organizations need to incorporate young people's use of technology into their service provision if they want to provide an age-relevant service.

The Samaritans, who were the first to offer emotional support by email in 1994, piloted an SMS (short message service, also known as text messaging) service in April 2006 to distressed young people in the UK and Ireland, which aims to provide emotional support by text at any time of day or night. This SMS service came about as a result of a report carried out by the Samaritans (2002) on young people's use of text messaging. The report showed that 94 per cent of 18–24-year-olds send personal text messages. A text service offers another means for a suicidal young person to reach out, a means that may be less daunting than making a phone call, and may be a preferred option for young people who may feel uncomfortable expressing themselves verbally. A Samaritans' volunteer will reply to anyone who sends a text with a confidential, non-judgemental text reply, giving emotional support, aiming to respond within 10 minutes.

The South African Depression and Anxiety Group have also launched a new SMS service for depressed teenagers. The initiative aims to help curb the high levels of teen suicide in the country. Suicide is said to account for around 9 per cent of all teenage deaths in South Africa.

## Internet online therapy

Online therapy is a growing area in psychology. There are an increasing number of websites offering online therapy for issues ranging from anxiety to sport psychology, from drug and alcohol misuse to obsessive–compulsive disorder (OCD), from depression to post-traumatic stress disorder (PTSD).

This is of particular relevance to young people, who are competent and frequent users of the Internet. One of the most significant advantages of online therapy is the potential to provide far greater access to treatment than would otherwise be obtainable, thereby enabling greater numbers of people in psychological distress to avail themselves of some form of therapy.

This accessibility is particularly pertinent to people outside of the major urban centres that may have restricted access to specialist mental health services. By delivering therapy via the Internet, greater access can be provided to those who are disadvantaged due to geographical isolation, physical impairment or other mobility, time and/or financial restrictions.

Another key advantage of Internet-based interventions for common mental health problems is that they appear to be cost-effective; with costs reduced to between one-third and one-sixth of other psychological treatments (Crone *et al.* 2004).

Contrary to popular belief, the research indicates that Internet therapy can enhance some clinical processes. For example, Internet interventions involving email correspondence between therapist and client provide both parties with a permanent record of the therapy. This can facilitate evaluation of the client's progress over time. Clients are able to revisit the techniques previously used or guidelines on how to approach 'homework', set goals, etc.

There is also substantial evidence that the act of writing one's thoughts and emotions is itself therapeutic (Pennebaker 2005), and that many clients are more candid in their responding via email or online than when speaking face-to-face (Fiegelson and Dwight 2000). Furthermore, email therapy allows people to interact at their own convenience without the need for appointment times.

Research continues into the impact of the Internet on therapeutic process and whether certain people in the population are more suited to Internet therapy than others. This research needs to include young people to examine whether it is possible to harness young people's ease with Internet-based technology as a tool in suicide prevention programmes.

### Computerized therapy packages

The related area of computerized therapy, already in wide usage throughout the UK, may have much to offer to young people in particular. Proudfoot *et al.* (2004) conducted a randomized controlled trial investigating the efficacy of a computerized cognitive behavioural therapy (CBT) package for patients with anxiety and depression in primary care. The treatment condition consisted of an interactive, multimedia, computerized CBT therapy package consisting of a 15-minute introductory video, followed by eight therapy sessions with allocated homework. Sessions and homework were customized to the patient's specific needs. Results showed that the treatment condition showed significant improvement on all response variables measured: depression and anxiety decreased, work and social adjustment improved, negative attributions decreased, positive attributions increased and satisfaction with treatment was enhanced.

An Australian study by Christensen *et al.* (2004) conducted a randomized controlled trial investigating interventions for depression using the Internet. This study examined two interventions—a psychoeducation website offering information about depression, and an interactive website offering CBT for the prevention of depression. This study was carried out with an adult population (mean age 36.43 years) with increased depressive symptoms were recruited by survey. Results showed that both web-based interventions were effective in reducing symptoms of depression. There is a need for further investigation of the efficacy of web-based packages to be carried out with young people.

### Dangers of the Internet

There has been increasing media attention on the dangers of so-called suicide sites. Such websites encourage and provide information on the most effective means of suicide to vulnerable young people. Dobson (1999) reported that over 100,000 sites about suicide now appear on the World Wide Web. Dobson highlights the dangers of Internet suicide groups and bulletin boards, which advocate suicide and discourage individuals from seeking psychiatric help. The dangers of Internet suicide sites are particularly pertinent to the problem of youth suicide as most web users fall in to the 14–24 age group, the very group with a high suicide rate and low peer support (Dobson 1999). The report further describes the profile of web users as qualitatively different to other individuals, being psychologically more vulnerable with higher risk-taking behaviour, substance abuse, and depression scores than control subjects.

## Conclusions and recommendations

First, we need to examine how we define young people, and the implications this has for the treatment available to young people.

### Research

◆ Only a small proportion of psychological autopsies conducted worldwide focus specifically on youth suicide. From psychological autopsies to randomized controlled trials, research needs to focus on young people as a group with identities, problems, and psychosocial habits different from older adults.

◆ More longitudinal studies investigating the complexities behind youth suicide are needed.

◆ Further research is clearly necessary to find effective interventions for suicidal young people including psychosocial rehabilitation. It is highly unlikely that there is a 'one size fits all' type intervention waiting to be developed, different countries and communities having different challenges and strengths.

◆ Research also needs to explicitly seek out the views of the young people in how services can meet their needs. Further research like the Irish Reaching Out study is needed to ensure that the voices of our young people in distress are heard.

◆ Community-based studies that examine micro-climates of subcultures of suicides are invaluable in teasing out and examining the complex causes behind suicide, many of which are culturally and historically bound. We need to learn from any programmes that have tailored their approach to the population, be that tailored to culture or age, to fully grasp the complexities of suicide and how to best address it.

### Services

◆ The lack of youth-specific research is mirrored in the lack of psychosocial interventions carried out with exclusively adolescent populations. Interventions and services aimed at suicidal young people need to take the young people's wishes into account, and find ways to be relevant, accessible and sensitive to young people. These interventions need to be evaluated and evidence-based.

◆ Cross-disciplinary dialogue is needed to set up multidisciplinary teams that provide psychosocial rehabilitation across age groups covering the domains of skills training, peer support, vocational services, and community resource development. These teams need to have the flexibility to meet the needs of suicidal young people from the pre-teen age group right up to young adults in their twenties.

◆ The response to suicidal young people must strive to meet the needs of high-risk subpopulations of young people with complex needs such as psychosis and/or substance misuse.

◆ The adult services could learn a lot from the Early Intervention for Psychosis Programme, a tailored programme for young people vulnerable to developing psychosis. By drawing on the core elements and approach of this programme, the adult services would be better placed to provide tailored care and crucial early intervention to its suicidal young people.

◆ Researchers and service providers need to learn from culturally tailored youth suicide programmes. We need to move away from a generic approach to suicide prevention, and adapt research to fully explore ethnic subcultures of suicide, the subculture of youth and the underlying factors. Such specific research is needed to inform how best to respond to youth suicide in an age-appropriate, culturally specific fashion.

◆ Adapting therapeutic practice to incorporate mobile phone technologies and Internet technology may be an effective way of reaching out to and connecting with suicidal young people.

◆ To tackle the complex problem of suicide, mental health professions need to adopt the language of recovery to empower suicidal young people and help young people to attain meaningful roles in the society. We need to foster a sense of belonging in them by reconnecting them to the community, and connecting them with a peer support network.

## References

Australian Institute for Suicide Research and Prevention (2003). *International Suicide Rates—Recent Trends and Implications for Australia*. Australian Government Department of Health and Ageing, Canberra.

Barton R (1999). Psychosocial rehabilitation services in community support systems: a review of outcomes and policy recommendations. *Psychiatric Services*, **50**, 525–534.

Bolger S, O'Connor P, Malone K *et al.* (2004). Adolescents with suicidal behaviour: attendance at AandE and six month follow-up. *Irish Journal of Psychological Medicine*, **21**, 78–84.

Brent DA, Perper JA, Moritz G *et al.* (1993). Firearms and adolescent suicide: a community case–control study. *American Journal of Diseases of Children*, **147**, 1066–1071.

Burns JM and Patton GC (2000). Preventive interventions for youth suicide: a risk factor-based approach. *Australia and New Zealand Journal of Psychiatry*, **34**, 388–407.

Christensen H, Griffiths KM, Jorm AF (2004). Delivering interventions for depression by using the Internet: randomised controlled trial. *British Medical Journal*, **328**, 265–275.

Comtois KA and Linehan MM (2006). Psychosocial treatments of suicidal behaviours: a practice-friendly review. *Journal of Clinical Psychology*, **62**, 161–170.

Cotgrove A, Zirinsky L, Black D *et al.* (1995). Secondary prevention of attempted suicide in adolescence. *Journal of Adolescence*, **18**, 569–577.

Crone P, Knapp M, Proudfoot J *et al.* (2004). Cost-effectiveness of computerized cognitive-behavioural therapy for anxiety and depression in primary care: randomised controlled trial. *The British Journal of Psychiatry*, **185**, 55–62.

Dobson R (1999). News: Internet sites may encourage suicide. *British Medical Journal*, **319**, 337.

Fiegelson ME and Dwight SA (2000). Can asking questions by computer improve candidness of responding? A meta analytic perspective. *Consulting Psychology Journal: Practice and Research*, **52**, 248–255.

Greenhill LL and Waslick B (1997). Management of suicidal behaviour in children and adolescents. *The Psychiatric Clinics of North America*, **20**, 641–666.

Harrington R, Kerfoot M, Dyer E *et al.* (1998). Randomized trial of a home-based family intervention for children who have deliberately poisoned themselves. *Journal of the American Academy of Child and Adolescent Psychiatry*, **37**, 512–518.

Hawton K, Arensman E, Townsend E *et al.* (1998). Deliberate self-harm: systematic review of efficacy of psychosocial and pharmacological treatments in preventing repetition. *British Medical Journal*, **317**, 441–447.

Hawton K, Rodham K, Evans E *et al.* (2002). Deliberate self-harm in adolescents: self-report survey in schools in England. *British Medical Journal*, **325**, 1207–1211.

Health Canada (2003). *Acting on What we Know: Preventing Youth Suicide in First Nations*. Health Canada, Ottawa.

Irish College of Psychiatrists (2005). *OP60: A Better Future Now: Position Statement on Psychiatric Services for Children and Adolescents in Ireland*. Retrieved on 12 May 2006 http://www.rcpsych.ac.uk/publications/collegereports/op/op60.aspx.

Kapur N, House A, Dodgson K *et al.* (2002). Effect of general hospital management on repeat episodes of deliberate self-poisoning: cohort study. *British Medical Journal*, **325**, 866–867.

LaFramboise TD and Howard-Pitney B (1995). The Zuni life skills development program: description and evaluation of a suicide prevention program. *Journal of Counselling Psychology*, **42**, 479–486.

Linehan MM (1995). *Understanding Borderline Personality Disorder: The Dialectic Approach Program Manual*. Guilford Press, New York.

May PA, Serna P, Hurt L *et al.* (2005). Outcome evaluation of a public health approach to suicide prevention in an American Indian Tribal Nation. *American Journal of Public Health*, **95**, 1238–1244.

Miller AL and Glinski J (2000). Youth suicidal behaviour: assessment and intervention. *Journal of Clinical Psychology*, **56**, 1131–1152.

Pennebaker J (2005). Two decades of expressive writing and health: the current state of the field. Keynote address delivered at the 19th annual conference of the European Health Psychology Society. In C Pier, B Klein, D Austin D *et al.* (2006). *Reflections on Internet Therapy: Past, Present and Beyond*. In psychological highlights. Retrieved 17 May 2006 from http://www.psychology.org.au/publications/inpsych/12.2_140.asp.

Power PJR, Bell RJ, Mills R *et al.* (2003). Suicide prevention in first-episode psychosis: the development of a randomised controlled trial of cognitive therapy for acutely suicidal patients with early psychosis. *Australian and New Zealand Journal of Psychiatry*, **37**, 314–420.

Proudfoot J, Ryden C, Everitt B *et al.* (2004). Clinical efficacy of computerised cognitive behavioural therapy for anxiety and depression in primary care. *The British Journal of Psychiatry*, **185**, 46–54.

Samaritans (2008). *Case Study: Samaritans SMS Text Messaging Project*. http://www.publictechnology.net/print.php?sid=13843. Retrieved 28 April 2008.

Shaffer D, Gould M, Fisher P *et al.* (1988). Preventing teenage suicide: a critical review. *Journal of the American Academy of Child and Adolescent Psychiatry*, **27**, 675–687.

Shaffer D, Gould MS, Fisher P *et al.* (1996). Psychiatric diagnosis in child and adolescent suicide. *Archives of General Psychiatry*, **53**, 339–348.

Shafii M, Carrigan S, Whittinghill JR, Derrick A (1985). Psychological autopsy of completed suicide in children and adolescents. *American Journal of Psychiatry*, **142**, 1061–1064.

Sheth HC (2005). Common problems in psychosocial rehabilitation. *International Journal of Psychosocial Rehabilitation*, **10**, 53–60.

Vassilas CA and Morgan HG (1997). Suicide in Avon. Life stress, alcohol misuse and use of services. *British Journals of Psychiatry*, **170**, 453–455.

Volkmar FR and Woolston JL (1997). Comorbidity of psychiatric disorders in children and adolescents. In AL Miller and J Glinski, eds (2000). Youth suicidal behaviour: assessment and intervention. *Journal of Clinical Psychology*, **56**, 1131–1152.

Zametkin AJ, Alter MR, Yemini T (2001). Suicide in teenagers: assessment, management, and prevention. *Journal of the American Medical Association*, **286**, 3120–3125.

# PART 13

# Elderly People and Suicide

# CHAPTER 94

# Suicidal behaviours on all the continents among the elderly

Diego De Leo, Karolina Krysinska,
José M Bertolote, Alexandra Fleischmann
and Danuta Wasserman

## Abstract

Despite tremendous variability across countries, suicide rates among the elderly, especially elderly males, remain globally the highest. On average, suicide rates increase with age, with the global suicide rate among those aged 75 and over being approximately three times higher than the rate among youth under 25 years of age. This chapter gives an overview of the epidemiology of fatal and non-fatal suicidal behaviour among people over 65 years of age on the five continents. The purpose is to facilitate a better appreciation of the extent of the differences among nations (where possible data from continents are provided), collectively with an example from a country from each of the continents: South Africa, China, Australia, Italy, and Brazil.

## Suicide

Lack of epidemiological data from many nations on mortality and morbidity makes cross-cultural comparisons regarding suicidal behaviours in the elderly a challenging task. Estimation of the actual prevalence of suicide among the older persons should be approached with particular caution due to high frequency of under-reporting, and lack of formal recognition of passive suicidal behaviours (e.g. self-starvation, refusal to take life-sustaining medication, etc.) in reported suicide statistics (De Leo and Diekstra 1990).

However, available data indicates that, despite tremendous variability across countries, suicide rates in the elderly remain globally the highest (Bertolote and Fleischman 2005). On average, suicide rates increase with age, with the global suicide rate among those aged 75 and over being approximately three times higher than the rate among youth under 25 years of age.

However, the pattern of suicide rates increasing with age is not found in every nation. Today, approximately one-third of the countries reporting mortality data to the World Health Organization present higher rates in young adults (males) than in subjects over 65 years of age. In addition, over the last thirty years, countries of different cultures have registered an increase in youth and young adults' suicide that has been paralleled by a decline in elderly rates (Alte da Veiga and Saraiva 2003; De Leo and Evans 2004; Pritchard

and Hansen 2005). The decrease has been particularly relevant in Anglo-Saxon countries, possibly in relation to increased economic security of the elderly, changing attitudes toward retirement, improved social services and better psychiatric care (De Leo 1998, 1999; De Leo and Spathonis 2003). The decline has not been confined to elderly males only. For example, in Australia, women who are aged 65–74 years today, have rates of suicide that are four times lower than those in 1965 (De Leo 2006). In a number of Latin American countries, as well as in some Asian nations, suicide rates in old age present less favourable trends. In these countries, economic, social changes and the collapse of traditional family structures may have contributed to the high elderly suicide rates (Pritchard and Baldwin 2000; De Leo 2003; Rudmin et al. 2003).

Worldwide, suicide is most prevalent among male subjects in the 75 years and older age group (De Leo and Heller 2004). Particularly in the Western world, this seems to contrast with the poor health and social status experienced by elderly women that result from more compromised psychophysical conditions secondary to greater longevity, poverty, widowhood, and abandonment. To explain this difference, it has been suggested that women might benefit from better established social networks, grater self-sufficiency in activities of daily living, and commitment to children and grandchildren (De Leo 2003).

Fatal and non-fatal suicidal behaviour exhibit opposite tendencies with respect to age; while suicide rates peak in the elderly in most nations, attempted suicide decreases with advancing age virtually everywhere else (De Leo et al. 2001; De Leo and Spathonis 2004). In the elderly, estimated ratios between attempts and completions vary from 4:1 (McIntosh 1992) to 2:1 (De Leo et al. 2001), whereas in young persons, they can reach the level of 100–200:1 (McIntosh 1992). Results of the WHO/EURO Multicentre Study on Suicidal Behaviour indicated the highest prevalence of suicide attempts in younger age groups, with the frequency decreasing with age for both sexes. In fact, subjects between the age of 15 and 34 years accounted for 50 per cent of all attempts recorded in hospitals, while the elderly (65+) comprised only 9 per cent of all suicide attempters (De Leo et al. 2001; Schmidtke et al. 2004). Similar age-related trends in non-fatal suicidal behaviour were observed in the recent WHO/ SUicide PREvention-Multisite Intervention Study on Suicidal

Behaviours (WHO/SUPRE-MISS) (Fleischmann *et al.* 2005). In this investigation only 1 per cent of all attempters were over the age of 65.

Literature converges in depicting the elderly as subjects whose suicide attempts usually involve the highest suicide intent scores; their acts are often carefully planned and are less impulsive than in younger individuals. Methods tend to be more violent, in general, and therefore have less opportunity for rescue (Pearson and Brown 2000; Caine and Conwell 2001; De Leo *et al.* 2001, 2002; Conwell *et al.* 2002). Also, alcohol is less involved in elderly suicidal behaviours compared to their younger counterparts (Neulinger and De Leo 2001). It has been reported that in old age, 85 per cent of subjects take their own lives on the first attempt (Suominen *et al.* 2004). Among factors contributing to the high rate of death subsequent to an attempt are: decreased healing abilities, frailty compounded by inability to survive the physical injury, and social isolation (Conwell *et al.* 2002).

There have been relatively few population studies looking at the prevalence of suicidal ideation in old age. Differences in methodology (e.g. timeframe, type of questions, and age of surveyed participants) make comparisons difficult (Forsell *et al.* 1997; Scocco *et al.* 2001). However, results indicate that between 2.3 per cent (Jorm *et al.* 1995) and 15.9 per cent (Skoog *et al.* 1996) of individuals over the age of 65 had experienced suicidal ideation in the month preceding the interview. In an Italian study by Scocco and De Leo (2002), almost one in ten participants over the age of 65 reported death wishes or suicidal ideation over the last 12 months. In the Gold Coast Survey on Suicidal Behaviour (De Leo *et al.* 2005), the lifetime prevalence of suicide ideation was 5.3 per cent in subjects aged 65–74 years, and 5.6 per cent in those aged 75+, percentages that are approximately half the frequency expressed by people below the age of 55 (in the 55–64 group the percentage was 8.1). In Taiwan, Yen *et al.* (2005) found that 16.7 per cent of respondents (65–74 years old) had thoughts of suicide within the past week. This study is of special interest, given that the majority of research on the subject has been conducted in Western countries, and there is scarcity of data regarding the prevalence of suicidal ideation among the elderly in other cultures (Chou *et al.* 2005; Fujisawa *et al.* 2005).

## Suicide in countries from five continents

International studies of the prevalence of suicidal ideation and suicide attempts across the lifespan lead to the conclusion that social and cultural factors might contribute to the observed variations in suicide rates among nations (De Leo and Spathonis 2003). Differences in socio-economic status, social systems, and types of health care, as well as ethnicity, religion, and traditions, can provide important insights to a better understanding of suicide and its prevention (Hawton *et al.* 2001; Rudmin *et al.* 2003; Berk *et al.* 2005; Wu and Bond 2006).

In order to facilitate a better appreciation for the extent of the differences in suicide rates among nations, data from all continents are given where available (Table 94.1), as well as an example from a country from each of the five continents. Data on elderly suicide rates in China are reported and discussed here due to the unique gender-, age- and urban/rural patterns of suicide in the country. The brief discussion on elderly suicide in South Africa underlines the role of sociocultural and political factors contributing to suicidal behaviour among the elderly.

Furthermore, data from the WHO/ SUPRE-MISS investigation allows for some unique insight regarding the prevalence of non-lethal suicidal behaviours among the elderly in participating countries.

## Africa

Injuries, including suicide, are common and increasing in many developing countries, including Africa; however, their incidence and trends are understudied and poorly known (Nordberg 2000). Most countries in Sub-Saharan Africa do not have compulsory registration of deaths, and in many cultures in the region, suicide remains a taboo subject, making it unlikely that the relatives of people dying by suicide will report the true cause of death (Gureje *et al.* 2007). Several studies have looked at suicide among the elderly in South Africa (which are reviewed below), and there is survey data regarding the prevalence of suicide ideation and attempts across the lifespan in the general populations of Ethiopia (Alem *et al.* 1999; Kebede and Alem 1999) and Nigeria (Gureje *et al.* 2007). Studies conducted in Ethiopia indicated that the majority of self-reported suicide attempts occurred when the respondents were between 15 and 24 years of age, with the frequency of such behaviour decreasing with age (Alem *et al.* 1999). Moreover, the lifetime prevalence of suicide ideation was decreasing with age; for example, suicide ideation among individuals aged 60 years and older was 68 per cent lower than young adults under the age of 25 (Kebede and Alem 1999). Gureje and his colleagues (2007) found that in Nigeria, respondents in the youngest age group (18–34 years old) were significantly more likely to have ever thought about suicide, made a suicide plan or attempted suicide than respondents over the age of 65.

### South Africa as an example

About 10,000 people die by suicide in South Africa every year, and the problem of suicide is increasing, especially among young people (Meel 2006). In the first national longitudinal study of suicide trends in the country over the period of 1968–1990, Flisher *et al.* (2004) reported that 1.1 per cent of all deaths were attributable to suicide, with the white males having the highest suicide rate in the country (33.1 per 100,000). Suicide rates in the elderly showed a significant variation depending on sex and race: the white male suicide rate was the highest (41.2 per 100,000), while the rate among the male Coloureds of Asian and African ancestry was significantly lower (7.7 per 100,000). Similarly, the elderly female suicide rate was the highest among Whites (7.1 per 100,000) and the lowest among the Coloureds (0.9 per 100,000).

To date, there is scarcity of data on the epidemiology of non-fatal suicidal behaviour in the general population in South Africa, and among the elderly in particular. Data from the WHO/ SUPRE-MISS study showed a trend similar to the one found in other countries; the majority of suicide attempters in Durban were young, and the elderly only accounted for 0.3 per cent of all attempters (Fleishmann *et al.* 2005).

Since the 1990s, South Africa has been undergoing serious political transition, transforming the social world of the country, with the elderly appearing as the least adaptable to these challenges. Due to the ethnic variation of the South African population, any analysis of suicide trends in the country, including elderly suicide, has to take into consideration the relevant cultural and socio-economic factors, including decreased resilience and unmet expectations

**Table 94.1** Elderly suicide rates in selected countries by age and sex

| Country | Year | Age 65–74 years | | | Age 75+ years | | |
|---|---|---|---|---|---|---|---|
| | | M | F | All | M | F | All |
| **Africa** | | | | | | | |
| Mauritius | 2003 | 9.5 | 7.6 | 8.4 | 8.9 | 0.0 | 3.4 |
| Zimbabwe | 1990 | Data available for aggregated 65+ age group only: 33.6 8.3 19.9 | | | | | |
| **Asia** | | | | | | | |
| China (Hong Kong SAR) | 2002 | 26.1 | 12.9 | 19.5 | 44.0 | 31.9 | 36.8 |
| China (mainland, selected rural and urban areas) | 1999 | 43.7 | 39.2 | 41.3 | 84.2 | 61.2 | 70.7 |
| China (mainland, selected rural areas) | 1999 | 83.8 | 70.4 | 76.8 | 139.7 | 102.2 | 117.6 |
| China (mainland, selected urban areas) | 1999 | 16.5 | 17.1 | 16.8 | 39.9 | 27.7 | 32.8 |
| Georgia | 2001 | 9.0 | 2.4 | 5.1 | 5.2 | 5.2 | 5.2 |
| Iran | 1991 | 0.4 | 0.2 | 0.3 | 2.0 | 0.0 | 1.1 |
| Japan | 2003 | 44.9 | 20.9 | 32.1 | 45.2 | 24.6 | 32.1 |
| Kazakhstan | 2003 | 69.5 | 16.2 | 37.2 | 60.5 | 23.1 | 33.4 |
| Kuwait | 2002 | 0.0 | 0.0 | 0.0 | 0.0 | 0.0 | 0.0 |
| Kyrgystan | 2004 | 29.0 | 0.0 | 12.4 | 32.7 | 12.1 | 18.7 |
| Philippines | 1993 | 1.5 | 0.8 | 1.2 | 3.2 | 2.8 | 3.0 |
| Republic of Korea | 2002 | 66.2 | 26.1 | 42.6 | 130.5 | 61.4 | 83.4 |
| Singapore | 2003 | 19.0 | 17.1 | 18.0 | 57.5 | 29.7 | 41.2 |
| Sri Lanka | 1991 | Data available for aggregated 65+ age group only: 87.0 21.0 | | | | | |
| Tajikistan | 2001 | 2.4 | 3.4 | 2.9 | 3.7 | 4.6 | 4.3 |
| Thailand | 2002 | 17.2 | 4.6 | 10.3 | 16.1 | 5.0 | 9.6 |
| Turkmenistan | 1998 | 10.6 | 4.1 | 6.9 | 12.9 | 17.5 | 16.1 |
| Uzbekistan | 2002 | 9.3 | 4.0 | 6.4 | 13.7 | 6.1 | 8.7 |
| **Australia and Western Pacific** | | | | | | | |
| Australia | 2002 | 17.6 | 5.1 | 11.1 | 22.1 | 5.2 | 11.9 |
| New Zealand | 2000 | 20.7 | 1.5 | 10.8 | 20.7 | 3.2 | 9.9 |
| **Europe** | | | | | | | |
| Albania | 2003 | 3.7 | 3.7 | 3.7 | 3.1 | 12.2 | 8.6 |
| Armenia | 2003 | 4.1 | 1.5 | 2.6 | 9.2 | 4.8 | 6.3 |
| Austria | 2004 | 47.6 | 16.0 | 30.3 | 93.1 | 17.5 | 42.2 |
| Azerbaijan | 2002 | 5.2 | 2.3 | 3.6 | 4.4 | 1.1 | 2.2 |
| Belarus | 2003 | 91.0 | 18.3 | 45.2 | 81.1 | 20.8 | 36.5 |
| Belgium | 1997 | 35.5 | 13.6 | 23.4 | 86.8 | 15.6 | 39.7 |
| Bosnia and Herzegovina | 1991 | 12.9 | 6.5 | 9.0 | 32.7 | 11.1 | 19.8 |
| Bulgaria | 2004 | 28.6 | 15.5 | 21.2 | 68.9 | 17.9 | 37.7 |
| Croatia | 2004 | 63.9 | 18.0 | 37.5 | 125.3 | 23.2 | 56.2 |
| Czech Republic | 2004 | 31.0 | 10.2 | 19.1 | 58.0 | 15.1 | 29.5 |
| Denmark | 2001 | 25.4 | 16.7 | 20.8 | 58.7 | 20.0 | 34.3 |
| Estonia | 2002 | 62.9 | 11.0 | 30.4 | 81.5 | 23.1 | 38.1 |
| Finland | 2004 | 44.0 | 8.5 | 24.6 | 39.6 | 8.0 | 18.4 |
| France | 2002 | 38.2 | 13.4 | 24.6 | 72.4 | 16.4 | 36.5 |
| Germany | 2004 | 28.3 | 10.1 | 18.6 | 55.8 | 17.1 | 29.7 |
| Greece | 2003 | 7.4 | 1.9 | 4.4 | 10.1 | 1.2 | 5.0 |
| Hungary | 2003 | 78.5 | 20.1 | 43.2 | 110.4 | 36.1 | 60.4 |
| Iceland | 2003 | 11.4 | 0.0 | 5.5 | 0.0 | 0.0 | 0.0 |
| Ireland | 2002 | 19.7 | 3.1 | 11.0 | 9.7 | 2.5 | 5.3 |

**Table 94.1** (Continued) Elderly suicide rates in selected countries by age and sex

| Country | Year | Age 65–74 years | | | Age 75+ years | | |
|---|---|---|---|---|---|---|---|
| | | M | F | All | M | F | All |
| Israel | 2003 | 18.5 | 6.4 | 11.8 | 23.3 | 5.6 | 12.7 |
| Italy | 2002 | 18.5 | 5.0 | 11.1 | 31.9 | 5.8 | 15.2 |
| Latvia | 2004 | 64.7 | 8.4 | 29.3 | 73.2 | 22.4 | 35.4 |
| Lithuania | 2004 | 91.9 | 14.6 | 43.9 | 80.2 | 27.8 | 42.9 |
| Luxemburg | 2004 | 18.0 | 20.5 | 19.4 | 72.6 | 16.2 | 35.5 |
| Macedonia FYR | 2003 | 22.1 | 8.8 | 14.9 | 41.2 | 17.8 | 27.8 |
| Malta | 2004 | 14.4 | 0.0 | 6.4 | 23.8 | 15.3 | 18.6 |
| Netherlands | 2004 | 11.6 | 5.2 | 8.2 | 22.6 | 9.1 | 14.0 |
| Norway | 2003 | 17.3 | 5.8 | 11.2 | 20.6 | 5.0 | 10.8 |
| Poland | 2003 | 32.7 | 6.6 | 17.4 | 29.4 | 6.0 | 13.5 |
| Portugal | 2003 | 33.1 | 7.7 | 19.0 | 68.9 | 12.5 | 34.0 |
| Republic of Moldova | 2004 | 40.5 | 9.4 | 21.7 | 38.1 | 10.8 | 20.0 |
| Romania | 2004 | 31.2 | 7.9 | 17.9 | 29.1 | 7.7 | 15.8 |
| Russian Federation | 2004 | 80.9 | 15.4 | 39.3 | 88.9 | 26.0 | 41.7 |
| Serbia and Montenegro | 2002 | 59.6 | 20.9 | 38.2 | 101.9 | 36.3 | 61.3 |
| Slovakia | 2002 | 28.4 | 4.1 | 13.9 | 60.9 | 9.1 | 26.5 |
| Slovenia | 2003 | 88.7 | 25.1 | 52.2 | 115.1 | 27.9 | 53.8 |
| Spain | 2003 | 20.9 | 6.0 | 12.8 | 42.9 | 8.1 | 21.3 |
| Sweden | 2002 | 28.8 | 8.4 | 18.0 | 36.5 | 10.1 | 20.3 |
| Switzerland | 2002 | 42.9 | 16.8 | 28.6 | 82.6 | 31.0 | 49.7 |
| Ukraine | 2004 | 58.4 | 11.1 | 29.2 | 66.5 | 18.1 | 31.2 |
| United Kingdom | 2002 | 8.7 | 3.4 | 5.9 | 10.4 | 3.7 | 6.1 |
| **North and South America** | | | | | | | |
| Argentina | 1996 | 22.2 | 5.2 | 12.6 | 42.4 | 7.7 | 20.5 |
| Belize | 1995 | 0.0 | 0.0 | 0.0 | 50.0 | 0.0 | 25.0 |
| Brazil | 1995 | 15.6 | 3.2 | 8.8 | 18.3 | 3.1 | 9.5 |
| Canada | 2002 | 19.1 | 3.4 | 10.9 | 23.7 | 2.7 | 10.7 |
| Chile | 1994 | 20.2 | 1.8 | 9.8 | 26.7 | 1.4 | 10.9 |
| Colombia | 1994 | 9.7 | 1.5 | 5.3 | 13.4 | 0.7 | 6.3 |
| Costa Rica | 1995 | 9.5 | 0.0 | 4.6 | 8.4 | 0.0 | 3.7 |
| Cuba | 1996 | 62.6 | 26.0 | 43.8 | 113.2 | 27.3 | 68.0 |
| Ecuador | 1995 | 9.1 | 2.4 | 5.6 | 10.7 | 1.0 | 5.2 |
| El Salvador | 1993 | 9.3 | 3.3 | 6.0 | 19.9 | 8.8 | 13.2 |
| Guyana | 1994 | 20.0 | 8.3 | 13.6 | 25.0 | 0.0 | 10.0 |
| Mexico | 1995 | 9.7 | 1.2 | 5.1 | 18.0 | 1.0 | 8.6 |
| Nicaragua | 1994 | 7.3 | 0.0 | 3.3 | 18.8 | 4.2 | 10.0 |
| Paraguay | 1994 | 17.4 | 4.9 | 10.3 | 9.0 | 5.7 | 7.0 |
| Puerto Rico | 1992 | 31.6 | 4.5 | 17.0 | 24.3 | 2.4 | 16.7 |
| Suriname | 1992 | 0.0 | 16.7 | 9.1 | 0.0 | 0.0 | 0.0 |
| Trinidad and Tobago | 1994 | 38.9 | 12.1 | 25.5 | 21.2 | 0.0 | 10.0 |
| United States | 2002 | 24.7 | 4.1 | 13.5 | 40.7 | 4.1 | 17.8 |
| Uruguay | 1990 | 29.2 | 16.8 | 22.7 | 71.2 | 10.0 | 32.4 |
| Venezuela | 1994 | 24.8 | 2.9 | 13.0 | 28.6 | 2.0 | 13.2 |

Source: World Health Organization, 2006.

regarding quality of life among the Whites, cultural taboos against suicide among the Blacks, and religious sanctions against suicide among the Asians and the Coloureds (Flisher and Parry 1994; Flisher *et al.* 1997; Scribante *et al.* 2004).) Also, the high suicide rates may be related to the increase in the elderly population, leading to reduced resources available for this age group, paralleled by lack of suicide prevention initiatives, discrepancies in government expenditures on healthcare resources and social security (Burrows *et al.* 2003; Flisher *et al.* 2004).

## Asia

Given the geographical, cultural, political and socio-economic diversity of Asian countries, often accompanied by scarcity of research and epidemiological data on suicide in many nations, it is difficult to give a concise overview of elderly suicide in the continent. Available evidence suggests that there are significant differences in age-related suicide patterns between Asian and Western countries. In Western countries, rates of suicide are high in the 15–25 age groups and highest in the elderly, while in Asia those under the age of 30 often have the highest suicide rates (Vijayakumar 2005; Vijayakumar *et al.* 2005a, b). Nonetheless, for the period 1999–2001, suicide rates among elderly males in China (59.2 per 100,000 in 1999) and South Korea (55.4 per 100,000 in 2000), and elderly females in China (63.1 per 100,000 in 1999), Hong Kong, SAR (26.6 per 100,000 in 1999), Japan (26.0 per 100,000 in 1999) and South Korea (23.0 per 100,000 in 2000) were among the highest globally (De Leo and Evans 2004). Given the unique suicide patterns of China, with regard to gender, age and urban/rural characteristics, a detailed analysis of elderly suicide in the country is presented in the next section.

### China as an example

China accounts for more than 30 per cent of the world's number of suicides; however, national suicide mortality rates have been decreasing from 22.9 per 100,000 in 1991 to 15.4 per 100,000 in 2000 (Yip 2001; Yip *et al.* 2005). When compared to Western nations, China displays significant disparities in age- and sex-specific rates in rural and urban parts of the country (Phillips *et al.* 2002). There are reported similarities among Chinese elderly suicides of Beijing, Taiwan, Singapore and Hong Kong, SAR; however, the urban suicide rate is lower in Beijing than in other Asian cities (Yip and Tan 1998; Yip *et al.* 1998; Tsoh *et al.* 2005; Chan *et al.* 2006).

A study of the epidemiological profile of suicides in Beijing over the period of 1987–1996 indicated that suicide rates were increasing with age. Rural males over the age of 75 had the highest suicide rates (109.1 per 100,000), twelve times higher than among rural youths (15–24 years old) (Yip 2001). Among urban males of 75 years of age and older, rates were approximately three times lower (38.3 per 100,000).

In parallel with age trends in non-fatal suicidal behaviour observed in other countries, the WHO/SUPRE-MISS study results showed that the majority of suicide attempters in the Chinese site (i.e. Yuncheng) belonged to the younger age groups (the mean age of females was 30 and 33 for males) (Fleischmann *et al.* 2005), while the older attempters over the age of 65 accounted for 4.2 per cent of all recorded cases.

In China, the problem of elderly suicide is particularly serious, due to the lack of effective welfare systems (including pension programmes), increasing poverty of the elderly, and sociocultural

transitions taking place in the country (He and Lester 2001; Ji *et al.* 2001; Yip *et al.* 2005). Traditionally, the younger generations respect and take care of the elderly; however, the one-child policy introduced in the 1970s, and the ongoing disintegration of the three-generational family in most parts of the country, have led to increasing social isolation among the elders.

## Australia and the Western Pacific

In Australia and New Zealand, similarly to the other countries in the New World (i.e. Canada and United States), suicide mortality among males 65 years of age has been declining since the late 1980s, following an increase in the early 1980s (De Leo and Evans 2004). Suicide rates of elderly females have been steadily declining over the last two decades, with the trend most notable in New Zealand. In both countries, suicide rates among the elderly males and females are relatively low compared to the elderly suicide rates (65–74 and 75+ age groups) in other parts of the world (for details see Table 94.1, and a detailed analysis of elderly suicide in Australia is presented in the next section). Unfortunately, due to the lack of suicide mortality and morbidity data in the Pacific Island countries, it is not possible to ascertain the incidence of elderly suicide in that region. However, data available from Fiji, Guam and Western Samoa indicates that from 1988–1992, suicide rates were the highest in the 15–24 age group in both males and females, and declining with age (Booth 1999). A similar pattern was also reported in Micronesia from 1960–1987 (Booth 1999).

### Australia as an example

According to official data in 2005, Australia's national suicide rate was 10.3 per 100,000, and suicide comprised 1.6 per cent of all deaths (ABS 2007). In 2005, the suicide rate among the elderly in the 65–74-year-old group was below the national rate (i.e. 9.6 per 100,000), and the suicide rate in those aged 75+ was higher (11.8 per 100,000). However, from the mid-1960s to 2002, mortality rates for those 75+ years of age in both genders have halved (De Leo and Heller 2004).

In Australia, among other New World Anglo-Saxon countries, suicide mortality rates in older males (75+) have been in decline since late 1980s, but sharper declines have been observed in elderly females, especially those aged 65–74 (Cantor *et al.* 1999; De Leo and Evans 2004). Simultaneously, there has been an increase in youth and young adult suicides (Snowdon and Hunt 2002; Pritchard and Hansen 2005).

Apart from improved financial status and psychosocial assistance, the decrease in elderly suicide rates in Australia and other Anglo-Saxon countries has been attributed to improved health, increased life expectancy, and higher levels of activity, as well as to reduced feelings of redundancy among the older generation. Today, 'the over 65s, relative to previous generations, are more affluent and healthier than ever before' (Pritchard and Hansen 2005, p. 22). It has also been speculated that limited access to lethal means used in suicide could have played a role in this process (Pritchard and Hansen 2005; De Leo 2006).

Results from a large population survey conducted in Queensland indicated that the lifetime prevalence of suicidal ideation and behaviour was the highest in the 25–44-year-old group, and declined with increasing age (De Leo *et al.* 2005), a result similar to studies performed in Europe and the US (e.g. Diekstra and Gulbinat 1993; Kessler *et al.* 1999). In the survey, 6.1 per cent of respondents in the age group 65–74 years reported having seriously considered suicide in the course of their lives, 2.4 per cent reported having planned it, and 2.3 per cent reported having attempted suicide (results for the 75+ age group were 6.9, 0.3 and 1.6 per cent, respectively) (De Leo *et al.* 2005).

## Europe

A recent analysis of epidemiology of suicide among the elderly in 19 European countries between 1999 and 2001 has revealed similar rates and trends in nations clustered according to their sociopolitical and geographical similarities (De Leo and Evans 2004, also see Table 94.1 for the most recent data available to the WHO). The highest suicides rates among males 65 years and over were found in Eastern European nations (i.e. Lithuania, Latvia, Russian Federation, Hungary and Bulgaria; between 56.8 and 94.8 per 100,000 in Bulgaria and Russia in 2000, respectively), and some parts of Western Europe (i.e. 61.3 per 100,000 in 2001 in Austria, 55.6 per 100,000 in 1999 in France, and 55.4 per 100,000 in 1999 in Switzerland). The lowest elderly male rates were reported in the Old World countries: Northern Ireland (7.8 per 100,000 in 2000), England and Wales (11.6 per 100,000 in 2000), Scotland (13.2 per 100,000 in 2000) and Ireland (17.6 per 1000,000 in 1999). The pattern of suicide rates in elderly females was somewhat different; although, the highest rates in Europe were still found in Eastern European countries (e.g. 28.2 per 100,000 in Hungary in 2002 and 24.5 per 100,000 in Lithuania in 2000), the lowest rates were reported in southern Europe: Greece (2.9 per 100,000 in 1999), Portugal (5.5 per 100,000 in 2000), and Italy (6.1 per 100,000 in 1999).

### Italy as an example

Suicide rates in Italy have been rather stable over the last two decades, with overall rates around 6 cases per 100,000 (ISTAT 2004). A detailed analysis of suicide trends over the period of 1887–1993 indicated a significant decrease in suicide rates for young people (15–24 years old), especially in females, and a rise in suicide among individuals over the age of 55 (De Leo *et al.* 1997). Over the last century, suicide rates of the elderly exhibited a rather stable trend with a marked increase at the end of the 1970s (with a peak of 23.1 per 100,000 in 1985), followed by relatively stable high rates of over 20 per 100,000 from 1985 onwards (ISTAT 2004).

Tatarelli *et al.* (1999) pointed out the non-uniformity of the nationwide distribution of suicides in Italy, an observation confirmed by recent analyses of elderly suicide mortality in the southern (Pavia *et al.* 2005) and northern parts of the country (Zeppegno *et al.* 2005).

De Leo *et al.* (1997) noted a discrepancy between the recent increase in the ageing Italian population and a relative lack of public health and social services to meet the needs of this group. The changing family structure, by moving away from the traditional patriarchal three-generational model providing protection, and emotional and economic stability, has resulted in loss of spontaneous support for the elderly. Conversely, the development of institutionalized social and health facilities, which is able to compensate at least in part for the loss of traditional support, is slow (Pritchard and Baldwin 2000). The structural changes in society and the family resulting from industrialization and urbanization (including lack of job opportunities) led to an altering in the social role played by the elderly, both for males and females, and their increasing isolation. As a result, the elderly males find that taking care of themselves has become increasingly challenging (as in other Latin American countries), while ageing females lose their traditional function in the family, and share the fate of loneliness and institutionalization with men.

## South and North America

The elderly suicide rates for both genders in Canada and United States have been declining since the end of the 1980s, and although suicide rates in elderly females in both North American countries are among the lowest globally, the male rates are elevated (De Leo and Evans 2004). Furthermore, suicide rates among the elderly (especially males) are among the highest across the lifespan, for example, 15.6 per 100,000 in 2002 for the 65+ age group (both males and females) in the US (McKeown *et al.* 2006), and 26.9 and 7.5 per 100,000 (for males and females, respectively) in British Columbia, Canada during 1981–1991 (Agbayewa *et al.* 1998). Unfortunately, there seems to be a scarcity of research and updated epidemiological data regarding suicide, including elderly suicide, in many South American countries.

### Brazil as an example

Brazil has one of the lowest suicide rates in the world (4 per 100,000 in 2000); however, in terms of absolute numbers of deaths, Brazil is among the ten countries with the highest number of suicides—over 6,000 per year (De Mello-Santos *et al.* 2005).

The analysis of suicide trends in Brazil during 1980–2000 shows that suicide rates have increased from the 45–54 age group onward, with individuals over the age of 65 representing the subpopulation with the highest suicide rates (De Mello-Santos *et al.* 2005). In 2000, the suicide rate for the age range 65–74 was 6.9 per 100,000 (12.1 in males and 2.5 in females), and 7.2 per 100,000 in people of 75+ years of age (14.2 in males and 2.1 in females).

While rates of fatal suicidal behaviour in Brazil follow the pattern characteristics for Latin American countries (i.e. the risk for suicide increasing with age), data from the WHO/SUPRE-MISS study showed that suicide attempters (in the catchment area of Campinas) concentrate mostly among young adults of both sexes. The elderly recorded only 1.2 per cent of all cases of non-fatal suicidal behaviour (Fleischmann *et al.* 2005).

Rodrigues and Werneck (2005) reported that, compared to younger generations, older Brazilian cohorts are at higher risk of suicide, in both genders. Worse, early life conditions experienced by today's elderly people (wars, urbanization, industrialization, and serious political changes) were suggested as a possible explanation for this phenomenon (Rodrigues and Werneck 2005).

# Conclusions

Understanding suicide and suicidal processes poses specific challenges at different stages across the lifespan; it appears more difficult in the elderly, due to the relatively limited numbers of behaviours (i.e. less suicide attempts, less repeats, more masked intent), and to a perhaps increasing attitudinal divide between the old and the young (De Leo *et al.* 2001). The task of deepening the knowledge on elderly suicide and its prevention is even more challenging in the global perspective, given the lack of epidemiological data from many countries, the complexity of cultural, ethnic and socio-economic factors involved, and the generally insufficient attention that elderly suicide has attracted so far.

Most research on suicide in older adults has been conducted in Western countries, and only a few studies have tried to examine this phenomenon and its correlates across the five continents. Recently, this situation has been slowly changing with new information deriving from studies conducted in Asian countries, including China (Tsoh *et al.* 2005), Hong Kong, SAR (Chiu *et al.* 2004), India (Abraham *et al.* 2005), Japan (Awata *et al.* 2005), and Taiwan (Yen *et al.* 2005). Results of these investigations show that there are a number of similarities between the Western and Asian countries in regard to risk factors, including depression, physical illness and previous history of suicidal behaviour (De Leo *et al.* 2002; Snowdon and Baume 2002). However, other studies indicate that the psychosocial dynamics of suicide outside the Western context are different (Chan *et al.* 2004), but seem to be rapidly changing as a result of the Westernization of traditional cultures (Pritchard and Baldwin 2000, 2002; Chiu *et al.* 2004; Yip *et al.* 2005).

Cultural values and attitudes, as well as the legal and political context in many countries, lead to methodological problems in the study of elderly suicide, as it is a case of criminalization of suicide as well as of attempted suicide, for example in India (Fleischmann *et al.* 2005). Suicide remains a taboo subject, not only in Hong Kong, SAR (Chiu *et al.* 2004), but also in many other countries where negative attitudes towards persons with suicidal behaviours continue to exist (see Part 1 of this book).

Despite an epidemiological dimension that should not permit any neglect, suicide in old age still attracts very little attention from media (which focuses much more on youth suicide) and public health planners. As a consequence, elderly suicidal behaviour has been the target of a small and barely relevant number of preventive programmes. This may reflect some of the many nihilistic aspects of the ageism culture, which, for example, considers depression as a normal/natural feature of the old age, elderly suicide as understandable, rational, and unpreventable (Draper 2006), and older adults as second or third rank citizens. In the words of Snowdon and Baume: 'it may be that the health strategists have formed a view that suicides in late life are often understandable, and little can be done to prevent them' (2002, p. 261). Clearly, elderly suicide prevention should start from fighting this very perspective.

## References

Abraham VJ, Abraham S, Jacob S (2005). Suicide in the elderly in Kaniyambadi block, Tamil Nadu, South India. *International Journal of Geriatric Psychiatry*, **20**, 953–955.

ABS (2007). *Suicides 2005*. 3309.0. Australian Bureau of Statistics, Canberra.

Agbayewa MO, Marion SA, Wiggins S (1998). Socioeconomic factors associated with suicide in elderly populations in British Columbia: an 11-year review. *Canadian Journal of Psychiatry*, **43**, 829–836.

Alem A, Kebede D, Jacobsson L *et al.* (1999). Suicide attempts among adults in Butajira, Ethiopia. *Acta Psychiatrica Scandinavica Suppl*, **397**, 70–76.

Alte da Veiga F and Saraiva CB (2003). Age patterns of suicide: identification and characterisation of European clusters and trends. *Crisis*, **24**, 56–67.

Awata S, Seki T, Koizumi Y *et al.* (2005). Factors associated with suicidal ideation in an elderly urban Japanese population: a community-based, cross-sectional study. *Psychiatry and Clinical Neuroscience*, **59**, 327–336.

Berk M, Dodd S, Henry M (2005). The effect of macroeconomic variables on suicide. *Psychological Medicine*, **36**, 181–189.

Bertolote JM and Fleischman A (2005). Suicidal behaviour prevention: WHO perspectives on research. *American Journal of Medical Genetics Part C: Seminar in Medical Genetic*s, **133**, 8–12.

Booth H (1999). Pacific Island suicide in comparative perspective. *Journal of Biosocial Science*, **31**, 433–448.

Burrows S, Vaez M, Butchart A *et al.* (2003). The share of suicide in injury deaths in the South African context: sociodemographic distribution. *Public Health*, **117**, 3–10.

Caine ED and Conwell Y (2001). Suicide in the elderly. *International Clinical Psychopharmacology*, **16**, S25–S30.

Cantor CH, Neuringer K, De Leo D (1999). Australian suicide trends 1964–1997: youth and beyond? *Medical Journal of Australia*, **171**, 137–141.

Chan CY, Beh SL, Broadhurst RG (2004). Homicide-suicide in Hong Kong, 1989–1998. *Forensic Science International*, **140**, 261–267.

Chan SMS, Chiu FKH, Lam CWH *et al.* (2006). Elderly suicide and the 2003 SARS epidemic in Hong Kong. *International Journal of Geriatric Psychiatry*, **21**, 113–118.

Chiu HF, Yip PS, Chi I *et al.* (2004). Elderly suicide in Hong Kong: a case-controlled psychological autopsy study. *Acta Psychiatrica Scandinavica*, **109**, 299–305.

Chou K-L, Jun LW, Chi I (2005). Assessing Chinese older adults' suicidal ideation: Chinese version of the Geriatric Suicide Ideation Scale. *Aging and Mental Health*, **9**, 167–171.

Conwell Y, Duberstein PR, Caine ED (2002). Risk factors for suicide in later life. *Biological Psychiatry*, **52**, 193–204.

De Leo D (1998). Is suicide prediction in old age really easier? *Crisis*, **19**, 60–61.

De Leo D (1999). Cultural issues in suicide and old age. *Crisis*, **20**, 53–55.

De Leo D (2003). Suicide over the lifespan: the elderly. In R Kastenbaum, ed., *Macmillan Encyclopedia of Death and Dying*, pp. 837–843. Thomson Gale, New York.

De Leo D (2006). Suicide in Australia. What we know and are seeking to discover. In D De Leo, H Herrman, S Ueda *et al.*, eds, *An Australian-Japanese Perspective on Suicide Prevention: Culture, Community, and Care*, pp. 17–35. Commonwealth of Australia, Department of Health and Aging, Canberra.

De Leo D and Diekstra RFW (1990). *Depression and Suicide in Late Life*. Hogrefe and Huber, Goettingen.

De Leo D and Evans R (2004). *International Suicide Rates and Prevention Strategies*. Hogrefe and Huber, Goettingen.

De Leo D and Heller T (2004). *Suicide in Queensland, 1999–2001. Mortality Rates and Related Data*. Australian Institute for Suicide Research and Prevention, Brisbane.

De Leo D and Spathonis K (2003). Culture and suicide in late life. *Psychiatric Times*, **20**, 14–17.

De Leo D and Spathonis K (2004) Suicide and suicidal behaviour in late life. In D De Leo, U Bille-Brahe, A Kerkhof *et al.*, eds, *Suicidal Behaviour. Theories and Research Findings*, pp. 253–286. Hogrefe and Huber, Goettingen.

De Leo D, Cerin E, Spathonis K *et al.* (2005). Lifetime risk of suicide ideation and attempts in an Australian community: prevalence, suicidal process, and help-seeking behaviour. *Journal of Affective Disorders*, **86**, 215–224.

De Leo D, Conforti D, Carollo G (1997). A century of suicide in Italy: a comparison between the old and the young. *Suicide and Life-Threatening Behaviour*, **27**, 239–249.

De Leo D, Padovani W, Lonnqvist J *et al.* (2002). Repetition of suicidal behaviour in elderly Europeans: a prospective longitudinal study. *Journal of Affective Disorders*, **72**, 291–295.

De Leo D, Padovani W, Scocco P *et al.* (2001). Attempted and completed suicide in older subjects: RESULTS from the WHO/EURO Multi-centre Study of Suicidal Behaviour. *International Journal of Geriatric Psychiatry*, **16**, 1–11.

De Mello-Santos C, Bertolote JM, Wang Y-P (2005). Epidemiology of suicide in Brazil (1980–2000): characterization of age and gender rates of suicide. *Revista Brasileira de Psiquiatria*, **27**, 131–134.

Diekstra RFW and Gulbinat W (1993). The epidemiology of suicidal behaviour: a review of three continents. *WHO Statistical Quarterly*, **46**, 52–68.

Draper B (2006) Suicide in the elderly. Prevention from an Australian context. In D De Leo, H Herrman, S Ueda *et al.*, eds, *An Australian-Japanese Perspective on Suicide Prevention: Culture, Community, and Care*, pp. 81–87. Commonwealth of Australia, Department of Healt and Aging, Canberra.

Fleischmann A, Bertolote JM, De Leo D *et al.* (2005). Characteristics of attempted suicides seen in emergency-care settings of general hospitals in eight low- and middle-income countries. *Psychological Medicine*, **35**, 1467–1474.

Flisher AJ, Liang H, Laubscher R *et al.* (2004). Suicide trends in South Africa, 1968–1990. *Scandinavian Journal of Public Heath*, **32**, 411–418.

Flisher AJ and Parry CD (1994). Suicide in South Africa. An analysis of nationally registered mortality date for 1984–1986. *Acta Psychiatrica Scandinavica*, **90**, 348–353.

Flisher AJ, Parry CD, Bradshaw D *et al.* (1997). Seasonal variation of suicide in South Africa. *Psychiatry Research*, **66**, 13–22.

Forsell Y, Jorm AF, Winblad B (1997). Suicidal thoughts and associated factors in an elderly population. *Acta Psychaitrica Scandinavica*, **95**, 108–111.

Fujisawa D, Tanaka E, Sakamoto S *et al.* (2005). The development of brief screening instrument for depression and suicidal ideation for elderly: The Depression and Suicide Screen. *Psychiatry and Clinical Neuroscience*, **59**, 634–638.

Gureje O, Kola L, Uwakwe R *et al.* (2007). The profile and risks of suicidal behaviours in the Nigerian Survey of Mental Health and Well-being. *Psychological Medicine*, **37**, 821–830.

Hawton K, Harriss L, Hodder K *et al.* (2001). The influence of the economic and social environment on deliberate self-harm and suicide: an ecological and person-based study. *Psychological Medicine*, **31**, 827–836.

He ZX and Lester D (2001). Elderly suicide in China. *Psychological Reports*, **89**, 675–676.

ISTAT (2004). *Suicidi e Tentativi di Suicidio. Rapporto 2004.* [Suicides and Attempted Suicide. 2004 Report]. Istituto Italiano di Statistiche, Roma.

Ji J, Kleinman A, Becker AE (2001). Suicide in contemporary China: a review of China's distinctive suicide demographics in their sociocultural context. *Harvard Review of Psychiatry*, **9**, 1–12.

Jorm AF, Henderson AS, Scott R *et al.* (1995). Factors associated with the wish to die in elderly people. *Age and Ageing*, **24**, 389–392.

Kebede D and Alem A (1999). Suicide attempts and ideation among adults in Addis Ababa, Ethiopia. *Acta Psychiatrica Scandinavica Suppl*, **397**, 35–39.

Kessler R., Borges G, Walters M (1999). Prevalence of and risk factors for lifetime suicide attempts in the national comorbidity survey. *Archives of General Psychiatry*, **56**, 617–626.

McIntosh JL (1992). Epidemiology of suicide in the elderly. *Suicide and Life-Threatening Behaviour*, **22**, 15–35.

McKeown R, Cuffe SP, Schulz R (2006). US suicide rates by age group, 1970–2002: an examination of recent trends. *American Journal of Public Health*, **96**, 1744–1751.

Meel B (2006). Epidemiogy of suicide by hanging in Transkei, South Africa. *American Journal of Forensic Medicine and Pathology*, **27**, 75–78.

Neulinger K and De Leo D (2001) Suicide in elderly and youth populations. How do they differ? In D De Leo, ed., *Suicide and Euthanasia in Older Adults*, pp. 137–153. Hogrefe and Huber, Goettingen.

Nordberg E (2000). Injuries as a public health problem in sub-Saharan Africa: epidemiology and prospects for control. *East African Medical Journal*, **77**, S1–43.

Pavia M, Nicotera G, Scaramuzza G *et al.* (2005). Suicide mortality in Southern Italy: 1998–2002. *Psychiatry Research*, **134**, 275–279.

Pearson JL and Brown JK (2000). Suicide prevention in late life: directions for science and practice. *Clinical Psychology Review*, **20**, 685–705.

Phillips M, Li X, Zhang Y (2002). Suicide rates in China, 1995–99. *Lancet*, **359**, 835–840.

Pritchard C and Baldwin DS (2000). Effects of age and gender on elderly suicide rates in Catholic and Orthodox countries: an inadvertent neglect? *International Journal of Geriatric Psychiatry*, **15**, 904–910.

Pritchard C and Baldwin DS (2002). Elderly suicide rates in Asian and English-speaking countries. *Acta Psychiatrica Scandinavica*, **105**, 271–275.

Pritchard C and Hansen L (2005). Comparison of suicide in people aged 65–74 and 75+ by gender in England and Wales and the major Western countries 1979–1999. *International Journal of Geriatric Psychiatry*, **20**, 17–25.

Rodrigues NCP and Werneck GL (2005). Age-period-cohort analysis of suicide rates in Rio de Janeiro, Brazil, 1979–1998. *Social Psychiatry and Psychiatric Epidemiology*, **40**, 192–196.

Rudmin FW, Ferrada-Nolli M, Skolbekken J-A (2003). Questions of culture, age and gender in the epidemiology of suicide. *Scandinavian Journal of Psychology*, **44**, 373–381.

Schmidtke A, Bille-Brahe U, De Leo D *et al.* (2004). Sociodemographic characteristics of suicide attempters in Europe. In A Schmidtke, U Bille-Brahe, D De Leo *et al.*, eds, *Suicidal Behaviour in Europe*, pp. 29–43. Hogrefe and Huber, Goettingen.

Scocco P and De Leo D (2002). One-year prevalence of death thoughts, suicide ideation and behaviours in an elderly population. *International Journal of Geriatric Psychiatry*, **17**, 842–846.

Scocco P, Meneghel G, Caon F *et al.* (2001). Death ideation and its correlates: survey of an over-65-year-old population. *Journal of Nervous and Mental Disease*, **189**, 210–218.

Scribante L, Blumenthal R, Saayman G *et al.* (2004). A retrospective review of 1018 suicide cases from the capital city of South Africa for the period 1997–2000. *American Journal of Forensic Medicine and Pathology*, **25**, 52–55.

Skoog I, Aevarsson O, Beskow J *et al.* (1996). Suicidal feelings in a population sample of non-demented 85-year-olds. *American Journal of Psychiatry*, **153**, 1015–1020.

Snowdon J and Baume P (2002). A study of suicides of older people in Sydney. *International Journal of Geriatric Psychiatry*, **17**, 261–269.

Snowdon J and Hunt GE (2002). Age, period and cohort effects on suicide rates in Australia, 1919–1999. *Acta Psychiatrica Scandinavica*, **105**, 265–270.

Suominen K, Isometsa E, Lonnqvist J (2004). Elderly suicide attempters with depression are often diagnosed only after the attempt. *International Journal of Geriatric Psychiatry*, **19**, 35–40.

Tatarelli R, Mancinelli, I Comparelli A *et al.* (1999). Suicide among elderly in Italy: a descriptive epidemiological study (1969–1994). *Comprehensive Psychiatry*, **40**, 253–260.

Tsoh J, Chiu HF, Duberstein PR *et al.* (2005). Attempted suicide in elderly Chinese persons: a multi-group, controlled study. *American Journal of Geriatric Psychiatry*, **13**, 562–571.

Yen YC, Yang MJ, Yang MS *et al.* (2005). Suicidal ideation and associated factors among community dwelling elders in Taiwan. *Psychiatry and Clinical Neuroscience*, **59**, 364–371.

Yip PSF (2001). An epidemiological profile of suicides in Beijing, China. *Suicide and Life-Threatening Behaviour*, **31**, 62–70.

Yip PSF, Chi I, Yu KK (1998). An epidemiological profile of elderly suicides in Hong Kong. *International Journal of Geriatric Psychiatry*, **13**, 631–637.

Yip PSF, Liu KY, Hu J *et al.* (2005). Suicide rates in China during a decade of rapid social changes. *Social Psychiatry and Psychiatric Epidemiology*, **40**, 792–798.

Yip PS and Tan RC (1998). Suicides in Hong Kong and Singapore: a tale of two cities. *International Journal of Social Psychiatry*, **44**, 267–279.

Vijayakumar L (2005). Suicide and mental disorders in Asia. *International Review of Psychiatry*, **17**, 109–114.

Vijayakumar L, Nagaraj K, Pirkis J *et al.* (2005a). Suicide in developing countries (1): Frequency, distribution, and association with socioeconomic indicators. *Crisis*, **26**, 104–111.

Vijayakumar L, Sujit J, Pirkis J *et al.* (2005b). Suicide in developing countries (2): Risk factors. *Crisis*, **26**, 112–119.

World Health Organization (2006). *Figures and Facts About Suicide.* Updated country charts retrieved 31 March 2007 from http://www. who.int/mental_health/prevention/suicide/country_reports/en/

Wu WCH and Bond MH (2006). National differences in predictors of suicide among young and elderly citizens: linking societal predictors to psychological factors. *Archives of Suicide Research*, **10**, 45–60.

Zeppegno P, Manzetti E, Valsesia R *et al.* (2005). Differences in suicide behaviour in the elderly: a study in two provinces in Italy. *International Journal of Geriatric Psychiatry*, **20**, 769–775.

# CHAPTER 95

# Suicidal elderly people in clinical and community settings

## Risk factors, treatment and suicide prevention

Diego De Leo, Brian Draper and Karolina Krysinska

## Introduction

Suicide in old age is still exposed to misunderstandings and controversies. From one side, in fact, it is the object of idiosyncratic interpretations (e.g. if subjects of advanced age are so close to their natural exit from life, why should they decide to hasten it?). From the other, the very answers to this question have fed a rationalistic view of elderly suicide that is widespread among community members: that self-killing may become an acceptable solution when facing the pains and miseries of old age (De Leo 1988).

This common view is tragically reflected by the suicide note left by James Whale, a popular film director (*Frankenstein, The Invisible Man*), who died in 1957 at the age of 60. In his final message he wrote, '*The future is just old age and illness and pain. I must have peace and this is the only way.*' Similar logic can be seen by the note left by George Eastman, the genial founder of Kodak, who shot himself with a firearm at the age of 77 and wrote: '*To my friends: My work is done. Why wait?*' (Suicide notes of famous people are condensed in a lay-book by Etkind 1997.)

The cases of Whale and Eastman actually speak for the non-paradoxical nature of suicide in old age. In fact, Whale was tired of fighting the homophobic attitudes of the Hollywood environment; he was depressed and abusing drugs and alcohol. Eastman was suffering from terrible pain, probably in relation with a spinal stenosis; he was also very depressed and fearing to be confined in a wheelchair.

Consequently, 'rationality' and 'logical thinking' in these behaviours are not sufficient explanations, but rather concepts that need to be broadened to encompass depression, physical illness, unbearable pain, alcohol and drug abuse, which are all well-known risk factors for suicidal behaviour in the general population. After many years of neglect from the scientific community, their role in elderly suicide today has finally found a less blurred allocation.

Certainly old age is a difficult period of life. Hopes and ideals have to be largely replaced by realism and concreteness, in order to better cope with the many challenges that fill the days of most elderly persons. Older adults, when ill, also constitute a special challenge in terms of treatability: the frequency of comorbidities, and the problems connected with polypharmacy require an appropriate and specific training by medical professionals. Even their psychological problems seem difficult to treat. For example, early psychoanalysts, such as Abraham (1949) and Fenichel (1951), were reluctant in acknowledging the fruitfulness of interventions with patients of advanced age.

The dialogue between individuals of different generations has always been problematic, and it will almost certainly continue to be so. Therefore, understanding elderly people (their world, needs, concerns, and expectations) may represent a too ambitious task for younger individuals. The American writer Philip Roth is far more resolute. In his beautiful novel *The Dying Animal* (2002), he writes:

> No, you can't understand. The only thing you understand about the old when you are not old is that they have been stamped by their time. But understanding only that freezes them in their time, and so amounts to no understanding at all.
>
> (2002, p. 36)

Suicidal behaviour clashes with the survival instinct. As such, for many people, it represents an unnatural act, for some an extreme choice, for others something that has to be condemned unconditionally, whatever its genesis. From this point of view, suicide in old age is not dissimilar from suicide in other age groups. It elicits the same reactions, but with a few significant additions, mostly routed by the culture of ageism: that suicide in the elderly is the product of a careful balancing of pros and cons; that is 'rational'; that is understandable and, consequently, excusable (De Leo and Marietta 1997).

The following sections will provide arguments to counteract these stereotyped views. Unfortunately, the available literature is not reflective of contributions equally representative of the different nations, but derives mostly from Western scholars (in the majority of cases of English mother tongue). This constitutes a serious bias, which not only concerns the East and West of the world, but also countries of established economies. For example, there are important differences among the elderly people of Italy or Spain and their peers from the UK or the USA. These differences have a certain impact on type and role of local risk factors for suicide; however, their extent has yet to be satisfactorily understood.

Moreover, there are no internationally operating agreements on the demographic boundaries for belonging to the 'elderly persons' category. This chapter is based on scientific contributions that consider, for once, 'older adults', individuals of 'advanced age', 'elderly people', 'old-olds', etc. Although there appears to be substantial consensus on the threshold of 65 years to define the beginning of old age, the improved conditions in quality of life, general health, and subsequent increased longevity render less acceptable today large aggregations of people of different age groups. This implies that individuals of 55–64 years of age should not be clustered with subjects of 85+ because the differences between them, just in terms of basic characteristics, are enormous (it would be similar to group together themes and behaviours of adolescents with those of 40-year-olds). Differences are getting important also between subjects in the age group 65–74 and those immediately succeeding, the 75–84, to the point that they originated the (medically/sociologically oriented) subdivision in 'young-old' and 'old-old'. In addition, it is well known that the differences in the ratio males/females change dramatically with the increasing of age, producing disproportionately higher rates in male subjects compared to their female counterparts (e.g. De Leo and Heller 2004). This suggests that some risk factors might be particularly age-sensitive, at least in males.

## Risk factors for suicide in the elderly

Factors that increase the risk of suicide in old age include demographic characteristics, psychopathology, personality traits, previous suicidal behaviour, physical illness and disability, life events, and access to lethal methods (De Leo and Spathonis 2004, Heisel 2006, O'Conell et al. 2006). There have also been indications that genetic factors interacting with physiological changes during ageing might play an important role in the aetiology of violent elderly suicide (Stefulj et al. 2006). Although there is a considerable overlap between suicide risk factors in the elderly and other age groups, for example, 'late life suicide is characterised by less warning, higher lethality and greater prevalence of depression and physical illness' (Salib et al. 2005, p. 71).

There is a dearth of studies on protective factors in elderly suicide; however, the perceived levels of quality of life, including satisfactory social relationships, good physical health, and optimism have been identified as correlates of longevity and good mental health in the older populations (Colombo et al. 2006; Dello Buono et al. 1998).

### Demographic characteristics

Despite considerable variations in suicide rates between countries, fatal suicidal behaviours are more prevalent among elderly males than females virtually everywhere (De Leo and Evans 2004; Pritchard and Baldwin 2002; Pritchard and Hansen 2005). With advancing age, the ratio of males:females also increases, with data from Italy verifying rates in males of 80+ years of age 12 times higher than in females (De Leo 1997a) and in Australia, for the same age group, more than 9 times higher (De Leo and Heller 2004).

Studies of the prevalence of non-fatal suicidal behaviour indicate recent increases in numbers of this type of behaviours among older males (Lamprecht et al. 2005), as well as the convergence of gender rates with increasing age (De Leo et al. 2001).

Studies in multicultural societies, including Singapore (Kua et al. 2003), South Africa (Flisher et al. 2004), and the United States (Oquendo et al. 2004), point out the role of factors related to ethnicity. For example, in a longitudinal study of suicide trends in South Africa over the period 1968–1990 (Flisher et al. 2004), the highest suicide rates were reported among the White elderly population, while the rate among the Asians and Coloureds of Asian and African ancestry was significantly lower for both sexes.

Also, low socio-economic status has been reported as a risk factor for elderly suicide in many nations worldwide (Berk et al. 2005; Wu and Bond 2006). Yip (2001) suggested that the high suicide rate among the elderly in rural China (i.e. 109 per 100,000 in males over the age of 75) might be related to limited access to health care facilities, along with the experience of serious hardships in everyday living, including lack of pensions and very limited government support.

### Psychopathology

Psychopathology is the most important risk factor for late-life suicide, and between 75 per cent (Conwell 1997) and 97 per cent (Waern et al. 2002) of elderly suicide victims are diagnosed with at least one mental disorder. Major depressive disorder is the strongest predictor of both non-fatal (Draper 1996; De Leo et al. 2001; Ruths et al. 2005) and fatal suicidal behaviour in old age (Harwood et al. 2001; Snowdon and Baume 2002; Turvey et al. 2002; Preville et al. 2005), as well as suicidal ideation (Barnow et al. 2004; Awata et al. 2005; Yen et al. 2005). Barnow and Linden (2002) found that a diagnosis of major depression was associated with a 40-fold increased risk of suicidality; however it was only 3 times higher when a psychiatric illness, other than major depression, was present.

A significant number of elderly with dysthymia, minor depression (Waern et al. 2002) and amidst a first episode of major unipolar depression (Conwell 1994; Waern et al. 2002), complete suicide. Unremitting hopelessness after recovery from a depressive episode can also pose a risk for older adults (Szanto et al. 2002), and severity of depression has been found to correlate with levels of suicidal ideation in the elderly (Alexopoulos et al. 1999; Heisel et al. 2005) and an increased risk of suicide (Kessing 2004).

In a study of psychiatric disorders and personality factors in suicide (Harwood et al. 2001), over 77 per cent of the suicides had a psychiatric disorder at the time of their death, with approximately 66 per cent suffering from depression. Conwell and colleagues (1991) found that 67 per cent of a sample of suicides were completed by individuals aged 50 years and over, with a diagnosis of major depression. In a 10-year longitudinal study of almost 15,000 subjects aged 65 years and older, Turvey et al. (2002) found that the presence of depressive symptoms was the strongest risk factor predicting eventual suicide. Preville and his colleagues (2005), in a case–control psychological autopsy study in Canada, reported that 75 per cent of suicides over the age of 60 could be diagnosed with minor and subthreshold depression compared with 13 per cent in the control group. Similar results were obtained in studies in Hong Kong, SAR; 76 per cent of elderly suicides were diagnosed with depressive disorders (Chiu et al. 2004), and 68 per cent of suicide attempters suffered from current major depression (Tsoh et al. 2005). Also, Yen et al. (2005) in Taiwan, China and Awata et al. (2005) in Japan found that depression was among the risk factors for suicidal ideation in the elderly. Unremitting hopelessness after recovery from a depressive episode can also pose a risk for older adults (Szanto et al. 2002).

Although depression has been identified as a risk of suicidality among the elderly in both Western and Asian countries, cultural factors might influence the way depressive psychopathology affects the levels of suicide risk and identification of the 'at-risk' individuals. In Asian cultures, depression tends to be manifested by somatization and hypochondriacal complaints rather than obvious psychopathological symptoms (Chiu et al. 2003). Also, depression plays an important aetiological role in elderly suicide-homicide in Western countries (Malphurs and Cohen 2005); however, a study of suicides-homicides in Hong Kong, SAR (Chan et al. 2004) has found an absence of mercy killings among elderly couples and a high relevance of economic factors in the aetiology of the behaviour.

Although there is paucity of data regarding suicide amongst elderly patients diagnosed with bipolar disorder (Aizenberg et al. 2006) and schizophrenia (Barak et al. 2004); the suicidal elderly constitute a heterogenous group and comorbidity plays an important role in suicide in this age population (Waern et al. 2002). Schizophrenia has been reported in approximately 6–17 per cent of elderly suicide deaths (Shah and De 1998). To a lesser extent, anxiety disorders in older age may present an associated high suicide risk (Waern et al. 2002), especially in cases of anxiety–depression syndrome (De Leo 1997a; Shah and De 1998).

Personality disorders may also be associated with suicidal thoughts and behaviours among elderly individuals (Harwood et al. 2001); however, the condition is more frequently encountered in younger suicidal individuals (Krysinska et al. 2006; Neulinger and De Leo 2001). Mostly in Anglo-Saxon and Scandinavian countries, alcohol abuse constitutes an important risk factor in elderly suicide (Kolves et al. 2006b), as well as for both males and females (Waern 2003). A concomitant alcohol abuse and depressive disorder may also present a specific risk for suicide in late life; however, it is not clear whether alcohol abuse results in depression, or whether it is used as a mechanism to cope with the symptoms of the affective disorder (McIntosh et al. 1994).

In general, dementia is not regarded as a risk factor for suicide (De Leo 1996; Conwell et al. 2002). When dementia is present, it is usually mild with comorbid depression. In some, frontal lobe impairments may lead to impulsive, poorly planned attempts. It is unclear whether insight into the dementing process is a factor that increases the risk of suicidality, since in patients unaware of the disease lessened insight may accompany the impairment in cognition (Padoani et al. 2001). However, one study has found a significantly increased rate of Alzheimer's neuropathology in the brains of older suicide victims. As depression may be the prodrome of dementia in late life, this evidence calls for further research (Rubio et al. 2001).

## Previous suicidal behaviour

Non-fatal suicidal behaviour, both first attempts and repetitions, are much more frequent in younger individuals than in elderly subjects (De Leo et al. 2001; Neulinger and De Leo 2001; Schmidtke et al. 2004), but a history of suicidal behaviour is a risk factor for repetition and completed suicide in the elderly (Hawton and Harriss 2006; Lamprecht et al. 2005; Ruths et al. 2005). Studies in Hong Kong, SAR (Chiu et al. 2004; Tsoh et al. 2005) confirmed that a history of suicide attempt is also a predictor for eventual completed suicide in Asian populations.

Based on the data from the WHO/EURO Multicentre Study on Suicidal Behaviour, De Leo and his colleagues (2002b) reported that over a 12-month follow-up period, 13 per cent of the elderly admitted to a hospital after a suicide attempt died by suicide, and 11 per cent repeated their non-fatal suicidal behaviour. Comparison of repeaters and non-repeaters showed that future suicides made significantly higher number of consultations with general practitioners in the year prior to the index attempt, and there was a higher presence of bereavement of the father in childhood among repeaters. The study results also showed that the mean suicide intent score for the index episode was higher among non-repeaters.

The phenomenon of 'elderly adolescentism' has been observed when comparing the epidemiology of non-fatal and fatal suicidal behaviour among the 'young-old' (65–74) and the 'old-old' (75 and over) (De Leo 1998b; De Leo and Scocco 2000). In the demographically 'rejuvenated' 65–74-year-old populations (who undoubtedly benefit from better overall physical health than previous generations, but still have to cope with the usual psychosocial problems of aging), stress-related phenomena typical of younger age groups have begun to emerge, such as 'cry-for-help' or frankly manipulative suicidal behaviour. The elderly adolescentism seems to be associated with an increase in prevalence of non-fatal suicidal behaviour, in contrast to the stabilization or decline in fatal acts in this age population as compared to the 'old-old' (De Leo 1998b).

## Physical illness and disability

Physical illness and resulting hospitalization has been associated with significantly higher suicide risk in all age groups (Hawgood et al. 2004), but more so among the older populations (Harwood et al. 2006a, b; Juurlink et al. 2004; Quan et al. 2002). However, the impact of physical illness upon suicidality is not completely understood as the majority of the elderly population experiences a physical illness, and only a small minority actually engages in suicidal behaviours. The influence of other risk factors, including depression and substance abuse, may relegate physical illness to the place of a secondary contributing factor; and in fact, comorbid somatic and depressive syndromes have been found in most suicidal elderly people (Draper 1996; Snowdon and Baume 2002).

Although there have been studies focusing on suicide risk in the elderly related to particular diagnoses, e.g. coronary artery disease (Artero et al. 2006) and cancer (Labisi 2006), including prostate cancer (Llorente et al. 2005), Juurlink et al. (2004) and Erlangsen et al. (2005) reported that treatment for multiple illnesses is strongly related to a higher risk of suicide. A psychological autopsy study in the UK (Harwood et al. 2006a, b) indicated that physical illness is among the three most frequent life problems associated with suicide in people over the age of 60, and over half of the study informants perceived the physical disease as a contributory factor to suicide of the next of kin; especially the pain, breathlessness, and functional limitations related to the illness.

## Personality characteristics

Certain pre-existing personality traits, particularly in comorbidity with psychiatric illness, especially depression (Kohn and Epstein-Lubow 2006), and hopelessness (Lynch *et al.* 2004; Dennis *et al.* 2005), are often associated with an increased suicide risk in late life. A psychological autopsy study of older people without psychiatric disorder (Harwood *et al.* 2006a) showed that 44 per cent of subjects had significant abnormal personality traits, including inflexible thinking and lack of adaptability. Other studies pointed out anancastic, anxious and low 'openness to experience' personality traits (Harwood *et al.* 2001), and aggression (Conner *et al.* 2004) as risk factors in late-life suicide. Artero *et al.* (2006) showed that in the elderly over the age of 65 coronary artery disease is associated with lifetime history of suicidal behaviour independently of depression, indicating the links between somatic and psychopathological factors, including anger/hostility and impulsivity. Depression, anxiety and hostility have also been identified as risk factors for suicidal ideation in the elderly (Scocco *et al.* 2001; Scocco and De Leo 2002).

Although worldwide suicide is most prevalent among male subjects (De Leo and Evans 2004), this seems to contrast with the poor health and low social status experienced by elderly women, which result from more compromised psychophysical conditions secondary to greater longevity, widowhood, abandonment, and poverty. To explain this difference, it has been suggested that women may posses personality characteristics protecting against suicide in late life, including a greater capacity to adjust to change and to be self-sufficient in activities of daily living, better ability to establish and preserve social networks, and more commitment to children and grandchildren (Canetto 1992).

## Life conditions and events

In older age, particularly after the age of 75 years, the concentration of less favourable life circumstances may contribute to elevated risk of suicide (McIntosh *et al.* 1994). The decline in physical health, lower degree of autonomy and more frequent losses can precipitate suicidal ideation and behaviour. However, such changes are common in older age, and it is not entirely clear why some individuals are better equipped to cope than others (De Leo 1998a).

Both recent and early-life experiences might be associated with increased levels of suicidality among the elderly. Studies show that physical illness, interpersonal problems, and recent bereavement and/or bereavement in last 12 months, as well as long-term bereavement related problems, are among most frequent events associated with completed suicide (De Leo *et al.* 2002b; Harwood *et al.* 2006a, b) and non-fatal suicidal behaviour (Hawton and Harriss 2006). Problems related to financial status, living arrangements, employment change and retirement also might contribute to the increased risk of suicidal behaviour (Duberstein *et al.* 2004b; Harwood *et al.* 2006a, b). Anticipation of, or a recent placement in a nursing home, has been considered to be a precipitating factor, particularly amongst those elderly who were married at the time of their suicide (Loebel *et al.* 1991).

Elderly survivors of offspring suicides might also be at increased risk (Waern 2005). The subjective feeling of being a burden to others

(Foster 2003) and psychiatric and developmental vulnerabilities (including early separation and loss) might play a moderating role between negative life events and suicidal ideation and behaviour (De Leo *et al.* 2002b; Duberstein *et al.* 1998). Studies of elderly Holocaust survivors indicate that the long-term impact of traumatic events includes increased risk for late-life suicidal ideation and depression (Clarke *et al.* 2004, 2006), suicide attempts (Barak *et al.* 2005), and fatal suicidal behaviour (Lester 2005).

Levels of social integration and social relationships are important mediators of suicidality in late-age (Hawton and Harriss 2006; Vanderhorst and McLaren 2005). A study by Dennis *et al.* (2005) indicated that poorly integrated social networks and higher levels of hopelessness were the only clinical factors which differentiated between older adults with depression who were at risk of suicide and the non-suicidal depressed elderly. Duberstein *et al.* (2004a) showed a positive association between family and social/community indicators of poor social integration and suicide; people who died by suicide were less likely to be married, have children or live with family; had lower levels of social interaction and were less engaged in religious practices or community activities.

Little information is available on suicide in nursing homes and there is inconsistent data regarding its prevalence as compared to the general population rates. Although some studies indicate that suicide rates in nursing homes are lower than the general population (Osgood *et al.* 1991), an Italian study by Scocco *et al.* (2006) showed a higher rate than the general population elderly suicide rate (29.7 per 100,000 vs 18.6 per 100,000, respectively). The authors indicated that the majority of elderly residents who attempted or completed suicide were suffering from a mental disorder, especially major depression. A psychological autopsy study of nursing home suicides in Finland (Suominen *et al.* 2003) reported similar results, pointing out the role of somatic and mental disorders (particularly depression) in this type of behaviour.

Australian studies by Draper and his colleagues (2002a, b, 2003) looked at the prevalence and risk factors for direct and indirect self-destructive behaviours (e.g. refusal to eat and/or take medication, lack of cooperation with staff) in nursing home residents. The results showed high prevalence of both types of behaviours; the reported weekly prevalence of indirect self-destructive behaviour was 61 per cent, and 14 per cent of residents engaged at least once during the previous week in direct self-harming behaviours (Draper *et al.* 2002a). Indirect self-destructive behaviours were found to be reliable predictors of mortality in the resident population (Draper *et al.* 2003), and appeared to be related to dementia rather than depression (Draper *et al.* 2002b).

## Family discord

Family conflicts are among life events closely related to increased suicide risk in individuals of all ages (Heikkinen *et al.* 1992; Kolves *et al.* 2006a), and Richman reported (1994) that conflicts were present in families of over 90 per cent of clients under 40 years of age and 70 per cent of the older individuals (including people over the age of 60) in therapy for suicidal behaviour or ideation. Rubenowitz and her colleagues (2001) indicated that family discord was a significant risk factor in late-life suicide in almost half of suicides and 6 per cent of elderly controls. Although the problems often had a chronic dimension, there were significant differences between the elderly females and males: in females the frequency of family discord was at a constant level during the last 2 years preceding death, while in men the frequency increased by almost 50 per cent during the last 6 months.

Similar results were obtained in other studies. For example, Duberstein *et al.* (2004b) found family discord to be present in the lives of 30 per cent of elderly suicides (versus 9 per cent of controls), and Waern *et al.* (2003) reported that 48 per cent of suicides in the age group 65–74 years and 42 per cent of the 'old-old' suicides (over 75 years of age), experienced family conflicts within 12 months prior to suicide (versus 6 per cent and 1.4 per cent of controls, respectively).

In a case–control psychological autopsy study of elderly suicide, Harwood *et al.* (2006) found that interpersonal and bereavement-related problems were the second most frequent difficulties experienced by the elderly in the year before death (physical illness being the major stressor). Interpersonal conflicts and poor relationship were reported in 32 per cent of suicides and were perceived as contributory to death in 23 per cent of cases. However, unlike the results of the studies discussed earlier (Rubenowitz *et al.* 2001; Waern *et al.* 2003; Duberstein *et al.* 2004b), interpersonal problems were common in both suicide and control groups, and did not emerge as a risk factor for suicide in a logistic-regression model. The authors attributed the disparity of results to the differences in coding systems between their study and other research—inclusion of problems of lesser severity in the category of interpersonal problems.

In spite of evidence that family discord and problems are contributory factors in many suicides of older people, their relationship with other risk factors, including psychopathology, physical illness, socio-economic strain, and caregiving stressors, is unclear. There are still unanswered questions regarding the nature, duration, dynamics, and content of the disagreements within families that may increase suicide risk (Duberstein *et al.* 2004b). The subjective feeling of being a burden to others, and accumulation of family problems compounded by unresolved conflicts from the past, may be important factors playing a mediating role (Foster 2003; Richman 1994). Elderly males may be more vulnerable to the impact of family discord, interpersonal loss and a feeling of abandonment in a relationship than their female peers (Canetto 1992; De Leo *et al.* 2001), and 'unsatisfied and frustrated need for attachment, within the context of long-term instability, often allows the older male to feel despair and choose death' (Leenaars 1997, p. 78).

### Access to lethal means of suicide

The elderly tend to perform carefully planned suicidal acts; they pay particular attention to avoid external interferences and the possibility of being rescued, and generally use highly lethal means (Conwell *et al.* 2002; De Leo *et al.* 2001, 2002b). Access to these lethal methods is then among the risk factors for elderly suicide.

Studies looking at methods of suicide among the elderly show the fall from high buildings where they live as a method frequently used by urban residents in the Western (Abrams *et al.* 2005) and Asian (Kua *et al.* 2003; Yip *et al.* 1998) countries. Kua *et al.* (2003) reported that in Singapore, 65 per cent of the elderly suicides died as result of jumping from high-rise buildings, and Yip *et al.* (1998) observed an increase in jumping as means of elderly suicide in Hong Kong, SAR, from 29 per cent of all suicides to 52 per cent over the period 1981–1995. Easy access to other means of suicide,

including firearms in the USA (Conwell *et al.* 2002; Oslin *et al.* 2004) and pesticides in India (Abraham *et al.* 2005) also has been related to increased risk of elderly suicide.

### Protective factors in elderly suicide

There has been a paucity of research on protective factors against suicide among the older generations. The protective effect of having children appears to diminish in old age (Salib *et al.* 2004), and gender-role orientation and attitudes affect the levels of suicide ideation across generations (Hunt *et al.* 2006). A study of trends in elderly suicide in Singapore (Kua *et al.* 2003) has reported significant differences in suicide among different ethnic groups (i.e. Chinese, Indian and Malay), with the Malays (devout Muslims) having the lowest prevalence of suicide. The authors have concluded that 'spirituality in the three ethnic groups may influence their attitude to life and suicidal tendency' (p. 536).

Studies on the quality of life in the elderly (De Leo *et al.* 1998; Condello *et al.* 2003), including a study on quality of life in the centenarians (Dello Buono *et al.* 1998), indicate that intellectual stimulation, good physical conditions, satisfactory social relationships, religiosity, optimisms, and financial security correlate with high levels of satisfaction with life. Other studies (e.g. Awata el al. 2005; Yen *et al.* 2005; Kissane and McLaren 2006) indicate that religious belief, satisfactory interpersonal relations and support, as well as community activity are among factors that can decrease the risk of suicide in the older individuals.

## Suicide notes in the elderly

Approximately 30–40 per cent of the elderly suicides leave notes (Neulinger and De Leo 2001, Salib *et al.* 2002a); a figure similar to the range of 15–42 per cent for suicides of all ages (Salib *et al.* 2002a). Although it has been suggested that leaving a suicide note is an indication of the seriousness of intent to die (Rosenberg *et al.* 1988), absence of a suicide note should not be considered as an sign of a less serious attempt, especially among the older suicides (Salib *et al.* 2002b). Many older people who commit suicide might have lost their ability to express themselves or may be lonely and isolated, having no one to write to (Salib *et al.* 2002a).

Although only a few studies have focused on late-life suicide notes, with some research showing a lack of differences between notes left by suicides in different age groups (Leenaars 1996), however several commonalities have been identified. Leenaars (1992, 1997) found four common themes in the elderly suicide notes: ageing (the fear of the diminished capacity to cope with the demands of adaptation, including physical illness, mental deterioration, and dependency), long-term instability (e.g. multiple losses, a history of psychiatric hospitalization), a non-ambivalent wish to die, and a feeling of total abandonment (especially in older males; also Salib *et al.* 2002a). Linn and Lester (1996) reported that elderly suicide notes contained fewer feelings of inadequacy and more indications of illness and grief over widowhood, and Foster (2003) found that the elderly suicides over the age of 65 were significantly more likely than younger suicides to express the feeling of being a burden to others (40 versus 3 per cent). A study in Hong Kong, SAR (Ho *et al.* 1998) showed that suicide notes of the elderly were shorter, contained specific instructions, and were less emotional than notes left by younger victims.

# Treatment and prevention of suicidal behaviour in the elderly

Traditionally, there are three levels of prevention with regard to suicidal behaviour in late life: universal, selective, and indicated (Mrazek and Haggerty 1994). Universal prevention refers to activities targeted at the general population, including health promotion and education, which may improve the overall emotional and social well-being of the elderly population, and may target suicide risk factors. Selective prevention refers to interventions aimed at populations identified as being at risk of suicide, while indicated strategies address specific high-risk individuals showing early signs of suicidality.

The majority of elderly suicide prevention programmes, as well as psychosocial and pharmacological interventions for the older people at risk of suicide, have been developed in Western countries (Lester and Tallmer 1994; McIntosh 1995; Scocco and De Leo 2002; Vijayakumar et al. 2002). Recently, studies have been conducted regarding the effectiveness of suicide prevention activities targeted at the elderly in East Asia, including Hong Kong, SAR, Japan and Republic of Korea (Chiu et al. 2003; Shiho et al. 2005). The major approach to suicide prevention in late age in these countries has been the screening of depression, and development of group activities and social networks (Ono 2004; Fujisawa et al. 2005; Oyama et al. 2005, 2006).

## Universal strategies: welfare and social support networks

Universal preventative initiatives targeted at the elderly include the introduction of social security programs, development of flexible retirement schemes, and improved health care availability (De Leo 2003). McCall (1991) used a time-series regression model to determine the extent of the association between age-, race-, and sex-specific suicide rates and social factors (i.e. health care availability, impoverishment and government expenditure). The results suggested that the elderly white male population has benefited from growing societal affluence, represented as the reduction in the percentage of the older persons living below the poverty line, increased financial/social security, and improved availability of health care services represented by levels of Medicare enrolment and numbers of doctors per capita. A systematic monitoring of physical health seems to be particularly important, in the light of its possible impact on suicidal behaviour (De Leo 2003).

Greater opportunities for relationships with peers and better access to recreational facilities, including community-based programmes (e.g. senior centres, volunteer organizations and adult daycare activities) may provide support for elderly people (Vanderhorst and McLaren 2005) and facilitate role transition typical of old age, including retirement and children leaving home. The effectiveness of a community-based suicide prevention programme aimed at the elderly was evaluated in Yuri, Japan (Oyama et al. 2005). The 8-year programme (1995–2000), based on population strategies involving psychoeducation, group activities, and self-assessment of depression, proved to be effective in elderly females only: the risk of suicide among females in Yuri was reduced by 76 per cent, however, there was no change in male suicide rates.

## Universal strategies: restricting access to means

Controlling access to lethal means of suicide in the general population represents one of the most effective suicide prevention approaches (Clarke and Lester 1989; Mann et al. 2005). Shah and Lodhi (2005) showed that changes in prescribing psychotropic medication, possibly resulting from more accurate diagnostic-specific prescriptions of drugs, have had an impact of trends in the suicide methods in the elderly.

In Australia, substitution of barbiturates with less toxic drugs could have had an important role in contributing to the decline in rates of suicide in older adults, particularly in female subjects, for whom overdosing with medication was a traditional suicide method (De Leo 2006).

## Selective/indicated strategies: helplines and community support programs

Only a small proportion of callers to agencies such as the Samaritans are elderly, and the aged are under-represented in the clientele of suicide prevention programmes and general mental health facilities (McIntosh et al. 1994). The reasons for such low utilization of services by the elderly are numerous, and range from poor information available to them, belief that these services are costly, and the low credibility given by older adults to most types of agencies and institutions (McIntosh et al. 1994). Negative attitudes towards mental health services (often along with lack of such services) have also been recognized among the elderly in Asian counties (Chiu et al. 2003). In addition, especially in Western cultures, men are less willing to express their emotions and, as a result, males at risk of suicide are more often under-diagnosed and under-treated, especially by general practitioners, than their female counterparts (De Leo 1998b).

In an attempt to overcome the elderly people's unwillingness to use phone-based services, a pioneering Tele-Help/Tele-Check programme was established in the Veneto region of Italy (De Leo et al. 1995). Tele-Help is a portable device that lets users send alarm signals activating a pre-established network of help and assistance. In Tele-Check, trained staff members contact each client at least twice a week to offer emotional support and monitor the clients' condition through a short, informal interview. If needed, the client may also contact the centre at any time. Clients are enrolled in the service after a standardized screening from general practitioners or social workers. This service appears to provide support of relevance for the prevention of late-life suicide: even 10 years after its introduction, a significantly lower than expected number of suicidal deaths was observed among the 20,000 service users compared to the general population (De Leo et al. 2002a). The positive results reported in this experience have lead to the implementation of similar initiatives in different countries, among them a comprehensive prevention project in Hong Kong, SAR (Chiu et al. 2003).

## Selective/indicated strategies: the family setting

Relatives are among the most frequently sought for help by the elderly (De Leo et al. 2002b). The mobilization of relatives and friends to monitor the emotional and psychological status of old-age individuals may assist in preventing suicidal ideation from progressing towards the action. This strategy may not only increase social contacts with older persons, but may also enhance the chances of discovery and assistance in the event of a suicide attempt for the elderly who live on their own.

Family members may be more effective than primary care physicians in detecting suicidality. Waern *et al.* (1999) examined the suicidal feelings and behaviours of the elderly who died by suicide as noted by doctors and relatives during the year preceding death. Results indicated that relatives were more proficient in detecting suicidal feelings (73 per cent), particularly in the case of female suicides, compared to doctors (39 per cent).

Family and relatives may also play an important role in the development and implementation of a treatment plan for an elderly person at risk of suicide, and several therapeutic approaches, including the reasons-for-living approach, behavioural contracting, and availability of social support are influenced by the family environment (McIntosh *et al.* 1994). Richman (1994) observes:

> The family can be a source of the tension that actually instigates the suicidal act, but they can also play a very important role in helping the potential suicide. Family therapy conducted by a properly trained therapist is [in the author's opinion] the treatment of choice for suicidal patients.
>
> Richman (1994, p. 73)

According to Richman, the foundations of family therapy for suicidal individuals are the potential presence of love, growth, and healing forces in the family (even if they are absent during the suicidal crisis), and the helping role of the therapist assisting in uncovering the positive resources, as well as helping to establish or re-establish satisfactory relationships between the elderly and their relatives (Leenaars 1997).

As family conflict is a risk factor for late-life suicide (Rubenowitz *et al.* 2001; Duberstein *et al.* 2004b), family discord could be a target of treatment efforts in older adults. Problem-solving (Williams *et al.* 2001) and interpersonal therapies (Reynolds *et al.* 1999) have proven effective in treatment of older individuals suffering from depression, and they may also be applicable for addressing the family issues that undermine mental health and suicide risk in old age (Duberstein *et al.* 2004b).

## Selective/indicated strategies: religious and spiritual settings

The impact of religious affiliation and spirituality upon suicide in older age should also be considered. Older people who practice their faith frequently have lower rates of depression, alcoholism and hopelessness than their non-religious peers (Koenig 1994), and spirituality was found to correlate with a positive self-appraisal of physical health (Daaleman *et al.* 2004). Religious communities may serve to moderate isolation and loneliness in old age by providing an active support network and meaningful volunteer work, which promote feelings of purpose and usefulness and enhance well-being (Krause and Shaw 2000; Krause 2006).

In many cultures and societies the clergy are often sought by older individuals for counselling in crisis situations, such as bereavement, physical illness, injury, divorce or marital separation and other traumatic events (Everly 2000). People over the age of 65 are more likely to seek the help of clergy rather than mental health specialists (Hohmann and Larson 1993). The role of clergy is particularly important for seniors in rural and small communities where mental health services are scarce, and religious groups and the clergy function as the counselling resources (Weaver and Koenig 1996).

Although clergy might be in a particularly useful position to help suicidal seniors, there has been a scarcity of published research on their role in responding to the needs of suicidal elderly people (Weaver and Koenig 1996). Also, often clergy are inadequately prepared to recognize the suicide potential of persons who seek their assistance and have insufficient knowledge concerning referral skills needed to effectively network with mental health professionals (Leane and Shute 1998). A literature review regarding the referral patterns among the clergy over a 20-year span showed that less than 10 per cent of individuals who were seeking the pastoral assistance for psychological problems were referred to mental health services (Meylink and Gorsuch 1987). At the same time, mental health specialists very seldom make referrals to religious sources of support and very rarely consider this type of counselling in treatment planning (Weaver and Koenig 1996).

Although the majority of clergy receive some training in counselling, albeit not specific to suicidality in older age, very few mental health professionals are trained in the subject of spirituality or religious issues and often have a tendency to 'psychologize' or 'medicalize' the important existential or spiritual issues that might be correlated with a suicidal crisis (Weaver and Koenig 1996). An alliance between the mental health and religious counselling resources for the elderly is likely to occur only after the first step of purging attitudinal barriers, fears, and concerns about collaborative links is achieved (Upanne 2001).

## Detection of suicidal ideas

Identifying suicidal ideas and tendencies among the elderly is the first goal of fundamental importance. Abilities to detect psychological and physical suffering should be improved by appropriate training and educational programmes, addressed particularly to general practitioners and other health professionals, such as nurses and social workers (De Leo 2003).

The identification of elderly at risk of suicide is a challenging task. General practitioners (GPs) have difficulties in the identification, assessment and management of depression and suicide risk in old age (Shah and Harris 1997; Suominen *et al.* 2004). This is accentuated where there is comorbid physical illness. The majority of depressed physically ill older people are undiagnosed, misdiagnosed or untreated (Borson *et al.* 1986; Koenig *et al.* 1992; Jackson and Baldwin 1993; Snowdon *et al.* 1996; Koenig *et al.* 1997a; Crawford *et al.* 1998). This fact may be partly due to the misattribution by both clinicians and patients of depressive symptoms to physical illnesses (Knauper and Wittchen 1994; Koenig *et al.* 1997b; Booth *et al.* 1998).

Older suicide victims have frequently been in contact with health professionals, particularly GPs, in the months before death. One study found that 58 per cent of those aged 55 years and over had seen a GP in the month before death (Luoma *et al.* 2002), and over a third have seen a GP within the week of their suicide (Pearson *et al.* 1997). This has been noted in various countries. For example, in Denmark 66 per cent had consulted a GP in the month before death (Andersen *et al.* 2000), in Hong Kong, SAR, 77 per cent had consulted a doctor within a month of their suicide (Chiu *et al.* 2004), and in Canada almost half had visited a physician in the previous week (Juurlink *et al.* 2004). It is unclear how often these contacts represent an opportunity for suicide prevention. It has been calculated that between 42–70 per cent of these contacts are due to psychosocial reasons, and 30–58 per cent to physical reasons (Van Casteren et al. 1993; Obafunwa and Busuttil 1994; Vassilas and Morgan 1994; Isometsä et al. 1995). The communication of suicidal intent has been found to happen during 22–45 per cent of last clinical contacts, though it has been reported to occur in only 11 per cent of GP contacts (Obafunwa and Busuttil 1994; Isometsä et al. 1995). Males are less likely to communicate suicidal intent than females (Isometsä et al. 1995), and older victims are less likely to communicate than younger victims (Conwell et al. 1998).

## Gatekeeper training

Education of at-risk older people, gatekeepers, and health professionals involved in their care is of crucial importance in addressing the problem. GPs education about depression and suicide in older people increases their detection capabilities for depressive and suicidal symptoms (Pfaff and Almeida 2003). There is modest evidence that suicidal ideation is a proxy end point for suicide in old age, hence providing some support to this approach (Links et al. 2005). But recognition needs to be linked to an intervention to improve the effectiveness, with strategies that might include the removal of barriers to care, depression screening, and the use of treatment guidelines.

There are several studies that lend support to this approach. Oyama et al. (2004) evaluated the outcome of a community-based suicide prevention programme for older people in the Japanese rural town of Joboji using a quasi-experimental design with two neighbouring control areas. The 10-year programme was based on strategies including screening for depression; follow-up with mental health care or psychiatric treatment; and health education on depression. The study found that when compared with a regional historical trend, the relative risks estimated by the age-adjusted odds ratios for both males and females were reduced to almost 25 per cent, with a better response to education for females than for males. In Sydney, Australia, an intervention that included multidisciplinary consultation and collaboration, training of GPs and carers in detection and management of depression, and depression-related health education and activity programmes was compared with routine care in a RCT of 220 older patients with depression in a residential care setting. At the nine-and-a-half-month follow-up, the intervention group had significantly greater improvement on the Geriatric Depression Scale and more use of antidepressants than the control group; though specific measures of suicidal ideation were not included (Llewellyn-Jones et al. 1999).

A community-based gatekeeper programme to identify socially isolated and economically disadvantaged at-risk elderly was introduced in mid 1990s at the Spokane Mental Health Center in the US (Florio et al. 1997). The initiative aimed at training employees of community businesses and corporations, including meter readers, utility workers, bank personnel, postal carriers, apartment managers, and pharmacists, to be able to identify and refer community-dwelling older adults who may be in need of geriatric and mental health services, but unlikely to be found by more traditional referral resources. Results of the study indicated that the trained gatekeepers were responsible for 40 per cent of referrals to the local Elder Services (Florio et al. 1996). Although over the period of 12 months, the adoption of the community gatekeeper programme did not result in high service utilization, the programme was inexpensive to implement and benefited the community via increased collaboration among providers of services (Florio et al. 1998).

In Germany, over the period 2001–2002, the Nuremberg Alliance against Depression introduced a four-level education programme to improve the care of depressed patients, including the elderly (Ziervogel et al. 2005; Hegerl et al. 2006). The project included an information campaign for the general public, support for self-help activities, and intensive 4-hour training for geriatric caregivers in nursing homes in order to improve knowledge and attitudes concerning depression and suicidality in old age and encouraging communication between the elderly in nursing homes, their relatives and the general practitioners. The advanced training for geriatric caregivers proved effective in increasing the caregivers' knowledge and attitudes towards old-age depression, including a better understanding of the link between depression and suicide, and pharmacological treatments for affective disorders (Ziervogel et al. 2005).

Hegerl and his colleagues (2006) reported that the 2-year evaluation of the programme showed a reduction in the prevalence of non-fatal suicidal behaviour in the general population in the Nuremberg region, especially in relation to high-risk methods (e.g. shooting, hanging, jumping). However, the authors did not present data regarding the impact of the same programme on suicide morbidity and mortality in the elderly.

## Assessment and management of a suicidal elder

One important component of health professional education is the assessment of suicide risk and management of older people at high risk. Even when depression is suspected, the assessment of suicide risk is often missed in older patients. Stoppe et al. (1999) surveyed 170 GPs using two case vignettes: Case 1 had mild depression in a healthy elder and Case 2 had severe depression with somatic comorbidity. Over 90 per cent considered depression in the differential diagnosis of Case 1 and 70 per cent in Case 2, yet only 2.4 per cent spontaneously indicated that they would ask about suicidal ideation. At the end of the interview, the GPs were directly asked about suicide and nearly 77 per cent indicated they would talk about suicide. The rest either indicated that they thought the patient would communicate suicidal thoughts themselves or that they feared that they might induce suicide by asking directly (Stoppe et al. 1999). Suominen et al. (2004) investigated health care contacts before and after a suicide attempt in a group of elderly (≥60 years) and others (<60 years) in Helsinki. Elderly suicide attempters had contacts more frequently; unfortunately, recognition and diagnosis of mood disorders by GPs was quite poor, with only 4 per cent of elderly attempters receiving a diagnosis of mood disorder prior to the attempt, and 57 per cent of them being diagnosed with a mood disorder after the attempt.

So, when should a clinician consider that an older patient might be at risk of suicide? There is no clear answer to this even in the obvious circumstance of the presence of clinical depression. While all depressed older persons should have at least an initial assessment of suicide risk, how often this should be repeated during the course of the illness is unclear. If enquiries about suicide risk are repeated too often, therapeutic rapport might be undermined. This is particularly true when no suicide risk is detected at the initial assessment and there are no other significant risk factors. Pilot data from a study of the last contact that suicide victims have with a health professional suggest that many older depressed patients were assessed by GPs to be improving in the weeks before death (Draper *et al.* 2008). Thus, improvement in the depression can be deceptive in terms of suicide risk, which is a clinical feature that has been noted for nearly 200 years (Goldney 2006). In addition, with increasing age, there is a lower rate of suicidal ideation reported before suicide attempts (Duberstein *et al.* 1999).

In the absence of clinical depression, there are some other situations that might warrant a suicide risk assessment. While there are other mental disorders in late life that have been reported to be associated with suicidal behaviour (including late-life psychoses, substance abuse, and anxiety disorders), this needs to be taken in context of the older person's life circumstances and personality type. Suicide risk is increased in older people with obsessional, anxious and low 'openness to experience' personality traits (Duberstein *et al.* 1994; Harwood *et al.* 2006a). Such individuals may have a restricted capacity to adapt to change and the various challenges associated with ageing. Recent life stressors, including the diagnosis of cancer or other serious conditions such as loss of sight and death of a spouse or close friend, may be overwhelming to some people. Chronic stressors such as pain, loneliness, complicated grief or severe disability, especially in the absence of adequate social support, are all circumstances that might lead to a suicidal behaviour in the vulnerable person, especially if there has been a history of previous suicide attempts.

In spite of evidence that physical illness is a contributory factor in a majority of suicides of older people, its role is unclear. Terminal illness is present in only 5–10 per cent, with many having a treatable depression or inadequate pain control (Leibenluft and Goldberg 1988; Draper 1995). Chronic physical disability with dependence on carers, loss of dignity, chronic pain and the fear of institutionalization may contribute to demoralization, depression and suicidality. A threshold phenomenon may exist whereby the physically ill may become suicidal with milder degrees of depression (Draper 1996), or put another way, physical illnesses may amplify suicide risk in those with premorbid vulnerability (Duberstein *et al.* 2004b). Psychological reactions occur, with some people feeling overwhelmed by the knowledge of an acute illness and others convincing themselves that they have cancer after minor symptoms are experienced, often ignoring reassurances by their doctor (Conwell *et al.* 1991; De Leo 1997a; De Leo *et al.* 1999; Snowdon and Baume 2002). The coping strategies chosen by an older person with a chronic illness have an effect on their emotional well-being (Felton *et al.* 1984; Ormel *et al.* 1997). Worries related to functional impairment may be a final common pathway to depression and suicidal ideation in physically ill elders (Gallo *et al.* 1997).

There are some types of behaviour that might alert the clinician to suicidal preoccupation. These include the giving away of possessions, changing of will, stockpiling of pills and passive indirect self-destructive behaviour such as refusal to eat and medication non-compliance. Indirect self-destructive behaviour has been defined as an act of omission or commission that causes self-harm leading indirectly, over time, to the patient's death (Conwell *et al.* 1996) and is particularly relevant to the institutionalised elderly where they have been found to be associated with increased mortality (Draper *et al.* 2003). It has also been reported to occur in 29 per cent of individuals with complicated grief (Szanto *et al.* 2006).

Assessment of suicide risk in older people requires the health professional to be attentive, calm and non-threatening; to give the patient space and time to vent; to work in collaboration with the patient; and to use the word suicide without flinching (Brown *et al.* 2001). The use of open-ended questions followed up by specific questions about the nature, timing and context of suicidal thoughts is recommended. Although it would not be feasible to screen all older primary care patients for suicidality, physicians should ask about suicidal thoughts in all older patients who present symptoms of depression. There should be no reluctance to question patients about suicidal ideation, because there is no evidence that such questions can increase the likelihood of suicidal behaviour (Callahan *et al.* 1996; Alexopoulos 1999).

Direct questioning might be aided by the use of a brief depression scale that includes items on suicidal ideation (Dombrovski and Szanto 2005). Options include the self-administered Beck Depression Inventory (Beck *et al.* 1961), the rater-administered Hamilton Rating Scale for Depression (Hamilton 1960) or the eight-item rater-administered Even Briefer Assessment Scale for Depression (Allen *et al.* 1994), the latter being particularly useful in primary care. Unfortunately, the Geriatric Depression Scale (GDS), the scale that is frequently used for depression screening in older people, does not have a specific item on suicide, which is a significant weakness of the instrument (Yesavage *et al.* 1983). However, five internally consistent GDS items assessing hopelessness, worthlessness, emptiness, an absence of happiness and absence of the perception it is 'wonderful to be alive' have been found to be highly associated with suicidal ideation (Heisel *et al.* 2005).

Deterrents to suicidal behaviour need to be determined. Common deterrents include religion and fear of upsetting family or friends. It is also important to obtain collateral information from family and friends if there is any concern about suicide risk (Dombrovski and Szanto 2005). Furthermore, the American Psychiatric Association's Practice Guideline for the Assessment and Treatment of Patients with Suicidal Behaviors states that family and friends can be contacted without the patient's consent if suicidality is suspected (APA 2003).

## High-risk management guidelines for older suicidal patients

High-risk management guidelines for older suicidal patients in primary care settings were developed for the Prevention of Suicide in Primary Care Elderly: Collaborative Trial (PROSPECT) (Brown *et al.* 2001). Short-term management of the older suicidal patient should take into account a number of clinical factors that need to be elicited in the assessment. Most importantly, the intensity of the suicidal ideation, clarity of plans and access to means should determine the location of care. There might be circumstances where a frail elder with intense suicidal preoccupation can be safely managed at home, as long as adequate supervision is provided and access to means removed. But hospitalization is often indicated, particularly when there is severe depression with features of psychosis, agitation, hopelessness, refusal to eat, poor insight, ruminating insomnia or where there is comorbid substance abuse. Impulsivity, especially in association with impairments of executive function, is another feature that might require short-term hospitalization (King *et al.* 2000; Keilp *et al.* 2001; Marzuk *et al.* 2005). A past history of suicidal behaviour has been identified as a risk factor for further suicide attempts in older people (Draper 1996; De Leo *et al.* 2001; Chan *et al.* 2007) and will need to be factored into assessment of future risk. Other reasons for hospitalization include the lack of social support, presence of concurrent medical issues (such as pain, cardiac problems, dehydration), and associated functional impairment that impact upon safe outpatient treatment, a history of poor compliance with treatment, or where the older person appears to have 'given-up'.

The type of hospitalization that is most effective in the treatment of older patients with depression has not been firmly established, though the limited evidence suggests that better outcomes occur in specialized acute old age psychiatry units as compared with acute general adult psychiatry units, while both appear to have better outcomes than general medical wards (Draper and Low 2004). Outcomes related to suicidal behaviour have not been specifically studied. Discharge planning for the older suicidal patient should be influenced by a number of factors. Most importantly the resolution of suicidal ideation is paramount and the clinician needs to be aware that the intensity of suicidal thoughts can fluctuate from day to day in the context of major depression (Szanto et al. 1996). Furthermore, the patient may only communicate their suicidal thoughts with certain people, for example, personal nurse, family or friends; thus, it is essential to have open communication within the treatment team and to check with the family or friends about it. Integration of hospital and post-discharge community care improves the outcomes of older depressed patients (Draper and Low 2004), though it is not clear whether it specifically reduces suicide risk. Such integration might include having the community nurse get to know the patient before discharge, a pre-discharge home visit to check on functional needs and remove any guns or stockpiled medications, continuity of medical care post-discharge, and members of the multidisciplinary inpatient team having a transitional role to help the older patient and the family settle in at home.

The style of management of the older suicidal patient in the community is the same whether it is following a hospital admission or the initial approach to treatment. The development of a therapeutic alliance is critical and is often best achieved by ensuring that alleviation of the patient's suffering—physical, psychological and spiritual—is central to the package of care being provided. Important components of community treatment include an individualized case management approach with ongoing care, home-based assessments to improve attendance and carer education (Draper and Low 2004). It should include explicitly written instructions to the older patient and family about what to do if suicidal thoughts recur and the provision of an emergency contact. Medication monitoring is also important and is often aided by having a medication blister pack that is filled out each week. At least weekly contact with a mental health professional psychiatrist/psychologist or a member of the multidisciplinary community team, until the patient has had clear resolution of their suicidal thoughts and feelings of hopelessness, is required. Psychoeducation about depression and any other relevant mental disorder should be provided to the older patient and family. Avoidance of alcohol and illicit drugs should be stressed (Brown et al. 2001).

## Pharmacological treatments

Earlier psychological autopsy studies found that many depressed suicide victims were untreated, or inadequately treated with benzodiazepines for associated insomnia (Cattell 1988; Conwell et al. 1990), though more recent studies have found higher rates of antidepressant prescription (Waern et al. 1996). It is not simply a failure by the GP to recognize or treat the depression appropriately. Patients may refuse treatment due to their conviction that the symptoms are secondary to their physical condition (Knauper and Wittchen 1994). The elderly are more likely to 'give up' and request euthanasia when depressed, possibly through subconscious suicide motivation (Koenig and Breitner 1990; Hooper et al. 1996). Refusal to accept life-saving treatments has been noted to more frequently occur in older individuals with high levels of hopelessness and may affect their decision-making capacity (Menon et al. 2000). Depression and pain have the capacity to affect judgement temporarily by subtly distorting the patient's perceptions in a manner that may convince family, friends and doctor of the 'rationality' of suicide. Yet the wish to die usually resolves once depression, pain and insomnia are treated (Szanto et al. 2003), though hopelessness might persist after depression resolves in older patients with a history of suicide attempts, and this may require specific attention in therapy to reduce future suicide risk (Szanto et al. 1998). Persistent hopelessness, substance abuse and personality disorder increase the risk of treatment non-compliance and disengagement from services (Rifai et al. 1994; Hunt et al. 2006).

There is consensus that antidepressant medication (Wilson et al. 2003), cognitive therapies (Koder et al. 1996), and electroconvulsive therapy (ECT) (Chiu et al. 2002) are effective in the short-term treatment of geriatric major depression. Age alone does not appear to significantly affect the general efficacy of antidepressant medication in the acute treatment of uncomplicated major depression. Selective serotonin reuptake inhibitors (SSRIs) and serotonin-noradrenaline reuptake inhibitors are the antidepressants of choice in older people (Alexopoulos 2005). Effectiveness of treatment with SSRIs is most likely enhanced by the greater likelihood of maintaining an adequate dose than with other antidepressants (Shasha et al. 1997).

The available evidence suggests that ECT is the most effective treatment available for severe depression in late life, particularly when there are psychotic features or with high acute suicide risk (Chiu et al. 2002). There is also indirect evidence that suggests ECT might offer a short-term protection from suicide (Isometsä et al. 1996), but no evidence that there is long-term protection (Schifano 1994).

However, while antidepressant treatments remain effective for major depression comorbid with chronic physical illness (Draper 2000), effectiveness is reduced both in terms of acute response and in maintaining remission (Alexopoulos et al. 2005; Reynolds et al. 2006). Other factors that reduce acute treatment response in older people include comorbid anxiety, cerebrovascular disease and age of onset before the age of 60 (Flint and Rifat 1997; Simpson et al. 1997; Reynolds et al. 1998).

There is now good evidence that maintenance treatment with antidepressants for major depression in old age should be continued for two years to prevent recurrence (Reynolds et al. 2006). It is uncertain whether there is added benefit of combining psychotherapy with pharmacotherapy. Two RCTs have shown that the addition of either cognitive behavioural therapy (Wilson et al. 1995) or interpersonal psychotherapy (Reynolds et al. 1992) to a pharmacotherapy regimen improved older depressed patients' outcomes at one-year follow-up. However, more recently no added benefit was found when interpersonal psychotherapy was combined with the SSRI paroxetine over a two-year period (Reynolds et al. 2006).

Do the improved depression outcomes in older patients on antidepressants translate into lower suicide rates? At present, pooled data from RCTs of antidepressants have not shown a reduction in suicide, but the short duration of most drug studies means that this is a question difficult to address from those datasets (Isacsson and Rich 2005). Naturalistic studies of population data, mainly from the 1990s, tend to support the hypothesis that antidepressants prevent suicide, but the presence of many confounding variables needs to be acknowledged (Isacsson and Rich 2005). For example, in Sweden, a 3.5-fold increase in use of antidepressants has been accompanied by a fall in suicide rates (Isacsson 2000), while in Australia an association between the exposure to antidepressants (mainly SSRIs) and reduction in suicide rates in older age groups between 1991–2000 has been reported (Hall et al. 2003). These latter findings are of particular interest for older people, but it is worth noting that there were much greater reductions in suicide rates in older Australians in the 30 years before the introduction of SSRIs (De Leo and Cerin 2003; Draper 2003).

There is stronger evidence that lithium prophylaxis has specific anti-suicide effects apart from its prophylactic efficacy in affective disorders (Müller-Oerlinghausen et al. 2003), but there are no studies that have specifically examined whether this occurs in old age. In addition, there are problems in using lithium in older people. The therapeutic range for lithium reduces with age, which, together with declining renal function, means that a lower lithium dosage is required in the elderly (von Moltke et al. 1993). When compared with younger populations, response to lithium augmentation in older people has been reported to be lower (Zimmer et al. 1991; Flint and Rifat 1994). Dose-limiting side-effects, particularly neuromuscular or neurologic, are a major factor (Flint and Rifat 1994). The poor tolerability of lithium may be enhanced in the physically ill elderly, with 76 per cent of patients in one series discontinuing due to adverse effects (Stoudemire et al. 1998). A dedicated lithium monitoring service for older people using a computerized database improves the quality of monitoring and reduces the risk of adverse events (Fielding et al. 1999). Hence, at this stage there are practical limitations in the use of lithium in the older population that might outweigh the theoretical benefit.

### Treatment of late-life depression and suicidality in primary care

One of the problems that need to be addressed is the effectiveness of the treatment of depression in primary care. Mental health specialists obtain better outcomes for depression in old age compared with GPs. An RCT of the treatment of depression in the frail elderly living at home in the UK by a community multidisciplinary old age psychiatry team showed that significantly more of the intervention group (58 per cent), than the GP-managed control group (25 per cent), had recovered after six months (Banerjee et al. 1996). However, there is mounting evidence through two RCTs in the US that collaborations between primary care and mental health professionals might be effective in preventing suicide, largely through more effective assessment and management of depression. The care is shared but the primary care health workers are in charge and are responsible for screening their patients. The collaboration involves a significant educational and supervisory approach by the mental health professionals.

In the multi-centre IMPACT (Improving Mood-Promoting Access to Collaborative Treatment) study, the primary care physician had access to a depression case manager (a nurse or psychologist) who was supervised by a psychiatrist and a primary care expert. It provided an intervention that included education, care management, and either support of antidepressant management by the patient's primary care physician or brief psychotherapy for depression provided by the depression case manager. The intervention patients had a significantly better outcome at 12 months with 45 per cent having a 50 per cent or greater reduction in depressive symptoms as compared to 19 per cent in the usual care group (Unützer et al. 2002). There were also significant reductions in suicidal ideation up to 24 months after the intervention (Unützer (2005).

The previously mentioned multi-centre PROSPECT study had twenty primary care practices in New York, Pittsburgh and Philadelphia randomly assigned to usual care or a high-intensity intervention. Both interventions received screening and assessment services for identification of diagnosis, however only the high-intensity intervention had a depression health specialist assigned to assist the primary care physician with guideline management based on an algorithm that included the SSRI antidepressant citalopram and/or interpersonal psychotherapy. Rates of suicidal ideation declined faster in the intervention patients compared with usual care after 4 months of treatment (Bruce et al. 2004). First remission of depression occurred earlier and was more common in the intervention group, and patients experiencing hopelessness were more likely to achieve remission in the intervention group (Alexopoulos et al. 2005).

## Conclusions

Current trends in suicide rates disprove that ageing societies have increasing elderly suicide rates (Erlangsen et al 2004). This fact, though poorly investigated, seems to indicate the existence of some abilities of societies (particularly the Western ones) to react and adapt to increased numbers of elderly citizens and their augmented longevity by creating acceptable living conditions even at very advanced ages. As a matter of fact, in many countries, suicide rates have fallen among the elderly who very rarely have been the target of specific anti-suicide strategies, but have received only the improvement in health and social care available to the whole population. In addition, trends in the so-called managed care, involving reduced hospital stays and reduction in hospital resources could have had an adverse effect on elderly suicide rates, although this was not the case. Not even the diffusion of right to end one's life movements seems to have had any appreciable impact so far.

Research data showing gender- and age-specific factors in elderly suicide, e.g. differences in suicide risk factors among the 'young-old' and 'old-old' (Erlangsen et al. 2004, 2005), and older males and females (De Leo 1997; Hunt et al. 2006), has called for development of suicide prevention initiatives and treatments suited to the particular needs of these subpopulations. Available data indicates that certain programmes, for example a community-based suicide prevention programme aimed at the elderly in Yuri, Japan (Oyama et al. 2005) and the Tele-Help/Tele-Check service for the elderly at home in Italy (De Leo et al. 2002) proved to be more effective for elderly females than males. This fact clearly calls for further research on elderly males, particularly of very advanced age, in which suicide rates are usually the highest.

Once more, elderly males (especially if 80+ years old) seem to remain the least adaptable individuals. Available evidence teaches us that women adjust better (see also Chapter 89 in this volume), and where situations in life become particularly critical, strategies in use to counteract them carry a more visible effect with female subjects. This may be due to women's attitude to more easily communicate their inner feelings, thus attracting and receiving emotional support. Men (especially today's elderly men) are less willing to express their emotions, and consequently, appear much less responsive to therapeutic projects based on the verbalization of their suffering. Apart from better education of health care providers in managing those problems that may trigger suicidal behaviour (depression, alcohol abuse, hypochondriacal preoccupations, somatic conditions), and the provision of those elements of security and personal growth that may characterize processes of successful ageing, there still is the need for more innovative strategies for fighting suicide in old age, particularly in elderly males. Even if we were to humbly accept the words of Philip Roth (2002) that we 'can't understand' the old when 'you are not old', we are anyway committed to try. Of course, that is, with the help of the elderly.

## References

Abraham K (1949). The applicability of psychoanalytic treatment to patients at an advanced age. In *Selected papers on Psychoanalysis*, pp. John and Hogart Press, London.

Abraham VJ, Abraham S, Jacob S (2005). Suicide in the elderly in Kaniyambadi block, Tamil Nadu, South India. *International Journal of Geriatric Psychiatry*, **20**, 953–955.

Abrams RC, Marzuk PM, Tardiff K *et al.* (2005). Preference for fall from height as a method of suicide by elderly residents of New York City. *American Journal of Public Health*, **95**, 1000–1002.

Aizenberg D, Olmer A, Barak Y (2006). Suicide attempts amongst elderly bipolar patiens. *Journal of Affective Disorders*, **91**, 91–94.

Alexopoulos GS (2005). Depression in the elderly. *Lancet*, 365, 1961–1970.

Alexopoulos GS, Bruce ML, Hull J *et al.* (1999). Clinical determinants of suicidal ideation and behaviour in geriatric depression. *Archives of General Psychiatry*, **56**, 1048–1053.

Alexopoulos GS, Katz IR, Bruce ML *et al.* (2005). Remission in depressed geriatric primary care patients: A report from the PROSPECT study. *American Journal of Psychiatry*, **162**, 718–724.

Allen N, Ames D, Ashby D *et al.* (1994). A brief sensitive screening instrument for depression in late life. *Age and Ageing*, **23**, 213–218.

APA (American Psychiatric Association) (2003). Practice guideline for the assessment and treatment of patients with suicidal behaviors. *American Journal of Psychiatry*, **160**(Suppl), 11.

Andersen UA, Andersen M, Rosholm JU *et al.* (2000). Contacts to the health care system prior to suicide. *Acta Psychiatrica Scandinavica*, **102**, 126–134.

Artero S, Astruc B, Courtet P *et al.* (2006). Life-time history of suicide attempts and coronary artery disease in community-dwelling elderly population. *International Journal of Geriatric Psychiatry*, **21**, 108–112.

Awata S, Seki T, Koizumi Y *et al.* (2005). Factors associated with suicidal ideation in an elderly urban Japanese population: a community-based, cross-sectional study. *Psychiatry and Clinical Neuroscience*, **59**, 327–336.

Banerjee S, Shamash K, Macdonald A *et al.* (1996). Randomised controlled trial of effect of intervention by psychogeriatric team on depression in frail elderly people at home. *British Medical Journal*, **313**, 1058–1061.

Barak Y, Aizenberg D, Szor H *et al.* (2005). Increased risk of attempted suicide among ageing Holocaust survivors. *American Journal of Geriatric Psychiatry*, **13**, 701–704.

Barak Y, Knobler CY, Aizenberg D (2004). Suicide attempts amongst elderly schizophrenia patients: a 10-year case–control study. *Schizophrenia Research*, **71**, 77–81.

Barnow S and Linden M (2002). Psychosocial risk factors of the wish to be dead in the elderly. Results from the Berlin Aging Study (BASE). *Fortschritte der Neurologie-Psychiatrie*, **70**, 185–191.

Barnow S, Linden M, Freyberger HJ (2004). The relation between suicidal feelings and mental disorders in the elderly: results from the Berlin Aging Study (BASE). *Psychological Medicine*, **34**, 741–746.

Beck AT, Ward CH, Mendelson M *et al.* (1961) An inventory for measuring depression. *Archives of General Psychiatry*, **4**, 561–571.

Berk M, Dodd S, Henry M (2005). The effect of macroeconomic variables on suicide. *Psychological Medicine*, **36**, 181–189.

Booth BM, Kirchner JE, Hamilton G *et al.* (1998). Diagnosing depression in the medically ill: validity of a lay-administered structured diagnostic interview. *Journal of Psychiatric Research*, **32**, 353–360.

Borson S, Barnes RA, Kukull WA *et al.* (1986). Symptomatic depression in elderly medical outpatients. I. Prevalence, demography, and health service utilization. *Journal of the American Geriatrics Society*, **34**, 341–347.

Brown, GK, Bruce ML, Pearson JL (2001). High-risk management guidelines for elderly suicidal patients in primary care settings. *International Journal of Geriatric Psychiatry*, **16**, 593–601.

Bruce ML, Ten Have TR, Reynolds CF *et al.* (2004). Reducing suicidal ideation and depressive symptoms in depressed older primary care patients: a randomized controlled trial. *Journal of American Medical Association*, **9**, 1081–91.

Caine ED and Conwell Y (2001) Suicide in the elderly. *International Clinical Psychopharmacology*, **16**, S25–S30.

Callahan CM, Hendrie HC, Nienaber NA *et al.* (1996). Suicidal ideation among older primary care patients. *Journal of the American Geriatrics Society*, **44**, 1205–1209.

Canetto SS (1992). Gender and suicide in the elderly. *Suicide and Life-Threatening Behavior*, **22**, 80–97.

Chan CY, Beh SL, Broadburst RG (2004). Homicide-suicide in Hong Kong, 1989–1998. *Forensic Science International*, **140**, 261–267.

Chan J, Draper B, Banerjee S (2007). Deliberate self-harm in older adults: A review of the literature from 1995 to 2004. *International Journal of Geriatric Psychiatry*, **22**, 720–732.

Cattell, HR. (1988). Elderly suicide in London: an analysis of coroners' inquests. *International Journal of Geriatric Psychiatry*, **3**, 251–261.

Chiu E, Ames D, Draper B *et al.* (2002). Depressive disorders in the elderly: a review. In M Maj and N Sartorius, eds, *Depressive Disorders*, pp. 313–363. John Wiley & Sons, Chichester.

Chiu HF, Takahashi Y, Suh GH (2003). Elderly suicide prevention in East Asia. *International Journal of Geriatric Psychiatry*, **18**, 973–976.

Chiu HF, Yip PS, Chi I *et al.* (2004). Elderly suicide in Hong Kong: a case-controlled psychological autopsy study. *Acta Psychiatrica Scandinavica*, **109**, 299–305.

Clarke DE, Colantonio A, Heslegrave R *et al.* (2004). Holocaust experience and suicidal ideation in high-risk older adults. *American Journal of Geriatric Psychiatry*, **12**, 65–74.

Clarke DE, Colantonio A, Rhodes A *et al.* (2006). Differential experiences during the Holocaust and suicidal ideation in older adults in treatment for depression. *Journal of Traumatic Stress*, **19**, 417–423.

Clarke RV and Lester D (1989). *Suicide: Closing the Exits*. Springer-Verlag, New York.

Colombo G, Dello Buono M, Smania K *et al.* (2006). Pet therapy and institutionalized elderly: a study on 114 cognitively unimpaired subjects. *Archives of Gerontology and Geriatrics*, **42**, 207–216.

Condello C, Padoani W, Uguzzoni U *et al.* (2003). Personality disorders and self-perceived quality of life in an elderly psychiatric outpatient population. *Psychopathology*, **36**, 78–83.

Conner KR, Conwell Y, Duberstein PR *et al.* (2004). Aggression and suicide among adults age 50 and over. *American Journal of Geriatric Psychiatry*, **12**, 37–42.

Conwell Y (1994). Suicide in elderly patients. In LS Schneider, CF Reynolds, BD Lebowitz *et al.*, eds, *Diagnosis and Treatment of Depression in Late Life*, pp. 397–418. American Psychiatric Press, Washington.

Conwell Y (1997). Management of suicidal behaviour in the elderly. *Psychiatric Clinics of North America*, **20**, 667–683.

Conwell Y, Duberstein PR, Caine ED (2002). Risk factors for suicide in later life. *Biological Psychiatry*, **52**, 193–204.

Conwell Y, Duberstein PR, Cox C *et al.* (1998). Age differences in behaviors leading to completed suicide. *American Journal of Geriatric Psychiatry*, **6**, 122–126.

Conwell Y, Duberstein PR, Cox C *et al.* (2002). Access to firearms and risk for suicide in middle-aged and older adults. *American Journal of Geriatric Psychiatry*, **10**, 407–416.

Conwell Y, Olsen K, Caine ED *et al.* (1991). Suicide in later life: psychological autopsy findings. *International Psychogeriatrics*, **3**, 59–66.

Conwell Y, Pearson J, DeRenzo EG (1996). Indirect self-destructive behavior among elderly patients in nursing homes. A research agenda. *American Journal of Geriatric Psychiatry*, **4**, 152–163.

Conwell Y, Rotenberg M, Caine ED (1990). Completed suicide at age 50 and over. *Journal of American Geriatric Society*, **38**, 640–644.

Crawford MJ, Prince M, Menezes P *et al.* (1998). The recognition and treatment of depression in older people in primary care. *International Journal of Geriatric Psychiatry*, **13**, 172–176.

Daaleman TP, Perera S, Studenski SA (2004). Religion, spirituality, and health status in geriatric outpatients. *Annals of Family Medicine*, **2**, 49–53.

De Leo D (1988). Sunset depression. Doctoral dissertation, Department of Social and Behavioural Sciences, University of Leiden.

De Leo D (1996). Dementia, insight and suicidal behavior. *Crisis*, **17**, 147–148.

De Leo D (1997). I comportamenti suicidari negli anziani: fattori demografici, psicosociali, malattie croniche [Suicidal behaviours in old age: demographic and psychosocial factors, and chronic illness]. *Geriatria* **9**, 277–290.

De Leo D (1997b). Note su comportamenti suicidari di anziani in ospedale generale [Observations on suicidal behaviour of elderly subjects within a general hospital]. *Italian Journal of Suicidology*, **7**, 49–52.

De Leo D (1998a). Reasons for living and the paradox of suicide old age. *Crisis*, **19**, 147–149.

De Leo D (1998b). Is suicide prediction in old age really easier? *Crisis*, **19**, 60–61.

De Leo D (2003). Suicide over the lifespan: the elderly. In R Kastenbaum, ed., *Macmillan Encyclopaedia of Death and Dying*, pp. 837–843. Thomson Gale, New York.

De Leo D (2006). Suicide in Australia. What we know and are seeking to discover. In D De Leo, H. Herrman, S Ueda *et al.*, eds, *An Australian-Japanese Perspective on Suicide Prevention: Culture, Community, and Care*, pp. 17–35. Commonwealth of Australia, Department of Health and Aging, Canberra.

De Leo D and Marietta P (1997). Suicide: determinism or freeedom? *Italian Journal of Suicidology*, **7**, 99–110.

De Leo D and Scocco P (2000). Treatment and prevention of suicidal behaviour in the elderly. In K Hawton and K van Heeringen, eds, *The International Handbook of Suicide and Attempted Suicide*, pp. 555–570. John Wiley & Sons, Chichester.

De Leo D and Cerin E (2003). More than antidepressants are needed to avert suicide. *British Medical Journal*, **326**, 1008.

De Leo D and Evans R (2004). *International Suicide Rates and Prevention Strategies*. Hogrefe & Huber, Göttingen.

De Leo D and Heller T (2004). *Suicide in Queensland, 1999–2001*. Australian Institute for Suicide Research and Prevention, Brisbane.

De Leo D and Spathonis K (2004). Suicide and suicidal behaviour in late life. In D De Leo, U Bille-Brahe, A Kerkhof *et al.*, eds, *Suicidal Behaviour. Theories and Research Findings*, pp. 253–286. Hogrefe & Huber, Göttingen.

De Leo D, Carollo G, Dello Buono M (1995). Lower suicide rates associated with a Tele-Help/Tele-Check service for the elderly at home. *American Journal of Psychiatry*, **152**, 632–634.

De Leo D, Diekstra RF, Lonnqvist J *et al.* (1998). LEIPAD, an internationally applicable instrument to assess quality of life in the elderly. *Behavioural Medicine*, **24**, 17–24.

De Leo D, Hickey P, Meneghel G *et al.* (1999). Blindness, fear of sight loss, and suicide. *Psychosomatics*, **40**, 339–344.

De Leo D, Padoani W, Scocco P *et al.* (2001) Attempted and completed suicide in older subjects: results from the WHO/EURO Multicentre Study of Suicidal Behaviour. *International Journal of Geriatric Psychiatry*, **16**, 300–310.

De Leo D, Dello Buono M, Dwyer J (2002a). Suicide among the elderly: the long-term impact of a telephone support and assessment intervention in northern Italy. *British Journal of Psychiatry*, **181**, 226–229.

De Leo D, Padovani W, Lonnqvist J *et al.* (2002b). Repetition of suicidal behaviour in elderly Europeans: a prospective longitudinal study. *Journal of Affective Disorders*, **72**, 291–295.

Dello Buono M, Urciuoli O, De Leo D (1998). Quality of life and longevity: a study of centenarians. *Age and Ageing*, **27**, 206–210.

Dennis M, Wakefield P, Molloy C *et al.* (2005). Self-harm in older people with depression. Comparison of social factors, life events and symptoms. *British Journal of Psychiatry*, **186**, 538–539.

Dombrovski AY and Szanto K. (2005). Prevention of suicide in the elderly. *Annals of Long-Term Care*, **13**, 25–32.

Draper B (1995). Prevention of suicide in old age. *Medical Journal of Australia*, **162**, 533–534.

Draper B (1996). Attempted suicide in old age. Editorial review. *International Journal of Geriatric Psychiatry* **11**, 577–587.

Draper B (2000). The effectiveness of the treatment of depression in the physically ill elderly. *Aging and Mental Health*, **4**, 9–20.

Draper B (2003). Antidepressant prescribing and suicide. Associations attribute possible causality inappropriately. *British Medical Journal*, **327**, 288.

Draper B, Brodaty H, Low LF (2002a). Types of nursing home residents with self-destructive behaviours: analysis of the Harmful Behaviours Scale. *International Journal of Geriatric Psychiatry*, **17**, 670–675.

Draper B, Brodaty H, Low LF. *et al.* (2002b). Self-destructive behaviours in nursing home residents. *Journal of the American Geriatrics Society*, **50**, 354–358.

Draper B, Snowdon J, Wyder M (2008) A pilot study of a suicide victim's last contact with a health professional. *Crisis*, **29**, 96–101.

Draper B, Brodaty H, Low LF *et al.* (2003). Prediction of mortality in nursing home residents: impact of self-destructive behaviours. *International Psychogeriatrics*, **15**, 187–196.

Draper B and Low LF (2004). *What is the effectiveness of old-age mental health services?* World Health Organisation Regional Office for Europe Health Evidence Network, Copenhagen.

Duberstein P, Conwell Y, Caine ED (1994). Age differences in the personality traits of suicide completers: preliminary findings from a psychological autopsy study. *Psychiatry*, **57**, 213–224.

Duberstein PR, Conwell Y, Conner KR *et al.* (2004a). Poor social integration and suicide: fact or artefact? A case–control study. *Psychological Medicine*, **34**, 1331–1337.

Duberstein P, Conwell Y, Conner KR *et al.* (2004b). Suicide at 50 years of age and older: perceived physical illness, family discord and financial strain. *Psychological Medicine*, **34**, 137–146.

Duberstein PR, Conwell Y, Cox C (1998). Suicide in widowed persons: a psychological autopsy comparison of recently and remotely bereaved older subjects. *American Journal of Geriatric Psychiatry*, **6**, 328–334.

Duberstein PR, Conwell Y, Seidlitz L *et al.* (1999). Age and suicidal ideation in older depressed inpatients. *American Journal of Geriatric Psychiatry*, **7**, 289–296.

Erlangsen A, Jeune B, Bille-Brahe U *et al.* (2004). Loss of partner and suicide risk among oldest old: a population-based register study. *Age and Ageing*, **33**, 378–383.

Erlangsen A, Vach W, Jeune B (2005). The effect of hospitalization with medical illnesses on the suicide risk in the oldest old: a population-based register study. *Journal of the American Geriatrics Society*, **53**, 771–776.

Etkind M (1997). *… Or note to be? A Collection of Suicide Notes.* Riverhead Books, New York.

Everly GS (2000). 'Pastoral crisis intervention': toward a definition. *International Journal of Emergency Mental Health*, **2**, 69–71.

Fenichel O (1951). *Trattato di Psicanalisi* [Treatise of Psychoanalysis], Astrolabio, Rome.

Felton BJ, Revenson TA, Hinrichsen GA (1984). Stress and coping in the explanation of psychological adjustment among chronically ill adults. *Social Science and Medicine*, **18**, 889–898.

Fielding S, Kerr S, Godber C (1999). Lithium in the over-65s—a dedicated monitoring service leads to a better quality of treatment supervision. *International Journal of Geriatric Psychiatry*, **14**, 985–987.

Flint AJ and Rifat SL (1994) A prospective study of lithium augmentation in antidepressant-resistant geriatric depression. *Journal of Clinical Psychopharmacology*, **14**, 353–356.

Flint AJ and Rifat SL (1997). Effect of demographic and clinical variables on time to antidepressant response in geriatric depression. *Depression and Anxiety*, **5**, 103–107.

Flisher AJ, Liang H, Laubscher R *et al.* (2004). Suicide trends in South Africa, 1968–1990. *Scandinavian Journal of Public Heath*, **32**, 411–418.

Foster T (2003). Suicide note themes and suicide prevention. *International Journal of Psychiatry in Medicine*, **33**, 323–331.

Florio ER, Hendryx M, Jensen JE *et al.* (1997). A comparison of suicidal and nonsuicidal elders referred to a community mental health centre program. *Suicide and Life-Threatening Behavior*, **27**, 182–193.

Florio ER, Jensen JE, Hendryx M *et al.* (1998). One-year outcomes of older adults referred for aging and mental health services by community gatekeepers. *Journal of Case Management*, **7**, 74–83.

Florio ER, Rockwood TH, Hendryx MS *et al.* (1996). A model gatekeeper program to find the at-risk elderly. *Journal of Case Management*, **5**, 106–114.

Fujisawa D, Tanaka E, Sakamoto S *et al.* (2005). The development of a brief screening instrument for depression and suicidal ideation for elderly: The Depression and Suicide Screen. *Psychiatry and Clinical Neuroscience*, **59**, 634–638.

Gallo JJ, Rabins PV, Iliffe S (1997). The 'research magnificent' in late life: psychiatric epidemiology and the primary health care of older adults. *International Journal of Psychiatry in Medicine*, **27**, 185–204.

Goldney RD (2006). Suicide and antidepressants: what is the evidence? *Australian and New Zealand Journal of Psychiatry*, **40**, 381–385.

Hall WD, Mant A, Mitchell PB *et al.* (2003). Association between antidepressant prescribing and suicide in Australia; 1991–2000: Trend analysis. *British Medical Journal*, **326**, 1008.

Hamilton M (1960). A rating scale for depression. *Journal of Neurology, Neurosurgery and Psychiatry*, **23**, 56–62.

Harwood D, Hawton K, Hope T *et al.* (2001). Psychiatric disorder and personality factors associated with suicide in older people: a descriptive and case–control study. *International Journal of Geriatric Psychiatry*, **16**, 155–165.

Harwood D, Hawton K, Hope T *et al.* (2006a). Suicide in older people without psychiatric disorder. *International Journal of Geriatric Psychiatry*, **21**, 363–367.

Harwood D, Hawton K, Hope T *et al.* (2006b). Life problems and physical illness as risk factors for suicide in older people: a descriptive and case–control study. *Psychological Medicine*, in press.

Hawgood J, Spathonis K, De Leo D (2004). Physical illness and suicidal behaviour. In D De Leo, U Bille-Brahe, ADJF Kerkhof *et al.*, eds, *Suicidal Behaviour. Theories and Research Findings*, pp. 139–163. Hogrefe & Huber, Göttingen.

Hawton K and Harriss L (2006). Deliberate self-harm in people aged 60 years and over: characteristics and outcome of a 20-year cohort. *International Journal of Geriatric Psychiatry*, 21, 572–581.

Hegerl U, Althaus D, Schmidtke A *et al.* (2006). The alliance against depression: 2-year evaluation of a community-based intervention to reduce suicidality. *Psychological Medicine*, **17**, 1–9.

Heikkinen M, Aro H, Lonnqvist J (1992). The partners' views on precipitant stressors in suicide. *Acta Psychiatrica Scandinavica*, **85**, 380–384.

Heisel MJ (2006). Suicide and its prevention among older adults. *Canadian Journal of Psychiatry*, **51**, 143–154.

Heisel MJ, Flett GL, Duberstein PR *et al.* (2005). Does the geriatric depression scale distinguish between older adults with high versus low levels of suicidal ideation? *American Journal of Geriatric Psychiatry*, **13**, 876–883.

Ho TP, Yip PS, Chiu CW *et al.* (1998). Suicide notes: What do they tell us? *Acta Psychiatrica Scandinavica*, **98**, 467–473.

Hohmann AA and Larson DB (1993). Psychiatric factors predicting use of clergy. In WEL Worthington Jr, ed., *Psychotherapy and Religious Values*, pp. 71–84. Baker Book House, Grand Rapids.

Hooper SC, Vaughan KJ, Tennant CC *et al.* (1996). Major depression and refusal of life-sustaining medical treatment in the elderly. *Medical Journal of Australia*, **165**, 416–419.

Hunt IM, Kapur N, Robinson J *et al.* (2006). Suicide within 12 months of mental health service contact in different age and diagnostic groups: national clinical survey. *British Journal of Psychiatry*, **188**, 135–142.

Hunt K, Sweeting H, Keoghan M *et al.* (2006). Sex, gender role orientation, gender role attitudes and suicidal thoughts ion three generations: a general population study. *Social Psychiatry and Psychiatric Epidemiology*, **41**, 641–7.

Isacsson G (2000). Suicide prevention—a medical breakthrough? *Acta Psychiatrica Scandinavica*, **102**, 113–117.

Isacsson G, Rich CL (2005). Antidepressant drug use and suicide prevention. *International Review of Psychiatry*, **17**, 153–162.

Isometsä ET, Heikkinen ME, Marttunen MJ *et al.* (1995). The last appointment before suicide: is suicide intent communicated? *American Journal of Psychiatry*, **152**, 919–922.

Isometsä ET, Henriksson MM, Heikkinen ME *et al.* (1996). Completed suicide and recent electroconvulsive therapy in Finland. *Convulsive Therapy*, **12**, 152–155.

Jackson R and Baldwin B (1993). Detecting depression in elderly medically ill patients: the use of the Geriatric Depression Scale compared with medical and nursing observations. *Age and Ageing*, **22**, 349–353.

Juurlink DN, Herrmann N, Szalai JP *et al.* (2004). Medical illness and the risk of suicide in the elderly. *Archives of Internal Medicine*, **164**, 1179–1184.

Keilp JG, Sackheim HA, Brodsky BS *et al.* (2001). Neuropsychological dysfunction in depressed suicide attempters. *American Journal of Psychiatry*, **158**, 735–741.

Kessing LV (2004). Severity of depressive episodes according to ICD-10: prediction of risk of relapse and suicide. *British Journal of Psychiatry*, **184**, 153–156.

King DA, Conwell Y, Cox C *et al.* (2000). A neuropsychological comparison of depressed suicide attempters and nonattempters. *Journal of Neuropsychiatry and Clinical Neurosciences*, **12**, 64–70.

Kissane M and McLaren S (2006). Sense of belonging as a predictor of reasons for living in older adults. *Death Studies*, **30**, 243–258.

Knauper B and Wittchen HU (1994). Diagnosing major depression in the elderly: evidence for response bias in standardized diagnostic reviews? *Journal of Psychiatric Research*, **28**, 147–164.

Koder DA, Brodaty H, Anstey KJ (1996). Cognitive therapy for depression in the elderly. *International Journal of Geriatric Psychiatry*, **11**, 97–107.

Koenig HG (1994). *Aging and God.* Haworth Press, New York.

Koenig HG and Breitner JCS (1990). Use of antidepressants in medically ill older patients. *Psychosomatics*, **31**, 22–32.

Koenig HG, Goli V, Shelp F *et al.* (1992). Major depression in hospitalized medically ill older men: documentation, management, and outcome. *International Journal of Geriatric Psychiatry*, **7**, 25–34.

Koenig HG, George LK, Meador KG (1997a). Use of antidepressants by nonpsychiatrists in the treatment of medically ill hospitalized depressed elderly patients. *American Journal of Psychiatry*, **154**, 1369–1375.

Koenig HG, George LK, Peterson BL *et al.* (1997b). Depression in medically ill hospitalized older adults: prevalence, characteristics, and course of symptoms according to six diagnostic schemes. *American Journal of Psychiatry*, **154**, 1376–1383.

Kohn R and Epstein-Lubow G (2006). Course and outcomes of depression in the elderly. *Current Psychiatry Reports*, **1**, 34–40.

Kolves K, Varnik A, Schneider B *et al.* (2006a). Recent life events and suicide: a case–control study in Tallinn and Frankfurt. *Social Science and Medicine*, **62**, 2887–2896.

Kolves K, Varnik A, Tooding LM *et al.* (2006b). The role of alcohol in suicide: a case–control psychological autopsy study. *Psychological Medicine*, **36**, 923–930.

Krause N (2006). Church-based social support and mortality. *Journal of Gerontology*, **61B**, 140–146.

Krause N and Shaw BA (2000). Giving social support to others, socioeconomic status, and changes in self-esteem in late life. *Journal of Gerontology*, **55B**, 323–333.

Krysinska K, Heller TS, De Leo D (2006). Suicide and deliberate self-harm in personality disorders. *Current Opinion in Psychiatry*, **19**, 95–101.

Kua E-H, Ko S-M, Ng T-P (2003). Recent trends in elderly suicide rates in a multi-ethnic Asian city. *International Journal of Geriatric Psychiatry*, **18**, 533–536.

Labisi O (2006). Assessing for suicide risk in depressed geriatric cancer patients. *Journal of Psychosocial Oncology*, **24**, 43–50.

Lamprecht HC, Pakrasi S, Gash A *et al.* (2005). Deliberate self-harm in older people revisited. *International Journal of Geriatric Psychiatry*, **20**, 1090–1096.

Leane W and Shute R (1998). Youth suicide: the knowledge and attitudes of Australian teachers and clergy. *Suicide and Life-Threatening Behavior*, **28**, 165–173.

Leenaars AA (1992). Suicide notes of the older adult. *Suicide and Life-Threatening Behavior*, **22**, 62–79.

Leenaars AA (1996). Suicide notes at symbolic ages. *Psychological Reports*, **78**, 1034.

Leenaars AA (1997). Suicide notes of the elderly and their implications for psychotherapy. *Clinical Gerontologist*, **17**, 76–79.

Leibenluft E and Goldberg RL (1988). The suicidal terminally ill patient with depression. *Psychosomatics*, **29**, 379–386.

Lester D (2005). *Suicide and the Holocaust*. Nova Science Publishers, New York.

Lester D and Tallmer M (1994). *Now I Lay me Down. Suicide in the Elderly*. Charles Press, Philadelphia.

Links PS, Heisel MJ, Quastel A (2005). Is suicide ideation a surrogate endpoint for geriatric suicide? *Suicide and Life-Threatening Behavior*, **35**, 193–205.

Linn M and Lester D (1996). Content differences in suicide notes by gender and age: serendipitous findings. *Psychological Reports*, **78**, 370.

Llewellyn-Jones RH, Baikie KA, Smithers H *et al.* (1999). Multifaceted shared care intervention for late life depression in residential care: randomised controlled trial. *British Medical Journal*, **319**, 676–682.

Llorente MD, Burke M, Gregory GR *et al.* (2005). Prostate cancer: a significant risk factor for late-life suicide. *American Journal of Geriatric Psychiatry*, **13**, 195–2001.

Loebel JP, Loebel JS, Dager SR *et al.* (1991). Antiicpation of nursing home placement may be a precipitant of suicide among elderly. *Journal of the American Geriatrics Society*, **39**, 407–408.

Luoma JB, Martin CE, Pearson JL (2002). Contact with mental health and primary care providers before suicide: a review of the evidence. *American Journal of Psychiatry*, **159**, 909–916.

Lynch TR, Cheavens JS, Morse JQ *et al.* (2004). A model predicting suicidal ideation and hopleessnes in depressed older adults: the impact of emotion inhibition and affect intensity. *Aging and Mental Health*, **8**, 486–497.

Malphurs JE and Cohen D (2005). A statewide case–control study of spousal homicide-suicide in older persons. *American Journal of Geriatric Psychiatry*, **13**, 211–217.

Mann JJ, Apter A, Bertolote J *et al.* (2005). Suicide prevention strategies: a systematic review. *Journal of the American Medical Association*, **294**, 2064–2074.

Marzuk PM, Hartwell N, Leon AC *et al.* (2005). Executive functioning in depressed patients with suicidal ideation. *Acta Psychiatrica Scandinavica*, **112**, 294–301.

McCall PL (1991). Adolescent and elderly white male suicide trends: evidence of changing well-being? *Journal of Gerontology*, **46**, 43–51.

McIntosh JL (1995). Suicide prevention in the elderly (age 65–99). *Suicide and Life-Threatening Behavior*, **25**, 180–192.

McIntosh JL, Santos JF, Hubbard RW *et al.* (1994). *Elder Suicide: Research, Theory and Treatment*. American Psychological Association, Washington.

Menon AS, Campbell D, Ruskin P *et al.* (2000). Depression, hopelessness, and the desire for life-saving treatments among elderly medically ill veterans. *American Journal of Geriatric Psychiatry*, **8**, 333–342.

Meylink W and Gorsuch R (1987). Relationship between clergy and psychologists: the empirical data. *Journal of Psychology and Christianity*, **7**, 56–72.

Mrazek PJ and Haggerty RJ (1994). *Reducing the Risks for Mental Disorders: Frontiers for Preventive Intervention Research*. National Academy Press, Washington.

Müller-Oerlinghausen B, Berghöfer A, Ahrens B (2003). The antisuicidal and mortality-reducing effect of lithium prophylaxis: consequences for guidelines in clinical psychiatry. *Canadian Journal of Psychiatry*, **48**, 433–439.

Neulinger K and De Leo D (2001) Suicide in the elderly and youth populations: how do they differ? In D De Leo, ed., *Suicide and Euthanasia in Older Adults*, pp. 135–154. Hogrefe & Huber, Göttingen.

Obafunwa JO and Busuttil A (1994). Clinical contact preceding suicide. *Postgraduate Medical Journal*, **70**, 428–432.

O'Conell H, Chin A-V, Cunningham C, Lawlor BA (2006). Recent developments: suicide in older people. *British Medical Journal*, **329**, 895–899.

Ono Y (2004). Suicide prevention program for the elderly: the experience of Japan. *Keio Journal of Medicine*, **53**, 1–6.

Oquendo MA, Lizardi D, Greenwald S *et al.* (2004). Rates of lifetime suicide attempt and rates of lifetime major depression in different ethnic groups in the United States. *Acta Psychiatrica Scandinavica*, **110**, 446–451.

Ormel J, Kempen GIJM, Penninx BWJH *et al.* (1997). Chronic medical conditions and mental health in older people: disability and psychosocial resources mediate specific mental health effects. *Psychological Medicine*, **27**, 1065–1077.

Osgood NJ, Brant BA, Lipman A (1991). *Suicide Among the Elderly in Long-term Care Facilities*. Greenwood Press, New York.

Oslin DW, Zubritsky C, Brown G *et al.* (2004). Managing suicide risk in old life: access to firearms as a public health risk. *American Journal of Geriatric Psychiatry*, **12**, 30–36.

Oyama H, Koida J, Sakashita T *et al..* (2004). Community-based prevention for suicide in elderly by depression screening and follow-up. *Community Mental Health Journal*, **40**, 249–263.

Oyama H, Ono Y, Watanabe N *et al.* (2006). Local community intervention through depression screening and group activity for elderly suicide prevention. *Psychiatry and Clinical Neurosciences*, **60**, 110–114.

Oyama H, Watanabe N, Ono Y *et al.* (2005). Community-based suicide prevention through group activity for the elderly successfully reduced the high suicide rate for females. *Psychiatry and Clinical Neurosciences*, **59**, 337–344.

Padoani W, Marini M, De Leo D (2001). Cognitive impairment, insight, depression and suicidal ideation. *Archives of Gerontology and Geriatrics*, **7**, 295–298.

Pearson JL, Conwell Y, Lyness JM (1997). Late-life suicide and depression in the primary care setting. *New Direction for Mental Health Services*, **76**, 13–38.

Pfaff J and Almeida O (2003). *Identifying and Managing Suicidal Risk in Older Adults: A Desktop Reference Guide for General Practice.* Commonwealth Department of Health and Ageing, Advance Press, Perth.

Preville M, Hebert R, Boyer R *et al.* (2005). Physical health and mental disorder in elderly suicide: a case–control study. *Aging and Mental Health*, **9**, 576–584.

Pritchard C and Baldwin DS (2002). Elderly suicide rates in Asian and English-speaking countries. *Acta Psychiatrica Scandinavica*, **105**, 271–275.

Pritchard C and Hansen L (2005). Comparison of suicide in people aged 65–74 and 75+ by gender in England and Wales and the major Western countries 1979–1999. *International Journal of Geriatric Psychiatry*, **20**, 17–25.

Quan H, Arboleda-Florez J, Fick GH *et al.* (2002). Association between physical illness and suicide among the elderly. *Social Psychiatry and Psychiatric Epidemiology*, **37**, 190–197.

Reynolds III CF, Dew MA, Frank E *et al.* (1998). Effects of age at onset of first lifetime episode of recurrent major depression on treatment response and illness course in elderly patients. *American Journal of Psychiatry*, **155**, 795–799.

Reynolds III CF, Frank E, Perel JM *et al.* (1999). Nortriptyline and and interpersonal psychotherapy as maintenance therapies for recurrent major depression: a randomised controlled trial in patients older than 59 years. *Journal of American Medical Association*, **281**, 39–45.

Reynolds III CF, Dew MA, Pollock BG, *et al.* (2006). Maintenance treatment of major depression in old age. *New England Journal of Medicine*, **354**, 1130–1138.

Reynolds III CF, Frank E, Perel JM *et al.* (1992). Combined pharmacotherapy and psychotherapy in the acute and continuation treatment of elderly patients with recurrent major depression: a preliminary report. *American Journal of Psychiatry*, **149**, 1687–1692.

Richman J (1994). Family therapy for the suicidal elderly. In D Lester and M Talmer, eds, *Now I Lay me Down. Suicide in the Elderly*, pp. 73–87. Charles Press, Philadelphia.

Rifai AH, George CJ, Stack JA *et al.* (1994). Hopelessness in suicide attempters after acute treatment of major depression in late life. *American Journal of Psychiatry*, **151**, 1687–1690.

Rosenberg M, Davidson L, Smith J *et al.* (1988). Operational criteria for the determination of suicide. *Journal of Forensic Science*, **33**, 1445–1456.

Roth P (2002). *The Dying Animal*. Vintage, London.

Rubenowitz E, Waern M, Wilhelmson K *et al.* (2001). Life events and psychosocial factors in elderly suicides: a case–control study. *Psychological Medicine*, **31**, 1193–1202.

Rubio A, Vestner AL, Stewart JM *et al.* (2001). Suicide and Alzheimer's pathology in the elderly: a case–control study. *Biological Psychiatry*, **49**, 137–145.

Ruths FA, Tobiansky RI, Blanchard M (2005). Deliberate self-harm (DSH) among older people: a retrospective study in Barnet, North London. *International Journal of Geriatric Psychiatry*, **20**, 106–112.

Salib E, Cawley S, Healy R (2002a). The significance of suicide notes in the elderly. *Aging and Mental Health*, **6**, 186–190.

Salib E, El-Nimr G, Yacoub M (2002b). Their last words: a review of suicide notes in the elderly. *Medicine, Science, and the Law*, **42**, 334–338.

Salib E, El-Nimr G, Habeeb B *et al.* (2004). Childlessness in elderly suicide: AN analysis of coroner's inquests of 200 cases of elderly suicide in Cheshire 1989–2001. *Medicine, Science and Law*, **44**, 207–212.

Salib E, Rahim S, El-Nimr G *et al.* (2005). Elderly suicide: an analysis of coroner's inquests into 200 cases in Cheshire 1989–2001. *Medicine, Science and Law*, **45**, 71–80.

Schifano F (1994). Pharmacological strategies for preventing suicidal behaviour. *CNS Drugs*, **1**, 16–25.

Schmidtke A, Bille-Brahe U, De Leo D *et al.* (2004). Sociodemographic characteristics of suicide attempters in Europe. In A Schmidtke, U Bille-Brahe, D De Leo *et al.*, eds, *Suicidal Behaviour in Europe*, pp. 29–43. Hogrefe & Huber, Göttingen.

Scocco P and De Leo D (2002). One-year prevalence of death thoughts, suicide ideation and behaviours in an elderly population. *International Journal of Geriatric Psychiatry*, **17**, 842–846.

Scocco P, Meneghel G, Caon F *et al.* (2001). Death ideation and its correlates: survey of an over-65-year-old population. *Journal of Nervous and Mental Disease*, **189**, 210–218.

Scocco P, Rapattoni M, Fantoni G *et al.* (2006). Suicidal behaviour in nursing homes: a survey in a region of north-east Italy. *International Journal of Geriatric Psychiatry*, **21**, 307–311.

Shah AK and De T (1998). Suicide and the elderly. *International Journal of Psychiatry in Clinical Practice*, **2**, 3–17.

Shah S and Harris M (1997). A survey of general practitioners' confidence in their management of elderly patients. *Australian Family Physician*, **26**(Suppl. 1), S12–S17.

Shah A and Lodhi L (2005). The impact of trends in psychotropic prescribing on the methods of suicide in the elderly. *Medicine, Science and Law*, **45**, 115–120.

Shasha M, Lyons JS, O'Mahoney MT *et al.* (1997). Serotonin reuptake inhibitors and the adequacy of antidepressant treatment. *International Journal of Psychiatry in Medicine*, **27**, 83–92.

Shiho Y, Tohru T, Shinji S *et al.* (2005). Suicide in Japan: present conditions and prevention measures. *Crisis*, **26**, 12–19.

Simpson SW, Jackson A, Baldwin RC *et al.* (1997). Subcortical hyperintensities in late-life depression: acute response to treatment and neuropsychological impairment. *International Psychogeriatrics*, **9**, 257–275.

Snowdon J and Baume P (2002). A study of suicides of older people in Sydney. *International Journal of Geriatric Psychiatry*, **17**, 261–269.

Snowdon J, Burgess E, Vaughan R *et al.* (1996). Use of antidepressants, and the prevalence of depression and cognitive impairment in Sydney nursing homes. *International Journal of Geriatric Psychiatry*, **11**, 599–606.

Stefulj J, Kubat M, Balija M *et al.* (2006). TPH gene polymorphism and aging: indication of combined effects on the predisposition to violent suicide. *American Journal of Medical Genetics Part B: Neuropsychiatric Genetics*, **141**, 139–141.

Stoppe G, Sandholzer H, Huppertz C *et al.* (1999). Family physicians and the risk of suicide in the depressed elderly. *Journal of Affective Disorders*, **54**, 193–198.

Stoudemire A, Hill CD, Lewison BJ *et al.* (1998). Lithium intolerance in a medical-psychiatric population. *General Hospital Psychiatry*, **20**, 85–90.

Suominen K, Henriksson M, Isometsä E *et al.* (2003). Nursing home suicides: a psychological autopsy study. *International Journal of Geriatric Psychiatry*, **18**, 1095–1101.

Suominen K, Isometsä ET, Lönnqvist JK (2004). Elderly suicide attempters with depression are often diagnosed only after the attempt. *International Journal of Geriatric Psychiatry*, **19**, 35–40.

Szanto K, Mulsant BH, Houck P *et al.* (2003). Occurrence and course of suicidality during short-term treatment of late-life depression. *Archives of General Psychiatry*, **60**, 610–617.

Szanto K, Reynolds III CF, Conwell Y *et al.* (1998). High levels of hopelessness persist in geriatric patients with remitted depression and a history of attempted suicide. *Journal of the American Geriatrics Society*, **46**, 1401–1406.

Szanto K, Gildengers A, Mulsant BH *et al.* (2002). Identification of suicidal ideation and prevention of suicidal behaviour in the elderly. *Drugs and Aging*, **19**, 11–24.

Szanto K, Reynolds III CF, Frank E *et al.* (1996). Suicide in elderly depressed patients. Is active vs passive suicidal ideation a clinically valid distinction? *American Journal of Geriatric Psychiatry*, **4**, 197–207.

Szanto K., Shear MK, Houck PR *et al.* (2006). Indirect self-destructive behaviour and overt suicidality in patients with complicated grief. *Journal of Clinical Psychiatry*, **67**, 233–239.

Tsoh J, Chiu HF, Duberstein PR *et al.* (2005). Attempted suicide in elderly Chinese persons: a multi-group, controlled study. *American Journal of Geriatric Psychiatry*, **13**, 562–571.

Turvey CL, Conwell Y, Jones MP *et al.* (2002). Risk factors for late-life suicide: a prospective community-based study. *American Journal of Geriatric Psychiatry*, **10**, 398–406.

Unutzer J (2005). Effects of treatment for late life depression on suicidal ideation: the IMPACT Trial. Presented at the Annual Meeting of the American Association for Geriatric Psychiatry; March 3–6, 2005, San Diego, Ca.

Unützer J, Katon W, Callahan CM *et al.* (2002). Collaborative care management of late-life depression in the primary care setting: a randomized controlled trial. *Journal of American Medical Association*, **288**, 2836–2845.

Upanne M (2001). A model-based analysis of professional practices in suicide prevention. *Scandinavian Journal of Public Health*, **29**, 292–299.

Van Casteren V, Van der Veken J, Tafforeau J *et al.* (1993). Suicide and attempted suicide reported by general practitioners in Belgium, 1990–1991. *Acta Psychiatrica Scandinavica*, **87**, 451–455.

Vanderhorst RK and McLaren S (2005). Social relationships as predictors of depression and suicidal ideation in older adults. *Aging and Mental Health*, **9**, 517–525.

Vassilas CA and Morgan HG (1994). Elderly suicides' contact with their general practitioner before death. *International Journal of Geriatric Psychiatry*, **9**, 1008–1009.

Vijayakumar L, Pirkis J, Whiteford H (2002). Suicide in developing countries (3): Prevention efforts. *Crisis*, **26**, 120–124.

von Moltke LL, Greenblatt DJ, Shader RI (1993). Clinical pharmacokinetics of antidepressants in the elderly. Therapeutic implications. *Clinical Pharmacokinetics*, **24**, 141–160.

Waern M (2003). Alcohol dependence and misuse in elderly suicides. *Alcohol and Alcoholism*, **38**, 249–254.

Waern M (2005). Suicides among family members of elderly suicide victims: an exploratory study. *Suicide and Life-Threatening Behavior*, **35**, 356–364.

Waern M, Beskow J, Runeson B *et al.* (1996). High rate of antidepressant treatment in elderly people who commit suicide. *British Medical Journal*, **313**, 1118.

Waern M, Beskow J, Runeson B *et al.* (1999). Suicidal feelings in the last year of life in elderly people who commit suicide. *Lancet*, **354**, 917–918.

Waern M, Rubenowitz E, Wilhelmson K (2003). Predictors of suicide in the old elderly. *Gerontology*, **49**, 328–334.

Waern M, Runeson BS, Allebeck P *et al.* (2002). Mental disorder in elderly suicides: case–control study. *American Journal of Psychiatry*, **159**, 450–455.

Weaver AJ and Koenig HG (1996). Elderly suicide, mental health professionals, and the clergy: a need for clinical collaboration, training, and research. *Death Studies*, **20**, 495–508.

Williams JW, Barrett J, Oxman T *et al.* (2001). Treatment of dysthymia and minor depression in primary care: a randomised controlled trial in older adults. *Journal of American Medical Association*, **284**, 1519–1526.

Wilson K, Mottram P, Sivanranthan A *et al.* (2003). *Antidepressants Versus Placebo for the Depressed Elderly* (Cochrane Review). In The Cochrane Library. John Wiley & Sons, Chichester.

Wilson KCM, Scott M, Abou-Saleh M *et al.* (1995). Long-term effects of cognitive-behavioural therapy and lithium therapy in depression in the elderly. *British Journal of Psychiatry*, **167**, 653–658.

Wu WCH and Bond MH (2006). National differences in predictors of suicide among young and elderly citizens: linking societal predictors to psychological factors. *Archives of Suicide Research*, **10**, 45–60.

Yen YC, Yang MJ, Yang MS *et al.* (2005). Suicidal ideation and associated factors among community dwelling elders in Taiwan. *Psychiatry and Clinical Neuroscience*, **59**, 364–371.

Yesavage JA, Brink TL, Rose TL *et al.* (1983). Development and validation of a Geriatric Depression Scale: a preliminary report. *Journal of Psychiatric Research*, **17**, 37–49.

Yip PSF (2001). An epidemiological profile of suicides in Beijing, China. *Suicide and Life-Threatening Behavior*, **31**, 62–70.

Yip PSF, Chi I, Yu KK (1998). An epidemiological profile of elderly suicides in Hong Kong. *International Journal of Geriatric Psychiatry*, **13**, 631–637.

Yip PSF, Liu KY, Hu J *et al.* (2005). Suicide rates in China during a decade of rapid social changes. *Social Psychiatry and Psychiatric Epidemiology*, **40**, 792–798.

Ziervogel A., Pfeiffer T, Hegerl U (2005). How effective is advanced training concerning depression and suicidality among the elderly? Results of a pilot study. *Archives of Suicide Research*, **9**, 11–17.

Zimmer B, Rosen J, Thornton JE *et al.* (1991). Adjunctive lithium carbonate in nortriptyline-resistant elderly depressed patients. *Journal of Clinical Psychopharmacology*, **11**, 254–257.

# PART 14

# Networking in Suicide Research and Prevention

# CHAPTER 96

# The World Health Organization's role in suicide prevention

Benedetto Saraceno

## Introduction

Suicide is not only a personal tragedy, but a serious international public health problem. The majority of suicides in the world (85 per cent) occur in low- and middle-income countries (Krug *et al.* 2002). Suicide is among the top three causes of death in the young population aged 15–34 (World Health Organization 2001).

Whereas national data about *completed* suicide exists for many countries, similar statistics on *attempted* suicide are largely missing, reflecting a lack of official or systematic national data collection. Hence, the scale of suicide attempts is not clearly known. Relying on hospital records and population surveys, it is estimated that attempted suicides are 10–20 times more frequent than completed suicides (Wasserman 2001).

The Secretary-General of the United Nations in his report to the General Assembly in 1991 drew attention to the fact that suicide was a significant and growing problem, particularly among youth. The ensuing monitoring process revealed a lack of comprehensive national strategies for preventing suicide and, in many countries, rapidly rising suicide rates. In 1993, a United Nations (UN) and World Health Organization (WHO) International Expert Meeting on Guidelines for the Formulation and Implementation of Comprehensive National Strategies for the Prevention of Suicidal Behaviour was held in Canada, which culminated in a report (United Nations 1996) that included a comprehensive set of guidelines, together with a case study of the Finnish national strategy. These guidelines encouraged the development of national suicide-prevention strategies around the world, for instance, in the United States (US Department of Health and Human Services 2001), where suicide was recognized as a national problem, and suicide-prevention as a national priority, as well as in Europe (WHO 2002b; Wasserman *et al.* 2004). In 1999, WHO launched the worldwide initiative for suicide prevention (SUPRE) with the overall goal of reducing the mortality and morbidity of suicidal behaviours.

The WHO, a specialized agency of the UN, is an intergovernmental organization, established by the formal agreement of, and ultimately governed by, 193 Member States. As the directing and coordinating authority on international health work, WHO stimulates international action on health issues of global concern with the ultimate objective of the attainment by all people of the highest possible level of health (WHO 2003). The WHO's normative function and advocacy role, as well as its convening power in establishing global partnerships, places it in a unique position to provide leadership at global, regional and country levels.

## The WHO worldwide initiative for the prevention of suicide

The activities of the WHO suicide-prevention initiative reflect core functions of the WHO Department of Mental Health and Substance Abuse and of the organization as a whole.

### Partnership

The suicide-prevention initiative is building global partnerships and collaborating with governments, international non-governmental organizations, professional associations, academic institutions, and relevant UN agencies. Early on, a WHO advisory network for the prevention of suicide was established to draw from the knowledge and experience of experts in the field around the world. Regional and national workshops on suicide-prevention brought together representatives of countries with a high burden of suicidal behaviours with the aims of:

1  Raising awareness of the magnitude of the problem;

2  Identifying cost-effective strategies for training workers in health and related sectors to identify people at risk;

3  Proposing cost-effective strategies for the reduction of methods of suicide;

4  Promulgating cost-effective interventions for the management of people at risk of suicidal behaviours; and finally,

5  Identifying relevant partners across sectors.

In its efforts, the WHO Department of Mental Health and Substance Abuse works closely with Ministries of Health of Member States, WHO Regional and Country Offices, and with WHO Collaborating Centres.

## Information

The WHO plays a key role in the collection, compilation and dissemination of essential epidemiological data on suicide. By providing a reliable information base in this area, it has become a widely used source of such data in the world. Information is not only furnished on the magnitude of the problem (World Health Organization 1999), but also on risk and protective factors associated with suicidal behaviours, on preventive measures and effective interventions. A relevant research agenda has been proposed.

In the mid-1980s, the WHO European multi-centre study on suicidal behaviour was established. It monitored trends of attempted suicides for nearly 15 years (De Leo *et al.* 2004). This study was a collaborative, coordinated, multinational project with up to twenty-one participating centres, which provided an unprecedented picture of attempted suicide in Europe. At the global level, the WHO Multisite Intervention Study on Suicidal Behaviours (SUPRE-MISS) was launched in 2002 to:

1 Evaluate different treatment strategies for suicide attempters through a randomized clinical trial (treatment as usual versus brief intervention) in a defined catchment area;

2 Conduct a community survey of suicidal behaviours in the same catchment area; and

3 Describe basic sociocultural characteristics of the communities (World Health Organization 2002a; Bertolote *et al.* 2005; Fleischmann *et al.* 2005).

These data provide, in most cases for the first time, comprehensive information on suicide attempters in eight low- and middle-income countries (i.e. Brazil, Estonia, India, Islamic Republic of Iran, People's Republic of China, South Africa, Sri Lanka, and Vietnam).

## Guidance

WHO Member States need scientifically sound, clear, and reliable technical guidance for suicide-prevention programmes, the management of those at risk of suicide or those who attempted suicide, and for the development and implementation of national strategies for suicide-prevention. Examples of countries receiving technical assistance include Brazil, Estonia, Mauritius, Guyana, India, Islamic Republic of Iran, Lithuania, People's Republic of China, South Africa, Sri Lanka, Thailand, Trinidad and Tobago, Uruguay, and Vietnam.

To this end, WHO has prepared a series of resources (World Health Organization 2000a–f; 2006a, b) addressed to specific social and professional groups particularly relevant to the prevention of suicide (i.e. general physicians, media professionals, teachers, primary health care workers, prison officers, counsellors, workplaces). Another resource targets survivors (those who are left behind after a completed suicide) to help them start a survivors' group. These resources have been translated into many languages and are widely used.

The WHO has produced an updated inventory of national strategies for suicide-prevention in WHO's European Member States (World Health Organization 2002b; Wasserman *et al.* 2004). It advocates for the development of national strategies for suicide-prevention and provides technical support in their preparation and implementation.

## Systems and services

The WHO encourages the establishment of effective and innovative services, and proposes cost-effective interventions for preventing suicidal behaviours and treating those at risk for or having attempted suicide. All efforts to assist governments of Member States in strengthening mental health systems follow the principles of equity, sustainability and involvement of all stakeholders.

## Conclusion

As suicide is a complex, multifactorial phenomenon, resulting from the interaction of biological, psychological, social and environmental factors, an equally complex approach is needed for its prevention. It is the WHO's role not only to generate political will and to raise the awareness among policy-makers to have suicide-prevention placed as a priority in the public health agenda, but also to reach beyond the health sector and to advocate for mainstreaming the issue of suicide-prevention in non-health sectors, such as education, jurisdiction, economics, media, legislation, and agriculture.

Even though the WHO has an important role to play in the prevention of suicide, it is ultimately the governments who have a responsibility for the health of their people.

## References

Bertolote JM, Fleischmann A, De Leo D *et al.* (2005). Suicide attempts, plans, and ideation in culturally diverse sites: the WHO SUPRE-MISS community survey. *Psychological Medicine*, **35**, 1457–1465.

De Leo D, Bille-Brahe U, Kerkhof A *et al.* (eds) (2004). *Suicidal Behaviour: Theories and Research Findings*. Hogrefe and Huber, Göttingen.

Fleischmann A, Bertolote JM, De Leo D *et al.* (2005). Characteristics of attempted suicides seen in emergency-care settings of general hospitals in eight low- and middle-income countries. *Psychological Medicine*, **35**, 1467–1474.

Krug EG, Dahlberg LL, Mercy JA *et al.* (eds) (2002). *World Report on Violence and Health*. World Health Organization, Geneva.

United Nations (1996). *Prevention of Suicide: Guidelines for the Formulation and Implementation of National Strategies*. United Nations, New York.

US Department of Health and Human Services (2001). *National Strategy for Suicide Prevention: Goals and Objectives for Action*. US Department of Health and Human Services, Rockville.

Wasserman D (2001). *Suicide: An Unnecessary Death*. Martin Dunitz, London.

Wasserman D, Mittendorfer-Rutz E, Rutz W *et al.* (2004). *Suicide Prevention in Europe. The WHO European Monitoring Survey on National Suicide Prevention Programmes and Strategies*. National Prevention of Suicide and Mental Ill-Health (NASP) at Karolinska Institute and Stockholm County Council's Centre for Suicide Research and Prevention.

World Health Organization (1999). *Figures and Facts about Suicide*. World Health Organization, Geneva.

World Health Organization (2000a). *Preventing Suicide: A Resource for General Physicians*. World Health Organization, Geneva.

World Health Organization (2000b). *Preventing Suicide: A Resource for Media Professionals*. World Health Organization, Geneva.

World Health Organization (2000c). *Preventing Suicide: A Resource for Teachers and Other School Staff*. World Health Organization, Geneva.

World Health Organization (2000d). *Preventing Suicide: A Resource for Primary Health Care Workers*. World Health Organization, Geneva.

World Health Organization (2000e). *Preventing Suicide: A Resource for Prison Officers*. World Health Organization, Geneva.

World Health Organization (2000f). *Preventing Suicide: How to Start a Survivors' Group*. World Health Organization, Geneva.

World Health Organization (2001). *The World Health Report: Mental Health: New Understanding, New Hope*. World Health Organization, Geneva.

World Health Organization (2002a). *Multisite Intervention Study on Suicidal Behaviours: Protocol of SUPRE-MISS*. World Health Organization, Geneva.

World Health Organization (2002b). *Suicide Prevention in Europe: The WHO European Monitoring Survey on National Suicide Prevention Programmes and Strategies*. World Health Organization, Copenhagen.

World Health Organization (2003). *The World Health Report: Shaping the Future*. World Health Organization, Geneva.

World Health Organization (2006a). *Preventing Suicide: A Resource for Counsellors*. World Health Organization, Geneva.

World Health Organization (2006b). *Preventing Suicide: A Resource at Work*. World Health Organization, Geneva.

# CHAPTER 97

# The World Psychiatric Association Section of Suicidology

Marco Sarchiapone, Jean-Pierre Soubrier and Danuta Wasserman

## The World Psychiatric Association

The World Psychiatric Association (WPA) was formally founded in 1961, but in fact started already in 1950, as the 'Organisation of the World Congress of Psychiatry' with Jean Delay as President and Henry Ey as Secretary General, both illustrious French psychiatrists. The goal was to implement regional conferences between world congresses, but also to build bridges between psychiatry and human sciences.

The establishment of Scientific Sections within the WPA was a critical factor ensuring the continuity of activities in the WPA between World congresses'. In the year 2007, there were sixty-five Sections.

## The Suicidology Section

The WPA Section on Suicidology was established on the eve of the third millennium, and has a quite recent history compared to other Sections. The path of suicidology is transdisciplinary, rather than having a definite location: its study was, at first, the object of philosophy, then of literature, theology, social sciences, only in the last two centuries has it acquired a medical character, specifically in psychiatry. Also in the psychiatric area, suicidology settled in a 'trans' fashion, namely acquiring a 'trans-nosographical' characterization, cutting across several psychiatric diagnoses. Possibly for this reason, a Section on suicidology within the World Psychiatric Association was necessary, serving as a vessel for a fluid entity as the study of suicidal behaviours.

The World Psychiatric Association and the International Association for Suicide Prevention (IASP) met in 1971 in Mexico together at the behest of Erwin Stengel, president of IASP at the time. Meanwhile, research in suicidology and suicide prevention developed with a collaboration between psychiatrists, mental health professionals and volunteers.

Discussions on the necessity for a Section on suicidology started with the initiative of Sergio Perez Barrero from Cuba, supported by José Manuel Bertolote, who was a WHO Officer in the Department of Mental Health and Substance Abuse in Geneva. The Section was confirmed by the WPA Executive Board during the international congress and Jubilee of WPA in Paris, France, in 2000.

It is a rule of the WPA that a Section cannot start before having the election of an executive board during the triennial world congress. Therefore, in 2002 in Yokohama, the WPA asked J.M. Bertolote to organize and chair the election. The first elected Chairman of the Section was Jean-Pierre Soubrier (France), former President of IASP during 1995–1997. The three elected executive board members included Co-Chair Nicoletta Tataru (Romania) and Secretary General Alexander Botsis (Greece). The five other board members were Danuta Wasserman (Sweden), editor of the Suicidology Section newsletter, Sylvia Pelaez (Uruguay), co-editor of the suicidology Section newsletter, Sergio De Risio (Italy), Nelson Moreno Ceballos (Dominican Republic), and Sergio Perez Barerro (Cuba): eight members in all.

At the WPA World Congress in Cairo 2005, the general assembly of the Section voted for the re-election of J-P Soubrier as Chairman, and Danuta Wasserman (Sweden) was elected as Co-Chair, Marco Sarchiapone (Italy) as Secretary General, and José Manuel Bertolote (Switzerland and Brazil), Julio Bobes (Spain), Jean Pierre Kahn (France), Alec Roy (USA) and Wolfgang Rutz (Sweden) as board members. In 2008, during the WPA meeting in Prague, Danuta Wasserman was elected Chair of the Section. Alec Roy was then elceted Co-chair of the Section, and Marco Sarchiapone was re-elected Secretary General; Jean-Pierre Soubrier was appointed as the Honorary Member of the Section.

From its inception, the WPA Section on Suicidology had the exciting task of bringing together different scientific personalities conducting research from divergent perspectives on suicidology, with a common interest in suicide prevention, which has been the main focus of efforts from the WPA Section on Suicidology. One of the first activities of the Section was to support dissemination of the publications stemmed from the WHO multisite intervention study on suicidal behaviours (SUPRE-MISS) programme. From this programme, several resource booklets were produced, addressing specific social groups and professionals, which are particularly relevant for the prevention of suicide, including health professionals, educators, social organizers, governments, law-makers, social communicators, law forces, families and communities (WHO 2000a–c, 2006a, b, 2007, 2008a, b).

## Activities

Since 2002, the Section has participated and given symposia (usually two at each conference or congress) in all major WPA regional and international conferences: Vienna in 2003, Florence in 2004, Cairo in 2005, Athens in 2005, Madrid in 2006, Prague in 2008 and Florence in 2009.

In 2005, at the thirteenth World Congress of WPA, in Cairo, Egypt, a joint symposium with the Section on Religion, Spirituality and Psychiatry chaired by Herman van Praag on 'Religion and Suicide' was given.

The Section has also sponsored other conferences, with the goal of implementing research in suicidology and suicide prevention, such as the First Latin-American International Meeting for Suicide Prevention on the theme 'A culture for life in the twenty-first century' in May 2004 in Montevideo, Uruguay and the First Mental Health International Conference on the theme of 'Direct and Indirect Self-Destructive Behaviours and Mental Disorders—Transcultural Differences', in collaboration with Emirates Psychological Association, in June 2007 in Dubai.

During workshops and symposia organized by the Section, nearly all the topics related to self-destructive behaviours and suicide have been discussed, from biology and genetics to psychology, religion and spirituality.

## Awards

The Section established an award in honour of the late Professor Sergio De Risio, an illustrious Italian psychiatrist with a deep and genuine interest in the field of suicidology, founder of a group of Italian suicidologists active in the WPA Section on Suicidology, who passed away in 2004. The De Risio Award, which is meant to be conferred to the author of the best poster in suicidology presented at a World Congress of Psychiatry, was approved by the WPA Executive Committee in 2006, thus allowing for the support of young researchers in the field of suicidology, to whom Sergio De Risio had devoted his utmost efforts and unforgettable teaching. In 2008, in Prague, the first award was given to Bruno Mendonça Coêlho, a young brazilian suicidologist.

Information about the Section can be found at the website http://www.wpanet.org.

## References

World Health Organization (2000a). *Preventing Suicide: A Resource for General Physicians*. World Health Organization, Geneva.

World Health Organization (2000b). *Preventing Suicide: A Resource for Teachers and Other School Staff*. World Health Organization, Geneva.

World Health Organization (2000c). *Preventing Suicide: A Resource for Primary Health Care Workers*. World Health Organization, Geneva.

World Health Organization (2006a). *Preventing Suicide: A Resource for Counsellors*. World Health Organization, Geneva.

World Health Organization (2006b). *Preventing Suicide: A Resource at Work*. World Health Organization, Geneva.

World Health Organization (2007). *Preventing Suicide in Jails and Prisons (Update 2007)*. World Health Organization, Geneva.

World Health Organization (2008a). *A Resource for Media Professionals (Update 2008)*. World Health Organization, Geneva.

World Health Organization (2008b). *Preventing Suicide: How to Start a Survivors' Group*. World Health Organization, Geneva.

# The International Association for Suicide Prevention

Lars Mehlum

## History of IASP

The International Association for Suicide Prevention (IASP) was founded by the Austrian suicidologist Erwin Ringel in Vienna in 1960, with the aim of preventing suicidal behaviour, to alleviate its effects, and to provide a forum for academicians and mental health professionals, later embracing also crisis workers, volunteers, and suicide survivors. Today, IASP has grown to become the leading international organization concerned with suicide prevention. It is in official relations with the World Health Organization (WHO), and as an umbrella organization, embraces members from nearly fifty national and international organizations on all continents. In its first decade, IASP held its conferences mainly in Europe and North America, but gradually, countries in other regions have been involved in hosting these world conferences. IASP and its international network of people, activities and resources has an important role to fill in a world that seems to be becoming gradually more aware of suicide as the huge societal problem it indeed is. Members from more than sixty different countries, with extensive knowledge and diverse experience, form a truly unique network that will be indispensable for the development of suicide preventive work worldwide.

## IASP structures

As in most similar organizations, IASP has its governing bodies, such as its General Assembly, which convenes every two years. An executive committee leads the organization in the interval between these general meetings. For many years, IASP had its central administrative office in Vienna, under the supervision of professor Ringel and his successors, but in 1995, moved to Chicago and later on to France. The IASP website, http://www.iasp.info, is hosted by the National Centre for Suicide Research and Prevention Unit at the University of Oslo and brings information about suicide and its prevention to the membership and to the public. On the website, members have online access to a worldwide directory of IASP members and organizations involved in suicidology.

IASP has always heavily depended on well-meaning cooperation and donations of time, office space, and additional resources from its elected officers and others involved. The organization is thus, in reality, a large working party where value is added through synergetic effects and coordinated action from many individuals, groups and organizations.

## IASP activities

IASP provides several forums for interchange of experience and knowledge. The journal *Crisis* is published quarterly, and contains research articles on the topics of suicide prevention and crisis intervention. A monthly news bulletin is also distributed to all members, keeping them informed about new developments and organization business.

To those who have contributed in a significant way to the development of the field of suicidology, IASP awards three different prizes biennially. The oldest is the Stengel Research Award, named after Erwin Stengel, the IASP's second president, and among the most prominent of suicide researchers in the twentieth century. The award has been given to M Bolt (1977), R Diekstra (1979), J-P Soubrier (1981), J Lönnqvist (1983), G Sonneck/J Beskow (1985), R Goldney/C Pfeffer (1987), P Cosyns/J Wilmotte (1989), D De Leo (1991), D Wasserman (1993), K Hawton (1995), A Schmidtke (1997), A Roy (1999), A Leenaars (2001), I Orbach (2003), K van Heeringen (2005) and JJ Mann (2007).

The Ringel Service Award, named after the IASP founding first president, is given for innovations in suicide prevention, and has been given to Zhai Shu Tao (1995), Y Saito (1997), V Scott (1999), L Mehlum (2001), J Nagdimon (2003) and L Ratnayeke (2007). The Farberow Award, named after the IASP's third president, Norman Farberow, a pioneer in our understanding of suicide bereavement and survivorship, is given for outstanding contributions to the field of post-vention. The award has so far been given to O Grad (1997), K Dunne Maxim/E Dunne (1999), S Clarke (2001), GH and E Weyrauch (2003), K Andriessen (2005) and K Dyregrov (2007).

## International conferences

One of the major tasks of IASP is to host international conferences. They are more important than ever because they enable people to interact, not only in the ever increasing cyberspace, but directly. Conferences bring people together to share knowledge, experiences, views and visions. They are also politically important and may give rise to policy changes in suicide prevention regionally, nationally and internationally. The selection of conference sites is important in this connection. IASP has, therefore, chosen to move its conferences to new continents and venues, such as Chennai in India, Durban, South Africa, and Montevideo, Uruguay.

## Regional conferences

From 2004 and onwards, IASP has increased its conference activities by also organizing regional conferences. Three Asia-Pacific Regional Conferences of the IASP have been organized in Bangkok (2004), Singapore (2006) and Hong Kong (2008), in collaboration with local organizations and authorities. Several regions of the world are interested in similar conferences, and the European biennial conferences are now held under the auspices of IASP. Whereas, world congresses remain important as arenas for global collaboration and development, it is probably more useful to discuss regional perspectives, problems and solutions within a culture-sensitive framework at regional conferences. Furthermore, since regional conferences may require fewer investments in terms of time and money from the individual delegate, they are often more easily accessible to local audiences, and may, thus, have a larger impact on national policies and practices.

## IASP as a multicultural, multi-language association

To further the wish of moving away from a situation where European and North American perspectives will continue to dominate the association, IASP has sought to foster multicultural and multi-language meeting places. Thus, sessions in different world languages have been organized at IASP conferences. With the help of suicide research and prevention centres at universities in Montreal, Canada and SAR Hong Kong, the IASP website has been developed in English, French, Spanish and Chinese versions, including information materials, which are provided in even more languages. These measures are necessary to make IASP more relevant and available to people in diverse cultures, and help mobilize more people to collaborate internationally.

## 10 September—World Suicide Prevention Day

With the goal of increasing public awareness of the problem of suicide, and the need for preventive measures, the IASP has pursued several lines of action. One of them has been to promote 'The World Suicide Prevention Day'. The day is an opportunity for the IASP to promote awareness about suicide, and its prevention, in a culture-sensitive and locally adapted fashion throughout the world. IASP received the co-sponsorship from the World Health Organization for the first time in 2003, and organized the first Day the same year in a very successful way. The following year, IASP launched the World Suicide Prevention Day under the motto 'Saving lives, restoring hope' at the WHO Headquarters in Geneva, Switzerland, through a special event attended by a large number of officials from WHO, other UN branches and major NGOs. The World Suicide Prevention Day message spread to every corner of the world over the next couple of days, and the media impact of this event showed a high response in broadcasting media,

newspapers and Internet sites. IASP also used its global network of national representatives, national branches of its organization, and other member organizations, to reach out to the public, authorities, professional associations, clinicians and volunteers, to use the World Suicide Prevention Day as an instrument for promoting increased awareness of the problem of suicide, and the many ways in which suicide rates can be reduced. The experiences with the World Suicide Prevention Day project, so far, indicate that:

- The main messages get substantial attention from local, national and international mass media;
- There seems to have been hardly any negative or harmful media coverage linked to the World Suicide Prevention Day;
- The World Suicide Prevention Day concept (international profile, message, materials, inspirational information, etc.) helps NGOs, institutions, groups and individuals to organize wide-ranging national and local events.

## Task forces

In order to strengthen the focus on specific fields of interest, or to provide recommendations, or other products important to the activity of the organization, IASP has established several task forces. These groups work according to specific mandates given to them, either by the General Assembly meeting, or by the Executive Committee. A task force on 'Cross-national systems for certifying suicidal deaths' has worked to establish a database for how a suicidal death is certified from a death certificate in different countries, in order to establish how we can best explain the way suicides are tabulated in national database/vital registry systems, and to provide the basis for case–control, cross-national studies to identify reasonably equivalent national systems. A task force on 'Suicide and terrorism' has collected available data about suicidal terrorist acts, and studied the processes that lead to suicidal acts of terrorism, with the aim of formulating prevention and intervention strategies to discourage suicidal terrorism. A task force on 'Post-vention' has organized meetings and promoted the field of post-vention actively, both within the organization and outside of IASP. Furthermore, they have compiled data on bereavement services, and made these available online to the public at the IASP website. The IASP task force on 'Genetics of suicidal behaviour' has promoted studies on genetic aspects of suicidal ideation and behaviour, both among suicidologists and behavioural geneticists, through organizing conferences on this topic.

## Collaboration with the WHO

For many years, IASP has enjoyed a very favourable working alliance with the WHO. The relationship is probably of mutual benefit, but no doubt of the utmost importance to IASP. In both scientific and policy matters, WHO and IASP have often made joint initiatives, such as the World Suicide Prevention Day project, and the prevention of suicide through restricting the access to pesticides. The WHO has formed a strategy for prevention of pesticide suicides (World Health Organization 2004) in collaboration with IASP.

IASP devotes a great deal of attention to the maintenance of its interdisciplinary and international independent profile. While this puts clear restrictions to the extent to which IASP can allow itself to receive support from commercial sponsors, it does have the great advantage of maintaining IASP as a forum for collaboration in a non-profit and independent context.

## Conclusion

Politicians and the public needs to be made aware that suicide is a largely preventable public health problem. It is equally important that myths and stigma associated with suicide and being suicidal are reduced. To help this happen, we need IASP, both nationally and internationally, to bring together the available knowledge and expertise for effective action in the field of suicide prevention.

As I have attempted to indicate, IASP is an organization with a great diversity of resources and activities. It is an organization in the process of growing, and it is developing to accommodate the need for competent contributions in suicide prevention throughout the world.

## Reference

World Health Organization (2004). *Pesticides and Health*. World Health Organization, Geneva.

# CHAPTER 99

# The International Academy of Suicide Research

Danuta Wasserman and J John Mann

## The IASR objectives

The International Academy of Suicide Research (IASR) was established in Bologna on 29 September 1990, at Padua University (De Leo and Schmidtke 2001). In his inauguration speech, the late Professor Nils Retterstøl from Oslo, Norway, welcomed this association of the world's leading researchers in suicidology and suicide prevention as an essential step forward in the field (IASR 2004a).

The overall aim of the Academy is to reduce the mortality and morbidity of suicide-related incidents by promoting the highest standard of suicide research and fostering communication and collaboration among scholars in the field of suicidology.

Traditionally, suicide research has focused on the psychological and behavioural characteristics of suicide attempters. However, promising evidence of the biology of suicide has emerged and, accordingly, the IASR now aims to promote more research in this specific area of suicidology. Another of IASR's objectives is to promote research on evaluation of preventive interventions and of suicide-prevention programmes under way in various countries. Examining the effects of various prevention programmes in different countries and cultures makes it possible to identify which components of an intervention are effective, and thus draw up better strategies for future suicide-preventive programmes (Mann *et al.* 2005).

## The IASR constitution

The constitution outlines the Academy's principles, bylaws and rules (IASR 2004b). The Academy is a non-profit organization, headed by a Board of Directors comprising a President-Elect, the current President, the immediate Past President and a Secretary-Treasurer. The first president, Professor René Diekstra (The Netherlands), was followed by Professor Diego De Leo (Italy), Professor Armin Schmidtke (Germany), Professor John Mann (USA), Professor Danuta Wasserman (Sweden), Professor Jouko Lönnqvist (Finland) and Professor David Shaffer (USA).

Under the Academy's bylaws, there are two categories of membership: member and associate. Member status is for individuals who have consistently established 'an enduring reputation as a distinguished scholar in the field of suicidal behaviour', while the associate category comprises individuals who have not yet established an 'enduring reputation' but currently hold academic posts in suicide research. Every candidate wishing to become a member must be nominated by one Academy member and seconded by another. Nominees are then accepted or rejected by a committee appointed by the Academy's current President and approved by the Board of Directors.

## Archives of Suicide Research

*Archives of Suicide Research* (ASR) is the official journal of the Academy. Under the direction of the editor-in-chief Professor Barbara Stanley (USA) and her co-editors Professor Alan Apter (Israel) and Professor Thomas Bronisch (Germany), ASR is emerging as the leading journal in suicide research.

Articles published in ASR represent a wide range of disciplines, including biology, epidemiology, psychiatry, psychology and sociology. It also publishes book and research reviews, suicidology news and notes, and case studies (Taylor and Francis, Archives of Suicide Research 2008).

## Morselli Award

The Academy's lifetime achievement award is named in honour of Enrico Morselli (1852–1929), an epidemiologist at the University of Genoa School of Medicine. Morselli, a predecessor of Emile Durkheim, was a pioneer of the application of statistical methods to suicidology, and addressed the influence of society on suicide rates. This biennial award, in the form of the Morselli Medal, is given by the Academy to an individual who has made an outstanding contribution to the study of suicidal behaviour and/or suicide prevention. The Morselli Medal was awarded to Professor Marie Åsberg of Karolinska Institute in Stockholm, Sweden in 2003; Professor Aaron Beck of Pennsylvania University, USA, in 2005; and Professors Edwin Shneidman (USA) and Norman Farberow (USA), both previously active at the Los Angeles Suicide Prevention Center, in 2007. Letters from Professor Shneidman and Professor Farberow, models for many generations of scientists, to the IASR members are presented in Figures 99.1 and 99.2.

## IASR meetings and Nobel Conference in Stockholm, June 2009

The Academy has held annual meetings for members since 1990. The most recent took place in Stockholm, Sweden in 2003;

Dear all

     I am looking forward to receiving the Morselli Medal. I have seen a picture of it and it appears to be both gracious and impressive, well representing the prestige it bears.

     My thoughts upon receiving notification of the award were more or less reflective. As you are probably aware, I have always been interested in the history of suicide, and indeed wrote an introductory chapter on it in our Encyclopedia of Suicide (Evans and Farberow 2003). I felt it was important that people know of the fascinating changes in attitude that and concern about suicide had existed in previous eras in different parts of the world. As a result I was well aware of the contribution on suicide by Morselli. I was also aware of the relative lack of awareness and appreciation among students of suicide for the encyclopedic task accomplished by Morselli. Indeed, his work, entitled Suicide: An Essay of Comparative Moral Statistics, has been described by Goldney and Schioldann, (2002) as 'arguably the most important work of 19th century suicidology'. Incidentally, Morselli was only 27 years old when he published his book in 1879. His work shines like a beacon, several decades before the seminal work of Durkheim, indicating the significance of suicide for concern as an important public health, mental health, medical, sociological, psychiatric, psychological, philosophical, and cultural event. Unfortunately, however, interest and research in the area lapsed in the ensuing decades, although they did see the monumental work of Durkheim and Freud in this period. To some degree, I feel a kind of kinship to Morselli in respect to the feeling that our work seems to have also served to restimulate interest and activity both worldwide and nationwide in the problem of suicide and its prevention. The increase in interest and involvement in the field from the time we started to the present is remarkable, as evidenced by the huge increase in both government activities and policies and in professional clinical and research programs.

     I am very pleased to receive this Award, for it represents recognition and acknowledgment, especially by our peers, of the significance of our contribution to the field. I am also very proud and grateful for the feeling that it allows me to join a list of very distinguished previous recipients of the Award.

     Please use whatever of the above in any way that you wish.


Dr Norman Farberow

**Fig. 99.1** Letter from Norman Farberow, 2007 Morselli Medal recipient.


Dear Dr. Wasserman,

     For years my favorite 19th century European suicidologist was Enrico Morselli. (I once owned a first edition of *Il Suicidio*). And so I am especially thrilled to be honored with the Morselli medal.

     This treasured award reflects, in my mind, my founding of the American Association of Suicidology, my heading the first national program in suicide prevention, my adding to the working vocabulary in our field—suicidology, psychological autopsy, postvention, psychache. I believe that, in some arcane way, my concept of psychache is the indirect heir of Morselli's ideas about moral pain, perturbations in the mind.

     I have had a wonderful run as a suicidologist and the Morselli medal is a capstone to my long career. And I am immensely grateful to the IASR for this signal recognition and honor. You have brought much pleasure to a ninety-year-old heart.

Thank you.

                      Sincerely,
                      Edwin S. Shneidman, Ph.D. Lett. D.
                      Professor of Thanatology Emeritus

**Fig. 99.2** Letter from Edwin Shneidman, 2007 Morselli Medal recipient.


New York, USA 2004 and 2005; Portoroz, Slovenia in 2006; Killarney, Ireland in 2007; and Glasgow, Scotland in 2008.

    The Academy's ultimate goals of broadening communication among researchers and scholars in the field of suicide and setting the highest standards for suicide research were attained during the Nobel Conference entitled 'The Role of Genetics in Promoting Suicide Prevention and Mental Health of the Population', which was organized by the National Swedish Prevention of Suicide and Mental Ill-Health (NASP) at Karolinska Institute in Stockholm, Sweden, in 2009. The conference was funded by the Nobel Foundation and the Association of the Nobel Assembly at Karolinska Institute. The most prominent researchers in the field from all over the world attended this event.

# Conclusion

Since the creation of the International Academy of Suicide Research in 1990, the organization has contributed a great deal of knowledge in the field of suicidology. The IASR has focused on crucial elements of suicide research including suicide prevention programmes and interventions. Suicidology is a complex multidisciplinary field because suicidal behaviour is the outcome of factors in the individual, their immediate family and friends and society. It is the unique interaction of these many factors in each individual patient that determines their risk for suicide, thus making it difficult to predict and prevent. The IASR provides a crucial forum for the discussion of research by researchers in the many disciplines united by the goal of understanding the causes of suicide and determining how to prevent it. Such scientific attention also helps to break the stigma associated with suicide and gives hope to the many families affected by this tragedy. Focused academic suicide organizations, such as the IASR are vital sources of greatly needed knowledge as to how to reduce suicide mortality and morbidity.

## References

*Archives of Suicide Research* (ASR) (2008). *Aims and Scope*. Retrieved 27 May 2008 from http://www.informaworld.com.proxy.kib.ki.se/smpp/title~db=all~content=t713667420~tab=summary.

De Leo D and Schmidtke A (2001). International organizations: The International Academy of Suicide Research. In D Lester, ed., *Suicide Prevention: Resources for the Millennium*, pp 304–311. Routledge, Philadelphia.

Evans G and Farberow NL (2003). *The Encyclopedia of Suicide*. Fact On File, New York.

Goldney RD and Schioldann JA (2002). *Pre-Durkhim Suicidology: The 1892 Reviews of Tuke and Savage*. Adelaide Academic Press, Adelaide.

International Academy of Suicide Research (IASR) (2004a). *History of the Academy*. Retrieved 22 May 2008 from http://www.depts.ttu.edu/psy/iasronline//history.html.

International Academy of Suicide Research (IASR) (2004b). *Constitution*. Retrieved 26 May 2008 from http://www.depts.ttu.edu/psy/iasronline//constitution.html.

Mann JJ, Apter A, Bertolote J *et al.* (2005). Suicide prevention strategies: a systematic review. *JAMA*, **294**, 2064–74.

Taylor and Francis (2008). *Archives of Suicide Research. Journal Details*. Retrieved 28 May 2008 from http://www.tandf.co.uk/journals/authors/usuiauth.asp.

# CHAPTER 100

# The European Psychiatric Association Section on Suicidology and Suicide Prevention

Danuta Wasserman, Marco Sarchiapone and Vladimir Carli

## Suicide research in Europe

European scholars historically pioneered research on suicide. Attitudes towards suicide dramatically changed during nineteenth and twentieth centuries, mainly due to the recognition of psychiatry as an autonomous discipline, which allowed treatment for disorders causing suicide, such as 'melancholy' or 'hysteria', for instance, and thanks to the original contribution of illustrious scientists such as Enrico Morselli (1882) and Emile Durkheim (1897/1951). As Durkheim, in his work, regarded suicide as a social illness reflecting alienation, anomy and other side-effects of modern times, Morselli, in his earlier moral statistics comparative essay, had already stressed the influence of biological, individual, and social factors on the development of suicide, and emphasized the importance of treatment, and the role of psychic suffering in suicidal persons.

As the study of suicidal behaviours in the twenty-first century has been engaging with the novel impulse of the biological trajectory of causation, taking advantage of new perspectives which stem from recent advances in scientific technology, European psychiatrists still achieve notable results: European contribution to scientific knowledge on suicide parallels with the huge commitment in the field by North America and the recent involvement of nations from other continents. With the aim of highlighting European contribution to this specific area of psychiatry, providing cohesion and coordinating individual European researchers, a new Section on Suicide and Suicide Prevention within the European Psychiatric Association (EPA), previously known as the Association of European Psychiatrists (AEP), was conceived and established by the General Assembly during the Annual Congress held in March 2006 in Nice.

## Section goals

The EPA Section on Suicidology's goal is to adhere to the highest scientific standards in order to keep pace with advances of scientific knowledge in psychiatry applied to suicidology. The original impulse for the creation of an EPA Section on Suicidology was to give a logistic frame and reference to the scientific activity of European psychiatrists, with the intent of conferring stability and prestige to the work of each member. It was, therefore, significant that scientists sharing a clear common historical, cultural and methodological matrix could merge their competences in such an association, joining their forces at a time when advances in scientific technology require enhanced means and huge numbers of patients to study.

In 2007, during the Section Meeting held within the XV European Congress of Psychiatry in Madrid, Section members reformulated the objectives of the Section's establishment, and decided that a part of the Section's work should be addressed to the prevention of suicide, as an essential duty of the psychiatrist working in the field of suicidology. For this reason, the title of Section was changed into 'EPA Section on Suicidology and Suicide Prevention'. Specific tasks of the Section would then be to increase awareness and early recognition of problems leading to suicidal risk, to develop specific guidelines for the treatment of suicidal patients, and to organize educational events and specialist courses for psychiatrists.

The Section has an Executive Board: Danuta Wasserman (Sweden), Chair, Marco Sarchiapone (Italy), Co-Chair, Dan Rujescu (Germany), Secretary General, and Vladimir Carli, (Italy) Treasurer. The development of the section can be followed by visiting http://www.aep.lu/

## Scientific activities

Basic scientific activity of the Section is the organization of the Section's symposia at the EPA's Congresses.

Symposia were organized at the EPA Congresses: in March 2007 in Madrid, in April 2008 in Nice, and in January 2009 in Lisbon, as well as at other meetings: in September 2006 in Portoroz, Slovenia, within the fifth International Meeting on 'Suicide: Interplay between Genes and Environment'.

As suicide research and prevention are a founding basis of the suicidologist's and Section member's identity, the Section specifically addresses the promotion of joint research and also intends to encourage the sharing of expertise and data among its researchers: one way of realizing this objective will be to implement the standardization of research methodology.

An example of joint European research is the SEYLE project (Saving and Empowering Young Lives in Europe) run by the consortium of twelve European Countries: Austria, Estonia, France, Germany, Hungary, Ireland, Israel, Italy, Romania, Slovenia, Spain, with Sweden as a coordinator. The main objectives of this project, funded by the European Commission, are to promote health of adolescents through decreased risk taking and suicidal behaviours, to evaluate outcomes of professionally, gate-keeper and student-guided preventive interventions and to recommend effective culturally adjusted models for promoting health of adolescents in different European countries. Data on lifestyles and values of European adolescents are also gathered.

## Teaching

Attention to clinical activity is guaranteed by giving training courses in collaboration with local university centres, and Continuing Medical Education (CME) courses during the EPA Congresses on 'Prevention and treatment of suicidal behaviours'. Currently, the initiative of the Section is the organization of an International collaboration of PhD training in Suicidology, a proposal by late Professor Andrej Marušič, from University of Primorska, Portoroz, Solvenia to be held in two or three European universities, with faculty members recruited among the Section's members.

The development of the Section can be followed by visiting http://www.epa.lu.

## References

Durkheim E (1897/1951). *Suicide: A Study in Sociology*, J Spaulding and G Simpson, trans. The Free Press, New York.

European Psychiatric Association accessible at http://www.aep.lu/.

Morselli E (1882). *Suicide: An Essay on Comparative Moral Statistics.* Appleton-Century-Croft, New York.

Saving and Empowering Young Lives in Europe, accessible at http://www.seyle.org.

# CHAPTER 101

# The American Association of Suicidology

Lanny Berman

## History of AAS

The American Association of Suicidology (AAS) (http://www.suicidology.org) was founded by clinical psychologist Edwin S. Shneidman, PhD, in 1968. After co-directing the Los Angeles Suicide Prevention Center (LASPC) since 1958 with Norman Farberow, PhD, Dr Shneidman was appointed Chief of The Center for Suicide Prevention at the National Institute of Mental Health (NIMH). There he had the opportunity to closely observe the limited available knowledge-base regarding suicide. Consequently, with the support of the NIMH, he organized a meeting of several world-renowned scholars, determined the need for and fathered a national organization devoted to research, education, and practice in suicidology, and advancing suicide prevention.

Given his leadership at the LASPC Shneidman was quick to recognize the contemporaneous and rapid expansion of the crisis centre/hotline movement across the United States. The newly established AAS embraced these centres as sources of research information on suicidal clients. Soon, the relationship between the AAS and these centres was symbiotic. AAS became the central clearing house for support and the hub of a many-spoked wheel, networking these centres to common needs, training materials, and goals.

As a result of this marriage of research and crisis counselling, the AAS developed a set of standards and criteria for certification of crisis centers throughout the United States and Canada. Since certifying its first center in 1976, the AAS has accredited more than 160 centres meeting what has been described as 'the gold standard' of service and training accreditation programmes. In 1989, the AAS began a certification programme for individual crisis workers as well. More than 400 individuals to date have passed a rigorous examination of their knowledge and application of crisis theory to their work

## The structure of the AAS

AAS membership includes researchers, mental health clinicians, public health specialists, school districts and emergency services, and survivors of suicide from America and across the globe. It networks these diverse constituencies through its annual conference, newsletters, listserv, and journal.

Since 1968 the AAS conference of research presentations and panels, training workshops, and interactive discussions annually has attracted more than 700 registrants. Parallel and concurrent conferences are sponsored by AAS for survivors and professionals who work with them (Healing after Suicide) and crisis centres (Collaborative Crisis Center conference). AAS also sponsors regional conferences and training workshops. Major papers from the AAS annual meeting, in addition to independently submitted research and case studies, appear in the Association's peer-reviewed, journal *Suicide and Life-Threatening Behaviour*, which has been published every two months continuously since 1971. Two quarterly newsletters are published by the AAS. *Newslink* presents articles and information of current interest on suicide and suicide prevention activities as well as organizational communications. *Surviving Suicide* similarly focuses on information of support to survivors and those who work with them.

In January 1995 a renewed commitment toward intellectual and proactive leadership was made by the association's board of directors. An active programme of externally supported research and prevention programming began and complemented the AAS's ongoing investment in setting standards for and upgrading the skills and understandings of those who work with at-risk individuals. In recent years AAS has secured several federal grants and subcontracts and grants from private foundations to work on such diverse issues as upgrading the suicide prevention programmes of the US Navy and the US Army, establishing recommendations for the prevention of youth suicide by firearms, teaching professionals about bipolar disorder and suicide risk among children, defining best practices in suicide prevention, and seeking ways to motivate help-seeking behaviour among males at risk for suicide (Berman 2006).

Notably, the AAS has invested in education and training as its primary mission. Core competency curricula have been developed for individuals developing and implementing suicide-prevention initiatives in states and communities, for primary care physicians, and for clinical professionals tasked with assessing and managing persons with suicide risk. These curricula are designed to teach clinical and practice skills typically not achieved in graduate mental health and public health training programmes.

Recognizing the lack of consensus in what was being disseminated across the globe as warning signs of suicide, AAS brought together an international task force of clinician-researchers in 2003 to review the research and come to agreement on a consensus list of empirically supported warning signs of suicide (Rudd *et al.* 2006).

AAS has since actively supported follow-up research, training, and dissemination of these warning signs to both the public and professional caregivers.

The AAS has also been instrumental in taking leadership positions in the development of the US Surgeon General's National Strategy for Suicide Prevention (US Public Health Service 2001), the US Centers for Disease Control and Prevention's Suicide Prevention Research Center, and the Department of Health and Human Services (DHHS)-supported Suicide Prevention Resource Center. Further, AAS task forces and sponsored work groups have produced and disseminated or published inpatient discharge guidelines for clinical aftercare, resources for clinicians as survivors of suicide, school suicide prevention and post-vention guidelines, and media reporting guidelines; in addition to performing ongoing sponsored research and prevention projects in areas as diverse as trespass suicides on the railroads and suicide among Alaskan Natives.

AAS produces a referral directory of more than 600 suicide prevention and crisis centres nationwide and a directory of almost 300 survivor support groups. Thousands of calls are received annually in the AAS Central Office from the public and the media regarding referrals and information needs. Public education and information have become core functions of the AAS. To that end the AAS has produced a variety of annually updated fact sheets, brochures, statistical reports, books, and resources offered to the public and professional communities.

## Awards

The AAS annually bestows several awards to recognize those who have significantly impacted the field of suicidology and suicide prevention through their work.

The Louis I. Dublin Award is the association's most prestigious honour and is given in recognition of distinguished contributions in the area of Suicidology. The first recipient of the Dublin Award, in 1971, was Dr Karl Menninger. Among the 36 recipients of the Dublin Award since 'Dr Karl' are luminaries such as Edwin Shneidman, Norman Farberow, Chad Varah, Aaron Beck, Norman Kreitman, Marie Asberg, Marsha Linehan, and Keith Hawton.

The Edwin S Shneidman Award, first named the Young Contributor Award, is presented to an individual who has made significant early career contributions to suicidology. This ward, first given in 1973, has recognized such individuals as Albert Cain, Cynthia Pfeffer, Madelyn Gould, David Rudd, and Thomas Joiner.

## Conclusion

As an active member of the international suicide prevention community and movement, AAS increasingly seeks and develope collaborations with both institutions and individuals across the globe, working in partnerships to reduce rates of suicide and improve the well-being of all peoples. AAS is a membership organization for all those involved in suicide prevention and intervention, or touched by suicide. AAS leads the advancement of scientific and programmatic efforts in suicide prevention through research education and training, the development of standards and resources, and survivor suport services.

## References

Berman AL (2006). Help-seeking in men: implications for suicide prevention. *Pogled: the View III*, **1–2**, 36–51.

Rudd MD, Berman L, Joiner T et al. (2006). Warning signs for suicide: theory, research, and clinical application. *Suicide and Life-Threatening Behaviour*, **36**, 255–262.

US Public Health Service (2001). *National Strategy for Suicide Prevention: Goals and Objectives for Action*. Department of Health and Human Services, Washington.

# CHAPTER 102

# The American Foundation for Suicide Prevention

Ann P Haas, Robert Gebbia and Paula J Clayton

## History of AFSP

In 1987, leading experts on suicide joined with families who had lost a loved one to suicide to form the American Foundation for Suicide Prevention (AFSP) (see http://www.afsp.org).

Following the approach that had proven to be effective in advancing the treatment and prevention of heart disease, cancer and diabetes, AFSP began with the goals of furthering the research necessary to understand and prevent suicide, and educating mental health professionals and the public about effective treatment and suicide-prevention strategies. From its inception, the work of the Foundation aimed to lower suicide rates, increase the public and private resources available for suicide prevention, and develop and support programmes to assist survivors of suicide loss. Over time, AFSP's focus broadened to include representatives from the civic and business communities, as well as people suffering from depression and other mood disorders that convey suicide risk.

More than 20 years later, AFSP remains the leading national non-profit organization in the US, exclusively dedicated to understanding and preventing suicide through research and education, and to reaching out to people with mood disorders and those impacted by suicide. From a single national office in New York City, the Foundation has expanded to include twenty-eight Chapters throughout the United States that bring AFSP programmes to states and communities and play an important role in focusing public attention on suicide.

## AFSP's activities are focused within five areas

1   *Research.* AFSP is the leading private supporter of suicide research, providing over $2 million annually in grants to researchers from all disciplines both in the US and abroad. Through its grants programme, AFSP encourages established investigators to explore new directions in suicide research, attracts talented new investigators to suicide research and helps them obtain advanced training and mentoring, and provides seed money for pilot projects that show promise in opening up new areas of study. Applications for research grants are reviewed by AFSP's Scientific Advisors who include over 120 leading scientists from all over the world with expertise on the genetic, neurobiological, epidemiological, clinical and psychosocial aspects of suicide. Grants have supported studies in Australia, Israel, China, Ireland, Great Britain, Sweden, Spain, Italy, Mexico and Canada, in addition to the US.

2   *Suicide-prevention projects.* AFSP initiates and plays a leadership role in implementing demonstration projects in areas where its interests and expertise can fill an existing gap. One such project is a web-based, interactive method of outreach to university students at risk for suicide, which is showing considerable promise in encouraging previously untreated students to get help. In separate projects, the outreach method is now targeting other at-risk groups including medical students and physicians. Another project is bringing together experts from countries around the world to critically examine one another's national suicide prevention strategies and encourage developing countries to replicate strategies for which there is evidence of effectiveness. AFSP is also engaged in a partnership with the National Institute of Mental Health (NIMH) and other US federal agencies to launch and support the Developing Centers on Interventions for the Prevention of Suicide (DCIPS), a network of collaborative research centres that are testing promising treatments and other interventions to prevent suicide.

3   *Educational resources.* AFSP's films, slide presentations, public service ads, and print materials provide needed education about suicide causation and prevention for both professionals and the public. The Foundation's documentary film, *Struggling in silence: physician depression and suicide*, has been shown extensively on public television in the US, and a companion film, *Out of silence: medical student depression and suicide*, has been widely distributed to medical schools. These films and related resource materials can be found on the website http://www.doctorswithdepression.org. Other AFSP films, including *More than sad: help for teen depression* and *The truth about suicide: real stories of depression in college*, alert students, faculty and other school personnel to depression and suicide risk among adolescents and young adults. In another educational initiative, AFSP partnered with the Annenberg Public Policy Center and other organizations to develop and disseminate *Reporting on suicide: recommendations for the media. These guidelines have*

*been found to significantly improve how* journalists portray suicide in their news stories.

4   *Survivor support.* AFSP reaches out to survivors of suicide loss to offer education, information and understanding, as well as opportunities to become involved in the Foundation's work. One major programme is an annual Survivors of Suicide Day Teleconference that is broadcast to over 100 sites and can be viewed worldwide on the AFSP website. Other programs include a Survivor Outreach Programme for families recently bereaved by suicide loss, and a Support Group Facilitator Training Programme.

5   *Advocacy.* AFSP works closely with other suicide prevention organizations and the broader mental health community to advocate for national and state policies and legislation that increase resources for suicide prevention programmes, expand access to mental health treatment and other initiatives that further the goal of preventing suicide. In its advocacy activities, AFSP mobilizes survivors, people with depression and other interested members of the lay public to help end the stigma and discrimination surrounding psychiatric disorders that can lead to suicide. AFSP researchers provide the scientific basis for the positions taken by the Foundation.

In addition to its formal programmes and activities, AFSP is widely recognized by the media and the public as the leading source in the US of accurate, up-to-date information about suicide. Foundation staff and affiliated scientists are also widely consulted for commentary and opinion on current events that involve suicidal behaviour.

## Fundraising

Since 2003, AFSP's annual budget has more than doubled to over $8 million. An increasing proportion of the Foundation's funds are raised by individual participants in its signature Out of the Darkness Overnight Walk, held annually each summer in different US cities, and the Out of the Darkness Community Walks that take place each autumn in locations throughout the country. Over 30,000 people participate in one or more of these events each year, bringing increased attention to the problem of suicide and involving thousands of new participants in the cause of suicide prevention. The walks and other AFSP fundraising events represent approximately 60 per cent of total revenue. Other sources of support include individual private donors through annual appeals, memorial gifts and bequests, as well as corporate, foundation and government grants.

AFSP brings together the scientists who provide the knowledge, the lay constituencies who bring the passion, and the business and community leaders who bring the resources and credibility.

# CHAPTER 103

# Suicide Prevention International

Herbert Hendin

## Introduction

With one million suicides a year and several hundred million people suffering from serious depression worldwide, depression and suicide are now recognized as major global health problems. Our ability to treat depression and prevent suicide has improved significantly over the past few decades, but proven suicide prevention measures have still not reached people both in developing countries and in large areas of many industrialized countries. Suicide Prevention International is uniquely positioned to address this problem.

Utilizing its international network of experts, Suicide Prevention International (SPI) undertakes projects that are most likely to prevent suicide, selects qualified investigators, and works with them in developing and implementing the projects from beginning to end. SPI's focused approach and broad base of expertise are at work implementing a wide range of projects. The following are a few examples.

## Recognizing an Imminent Suicide Crisis

The inability to know when patients are in a suicide crisis, i.e. at acute as opposed to long-term risk for suicide, has been a major handicap to therapists treating these patients. Based on over a decade of study with therapists of patients who killed themselves while in treatment, scientists in SPI's Recognizing an Imminent Suicide Crisis (RISC) project have developed an instrument, the Affective States Questionnaire (ASQ), that holds the promise of being able to do just that. Past work on the project has demonstrated the role of intense affective states such as desperation, rage, guilt, hopelessness, and anxiety in triggering a suicide crisis. It has validated these findings with a comparison group that was comparably depressed but was never seriously suicidal. Major medical centres have completed encouraging tests of the ASQ's ability to recognize a suicide crisis and are now prospectively implementing and testing the ASQ with large populations. Confirmation of the findings would be of enormous value in informing us when to intervene actively because patients are at imminent risk for suicide (Hendin *et al.* 2007).

## Global support for survivors of suicide

Support groups for survivors of suicide can be effective, but in general they provide limited services and suffer from a lack of professional leadership. Suicide Prevention International has developed a model programme for survivors of suicide that trains qualified mental health professionals to organize and operate survivor support groups and programmes in the United States and abroad. The programme includes weekly sessions for the recently bereaved, individual help for those who need it, monthly support groups, and support for children as well as adults who are survivors of suicide. The training and programme are underway at social service and health care agencies in New York City (see http://www.suicideprevention-internatinal.org).

## Suicide prevention in rural China

With 21 per cent of the world's population, China has between 30–40 per cent of the world's suicides. Suicide is the leading cause of death for young people in China between 15–34 years of age. Three-quarters of the suicides are in rural China where the suicide rates are three times the urban rates. Suicide prevention and treatment services are generally not available in the rural areas of China, largely due to a shortage of doctors and trained health care providers in the villages and towns. SPI is helping to implement two projects in rural China that address this problem (Hendin *et al.* 2008).

### Developing a mental health service network in rural China

This project's investigators are building on the existing health care system in rural China to develop a mental health service network. The network is based on training personnel in the villages and towns in Hunan province to recognize and refer individuals with depression, and/or risk for suicide to a county mental hospital for specific treatment and subsequently to provide community mental health care for these patients. Specialized training will also be provided to the county psychiatrists. The network will be evaluated based on comparison to a control region. More people who are at high suicide risk will receive adequate treatment/intervention and it is expected there will be a significant reduction in suicide and attempted suicide. A major goal of the project is to establish a cost-effective model for providing care for these patients that could be adopted by the Chinese government for rural areas throughout China. With this in mind, SPI is consulting with Chinese officials in the Ministry of Health and is keeping them informed of our progress during the course of this project (Hendin *et al.* 2008).

### Social intervention with suicide attempters in rural China

Because of the large role that social factors play in contributing to suicide in China, the development of social support networks for individuals who make an initial suicide attempt is another potential approach to reduce the suicide rate in rural China. SPI is working with Chinese investigators in Beijing on a project in Shandong province designed to help patients who attempt suicide—identified at the time of their treatment in hospital emergency rooms—find alternative ways of dealing with interpersonal conflicts and other stresses. These patients are randomly assigned to an intervention group or to a control group. The intervention group receives home visits over a 12-month period by either a psychiatrist or an emergency room doctor from the county hospital. They meet with the patients and with a family member or close friend who has been identified as someone the subject can trust. They discuss interpersonal conflicts and other stresses experienced by the subject, mobilize social support in the family and the village to help the subject, discuss different methods of reducing stress, and establish a 'crisis warning system' to ensure that they are notified if the subject starts to deteriorate psychologically. The project is designed to demonstrate that, with minimal input of mental health professionals, it may be possible to reduce suicide attempts and suicide in rural areas where medical services are lacking (Hendin *et al.* 2008).

## SPI's structure

SPI is funded by private foundations, individual donors interested in suicide prevention, and international corporations concerned about the health and well-being of people in the countries in which they operate. Collaborating professional organizations range from the American Medical Association, the American Psychiatric Association, and the Milbank Memorial Fund, an organization concerned with health care policy, to the World Health Organization, the World Psychiatric Association, and the Swedish National Prevention of Suicide and Mental Ill-Health at Karolinska Institute.

SPI's Scientific Advisory Council includes representatives from twenty-two countries with expertise in suicide prevention, public health, health care economics social medicine, youth suicide, suicide in the elderly, and in the problems of those who have lost a loved one to suicide.

SPI brings them together for workshops—in Hong Kong in 2006 and in Helsinki in 2007—that help us to determine where suicide prevention needs are greatest and which projects can best meet them.

Our international collaborative network is permitting us to implement the projects in which SPI is currently engaged on a large scale and in a variety of cultural settings. The progress we have made so far encourages us to believe that we are on a path to make a significant contribution to reducing the global public health problem that suicide represents.

## References

Hendin H, Maltsberger JT, Szanto K (2007). The role of intense affective states in signaling a suicide crisis. *Journal of Nervous and Mental Disease*, **195**, 363–368.

Hendin H, Wang H, Hegerl U *et al.* (2008). Suicide prevention in Asia: future directions. In H Hendin, M Phillips, L Vijayakumar *et al.*, eds, *Suicide and Suicide Prevention in Asia*, pp. 97–108. World Health Organization, Geneva.

# CHAPTER 104

# The role of volunteer organizations in suicide prevention

Karl Andriessen

## Abstract

Contemporary suicide prevention emerged, to a large extent, as a result of groundwork conducted by volunteers. This chapter focuses on the involvement of volunteers in suicide prevention organizations throughout history and across the world, without forgetting the involvement of volunteers in suicide bereavement support. The characteristics of volunteers and volunteer organizations are presented. The question regarding the effectiveness of volunteer organizations is addressed, e.g. the available evidence regarding the positive effects of telephone crisis lines, online chat, and 'befriending' in rural areas are discussed. However, further research is needed given the shortage of studies. The chapter concludes with a plea for increased cooperation between volunteer and professional organizations, and integration of volunteer work in national suicide prevention policies in order to provide optimal care to the people in need.

## Introduction

A volunteer is a person who provides 'an unpaid direct service [to people] to whom the volunteer is not related' (Scott and Armson 2000, p. 700). The services are provided via 'some kind of formal scheme' (Scott and Armson 2000, p. 700). As such, volunteer work derives from kindness between relatives and friends, and consists of services provided to other third persons in a (semi-)structured framework.

This chapter focuses on the important role of volunteers in suicide prevention, as well as what is known about the effectiveness of volunteer organizations.

## Involvement of volunteers

The development of contemporary organized suicide prevention is relatively due to volunteer work. The eldest records of volunteer organizations involved in suicide prevention go back to the end of the nineteenth century. A survey conducted by Farberow and Shneidman (1961) found a local German volunteer rescue organization that operated from 1893 to 1906. The survey also showed a similar organization in Budapest. In 1906, the Anti Suicide Bureau of the Salvation Army was established in London; simultaneously, the National Save-a-Life League emerged in New York, and both organizations relied on voluntary donations and some volunteer involvement.

Among the services started up in Vienna, during the first half of the twentieth century, the Lebensmüdenstelle der Ethischen Gemeinde (Ethical Community for Suicidal Persons) started in 1927 with a staff of volunteer counsellors and social workers. The organization did rather well in attracting suicidal persons from the community. In 1928, Victor Frankl initiated a youth counselling service for suicide prevention, with various professionals providing counselling in their own houses (Farberow and Shneidman 1961). However, these, as well as other promising services, were closed due to the Second World War (Dublin 1963).

After the war, a few new suicide prevention organizations emerged, including three influential organizations involving volunteers:

1 *The Suicide Prevention Agency*: in 1947, Dr Erwin Ringel started the Lebensmüdenfürsorgestelle in the University Neuropsychiatric Clinic in Vienna. Most of the multidisciplinary staff were volunteer members. The agency successfully established cooperation with police departments and hospitals to reach those who attempted suicide. Prevention methods included outreach, social support, psychotherapy and follow-up. Apparently, only a very small minority of those treated repeated their attempt with a non-fatal or fatal suicide attempt (Farberow and Shneidman 1961; Dublin 1963).

2 *The Samaritans*: 'When I made it known to the press that from 2 November 1953 people contemplating suicide were invited to telephone me ... I did not think of myself as founding an organization, still less a world movement' (Varah 1973, p. 15). Starting as a private initiative of one Reverend in London, the Samaritans has become a worldwide organization providing 24-hour telephone crisis lines, online support, home visits and drop-in centres. Emphasis is put on direct human contact between a volunteer and the person in need, known as 'befriending'. The principles of befriending can be applied in various settings, e.g. prisons (Hall and Gabor 2004).

3 *The Los Angeles Suicide Prevention Center*: the centre was founded in 1958 (Shneidman *et al.* 1961; Shneidman and Farberow 1965). The centre became a pioneer for contemporary suicide prevention by integrating three complementary aspects: clinical work, community (public health) involvement and research. The professional multidisciplinary staff provides treatment for the people who come to the centre (located in the Los Angeles Hospital). Simultaneously, a 24-hour suicide

crisis line is maintained by trained and supervised volunteers. If necessary, callers are invited to come to the centre or referred to community resources. In addition to the clinical programme, meetings and conferences were held with various community and governmental organizations (e.g. hospitals, police, welfare organizations, etc.) in order to raise awareness, improve collaborations, and facilitate training for these organizations. Research programmes were also included from the outset, resulting in influential publications, which included the operation of a suicide prevention centre. This particular centre, amid the volunteer staff and suicide prevention crisis line, has inspired several centres throughout the world.

Currently, similar organizations such as Befrienders, International Federation of Telephonic Emergency Services (IFOTES), Lifeline, American Association of Suicidology (AAS), and The International Association of Suicide Prevention (IASP) are well-respected suicide prevention organizations, representing thousands of centres that apply high-quality standards for volunteers and care given from telephone support.

It is estimated that 100,000 volunteers worldwide are directly involved in suicide prevention (Vijayakumar and Armson 2005). In addition, volunteers are active in less developed or rural regions (e.g. African and Asian countries) with low health resources for mental health care (Ratnayeke 1996; Gulvady 2001).

Worldwide, thousands of volunteers are involved in suicide bereavement services. In fact, given that suicide-bereaved relatives have a 2–3 times elevated risk for suicidal behaviour (Qin *et al.* 2002), post-vention is prevention (Andriessen 2006). By far, the majority of suicide support groups are facilitated by survivors and/or by a duo of a survivor and a paid professional (Farberow 1998; Andriessen 2004).

## Characteristics of volunteers

In a suicide-prevention organization, volunteers are selected, trained, and supervised to provide services for telephone, online, or face-to-face support. They need qualities rather than qualifications (Scott and Armson 2000). Experienced volunteers are a valuable resource for training and supervising new volunteers (Mishara and Giroux 1993).

The volunteer is primarily interested in the person rather than the problem, i.e. 'tell me who you are' rather than 'what is your diagnosis?' The volunteer provides active, empathic and non-judgemental listening. The focus of the exchange is predominantly on the here and now and crisis situation, as well as the related experiences of distress, hopelessness, anger, anxiety, etc., rather than causal and distal factors. Volunteers (and paid clinicians) should inquire about suicidal ideation as a regular part of the risk assessment, and certainly become more directive in acute life-threatening situations when, for example, a caller threatens or attempts suicide during the conversation.

The work of volunteers is demanding. Suicide-prevention training, coping skills education, limiting volunteer working hours, and psychological debriefing could prevent compassion fatigue and vicarious traumatization (Kinzel and Nanson 2000).

One study of volunteers in a suicide prevention centre found that up to 50% of the volunteers have had suicidal ideation, 13% had attempted suicide, and some were bereaved by suicide (Mishara and Giroux 1993). These figures are significantly higher than in non-suicide specific crisis lines (Vijayakumar and Armson 2005). Perhaps the close experience of suicidal behaviour contributes to an openness of mind and motivation necessary for suicide-prevention volunteer work. The question remains open for further research.

## Characteristics of volunteer organizations

Scott (1996) and Scott and Armson (2000) identified four characteristics of volunteer organizations: availability, accessibility, acceptability, and adaptability. Here, we summarize and update these characteristics.

### Availability

In Western countries, volunteers complement the work of the professional sector by the type of work (befriending versus psychotherapy) and the timing, e.g. 24-hours and during weekends. Volunteers may reach people in need who are unable or reluctant to visit a professional clinician, where, otherwise, would not receive support. As such, they bridge the gap between receiving professional care or no care whatsoever. In regions with few professionals, volunteers may be the only caregivers available (Ratnayeke 1996; Marecek and Ratnayeke 2001; Gulvady 2001).

### Accessibility

Volunteer organizations have become active throughout the world, with the ability to reach people in need via various channels, i.e. telephone, online, drop-in centres, home visits, etc. Help-seeking and mental health problems are taboo subjects in many cultures. The threshold to anonymously contact a volunteer organization might be lower than immediately stepping into a clinical setting.

### Acceptability

Historically, some cultures are not familiar with seeking help from third persons. Scott and Armson (2000) gave an example of the role of the extended family in Africa. The more such traditional support mechanisms weaken, the more alternative support systems should be developed.

### Adaptability

Volunteer work is often grass-rooted. It emerges as a response to local needs. Volunteer organizations may adopt formulas, procedures, and quality criteria that were developed elsewhere; still, these formats/programmes need to be evaluated against the local culture, the identified needs and resources. In addition, as society evolves, the programme should be flexible to allow for modifications when necessary. This implies that evaluation should be included from the onset of the implementation process.

## Effectiveness of volunteer organizations

Since their inception, there has been a debate on the effectiveness of suicide-prevention centres (mostly staffed by volunteers) in reducing suicide and attempted suicide. Vijayakumar and Armson (2005) listed a few ecological and time-series studies respectively, with the focus on suicide mortality. The findings of these studies conflict with other study results, as some discovered a preventive effect, whereas others did not.

Lester (1997) reviewed fourteen studies that reported suicide rates of the regions served by suicide-prevention centres. The results of the meta-analysis provided a significant preventive effect, though the effect was small. Leenaars and Lester (2004) looked at changes in suicide rates in the Canadian provinces correlated with the establishment of suicide-prevention centres over time, and found a preventive, but not significant, effect. Though the effect sizes are not impressive, the findings are encouraging. Questions that remain to be answered include the potential *causal* relation between the centres and suicide rates, the effectiveness on certain subgroups (rather than on the overall population), and effects on attempted suicide rates, e.g. on hospital admissions for suicide attempts.

Other important questions are related to proximal factors, such as what happens during a call to a crisis line and its short-term outcomes. That was the focus of a series of studies conducted by Mishara *et al.* (2007a) who silently monitored 2611 calls to 14 US suicide-prevention centres. A surprising finding was that the majority of the volunteers didn't systematically assess suicide risk. The implementation of risk-assessment guidelines seems highly necessary (Joiner *et al.* 2007). Furthermore, Mishara *et al.* (2007b) reported that empathy and respect, supportive approach, good contact and collaborative problem-solving were related to positive endings of a call. A 3-week follow-up study of 800 non-suicidal callers found decreased levels of crises and hopelessness. One-third of the callers who had received a mental health referral had complied (Kalafat *et al.* 2007), and a 3-week follow-up study of suicidal callers found that the levels of hopelessness and psychological pain had decreased, but the intensity of the intent did not continue to decrease after the call. The results illustrated that 43% kept feeling suicidal and 3% had made a suicide attempt, 30% called the centre again, and only 16% of those who received a mental health referral had complied with the referral (Gould *et al.* 2007).

This landmark study provides evidence for the potential effectiveness of suicide-prevention centres. At the same time, the necessity of thorough selection, training, and supervision of volunteers is apparent.

Barak and Bloch (2006) reported promising results regarding the perceived helpfulness of an online chat programme provided by trained volunteers. Depth and smoothness of the writing were significantly related to improved client mood at the end of the chat, which was not the case in bumping and shallow conversations. The length of the helper's and client's writing contributed to the positive effect.

Responding to alarmingly high suicide rates in rural villages in Sri Lanka, the local Befrienders branch Sumithrayo, started a controlled outreach programme in 1996 (Ratnayeke 1996; Marecek and Ratnayeke 2001). Trained volunteers made themselves available in one village by visiting the leaders, facilitating community meetings, and visiting every household. Special attention was given to families where suicides or attempted suicides had occurred as well as economic hardship or violence. Before the project, the number of suicides and attempted suicides were similar in the intervention village and the comparison village. During the next four-and-a-half-years, the number of suicides and attempted suicides dropped to zero in the intervention village, whereas the numbers remained stable in the comparison village (three suicides and ten attempts during two observation years, after which the project was expanded to this comparison village) as well as in the whole district. Though it concerns a small-scale project, the results are impressive, and show the impact of this pioneer volunteer initiative.

## Concluding remarks

Given the extent of volunteer involvement in suicide prevention, the shortage of qualitative and empirical studies regarding effectiveness is striking, and research on the effects of volunteerism on volunteers is notably absent. As telecommunication and its use by volunteers in suicide prevention evolves rapidly (Krysinska and De Leo 2007), this warrants research regarding effectiveness of volunteer organizations in well-defined populations, cost-efficiency, sustainability, and psychological impact on the volunteers.

Sufficient funding would be a prerequisite to develop comprehensive long-term coordinated programmes (Wasserman 2004). This is as much true for suicide prevention, in general, as for volunteer organizations specifically. Volunteer organizations could benefit from community linkages and professional marketing by raising governmental and corporate funding.

Volunteers are available and accessible. Their actions are culture-sensitive and have low threshold for contact. Thoroughly selected, trained and supervised volunteers provide unique services to the persons in need. They develop support complementary to paid professionals; alternatively, they are the major service providers in the absence of professionals. As such, volunteer and professional organizations should join hands in a win–win situation for optimal service delivery. Moreover, the work of volunteer organizations should be integrated in national and regional suicide prevention programmes and policies, guarding quality levels and programme sustainability.

## References

Andriessen K (2004). Suicide survivor activities: an international perspective. *Suicidologi* (Norwegian Journal of Suicidology), **9**, 26–31.

Andriessen K (2006). Can postvention be prevention? *Psychiatria Danubina*, **18**, 125.

Barak A and Bloch N (2006). Factors related to perceived helpfulness in supporting highly distressed individuals through an online support chat. *CyberPsychology and Behavior*, **9**, 60–68.

Dublin L (1963). *Suicide. A Sociological and Statistical Study*. The Ronald Press Company, New York.

Farberow N (1998). Suicide survivor programs in IASP member countries. In R Kosky, H Eshkevari, R Goldney *et al.*, eds, *Suicide Prevention: The Global Context*, pp. 293–297. Plenum Press, New York/London.

Farberow N and Shneidman E (1961). A survey of agencies for the prevention of suicide. In N Farberow and E Shneidman, eds, *The Cry for Help*, pp. 136–149. McGraw-Hill, New York.

Gould M, Kalafat J, Munfakh J *et al.* M (2007). An evaluation of crisis hotline outcomes, part 2: suicidal callers. *Suicide and Life-Threatening Behavior*, **37**, 338–352.

Gulvady M (2001). Befriending in developing countries. In L Vijayakumar, ed., *Suicide Prevention: Meeting the Challenge Together*, pp. 191–197. Orient Longman, Chennai.

Hall B and Gabor P (2004). Peer suicide prevention in a prison. *Crisis*, **25**, 19–26.

Joiner T, Kalafat J, Draper J *et al.* (2007). Establishing standards for the assessment of suicide risk among callers to the National Suicide Prevention Lifeline. *Suicide and Life-Threatening Behavior*, **37**, 353–365.

Kalafat J, Gould M, Munfakh J *et al.* (2007). An evaluation of crisis hotline outcomes, part 1: nonsuicidal crisis callers. *Suicide and Life-Threatening Behavior*, **37**, 322–337.

Kinzel A and Nanson J (2000). Education and debriefing: strategies for preventing crises in crisis-line volunteers. *Crisis*, **21**, 126–134.

Krysinska K and De Leo D (2007). Telecommunication and suicide prevention: hopes and challenges for the new century. *Omega*, **55**, 237–253.

Leenaars A and Lester D (2004). The impact of suicide prevention centers on the suicide rate in the Canadian provinces. *Crisis*, **25**, 65–68.

Lester D (1997). The effectiveness of suicide prevention centres: a review. *Suicide and Life-Threatening Behavior*, **27**, 304–310.

Marecek J and Ratnayeke L (2001). Suicide in rural Sri Lanka: assessing a prevention programme. In OT Grad, ed., *Suicide Risk and Protective Factors in the New Millennium*, pp. 215–219. Cankarjev dom, Ljubljana.

Mishara B, Chagnon F, Daigle M *et al.* (2007a). Comparing models of helper behaviour to actual practice in telephone crisis intervention: a silent monitoring study of calls to the US 1–800-SUICIDE Network. *Suicide and Life-Threatening Behavior*, **37**, 291–307.

Mishara B, Chagnon F, Daigle M *et al.* (2007b). Which helper behaviors and intervention styles are related to better short-term outcomes in telephone crisis interventions? Results from a silent monitoring study of calls to the US 1–800-SUICIDE Network. *Suicide and Life-Threatening Behavior*, **37**, 308–321.

Mishara B and Giroux G (1993). The relationship between coping strategies and perceived stress in telephone interventions volunteers in a suicide prevention centre. *Suicide and Life-Threatening Behavior*, **23**, 221–229.

Qin P, Agerbo E, Mortensen P (2002). Suicide risk in relation to family history of completed suicide and psychiatric disorders: a nested case–control study based on longitudinal registers. *Lancet*, **360**, 1126–1130.

Ratnayeke L (1996). Suicide and crisis intervention in rural communities in Sri Lanka. *Crisis*, **17**, 149–154.

Scott V (1996). Reaching the suicidal: the volunteer's role in preventing suicide. *Crisis*, **17**, 102–104.

Scott V and Armson S (2000). Volunteers and suicide prevention. In K Hawton and K Van Heeringen, eds, *The International Handbook of Suicide and Attempted Suicide*, pp. 699–711. Wiley and Sons, Chichester.

Shneidman E and Farberow N (1965). The Los Angeles Suicide Prevention Center: a demonstration of public health feasibilities. *American Journal of Public Health*, **55**, 21–26.

Shneidman E, Farberow N, Litman R (1961). The Suicide Prevention Center. In N Farberow and E Shneidman, eds, *The Cry for Help*, pp. 6–18. McGraw-Hill, New York.

Varah C (1973). *The Samaritans in the '70s. To Befriend the Suicidal and Despairing*. Constable, London.

Vijayakumar L and Armson S (2005). Volunteer perspectives on suicide prevention. In K Hawton, ed., *Prevention and Treatment of Suicidal Behaviour, from Science to Practice*, pp. 335–349. Oxford University Press, Oxford.

Wasserman D (2004). Evaluating suicide prevention: various approaches needed. *World Psychiatry*, **3**, 153–154.

# PART 15

# Examples of How to Develop Suicide Prevention on all the Continents

# Examples of How to Develop Suicide Prevention on all the Continents: Africa

# CHAPTER 105

# Suicide Prevention in South Africa

Stephanie Burrows and Lourens Schlebusch

## Framework for a national suicide preventive programme

Suicidal behaviour is an increasingly significant public health concern on the African continent. Although there is an obvious, urgent need for comprehensive national suicide prevention programmes, only a handful of local or regionalized efforts exist and to the best of our knowledge there are no national programmes. In South Africa, a framework for a national suicide prevention programme has been proposed (Schlebusch 2005; Burrows and Schlebusch 2008), and a statement of intent to implement such plans has been issued by government representatives and South African suicidologists (Burrows 2005).

In some ways, South Africa has set the lead in contemporary suicide research in Africa (Kinyanda and Kigozi 2005; Schlebusch 2005). For example, the twenty-third World Congress of the International Association for Suicide Prevention (IASP) was held for the first time on the African continent and hosted in Durban (a major harbour city on the east coast of South Africa) in 2005. South Africa has unique features compared to many other countries on the continent in that it is fairly prosperous with many well-established universities, research institutes and research infrastructures. It is one of the few countries in the African region to regularly monitor and update data on suicidal behaviour (Matzopoulos 2005; Schlebusch 2005) and researchers have developed a framework for the management (Schlebusch 2005) and prevention of suicidal behaviour (Burrows and Schlebusch 2008).

## Data collection and collaborative research

Little is known about the suicidal behaviour profile of many African countries or regions. Early publications were frequently by visiting scientists and expatriates mostly from Europe, although indigenous publications gradually emerged. More recently, collaborative work between indigenous and Western scientists has led to significantly more publications. In a sense, then, the development of research on suicidal behaviour in a particular country on the continent reflects that country's history.

The prevention of suicidal behaviour depends on a thorough understanding of its complexity/magnitude, aetiology and comorbid factors in different African contexts and cultures. In South Africa alone, there are eleven different official languages.

As pointed out by authorities, different strategies are required in different groups (Wasserman 2001). Systematic data collection and research, although limited in Africa, are critical to this process. Three major research programmes in South Africa are noteworthy. The first is the National Injury Mortality Surveillance System (NIMSS), developed in response to the lack of detailed epidemiological data on injury mortality (Butchart et al. 2001). The NIMSS collates information that arises from existing medico-legal investigative procedures, as a collaborative effort between different research groups and government bodies in South Africa. Demographic variables of the deceased, spatial and temporal details of the injury event, the manner and external cause of death, and the involvement of alcohol are recorded (Matzopoulos 2005).

The second is the WHO worldwide initiative for the prevention of suicide, the Suicide Prevention Multisite Intervention Study on Suicidal Behaviours (SUPRE-MISS), launched in 2000 to address the public health problem of attempted suicide and to reduce mortality and morbidity associated with suicidal behaviour (Bertolote et al. 2005). Durban serves as the Africa SUPRE-MISS study site. The third is the Durban Parasuicide Study (DPS) that originated in 1978 (Schlebusch 2005) under the leadership of the second author (LS). The initial impetus for the DPS research group came from a growing awareness that only medical stabilization was being provided to patients admitted to hospital for suicidal behaviour. Consequently, a referral protocol was established, allowing all patients admitted for medical treatment of suicidal behaviour to be comprehensively assessed psychologically. An ongoing research programme on suicidal behaviour was established which has resulted in numerous publications and several Southern African conferences on suicidal behaviour.

Significantly more suicidology research data are available from South Africa (Schlebusch 2005) and from Uganda (Ovuga 2005). Nevertheless, there needs to be renewed awareness of the problem and wide dissemination and exchange of data, research tools and methods. A greater understanding can be enhanced with inter-African collaborative research, networking and global cooperation and access to the latest information about suicide prevention. The several Southern African conferences, stemming from the work of the long-standing Durban Parasuicide Study (Schlebusch 2005), and the International Association for Suicide Prevention's Congress, have assisted in this process (Burrows 2005).

## Primary health care

Because psychiatric/psychological conditions and substance dependence/abuse have been associated with increased suicidal behaviour risk in many African settings (Eferakeya 1984; Ndosi and Waziri 1997; Alem *et al.* 1999; Schlebusch *et al.* 2003; Kinyanda *et al.* 2004; Schlebusch 2005; Kinyanda 2006; Gureje *et al.* 2007), more attention should be given to their early detection and effective treatment. Treatment strategies must be holistic and culturally relevant and incorporate traditional healers and beliefs (Schlebusch and Rugieri 1996; Freeman 2003; Mkize 2005; Ovuga 2005). The aim should be to create uniquely African strategies, not simply to transplant knowledge on suicide prevention into Africa from the Western world (Schlebusch 2005).

Many suicidal patients consult health-care workers complaining of somatic symptoms in the days, weeks or months preceding the suicidal act. As the majority of the population in rural areas have limited access to mental health services, individuals in a suicidal crisis are often more likely to visit a general practitioner or traditional healer than a mental health specialist. These primary health-care providers can play a critical role in the prevention of suicidal behaviour if trained to recognize, monitor and treat underlying psychopathology (Schlebusch 2005; Ovuga *et al.* 2007). Practitioners dealing with somatic diseases associated with depression and suicidal behaviour need to be made aware of the impact of disease processes on such behaviour. For example, in light of the increase in HIV/AIDS infections in sub-Saharan Africa and especially South Africa, provision for pre- and post-test counselling is mandatory to minimize the risk of suicidal behaviour during crisis/high-risk periods (Schlebusch 2005, 2006).

## Community-based efforts

Given the limited numbers of mental health professionals, community-based initiatives such as mental health centres, self-help support groups and education/training programmes play an essential role in the prevention of suicidal behaviour. Suicide crisis centres provide much needed immediate emotional support to suicidal people. Helplines like Lifeline Southern Africa and Samaritans/Befrienders Worldwide operate in several African countries such as Botswana, Ghana, Mauritius, Namibia, Sudan and Zimbabwe. In South Africa such facilities and other organizations are extensively available. Depending on the needs of the communities they serve, these facilities also provide specific help in dealing with many other factors associated with suicidal behaviour such HIV/AIDS, rape, abuse and trauma. Telephonic counselling is usually the main focus, but face-to-face counselling, a referral service to community-based services, information and educational materials, and outreach work may be available. Although South African studies show these centres are helpful (Stein *et al.* 1997; Meehan and Broom 2007), more evaluative studies are needed and it is important to monitor patterns of suicidal behaviour on an ongoing basis because it changes across time in different groups (Burrows and Schlebusch 2008).

Help for families following their bereavement after a suicide is essential. Self-help support groups are powerful, inexpensive, constructive ways for people to help themselves and others. Likewise, such groups exist in South Africa.

Further education and training programmes have been recommended (Schlebusch 2005; Burrows and Schlebusch 2008) for those who come into contact with suicidal individuals to help eliminate myths surrounding suicidal behaviour, provide information about the clues to suicidal behaviour for early recognition, and promote skills development on how to support and assist suicidal patients and their families in obtaining help. Such training should target the police, the legal profession, the clergy and others, but given the high levels of suicidal behaviour among youth in South Africa, the education of school personnel and parents is of particular importance (Madu and Matla 2003; Schlebusch 2005). Liaison between the various clinical services and education departments is required for referral of at-risk pupils to appropriate professional help. Additionally, interventions for pupils involving crisis management, self-esteem enhancement and the development of coping/psychosocial skills and healthy decision-making have been emphasized, not only to reduce the risk of suicidal behaviour among youth, but also other risk factors such as aggressiveness and alcohol/drug dependence/abuse (National Institute of Public Health of Québec 2004). Following WHO guidelines (WHO 2000), the important role of the media has been highlighted in de-stigmatizing mental illness and providing information on helplines and community resources, risk factors and warning signs (Schlebusch 2005).

## Restricting access to methods of suicide

Internationally, there is evidence that controlling the availability of suicide methods can be effective in suicide prevention (Leenaars 2001; Hawton 2005). In South Africa, pesticides, common household utilities (paraffin, poisons, etc.), over-the-counter medications and firearms are among the most frequently used methods in suicidal behaviour (Schlebusch 2005). In parts of Africa pesticides typically can be bought in lethal doses from markets and street vendors without any restrictions (Abebe 1991; Tagwireyi *et al.* 2006). Modifying policies to control their production, distribution and sales; promoting their safer storage; improving the medical management of pesticide ingestion; and educating the community are recommended as they may have dramatic effects on reducing the risk of suicidal behaviour. Legislation can also be changed to further restrict the maximum size of prescriptions for lethal medications, although experience such as in Tanzania, because of inadequate supervision over dispensation of medication (Ndosi *et al.* 2004), shows that legislation is not sufficient without enforcement. Similarly, legislation regarding firearm sales/ownership and gun safety (education and training, safe storage of firearms) is important. In Cameroon, where ownership of firearms is restricted to registered hunters, no suicides by firearms were reported in the two largest cities over a 5-year period (Bahebeck *et al.* 2005).

## Conclusions

There is an obvious need to prioritize suicide prevention in Africa. Although comparisons between different African countries are difficult, the recommended South African national programme for suicide prevention can be adapted for use in other African countries as it provides for a strategic framework for action at all levels (national, provincial and local) and in all groups of the population, with a particular focus on high-risk groups. This is an evolving, long-term, research and evidence-based strategy whose ultimate goal is the prevention of suicidal behaviour. It is essential that the strategy is research-based with evaluation as an integral part; and that it is appropriate and responsive to the social and cultural needs of the populations they serve. Strengthened collaborations within Africa and beyond are also essential.

## References

Abebe M (1991). Organophosphate pesticide poisoning in 50 Ethiopian patients. *Ethiopian Medical Journal*, **29**, 109–118.

Alem A, Kebede D, Jacobsson L et al. G (1999). Suicide attempts among adults in Butajira, Ethiopia. *Acta Psychiatrica Scandinavica*, **397**, 70–76.

Bahebeck J, Atangana R, Mboudou E et al. (2005). Incidence, case-fatality rate and clinical pattern of firearm injuries in two cities where arms owning is forbidden. *Injury, International Journal of the Care of the Injured*, **36**, 714–717.

Bertolote JM, Fleischmann A, De Leo D et al. (2005). Suicide attempts, plans, and ideation in culturally diverse sites: the WHO SUPRE-MISS community survey. *Psychological Medicine*, **35**, 1457–1465.

Burrows S (2005). Suicide mortality in the South African context: exploring the role of social status and environmental circumstances. Doctoral dissertation. Karolinska Institutet, Sweden.

Burrows S and Schlebusch L (2008). Priorities and Prevention Possibilities for Reducing Suicidal Behaviour in South Africa. In a Van Niekerk, S Suffla, M Seedat, eds., *Crime, violence and injury prevention in South Africa: Developments and challenges*, p. 190–210. Medical Research Council, Cape Town.

Butchart A, Peden M, Matzopoulos R et al. (2001). The South African national non-natural mortality surveillance system: rationale, pilot results and evaluation. *South African Medical Journal*, **91**, 408–417.

Eferakeya AE (1984). Drugs and suicide attempts in Benin City, Nigeria. *British Journal of Psychiatry*, **145**, 70–73.

Freeman M (ed.) (2003). *Mental Health and HIV/AIDS: Proceedings of the Round-table Meeting*. HSRC Publishers, Cape Town.

Gureje O, Kola L, Uwakwe R et al. (2007). The profile and risks of suicidal behaviours in the Nigerian Survey of Mental Health and Well-Being. *Psychological Medicine*, **37**, 821–830.

Hawton K (2005). Restriction of access to methods of suicide as a means of suicide prevention. In K Hawton, ed., *Prevention and Treatment of Suicidal Behaviour. From Science to Practice*, pp. 279–292. Oxford University Press, Oxford.

Kinyanda E (2006). Deliberate self-harm in urban Uganda: a case–control study. Doctoral dissertation. Norwegian University of Science and Technology, Norway.

Kinyanda E and Kigozi F (2005). Epidemiology of suicide in Africa. Paper presented at the XXIII World Congress of the International Association for Suicide Prevention, 13–16 September 2005, Durban, South Africa.

Kinyanda E, Hjelmeland H, Musisi S (2004). Deliberate self-harm as seen in Kampala, Uganda—a case–control study. *Social Psychiatry and Psychiatric Epidemiology*, **39**, 318–325.

Leenaars A (2001). Controlling the environment to prevent suicide. In D Wasserman, ed., *Suicide: An Unnecessary Death*, pp. 259–263. Martin Dunitz, London.

Madu SN and Matla MP (2003). The prevalence of suicidal behaviours amongst secondary school adolescents in the Limpopo Province, South Africa. *South African Journal of Psychology*, **33**, 126–32.

Matzopoulos R (ed.) (2005). *A Profile of Fatal Injuries in South Africa: Sixth Annual Report of the National Injury Mortality Surveillance System*. Medical Research Council–University of South Africa, Crime, Violence and Injury Lead Programme, Tygerberg.

Meehan SA and Broom Y (2007). Analysis of a national toll-free suicide crisis line in South Africa. *Suicide and Life-Threatening Behavoir*, **37**, 66–78.

Mkize DL (2005). Traditional healers and suicide in South Africa. Paper presented at the XXIII World Congress of the International Association for Suicide Prevention, 13–16 September 2005, Durban, South Africa.

National Institute of Public Health of Quebec (2004). *Suicide Among Young People: Scientific Advice*. National Institute of Public Health of Quebec, Montréal.

Ndosi NK and Waziri MC (1997). The nature of parasuicide in Dar es Salaam, Tanzania. *Social Science and Medicine*, **44**, 55–61.

Ndosi NK, Mbonde MP, Lyamuya E (2004). Profile of suicide in Dar es Salaam. *East African Medical Journal*, **81**, 207–211.

Ovuga E (2005). Depression and suicidal behaviour in Uganda: Validating the Response Inventory for Stressful Life Events (RISLE). Doctoral dissertation. Karolinska University Press, Stockholm.

Ovuga E, Boardman J, Wasserman D (2007). Integrating mental health into primary health care: local initiatives from Uganda. *World Psychiatry*, **6**, 60–61.

Schlebusch L (2005). *Suicidal Behaviour in South Africa*. University of Kwa-Zulu Natal Press, Pietermaritzburg.

Schlebusch L (2006). HIV/Aids og risikoen for selvmordsatferd (trans. HIV/AIDS and the risk for suicidal behaviour). *Suicidologi*, **11**, 30–32.

Schlebusch L and Ruggieri G (1996). Health beliefs of a sample of black patients attending a specialised medical facility. *South African Journal of Psychology*, **26**, 35–38.

Schlebusch L, Vawda N, Bosch BA (2003). Suicidal behaviour in black South Africans. *Crisis*, **24**, 24–28.

Stein DJ, Wessels C, Van Kradenberg J et al. (1997). The Mental Health Information Centre: a report of the first 500 calls. *Central African Journal of Medicine*, **43**, 244–246.

Tagwireyi D, Ball DE, Nhachi CFB (2006). Toxicoepidemiology in Zimbabwe: pesticide-poisoning admissions to major hospitals. *Journal of Toxicology and Clinical Toxicology*, **44**, 59–66.

Wasserman D (ed.) (2001). *Suicide: An Unnecessary Death*. Martin Dunitz, London.

World Health Organization (2000). *Preventing Suicide: A Resource for Media Professionals*. Department of Mental Health, World Health Organization, Geneva.

# CHAPTER 106

# Suicide prevention in Uganda

Emilio Ovuga and Jed Boardman

## The challenge

Suicide is a global public health problem across the world: about 1 million people kill themselves each year and rates have increased over the past 50 years (World Health Organization 2001). Significant increases have been seen in young people (Wasserman *et al.* 2005) and suicide remains one of the leading causes of death among youth. Yet for many countries there are no reliable suicide statistics (Khan 2005). This is the case in sub-Saharan Africa where few published studies exist (e.g. Dong and Simon 2001; Nwosu and Odesanmi 2001; Kinyanda *et al.* 2004; Ndosi *et al.* 2004; Kinyanda *et al.* 2005; Ovuga *et al.* 2005a). Given the poverty, military unrest, psychological trauma, burden of neuropsychiatric disorders, alcoholism and AIDS, and the rapid rate of social change, these global trends are likely to be present in Africa.

In this chapter we examine briefly a background model and factors linked to suicide and a public health approach to its prevention. An example of efforts to tackle suicide in one district of Uganda is provided.

## Theory

The stress–diathesis model of suicide postulates an interaction of stressful experiences with vulnerability factors (Wasserman 2001). Vulnerability factors include genetic predisposition, personality traits, presence of mental disorder and social isolation. Factors that precipitate suicidal acts include property loss, the diagnosis of life-threatening illness, bereavement, rejection and interpersonal disputes within families. The stress–diathesis model may be universally plausible, but it may omit the background importance of poverty and the details of individual factors may differ between cultural and social groups. For example, while in industrialized countries suicide may occur in the context of social isolation, in developing countries, where many people have close family ties, it commonly occurs in the context of family disputes. In addition, the nature of depression in Africans is in need of re-evaluation and the explanation of low levels of presentation owing to somatization should be questioned (Ovuga *et al.* 2005b).

From research conducted in Africa, Ovuga (2005) suggests that suicide occurs within the context of a triad of threat of fear of abandonment, shame, injury or death; loss of self-esteem; and suicide ideation as a coping strategy within the context of personal vulnerability, social adversity and recurrent negative life events that evoke the experience of life as meaningless. Under the circumstances suicide presents itself as an attractive alternative to life full of suffering and misery. Suicidal persons place responsibility for their suicidal behaviour, irrespective of the nature of life difficulties, in their world of social support system and expect the family to solve their personal problems for them in order to survive. This approach assumes that suicide may not be entirely a personal matter and is a dynamic phenomenon that depends on the nature of one's social environment—once the quality of social relations improves suicidal ideation dissipates. Thus a supportive social network will militate against high-risk suicide behaviour while the fear of abandonment, shame, injury or death and emergence of low self-esteem will promote suicide.

## Public health approach to suicide prevention

The public health approach to prevention rests on the recognition of the interaction between agent, host and environment. Disease prevention involves boosting the immunity of host; modifying or eliminating potential risk factors; promoting healthy host lifestyle; improving the safety of the environment; and treatment for diseased individuals. For suicide prevention at a population level this requires the identification of protective factors and often complex multilevel socio-economic and cultural risk factors; improving the mental health and coping skills of communities and individuals; and promoting the safety of the environment. Though suicide is a rare event, the public health perspective holds that potential suicides arise from several members of the general population with low level of risk for suicide rather than from the few individuals with high levels of risk for suicide (Knox *et al.* 2004). Strategies for suicide prevention that have worked in developed countries include treatment of psychiatric disorders, control of alcohol and drugs of abuse, arms control, detoxification of domestic gas, detoxification of motor vehicle emissions, control of availability of toxic substances and the control of media reporting and portrayal of suicide (World Health Organization 1993).

However, developing countries give low priority to mental health services and access to these and their quality is low. There is little available research on suicide in Africa, but the little that does

**Table 106.1** Proposed suicide prevention strategy for Uganda based on public health approach

| Intervention | Approach | Target population | Aims | Examples of specific activities |
|---|---|---|---|---|
| Universal prevention | Population | Activities target entire communities<br><br>Programmes that reach asymptomatic individuals at low risk | Identify individuals with risk factors; reduce risk; reduce individual vulnerability; enhance mitigating factors | Population screening; promote and protect cultural activities that engender social cohesion in the face of negative life events; initiate programmes to reduce risk for suicide; provide public mental health education; promote accessibility, affordability and acceptability to health care; collaborate with other agencies; support policy reform; secure political support through lobbying and advocacy |
| Selective prevention | Medium risk | Identify vulnerable subgroups at increased risk of suicide | Identify people with increased risk of suicide, e.g. those with alcohol use problems; victims of war and violence, and the bereaved | Gatekeeper screening and first aid counselling; referral for further professional assessment; appropriate professional care for individuals with symptoms of psychiatric illness, with suicide wishes; liaise with other agencies in the community with relevant support |
| Indicated prevention | High risk | Identify persons with symptoms or are highly suicidal | Refer individuals for professional evaluation and possible treatment | Identify and treat accordingly: those with current psychiatric disorder; actively suicidal; have attempted suicide; those known to possess risk markers for suicide, e.g. persistent suicide ideation; those with persistent family disputes; those who have experienced severe loss |

exist suggests mental disorder plays a role (Ndosi *et al.* 2004). The methods employed often include hanging, firearms and the use of agricultural poisons, for example organophosphates (Dong and Simon 2001). Over-the-counter medicines, e.g. chloroquine and paracetamol, are also used. Suicide is illegal in many African countries but its designation as such does not act as a deterrent. Such anachronistic laws need repeal. Abuse of women and corporal punishment of children are common and there is a culture of shame and taboo associated with suicide that runs counter to open discussion.

To support the development of suicide prevention programmes there is an urgent need to record and monitor suicides nationally. Surveillance centres need to be established across Africa and robust research programmes created.

Table 106.1 provides a schematic presentation of suicide prevention strategies in low-income countries where suicide prevention activities are often not the priority of governments. A local initiative in the Adjumani district of north-west Uganda is described to illustrate the implementation of the scheme that views suicide prevention as the collective social responsibility of everyone.

## The case of Uganda

In Adjumani district (population 204,000) alcohol abuse, depression and suicide are common (Ovuga 2005). In 2004 the rate of suicide established from surveillance was 49.6 per 100,000. A sensitization seminar for district health, education, community, civic and political leadership, and police prisons and judiciary was held. Political support and commitment from area members of parliament and district political leaders have been given to combat the problems identified. The community established a body to coordinate health, political and community activities to combat the problems of suicide and alcohol abuse. Suicide and alcohol abuse were integrated within the overall health care package

of the district to ensure that they too attained priority health status. Primary health-care providers in the district were trained as were representatives of the community to act as gatekeepers for suicide prevention (Ovuga *et al.* 2007). Partnerships with overseas agencies (THET International and Sheffield Care Trust in the United Kingdom) were established to provide technical support for the development of psychosocial services in the district. Packages of mental health educational materials are being developed for use in public and school health education campaigns. Legal support has been secured in drafting regulations, bylaws and district policies to promote mental health and prevent suicide and mental ill-health. Research to determine the epidemiology of suicide behaviour, and develop effective and culturally sensitive psychosocial interventions, is underway. Although the initiative is less than two years old, several positive outcomes have already emerged. Suicide is now discussed openly by the public. The district criminal system no longer prosecutes people for attempting suicide, although it is a crime according to Uganda's constitution and penal code. Primary health care workers are more confident at identifying and providing whatever services they can for psychosocial problems.

## References

Dong X and Simon MA (2001). The epidemiology of organophosphate poisoning in urban Zimbabwe from 1995–2000. *International Journal of Occupational and Environmental Health*, **7**, 333–338.

Kinyanda E, Hjelmeland H, Musisi S *et al.* (2005). Repetition of deliberate self-harm as seen in Uganda. *Archives of Suicide Research*, **9**, 333–344.

Kinyanda E, Hjelmeland H, Musisi S (2004). Deliberate self-harm as seen in Kampala, Uganda. A case–control study. *Social Psychiatry and Psychiatric Epidemiology*, **39**, 318–325.

Khan MM (2005). Suicide prevention and developing countries. *Journal of Royal Society of Medicine*, **98**, 459–463.

Knox KM, Conwell Y, Caine ED (2004). If suicide is a public health problem, what are we doing to prevent it? *American Journal of Public Health*, **94**, 37–45.

Ndosi NK, Mbonde MP, Lyamuya E (2004). Profile of suicide in Dar es Salaam. *East African Medical Journal*, **81**, 207–211.

Nwosu SO and Odesanmi WO (2001). Pattern of suicides in Ile-Ife, Nigeria. *West African Journal of Medicine*, **20**, 259–262.

Ovuga E (2005). Depression and Suicidal Behaviors in Uganda. Validating the Response Inventory for Stressful Life Events (RISLE). PhD Thesis. Karolinska University Press, Stockholm.

Ovuga E, Boardman J, Wasserman D (2005a). Prevalence of suicide ideation in two districts of Uganda. *Archives of Suicide Research*, **9**, 321–332.

Ovuga E, Boardman J, Wasserman D (2005b). The prevalence of depression in two districts of Uganda. *Social Psychiatry and Psychiatric Epidemiology*, **40**, 439–445.

Ovuga E, Boardman J, Wasserman D (2007). Intgegrating mental health into primary health care: local initiatives from Uganda. *World Psychiatry*, **6**, 60–61.

Wasserman D (2001). A stress–vulnerability model and the development of the suicidal process. In D Wasserman, ed., *Suicide—An Unnecessary Death*, pp. 19–28. Martin Dunitz, London.

Wasserman D, Cheng Q, Jiang G-X (2005). Global suicide rates among young people aged 15–19. *World Psychiatry*, **4**, 114–120.

World Health Organization (2001). *The World Health Report 2001. Mental Health: New Understanding, New Hope.* World Health Organization, Geneva.

World Health Organization (1993). *Guidelines for the Primary Prevention of Mental, Neurological and Psychosocial Disorders; 4. Suicide.* Division of Mental Health, World Health Organization, Geneva.

# CHAPTER 107

# Suicide Prevention in Hong Kong

Paul Yip

## Introduction

Hong Kong, formerly a British Colony, returned to People's Republic of China and has been a special administrative region of that country since 1997. In 2006, Hong Kong had a population of 6.9 million people with a living area of about 1000 square kilometres: it is one of the most densely populated areas on Earth. Economic development in Hong Kong has been impressive during the past two decades with a GDP of about 25,000 US dollars per year. However, Hong Kong's suicide rate has increased from 9.6 to 18.6 deaths per 100,000 from 1981 to 2003, and is well above the global average of 14.5 per 100,000. In 2003, 1264 people committed suicide with an average of about 3.5 persons per day. It is the sixth leading cause of death, and has accounted for 3 per cent of the deaths annually. Moreover, suicide is the leading cause of death among the 15–24 age group, and the rate has increased by more than 70 per cent since 1997. Due to the increase in suicides among young people and adults, the proportion of life of years lost due to suicide has contributed to about 8 per cent of the total loss (Yip et al. 2005a). In 2003, the estimated loss of labour productivity on account of suicide was about US$175 million.

At present, the health authority has noted suicide as being a medical issue that is addressed primarily through clinical intervention; particularly the treatment of depression, by providing fast-track clinics in some publicly funded hospitals for older adults, and a crisis centre for providing a 24-hour service for suicidal persons (Yip 2005b). However, about two-thirds of all people who committed suicide did not receive any psychiatric care during the year before death (CSRP 2005). Among suicidal persons, less than 20 per cent had thought about calling telephone hotlines (CSRP 2005). Hence, it is important to adopt a population-based strategy that aims at actively reducing risks among the whole population (Lewis et al. 1997; Yip 2005). Countries in this region do not have the same resources as the West for preventing suicides. Therefore, it is even more important to be able to adopt a cost-effective public health approach for suicide prevention in Asia (Mann et al. 2005).

We like to use the term *flooding* as a metaphor to illustrate how to deal with suicide. When a flood occurs, we work hard to save those being affected, and mainly focus our attention on the victims who are swept downstream. However, some of the major causes of the flooding, including the deforestation and over-farming upstream, have often been overlooked. A public health approach should acknowledge the importance of both, the high risk and the population-based strategies for suicide prevention, and requires a multi-sector effort to tackle the problem at multiple levels. Figure 107.1 shows the effect of a shift in the mean suicidal risk of a population. If we can reduce the mean from $\mu_0$ to $\mu_1$, the overall number of suicide can be reduced substantially. It echoes the Rose Theorem: 'reducing a small risk for a large population is more effective than reducing a high risk for a small population'.

## Suicide prevention

The Government, non-governmental organizations (NGOs), and university research centres are playing different roles in suicide prevention in Hong Kong. All three strategies have been practiced by some stakeholders in the community. For example, the Hong Kong Government has provided fast-track clinics for older adults who have been diagnosed as depressed and suicidal. Some NGOs have provided help for those with financial problems and who are unemployed, factors that have been shown to increase suicidal risks when compared to the general population. Medical doctors have also improved their skills in detecting suicidal patients, and the university has been working with the media to improve suicide reporting, and conduct community-based suicide prevention efforts. However, integration and evaluation of these measures are not yet in place.

Nonetheless, the government has yet to commit itself to adopting a public health approach to deal with suicide prevention. The community has attempted to reorganize itself to meet the needs of people at risk in order to provide a concerted effort to reduce the number of suicides. Sometimes, the work overlaps, and there are some gaps which have yet to be filled.

A coalition of suicide prevention needs to be formed with a coordinated effort, not a duplication of effort. A critical mass in suicide prevention work, with the correct dosage, is needed. Evaluation, outcome assessment and monitoring are absolutely essential.

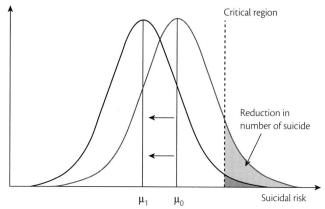

**Fig. 107.1**  A graphical representation of the Rose Theorem (1992).

$\mu_1$: Improved population mean
$\mu_0$: Original population mean

Based on overseas' experience, the commitment and support of the government, or its agency, is an essential ingredient for any successful suicide prevention programme. Suicide-prevention work in the community is meant to be continuous and remain sustainable.

In the past years, the increasing trend of Hong Kong suicide rates have reverted, and a 18 per cent reduction was achieved in 2004, including a further 8 per cent reduction in 2005, while leveling off in 2006 (CSRP 2005).

In Hong Kong, there is no tradition for conducting suicide prevention holistically; however, it is not impossible, provided the commitment and the support for suicide-prevention work are available. It is essential that any suicide-prevention effort to be evidence-based. The research centre in Hong Kong University has benefited from the support received from a group of esteemed suicide researchers around the globe, and it is strategically placed within the university so that the expertise from other disciplines are readily available. The centre is also partnering with society and serving the community, and planning to engage front-line workers and NGOs in the community. We provide a training programme, which trains the trainers, improves knowledge, and engages in evidence-based suicide-prevention programmes, with a vigorous evaluation. The centre has become a hub for suicide knowledge, and searches for best practice to benefit the community.

## Conclusion

Suicide is a complex and multifactorial problem, which involves psychological, social and biological aspects. It is important to advocate a multilayer intervention suicide-prevention programme. Hence, a public health approach for suicide prevention should be adopted and pursued actively in Hong Kong.

## References

CSRP (2005). *Hong Kong Jockey Club for Suicide Research and Prevention Findings into Suicide and its Prevention: Final Report.* The University of Hong Kong, Hong Kong.

Lewis G, Hawton K, Jones P (1997). Strategies for preventing suicide. *British Journal of Psychiatry*, **171**, 351–354.

Mann JJ, Apter A, Bertolote J *et al.* (2005). Suicide prevention strategies: a systematic review. *Journal of the American Medical Association*, **294**, 2064–2074.

Rose R (1992). *The strategy of preventive medicine*, p. 24. Oxford University Press, Oxford.

Yip PSF (2005). A public health approach to suicide prevention. *Hong Kong Journal of Psychiatry*, **15**, 29–31.

Yip PSF, Liu Ka, Song XM, Hu JP (2005a). Suicides in mainland China. *Social Psychiatric and Psychiatric Epidemiology*, **40**, 792–798.

Yip PSF, Yang KCT, Law FYW (2005b). Suicide in general hospitals in Hong Kong. *Hong Kong Medical Journal*, **11**, 70–71.

# CHAPTER 108

# Suicide prevention in India

## Considering religion and culture

Lakshmi Vijayakumar

## Introduction

India is the seventh largest country in the world and the largest democracy. The population of India is 1.08 billion, which means that one in every six human beings are Indian. There are twenty-eight states and seven Union Territories, eighteen official languages and eight hundred dialects. India is truly a multicultural, multilingual, multi-religious melting pot.

India is now emerging as an economic power. The software and IT sector, modernization of telecommunications and increased pace of privatization, has brought about a paradigm shift in the lifestyle of the urban Indian. However, the growth is not equitable, and the urban/rural divide is wide. There is also a huge disparity in the availability of infrastructure and resources, not only between the different states of India, but also within a state. As an illustration, there are only 60 doctors per 100,000 population, but there are 50 Internet users per 1000 population. Suicide is an important issue in this emerging Indian context.

## The epidemiology of suicide in India

More than one *lakh* (one hundred thousand) lives are lost every year due to suicide in India. During the last three decades (from 1975 to 2005), the suicide rate has increased by 43 per cent. The rates were approximately the same in 1975 and 1985, and from 1985 to 1995, there was an increase of 35 per cent, from 1995 to 2005, the increase was 5 per cent (Figure 108.1). However, the male:female ratio has been stable at around 1.4:1. There is a wide variation of suicide rates within the country. The southern states of Kerala, Karnataka, Andhra Pradesh and Tamil Nadu have a suicide rate of >15, while in the Northern States of Punjab, Uttar Pradesh, Bihar and Jammu and Kashmir, the suicide rate is <3. This variable pattern has been stable for the last twenty years. Higher literacy, a better reporting system, lower external aggression, higher socio-economic status and higher expectations are possible explanations for the higher suicide rates in the southern states.

The majority of suicides (37.8 per cent) in India are committed by those below the age of 30 years. The fact that 71 per cent of suicides in India (Ministry of Health Affairs 2005) are by persons below the age of 44 years imposes a huge social, emotional and economic burden on the society. Suicide rates are nearly equal among young men and women (Mayer and Ziaian 2002), with a consistently narrow male to female ratio at 1.4:1.

Statistics show that more Indian women die by suicide than their Western counterparts. Poisoning (36.6 per cent), hanging

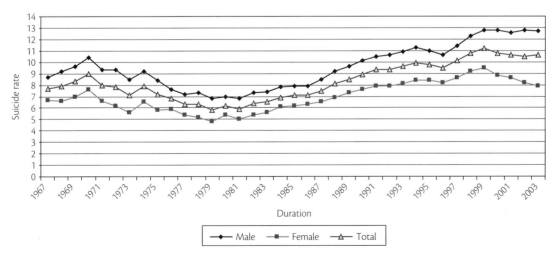

**Fig. 108.1** The suicide rate in India 1967–2003.

(32.1 per cent) and self-immolation (7.9 per cent) were the most common methods used to commit suicide (Ministry of Home Affairs 2005). However, two large epidemiological verbal autopsy studies, in rural Tamil Nadu, revealed that the annual suicide rate is six to nine times higher than the official rate (Joseph *et al.* 2003; Gajalakshmi and Peto 2007). If these figures are extrapolated, it suggests that there are at least half a million suicides in India every year. It is estimated that 1 in 60 persons are affected by suicide. It includes both those who have attempted suicide and those who have been affected by the suicide of a close family or friend. Thus, suicide is a major public and mental health problem, which demands urgent action.

Divorce, dowry, love affairs, cancellation or the inability to get married (according to the system of arranged marriages in India), illegitimate pregnancy, extra-marital affairs and other conflicts relating to the issue of marriage play a particularly crucial role in the suicide of women in India. A distressing feature is the frequent occurrence of suicide pacts and family suicides, which are mostly due to social reasons, and can be viewed as a protest against archaic societal norms and expectations. In a population-based study on domestic violence, it was found that 64 per cent of cases had a significant correlation between domestic violence of women and suicidal ideation (World Health Organization 2001). Domestic violence was also found to be a major risk factor for suicide in a study conducted in Bangalore (Gururaj *et al.* 2004). Poverty, unemployment, debts and educational problems are also associated with suicide. The recent spate of farmer suicides in India has raised societal and governmental concerns to address this growing tragedy.

Mental disorders occupy a premier position in the matrix of causation of suicide. Studies show that around 90 per cent of those who die by suicide have a mental disorder (Vijayakumar *et al.* 2005a). Two case–control studies, using the psychological autopsy technique, have been conducted in Chennai and Bangalore, in India (Vijayakumar and Rajkumar 1999; Gururaj *et al.* 2004), and among those who died by suicide, 88 per cent in Chennai and 43 per cent in Bangalore had a diagnosable mental disorder.

## Legal aspects of suicidal behaviour in India

In India, attempted suicide is a punishable offence. Section 309 of the Indian Penal Code states that 'whoever attempts to commit suicide and does any act towards the commission of such an offense shall be punished with simple imprisonment for a term which may extend to one year or with a fine or with both'.

However, the aim of the law to prevent suicide by legal methods has proved to be counterproductive. Emergency care to those who have attempted suicide is denied, as many hospitals and practitioners hesitate to provide the needed treatment, for fear of legal difficulties. The actual data on attempted suicides becomes difficult to ascertain as many attempts are described as accidental to avoid entanglement with the police and courts.

## Social and public health approaches for suicide prevention

India grapples with infectious diseases, malnutrition, infant and maternal mortality, and other major health problems; thus,

suicide is accorded as a low priority in the competition for meagre resources. The mental health services are inadequate for the needs of the country. For a population of over a billion, there are only about 3500 psychiatrists. Rapid urbanization, industrialization and emerging family systems are resulting in social upheaval and distress. The diminishing traditional support systems leave people vulnerable to suicidal behaviour. Hence, there is an emerging need for external emotional support. The enormity of the problem, combined with the paucity of mental health services, has led to the emergence of NGOs in the field of suicide prevention.

The primary aim of these NGOs is to provide support to suicidal individuals by befriending them. Often these centres function as an entry point for those needing professional services. Apart from befriending suicidal individuals, the NGOs have also undertaken education of gatekeepers, raising awareness in the public and media, as well as implementing some intervention programmes. However, there are certain limitations in the activities of the NGOs. There is a wide variability in the expertise of volunteers and in the services they provide. Quality-control measures are inadequate, and the majority of their endeavours are not evaluated (Vijayakumar and Armson 2005).

A social and public health response to suicide is crucial in India, and should complement a mental health response. Mental illness is a risk factor for suicide in India, just as it is in developed countries. However, additional risk factors are prominent in India. These tend to relate to societal structures and specific stressors. A social and public health approach acknowledges that suicide is preventable, and promotes a framework in an integrated system of interventions across multiple levels within society, which includes the individual, the family, the community, and the health-care system. A key step in such an approach involves modifying attitudes toward suicide, via educational efforts and, in some cases, legal levers (e.g. decriminalizing suicide) (Vijayajumar *et al.* 2005b).

The World Health Organization's suicide prevention multi-site intervention study on suicidal behaviour (SUPRE-MISS) was initiated in seven culturally different sites, in order to evaluate the effectiveness of brief interventions, and contacts for those who have attempted suicide and seen in the emergency care setting. The results from the Chennai, India site revealed that attempted suicide and completed suicide were significantly lower in the intervention group, signifying that low cost community interventions are effective in preventing suicidal behaviour (Fleischmann *et al.* 2008).

SNEHA (meaning 'friendship'), a premier NGO in suicide prevention, initiated a study to assess the usefulness of trained volunteer delivered befriending sessions for those bereaved by the Asian tsunami in 2004. A non-randomized control design, involving all adults aged 18 years and over who have lost at least one close family member during tsunami from two coastal areas in Chennai, was recruited. After baseline assessments, participants in the intervention site received monthly befriending support by volunteers. One year after the baseline assessment, all participants in the intervention and control group were interviewed. The results revealed that participants receiving consistent befriending intervention from trained volunteers were less likely to report depressive symptoms and general psychological disorders. Further suicide attempts were lower in the intervention group (Vijayakumar and Suresh Kumar 2008).

# Conclusion

Suicide prevention efforts are at a nascent stage of development in India. Active lobbying by NGOs has resulted in the inclusion of suicide prevention in the re-drafted national mental health policy. However, there is an urgent need to develop a national plan for suicide prevention in India. Suicide prevention initiatives in India should bring together traditional knowledge and modern science to develop acceptable, cost-effective and appropriate strategies, but above all, decriminalizing attempted suicide is an urgent need if any suicide prevention strategy is to succeed in the prevailing system.

# References

Fleischmann A, Bertolote JM, Wasserman D *et al.* (2008). Effectiveness of brief intervention and contact for suicide attempters: a randomized controlled trial in five countries. *Bulletin of the World Health Organization.* Accessed at http://www.who.int/bulletin/volumes/86/07–046995.pdf.

Gajalakshmi V and Peto R (2007). Suicide rates in Tamil Nadu, South India: verbal autopsy of 39,000 deaths in 1997–98. *International Journal of Epidemiology,* dol:10.1093/ije/dy11308.

Gururaj G, Isaac M, Subhakrishna DK *et al.* (2004). Risk factors for completed suicides: a case–control study from Bangalore, India. *Injury Control and Safety Promotion,* **11**, 183–191.

Joseph A, Abraham S, Mulliyil JP *et al.* (2003). Evaluaton of suicide rates in rural India using verbal autopsies, 1994–9. *British Medical Journal,* **326**, 1121–1122.

Mayer P and Ziaian T (2002). Suicide gender and age variations in India. Are women in Indian society protected from suicide? *Crisis,* **23**, 98–103.

Ministry of Home Affairs (2005). *Accidental Deaths and Suicides in India.* National Crime Research Bureau, Government of India.

Vijayakumar L and Armson S (2005). Volunteer perspective on suicides. In K Hawton, ed., *Prevention and Treatment of Suicidal Behaviour,* pp. 335–350. Oxford University Press, Oxford.

Vijayakumar L and Rajkumar S (1999). Are risk factors for suicide universal? A case–control study in India. *Acta Psychiatrica Scandinavica,* 99, 407–411.

Vijayakumar L and Suresh Kumar M (2008). Trained volunteer-delivered mental health support to those bereaved by the Asian tsunami: an evaluation. *International Journal of Social Psychiatry,* **54**, 293–302.

Vijayakumar L, John S, Pirkis J *et al.* (2005a). Suicide in developing countries (2): Risk factors. *Crisis,* **26**, 112–119.

Vijayakumar L, Pirkis J, Whiteford H (2005b). Suicide in developing countries (3): Prevention efforts. *Crisis,* **26**, 120–124.

World Health Organization (2001). *World Health Report. Mental Health. New Understanding, New Hope.* World Health Organization, Geneva.

# CHAPTER 109

# Suicide prevention in Japan

Chiaki Kawanishi and Yoshihiro Kaneko

## Mortality and suicide

Suicide has been an emerging problem for many years in Japan, especially amongst males of working age, young people and the elderly. A dramatic jump in the year-over-year number of suicides occurred in 1998 (32,863 victims compared to 24,391 in 1997). Since 1998, suicide numbers have exceeded 30,000 every year for ten consecutive years (MHLW 2008). According to the latest suicide rates, 37.7 per 100,000 males and 14.7 per 100,000 females completed suicide in Japan in 2007 (National Police Agency 2008). Seventy per cent of the victims are men and approximately a third are aged 60 years or over. Trigger factors for suicide are health and financial problems. The number of people who attempted or committed suicide in Japan due to work-related stress has doubled since 2003–2004. Due to cultural factors, Japanese men are not supposed to show weakness. The economic conditions of the elderly are worsening as the government restructures its budget and reduces the social security and pension budgets. There are not enough experts and psychiatrists available for consultations with people suicidal crisis.

## Governmental actions to promote suicide prevention

Ministry of Health, Labour and Welfare (MHLW) called a special committee and released a report on national suicide prevention strategies in 2002 (MHLW 2002). The Japanese Multimodal Intervention Trials for Suicide Prevention (J-MISP) were launched to develop effective suicide-prevention methods supported by the MHLW in 2006. J-MISP consists of two projects: a community intervention trial (NOCOMIT-J) and a randomized controlled trial of post-suicide attempt case management (ACTION-J). The Diet approved the Basic Law on Suicide Countermeasures, which came into force in 2006. In 2007, the Cabinet agreed on the National Suicide Prevention Measure Outline, and the Cabinet Office coordinates the implementation. MHLW have supported community intervention projects in twenty selected regions. The time course of developing suicide-prevention measures is shown in Table 109.1

The government has a goal to cut suicides by 20 per cent by 2016. Several prevention measures within public health and health care systems are supported by the government. In 2008, MHLW introduced a new scheme for the payment of treatment fees from the medical insurance system to medical institutions. Remuneration is paid for psychiatric consultation for suicide attempters at emergency departments, and for psychiatric referrals by primary care doctors.

## Suicide legislation in Japan

A new act on suicide prevention and supporting suicide survivors in Japan (Basic Law on Suicide Countermeasures, Law No 85 of 2006) was implemented on 28 October 2006. The intention of this legislation is that both national governmental and local authorities should be responsible for suicide prevention in the whole country. The fundamental concepts of suicide prevention in Japan are:

◆ Suicide should be recognized as an individual and social problem. Provision of some social policy can help this;

◆ Suicide-prevention and crisis management, with post-vention, is an important consideration in policy-making;

◆ Suicide has various and complicated backgrounds, therefore psychiatric and other services are required to prevent and support suicide attempters;

◆ Suicide-prevention activities should consider supporting families of victims and survivors, and in collaboration with the national governmental and local authorities, health care providers, businesses, schools and voluntary organizations.

Two examples of suicide preventive projects are presented below.

## Special focus on children and adolescents in suicide prevention

Suicide has been recognized as a problem for children and adolescents in Japan, and health care measures and promoting health care education for adolescents and children have been prioritized. It is suggested that measures to improve anonymous telephone counselling should be undertaken, along with lectures in schools for children, teachers and parents regarding how to prevent suicide, and to improve recognition of students who have suicidal thoughts or plans as early as possible (MHLW 2008).

Psychological problems are recognized as important associated problems for psychiatric disorders, and the government is stimulating provision of improvements to the systems, providing

**Table 109.1** Suicide prevention in Japan: time course of developing preventive measures

| | |
|---|---|
| 1998 | Suicide dramatically increased (24,391 in 1997→ 32,863 in 1998). The number of suicides has exceeded 30,000 for 10 consecutive years since then. Suicide rate (around 25 per 100 000 inhabitants) has been the worst among developed countries. |
| 2000 | The health initiative Health Japan 21 mentioned suicide prevention. |
| 2001 | The Ministry of Health, Labor, and Welfare (MHLW) prepared a budget for suicide prevention for the first time (support for a crisis help line, Federation of Inochi No Denwa). |
| 2002 | MHLW and the Special Committee on Suicide Prevention released the proposals for national suicide prevention strategies. |
| 2005 | MHLW established the Strategic Research Project; suicide associated with mental illness was targeted together with diabetes. Resolution to request urgent, effective promotion of integrated preventive measures concerning suicide, was carried in the inquiry by the commission of health, labor, and welfare at the House of Councillors. |
| 2006 | Japanese Multimodal Intervention Trials for Suicide Prevention (J-MISP) was launched in order to develop suitable and feasible preventive measure for suicide. J-MISP consists of two projects: (1) a community intervention trial (NOCOMIT-J) and (2) a RCT trial of post-suicide attempt case management (ACTION-J). The Diet approved the Suicide Prevention Law. |
| 2007 | The Cabinet set the National Suicide Prevention Measure Outline. MHLW have supported community intervention projects in selected 20 regions. A National Suicide Prevention Centre was established. |
| 2008 | MHLW and The special committee on suicide attempters' and survivors' care released the guideline 'Preparation guide' to encourage subsets of society to create active guidelines. MHLW set a new scheme of treatment fees paid to medical institutions under the medical insurance system. Remuneration is paid for psychiatric consultation for suicide attempters at emergency departments, and psychiatric referrals by primary care physicians. MHLW proposed and support the educational programme for primary care physicians on diagnosis and treatment of depression. |

psychiatric treatment for children and young people. This psychiatric treatment should be supported with a combination of different psychological and psychosocial treatments to strengthen suicide-preventative effects (Wasserman 2001).

The need to prevent suicide contagion and to protect children's mental states has led to a request to the media to take measures against publishing harmful information in an irresponsible way, although no specific guidelines are issued.

Some concrete suggestions for measures to prevent mental ill-health and suicide have been discussed by responsible authorities:

◆ Lowering of medical fees to facilitate health-seeking behaviours;

◆ Training child and adolescent psychiatrists and other professions working with mental health problems of children and adolescents in modern diagnostics and treatment;

◆ Appointing child psychiatrists at child guidance centres;

◆ Creating residential treatment centres for emotionally disturbed children;

◆ Giving open lectures for medical and affiliated staff at universities on topics to promote mental health and prevent suicide;

◆ Integrating knowledge about suicide prevention into school education.

## A decrease in suicide rates in a Japanese rural area after community-based intervention by the health promotion approach

A community-based suicide prevention programme was undertaken in the Akita Prefecture of Japan (Motohashi *et al.* 2007)

following a systematic review of recent strategies to prevent suicide (Mann *et al.* 2005). A health promotion approach was utilized including raising awareness and emphasizing empowerment of residents and civic participation. Welfare and community network measures were also taken. There was a significant drop in suicide rates in the area, from 70.8 per 100,000 inhabitants (1999) before the intervention to 34.1 per 100,000 after the intervention (2004). The study showed that empowering residents and increasing civic participation reduced the suicide rate in this rural area of Japan.

### References

Mann J J, Apter A, Bertolote J *et al.* (2005). Suicide prevention strategies: a systematic review. *Journal of the American Medical Association*, **294**, 2064–2074

MHLW (Ministry of Health, Labour and Welfare) (2002). *Japanese Multimodal Intervention Trials for Suicide Prevention*. http://www.jfnm.or.jp/itaku/J-MISP/index.html, last accessed 23 June 2008.

MHLW (Ministry of Health, Labour and Welfare) (2008). *Abridged Life Table for Japan 2006*. http://www.mhlw.go.jp, last accessed 23 June 2008.

Motohashi Y, Kaneko Y, Sasaki H *et al.* (2007). A decrease in suicide rates in Japanese rural towns after community-based intervention by the health promotion approach. *Suicide and Life-Threatening Behavior*, **37**, 593–599.

National Campaign for Maternal and Child Health until 2010 (2000). A *Report from the Sukoyaka Family 21 Planning Committee, Japan*. http://www.mhlw.go.jp/english/wp/other/councils/sukoyaka21/2.html, last accessed 23 June 2008.

National Police Agency (2008). *A Survey of Suicide During the Year 2007 in Japan*. http://www.npa.go.jp/toukei/chiiki10/h19-zisatsu.pdf in Japanese.

Wasserman D (2001). *Suicide: An Unnecessary Death*. Japanese translation and publishing Tuttle-Mori Agency, Inc., Tokyo.

# CHAPTER 110

# Suicide prevention in Pakistan

## Murad M Khan

Pakistan is a developing country located in South Asia, with a population of approximately 162 million, 97 per cent of which are Muslims. Suicide is a condemned act in Islam. Historically, suicide was rare, but over the last decade or so has become a major public health problem in Pakistan (Khan and Prince 2003).

Despite this, there are no official statistics from Pakistan. National rates are neither known nor reported to the World Health Organization (WHO) (World Health Organization 2001).

Under Pakistani law (based on the tenets of Islam), both suicide and deliberate self-harm (DSH) are illegal acts, which are punishable with a term in jail and a financial penalty. People avoid going to government hospitals, where suicidal acts are registered. Many seek treatment from private hospitals that neither diagnose suicide nor report them to police. Suicide and DSH are, therefore, under-reported in Pakistan (Khan and Reza 1998).

## Sources of information

Information on suicide in Pakistan comes from newspapers, non-governmental organizations (NGOs), volunteer and human rights organizations, and police departments of various cities (Khan and Prince 2003). Further information is available from hospital-based studies on acute intentional poisoning (Waseem *et al.* 2004), DSH (Kermani *et al.* 2006) and autopsies carried out by forensic medicine departments (Sultana 2002; Bashir *et al.* 2003).

## Where does suicide occur in Pakistan?

Suicide cuts across all ethnic, provincial and rural/urban boundaries. It has been reported from all major cities, including Karachi (Sultana 2002; Ahmed *et al.* 2003; Farooqi *et al.* 2004), Larkana (Aziz *et al.* 2006), Lahore (Aziz and Awan 1999), Multan (Ahmed *et al.* 2002), Bahawalpur (Suliman *et al.* 2006), Faisalabad (Saeed *et al.*2002), Rawalpindi (Khattak 2006) and Peshawar (Bashir *et al.* 2003). Suicide has been reported from the remote Ghizer District, in the northern areas of Pakistan (Ahmad and Khan 2005).

## Suicide rates in some cities of Pakistan

While official rates of suicide are lacking, it is possible to calculate rates in some cities and districts of Pakistan.

Crude rates vary from a low of 0.43/100,000 per year (average for 1991–2000) in Peshawar, to a high of 2.86/100,000 for Rawalpindi (in 2006), with other cities falling in between: Karachi, 2.1/100,000 (1995–2001); Lahore, 1.08/100,000 (1993–95); Faisalabad, 1.12/100,000 (1998–2001) and Larkana, 2.6/100,000 (2003–2004).

## Gender and age differences

Gender differences show that in all studies men outnumber women. Gender-specific rates show that for men, highest rates are 5.2/100,000 in Rawalpindi and Haripur, while for women the highest rates are 16.7/100,000 in the Ghizer District, located in northern areas of Pakistan.

In Pakistan, most suicides are committed by young people. The highest age- and gender-specific rates for both genders in the age group 20–40 years are: 7.03/100,000 in Larkana for men; and for women, 32/100,000 in the Ghizer District, northern Pakistan.

## Methods used

A review of seven studies, which list methods used in suicide (N = 5394), showed that poisoning (34 per cent) and hanging (26 per cent) to be the two most common methods, followed by firearms (16 per cent), drowning (11 per cent), self-immolation (5 per cent) and jumping from height or in front of trains or moving vehicles (1 per cent each) (Aziz and Awan 1999; Khalid 2001; Saeed *et al.* 2002; Ahmed *et al.* 2003; Bashir *et al.* 2003; Aziz *et al.* 2006; Khan and Hyder 2006). Use of medications for suicide featured in only four cases (one male and three female).

## Suicide prevention in Pakistan

A multisectoral approach is needed to address suicide prevention in Pakistan

1   *Community mental health programmes.* Almost 34 per cent of the Pakistani population suffer from common mental disorders (Mirza and Jenkins, 2004). Ideally, mental health and suicide prevention programmes should be integrated within the primary health care (PHC) system. In Pakistan, publicly funded PHC system is largely ineffective. Hence, training PHC staff to screen for suicidal patients would be impractical. Instead, low-cost community mental health programmes, using mental

**Table 110.1** Crude and gender-specific suicide rates in eight cities/districts of Pakistan

| City/Province | Years | Population[1] | No of suicides | Crude rates/ 100,000/annum | Rates men/ 100,000 | Rates women/ 100,000 | Ratio men:women |
|---|---|---|---|---|---|---|---|
| Faisalabad, Punjab | 1998–2001 | 2.11 M = 11.02 W = 10.17 | 95 M = 67 W = 28 | 1.12 | 1.51 | 0.68 | 2.3:1 |
| Lahore, Punjab | 1994–1995 | 4.54 M = 2.36 W = 2.17 | 100 M = 65 W = 35 | 1.08 | 1.3 | 0.79 | 1.8:1 |
| Karachi, Sindh | 1995–2001 | 9.3 M = 4.86 W = 4.49 | 1379 M = 863 W = 516 | 2.12 | 2.49 | 1.70 | 1.6:1 |
| Larkana, Sindh | 2003–2004 | 1.0 M = 0.52 W = 0.48 | 52 M = 35 W = 17 | 2.6 | 3.3 | 1.7 | 2:1 |
| Peshawar, NWFP[2] | 1991–2000 | 0.90 M = 0.47 W = 0.43 | 39 M = 29 W = 10 | 0.43 | 0.61 | 0.23 | 2.9:1 |
| Rawalpindi, Punjab | 2006 | 1.81 M = 0.94 W = 0.87 | 52 M = 49 W = 3 | 2.86 | 5.2 | 0.34 | 16:1 |
| Haripur, NWFP[2] | 2005 | 0.80 M = 0.34 W = 0.36 | 25 M = 18 W = 7 | 3.11 | 5.2 | 1.91 | 2.5:1 |
| Ghizer District, Northern Areas | 2000–2004 | 0.13 M = 0.07 W = 0.06 | 55 M = NA W = 55 | NA | NA | 16.7 | NA |

NA, not available; M, men; W, women.

[1] Mid-year average population for study years, in millions.

[2] North-West Frontier Province.

health care workers and lay counsellors, should be considered. Suicide prevention as part of the programme would be more meaningful.

2 *Psychological management of deliberate self-harm.* The WHO estimates there are 10–20 DSH acts for every suicide. In Pakistan, there would be in excess of 100,000 DSH acts annually. Most DSH acts are committed by young married women and young single men, using organophosphate insecticides (Khan 1998). The underlying psychological issues in DSH cases are rarely addressed. Every DSH subject, no matter how apparently innocuous the act, should receive a psychiatric assessment. Training emergency room personnel can contribute significantly to suicide prevention

3 *The legal status of suicide and attempted suicide.* The criminalization of DSH and suicide has lead to a stigma effect, avoidance of health-seeking help, and lack of involvement of professionals and limitations in programmes for suicide prevention. There is an urgent need to review and repeal the law regarding DSH and suicide in Pakistan.

4 *Restricting the availability of methods.* In Pakistan, the three most common methods are hanging, ingestion of insecticides

and firearms. While hanging is difficult to control, restricting availability of the latter two can potentially prevent 50 per cent of suicides in Pakistan. Public education campaigns to promote safe storage of insecticides and firearms are needed.

5 *Crisis intervention/suicide hotlines.* Crisis intervention centres, and suicide-prevention telephone hotlines, play an important role in helping suicidal people. There is an urgent need to establish such services in Pakistan.

6 *School-based programmes.* The majority of suicides in Pakistan are in younger age groups; and a school-based intervention, as recommended by the WHO's suicide-prevention strategies, should be initiated. This includes crisis management, self-esteem enhancement, social skills training and healthy decision-making.

7 *Social policies.* Most suicide victims belong to lower socio-economic strata of society, where poverty, unemployment and adverse social circumstances are high. The government needs to implement social policies that are equitable and fair, and address the problems of the common man. There is a need for increased spending on mental health, as well as proper utilization of available resources.

**8** *The need for more research.* Mortality statistics on suicides should be collected through a standard system of registration, recording and diagnosis of suicides, at all town/city, district and provincial levels. Information obtained can be used for epidemiological–analytical, intra-country and cross-national studies.

## Conclusion

The traditional low suicide rate, and the protective influence of Islam, has undergone a radical change, and suicide has become a major public health problem in Pakistan. Lack of resources, poorly established primary and mental health services, and weak political processes make suicide prevention a formidable challenge in Pakistan. Public and mental health professionals need to work with government and non-governmental organizations to take up this challenge.

## References

Ahmad A and Khan SR (2005). *Assessment of Root Causes of Suicide Cases among Women in Ghizer District of Northern Areas of Pakistan (during 2000–2004)*. Department for International Development, British Council, Islamabad.

Ahmed R, Ahad K, Iqbal R *et al.* (2002). Acute poisoning due to commercial pesticides in Multan. *Pakistan Journal of Medical Sciences*, **18**, 227–231.

Ahmed Z, Ahmed A, Mubeen SM (2003). An audit of suicide in Karachi from 1995–2001. *Annals of Abbasi Shaheed Hospital*, **8**, 424–428.

Aziz K and Awan NR (1999). Pattern of suicide and its relationship to socio-economic factors/depressive illness in the city of Lahore. *Pakistan Journal of Medical Sciences*, **15**, 289–294.

Aziz K, Afridi HK, Khichi ZH (2006). Psychological autopsy study of suicide pattern and its relationship to depressive illness. *Annals of King Edward Medical College*, **12**, 121–123.

Bashir MZ, Hussain Z, Saeed A *et al.* (2003). Suicidal deaths; assessment in Peshawar. *The Professional*, **10**, 137–141.

Farooqi AN, Tariq S, Asad F *et al.* (2004). Epidemiological profile of suicidal poisoning at Abbasi Shaheed Hospital. *Annals of Abbasi Shaheed Hospital*, **9**, 502–505.

Kermani F, Ather AA, Ara J (2006). Deliberate self-harm: frequency and associated factors. *Journal of Surgery Pakistan*, **11**, 34–36.

Khalid N (2001). Pattern of suicide: causes and methods employed. *Journal of the College of Physicians and Surgeons Pakistan*, **11**, 759–761.

Khan MM (1998). Suicide and attempted suicide in Pakistan. *Crisis*, **19**, 172–176.

Khan MM and Hyder AA (2006). Suicides in the developing world: case study from Pakistan. *Suicide and Life- Threatening Behavior*, **36**, 76–81.

Khan MM and Prince M (2003). Beyond rates: the tragedy of suicide in Pakistan. *Tropical Doctor*, **33**, 67–69.

Khan MM and Reza H (1998). Benzodiazepine self-poisoning in Pakistan: implications for prevention and harm reduction. *Journal of the Pakistan Medical Association*, **48**, 293–295.

Khattak I (2006). Poverty drove 52 to suicide last year. *The Dawn Newspaper*, p. 2 January 17.

Mirza I and Jenkins R (2004). Risk factors, prevalence, and treatment of anxiety and depressive disorders in Pakistan: systematic review. *BMJ*, **328**, 794.

Saeed A, Bashir MZ, Khan D *et al.* (2002). Epidemiology of suicide in Faisalabad. *Journal of Ayub Medical College Abbottabad*, **14**, 34–37.

Suliman MI, Jibran R, Rai M (2006). The analysis of organophosphates poisoning cases treated at Bahawal Victoria Hospital, Bahawalpur in 2000–2003. *Pakistan Journal of Medical Sciences*, **22**, 244–249.

Sultana K (2002). Proportion of suicidal deaths among autopsy. *Annals of Abbasi Shaheed Hospital*, **7**, 317–318.

Waseem T, Nadeem MA, Irfan K *et al.* (2004) Poisonings in patients of medical coma and their outcome at Mayo Hospital, Lahore. *Annals of King Edward Medical Colegel*, **10**, 384–386.

World Health Organization (2001). *The World Health Report 2001. Mental Health: New Understanding, New Hope*. World Health Organization, Geneva.

# CHAPTER 111

# Suicide prevention in Singapore

Chia Boon Hock

## Introduction

Singapore is a small island nation (pop: 3.3 million), which is centrally located in South East Asia. The resident population comprises a mixture of cultures including Chinese (77 per cent), Malay (14 per cent) and Indian (8 per cent). Over the last decades, suicide rates in Singapore have fluctuated between 8–10/100,000 populations per year (Chia and Chia 2008). Between 2000 and 2004, suicide accounted for 2.2 per cent of all deaths. These rates were highest in those aged >65 years (29.9/100,000); amongst ethnic Chinese (13.5/100,000), followed by ethnic Indians (13.2/100,000) and ethnic Malays (2.8/100,000). The male:female ratio of completed suicide was 1.5:1. The most common mode of suicide was by jumping from high-rise buildings, with 23 per cent having attempted suicide before. In 55 per cent of the cases, the victims had provided warnings that they were contemplating suicide.

## Risk factors

Risk factors for suicide in Singapore vary with age, relationships, education and stress, which is most prevalent among the younger age groups (<25 years); marital, financial problems and mental disorders peak in the middle age group (25–59 years); and physical illness is most common among the elderly (>60 years)(Chia et al. 2008). Overall, clinical depression and schizophrenia were associated with 34 and 14.5 per cent of all suicides, respectively. About 76.5 per cent of schizophrenic suicides had been recently discharged from a mental hospital. Other groups, with high risk for suicide, include those who are unemployed, and those with drug addiction and gambling problems (Chia and Chia 2008).

## Suicide prevention

Singapore has a well-developed medical and mental health care system, with a doctor:population and psychiatrist:population ratio of 1:500 and 1:32,000, respectively. It also has a small, but dedicated core of psychotherapists, counsellors and social workers. Although there is no formal national strategy for suicide prevention, there are a number of non-governmental organizations which provide assistance or support to groups known to be at high risk. These organizations, such as the Samaritan of Singapore (SOS),

Singapore Action Group for the Elderly (SAGE), Singapore Anti-narcotic Association, Alcoholics Anonymous and Gambling Anonymous, provide 24-hour counselling hotlines and specialized intervention programmes. The SOS organization, for example, organizes emergency support squads and counselling support. Together with other mental health-care professions, they help organize an annual suicide week, during which conferences and forums are held to raise awareness of suicide risk and behaviour in the community. In early 2005, the LOSS (Local Outreach to Suicide Survivors) programme was launched island-wide, with the active support of the Singapore Police and the Coroner's Court. When an incident of suspected suicide occurs, the police contact the SOS organization, who then dispatches a team to attend to the survivor (acknowledging the increased risk of suicide in survivors). Initial contact may occur at the scene of the incident, their residence, the mortuary or the funeral wake (Samaritans of Singapore 2008).

On the governmental level, initiatives have mostly been targeted at addressing general social problems within different age groups. In the young age groups, the problem of educational stress and relationship issues are addressed by encouraging schools to place less emphasis on academic results, developing more holistic approaches to education, introducing trained counsellors into schools, and training teachers to better identify students with emotional and social problems. Specific programmes have been developed to help unemployed adults to find jobs, undergo retraining, and to help them manage their finances. There are also governmental agencies that provide counselling for those undergoing marital, family or relationship difficulties.

There are also many publicized programmes, which are targeted at improving geriatric medical care, increasing discussion about how to better provide financial and physical support for the elderly, and improving awareness of psychological needs of the elderly. Although these programmes do not target suicide directly, they may help indirectly by decreasing the risk generally.

Raising awareness of mental illness, such as depression and schizophrenia, and their association with suicide, has taken many forms. The push has been spearheaded by the Institute of Mental Health (IMH), which is the primary mental health hospital in Singapore. For example, a recent study by IMH found that the rates of depression, anxiety disorder and dementia in Singapore are on a par with other developed countries (Chua et al. 2004a, b). They found that in their lifetime, an adult Singaporean has a 5.6 per cent chance of developing depression. This, in part, provides real evidence and helps raise awareness of the issue.

Governmental agencies, such as the Ministry of Health and the Health Promotion Board, have been coordinating the publicity regarding depression, schizophrenia and other mental illness. On the public front, they have distributed pamphlets, arranged public lectures/forums, organized hotline and e-mail services, TV advertisements and documentaries to educate the general public, and to encourage people to seek help and treatment, and to de-stigmatize mental illness. On the medical front, as an ongoing educational exercise, booklets on how to identify and treat mental illnesses are regularly distributed to all practising medical practitioners in Singapore.

## Conclusion

Overall, since the 1950s, the suicide rate among young adolescents (10–19) and young adults (20–29) in Singapore has remained relatively constant at 3 and 9 per 100,000 populations per year, respectively, while in the older adults (40–59) and the elderly (60±), suicide rates have fallen from 25 to 10 and 50 to 23 per 100,000 populations per annum, respectively. However, there is still much that needs to be done. Many suicide victims have had recent admission to mental and general hospitals, suggesting that improvements can be made

in mental health-care and post-discharge follow-up treatment (Thong *et al.* 2008). Almost 95 per cent of all Singaporeans live in high-rise buildings, and 72 per cent of all suicides are by jumping. Better design of these buildings, with higher barriers or break-fall devices, may help minimize the impulsive suicides. Finally, judicious use of the media in order to help educate the public about suicide (i.e. the risk factors, identifying signs and the help available, without sensationalizing the act or providing details about methods) may help minimize suicide and copy-cat incidents.

## References

Chia BH and Chia A (2008). Singapore. In Yip PSF, ed., *Suicide in Asia – causes and prevention*, Hong Kong University, Hong Kong.

Chia BH, Chia A, Tai BC (2008). Suicide letters in Singapore. *Archives of Suicide Research*, **12**, 74–81.

Samaritans of Singapore (2008). *Annual Report 2007/2008*. Samaritans of Singapore, Singapore.

Chua HC, Lim L, Ng TP, *et al.* (2004a). The prevalence of psychiatric disorders in Singapore adults. *Annals Academy of Medicine*, **33**, 102.

Chua HC, Ng TP, Mahendran R, Lee T (2004b). Risk factors for depressive disorders in Singapore adults. *Annals Academy of Medicine*, **33**, 102.

Thong JY, Su AHC, Chan YH, *et al.* (2008). Suicide in psychiatric patients: case-controlled study in Singapore, *Australian and New Zealand Journal of Psychiatry*, **42**, 509–519.

# CHAPTER 112

# Suicide prevention in Vietnam

Huong Tran Thi Thanh and
Duc Pham Thi Minh

## Suicidal behaviours in Vietnamese culture

Although the highest suicide rates are currently found in Eastern Europe, the largest number of suicides take place in Asia (Bertolote 2001). Unfortunately, in Vietnam, as in many other Asian countries, national strategies for suicide prevention have not yet been developed. Suicide was among the ten leading causes of death in Vietnam during 2002, and according to the Ministry of Health, the estimated suicide rate (based on hospital records of mortality is 0.98/100,000 (Ministry of Health in Vietnam 2002). The real suicide rate in Vietnam is still unknown, because the number of deaths reported by the Ministry of Health is based only on hospital data. However, most suicides occur outside the hospital system. There is no national system to monitor causes of death, including suicide, in Vietnam.

In 2000, the WHO multi-site intervention study along on suicidal behaviours (SUPRE-MISS) was launched in Vietnam, in collaboration with Hanoi Medical University and the National Swedish Prevention of Suicide and Mental Ill-Health (NASP) at Karolinska Institute, Sweden, and with WHO support. The study focused on revealing risk factors and characteristics of suicidal behaviour. The aim of the study was to find similarities and dissimilarities between suicidal behaviours in Vietnam and Western countries. Similarities can support the use of suicide preventive strategies in Vietnam that were successful in the West. However, given the dissimilarities between cultures, the Vietnamese culture requires more specific preventive approaches. Most Vietnamese people are strongly influenced by Buddhist practices, even if they do not openly admit that they are Buddhists (Nyguyen 1987). This cultural and religious tradition in Vietnam may explain the low level of suicidal thoughts and suicide attempts in comparison with other countries (Bertolote et al. 2005; Thanh et al. 2005; Thanh et al. 2006). However, in one study of self-evaluation of the seriousness of suicide attempts, it was found that in Vietnam, more people reported suicide attempts as being serious compared to the general population of other countries (Fleischmann et al. 2005).

In Vietnam, according to the results from the WHO SUPRE-MISS study, the ratio of suicidal thoughts:to suicide plans:to suicide attempts on a lifetime basis was calculated to be 22.3:2.8:1. The prevalence of suicidal thoughts was similar to other countries (Bertolote et al. 2005; Thanh et al. 2006), with only a small number of people who actually progressed from suicidal thoughts to suicidal plans. The gap between suicide plans and suicide attempts was quite small.

Suicide attempts are highest among the 15–24 age group. Suicide attempters in Vietnam seem to be younger than in other European studies (Schmidtke et al. 2004). There are no strong legal or religious prohibitions against self-destructive behaviour inVietnamese culture. In a cultural environment of this kind,family or other types of conflict (a well-known psychosocial stressor) can result in impulsive suicide attempts, especially among young persons, without any underlying psychiatric illness being present, when firm support from their various networks is simultaneously lacking (Wasserman et al. 2008).

Suicide attempts are more often seen among females, especially in rural areas. Some theories suggest that this occurs because of the low status of rural females in many developing countries, and females are often subjected to domestic violence due to family conflicts (World Health Organization 2002). This may also be valid for young suicide attempters in rural Vietnam. It seems that suicidal acts in Vietnam are often due to severe stress from acute life events, such as family or other conflicts.

Attempted suicide in urban areas are performed by means of analgesics and antipyretics, e.g. paracetamol and rotunda, a traditional medicine with an action similar to paracetamol (X60), and with tranquillizers (X61), which closely resemble Western patterns of suicide-attempt methods (Schmidtke et al. 2004), while pesticide and raticides are means of suicide attempts in rural areas. The existence of potent pesticides, which are in most people's homes, makes pesticides easily available and often cheaper than medications used for intoxications, which are used as a method of suicide and attempted suicide in Vietnamese urban areas.

There were no attempted suicides with firearms in Vietnam, since firearms are not accessible to the general population. Firearm possession is prohibited, except for military personnel and policemen.

Alcohol dependence and addiction, which are commonly found in Western studies among both males and females who attempt or commit suicide (Wasserman and Varnik 1998), are very rare in Vietnam (Fleischmann et al. 2005; Thanh et al. 2005). This probably mirrors cultural patterns, as attempting to escape conflicts and stressful situations by resorting to alcohol is less common in Vietnam than in the West.

Suicide attempters in Vietnam have a low prevalence of psychiatric disorders. Perhaps this differs from Western countries, because of help-seeking behaviour, stigma of mental disorders, and the reluctance to give a mental disorder diagnosis to young people by health professionals.

## Plan for the cultural specific prevention of suicide in Vietnam

Using some of the characteristics mentioned above, a plan for the prevention of suicide could be designed as follows:

- Surveillance and registration of suicide and other causes of death should be developed;

- Improving family roles in caring from family members;

- Improving communication between parents and children, and other family members;

- Developing training programmes on suicide prevention for teachers and students within the school system, which can be based on guidelines from the WHO (World Health Organization 2000; Wasserman and Narboni 2001);

- Enhancing the activity of community organizations (e.g. Women's Union and Youth Federation) in improving social life among its members;

- Involving pagodas and churches through religious talks in these venues;

- Establishing a counselling networks (e.g. hotline counselling);

- Making the health sector more active in suicide prevention, and stimulate the recording and follow-up of persons with suicide risk;

- Organizing suicide-preventive networks;

- Reducing accessibility to pesticides.

## References

Bertolole J (2001). Suicide in the world: an epidemiological overview, 1959–2000. In D Wasserman, ed., *Suicide: An Unnecessary Death*, pp. 3–10. Martin Dunitz, London.

Bertolote J, Fleischmann A, De Leo D *et al.* (2005). Suicide attempts, plans and ideation in culturally diverse sites: the WHO SUPRE-MISS community survey. *Psychological Medicine*, **35**, 1457–1465.

Fleischmann A, Bertolote J, De Leo D *et al.* (2005). Characteristics of attempted suicides seen in emergency care settings of general hospitals in eight low-and middle income countries. *Psychological Medicine*, **35**, 1467–1474.

Ministry of Health in Vietnam (2002). *Health Statistics Yearbook*. Ministry of Health, Vietnam.

Nguyen Khac Vien (1987). *Vietnam, A Long History*. The Gioi (The World), Hanoi.

Schmidtke A, Bille-Brahe U, De Leo D *et al.* (eds) (2004). *Suicidal Behaviour in Europe*. Hogrefe & Huber, Gottingen, Germany.

Thanh HT, Jiang GX, Van TN *et al.* (2005). Attempted suicide in Hanoi, Vietnam. *Soc Psychiatry Psychiatr Epidemiol*, **40**, 64–71.

Thanh HT, Tran NT, Jiang GX *et al.* (2006). Life time suicidal thoughts in an urban community in Hanoi, Vietnam. *BMC Public Health*, **6**, 76.

Wasserman D and Narboni V (2001). *Guideline for Suicide Prevention in Schools*. National Centre for Suicide Research and Prevention of Mental Ill-Health, Stockholm.

Wasserman D and Varnik A (1998). Suicide-preventive effects of perestroika in the former USSR: the role of alcohol restriction. *Acta Psychiatrica Scandinavica Supplementum*, **394**, 1–4.

Wasserman D, Tran Thi Thanh H, Pham Thi Minh D *et al.* (2008). Suicidal process, suicidal communication and psychosocial situation of young suicide attempters in a rural Vietnamese community. *World Psychiatry*, **7**, 47–53.

World Health Organization (2000). *Preventing Suicide: A Resource for Teachers and Other School Staff*. Department of Mental Health, World Health Organization, Geneva.

World Health Organization (2002). *World Report on Violence and Health*. World Health Organization, Geneva.

# Examples of How to Develop Suicide Prevention on all the Continents: Australia and New Zealand

# CHAPTER 113

# Suicide prevention in Australia

Diego De Leo and Karolina Krysinska

## Introduction

### Suicidality in Australia

Australia is among countries with a medium rate of suicide: 10.3 per 100,000, with the male:female suicide ratio of approximately 4 to 1, and suicide rates 16.4 per 100,000 and 4.3 per 100,000, respectively (ABS 2007). Young males in the age group of 25–34 are at the highest risk 25.1 per 100,000 (ABS 2007). Similarly to other countries with an Anglo-Saxon sociocultural background (De Leo 1999), the rates for males decrease with advancing age only to rise again among elderly males over the age of 75, to 21.6 per 100,000 (ABS 2007).

## Life framework and the future

Australia was one of the first countries to introduce a national strategy for the prevention of suicide. The initial programme, the National Youth Suicide Prevention Strategy, was implemented from 1995–1999, and was followed by the National Suicide Prevention Strategy which targeted all age groups. The strategy was based upon the Living is For Everyone (LIFE) Framework, which provided the overall structure and conceptual guidance for national and local initiatives and programmes (Commonwealth Department of Health and Aged Care 2000). The framework's aims were to prevent suicide and to promote resilience and mental health in the Australian population across all age groups, with a special focus on the youth and young adults. Specifically, six action areas were identified within the LIFE Framework:

1 Promoting resilience, well-being and community capacity;

2 Reducing risk factors and enhancing protective factors for suicide and self-harm;

3 Developing community services and support for high-risk groups;

4 Developing services for high-risk individuals;

5 Stimulating partnerships with Aboriginal and Torres Strait Islander communities; and

6 Progressing the evidence base for good practice and prevention of suicide (Commonwealth Department of Health and Aged Care 2000).

Over a period of seven years, 22 national and 156 state/territory projects were funded under the strategy, the majority of them being universal and selective suicide-prevention initiatives implemented in community-based settings (Headey *et al.* 2006; Robinson *et al.* 2006). The national initiatives included the development of the Australian Network for Promotion, Prevention and Early Intervention for Mental Health (Auseinet) and the Mindframe National Media Initiative, the introduction of the National Youth Participation Strategy, a range of activities for individuals bereaved by suicide, and publication of culturally appropriate information leaflets for the indigenous populations. Following the six areas of action, a wide range of at-risk groups was targeted by the strategy; however, at the local, state and territory levels, the three major target groups for interventions were the youth, Aboriginal and Torres Strait Islander populations and people in rural and remote areas (Headey *et al.* 2006).

Although the decrease in the overall suicide rate in Australia (from 14.7 per 100,00 in 1997 to 10.3 per 100,000 in 2005), especially among the young males aged 15–24 (from 31.0 per 100,000 in 1997 to 16.2 per 100,000 in 2005), has been attributed to the effectiveness of the National Suicide Prevention Strategy (Goldney 2006; ABS 2007; Morrell *et al.* 2007), problems related to the accuracy of national suicide mortality data call for caution in considering the strategy's impact (De Leo 2007).

Following extensive consultations with key suicide prevention stakeholders at the national and local levels, in August 2005, the Commonwealth Government Department of Health and Ageing recommended a review of the effectiveness, relevance and appropriateness of the LIFE Framework. The review acknowledged its importance and impact; however, it indicated the need to revise the framework in order to clarify its purpose and to ensure that the framework is reflective of a diverse Australia. Also, the need for greater integration of information presented in the framework documents and publications, as well as adding practical content with an implementation focus and presenting the material in a more visual and concise manner, was recommended. Consequently, the Redevelopment of the LIFE Framework Project commenced and a new framework—Life is for Living—has been developed with the implementation starting in 2008.

The Life is for Living Framework is based upon a vision 'that suicide prevention activities will reduce loss of life' and its purpose is that 'individuals, families and communities will have the support necessary to ensure that no one sees suicide as their only option' (Commonwealth of Australia 2007). Three fundamental principles, i.e. doing no harm, client-centred service delivery and community ownership and responsibility for action, apply to six action areas of the framework:

1 Improving the understanding of the key issues in suicide prevention;

2 Working collaboratively within and across government, service providers and communities;

3 Improving family and community awareness, understanding and capacity to respond;

4 Providing support to build individual resilience and the capacity for self-help in times of adversity;

5 Targeting the areas of greatest need; and

6 Knowing what works and communicating it effectively to the point of need.

These action areas were adapted through the process of stakeholders consultations from the original areas of action delineated in the LIFE framework, and each of them has a specific objective and expected implementation outcomes. The high-risk target groups under the new strategy are people who engage in self-injurious behaviours and/or have a history of suicide attempts, men, indigenous people, individuals living in rural and remote parts of Australia, and individuals from culturally and linguistically diverse backgrounds.

While the LIFE framework activities were based upon the spectrum of mental illness interventions model (adapted from Mrazek and Hagerty 1994)—i.e. prevention, treatment and continuing care—the new framework is founded upon the model of Pathways to Care for Suicide Prevention. This model, although also based upon the concepts of universal, selective and indicated prevention, includes a wider range of interventions, stresses more the role of clinicians, service providers, community and individuals in prevention of suicide, as well as the need to ensure that there are community-based 'safety nets' at the points of intervention handovers.

Reduction in suicide mortality is one of the effectiveness measures for the framework. Other suggested measures include increased awareness, interest and understanding of issues related to suicide and its prevention, increased application and understanding of effective suicide-prevention initiatives, higher capacity of communities and families to respond to individuals at risk of suicide, as well as improved resilience and well-being in people from high suicide risk populations.

The new framework is presented in a practical and user-friendly format on a website (http://www.lifeisforliving.net) and in a set of documents (including twenty-five fact sheets), which will be distributed among major stakeholders and individuals in the general community.

## References

ABS (2007). *Suicides 2005*. Document no. 3309.0. Australian Bureau of Statistics, Canberra.

Commonwealth of Australia (2007). *Life is for Living: A Framework for Prevention of Suicide in Australia*. Australian Government Department of Health and Ageing, Canberra.

Commonwealth Department of Health and Aged Care (2000). *Areas for Action, LIFE: A Framework for Prevention of Suicide and Self-harm in Australia*. Commonwealth Department of Health and Aged Care, Canberra.

De Leo D (1999). Cultural issues in suicide and old age. *Crisis*, **20**, 53–55.

De Leo D (2007). Suicide mortality data need revision. *Medical Journal of Australia*, **186**, 157.

Goldney R (2006). Suicide in Australia: some good news. *Medical Journal of Australia*, **185**, 304.

Headey A, Pirkis J, Merner B *et al.* (2006). A review of 156 local projects funded under Australia's National Suicide Prevention Strategy: overview and lessons learned. *Australian eJournal for the Advancement of Mental Health*, **5**, 3.

Morrell S, Page AN, Taylor R (2007). The decline in Australian young male suicide. *Social Science and Medicine*, **64**, 747–754.

Mrazek PJ and Haggerty RJ (1994). *Reducing the Risk of Mental Disorders: Frontiers for Preventive Intervention Research*. National Academy Press, Washington.

Robinson J, McGorry P, Harris MG *et al.* (2006). Australia's national suicide prevention strategy: the next chapter. *Australian Health Review*, **30**, 271–276.

# CHAPTER 114

# Suicide prevention in New Zealand

Annette Beautrais and Gregory Luke Larkin

## Introduction

Suicide rates and suicide prevention emerged as important *fin de siècle* social issues in New Zealand in the 1990s; they continue to be focal policy and public health concerns in New Zealand today and for the foreseeable future. This attention has been stimulated by two lines of evidence. First, international comparisons suggest that New Zealand has one of the highest rates of youth (15–24 age group) suicide in the developed world. Comparisons between countries of the Organization for Economic Co-operation and Development (OECD) consistently show New Zealand to share top ranking with Finland and Ireland (Ministry of Health 2006a) for male youth suicide rates, but New Zealand's high rates of female youth suicide are without peer. Secondly, suicide rates increased markedly among young New Zealanders from the mid-1980s to the mid-1990s, garnering national attention, yet fuelling public misperception that youth suicides account for most suicides in the country. Indeed, these data led the New Zealand government's early suicide prevention efforts to target youth explicitly. Forgotten, however, is the plight of those at highest risk: adults in later life. The reality is that youth suicides account for only 20 per cent of all suicides in New Zealand every year. Suicides in adult males account for half of all suicides, and the changing, ageing, population demographics suggest that numbers and rates of suicide in older adults will significantly increase in the next decade. If the suicide toll is to be meaningfully reduced, recognition of the epidemiologic facts and a corresponding alignment of resources are needed to adequately address suicide risk across the lifespan.

## Suicidal behaviour in New Zealand

At present (2008), there are approximately 500 suicides in New Zealand each year and over 10 times as many people (approximately 5500) are admitted to hospital for suicide attempts (Ministry of Health 2006b). These annual figures have remained substantially unchanged in the last few decades. Seemingly immune to the latest advances in aetiologic and prevention research, suicide remains the ninth leading cause of death in New Zealand, the second major cause of death for young people aged 15–24 and the leading cause of injury-related fatalities (Ministry of Health 2006a, b, 2007). Three times as many males as females die by suicide. Rates of suicide amongst

men aged 85 and older are three times those of teenaged males. (Among those who present to hospital emergency departments with suicide attempts or ideation, 10–20 per cent make a further attempt within one year, 1–2 per cent will die by suicide within the same year and 10–15 per cent will eventually die by suicide [Larkin and Beautrais submitted].)

New Zealand's first national mental health survey conducted, from October 2003 to December 2004, examined suicidal behaviour in a sample of 12,992 nationally representative participants aged 16 and older (Beautrais *et al.* 2006). Highest in women, overall lifetime prevalences for suicidal ideation, plan and attempt were 15.7, 5.5 and 4.5 per cent, respectively. Twelve-month prevalences for ideation, plan and attempt were 3.2, 1.0 and 0.4 per cent. Risk of ideation in the previous 12 months was higher in females, younger people, people with lower educational qualifications, and people with low household income. Risk of making a plan or attempt was higher in younger people and in people with low household income. After adjustment for sociodemographic factors there were no ethnic differences in ideation, although indigenous Māori, and Pacific people had elevated risks of plans and attempts compared with non-Māori non-Pacific people. Individuals with a mental disorder had elevated risks of ideation (11.8 per cent), plan (4.1 per cent) and attempt (1.6 per cent) compared with those without mental disorder. Less than half of those who reported suicidal behaviours within the past 12 months had made visits to health professionals within that period. Fewer than one-third of those who had made attempts had received treatment from a psychiatrist.

## Suicide research in New Zealand

Over the past two decades, New Zealand researchers have contributed a disproportionately large volume of published work to the world suicide literature. Research has explored risk and protective factors for suicidal and self-harm behaviours in people of all ages, the epidemiology of suicidal behaviours, methods of suicide, knowledge and attitudes about suicide, outcome after suicide attempts, gene–environment interactions, the media, and the contribution of social factors to suicide. For a comprehensive overview see Beautrais and Larkin (submitted). This body of research has informed opinion leaders and policy-makers domestically and abroad. It has helped underwrite the New Zealand Youth Suicide

Prevention Strategy (Ministry of Youth Affairs, Ministry of Health *et al.* 1998), the national Suicide Prevention Strategy for people of all ages (Associate Minister of Health 2006) and the associated Action Plan (Ministry of Health 2008). This evidence has been synthesized by Fergusson and Beautrais to develop a conceptual model of the complex processes and causal pathways that, at a population level, lead to suicidal behaviour (Associate Minister of Health 2006; Beautrais and Surgenor 2007) (Figure 114.1).

## Suicide prevention in New Zealand: status at the beginning of the twenty-first century

New Zealand's recent suicide-prevention efforts began with development of the national Youth Suicide Prevention Strategy in 1998 (Ministry of Youth Affairs, Ministry of Health *et al.* 1998). This strategy provided a national framework for developing a series of interventions including:

- Media reporting guidelines for suicide (Ministry of Health 1998);

- Guidelines for suicide prevention in schools ( Beautrais *et al.* 1998);

- By child youth and family workers (Child Youth and Family February 2005);

- Mental health services (Mental Health Services New Zealand 1993);

- Emergency departments (New Zealand Guidelines Group 2003); and

- Primary care providers (Royal New Zealand College of General Practitioners and Ministry of Youth Affairs 1999);

- A national suicide information and resource centre (www.spinz. org.nz); and

- Culturally specific programmes for Māori youth.

While the youth suicide prevention strategy was overseen by a minor ministry (The Ministry of Youth Affairs), a government interagency committee (involving education, justice, police, health, prisons, social welfare, child welfare, Māori and relevant other sectors) ensured a broader ownership of, and a collective focus for, youth suicide prevention.

Beginning in the late 1990s, some highly successful national programmes were initiated under the broad umbrella of mental health promotion and suicide prevention, including the national mental health de-stigmatization programme Like minds, Like mine (Vaughan 2004; Vaughan and Hasen 2004), begun in 1997, and the National Depression Initiative, begun in 2006 (http://www.moh. govt.nz/moh.nsf/indexmh/national-depression-initiative-faq). Beyond government-led suicide-prevention work, some innovative interventions were initiated by concerned professionals. Perhaps the most ambitious was the Towards Well-being (TWB) Project in the national child welfare system (Child, Youth and Family Services) (http://www.nzfvc.org.nz/accan/papers-presentations/ abstract266v.shtml) in which a small group of expert and highly experienced clinical psychologists and mental health social workers developed a national suicide assessment and monitoring programme for all young people who needed child welfare services.

Despite the potential generalizability of many of the guidelines documents and programmes developed under the Youth Suicide Prevention Strategy, it became apparent that a major limitation of

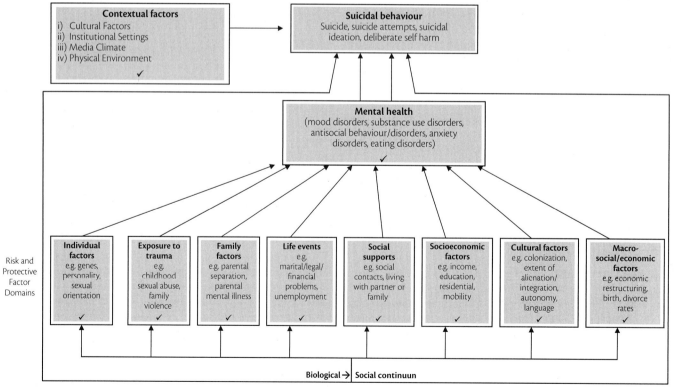

**Fig. 114.1** Pathways to suicidal behaviour.

the Strategy was, in fact, its focus on youth, which failed to provide an appropriate framework for developing suicide-prevention initiatives for people of all ages. In addition, increased knowledge about the aetiology of suicide and approaches to suicide prevention suggested it was timely to revise and extend the strategy to develop an explicit, all ages, perspective. This was done in 2006 with the development of the national Suicide Prevention Strategy (Associate Minister of Health 2006) and in 2008 with the associated implementation Action Plan (Associate Minister of Health 2006; Ministry of Health 2008) which includes goals for suicide prevention for the 2006–2016 decade. The overall aims of the strategy are to reduce mortality, morbidity and distress associated with suicidal behaviour, and to minimize social inequalities in the risk of suicide and suicide attempts.

## Challenges for current suicide prevention efforts

In conclusion, New Zealand's current national suicide prevention plan is generally evidence-based, and retains a public health perspective, consistent with strategies formulated in similar, developed countries. The strategy is valuable in that it compels government to do several important things: first, acknowledge the problem of suicide; second, increase national awareness about suicide; third, pass legislation that promotes suicide prevention; and fourth, increase funding for suicide prevention and research. Such political championship is highly effective, indeed vital, in maintaining a government focus on suicide prevention.

While the national Strategy articulates specific policy agendas for suicide prevention, the translation of those agendas requires effective implementation at the micro, meso, and macro levels. This process raises important issues about how broad policy directions by governments and ministries can be translated into effective programmes. Greater use of the principles of prevention science by community planners and service providers may help resolve these issues. A prevention science approach requires that broad policy action advocated by governments and ministries is carefully translated into service development (Beautrais 2007; Beautrais et al. 2007).

The macro-level challenges of translating knowledge into practice are best framed within the broad goals of knowledge translation (KT) and technology diffusion (Larkin et al. 2007). Optimal implementation of the latest evidence requires that attention be paid to the context of the candidate community and the key stakeholders therein. Ethical and equitable KT can help mitigate the global burdens of suicidal behaviour. Knowledge translation approaches account for the benefits of implementing innovations to ensure that disparities and gaps in health experienced by the least advantaged are prioritized. Suicide is an emotive issue for the public at large and for many stakeholders. Broad implementation and adoption of the latest science, new clinical practice guidelines, and best practice models can help meet many KT-related challenges. Adherence to the principles and ethics of KT provide the current best guide for researchers, politicians, economists, policy-makers and opinion leaders to address these challenges and more strongly promote a suicide-prevention strategy that is vertically and horizontally integrated, and responsive to the needs of New Zealanders from every generation, both living and in the future.

## References

Associate Minister of Health (2006). *The New Zealand Suicide Prevention Strategy*. Ministry of Health, Wellington.

Beautrais AL (2007). Translating knowledge into suicide prevention: the current challenge. *New Zealand College of Clinical Psychology Journal*, Spring, 1–10.

Beautrais AL and Larkin G (submitted). Status of suicide prevention in New Zealand on the edge of the 21st century.

Beautrais AL and Surgenor LJ (2007). Suicidal behaviour and practitioner issues. In IM Evans, M O'Driscoll, and JJ Rucklidge, eds, *Professional Practice of Psychology in Aotearoa New Zealand*, pp. 195–210. The New Zealand Psychological Society, Wellington.

Beautrais AL, Coggan CA et al. (1998). *Young People at Risk of Suicide: A Guide for Schools*. Ministry of Education and National Health Committee, Wellington.

Beautrais AL, Fergusson DM et al. (2007). Effective strategies for suicide prevention in New Zealand: a review of the evidence. *New Zealand Medical Journal*, **120**, 1–13.

Beautrais AL, Wells JE et al. (2006). Suicidal behaviour in Te Rau Hinengaro: The New Zealand Mental Health Survey (NZMHS). *Australian and New Zealand Journal ofPsychiatry*, **40**, 896–904.

Child Youth and Family (February 2005). *Towards Well-Being. Youth Suicide Prevention Programme. Request For Proposal*. Tender Document. Child, Youth and Family, Wellington.

Larkin G and Beautrais A (2008). The epidemiology of emergency department visits for suicide attempts in the South Pacific: New Zealand 1997–2006. *Annals of Emergency Medicine*, **51**, 277.

Larkin G, Hamann C et al. (2007). Knowledge translation at the macro level: legal and ethical considerations. *The Journal of Academic Emergency Medicine*, **4**, 1042–1046.

Mental Health Services New Zealand (1993). *Guidelines on the Management of Suicidal Patients*. Department of Health, Wellington.

Ministry of Health (1998). *Preventing Suicide: Guidelines for the Media on the Reporting of Suicide*. Ministry of Health, Wellington.

Ministry of Health (2006a). *Suicide Trends in New Zealand 1983–2003. Monitoring Report No. 6*. Ministry of Health, Wellington.

Ministry of Health (2006b). *New Zealand Suicide Trends. Mortality 1921–2003 Hospitalisations for Intentional Self-harm 1978–2004*. Ministry of Health, Wellington.

Ministry of Health (2007). *Suicide Facts*. Ministry of Health, Wellington.

Ministry of Health (2008). *New Zealand Suicide Prevention Action Plan 2008–2012: The Summary for Action*. New Zealand Ministry of Health, Wellington.

Ministry of Youth Affairs, Ministry of Health et al. (March 1998). *New Zealand Youth Suicide Prevention Strategy*. Ministry of Youth Affairs, Ministry of Health, Te Puni Kokiri, Wellington.

New Zealand Guidelines Group (2003). *The Assessment and Management of People at Risk of Suicide. People at Risk of Suicide*. Ministry of Health, New Zealand Guidelines Group, Wellington.

Royal New Zealand College of General Practitioners and Ministry of Youth Affairs (1999). *Guidelines for Primary Care Providers. Detection and Management of Young People at Risk of Suicide*. Ministry of Youth Affairs, Wellington.

Vaughan G (2004). Like minds, like mine. In S Saxena and PJ Garrison, *Mental Health Promotion. Case StudiesFrom Countries*, pp. 63–66. World Health Organization, Geneva.

Vaughan G and Hasen C (2004). Like minds, like mine: a New Zealand project to counter the stigma and discrimination associated with mental illness. *Australasian Psychiatry*, **12**, 113–117.

# Examples of How to Develop Suicide Prevention on all the Continents: Europe

# CHAPTER 115

# Suicide prevention in Estonia

Airi Värnik and Danuta Wasserman

## Estonian–Swedish Mental Health and Suicidology Institute (ERSI)

Mortality data on suicide were kept in secret behind the doors of statistical offices in the former Soviet Union. All the draft articles for scientific journals were censored in special ministerial departments, and information considered as state secrets or data liable to ruin the illusory image of consummate welfare, was deleted or rejected.

In 1988, during the Gorbachev reform era, permission was given to form a Suicide Research Group within the framework of the re-established Estonian Medical Association (EMA), and to have access to statistical data (Wasserman and Värnik 1998). According to calculations, the suicide rate was approximately 33–35 per 100,000 inhabitants.

The Baltic republics regained their independence in 1991, and were granted creative freedom. The assistance from the National Swedish Prevention of Suicide and Mental Ill-Health (NASP) resulted in the growth of the EMA Suicide Research Group into the Estonian-Swedish Institute of Suicidology (ERSI), in Tallinn, in 1993 (Estonian–Swedish Mental Health and Suicidology Institute 2008), with economic support from Stockholm Care, an agency of Stockholm County Council and the Swedish Eastern European Committee.

Immediately after the inauguration, courses on suicidology for medical staff began. To date, ERSI has transferred knowledge to thousands of people, specified by the following target groups.

- A basic course in suicidology, followed by courses and seminars on specific topics were prepared and performed for physicians, nurses, psychologists, social workers, schoolteachers and police officers.

- A group of trainers are continuously growing, and includes those who passed ERSI courses. In the training trainers' course, special emphasis is directed to the high quality of content and interactive methodology in conveying the message to the audience.

- Besides training trainers in Estonia, the project 'Suicidology and reforms in psychiatry' for Russian psychiatrists from St Petersburg and Kaliningrad, in collaboration with the Swedish East European Committee, was established to train a group of lecturers who will organize courses in their districts.

- The courses in suicidology and interventions in suicidal crisis are given to university students, and their diploma projects and papers in suicidology are supervised.

- Estonian 'Lifeline' was initiated by the ERSI in 1995, and enlarged to a crisis centre providing services. Volunteers are being trained by ERSI to work in different emergency crisis services.

- Consultations are provided in regards to special suicidological cases for medical staff and other specialists if needed.

## Integration of suicide awareness into Estonian society

Public-relation activities to integrate suicide awareness into Estonian society were an important component of ERSI work. Catching the attention of mass media helped to diminish the taboo and stigma concerning suicidal behaviours. Disseminating information that suicide is preventable to the public and authorities has also proven effective.

ERSI informed the Estonian politicians and decision-makers about the magnitude of suicidal behaviour as an important public health problem and economic burden. In response, the draft of a national suicide-prevention action plan was ordered from ERSI, which was forwarded to the Ministry of Social Affairs in 2001, and evaluated internationally. A chapter on suicide prevention will be incorporated in accordance with political decisions on National Mental Health Policy.

Several international conferences, and workshops on suicidology, were held in Tallinn, the capital of Estonia. The WHO regional workshop on suicide prevention was organized in Tallinn in 1999, and its conclusions were forwarded to governmental, municipal and social institutions, to various organizations, as well as the media (World Health Organization 1999). Translations of WHO resources into Estonian were published and delivered to target groups (World Health Organization 2008). The tenth anniversary of ERSI was celebrated with an international conference, in 2003 (Värnik 2003), and the fifteenth anniversary in 2008 (Värnik et al. 2008). An international conference was held in Tallinn on a European Commission project aimed at improving the mental health of Europeans called 'Implementation of Mental Health Promotion and Prevention Policies and Strategies in EU Member States and Applicant Countries' (EMIP 2008). In 2007, ERSI was awarded the 'European Health Forum Award' as one of the partner's of the European Commission project 'European Alliance Against Depression' (EAAD).

A representative from ERSI took part in the WHO European Ministerial Conference on Mental Health (World Health Organization 2005), as an expert on suicidal behaviours in societies of transition. The documents of the conference were widely disseminated to different target groups, which gave grounds for discussions of the European Commission Green paper 'Promoting the mental health of the population—towards a strategy on mental health for the European Union' (European Commission Green Paper 2005).

## The quest for knowledge and research for evidence-based strategies

Close contacts with NASP, colleagues from other countries and the WHO, have allowed ERSI to expand the knowledge and gain experience, which was essential in promoting the field. Teaching methods and models of suicide prevention have been developed and implemented. A library on suicidology has been created. Information and experience was gathered by participating in conferences, symposiums and workshops on suicidology.

Epidemiological and clinical research, such as surveys of the distribution and dynamics of suicide and suicidal behaviour among specific groups, risk and protective factors, availability, quality and capacity of public health services, with respect to assessment and treatment of suicidal patients, made it possible to use the results to establish country-specific prevention strategies.

There have been numerous publications and presentations at conferences, which stemmed from ERSI's local and international projects (Estonian–Swedish Mental Health and Suicidology Institute 2008).

## From rejection to appreciation

When suicide research and prevention began to be implemented in Estonia, there was very little interest in the work, and attitudes were sceptical or dismissive. Step by step, ERSI has spread knowledge about suicidology among the Estonian authorities, specialists and, through the mass media, the public. ERSI's work, and suicide-related topics, have a high profile in the media, with numerous interviews on TV, the radio, and in the press. A major increase in popular suicide awareness is taking place.

Judging the effectiveness of suicide prevention by suicide rates and trends, the suicide rate in Estonia has decreased steadily since 1995 from 41 to 19 per 100,000 inhabitants in 2005 and is now the lowest among the Baltic States and Russia, whereas Estonia started on the same level as these neighbouring countries.

ERSI's work has gradually shifted towards earlier stages of the suicidal process, and towards the promotion of mental health in general. Today, ERSI is a main expert for the Estonian Ministry of Social Affairs, in the field of suicide prevention and promoting mental health.

## References

EMIP (Implementation of Mental Health Promotion and Prevention Policies and Strategies in EU Member States and Applicant Countries) (2008). *EC project.* Accessed at http://www.emip.org/

European Commission Green paper (2005). *Promoting the Mental Health of the Population. Towards a Strategy on Mental health for the European Union.* Accessed at: http://europa.eu.int/comm/health/ph_determinants/life_style/mental/green_paper/consultation_en.htm.

Estonian–Swedish Mental Health and Suicidology Institute (ERSI) (2008). Accessed at http://www.suicidology.ee/index.php?page=3.

Värnik A (ed.) (2003). *Suitsiidiuuringud* [Suicide Studies]. *ERSI 10. Aastapäeva kogumik,* pp. 1–112. [ERSI 10th anniversary collected papers]. Iloprint, Tallinn.

Värnik A, Sisask M and Kõlves K (ed.) (2008). *Essential Papers on Suicidology 1993–2008. ERSI 15th anniversary collected papers.* pp. 1–340. Rebellis AS, Tallinn.

Wasserman D and Värnik A (1998). Suicide-preventive effects of perestroika in the former USSR: the role of alcohol restriction. *Acta Psychiatria Scandinavica Supplementum,* **394,** 1–4.

World Health Organization (1999). *Report on a workshop on Suicide Prevention for countries in the Baltic Region.* Department of Mental Health, World Health Organization, August 25–27. Tallinn, Estonia.

World Health Organization (2005). *Mental Health: Facing the Challenges, Building Solutions,* p. 180. Report from the WHO European Ministerial Conference. World Health Organization, Geneva.

World Health Organization (2008). *Mental Health.* WHO/Euro resources. Accessed at: http://www.who.int/mental_health/resources/suicide/en/index.html.

# CHAPTER 116

# Suicide prevention in Finland

Jouko Lönnqvist

## Suicide prevention and national health policy

Finland, with a population of 5.5 million people, forms a culturally homogeneous, well-educated and well-functioning modern Western society. The Finnish health care system is mainly public, and financed by taxes collected both by the state and the municipalities (http://www.vn.fi/stm/english/).

Suicide has been one of the leading causes of death for decades. Suicide mortality has had a general increasing trend from the early 1920s to the peak of suicide rate, 30 per 100,000, in 1990. Since then, however, the suicide rate has been decreasing, and was 18 per 100,000 in 2005.

The first parliamentary committee on suicide was launched in Finland in the mid-1970s. The reason for this was the heavily increasing trend of suicide mortality, and the increasing awareness of suicide as an important public health issue. In the early 1980s, the minister of Social Affairs and Health decided to launch a novel national suicide-prevention project. The project was accepted and started officially on 1 May 1986, after about two years of preliminary preparation. The ultimate aim was to reverse the increasing trend of suicide mortality, and to decrease the suicide rate by 20 per cent during the next ten years (Upanne M *et al.* 1999). The project was a part of the Finnish national strategy of the WHO's 'Health for All by the Year 2000' programme (Ministry of Social Affairs and Health 1987). The author of this chapter was appointed the leader of the project. A separate research unit was established at the National Public Health Institute to support the management and research activities of the project.

## Basic structure and characteristics of the national suicide prevention project

The basic principle of the project was to build national prevention activities on the reliable picture of the current Finnish suicide situation. Some longitudinal and trans-sectional epidemiological studies on suicide mortality, based on the available Finnish mortality statistics, were performed. In collaboration with the mass media, and by arranging local public meetings and lectures, a public awareness and discussion was raised. All suicides (N = 1397) committed during one year, throughout the country, were scrutinized by using a psychological autopsy method, combined with a normal and legal police investigation, and a routine medico-legal examination.

We believed that the best way to change attitudes of the various professionals, and to find common concepts to describe suicidal behaviours, would be 'learning by experience'. For this purpose, about 250 field researchers, mostly locally practising and experienced mental health workers (doctors, psychologists, social workers and nurses specializing in psychiatry), were trained for interviewing relatives, the next of kin and treating personnel, and for collecting other important data on every suicide case. Every suicide was discussed in the fifteen provincial project groups in the whole of Finland, including representatives of police, medico-legal experts, primary health care and social services, psychiatric services, and possibly other sectors of society. Every structured case report ended with concrete suggestions for suicide prevention, based on the findings from each individual case (Lönnqvist 1998). Altogether, about 1000 thousand people participated in the project, and more than 2000 relatives of the suicide victims, and approximately the same amount of the treating personnel interviewed in the connection of the project suicides were influenced by the project. All of them were also key suicide prevention agents in their own professional surroundings. The project had a direct impact on about 100,000 professionals and citizens, with an indirect impact through the 100,000 professionals and mass media on the whole society of Finland.

This ambitious programme extended suicide research and prevention efforts throughout the entire country. It was the first comprehensive effort of its kind anywhere (Wilson 2004).

More than one hundred scientific publications were published from the psychological autopsy sample. The major risk factors for suicide were depression, personality disorders, alcoholism, schizophrenia, and organic or other mental disorders (Henriksson *et al.* 1993; Lönnqvist *et al.* 1995). Two-thirds of suicide deaths occurred in people who were depressed, yet only 15 per cent had received appropriate treatment. Alcohol was found in the blood of half of the people who committed suicide, and one-third of all suicides were made by alcohol-dependent individuals. People who survived a previous suicide attempt were at very high risk for repeated attempts, and yet, they typically received little or no treatment or consistent follow-up.

## Developing a national suicide prevention strategy

After all suicide cases were collected and analysed, in 1987–88, the fifteen provincial project groups published their final reports in 1989–1990, with proposals for suicide prevention in their own region and province. The national strategy and action plan was worked through in 1991, by the national project group representing all main sectors of the Finnish society, and led by the director general of the National Board of Health. The national project group was supported by the project leader, secretariat and core planning team of the project group.

The national suicide prevention programme, 'Suicide Can Be Prevented' (National Research and Development Centre for Welfare and Health 1993) was based on the findings of a national psychological autopsy study of suicide deaths. The key targets were people with depression, substance use problems, in crisis situations, those in need of psychosocial support due to physical illnesses, and people who attempted suicide. The project focused mainly on actions that directly influenced the risk factors for suicidal behaviour. Younger generations were the main targets of the programme. Enhancing awareness and changing negative attitudes towards suicide were also in focus.

A booklet—'Suicide can be Prevented' (National Research and Development Centre for Welfare and Health 1993)—was distributed throughout the country to raise awareness among physicians, those working in health and social care, teachers, police officers, church leaders and other people, who all come in regular contact with potential individuals at risk for suicide. The most important advice was to take early signs of self-destructive behaviour seriously, and to always consider the possibility of suicide among people with mental disorders. Health and welfare workers were also advised to pay close attention to the well-being of patients with chronic illness or disability, who may be depressed, but do not acknowledge it.

Asking about depression and suicide should be as routine as checking for hypertension, and physicians should consider addressing these issues directly with patients. We found that patients who are feeling suicidal are likely to admit their feelings when asked by their physician, but they seldom spontaneously convey this information.

Alcohol was identified as a particularly relevant risk factor for suicide in Finland, and given priority in our suicide-prevention strategy.

Because the high rates of suicide were observed among young men in the 15–24 age group, the programme focused on this group. We launched mental health, depression and suicide awareness programmes in the school system. The military, which evaluates all 18-year-old men as part of the national Finnish draft, received special instructions on the identification and referral of at-risk youths.

The suicide preventive programme leaders also tried to train the media on appropriate suicide reporting, so that suicides did not receive sensational coverage that might encourage copy-cat suicides.

## Goal attainment

The Finnish government commissioned both an internal and external evaluation to assess the outcome of the strategy (Ministry of Social Affairs and Health 1999).

The principal aim of the Finnish National Suicide Prevention Project, launched in 1986, was to reduce suicide mortality by 20 per cent within ten years (Hakanen and Upanne 1966). Suicide rates were 26.6 in 1986, and actually increased during the years 1986–1990 to 30.0, which were higher than ever. The programme was not yet successful, with only a 9 per cent reduction in the incidence of suicide achieved over the entire official duration of the project (23.6 in 1996). From the beginning of the implementation phase (1991–92), the suicide rate has continuously decreased from the peak in 1990 (30.0 per 100,000) to a low point of 17.9 per 100,000, in 2005. The suicide rate, in 2005, was 40 per cent lower than in 1990.

The external evaluation of the Finnish national suicide prevention project in 1999 concluded that:

> Implementation was successful in putting suicide prevention on the social agenda and at large in promoting development in the chosen areas. It may already have contributed to the reversal of the increasing trend in suicide rates. It gave experiences of an interactive, participating working model and produced practical models and guidebooks for suicide preventive work. In these respects, the project has been both purposeful and appropriate and has produced good results.
>
> Kerkhof (1999, p. 63)

In 2001, the Government of Finland developed a new public health policy called the 'Governmental Resolution on the Health 2015 Public Program' (Ministry of Social Affairs and Health 2001). This programme, targeted at younger generations, has been developed to reduce accidental and violent death among young adult men by one-third of the level during the late 1990s. Finland has also been active in the development of a mental health strategy, of which suicide prevention is an elementary part, both in the WHO and the European Union.

## References

Hakanen J and Upanne M (1996). Evaluation strategy for Finland's suicide prevention projects. *Crisis*, **17**, 167–174.

Henriksson MM, Aro HM, Marttunen MJ et al. (1993). Mental disorders and comorbidity in suicide. *American Journal of Psychiatry*, **150**, 935–940.

Kerkhof AJ (1999). The Finnish national suicide prevention program evaluated. *Crisis*, **20**, 63.

Lönnqvist J (1988). National suicide prevention project in Finland. A research phase of the project. *Psychiatria Fennica*, **19**, 133–142.

Lönnqvist JK, Henriksson MM, Isometsä ET et al. (1995). Mental disorders and suicide prevention. *Psychiatry and Clinical Neuroscience*, **49**(Suppl 1), 111–116.

Ministry of Social Affairs and Health (1987). *Health for All by the Year 2000. The Finnish National Strategy*. Ministry of Social Affairs and Health, Helsinki.

Ministry of Social Affairs and Health (1999). *Suicide Prevention in Finland 1986–1996. External Evaluation by an International Peer Group*. Ministry of Social Affairs and Health, Helsinki.

Ministry of Social Affairs and Health (2001). *Government Resolution on Health 2015—Public Health Programme*. Edita, Helsinki.

National Research and Development Centre for Welfare and Health (1993). *Suicide can be Prevented. A Target and Action Strategy for Suicide Prevention*. National Research and Development Centre for Welfare and Health, Helsinki.

Upanne M, Hakanen J, Rantanen M (1999). *Can Suicide be Prevented? The Suicide Project in Finland 1992–1996. Goals, Implementation and Evaluation*. National Research and Development Centre for Welfare and Health, Helsinki.

Wilson J (2004). Finland pioneers suicide prevention. *Annals of Internal Medicine*, **140**, 853–856.

# CHAPTER 117

# Suicide prevention in France

Véronique Narboni and Jean-Pierre Soubrier

## The French paradox?

France has often been described as an ideal place to live: fine wining and dining, lovely villages and cities, where the pursuit of happiness defines the quality of life. Despite this positive image, another face of French society emerges in a country with one of the highest suicide rates in Europe.

Every year, more than 10,000 people commit suicide in France; representing 1 suicide every 50 minutes. However, recent publications from the High Level Committee on Public Health (*Haut comité de Santé publique*), state that these figures are underestimated by about 20 per cent. Reasons for underestimation are mainly due to the fact that most suicides are 'hidden' behind other more obvious causes of death, such as accidents and drug poisoning, or the simple fact that suicide is not identified as such.

After a significant increase in the 1980s, suicide rates in France have been gradually dropping since 1993. However, today, death by suicide remains high, which is double of that by car accidents. Furthermore, it has been reported that between 160,000 and 180,000 suicide attempts take place every year, representing 16–18 times the number of completed suicides.

In France, suicide is the first cause of death in the 35–44 age group, and the second cause of death in the 15–24 age group, according to the latest statistical analysis (INSERM 2005).

## Key milestones and the history of suicide in France

France gave birth to the human rights constitution. To better understand the process of suicide prevention in France, key historical dates are outlined below.

### Semantic background

The word suicide is Latin for *suicidium*, from *sui caedere*, to kill oneself. It was initially introduced in France in 1734 by Abbé Prevost, and later confirmed, in 1737, by Abbé Desfontaines (Soubrier 1999). In 1762, the French Academy officially accepted the inclusion of 'suicide' in its dictionary as 'to kill oneself'.

In 1810, Napoleon stated that the act of suicide is no longer a 'punishable act', however, socially, morally and politically, committing suicide has remained taboo (Minois 1995).

### Psychiatric, sociological and societal background

Jean Etienne Esquirol declared in 1838 that suicide was 'an act only committed by mental patients in a moment of delusion' (Esquirol 1838), which opened a wide-scientific discussion on suicide.

In 1888, Emile Durkheim was the first to provide a sociological explanation of suicide, linking social disintegration and suicide, and lending support to current assumptions that social capital is a protective factor in the mental health of the general population (Durkheim 1888). This was a big step in France, where the question of suicide was no longer a matter of morality or immorality, but rather a psychological or a social problem. In the twentieth century, Halbwachs (1930) and Baecheler (1975) further explored the sociological background of suicide, the latter discussing the challenge of suicide prevention: *L'illusion des spécialistes* (Baecheler 1975).

After the Second World War, the French Health Care System was created. Shortly after this, and using the English model of Chad Varad and the Samaritans (1953), associations in France such as Recherche and Rencontres (Research and Meetings, 1958) and telephone help lines such as SOS Amitié (the Friendship hotline) were initiated.

### Research background

In 1969, the Suicide Studies and Prevention Group (Groupement d'Etude et de Prevention du Suicide—GEPS), was founded by mainly intensive care psychiatrists and child/adolescent psychiatrists—Professors Pierre Pichot, Pierre Moron, Jacques Vendrinne and Jean-Pierre Soubrier—played a crucial role in disseminating information concerning suicide, and increasing public awareness on the issue. This group also developed surveys and research protocols in order to demonstrate the objective and the subjective importance of suicide within the society. GEPS also created forums (Vedrinne *et al.* 1981) to complete sensitization work; these forums were, and still are, a place of exchange between field experts and researchers, and contribute to suicide-prevention implementation.

### Legal background

In 1982, the Association Against Suicide Promotion (Association de Défense Contre l'Incitation au Suicide—ADIS) was created after publication of the book *Suicide: How to make it*. Following this publication, widespread political debate occurred, and in 1985, the National Academy of Medicine requested the government to take action (Soubrier 1985). The senate proposed a law against incitation to suicide. However, in 1987, a law against provocation to suicide was finally passed by the National Assembly.

### Political background

In 1992, the Economic and Social Council's Report 18 (Conseil économique et social 1993) issued a report in which suicide was the main topic. For the first time in France, this report acknowledged that suicide was a major public health concern. It triggered several initiatives, a major one being the snapshot of the French situation revealed by the data collected from the Regional Observatory between 1995 and 1997 (FNORS 2005).

## Suicide prevention in France today

### The network in place: from JNPS to UNPS

At the end of 1996, a new association titled the National Day for Suicide Prevention and celebrated on 5 February each year (Journée Nationale pour la Prévention du Suicide—JNPS), was created as the result of joint efforts of six associations working in the field of suicide prevention. Its goal is to increase awareness by informing the public that suicide, contrary to being taboo, should be discussed as a first step in prevention (Box 117.1). It also strengthens the need for multidisciplinary approach.

The year 2000 was an important development for the association, which became known as the National Union for Suicide Prevention (Union Nationale pour la prevention du suicide—UNPS), enlarging its scope of activities beyond the major communication event of 5 February and developing action in the regions.

---

**Box 117.1** Themes of the National Day of Suicide Prevention

1999 Suicide prevention, it's possible (Prévenir le suicide, c'est possible)

2000 Medical challenge, social challenge: I commit myself (Défi médical, défi social: je m'engage)

2001 Choosing life (Choisir la vie)

2002 Local policies, global policies (Politiques locales, politique globale)

2003 Suicide: human relations in question (Suicide: la relation humaine en question)

2004 Violence and suicide at work (Violence et suicide au travail)

2005 Regulations, ethics, suicide: prohibit, assist or prevent (Droit, éthique, suicide: interdire, assister ou prévenir)

2006 Certainty and uncertainty of prevention (Certitudes et incertitudes de la prévention)

2007 Wish to live: suicide is not a fate (Envie de la vie: Le suicide n'est pas une fatalité)

2008 Wish to live (Envie de la vie)

2009 Precariousness and suicide (Prévenir le suicide)

---

Today, UNPS includes over twenty associations, which are dedicated directly or indirectly to suicide prevention, and presently there is also a dedicated website 'Info suicide' (http://www.info-suicide.org).

## National policies: from guidelines to daily practices

In 1998, the first national prevention programme was launched and suicide became one of the top ten national public health priorities. In addition, The National Strategy for Suicide Prevention (2000–2005) was officially launched in September 2000 (Ministre délégué de la santé 2001). At this juncture, suicide prevention became a priority for public health services.

Part of this strategy was regionally implemented with a specific 'train the trainers' programme, organized by psychiatrists and psychologists for people interested or involved in suicide prevention. The French strategy closely followed the launch of the WHO worldwide SUPRE suicide prevention 'Live your Life' initiative in 1999 (World Health Organization 1999).

The French Federation of Psychiatry, in partnership with ANAES (Agence Nationale d'Accreditation et d'Evaluation de la Santé), organized a Consensus conference in October 2000, on suicide crisis (Conference de Consensus 2000). A model to assess and better manage suicidal people was created. Following this first consensus conference, other task force meetings elaborated more specific guidelines targeting children and adolescents (FFP 1998). Along with this conference, a French translation of the WHO's resource material *Preventing suicide: a resource for teachers and other school staff* (WHO 2000a), was disseminated to all public health professionals via the regional school system. Another of the WHO's resource materials, *Preventing suicide: a resource for prison officers* (WHO 2000b), was also translated into French and has been recognized as an ideal model in the official report on suicide prevention in prisons, which was written by JL Terra (Terra 2003).

For general practitioners, DepRelief and Lundbeck's initiatives, WHO resources (WHO 2000c), a CD-ROM on evaluation of suicide risk (Soubrier 2000) and interactive seminars were disseminated throughout France.

## Suicide prevention strategy with adolescents and children: a priority

Over the last 10 years, sensitizing school staff, as well as specific training for school doctors and nurses on-site, has been a major goal for prevention. Today, it is a requirement to assess all adolescents' and teenagers' mental health, and observe any changes in their behaviour or appearance. Referral to a specialist can be organized within the care network.

## Conclusion

First introduced as a mental health issue, suicide remains a public health priority in France. A lot has already been done, however, more efforts and continuous education of society and health care professionals will be needed to decrease the French suicide rate in the near future.

# References

Baecheler J (1975). *Suicides*. Calmann Levy, Paris

Conference de Consensus (2000). *La crise suicidaire: reconnaître et prendre en charge* [Suicide crisis: identify and manage], 19–20 Octobre 2000. Federation Française de Psychiatrie, ANAES.

Conseil économique et social (1993). *Le suicide* [Suicide]. Étude présentée par la section des Affaires Sociales sur le rapport de Monsieur Michel Debout, rapporteur, le 6 juillet 1993.

Durkheim E (1888). Suicide et natalité: étude de statistique morale. *Rev philisophique France l'etranger 1888*, **26**, 446–463.

Esquirol JED (1838). *Des maladies mentales [Mental Maladies]*. pp. 253–331. J.B. Baillière, Paris.

FNORS (Federation nationales des observatories regionaux de santé) (2005). *Prevention des suicides et tentatives de suicide. Etats des lieux 1995–1997. Bilans regionaux Aquitaine, Bretagne, Midi-Pyrennées, Nord Pas de Calais, Rhône Alpes* [Suicide prevention and suicide attempts. What's the reality from 1995–1997. Regional analysis Aquitaine, Bretagne, Midi-Pyrénnées, Nord Pas de Calais, Rhône Alpes]. Edition FNMF, Paris.

FFP (1998). *Guidelines for Clinical Practice in the Management of Adolescents after Suicide Attempts. ANAES, Recommandations professionnelles.* French Federation of Psychiatry, Paris.

Halbwachs M (1930). *Les Causes Du Suicide [The Causes of Suicide]*. Alcan, Paris

INSERM (2005). *Data for 2005*. Edition INSERM, Paris.

Ministre délégué de la santé (2001). *Relative à la stratégie nationale d'actions face au suicide (2000–2005): actions prioritaires pour 2001* [Strategic action plan against suicide (2000–2005): public health priority 2001], no. 2001–318 du 5 juillet 2001. Circulaire signée par Bernard Kouchner Ministre délégué de la santé 27p.

Minois G (1995). *Histoire du suicide: la société occidentale face à la mort volontaire*. Fayard, Paris.

Soubrier J-PS (1985). La prévention du suicide est-elle encore possible après la publication autorisée du livre suicide mode d'emploi [Is suicide prevention still possible since the authorized publication of the book *Suicide: How to Make it?*]. *Bulletin de l'Académie National de Médecine*.

Soubrier J-P (1999). Definition of suicide. In ES Shneidman, AA Leenaars and AL Berman, eds, *Suicidology: Essays in Honour of Edwin S. Shneidman*, pp. 35–44. Jason Aronson Inc.

Soubrier J-P (2000). *Evaluation du risque suicidaire* [Suicide risk assessment]. CD-ROM Impact Medecin, Paris and Lundbeck.

Terra JL (2003). *Prevention du suicide des personnes detenues. Rapport de mission Décembre 2003 [Suicide prevention among prisoners. Mission report december 2003]*. Ministére de la justice [Justice Ministry], France.

Vedrinne J, Quénard O, Weber D (1981). Suicide et conduites suicidaires [Suicide and suicidal behaviour]. *Médecine Légale et de Toxicologie Médicale*, 2 tomes, 1981–1982. Masson, Paris.

World Health Organization (1999). *Live Your Life. SUPRE Suicide Prevention*. World Health Organization, Geneva.

World Health Organization (2000a). *Preventing Suicide: A Resource for Teachers and other School Staff*. World Health Organization, Geneva.

World Health Organization (2000b). *Preventing Suicide: A Resource for Prison Officers*. World Health Organization, Geneva.

World Health Organization (2000c). *Preventing Suicide: A Resource for General Physicians*. World Health Organization, Geneva.

# CHAPTER 118

# Suicide prevention in Germany

Elmar Etzersdorfer

The suicide rate in Germany is around the European average; nevertheless, in Germany the third highest absolute number of suicides is committed in Europe (after France and Poland). In 2005, there were 10.260 suicides (7.523 males and 2.737 females; 18.7 and 6.5/100.000, respectively). There are marked regional differences that have been observed for many years, and the suicides reflect a Hungarian pattern (increasing rates with increasing age).

There are many initiatives, as well as institutions, all over the country, which cover a broad spectrum ranging from telephone services and crisis intervention centres to inpatient facilities. I will, therefore, focus on the most important and influential activity of the last years, i.e. the implementation of a national suicide prevention programme (NaSPro, Nationales Suizidpräventionsprogramm).

## NaSPro

Starting as an initiative of the German Association for Suicide Prevention (DGS) in 2002, the NaSPro has achieved increasing attention and cooperation in the country. It is chaired by Professor Armin Schmidtke (Würzburg), and the secretary is Georg Fiedler (Hamburg). From the first, NaSPro had been organized as a broad and integrative approach, acknowledging that suicidal behaviour is a multifaceted phenomenon, which necessitates including experts from different fields of science, as well as practitioners, relatives' organizations, representatives of political, religious and other organizations that might contribute to the task of suicide prevention.

The chosen structure of the NaSPro includes actions on a horizontal level, which means for certain target groups such as adolescents, elderly etc., as well as a vertical level, comprising specific interventions, e. g. media initiatives, reducing availability of means. An executive group consists of experts and interested people; an independent scientific board (consisting of national as well as international experts that are not directly involved in the activities) guarantees the scientific basis.

The next step was the formulation of working groups, who focus their suicide-prevention work on specific risk groups, settings or structures. Currently, there are seventeen working groups, with topics including addiction, the elderly, networking, specific risk groups, primary prevention, the workplace, and the armed forces.

The working groups work independently, so progress in the different groups varies, as do the focus and the approaches to the task of suicide prevention. In this work, the WHO guidelines are utilized (WHO 2009).

## Activities

More than eighty organizations support the NaSPro and participate in different activities; with members of very different backgrounds and affiliations cooperating. There have been several conferences, and general meetings each year, of the NaSPro-initiative to coordinate and stimulate ongoing projects. Press conferences are organized in connection with the World Suicide Prevention Day on 10 September.

Another focus is the attempt to comprehend different training activities: a German academy for suicide prevention has been founded, one working group collects material concerning different educational activities that are already in existence, and works to improve training courses for various types of training. The Academy also provides material for the training of specific professional groups, such as nurses in old people's homes.

Other activities focus on the availability of means to commit suicide, e.g. car exhaust fumes, medications, registering hotspots.

The number of activities is large and comprises an enormous variety. The NaSPro is embedded in national as well as international structures, thus guaranteeing a constant exchange of expert opinions on different projects, and the rapid integration of new developments in suicide prevention. There is also considerable political support, including the federal committee on health in the German Bundestag.

## Conclusion

It is too early for conclusions at the moment, but we can say that the NaSPro is a very promising initiative, which has already increased public awareness, the general interest in suicide prevention in Germany, and among particular groups, to a considerable degree, which hopefully will be of value for the task of suicide prevention.

## References

German Association for Suicide Prevention (2009). Accessed at: http://www. suizidprophylaxe.de

NaSPro (2009). Accessed at: http://www.suizidpraevention-deutschland.de

WHO (2009). Accessed at: http://www.who.int/mental_health/resources/ suicide/en/

# CHAPTER 119

# Suicide prevention in Israel

Alan Apter and Cendrine Bursztein

In Israel, approximately 400–500 people commit suicide each year. In 2000, the Ministry of Health reported an incidence of 8.7 per 100,000 in individuals aged 15 years or more (Ministry of Health 2005). By gender, the rate was four times higher in men (14.2 per 100,000) than women (3.7 per 100,000). In 2002, the average annual number of emergency department visits for suicide attempts was 3600 (Ministry of Health 2005). More than one-third of these registered suicide attempts were committed by youth in the 15–24 age group. The figures for attempted suicide, however, may be grossly underestimated, given the known bias associated with reports from emergency room facilities.

Although Israel has been slow to recognize the value of a national suicide prevention programme compared to many countries in Europe, North America, and Oceania (Australia and New Zealand), recent developments are encouraging. Several governmental and non-governmental initiatives have been instituted by the Inter-Ministerial Committee for Suicide Prevention, Path to Life, a parent–professional alliance (http://www.path-to-life.org), and the Ministries of Health, Welfare and Education. Together, these are expected to lead to a concerted unified nationwide effort to build a national suicide prevention plan.

Even though Israel has not yet adopted an official suicide prevention plan, the Israel Defence Force (IDF) has taken a significant step toward this goal. These activities will be described below.

## National suicide prevention plan

A first draft of action has been presented to the Israeli Ministry of Health which includes the following components. These are planned to be assessed in pilot interventions:

1 Updated and detailed epidemiological database on suicide and attempted suicide. These data will provide professionals in Israel grounds for the study of the characteristics of populations at risk, frequency of suicide, methods of suicide, and hotspots on which prevention efforts should focus. They are also essential for estimating the effectiveness of the various interventions available.

2 Mental health and suicide awareness campaigns for the public and gatekeeper training for target groups. The following elements are planned:

- ◆ Education about depression and suicide for primary care physicians.
- ◆ Education for other gatekeepers (other health care professionals, religious functionaries, counsellors, policemen, teachers).
- ◆ Cooperation with the media and actions to raise public awareness, such as posters, cinema spots, leaflets, brochures, public events, and Internet sites.
- ◆ Support for high-risk groups and their families by self-help campaigns, parents' associations, crises centers, and direct access to professional help during crises (for example, by using 'emergency cards').

3 School-based prevention programmes. In Israel, the following programmes will be evaluated in pilot studies:

- ◆ The TeenScreen programme, which screens for students at risk and refers them to mental health professionals for treatment (Shaffer et al. 2004).
- ◆ Question, Persuade and Refer (QPR), a programme for training teachers and other school staff in recognizing students at risk of suicide or suffering from mental illness and referring them to treatment resources (Wyman et al. 2008).
- ◆ A skills-training programme for students, which emphasizes problem-solving, coping, and ognitive skills, as well as the reduction of such suicide risk factors as depression, hopelessness, and drug abuse (Gould et al. 2003).

4 Assessment of psychotherapies targeting suicidal individuals and provision of a better chain of care. Studies of treatments that target suicidality specifically, such as cognitive behavioural therapy (CBT) and dialectical behaviour therapy (DBT), are in the planning stages. Better follow-up care of suicide attempters after hospitalization is also needed to prevent repeated attempts.

5 Lethal-means restriction. In Israel, the most common method of suicide is weapons. The IDF has implemented several programmes to restrict the availability of firearms and other weapons, which will be described in detail below.

## Established suicide prevention actions in the Israel Defence Forces

During times of peace, suicide is the leading cause of death in the military in Israel. Military service in Israel is compulsory for all Jews and male Druze aged 18 years (Bleich *et al.* 1986). According to the Israel Ministry of Health, the male suicide rate is higher in the 18–24 age group than in the 15–17 age group, and highest in the 19–20 age group (193 per 100,000) (Ministry of Health 2005). Since 1990 an average of 35 IDF soldiers committed suicide annually (http://www.nrg.co.il/online/43/ART1/052/775.html).

In response to this problem, the IDF launched a suicide-prevention programme in 2006. Dr Lubin, the IDF officer in charge of the programme, provided the information for this chapter (personal communication). The design of the programme was based on the experience acquired from suicide-prevention plans in the United States Air Force (Knox *et al.* 2003), the Norwegian Army (Mehlum 2001), and the findings of a series of clinical psychological autopsy studies of suicide cases.

1   Primary prevention. Twelfth-grade high school students attend lectures on what to expect during their upcoming military service in order to reduce anxiety and uncertainty.

♦ New recruits have regular access to mental health officers during basic training, which continues during service. The army also conducts lectures on the subject for soldiers, and offers assistance for those who might need it.

♦ Commanders are provided gatekeeper training in recognizing the signs and symptoms of mental distress and dealing with suicidal ideation.

♦ Commanders are provided counsel and advice from health professionals regarding specific soldiers who are at risk.

♦ The army computer network offers an Intranet site with theoretical information on mental health and relevant practical activities for commanders.

♦ Commanders have access to the army's computerized records database which includes relevant personal information on soldiers (with consideration of medical ethics and the laws of individual privacy).

♦ New rules and regulations restrict the availability of lethal weapons during basic training and following service; soldiers are discouraged from taking weapons home during leave.

2   Secondary prevention. The army's Mental Health Service advises commanding officers on how to handle individual soldiers or specific crisis situations. It also provides soldiers with psychotherapy and pharmacotherapy by trained and licenced psychiatrists, clinical psychologists, and social workers.

3   Tertiary prevention. The military has adopted specific interventions to be put into practice when an individual soldier in crisis is identified. These include an interview of mental health professionals with the soldier's commander, removal of lethal weapons from the environment of the soldier, and close observation of the soldier until he or she is brought for psychiatric evaluation. In addition, the army network is connected to civilian helplines which provide assistance to soldiers in crisis.

In 2006, the first year of the programme, 26 soldiers committed suicide, representing a 20 per cent decrease compared to previous years. In 2007, only 14 soldiers committed suicide, a drastic decrease of 60 per cent compared to the years prior to 2006.

It is interesting to compare this decrease with that found following the United States Air Force (USAF) prevention programme put into action in 1997. Preliminary investigation showed that during the years 1994–1998, the suicide rate among USAF members decreased significantly, from 16.4 suicides per 100,000 to 9.4 (Litts *et al.* 2000). A later study found that implementation of the programme was associated with a sustained decline in the rate of suicide over a period of 6 years (33 per cent relative risk reduction) (Knox *et al.* 2003).

Although in Israel it is too early to conclude if the drop in suicides was a direct result of the new IDF suicide-prevention programme, the results are certainly encouraging.

## References

Bleich A, Chen E, Levy A (1986). Conflictual areas in the interaction between the Israeli adolescent and compulsory military service: a possible source of crisis situations. *Israel Journal of Psychiatry and Related Science*, **23**, 29–37.

Gould M, Greenberg T, Velting D *et al.* D (2003). Youth suicide risk and preventive interventions: a review of the past 10 years. *Journal of the American Academy of Child and Adolescent Psychiatry*, **42**, 386–405.

Knox KL, Litts DA, Talcott GW *et al.* (2003). Risk of suicide and related adverse outcomes after exposure to a suicide prevention programme in the US Air Force: cohort study. *BMJ*, **327**, 1376.

Litts DA, Moe K, Roadman CH *et al.* (2000). Suicide Integrated Product Team, United States Air Force, Dept of Defense. Division of Violence Prevention, National Center for Injury Prevention and Control, CDC. Suicide Prevention among Active Duty Air Force Personnel—United States, 1990–1999, *JAMA*, **283**, 193–194.

Mehlum L (2001). Effective suicide prevention in the military. In N Retterstøl N and MS Mortensen, eds, *Disasters and After Effects. Disaster Psychiatry in a Troubled World*, pp. 31–37. Atlantic Press, Oslo.

Ministry of Health (2005). http://www.gov.il/pages/default.asp?maincat=2&catid=3968&pageid=2707. In Hebrew.

Shaffer D, Scott M, Wilcox H *et al.* (2004). Screening high-school students for suicide risk. *Journal of the American Academy of Child and Adolescent Psychiatry*, **43**, 71–79.

Wyman PA, Brown C, Hendricks IJ *et al.* (2008). Randomized trial of a gatekeeper program for suicide prevention: 1-year impact on secondary school staff. *Journal of Consulting and Clinical Psychology*, **76**, 104–115.

# CHAPTER 120

# Suicide prevention in Italy

Marco Sarchiapone

National statistics on suicide deaths in Italy have been collected systematically from 1950 to 2003, which shows that the overall suicide rate has increased from 6 to 7 suicides per 100,000, with a slight gender imbalance, i.e. the female rate has decreased instead. In 2004, 3265 persons died due to suicide in Italy (Preti and Cascio 2006; ISTAT 2008).

According to the most recent available data, in Italy, the age and gender group with the highest rates of completed suicides are males aged 18–64. Completed suicides appear to be associated primarily to psychiatric disorders, and secondarily to physical illness; while if controlling for marital status, unmarried individuals carry higher rates of suicide (De Risio and Sarchiapone 2002).

Evidence from worldwide experience shows that national government plans often result in effective suicide prevention. Nevertheless, national prevention strategies have not been developed in Italy, and suicide prevention is delegated to non-governmental organizations, such as private agencies or associations, psychiatric associations and universities.

Therefore, to date several initiatives which address specific topics in suicide prevention exist, albeit they may not attain the comprehensiveness of a national prevention strategy.

Reasons for failed governmental support to suicide prevention may be the seemingly low suicide statistics compared to other European countries, but also the moral stigma of suicide that has been often associated with strong Catholic beliefs, reinforced in Italy by the presence of the Holy See within the State Capitol.

## Public awareness of depression and suicide risk

Initiatives aimed at preventing suicide are often channelled through prevention and treatment of depression, which is a high risk factor for attempting and completing suicide.

Continuous Medical Education (CME) courses for general practitioners on the treatment of depression, and prevention of suicide, have been locally organized by the University of Molise in 2006 and 2007.

The European Alliance Against Depression (EAAD) is also present and active in Italy in the Trentino region.

## The role of the media

In Italy, national broadcasting morning programmes include general psychological reports, where issues related to suicide may occasionally arise, especially linked to recent news on suicidal events that affect public opinion. Also, commercial psychological magazines, sold in kiosks, sometimes deal with psychiatric topics and suicide.

## Suicide prevention in schools

Although specific school programmes, which target suicidal crises or other psychiatric issues have not been implemented so far in Italian schools. A General Psychological consultation service for pupils, which addresses problems related to suicidal behaviour is available; though, this service is usually provided on request by students or teachers only once or twice a week. Nonetheless local initiatives have been started, with the aim of empowering psychological and psychiatric services in schools through specific programmes for detection and treatment of youth-related problems. This is the case with the Lecce school district, in southern Italy, where a programme for youth in distress which includes suicidal behaviours has been recently implemented. In some cases, schools are reached by university programmes and research projects, thus taking advantage of them, as is the case with the school district of Cagliari, Sardinia.

## Youth and suicide

Suicide is a major concern among youth in Italy, where suicide ratio for adolescents has been rising since 1950. Youth is, therefore, a primary target for interventions by several organizations and agencies. A foundation has been recently established for supporting distress of the young: 'Amico Charlie'. Its main headquarters are in Milan, and its main goal is to take care of young patients who are admitted for attempting suicide to the Fatebenefratelli Hospital of Milan. It also consists of a crisis centre for adolescents who display self-harm behaviours, and offers a counselling service for parents, teachers and survivors of suicide. It has an efficient, updated and helpful website (http://www.amicocharlie.it) where advice can be found on the treatment of suicidal behaviours, including what has to be done in case a specific referral for suicidal youth is needed. The foundation also organizes seminars and courses for teachers and social workers on recognizing early signs of suicidal risk in adolescents.

## The elderly and suicide

In Trieste, a private organization called 'Progetto Amalia' has been established, with the aim of specifically managing the distress of the elderly. Among its manifold targets, prevention of suicidal behaviours of the elderly is pre-eminent, and includes the 'Telefono Speciale' programme, which provides a telephone helpline with a toll-free number that offers service 24 hours a day. Telephone operators are not mental health professionals, but have received specific training for managing suicidal individuals and referring them to local mental health facilities. The organization was established as a private initiative of a local television company, but it is currently funded by the Italian Ministry of Health.

## Reducing access to lethal means and methods of self-harm

In Italy, firearms are lawfully sold only to individuals with a specific licence, with a mandatory psychiatric consultation when requesting such a licence. Psychoactive drugs are only sold with a prescription, which expires after three provisions. These well-established rules are intended to restrict access to common methods used for suicidal and self-harming behaviours (World Health Organization 2002, 2007, 2008).

## Suicide units and associations

The WHO, through its WHO/EURO Network on Suicide Prevention and Research, has been collecting data on attempted suicide from the catchment area of Molise, and previously, in the catchment area of Padua and Rome. Recently in 2007, the WHO's resource material *Preventing suicide in jails and prisons* has been translated into Italian (World Health Organization 2000).

The Italian Psychiatric Association comprises a section for the 'Study and treatment of suicidal behaviour', and the psychiatric clinic of the University of Padua has established an Association for 'Study and Prevention of Suicide' linked to the Section. The association's scientific aims comprise of the promotion of knowledge on suicide among physicians and in society. A scientific journal, both in Italian and English—*Studies on aggression and suicide*—publishes research articles on the biology and psychopathology of aggression and suicidal behaviours.

## References

De Risio S and Sarchiapone M (2002). Il suicidio. *Aspetti biologici, psicologici e sociali.* [Suicide-Biological, Psychological and social aspects.] Masson Publishing, Milan, Italy.

ISTAT (Istituto Nazionale di Statistica)(2008). Statistiche giudiziarie penali, anno 2003 e 2004. *National Institute of Statistics (2008). Penal Judiciary Statistics, year 2003 and 2004.*

Preti A and Cascio MT (2006). Prison suicides and self-harming behaviours in Italy, 1990–2002. *Medical Science and Law*, **46**, 127–134.

World Health Organization (2000). *Preventing Suicide: A Resource for Prison Officers.* World Health Organization, Geneva.

World Health Organization (2002). *Suicide Prevention in Europe. The WHO European Monitor Survey on National Suicide Prevention Programmes and Strategies.* World Health Organization, Geneva.

World Health Organization (2007). *The Prevention of Suicide.* Accessed at: http://www.who.int/mental_health/resources/resource_jails_prisons_italian.pdf.

World Health Organization (2008). *Suicide Prevention (SUPRE).* Accessed at: http://www.who.int/mental_health/prevention/suicide/suicideprevent/en/.

# CHAPTER 121

# Suicide prevention in Romania

Doina Cozman

Romania, located in south-eastern Europe, has 41 counties and the District of Bucharest, with a population in 2000 of 21.7 millions, 45 per cent of whom reside in rural settings. Loss of financial stability during the transition to free market economy is a characteristic of contemporary Romanian society. Dramatic shifts within the 1990s have generated interest in mental health and prevention in psychiatry, which includes the legislative Mental Health Law, which was passed through Parliament in 2002 (Jané-Llopis and Anderson 2006). Reporting suicide statistics to the WHO, which was banned during the communist regime, became possible after the political changes in December 1989 (Schmidtke *et al.* 2004).

Suicide statistics were not reported to the international medical or political structures, a 'strategy', which was employed to cover up the sad reality that the totalitarian regime restricted human rights (Cozman 2004).

## Suicide rates

The National Institute of Forensic Medicine supplies statistics on suicidal behaviour and death by suicide. Since 1994, Romania has reported overall suicide rates to the WHO: in 1994 they were 12.7 per 100,000 population, (Schmidtke *et al.* 1999), 14.64 in 2006, and 13.38 in 2007 (National Institute of Forensic Medicine 'Mina Minovici' 1999, 2007, 2008).

## Geographical variations

The suicide rates differ from one region to another. In order to fully understand the specific significance of geographical variations in suicide rates within Romania, population data and the ethnic background of some counties (mainly in Transylvania), must be taken into consideration (Romanian National Institute of Statistics 2007). Thus, the Hungarian minority is well-represented in counties like Harghita and Covasna, where the rates of suicide, both for males and females, have constantly been the highest in Romania. Since 1993, in Harghita, which is regarded as the county with the highest incidence of fatalities by suicide, rates higher than 30 per 100,000 were recorded every year, with a peak of 38.45 per 100,000 in 1993 (Veress 1997); however, most counties with low suicide rates have a compact Romanian ethnic population (more than 95 per cent).

## Gender distribution

In 2007, the male:female ratio of suicide in Romania was 3.44:1 (National Institute of Forensic Medicine 'Mina Minovici' 2008). A continuous increase in male suicide rates (from 16.3 to 22.5 per 100,000) was reported between 1994 and 2003, both in urban and rural settings. This might originate in the dynamics of Romanian labor market—unemployment, insecure jobs, and unsuccessful emigration for employment—which may acccount for the increased suicide risk in subjects experiencing such pressures. Suicide among the 40–59 age group (from 26 to 39.9 per 100,000 populations) and the 60–79 age group (from 26.3 to 33.3 suicides per 100,000) underwent the most dramatic increase. Meanwhile, female suicides decreased slightly (from 5.5 to 4.6 per 100,000). Data from a study conducted during 1984–1998 in the county of Cluj suggests that suicide in elderly women is twice as frequent as in women under 40 (Cozman 2004).

The age group 65+ has the highest suicide rate in Romania, which derives from underlying social issues and ramifications (Cozman 2006).

Suicide among adolescents is an insufficiently known and poorly acknowledged issue. Recent Romanian epidemiological studies suggest that incidence of suicide in teenagers is approximately 3/100,000, which raises questions concerning the accuracy of reports on the causes of death in this age group (Cozman 1999).

According to data reported to the WHO within the last decade, total rates of suicide in Romanian population in the 15–29 age group remain relatively constant, i.e. 13.5 per cent of total suicide cases recorded per year, with a male:female ratio of 6:1. The gap between sexes is the highest in the 25–29 age group, and gradually decreases towards adolescence, with reported rates of female and male suicide as being almost equal for the 15–19 age group (Romanian Executive Authority for Youth 2005).

## Methods of suicide

Methods employed in 2007 were: hanging (79.75 per cent), self-poisoning (9.31 per cent), drowning (2.54 per cent), jumping (2.54 per cent), self-cutting (2.08 per cent), burning oneself (1.27 per cent), firearms (0.54 per cent), electrocution (0.35 per cent), etc. (National Institute of Forensic Medicine 'Mina Minovici' 2008).

## Suicide prevention in Romania

The Final Report of the European Review of Suicide and Violence Epidemiology Project provided post-communist Romania with state-of-the-art approach on adequate suicide reporting and monitoring, which is the first step in any effective national suicide-prevention programme (Stone *et al.* 2002).

The Law for Mental Health and Protection of persons with mental disorders includes provisions for suicide prevention, i.e. appropriate institutional structures for primary and secondary prevention of suicidal behaviour (mental health centres, daycare hospitals, crisis intervention centres), 72-hour emergency psychiatric treatment for persons with deliberate self-harm without consent of the patient, and assessment of the necessity for ongoing treatment by a commission of three psychiatrists after 72 hours (Official Monitor 2002).

Unfortunately, there is no specific suicide-prevention programme; however, current mental health prevention programmes have an indirect impact on suicide prevention in Romania (World Health Organization 2002, Jané-Llopis and Anderson 2006):

1 *Community mental health programmes.* The National Prevention Programme for psychiatric and psychosocial disorders and the National Health Insurance Fund are the two main mental health budget sources. Promoting reform of the health care system, improvement of health care services, diagnostic procedures, treatment, follow-up and rehabilitation in cases with psychiatric disorders of suicide attempters, and developing medical staff awareness on attitudes and taboos about suicide are all components of those programmes. Public health actions focus on social de-stigmatization and population/target-group training on early intervention in stress and psychiatric disorders.

2 *Crisis lines.* Independent crisis lines, based on volunteer work, started in Romania (The Anti Suicide Alliance in Cluj-Napoca, Cry for Help in Miercurea Ciuc) after the fall of the communist regime. They respond without discrimination, and provide counselling for negative life events, give confidentiality and specific information on suicidal risk and other mental health issues (drug and alcohol addiction), including raising awareness.

The non-governmental organization (NGO) Anti-Suicide Alliance (ASA) provides volunteer services (also at night) in suicide prevention and crisis intervention. A Suicide Crisis Centre in Cluj-Napoca was established to improve the quality of life in central Transylvania. The ASA ensures psychological counselling by phone using its LIFE LINE service. Cry for Help is an NGO with effective prevention activities for Harghita (the Romanian county with the highest suicide rates).

3 *Relationship with mass-media.* NGOs have initiated actions for implementing good practice standards for media coverage of suicide on 10 September, World Suicide Prevention Day. The topic has also been debated in Romanian psychiatric congresses and symposia within the past two years.

4 Local educational initiatives involve:

 ◆ parenting programmes;

 ◆ crisis management;

 ◆ promoting healthy lifestyles;

 ◆ the elderly;

 ◆ children with increased social vulnerability (institutionalized, abused, with parents in detention).

5 Restricting availability of suicide methods is extended by:

 ◆ controlling the prescription and selling of pharmaceuticals through regulations imposed by the Ministry of Health;

 ◆ laws restricting the possession and use of firearms and ammunition.

### Training for health care and mental health services

Various programmes, mostly for family practitioners, psychiatric personnel and volunteers, are designed to improve health care (World Health Organization 2002). Training of mental health personnel is provided by medical, psychology and social work colleges. There are 4.2 psychiatrists, approximately 1000 psychologists and 2000 nurses (including psychiatric nurses) per 100,000 inhabitants in Romania.

### Challenges and obstacles

Although a strategic and legislative background exists, adequate training and funding of effective infrastructure for implementing programmes are a challenging task. Effective prevention requires expanding training programmes. There is no National Institute to coordinate reporting, monitoring, assessment and research of suicide. The Romanian health care system can not yet provide effective management of patients, with increased suicide risk, who require long-term treatment in psychiatric units.

### Opportunities for progress

In the region of Transylvania, The Anti-Suicide Alliance is involved in preventive actions: e.g. crisis lines, volunteer training, crisis intervention and counselling, research, public information/awareness actions and workshops. The Centre for Psychological Counseling of the University Babes-Bolyai provides training in violence prevention for parents, teachers and health personnel. The Romanian League for Mental Health supports mental health promotion projects. Also, the Twinning Light Partnership Programme, between the Romanian and Dutch Ministries of Health, has improved the training programme for medical staff in mental health services.

## Conclusion

Some steps have been taken in Romania in order to ensure adequate monitoring, reporting and assessment of suicide behaviour. A legislative and strategic background has emerged, and comprehensive programmes have been developed in the field of mental health during the post-communist years. However, the vast majority of initiatives are mental health prevention strategies, with an indirect impact on suicide prevention. Direct approaches in suicide prevention are few, and mostly initiated locally by NGOs.

### References

Cozman D (1999). *Suicide. A Biopsychosocial study.* Risoprint Publishing House, Cluj-Napoca.

Cozman D (2004). Suicide in Romania. In E Sorel and D Prelipceanu, eds, *WPA: Images of Psychiatry in Romania. 21st Century Romanian Psychiatry*, pp. 84–95. Infomedica Publishing House, Bucharest.

Cozman D (2006). *Synopsis of Suicidology*, pp. 50–74. Science Book Publishing House, Cluj-Napoca.

Jané-Llopis E and Anderson P (eds) (2006). *Mental Health Promotion and Mental Disorder Prevention Across European Member States: A Collection of Country Stories.* European Communities, Luxembourg.

National Institute of Forensic Medicine 'Mina Minovici' (1999). *Report on the Activity of the Romanian Network of Forensic Medicine for the Year1998.* Accessed at: http://www.legmed.ro.

National Institute of Forensic Medicine 'Mina Minovici' (2007). *Report on the Activity of the Romanian Network of Forensic Medicine for the Year 2006.* Accessed at: http://www.legmed.ro.

National Institute of Forensic Medicine 'Mina Minovici' (2008). *Report on the Activity of the Romanian Network of Forensic Medicine for the Year 2007.* Accessed at: http://www.legmed.ro.

Official Monitor (2002). Law no. 487 of 11/07/2002 on Mental Health and the Protection of Individuals that Present Psychic Disorders. Accessed at: http://www.ms.ro.

Romanian Executive Authority for Youth (2005). *National Action Plan for Youth.* Accessed at: http://www.e-tineret.ro.

Romanian National Institute of Statistics (2007). *Romanian Statistical Annual for 2006.* Accessed at: http://www.insse.ro/cms/rw/pages/index.ro.do.

Schmidtke A, Weinacker B, Apter A *et al.* (1999). Suicide rates in the world: update. *Archives of Suicide Research*, **5**, 81–89.

Schmidtke A, Bille-Brahe U, DeLeo D *et al.* (eds) (2004). *Suicidal Behaviour in Europe. Results from the WHO/EURO Multicentre Study on Suicidal Behaviour.* Hogrefe and Huber Publishers, Gottingen.

Stone DH, Chishti P, Roulston C *et al.* (2002). *Final Report of the European Review of Suicide and Violence Epidemiology (EUROSAVE). Part of the Injury Prevention programme of the European Commission.* Agreement reference no. VS/1999/5300(99CVF3-316), project reference no. 1999/IPP/1021 (UK). Available at http://www.euro-save.com.

Veress A (1997). Epidemiological, clinical, therapeutical and preventive issues in suicide in Harghita County, Romania. Dissertation Thesis, University of Medicine, Targu Mures, Romania.

World Health Organization (2002). *Suicide Prevention in Europe. The WHO European Monitoring Survey on National Suicide Prevention Programmes and Strategies.* World Health Organization, Geneva.

# CHAPTER 122

# Suicide prevention in Russia

Valery Krasnov and Vladimir Voitsekh

## Introduction

The suicide rate is considered a statistically stable phenomenon for certain countries, regions and ethnicities. However, recently suicide rates have been increasing all over the world, especially among young people. Moreover, they are the prevalent cause of death in the 15–34 age group (World Health Organization 2001). In this sense, Russia is no different from other countries. Suicide is the fifth cause of all deaths in this country, and this fact calls for preventive measures.

On the basis of suicide rate, the WHO has recognized Russia as a country in an emergency situation, and the noticeable correlations between the prevalence of suicides and homicides seems to confirm this statement.

## Suicidality in Russia

At the end of the nineteenth century, different authors estimated the number of suicides in Russia as 3–3.3 per 100,000 inhabitants. At the beginning of the twentieth century, the suicide rate increased, which could be due to the political crisis at that time with protest actions and divisions within the society. In the 1920s, the suicide rate in Russia did not exceed 10 per 100,000, and was among the lowest in Europe during that time. After the 'Khrushchev Thaw', the suicide rate approached the average European level. Subsequently, during the period from the mid-1960s to the mid-1980s, the number of suicides increased, especially among men, and reached its maximum in 1984 ('the stagnation peak'), when Russia exhibited the second highest level of suicides after Hungary. At the time of Gorbachev's perestroika, the suicide rate decreased sharply, and coincided with his anti-alcohol campaign, as well as the country's recovery from economic, political and social stagnation. Wasserman and Varnik (Wasserman *et al.* 1994, Wasserman and Värnik 2001) connected this change principally with the reduced consumption of alcohol.

However, after 1988, the suicide rate gradually increased, and reached a peak in 1994 at 42.4 per 100,000. Those years were characterized by political, social and economic crises and unemployment, which were the risk factors mentioned in the WHO Report (World Health Organization 2001). Another peak of suicides coincided within the timeframe of the financial crisis in August 1998.

Late 1998 was not characterized so much by the increase of suicides committed, but rather by the pronounced increase in the number of suicide attempts (especially in Moscow) among the recently prosperous businessmen and their families (Figure 122.1).

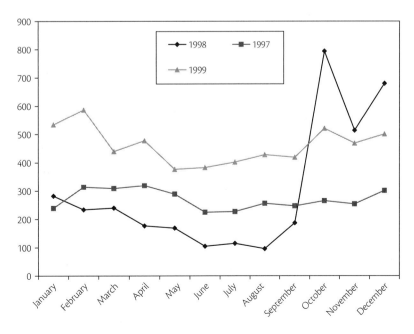

**Fig. 122.1** Suicide attempts in Moscow during the period of defaults.

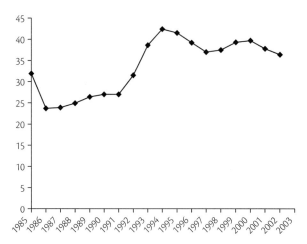

**Fig. 122.2** The suicide rate in Russia 1985–2003.

Furthermore, the number of suicide attempts among young people under 20 increased threefold.

Economic instability, significant impoverishment among majority of people, and disappointment in the state policy and authorities brought about psychological instability within society, which was accompanied by dramatic shifts in the number of suicides during the last two decades (Figure 122.2).

In the latter years, the total suicide rate in Russia shows a slight tendency to decrease.

However, suicide rates differ immensely among various regions. For example, in 2005, the suicide rate in Russia was 32.4 per 100,000 population. However, the figures in different regions broke down as follows: 9.3 in Moscow; 15.2 in St Petersburg; 24.4 in the Kursk region (Central Russia); 72.2 in the Chita region (Far East); 4.7 in Dagestan Republic (South Russia); and 51.1 in the Archangelsk region (North Russia). In general, suicide rates in Russia increase from the South to the North, and from the West to East. Moreover, the increased proportion of suicides in younger people in the 15–34 age group was registered during the last years.

The analysis of gender differences shows changes in the male:female suicide ratio, which seem to be associated with developments in the country, and is predominantly presented by changes in the male suicide rate. Thus, in 1924, the male:female ratio was 1.8:1, in 1975 it was at 4.5:1, followed by 4.9:1 in 1994, and 5.2:1 in 2004. In the city of Moscow, this ratio fluctuates within a range of 2.9:1 to 2.6:1.

## Social and economic factors

The male population of Russia reacts to social and economic changes by higher rates of suicide than women. According to Nemtsov (2001), a possible explanation could be an increasing rate of alcohol consumption (mainly in men). Though this correlation is pronounced, the matter seems to be more complicated than just direct impact of alcohol. Rapid changes in Russia, the aftermath of well-known ecological disasters (Chernobyl, for example), local military actions and ethnic conflicts, migration processes, disrupted social connections, changes in lifestyle, living circumstances, and unemployment, inevitably influence the mental health of the population and restrict individual capacities for social adjustment.

The high rate of suicides in the last decades coincided with very high mortality rates, especially from cardiovascular disorders.

The age structure of suicides in Russia differs significantly from the worldwide average. In Russia, the mortality curve has two age-related peaks: in the 45–55 and 80+ age groups, while the average suicide profile has one peak in the middle age.

## Suicide prevention

A methodological research centre for preventive suicidology was established during the former Soviet Union era, at the Moscow Research Institute of Psychiatry, in 1980. Its main task was to study the problem of suicide and prepare recommendations for clinical institutions. In 1995, the Ministry of Public Health issued an order for the organization of suicidology centres in large cities. Each of them should consist of: a 'phone of trust' (hotline), a crisis department within general hospitals, and units for social–psychological aid in outpatient clinics (general as well as psychiatric). However, the order was not financially supported. Due to the absence of a federal programme on suicide prevention, such centres were only established in some cities and regions, mostly without a number of recommended components. In some regions, the initiatives of specialists are supported by local authorities. For example, consequent work on suicide prevention was carried out in one of the biggest universities—Bauman Moscow Technical University—in cooperation between the Moscow Research Institute of Psychiatry and the administration of University (Voitsech 2007).

### References

Nemtsov A (2001). *Mortality caused by alcohol in Russia, 1980–90*, p. 60. (In Russian). Moscow Resarch Institute, Moscow.

Voitsech V (2007). *Suicidology*, p. 277. (In Russian). Miklosh, Moscow.

Wasserman D, Varnik A, Eklund G (1994). Male suicides and alcohol consumption in the former USSR. *Acta Psychiatrica Scandinavica*, **89**, 306–313.

Wasserman D and Varnik A (2001). Perestroika in the former USSR: history's most effective suicide-preventive programme for men. In D Wasserman, ed., *Suicide—An Unnecessary Death*, pp. 253–257. Martin Dunitz, London.

World Health Organization (2001). Mental *Health: New Understanding, New Hope. World Health Report*. World Health Organization, Geneva.

# CHAPTER 123

# Suicide prevention in Scotland

Jacki Gordon and Gregor Henderson

## Choose Life: Scotland's suicide preventive strategy

Choose Life (Scottish Executive 2002)—Scotland's 10-year suicide prevention strategy and action plan—was launched in December 2002 in direct response to national and local concerns over the increasing suicide rate at that time: while female rates had remained fairly stable over the preceding 30 years, male suicides had more than doubled (Platt *et al.* 2006).

By international standards, the suicide rate in Scotland is not exceptionally high (European age standardized rate of 15.1 per 100,000 over 2004–2006; population 5.12 million), but it is about twice as high as that for England and Wales (Platt *et al.* 2006).

Choose Life calls for suicide prevention activities to be undertaken as one core part of wider public health actions and policies and asserts suicide prevention to be the 'shared responsibility' of public, private and voluntary agencies. It endorses the importance of partnership-working, effective coordination and leadership, and the value of combining population approaches (to reduce the risk conditions that lead to heightened vulnerability and increase protective factors) with targeting of identified populations, groups and communities who are at heightened risk (Scottish Executive 2002). The strategy's original key objectives and priority groups are detailed in the Boxes below.

---

**Box 123.1** Choose Life's key objectives

- Early prevention and intervention
- Responding to immediate crisis
- Longer-term work to provide hope and support recovery
- Coping with suicidal behaviour and completed suicide
- Promoting greater public awareness and encouraging people to seek help early
- Supporting the media
- Knowing what works

---

**Box 123.2** Choose Life's priority groups

- Children (especially looked after children)
- Young people (especially young men)
- People with mental health problems
- People who have attempted suicide
- People affected by the aftermath of suicidal behaviour or completed suicide
- People who abuse substances
- People in prison

---

## Implementation of Choose Life

As part of its work on improving public health and well-being and on addressing inequalities and promoting social inclusion, the Scottish Government created a National Programme for Improving Mental Health and Wellbeing (http://www.wellscotland.info). Thus Choose Life is integrated within and complemented by a broader public health approach to mental health (Platt 2003).

It is recommended that national suicide-prevention strategies should have a body or agency to coordinate implementation (United Nations 1996). Accordingly, Choose Life has a National Implementation Support Team (NIST) which is responsible for supporting national and local agencies to achieve the Government's aims and objectives for suicide prevention.

Choose Life is being implemented in identifiable phases, the first spanning 2003–2006, the second from 2006–2008, with the third phase currently being planned for 2008–2011. From the outset, there was a clear vision for what should be achieved over the initial first three-year period.

In its first phase, £12 million was allocated to Choose Life activity. Of this, £3 million was reserved for national-led action, with the remaining £9 million dispersed across each of Scotland's 32 local authority (i.e. local government) areas to help support local suicide prevention action as part of community planning partnership activity.

The Government issued national guidance to local areas to direct their activity. This guidance stated that each area should: coordinate, develop and implement local suicide-prevention action plans tailored to local needs; engender engagement and innovation among local voluntary organisations, community-based and self-help initiatives; and develop and implement capacity building and training. In addition, each area was required to nominate (or appoint) a local suicide prevention coordinator to support and drive local action, and to be the key point of contact for NIST.

For its part, NIST has four key functions, broadly defined as information collection and dissemination, operational support, training, and marketing. Thus first, NIST provides national and local epidemiological data on suicides; collects and disseminates knowledge and evidence on research, practice and effectiveness of interventions; and has established a Suicide Information and Research Evidence Network (SIREN) so that researchers, policy planners and practitioners can learn from each other. Second, NIST draws on international, national and local thinking, evidence and experience and provides: development support to national and local organizations; and operational support to local areas (including giving feedback, encouragement, advice, and tangible support with action plans). Next, NIST coordinates a Scotland-wide training strategy to support the developments and national roll out of suicide prevention training. Finally, through its marketing and communication strategy, NIST raises public awareness and understanding about suicide prevention. As part of this, it has developed and maintains the Choose Life website (http://www.chooselife. net). This is an information and education resource for anyone with an interest in suicide and its prevention, and is Scotland's key portal for information on this issue.

## Evaluation of Choose Life

An extensive independent national evaluation of Choose Life was commissioned to monitor the progress being made over its first phase. Specifically, the Scottish evaluation aimed to identify whether a sustainable infrastructure was being developed to address the longer-term objectives set out in Choose Life, review progress in achieving its milestones and make recommendations to guide future implementation.

A defining feature of the national evaluation was its (deliberately) formative nature. Thus, the Scottish Government, NIST, together with identified local coordinators, and other key stakeholders worked collaboratively with the evaluation team. This meant that both Government and NIST were made aware of *emerging* findings (in part through the availability of an interim report) and consequently were able to reflect on the implications of these prior to the full report becoming available, and to use these to inform the next set of Government policy and guidance issued to local areas for phase two (when a further £3.2 million per year was provided for local activity, and £1 million per year for NIST-led support action).

In its final report, the evaluation concluded that considerable progress has been made towards establishing the kind of infrastructure which the Government and its partners set out to achieve.

> Choose Life has provided a powerful, unprecedented rallying call to bring partners together in order to expedite cross-sectoral planning and action to tackle suicide prevention as part of a (national) mental health improvement agenda.
>
> Platt *et al.* (2006, p. 142)

The evaluation was required to make recommendations to help guide future national and local activity. By and large these centred on:

- How suicide prevention might be sustained and mainstreamed more in the future;
- How action might be targeted in a more focused manner (e.g. to minimize duplication of effort);
- Ensuring an inequalities focus (as socio-economic deprivation and low socio-economic status are strongly associated with suicides in Scotland);
- Better local use of evidence and evidence-based approaches (and more use of evaluation); and
- Strengthened involvement of clinical and substance misuse services.

## Building on the findings from the evaluation

A number of steps were taken to ensure that the findings from this evaluation informed policy and practice. First, the Government's strategic advisor and National Programme Director prepared a written response to the evaluation which mapped out how the Scottish Executive (now the Scottish Government) would respond to each of the recommendations. In doing so, this document signalled Choose Life's direction of travel for its next phase, and crucially, specified how the suicide prevention agenda would become more integrated within and further advanced through existing and new government policies and plans, e.g. by including specific actions in Scotland's mental health service delivery plan (which sets out targets for the development of mental health services in Scotland for 2007–2010) including a commitment to educate and train 50 per cent of key front line mental health services, primary care and accident and emergency staff in suicide assessment and prevention by 2010 (Scottish Executive 2006). Second, a series of roadshows were run across the country to which Choose Life coordinators were invited along with a delegation of up to six local stakeholders who they considered pivotal to sustaining or mainstreaming suicide-prevention action in local areas. At each roadshow, these stakeholders considered the implications for local action of both the evaluation and the government response to it, and the issues they raised were summarized in a report. In this way, the responses of local stakeholders not only become part of the "national record", but also, part of the *process* that informs thinking about implementation in the future.

## Progress five years into the implementation of Choose Life

At the time of writing this chapter, we are at the halfway mark in the strategy's implementation. We believe that Choose Life has continued to build on the demonstrable progress that was evidenced by the evaluation, and that the combination of Government policy, and national and local action is maintaining a high profile for suicide prevention, and ensuring that activity is mainstreamed and sustained. For example: all local areas now have plans on how to continue their local suicide prevention actions in the future; there is agreement to integrate the NIST functions into Scotland's principal public health delivery organisation (NHS Health Scotland); international reviews have been commissioned on effective interventions and determinants of suicide and suicidal behaviours; NIST has created high quality marketing materials for local use; over 11,000 people in Scotland have now participated in Applied Suicide Intervention Skills Training (ASIST) and an evaluation of the impact of this is progressing; as previously mentioned, there is now a commitment across the National Health Service in Scotland to train half of key front line staff in suicide prevention over the next three years; SIREN is successfully bringing together an extremely diverse range of stakeholders to hear and discuss the evidence base for suicide prevention; and there is now evidence of improved linkage and involvement with clinical and substance misuse services at national and local levels.

Of course, what matters is whether Choose Life is effective in saving lives, and we know that Choose Life will have been cost saving if it saves five additional lives a year (Platt *et al.* 2006).

Between 2000–02 and 2004–06, Scotland's suicide rate fell by 13%. We hope that this marks the start of a sustained downward trend.

## References

Platt S (2003). Tackling suicide in Scotland: a national strategy and action plan. *Journal of Mental Health Promotion*, **2**, 40–48.

Platt S, McLean J, McCollam A et al. (2006). *Evaluation of the First Phase of Choose Life: The National Strategy and Action Plan to Prevent Suicide in Scotland*. Scottish Executive Social Research, Edinburgh.

Scottish Executive (2002). *Choose Life: A National Strategy and Action Plan to Prevent Suicide in Scotland*. Scottish Executive, Edinburgh.

Scottish Executive (2006). *Delivering for Mental Health*. Scottish Executive, Edinburgh.

United Nations (1996). *The Prevention of Suicide: Guidelines for the Formulation and Implementation of National Strategies*. United Nations, New York.

# CHAPTER 124

# Suicide prevention in Sweden

Danuta Wasserman, Ana Nordenskiöld,
Inga-Lill Ramberg and Camilla Wasserman

## Background

Suicide and attempted suicide are still surrounded by feelings of guilt, shame, fear and unease. These acts are often incorrectly perceived as being predestined and impossible to prevent. Suicide among men in the 15–44 age group is the most common cause of death in Sweden. For females in the same age group, suicide is the second most common cause of death after tumours.

A suicidal act is not only a drastic example of difficulties in coping with the hardships of life and mental problems, but it is also a frequent indicator of how the health care and public health systems and ordinary fellow human beings fail to respond in an adequate manner to suicidal people. The responses encountered by suicidal individuals seeking care are a measure of quality, not only of medical and psychological care services, but also of the psychosocial conditions in society.

Ambiguous attitudes towards preventive measures and the persistent taboo surrounding suicide, as well as the attitude that suicide is a human right, make suicide-preventive activities necessary. In 1993, the Riksdag (the Swedish Parliament) stated that a country wishing to embark on active efforts to prevent suicide needs to have a national programme, as well as an institution for activities of this kind.

## Sweden's first national suicide-prevention programme, 1995

Research in suicidology has always been strong in Sweden. It started with the activities of Ruth Ettlinger (Ettlinger 1975), who not only initiated research on suicide prevention in Sweden, but was also a co-founder of the organization that later became the International Association for Suicide Prevention (IASP). Many researchers provided a scientific basis for a Swedish National Programme:

- *Biological studies* performed at the Karolinska University Hospital by Marie Åsberg with co-workers, as well as at Lund University Hospital by Lil Träskman-Bendz with co-workers;

- *Sociomedical suicidological studies* by Jan Beskow and his Gothenburg group, using the psychological autopsy method;

- *Socio-epidemiological studies* conducted by Lars Jacobsson and his group at Umeå University;

- *Evaluation of the educational programme for GPs* on the island of Gotland by Wolfgang Rutz and co-workers;

- *Studies in child and adolescent psychiatry* by Anne-Liis von Knorring and co-workers at Uppsala University and by Per-Anders Rydelius and his co-workers at the Karolinska Institute;

- *Psychodynamic and genetic studies* carried out by Danuta Wasserman's research group at Karolinska Institute, in which studies of the suicidal process are performed within a broad concept of the stress–vulnerability model, including research on the role of interplay between genes and environment in suicidal behaviours.

Without this extensive scientific basis, the suicide-preventive measures undertaken in Sweden would not have been feasible.

A broad consensus prevails among Sweden's leading researchers that suicidal behaviour needs to be prevented, not only in biological terms, but also by psychosocial and psychological measures. This expert consensus led to a parliament resolution to meet the national need for knowledge and development in the field of suicide prevention, which in 1994, resulted in the creation of the National Centre for Suicide Research and Prevention of Mental Ill-Health (NASP) at the National Institute for Psychosocial Medicine (IPM), Karolinska Institute (KI) in Stockholm. NASP, headed by Danuta Wasserman, became integrated with Stockholm County Council's regional centre for suicide research and prevention, which was established in 1993. Danuta Wasserman holds the first European chair of psychiatry and suicidology at Karolinska Institute.

The first step in developing a first national strategy was to set up the Swedish National Council for Suicide Prevention. The Council for Suicide Prevention comprised of representatives from the Federation of County Councils, the Swedish Association of Local Authorities, the Armed Forces, the National Police Board, the Central Board of the Church of Sweden, and journalists, all under the auspices of the Swedish National Board of Health and Welfare, the National Institute of Public Health and NASP.

In 1995, the first Swedish national programme to develop suicide prevention, Support in Suicidal Crises, was published (National Council for Suicide Prevention 1995). The programme was inspired by the United Nations meeting in Canada in 1993, (Ramsay and Tanney 1996) at which NASP was represented, and the Finnish programme for suicide prevention (National Research and Development Centre for Welfare and Health 1993). NASP being the government's expert in suicide prevention, together with the Swedish National Board of Health and Welfare and the National Institute of Public Health, has been responsible for monitoring and evaluating the implementation of the Swedish programme. This first suicide-prevention programme in Sweden was a product of public authorities, but was never presented for ratification by the Swedish parliament. This was a drawback for the implementation process, since the preventive activities were limited to relying on the good will of individual people, organizations and authorities.

In December 1997, NASP initiated six regional networks for suicide prevention in Sweden. For each region, a management group whose composition reflected the ambition of cross-sectorial work in suicide prevention, was appointed. A national network conference for suicide prevention in various regions of Sweden is held biennially (in Stockholm in 1997, Umeå in 1999, Uppsala in 2001, Stockholm 2003, Jönköping 2005, Gothenburg 2007, and Malmö 2009). In each region, a professor of adult or child/adolescent psychiatry heads the steering group together with representatives of the public health, volunteer and survivor sectors.

NASP has been involved in the establishing of sister institutions in other countries. In February 1993, the Swedish–Estonian Institute (ERSI) in Tallinn was created. The same kind of collaboration has, since 2000, been ongoing with Ukraine (Mechnikov Odessa National University), Vietnam (Hanoi Medical University), and Uganda (Kampala, Makerere University and Gulu University) and with many other research groups throughout the world.

NASP has an advisory function in the WHO Multisite Intervention Study on Suicidal Behaviours (SUPRE-MISS), and is a WHO Europe Lead Collaborating Centre concerning Prevention of Suicide and Mental Ill-Health, and also acts as an advisor to European Union Programmes on Improving Mental Health (European Commission 2005).

## The second national suicide-prevention programme in Sweden, 2008

Following the WHO Mental Health Declaration 2005 (WHO 2005), the Swedish government decided in 2005 that a more comprehensive National Programme for Suicide Prevention to be ratified by the Swedish Parliament should be created.

Consequently, during 2006–2007, the National Board for Health and Welfare, the National Institute of Public Health, with support from NASP, and other regional suicide preventive networks in Sweden and relevant organizations, prepared a new programme with the following nine strategies (Socialstyrelsen [The National Board of Health and Welfare] and Statens Folkhälsoinstitut [Swedish National Public Health Institute] 2006):

1   To promote better life opportunities in order to support the groups that are most at need;

2   To minimize alcohol consumption in target and high-risk groups;

3   To reduce the availability of means to commit suicide;

4   To educate gatekeepers about effective management of persons with suicide risk;

5   To support medical, psychological and psychosocial services in preventing suicide;

6   To disseminate knowledge about evidence-based methods for reducing suicide;

7   To raise the competence of health care personnel;

8   To systematically analyse within the frame of the National Board for Health and Welfare, all suicides which occur in the health care system during care and 28 days after discharge from the hospital, so-called 'Lex Maria' regulation;

9   To support voluntary organizations.

In the spring of 2008, the Swedish government announced a 'Vision Zero' for suicide. The idea behind Vision Zero was that suicide prevention is everyone's responsibility, and first-aid training to help suicidal people should be given to every citizen. This policy sends a strong signal to the whole population that the topic is important, as well as lifting the stigma and taboo surrounding suicide.

The Second National Suicide Preventive Programme for Sweden, including both public health and health care strategies (Proposition of the Swedish Government 2007), was ratified by the Swedish parliament in June 2008 (Parliamentary Protocol 2008). This type of parliamentary ratification gives not only legal status to this suicide preventive programme, but also poses the legal requirements for action to be taken by different actors.

## Evaluation of the suicide preventive programme

A continuous evaluation of suicide preventive activities is performed with process oriented and epidemiological measures. Suicide rates decline markedly and continuously in Sweden, both for males and females in all age groups, with the exception of the 15–24 age group, in which suicide rates are stable.

## Conclusion

Viewing suicide as predestined and impossible to prevent or treat can still be encountered among laymen and health-care staff. Professionals should strive for a greater awareness concerning the strong negative emotions aroused by a patient's suicide or attempted suicide.

The evidence concerning effectiveness of suicide-prevention measures is now growing (Wasserman 2001), and national suicide-prevention programmes are helpful in disseminating this knowledge in a structured way (Wasserman et al 2004).

## References

Ettlinger R (1975). Evaluation of suicide prevention after attempted suicide. *Acta Psychiatrica Scandinavica, Supplementum 260*. Munksgaard, Copenhagen.

European Commission (2005). Green Paper: Improving the Mental Health of the Population: Towards a Strategy on Mental Health for the European Union. European Communities, Brussels.

National Council for Suicide Prevention (1995). *Support in Suicidal Crises. The Swedish National Programme to Develop Suicide Prevention*. Modin Tryck, Stockholm.

National Research and Development Centre for Welfare and Health (1993). *Suicide can be Prevented. A Target and Action Strategy for Suicide Prevention*. Stakes, Helsinki.

Parliamentary protocol regarding the acceptance of suicide prevention in Sweden (2008). *Självmordsprevention [Suicide Prevention]*. 2007/08:123 Accessible at: http://ki.se/suicide

Proposition of the Swedish Government (2007). *En ny folkhalsopolitik [A New Public Health Policy]*. Prop. 2007/08:110, 106–122. Accessible at: http://www.regeringen.se/download/2ee01484.pdf?major=1&minor=1 00978&cn=attachmentPublDuplicator_0_attachment

Ramsay R and Tanney B (1996). *Global Trends in Suicide Prevention: Toward the Development of National Strategies for Suicide Prevention.* Tata Institute of Social Sciences, Mumbai.

Socialstyrelsen [The National Board of Health and Welfare] and Statens Folkhälsoinstitut [Swedish National Public Health Institute] (2006). *Förslag till nationellt program för suicidprevention-befolkningsinriktade och individinriktade strategier och åtgärdsförslag [Proposal for the National Programme for Suicide Prevention-Public Health and individual oriented strategies and actions]*. Socialstryrelsen, Stockholm. Accessible at: http://www.socialstyrelsen.se/Publicerat/2006/9391/2006-107-23.htm

Wasserman D, Mittendorfer-Rutz E, Rutz W *et al.* (2004). *Suicide Prevention in Europe. The WHO European Monitoring Survey on National Suicide Prevention Programmes and Strategies.* The Swedish National Centre for Suicide Research and Prevention of Mental Ill-Health, Stockholm.

Wasserman D (ed.) (2001). *Suicide: An Unnecessary Death*. Martin Dunitz, London.

WHO (2005). *Mental Health Declaration for Europe—Facing the Challenges, Building Solutions.* WHO EUR/04/5047810/6. http://www.euro.who. int/mentalhealth/publications/20061124_.

# CHAPTER 125

# Suicide prevention in Ukraine

Vsevolod Rozanov and Alexander Mokhovikov

## Introduction

According to the WHO official data, for the period from 1986 to 1996, there was a dramatic rise in suicide rates in the Ukraine, from 18.47 to 29.43 per 100,000. Since 1997, there has been a steady lowering of suicide rates, and the latest available data, in 2006, is 19.54. per 100,000. Nevertheless, today, the Ukraine remains the country with 'high' suicide rates, where suicide in males is almost five times higher than in females, and in rural areas suicide rates are almost twice as high as in the urban environment.

## Suicide prevention

There is no national suicide-prevention programme in Ukraine (Suicide Prevention in Europe 2002). Suicide prevention is only mentioned in the National Health Promotion Plan and Conception of Mental Health Care, with crisis centre development as the main measure (European Network on Mental Health 2001). On the other hand, Ukraine has signed the Mental Health Declaration and Action Plan for Europe (European Ministerial Conference 2005), and recently a task-force under WHO liaison office was established to formulate how to reform the mental health care system in Ukraine for better integration into European context. As in many developing countries (Vijayakumar *et al.* 2005), suicide prevention activity in Ukraine is supported, mainly, by the so-called 'third sector', i.e. non-governmental organizations (NGOs) and volunteer organizations. While in the wider public domain, suicide remains stigmatized. The army, police (militia) and penitentiary system are implementing internal monitoring and preventive measures regarding suicide attempts and completed suicide, and have internal suicide-prevention plans of action.

Our experience in building prevention programmes started with research, accumulation of professional experience and hotline services, which were established in Odessa and all over the Ukraine, with the translation of several books by Western authors into Russian, and the publication of papers in suicidology during the 1990s. This was supported by the establishment of the academic course of suicidology at the Odessa National Mechnikov University. It was also important that Odessa NGO Human Ecological Health, presently also centre at Odessa University started actively participating in the WHO Europe suicide attempts monitoring study and prevention network, thus ensuring a methodological basis and international links. Practical work started in 1999, when Human Ecological Health was invited to implement prevention measures in one of the big Ukrainian Army units, which was facing suicidal crisis, with nine deaths of soldiers and officers during a 1-year period. From the very beginning, we have chosen the educational model of preventionstrategy, and after a series of seminars for commanders and medical staff, we were able to show that intensive education, together with prevention resources dissemination, can lower completed suicides in a given environment (Rozanov *et al.* 2002). But only sustainable activity can ensure success in prevention. It was a challenge, and the next step was to enhance efforts in fund-raising to sustain preventive measures.

Future expansion of education in suicide prevention, with financial support from the Swedish East European Committee, and with scientific and methodological support from the National Swedish Prevention of Suicide and Mental Ill-Health (NASP) at Karolinska Institute in Sweden, was connected with the penitentiary system of Ukraine, and later focused on other relevant groups, such as medical doctors (e.g. psychiatrists, family doctors, ambulance doctors, reanimation unit specialists), school teachers and psychologists, telephone hotline volunteers, HIV/AIDS rehabilitation centre volunteers, Red Cross patronage personnel, and mass media representatives. From the very beginning, the format of the seminars was based on 'training of trainers' methodology, providing to participants, using a variety of resources and electronic methodological material, further dissemination of the knowledge required, and encouraging them to start their own local programmes. Educational staff knowledge was enhanced through participation in NASP's KIRT courses (Karolinska Institute Research and Training). From the very beginning, one of the prerequisites was to cover not only Odessa but also other cities of Ukraine. An important achievement was that a network of suicide prevention specialists was created during the projects' implementation period, which now embraces twenty-six people in fifteen cities of Ukraine. A primary outcome of the projects was the successful enhancement of the participants' knowledge, and their confidence in dealing with the problem of suicide and suicide prevention. An important outcome was the preparation and dissemination of a number of high-quality suicide-prevention booklets. These included six WHO suicide prevention resources (World Health Organization 2000a–f, 2006a, b), which were translated into Russian, and other resources developed by the teaching group: about 4000 copies. The scientific skills of suicide prevention specialists were also promoted by the active involvement in a large project on gene–environmental interactions in suicidal behaviours (Wasserman *et al.* 2008)

As a result of those experiences, a new initiative was taken to formulate a proposal for the National Suicide-Prevention Strategy for the Ukraine. This was supported by the national network of trained specialists, establishment of relations and links to many ministries, interested agencies, nested programmes and volunteer groups. A proposal for the National Suicide-Prevention Plan was developed by the working group in Ukraine, and with active support from NASP and the International Steering Committee, which embraced suicidologists from Sweden, Germany, Estonia and Israel. The published document was discussed extensively in the professional and wide public auditoriums via meeting and round tables in the Ukraine, which provided a variety of suggestions on further implementation of the plan.

## Conclusion

In summary, it can be stated that education, especially 'training of trainers' technology, together with resource dissemination and network establishment, is a useful model for suicide prevention in countries without a national suicide-prevention strategy, and a good starting point for future system change towards building such a strategy and its implementation on the basis of wide discussion.

### References

European Network on Mental Health (2001). *Mental Health in Europe*, p. 97. *Country Reports from the WHO European Network on Mental Health.* World Health Organization, Geneva.

European Ministerial Conference (2005). *Mental Health: Facing the Challenges, Building Solutions*, p. 180. *Report from the WHO European Ministerial Conference.* World Health Organization, Geneva.

Rozanov VA, Mokhovikov AN, Stiliha R (2002). Successful model of suicide prevention in the Ukraine military environment. *Crisis*, **23**, 171–177.

Suicide Prevention in Europe (2002). *The WHO European Monitoring Survey on National Suicide Prevention Programmes and Strategies*, p. 24. World Health Organization, Geneva.

Vijayakumar L, Pirkis J, Whiteford H (2005). Suicide prevention in developing countries (3). Prevention efforts. *Crisis*, **26**, 120–124.

Wasserman D, Sokolowski M, Rozanov et al. (2008). The CRHR! gene—a marker for suicidality in depressed males exposed to low stress. *Genes, Brain and Behaviour*, 7, 14–19.

World Health Organization (2000a). *Preventing Suicide: A Resource for General Physicians.* World Health Organization, Geneva.

World Health Organization (2000b). *Preventing suicide: a resource for media professionals.* World Health Organization, Geneva.

World Health Organization (2000c). *Preventing Suicide: A Resource for Teachers and Other School Staff.* World Health Organization, Geneva.

World Health Organization (2000d). *Preventing Suicide: A Resource for Primary Health Care Workers.* World Health Organization, Geneva.

World Health Organization (2000e). *Preventing Suicide: A Resource for Prison Officers.* World Health Organization, Geneva.

World Health Organization (2000f). *Preventing Suicide: How to Start a Survivors' Group.* World Health Organization, Geneva.

World Health Organization (2006a). *Preventing Suicide: A Resource for Counsellors.* World Health Organization, Geneva.

World Health Organization (2006b). *Preventing Suicide: A Resource at Work.* World Health Organization, Geneva.

# Examples of How to Develop Suicide Prevention on all the Continents: North America

# CHAPTER 126

# Suicide prevention in Canada

Gustavo Turecki and Monique Séguin

## Abstract

Suicide is a major public health problem in Canada. While several different initiatives have been made since 2000 to develop and implement a national strategy, the Canadian Government still has no public suicide-prevention programme. However, a few Canadian provinces and/or jurisdictions currently have or previously had a defined and/or implemented suicide prevention programme or targeted strategy. This chapter describes the major points of these strategies and identifies areas of concern.

## Epidemiology

Suicide is a major public health problem in Canada. Over the last decade, total Canadian suicide rates have remained relatively stable, hovering between 11 and 14 per 100,000 individuals (Statistics Canada 2002 and 2008). However, substantial regional variation has been the norm, with significantly higher rates in provinces such as Quebec (18 per 100,000 in 2002) and Alberta (13.8 per 100,000 in 2002) and staggeringly high rates in some of the primarily Aboriginal northern regions, especially in Nunavut, where total rates were 79.8 per 100,000 in 2002 (142.1 per 100,000 among males) (Statistics Canada 2006).

## Suicide prevention programmes in Canada

The Canadian Government has been debating with the issue of implementing a comprehensive national strategy on suicide for decades (Leenaars 2000). A number of efforts have been made in order to foster interest and implementation of a national strategy on suicide. These include the development of a White Paper in 1970 (Health Canada 1970), which identified suicide as a major public health problem, as well as a series of other initiatives, such as a National Task Force on Suicide in 1980 (Health Canada 1980) and the production of the document *Suicide in Canada* (Health Canada 1987), both of which established a list of priorities for specific risk groups. More recently, suicide prevention efforts led to the creation of the report of the Royal Commission on Aboriginal Peoples (Health Canada 1995), and in addition, the Blueprint for a Canadian National Suicide Prevention (CASP 2004), which offered a proposed national outline for suicide prevention. Finally, in 2006, the report of Canada's Standing Committee on Social Affairs, Science and Technology, also known as the Kirby report and titled *Out of the shadows at last*, like many previous publications, called for federal, provincial and territorial governments to work with stakeholders to develop a truly Canadian suicide prevention strategy.

In parallel, a number of non-governmental national advocacy agencies, such as the Canadian Mental Health Association and the Canadian Association of Suicide Prevention, and several provincial organizations, such as the Center for Suicide Prevention in Alberta, the Association Québécoise de Prévention du Suicide in Québec, SAFER – the Suicide Attempt, Follow-up, Education and Research Program – in Vancouver, played and continue to play an important role in response to the promotion of suicide prevention in Canada. Yet the Canadian Government still has no public strategy in order to prevent suicide.

## Suicide prevention programmes in Canadian provinces

In Canada, the mandate to provide direct health services falls under the provincial jurisdiction. This explains the difference in the delivery of health policies between different Canadian regions. As such, a few Canadian provinces and or jurisdictions currently have or previously had a defined and/or implemented suicide-prevention programme or targeted strategy. The following paragraphs provide examples of the main points contained in some of these programmes.

In 2005, the Alberta Mental Health Board led a collaborative effort of provincial and federal government ministries, survivors, regional health authorities, and non-governmental organizations to create the Alberta Suicide Prevention Strategy. The following are the main goals and objectives of this strategy:

1 Secure targeted and sustainable funding to implement the Alberta Suicide Prevention Strategy.

2 Enhance mental health and well-being among Albertans.

3 Improve intervention and treatment for those at risk of suicide in Alberta.

4 Improve intervention and support for Albertans affected by suicide.

5   Increase efforts to reduce access to lethal means of suicide.

6   Increase research activities in Alberta on suicide, suicidal behaviour, and suicide prevention.

7   Improve suicide and suicidal behaviour-related surveillance systems in Alberta.

8   Increase evaluation and continuous quality improvement activities in Alberta for suicide prevention programmes.

In 1989, the New Brunswick government established a provincial committee to advise mental health services on strategies to be developed, implemented, or reviewed with regard to suicide prevention. It also worked with New Brunswick organizations to coordinate provincial efforts and to develop a common province-wide approach. As a result, a suicide prevention programme was developed aiming to reduce this province's suicide rates. As part of this programme, a provincial suicidologist has the key role of promoting province-wide leadership on suicide prevention. The service delivery is provided primarily at the community-based level. The New Brunswick Suicide Prevention Program mobilizes agencies and individuals who work provincially and locally. Thirteen community suicide prevention committees are in place throughout New Brunswick's health regions. They advise their local community mental health centre and the provincial suicide-prevention committee on the actions required in order to meet the programme's objectives. They also work with other regional organizations to coordinate their efforts.

As for the province of Québec, the provincial government launched in 1998 a province-wide strategy for suicide prevention called *Québec's strategy for preventing suicide: help for life* (MSSS 1998). Seven objectives were included in this five-year programme:

1   Provide and consolidate essential services and put an end to the isolation of caseworkers.

2   Increase professional skills in the identification and treatment of individuals affected with mental disorders.

3   Intervene with groups at risk, and more specifically, with men at risk of suicide, as well as individuals who attempted suicide.

4   Foster promotion-prevention programmes among young people, by improving personal and social skills.

5   Reduce access to and minimize risks associated with the means of suicide.

6   Counteract the trivialization and sensationalization of suicide by developing a sense of community and responsibility.

7   Intensify and diversify suicide-related research.

A number of actions reinforced by this strategy have been implemented and are functional, such as a 24-hour crisis line service, crisis intervention in all regions of the province, early prevention, post-vention services and information and support to family members.

The Québec strategy for suicide prevention, however, was not renewed when the initial five-year period ended. Instead, the Québec provincial government proposed a broad mental health plan that contained an unspecific and extremely general suicide intervention/prevention plan. Accordingly, in this three-year strategic plan, two objectives focused on suicide intervention: (1) Intervention and support for individuals in crisis, especially adult men, and (2) Intervention for high-risk individuals. This mental health action plan, however, has been difficult to implement,

having met stiff resistance from a large sector of mental-health-care professionals from this province, primarily because of resistance to changes imposed by the government in the structure of mental health-care delivery practices.

Other provinces have also proposed suicide prevention plans. Of note, the territory of Nunavut released its suicide prevention strategy on June 2007. In a territory where suicide rates are among the highest in the word, and where suicide has such a devastating social impact, a suicide prevention plan was long overdue. Unfortunately, this territorial government plan, which was noted for its lack of specifics, was built without input from the professional community, with no representative public consultation, and it was not evidence-based. Another province which has been criticized for its lack of a comprehensive suicide prevention plan is Ontario. This province has not defined and/or implemented a strategy addressing suicide, except for a province-wide, tool-free telephone and Internet counselling and referral service targeting youth. However, extensive condemnation has done little to change this long-standing situation.

## Blueprint of a Canadian national suicide prevention programme

In the midst of this regionally heterogeneous reality, Canada is still waiting for the Blueprint of a Canadian National Suicide Prevention to be pushed ahead. The Blueprint is the outline of a national suicide prevention strategy for Canada. It is also a policy agenda, a national task list, and tool for identifying best practices, and a roadmap to and integrated solution. The following guiding principles were used to guide the development of this blueprint:

◆ Suicide prevention is everyone's responsibility.

◆ Canadians respect their multicultural and diverse society and accept responsibility to support the dignity of human life.

◆ Suicide is an interaction of biological, psychological, social and spiritual factors and can be influenced by societal attitudes and conditions.

◆ Strategies must be humane, kind, effective, caring and should be evidence-based; active and informed; respectful of community and culture-based knowledge; inclusive of research, surveillance, evaluation and reporting, as well as reflective of evolving knowledge and practices.

Many suicides are preventable. A recent meta-analysis identified physician education in depression recognition and treatment, as well as restricting access to lethal methods, as the only two suicide prevention strategies with evidence of effectively reducing suicide rates (Mann *et al.* 2005). Realistic opportunities exist for saving many lives in Canada. With the development of a national suicide-prevention strategy that is based on evidence and contains specific plans of action we will be able to make substantial gains in the battle against suicide. Unfortunately, in Canada we are still waiting for such action to materialize.

## References

CASP (Canadian Association for Suicide Prevention (2004). *Blueprint for a Canadian National Suicide Prevention*. Canadian Association for Suicide Prevention, Winnipeg.

Canada's Standing Committee on Social Affairs, Science and Technology (2006) *Out of the Shadows at Last*. Canadian Senate, Ottawa.

Health Canada (1970). *National Strategy on Suicide: the White Paper on Suicide Prevention*. Health Canada, Ottawa.

Health Canada (1980) *National Task Force on Suicide*. Health Canada, Ottawa.

Health Canada (1987) *Suicide in Canada*. Health Canada, Ottawa.

Health Canada (1995) *Royal Commission on Aboriginal People*. Health Canada, Ottawa.

Leenaars, A. (2000). Suicide prevention in Canada: a history of a community approach. *Canadian Journal of Community Mental Health*, **19**, 57–73.

Mann JJ, Apter A, Bertolote J *et al.* (2005) Suicide prevention strategies: a systematic review. *Journal of the American Medical Association*, **294**, 2064–2074.

MSSS (Ministère de la Santé et des Services Sociaux) (1998). *Stratégie québécoise d'action face au suicide: s'entraider pour la vie*. Québec

Statistics Canada (2002) *Health Reports*, **13**, No. 2. Catalogue 82–003, Statistics Canada, Ottawa.

Statistics Canada (2006) *Catalogue 84F0209XIE*, Statistics Canada, Ottawa.

Statistics Canada (2008) *CANSIM*, table 102–0551 and Catalogue no. 84F0209X, Statistics Canada, Ottawa.

# CHAPTER 127

# Suicide prevention in the United States of America

## Jerry Reed and Morton M Silverman

## Introduction

In May 1993, the United Nations convened a meeting of fifteen experts from twelve countries (Australia, Canada, China, Estonia, Finland, Hungary, India, Japan, Netherlands, Nigeria, United Arab Emirates and the United States) to draft guidelines for the development of national strategies for the prevention of suicidal behaviours (Ramsay and Tanney 1996). These guidelines were subsequently published as *Prevention of suicide: guidelines for the formulation and implementation of national strategies* (United Nations 1996).

The UN Guidelines emphasized that the development of a national strategy required:

1   A government-initiated national policy that declares suicide prevention as a public health priority;

2   Broad involvement from different sectors and segments of society, and

3   The establishment of a coordinating body to formulate and implement the strategy (Ramsey 2001).

In 1997, following the United Nations Guidelines, advocates pressed for resolutions to be introduced in the 105th Congress of the United States to recognize suicide as a national problem, worthy of a national solution, and calling for the development of a national strategy. Both resolutions specifically urged the development of 'an effective national strategy for the prevention of suicide', and were critical steps in moving suicide prevention efforts in the United States forward.

## Suicide Prevention in the United States

In July 1997, the Centers for Disease Control and Prevention established two new injury control research centers, one to focus specifically on suicide. At approximately the same time, Dr David Satcher, the newly appointed Surgeon General of the United States, stated his intention to ensure that mental health and suicide prevention would be addressed during his tenure as the senior public health official in the USA. Soon thereafter, dedicated public servants and private individuals jointly organized and participated in the first National Suicide Prevention Conference held in 1998 in Reno, Nevada, to consolidate a scientific base for crafting a national suicide prevention strategy. Over 450 advocates,

researchers, public servants, policy-makers, clinicians, survivors and countless others gathered and made recommendations that led to the Surgeon General's *Call to action to prevent suicide*, published in 1999 (USPHS 1999).

The Call to Action proposed a conceptual foundation designated as 'AIM':

1   *Awareness*: broaden the public's awareness of suicide and its risk factors;

2   *Intervention*: enhance services and programmes, both population-based and clinical care; and

3   *Methodology*: advance the science of suicide prevention.

The AIM framework included 15 recommendations derived from consensus-based and evidence-based findings intended to serve as a foundation for a more comprehensive National Strategy for Suicide Prevention.

In 2001, the *National strategy for suicide prevention: goals and objectives for action*, was published by the US Department of Health and Human Services (USDHHS 2001). This document, containing eleven goals and sixty-eight objectives, became the roadmap for effectively addressing the public health problem of suicide in the United States. Calling on representatives from government, business and charitable organizations to work together to prevent suicide, multiple sectors, trade associations, industries, professional groups and others were identified as having a role to play. Among some of the key organizations that were already active in suicide prevention, and supported the Strategy, was the American Association of Suicidology, American Foundation for Suicide Prevention, Suicide Prevention Action Network USA (SPAN USA), The Jed Foundation, Yellow Ribbon, and the National Council for Suicide Prevention.

While the National Strategy (NSSP) did not mandate action, it served as a model for states to follow as efforts were advanced nationally to address suicide. Today, forty-six of fifty states have developed a state strategy to prevent suicide, and many state legislatures have passed laws or resolutions to prevent suicide in their state. Many have funded the establishment of State Offices of Suicide Prevention.

One of the first tangible results of the NSSP was a federal appropriation in 2002 of $7.5 million over three years to establish a National Suicide Prevention Resource Center (SPRC), in Newton,

**Table 127.1** History of Suicide Prevention in the USA

| |
|---|
| 1958: Los Angeles Suicide Prevention Center opens, funded by the US Public Health Service and directed by Edwin Shneidman, Ph.D. |
| 1966: Center for the Study of Suicide Prevention (later renamed the Suicide Prevention Research Unit) established at the National Institute of Mental Health. |
| 1968: American Association of Suicidology founded by Edwin Shneidman, Ph.D. |
| 1983: CDC Violence Prevention Unit (later subsumed into the National Center for Injury Prevention and Control) established; focuses public attention on an increase in the rate of youth suicide. |
| 1985: DHHS Secretary's Task Force on Youth Suicide established to review the problem of youth suicide and recommend actions. |
| 1987: American Foundation for Suicide Prevention founded. |
| 1989: *Report of the DHHS Secretary's Task Force on Youth Suicide* published by the US Department of Health and Human Services. |
| 1996: Suicide Prevention Advocacy Network (SPAN) founded with the goal of preventing suicide through public education, community action, and advocacy. Subsequently the name changed to the Suicide Prevention Action Network USA (SPAN USA). |
| 1996: *Prevention of Suicide: Guidelines for the Formulation and Implementation of National Strategies* published by the World Health Organization and the United Nations. |
| 1998: National Suicide Prevention Conference held in Reno, Nevada as a response to the WHO/UN publication. This public/private partnership created an expert panel that issued 81 recommendations. |
| 1999: *Surgeon General's Call to Action to Prevent Suicide* published, which consolidated the National Suicide Prevention Conference's recommendations, including the creation of a National Strategy for Suicide Prevention. |
| 2001: *National Strategy for Suicide Prevention: Goals and Objectives for Action* published by the US Department of Health and Human Services. It outlined a coherent national plan to enhance the suicide prevention infrastructure, including the creation of a technical assistance and resource centre. |
| 2002: Suicide Prevention Resource Center established at Education Development Center, Inc. with funding from the Substance Abuse and Mental Health Services Administration. |
| 2002: *Reducing Suicide: A National Imperative* published by the Institute of Medicine of the National Academies of Science. This publication examined and summarized the state of knowledge about suicide and the state of the art of suicide prevention. |
| 2003: *Achieving the Promise: Transforming Mental Health Care in America* published by the President's New Freedom Commission on Mental Health. |
| 2004: Garrett Lee Smith Memorial Act passed by the US Congress to support and enhance youth suicide prevention efforts in the states, among tribal nations and at colleges and universities. |
| 2004: National Suicide Prevention Lifeline (1–800–273-TALK) funded by the Substance Abuse and Mental Health Services Administration, US Department of Health and Human Services. |
| 2005: The Department of Labor, Heath and Human Services, and Education, and Related Agencies Appropriations Act of 2006 which appropriates a total of $30 million for suicide prevention was signed into law. |
| 2006: The SAMHSA Program Priority Matrix was updated to include suicide prevention as one of the matrix priorities. |
| 2006: Federal Working Group on Suicide Prevention established. Representatives from SAMHSA, Centers for Disease Control, National Institute on Mental Health, Indian Health Services, Department of Defense, Veterans Affairs and other federal agencies. |
| 2007: Joshua Omvig Veteran Suicide Prevention Act passed by Congress directing the Department of Veterans Affairs to reduce the incidence of suicide among veterans of military service. |

Massachusetts. The mission of the centre would be to provide technical assistance to stakeholders, gather information on best practices, and serve as a clearing house for suicide prevention information and programmes. SPRC promotes the implementation of the NSSP and enhances the nation's mental health infrastructure by providing states, government agencies, private organizations, colleges and universities, and suicide survivor and mental health consumer groups with access to the science and experience that can support their efforts to develop programmes, implement interventions, and promote policies to prevent suicide.

In 2002, the Institute of Medicine of the National Academies of Science published *Reducing suicide: A national imperative*, which called for more research into the causes of suicide and interventions that work to prevent suicide (IOM 2002). In 2003 the *President's New Freedom Commission on mental health report* was released and the very first recommendation focused on suicide prevention as a key element of a comprehensive mental health system (PNFCMH 2003). This acknowledgement ensured that suicide prevention had

carried from one presidential administration to another as a key item on the health public policy agenda.

On 21 October 2004, President Bush signed the Garrett Lee Smith Memorial Act (Public Law 108–355) providing an $82 million authorization for youth suicide prevention and early identification programmes. In addition to providing grants to states and tribal communities to advance their youth suicide-prevention efforts, grants would be made available to colleges and universities to enhance their behavioural health capacity to address campus suicide and its prevention. To date, 59 states and tribal communities have received federal grants up to $400,000 per year for youth suicide prevention efforts and, in addition, 64 colleges have received grants to develop campus-wide suicide prevention programmes. This law represented the first-ever federal funding for youth suicide-prevention in the United States.

In 2004 the federal government established a grant to launch a National Suicide Prevention Lifeline. This initiative supports a national network of local crisis centres that have the capacity to accept calls from those who may be in suicidal crisis. By dialling one national number callers are seamlessly connected to the crisis centre closest to where they are calling from. Once connected, crisis intervention is provided by trained staff and volunteers located in nationally certified crisis centres.

In 2006, the Administrator of the Substance Abuse and Mental Health Services Administration (SAMHSA), a federal agency under the Department of Health and Human Services, designated suicide prevention as a programme and policy priority for the agency. By doing so, suicide prevention would now be incorporated into the fabric of the agency and concrete steps to advance suicide-prevention efforts would be taken. In 2007, a similar effort was taken at the Department of Health and Human Services, when the Department's five-year strategic plan was amended to include suicide prevention as one of the Department's core prevention measures, and establishing the national goal of reducing suicide deaths by six per cent by 2012. With the annual toll of deaths by suicide at approximately 31,000, this translates to a reduction of nearly 2,000 suicide deaths by 2012.

In 2007, Congress passed the Joshua Omvig Veteran Suicide Prevention Act (Public Law 110–110), directing the Department of Veterans Affairs to reduce the incidence of suicide among veterans of military service, make available 24-hour mental health care for veterans found to be at risk, and develop an outreach and education programme for veterans and their families to identify readjustment problems and promote mental health. With data suggesting 20 per cent of suicidal deaths in the United States are veterans of all ages, public policy attention has shifted to include suicide prevention efforts for this at-risk population.

Since 1996, suicide-prevention efforts in the USA have been steadily advanced. With efforts focusing on youth suicide-prevention, veterans suicide-prevention and establishing a national resource centre and a national suicide-prevention lifeline, attention needs to be directed at better suicide-prevention research, older adult suicide-prevention, and the formation of a coordinating body called for in the United Nations guidelines to oversee the implementation and advancement of the NSSP. It is expected that the National Action Alliance for Suicide Prevention will be launched in 2009, bringing together representatives from the public, private and philanthropic sectors to bring focus, resolve and national attention to advancing the objectives in the NSSP. This initiative will move the NSSP objectives from paper to practice by monitoring, guiding, coordinating and promoting suicide prevention efforts across the country.

## Conclusion

Suicide prevention in the USA over the last decade has made significant progress. Our success is determined more by the collaborative approach we have taken, leveraging broad national investments to support local and grassroots efforts. No one sector, agency or non-governmental organization can single-handedly prevent suicide. Instead, it takes a community to prevent suicide and the work of all committed to saving lives through suicide-prevention efforts if we are to reduce the mortality and morbidity associated with the preventable public health problem of suicide. Our approach in the United States has not been to mandate or legislate action but to inspire and promote action at all levels. While our work is far from complete, the suicide-prevention movement in the United States continues to make progress.

## References

IOM (Institute of Medicine) (2002). *Reducing Suicide: A National Imperative.* National Academies of Science Press, Washington.

PNFCMH (President's New Freedom Commission on Mental Health) (2003). *Achieving the Promise: Transforming Mental Health Care in America.* Government Printing Office, Washington.

Ramsey R (2001). United Nations Impact on the United States National Suicide Prevention Strategy (NSPS). Paper presented at the American Association of Suicidology 34th Annual Conference, April 18, 2001.

Ramsay R and Tanney B (1996). *Global Trends in Suicide Prevention: Toward the Development of National Strategies for Suicide Prevention.* Tata Institute of Social Sciences, Mumbai.

United Nations (1996). *Prevention of Suicide: Guidelines for the Formulation and Implementation of National Strategies.* Department for Policy Coordination and Sustainable Development, New York.

USDHHS (US Department of Health and Human Services_ (2001). *The National Strategy for Suicide Prevention: Goals and Objectives for Action.* US Public Health Service, Rockville.

USPHS (US Public Health Service) (1999). *The Surgeon General's Call to Action to Prevent Suicide 1999.* Department of Health and Human Services, US Public Health Service, Washington.

# Examples of How to Develop Suicide Prevention on all the Continents: South America

# CHAPTER 128

# Suicide prevention in South America

## A serious problem—few solutions

Paulo Alterwain, Héctor Basile, Daniel Fränkel,
Jaime Greif, Silvia Hernandez and
María del Carmen Paparamborda

## Introduction

South America is a major region in the world, which includes many countries on the continent of South America, Central America and Mexico. The historic origin, cultural development, and various populations, which share similar characteristics, are reasons why this major region is also known as Latin America.

Psychosocial and economical related problems are prominent in South America. Diverse trauma including loss of cultural values and traditional beliefs, poverty, hunger, discrimination, violence, natural disasters, and poor working and social conditions are influencing mental health.

Suicide, as well as suicidal behaviour, is an individualistic phenomenon. However, suicidal actions are multifaceted and cluster-based, and often determined by poor social conditions. Accumulation of negative life events can be triggering factors for suicidal conditions.

Cultural differences with regard to style and characteristics can be found in suicides that are committed in both urban and rural areas. In South America particularly, the general beliefs and penalties regarding suicides are quite similar to those of the Judeo-Christian European cultural perspectives. Europe-originated legal features (mainly from The Netherlands and Italy) in the nineteenth century are maintained, and can be seen in their respective penal codes. Suicide is not penalized. Suicidal behaviours are referred to either psychiatric or psychological treatment. Uruguayan laws date from 1889, with some adjustments in 1934. The law recognizes and protects the right to life and any stimulus, cooperation or help to any person attempting suicide is punished.

In 2006, suicide rates in South America were 6.4/100,000 (Paparamborda 2007). Suicide rates for various countries within this region are illustrated in Figure 128.1. Suicides in different South American countries vary among age groups: adolescents, young people, and the elderly (Figures 128.2 and 128.3) (Granados 1977; World Health Organization 2000).

Epidemiologic information on completed suicide is still scarce in South and Central America, and the magnitude of so-called uncertain cases of suicide is not known (Bertolote and Fleischmann 2002).

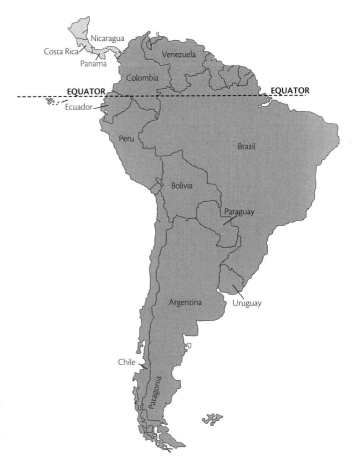

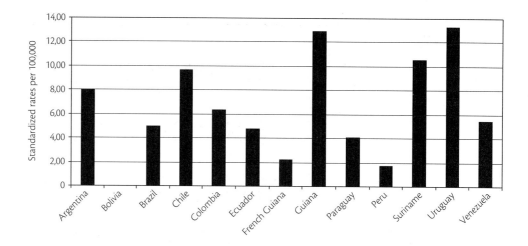

**Fig. 128.1** Distribution of suicide rates per country in South America, 1999–2003.

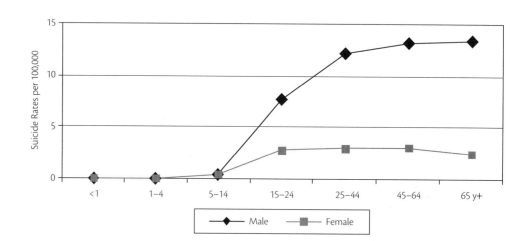

**Fig. 128.2** Distribution of suicide rates per age and gender, Brazil 2000–2002.

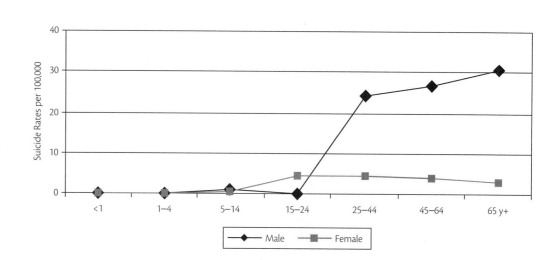

**Fig. 128.3** Distribution of suicide rates per age and gender, Chile 2001–2003.

In Figure 128.4, the comparison between suicide rates and rates for traffic accidents and homicides in countries of South America is shown.

Official records concerning suicidal ideation and suicide attempts are lacking, and gathering this information is difficult because people are prone to either keep strict confidence or conceal the fact.

## Methods of suicide

Arms, toxic substances and hanging are the predominant suicidal methods utilized. However, jumping from a window or drowning are methods increasingly used by juvenile suicides (10–24 age group). The predominant abuse of legal and illegal drugs, as well as alcohol, is frequently observed in those who committed suicide (Paparamborda and Rodriguez 2000; Vignolo and Paparamborda 2000).

## Care for suicide attempts

Care is provided at both general hospital emergency rooms and psychiatric outpatient departments. In general, inpatient care at either a general hospital or mental hospital is brief. Protocols for care, follow-up of suicide attempters and periodic controls are usually insufficiently performed. In a majority of cases, relapse often occurs.

## University teaching

Suicidology courses are given at university schools of medicine, nursing schools, and schools of psychology (both undergraduate and postgraduate levels). Currently, several curriculae have been introduced at universities, for example, in Argentina at the Universidad de Palermo (University of Palermo, Buenos Aries) and the Universidad Católica de Córdoba (The Roman Catholic University of the city of Cordoba). These universities have begun specific interdisciplinary courses on health promotion which focus on suicidal behaviour and care.

## Health and social policies

In many South American countries (e.g. Argentina, Chile Brazil and Uruguay), suicide has been acknowledged as a national health priority, and national programmes are in preparation. There are also several new specific legislations.

## Regional networking

Knowledge concerning suicide prevention in South America is similar to other regions that have been successful in exerting control, and reducing suicide risks. However, cultural conditions in the South American region have not been sufficiently acknowledged, and for that reason, cooperation and information exchanging networks have been created. The Asociación de Suicidología de Latinoamerica y el Caribe (ASULAC) (The Suicidology Network for Latin America and the Caribbean), founded in 2000, is linked to international organizations (http://www.ultimorecurso.com.uy).

In Argentina, Brazil, Colombia, Chile and Uruguay, national associations have been created. The Unión Nacional para la Prevención del Suicidio (The Suicide National Prevention Association), was founded in Uruguay in 2004 with the support of Professor J-P Soubrier from France, using the French National Union for Suicide Prevention (UNPS) as a model, which is adjusted

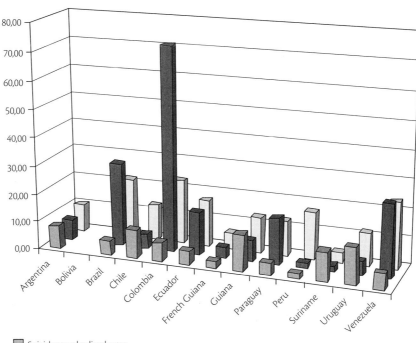

**Fig. 128.4** Distribution of standardized rates of suicide, homicide, and traffic accidents, South America 2006.

■ Suicide standardized rates

■ Standardized rate of homicide and injuries inflected by another person intentionally

□ Traffic accidents standardized rate

to Uruguayan needs. This national association is active in the following areas (Paparamborda and Alterwain 2000):

◆ Surveillance of the prevalence of violence and suicidal behaviour;

◆ Dissemination of information on suicide prevention;

◆ Training of interdisciplinary teams to specialize in prevention and care of suicidal persons in both urban and rural areas, including teaching teams that are specifically trained to deliver seminars, workshops and courses at schools, sport clubs, social clubs, and for the mass media;

◆ Improvements in care and follow-up of suicidal attempters through medical, district care centres, policemen and firemen;

◆ Lobbying of administration and political decision-makers in order to make necessary reforms so that an integrated, inter-sectional national programme for suicide prevention can be achieved.

It is high time for a change to take place in South America. Anthropological, cultural and social conditions require a change of the paradigms in approaching the problem of suicide. In this region, negative attitudes still exist, as well as prejudices, against suicidal individuals and their families.

A greater social consciousness needs to be achieved, stigma needs to be abolished, and important population oriented strategies need to be applied with the short-, medium- and long-term goals.

It is time for South America to be in a position to include suicide-prevention programmes within the social, technical and humanitarian agenda, in order to save lives through effective and efficient preventive activities.

## References

Bertolote JM and Fleischmann A (2002). A global perspective in the epidemiology of suicide. *Suicidology*, **7**, 2.

Granados B (1997). [Magnitude, Structure by Age and Gender, and Suicide in Costa Rica 1980–1994.] *Rev. Costarric. Sal. Púb.*, **6**, 11. Available at: http://www.scielo.sa.cr.

Paparamborda MC (2007). [Mental Health in the New Millenium: 2007. *Mental Health Journal*. (7) 3,7. Spanish. Montevideo, Uruguay, On Challenges Thereof, May 2007].

Paparamborda MC and Alterwain P (2000). Suicide in Uruguay, VII Workshop on Suicide Prevention PAHO/WHO, 22–24 February, 2000. Montevideo, Uruguay.

Paparamborda MC and Rodríguez M (2000). An Epidemiological Study of Psychiatric Emergencies. *Mental Health Journal*. (1) 2. Spanish. Montevideo, Uruguay. March 2000].

Vignolo JC and Paparamborda MC (2000). A Study on Suicide In Uruguay 1998–2000, and An Epidemiological Analysis for Year 2000. Epidemiological Bulletin (2828) Spanish. WHO/PAHO, Washington.

World Health Organization (2000). *Health Statistics in the Americas, Year 2000*. Available at: http://www.paho.org. World Health Organization, Geneva.

# CHAPTER 129

# Suicide prevention in Argentina

Carlos Martínez

The year 2007 will perhaps be a particularly meaningful year in the history of Argentina, because of the newly born Suicidology Discipline. The National Suicidology Congress has commerated the 40 years of Centro de Asistencia al Suicida de Buenos Aires (Buenos Aires Suicide Prevention Centre), which runs the oldest telephone helpline in the country, the creation of the Suicidology Section in the Argentinian Psychiatric Association, and the discussion about creating a Professorship in Suicidology at Universidad de Palermo, Buenos Aires.

These milestones were preceded by eight consecutive annual congresses organized by the Argentine Suicide Prevention Association from 1997 to 2004. In these congresses volunteers, therapists, teachers, students, civil servants, journalists, social workers, lawyers, researchers, survivors and those who have eventual interest in the subject participated.

This particular process of public awareness promoted the creation of the Expert Commission in the Health Department, in order to formulate the National Programme of Suicide Prevention. From 2008 to 2011, the work will focus on four main areas: collecting information, planning of preventive activities, training, and the evaluation of human resources available for suicide prevention. In 2005, the national suicide rate in Argentina was 8.2 per cent per 100,000 inhabitants, compared to 6 and 7 per cent per 100,000 inhabitants registered at the end of the twentieth century.

## Multisectorial programme with varied scope (PMVA)

The Argentine Association of Suicide Prevention has been able to implement local prevention programmes, which are available both in local towns and provinces, and are aimed at conducting epidemiological surveillance and the mitigation of negative social conditions influencing suicide trends in the same community in which epidemiological monitoring is conducted.

When the local community is involved, and the causes of the suicide are known, it is very important that the person managing the programme uses proper interventions. A modular programme with interactive possibilities, using evaluation and identification techniques from the Inventory of Suicide Orientations (ISO 30)

questionnaire (King and Kowalchuk 1994; Casullo *et al.* 2000) is used in this project. It is a self-applicable questionnaire, which allows administration for larger populations.

## Description of tasks in the PMVA project

### Sector I: Mental health professionals

- Receive patients who attempted suicide into the emergency care service;
- Give psychotherapeutic assistance for patients who report suicide events;
- Give family psychotherapeutic treatments;
- Coordinate support groups for patients with suicidal thoughts and suicide attempts;
- Evaluate suicidal risk by means of the ISO 30 questionnaire;
- Coordinate family groups for those affected by suicide;
- Develop community actions for rehabilitation work in order to prevent suicide relapse.

### Sector II: Teachers

- Inform about risk factors;
- Detect students and families at risk, and guide them on how to correctly manage a crisis situation;
- Evaluate suicide risks by means of ISO 30;
- Work with the student groups in educational facilities;
- Perform post-vention in cases where a suicide has taken place;
- Train and encourage students in the techniques of risk evaluation;
- Inform the family about the preventive activities;
- Restrain aggressive and impulsive students from outburst situations.

### Sector III: Health professionals

- Inform the population about risk aspects;
- Plan and collaborate with local organizations;

◆ Perform campaigns in schools, and in the press, in order to raise the public awareness and psychoeducation for target groups;

◆ Properly guide family training programmes on how to avoid suicide in high-risk populations.

### Sector IV: Telephone operators

◆ Evaluate the suicide potential of the caller;

◆ Solve crisis situations on the phone if possible;

◆ Record the information received from the telephone caller;

◆ Refer those cases that can not be resolved on the phone to the emergency care services;

◆ Complete a phone call file, update the statistics, and consequently, establish new points of view as the monitoring of the programme continues.

### Sector V: Monitoring, supporting the programme, and campaigning

These tasks are carried out by qualified professionals from different areas, who are trained in suicidology and suicide prevention. It is essential to involve qualified professionals from sectors I and II (as described above) when implementing a promotion and/or prevention campaign that is directed towards children and adolescents. If professionals are not well-prepared, the programme could be detrimental, thus producing a boomerang effect or simply a neutralized result, which can endanger future actions.

## School programme concerning identification of suicide risk

Interventions in larger organizations, at the level of school districts, are better accepted than those performed in an isolated school, as the authorities are prepared to assist the programme at any level in the organization. It also allows the training of teachers, which has implications in the practical work in the resolution of suicidal crises. If teachers take part in an intervention before formal training, thus lacking conceptual and practical tools, they feel exhausted, which can have an negative influence on students who need psychological help.

### Preparation stage
Schedule: 3 hours.

◆ Planning for teachers, teams and school authorities.

### Pre-intervention stage (identification of students at risk)
Schedule: number of hours depend on the size of the population to be evaluated.

◆ Use of ISO 30 questionnaire and complementary tests.

◆ Selection of cases;

◆ Allocation of students according to risk: high, moderate, low.

### Intervention stage (monitoring and assistance)

◆ 10 meetings/support groups for students with high and moderate risk;

◆ Students who have low risk are enrolled in the Institutional Campaign of Sensitizing on the value of life.

### Post-intervention stage (evaluation of effectiveness)
Schedule: number of hours depend on the size of the population to be evaluated

◆ Use of ISO 30 questionnaire and complementary tests;

◆ Refer cases identified in the intervention stage, if necessary to individual or family treatment.

### Communication stage and scheduling of the monitoring
Schedule: 4 hours.

◆ Teachers, teams and school authorities receive information about results;

◆ Design of follow-up activities to sustain the programme.

Interested professionals from the district are stimulated to participate in all stages of the programme in order to secure the sustainability of the programme when the development phase of the programme is finished.

Evaluation for both programmes were performed by the ISO 30 questionnaire in Argentina (Casullo and Fernández Liporace 1997; Casullo 1998, 2002, 2004a, b; Casullo *et al.* 2006), and at the intervention unit by the Support Group (Martínez and Pomares 2006; Martínez 2007).

### References

Casullo MM (1998). *Adolescentes en riesgo. Identificación y orientación psicológica* [Adolescents at risk. Identification and psychological guidance]. Paidós, Buenos Aires.

Casullo MM (2002). Narraciones de adolescentes con alto riesgo suicida [Reports of adolescents at risk for suicide]. *Psicodiagnosticar*, **12**, 43–52.

Casullo MM (2004a). *Ideaciones y comportamientos suicidas* [Suicidal ideation and behaviour]. Conferencia dictada en la Universidad de Córdoba. Argentina.

Casullo MM (2004b). *El diagnóstico psicológico. Psicología & Psicoanálisis & Salud Colectiva* [The psychological diagnosis. Psychology & Psychoanalysis & Public Health]. 1, 2004. Centro Internacional de Psicología y Psicoanálisis, Chile.

Casullo MM and Fernández Liporace M (1997). Investigación sobre riesgo suicida en adolescentes. Prácticas psicológicas en la escuela [Investigation into Adolescent Suicidal Risk. Psychological Practices]. *Investigaciones en Psicología*, **2**, 33–41.

Casullo MM, Bonaldi P, Fernández Liporace M (2000). *Comportamientos suicidas en la adolescencia. Morir antes de la muerte* [Suicidal Behaviours in Adolescence. Die before death]. Lugar, Buenos Aires.

Casullo MM, Fernández Liporace M, Contini de González N (2006). *Estudio comparativo sobre adolescentes en riesgo suicid.* [Comparative study of adolescents at risk for suicide]. *Revista de Investigaciones en Psicología*, **3**, 21–36.

King J and Kowalvchuk B (1994). *ISO-30. Inventory of Suicide Orientation.* National Computer Systems, Minnesota.

Martínez C (2007). *Introducción a la Suicidología. Teoría, intervenciones e investigación* [Introduction to suicidology. Theory, intervention and research]Editions Lugar, Buenos Aires.

Martínez C and Pomares A (2006). Las redes sociales de apoyo en la rehabilitación del proceso suicida. Trabajo presentado en el II Congreso Internacional de Suicidología, Setiembre de 2006 [Social networks to help the suicidal process of rehabilitation. Paper presented at the II International Congress of Suicidology]. Corrientes, Argentina.

# CHAPTER 130

# Suicide prevention in Brazil

Neury J Botega, Carlos Felipe Almeida D'Oliveira and José M Bertolote

## Introduction

Brazil is the largest, and most populous, country in South America (population estimated in 2005 at 185 million). The low suicide rate in Brazil (around 4 per 100,000 inhabitants/year) is similar to those of most South American countries; however, in some population groups, such as farmers and male adolescents in the Rio Grande do Sul state, and for youngsters living in urban areas and indigenous groups, the rates are considerably higher. In spite of the low national suicide rate, the total number of suicides in 2005 was 8550, which places Brazil amongst the countries with the highest number of suicide deaths (Souza *et al.* 2002; Oliveira and Lotufo Neto 2003; Brasil—Ministério da Saúde 2006a).

The increasing suicide rates in indigenous groups seem to be related to extreme pressure exerted by Western society, self-devaluation and alcohol misuse (Morgado 1992). The national mortality rate for indigenous youths aged 10–19 is 14.4, which is seven times higher than the rates among white and black youths. The proportional mortality, due to suicide, is higher among adolescents, corresponding to 3.8 per cent of all deaths in this age group (Mello-Santos *et al.* 2006; Brasil—Ministério da Saúde 2006a, 2007).

The Brazilian health service system consists of a network of health care providers, both from public and private sectors. Around 20 per cent of the population is covered by private health insurance plans. There is a heavy concentration of human resources in the most developed regions and in the state capitals, mainly in the south and south-east. Based on the membership of the Brazilian Psychiatric Association, estimates show that there are 2.5 psychiatrists per 100,000 persons. This estimate is low, as it only accounts for half of all physicians who work as psychiatrists. The number of psychiatric hospitalizations has decreased since the 1990s. A system of alternatives to psychiatric hospitalization based on day hospitals has been developed (Larrobla and Botega 2001).

Urban violence and high homicide rates have overshadowed the problem of suicide in Brazil. The need for violence- (including suicide-) prevention policies has gained government attention, and suicide behaviour has emerged as an important issue in the public health sector in Brazil (Botega and Garcia 2004; D'Oliveira 2004; Botega 2007).

## Suicide prevention

In 2006, the Health Ministry launched a national strategy for suicide prevention (Brasil—Ministério da Saúde 2006b). This document was prepared in collaboration with a task force composed of several representatives of the society. It reinforces the need to develop suicide-prevention strategies based on data derived from local research studies, such as epidemiological information on psychiatric disorders mostly associated with suicide behaviour: early detection and appropriate treatment of psychiatric disorders and improvement of psychosocial conditions, which are significantly associated with suicide. Furthermore, it advocates training of health care professionals in suicide prevention; increasing the availability of medication for treatment of both mood and schizophrenic disorders; restriction of access to means of suicide such as firearms and pesticides; appropriate treatment after a suicide attempt; and the reduction of stigma towards people with mental disorders and those who attempt suicide.

Non-governmental organizations have played an important role in promoting awareness about the risks of carrying firearms and supporting projects for violence prevention. More severe legislation to inhibit illegal gun ownership was adopted.

A series of booklets on suicide prevention, produced by the Health Ministry, was made available for general practitioners, mental health professionals, media professionals and survivor groups (Brasil—Ministério da Saúde 2006c; D'Oliveira and Ferrara 2006). Governmental special training programmes in suicide prevention for health personnel are a growing priority in Brazil (Berlim *et al.* 2007; Botega *et al.* 2007). These are especially relevant, since the primary care system services take care of an extremely high number of individuals with mental disorders. Nevertheless, a high proportion of these disorders, especially depression, goes unrecognized or is treated inadequately (Abas *et al.* 2003). A study carried out in a primary care setting showed that 12.2 per cent of the 1996 patients were diagnosed by general practitioners with major depression. A much higher number, 24.3 per cent, was found by the investigators to meet DSM-IV criteria. Of those individuals diagnosed by the general practi-tioners, only 16.5 per cent were given antidepressant medication (Levav *et al.* 2005).

Brazil was one of the countries participating in the World Health Organization (WHO) Multisite Intervention Study on Suicide Behaviour (SUPRE-MISS) (Bertolote *et al.* 2005). This was the first national survey about suicide behaviour, and was based on general population information: the data collected has guided preventive efforts. As part of this project, a community survey was carried out in Campinas, a city located in the most populous and industrialized region of the country. Life prevalence estimates in the general population were 17.1 per cent for suicide ideation, 4.8 per cent for suicidal plans and 2.8 per cent for suicide attempts (Botega *et al.* 2005a). A second SUPRE-MISS subproject involved the evaluation of a brief intervention and follow-up contacts versus treatment as usual for suicide attempters, in its effectiveness to reduce suicide mortality in a randomized controlled trial (Fleischmann *et al.* 2005, 2008). As a consequence of these results, the Health Secretariats of the cities of São Paulo and Campinas have launched a programme devoted to people who attempted suicide. It aims to collect a comprehensive database of all suicide attempters seen at the emergency departments, as well as provide support by means of a follow-up protocol, which comprises regular visits and phone calls to these patients. The adoption of this policy has involved a partnership among the federal and state governments, universities and a research sponsoring agency.

Academic interest in suicidology is growing in Brazil, with projects on the development and evaluation of the reliability of research instruments (Berlim *et al.* 2003; Werlang and Botega 2003; Botega *et al.* 2005b), measuring of attitude changes in nursing personnel after a training course on suicide prevention (Berlim *et al.* 2007; Botega *et al.* 2005b, 2007), and genetics in suicide (Correa *et al.* 2004, 2007).

## Conclusion

In November 2000, the Association of Suicidology of Latin America and Caribbean (ASULAC) was formally established. Its first two congresses, carried out in Montevideo, Uruguay in 2005, and in Belo Horizonte, Brazil in 2007, have been particularly fruitful as demonstrated by the growing interaction among professionals interested in suicide prevention, as well as the beginning of collaborative studies in suicidal behaviour.

## References

Abas M, Baingana F, Broadhead J *et al.* (2003). Common mental disorders and primary health care: current practice in low-income countries. *Harvard Review of Psychiatry*, **20**, 166–173.

Berlim MT, Mattevi BS, Pavanello DP *et al.* (2003). Psychache and suicidality in adult mood disordered outpatients in Brazil. *Suicide and Life-Threatening Behaviour*, **33**, 242–248.

Berlim MT, Perizzolo J, Lejderman F *et al.* (2007). Does a brief training on suicide prevention among general hospital personnel impact their baseline attitudes towards suicidal behaviour? *Journal of Affective Disorders*, **100**, 233–239.

Bertolote JM, Fleischmann A, De Leo D *et al.* (2005). Suicide attempts, plans, and ideation in culturally diverse sites: the WHO SUPRE-MISS community survey. *Psychological Medicine*, **35**, 1457–1465.

Botega NJ (2007). [Suicide: moving away umbrage towards a National Prevention Plan] (editorial). *Revista Brasileira de Psiquiatria*, **29**, 7–8.

Botega NJ and Garcia LSL (2004). Brazil: the need for violence (including suicide) prevention. *World Psychiatry*, **3**, 157–158.

Botega NJ, Barros MBA, Oliveira HB *et al.* (2005a). Suicide behaviour in the community: prevalence and factors associated to suicidal ideation. *Revista Brasileira de Psiquiatria*, **27**, 45–53.

Botega NJ, Reginato DG, Silva SV *et al.* (2005b) Nursing personnel attitudes toward suicide: the development of a measure scale. *Revista Brasileira de Psiquiatria*, **27**, 315–318.

Botega NJ, Silva SV, Reginato DG, *et al.* (2007) Maintained attitudinal changes in nursing personnel after a brief training on suicide prevention. *Suicide and Life-Threatening Behaviour*, **37**, 145–153.

Brasil—Ministério da Saúde (2006a). *Saúde Brasil 2006: uma análise da situação de saúde no Brasil* [Health in Brazil: an analysis of the present status]. Ministério da Saúde, Brasília.

Brasil—Ministério da Saúde (2006b). *Diretrizes Nacionais de Prevenção do Suicídio* [National guidelines for suicide prevention]. Portaria no 1.876. Diário Oficial 14 August 2006.

Brasil—Ministério da Saúde (2006c). *Prevenção do Suicídio: Manual dirigido a profissionais das equipes de saúde mental* [Suicide prevention: a manul for mental health staff]. Ministério da Saúde, Pan-American Health Organization, Universidade Estadual de Campinas, Brasília.

Brasil—Ministério da Saúde (2007). *Informações de Saúde—Estatísticas Vitais* [Information about the health system]. Sistema de Informações sobre Mortalidade/MS/SUS/DASIS. Available at: http://tabnet.datasus.gov.br. Accessed June 2007.

Correa H, Campi-Azevedo AC, De Marco L *et al.* (2004). Familial suicide behaviour: association with probands suicide attempt characteristics and 5-HTTLPR polymorphism. *Acta Psychiatrica Scandinavica*, **110**, 459–464.

Correa H, De Marco L, Boson W *et al.* (2007). Association study of T102C 5-HT(2A) polymorphism in schizophrenic patients: diagnosis, psychopathology, and suicidal behaviour. *Dialogues in Clinical Neurosciences*, **9**, 97–101.

D'Oliveira CFA (2004). Atenção a jovens que tentam o suicídio: é possível prevenir [Caring for teenagers who attempt suicide].In CA Lima, ed., *Violência faz mal à saúde*, pp. 177–184. Ministério da Saúde, Brasília.

D'Oliveira CFA and Ferrara AM (2006). *Suicídio, sobreviventes, família: Levantamento bibliográfico sobre os temas* [Suicide, survivors, family: a bibliographic review]. Ministério da Saúde, Brasília.

Fleischmann A, Bertolote JM, De Leo D *et al.* (2005). Characteristics of attempted suicides seen in emergency-care settings of general hospitals in eight low- and middle-income countries. *Psychological Medicine*, **35**, 1467–1474.

Fleischmann A, Bertolote JM, Wasserman D *et al.* (2008). Effectiveness of brief intervention and contact for suicide attempters: a randomized controlled trial in five countries. *Bulletin of the Word Health Organization*, **86**, 703–709.

Larrobla C and Botega NJ (2001). Restructuring mental health: a South American survey. *Social Psychiatry and Psychiatric Epidemiology*, **36**, 256–259.

Levav I, Kohn R, Montoya I *et al.* (2005). Training Latin American primary care physicians in the WPA module on depression: results of a multicenter trial. *Psychological Medicine*, **35**, 35–45.

Mello-Santos C, Bertolote JM, Wang YP (2006). Suicide trends and characteristics in Brazil. *International Psychiatry*, **3**, 5–6.

Morgado AF (1992). The Guarani-Kaiwa suicide epidemic: investigating its causes and suggesting the 'impossible return' hypothesis. *Cadernos de Saúde Pública*, **7**, 585–598.

Oliveira CS and Lotufo Neto F (2003). Suicide among indigenous people: a Brazilian statistical view. *Revista de Psiquiatria Clínica*, **30**, 4–10.

Souza E, Minayo M, Malaquias J (2002). Suicide among young people in selected Brazilian state capitals. *Cadernos de Saúde Pública*, **18**, 673–683.

Werlang BS and Botega NJ (2003). A semistructured interview for psychologycal autopsy: an inter-rater reliability study. *Suicide and Life-Threatening Behaviour*, **33**, 326–330.

# CHAPTER 131

# Suicide prevention in Chile

Marcello Ferrada-Noli, Rubén Alvarado
and Francisca Florenzano

## Introduction

In 2001, addressing the Council for Mental Health Seminar in Oslo, Norway, Gro Harlem Brundtland, at the time as the Director General of the World Health Organization, made a special mention of Chile's mental health care accomplishments.

> During a period of 10 years, Chile also has been able to make remarkable achievements: the number of psychiatrists working in public services has doubled; long stay beds have been decreased by over 30 per cent in favour of community-based care; and more than 40 consumer and family advocacy groups have been established.
>
> Harlem Bruntland (2001, http://www.who.int/director-general/
> speeches/2001/index.html)

## The epidemiology of suicide in Chile

Although the epidemiology of suicide is known to be highly correlated with psychiatric factors and advances in mental health issues, the suicide rate in Chile had risen from 5.6 per 100,000 in 1990, to 10.3 in 2005: the suicide rate increased for men in the same period from 9.7 to 17.4, and for women from 1.6 to 3.4. This phenomenon has placed the country among the countries with the highest suicide figures in South America (Ministry of Health 2008; WHO 2008).

The proportion of undetermined forensic diagnoses of the mode of death (e.g. deaths that could be suicide or accident, or unknown) has been estimated to be equally high in Chile. In a study comprising all deaths certified as caused by trauma, poisoning or violence in which case accidental or self-inflicted nature was ignored, the authors found that in 41.7 per cent of those deaths, no defined cause (accidental or self-inflicted) has been reported (Castillo et al. 1997).

The improvements that took place during 1997 in the Chilean registration system for causes of death resulted in a decrease of the undetermined cases. In return, this could partially explain the relative increase of suicide rates per 100,000 in Chile between 1997 (6.2) and 1998 (6.9) 1999 (6.8). However, this system change is not enough to explain the abrupt leap of the Chilean suicides that occurred in 2000 (9.6) or the increase of the suicide rate observed thereafter (10.4 in 2001, 10.2 in 2002, 10.4 in 2003, 10.8 in 2004, and 10.3 in 2005).

What mechanisms may lie beneath the 'unexpected' rise of the Chilean suicide rate? Due to the close associations between depressive disorders and suicidal behaviour, one aspect to consider would be the actual prevalence of depression that Chileans have in comparison to other countries in the region, and the reasons for its possible increase. Depression diagnoses in Chile (15 per cent) have been reported since the mid 1980s as having the highest prevalence among a sample of Latin American countries (García-Alvarez 1986), and later investigations report an increase of this prevalence (Carvajal 1994). With regard to lifetime prevalence of major depressive disorder, it has been found that Chile (9.2 per cent) remains at the same level as other Latin American countries (Vicente et al. 2006a). Also, other diagnoses and the comorbidity of depression—as well as trauma-related diagnoses—should be epidemiologically examined for identification of risk factors for suicide in certain populations. This may help to explain the observed increase of suicide incidence and aid in optimization of prevention programmes.

Yet another partial explanation may be the relatively drastic change of the Chilean demographic structure in recent years, characterized among other things by an increased longevity and life expectancy (Solimano and Mazzei 2007). Even if this can not explain the national suicide rates at large, we found in this analysis a significant increase in the suicide rates among the elderly (over 65) between the years 1990 (11.1) and 2000 (15.9).

Suicide is a leading cause of death for Chilean males of productive age, and the first cause of death in young women and men in the 15–24 age group (ranking first among the twenty-five countries in the Americas). The ratio of male:female in suicide deaths is the second highest, worldwide (the world's highest ratio is observed in Puerto Rico). The World Health Organization attributes this phenomenon to a general cultural contextual factor.

Notable regional variations are observed in the epidemiology of suicide in the country. The manifest dissimilarity in the epidemiology of suicide observed in various regions of Chile can be partly attributed to climatic aspects implicated in the seasonal variation of the suicide incidence. A Chilean study examining the seasonal distribution of suicides in zones of low latitude compared with regions of high latitude found 'the existence of a unimodal springtime peak of suicides in Chile, but not in the zone of low latitude' (Heerlein et al. 2006).

Regional variations could also be explained by the geographic distribution of ethnic groups in the Chilean territory, with higher rates of suicide in areas where indigenous populations inhabit. The phenomenon that ethnic minorities would share a higher burden of suicidal deaths is of a worldwide nature. For instance, immigrants in Sweden—which comprise minorities from Chile—have shown in general a higher suicide rate than both native Swedes and their counterparts in Chile (Ferrada-Noli 1997).

A psychiatric epidemiology study based on data from the Psychiatric Prevalence Study in Chile (a national household survey of 2987 persons aged 15 years and older conducted in 1992–1999) found partly significant regional differences in the rates for other major depressive disorder (a diagnosis likely associated with suicidal behaviour), but also with regard to health-service utilization (Vicente *et al.* 2006b). A possible conclusion to draw would be that the regional differences in the Chilean suicide incidence would, to some extent, depend on the difficulties in achieving contact with mental health services due to, for instance, long distances or difficult communications. This is likely to happen in larger geographical regions with low population density, a situation also observed in areas of Northern Europe. As a result, decreasing treatment opportunities in mental health settings lead to an increase in suicidal deaths (Ferrada-Noli *et al.* 1996).

## Suicide prevention

Within a general public-heath strategy, the Chilean Ministry of Health (MINSAL) has established various goals relevant to suicide prevention. According to a public presentation of the Mental Health Department in April 2008, one aim is to reduce the incidence of 'depressive episodes' for which a specific goal of 10 per cent reduction has been set. The prevalence of depressive episodes is expected to decrease to 6.8 per cent. Another specific goal is to reduce the age-adjusted suicide rate from 9.7 to 8.7 per cent. A National Plan for Suicide Prevention, engaging the public and private sector, will be implemented at regional levels. The design has considered, among other things education of specialized personnel, improvement of forensic diagnosing on self-inflicted-related deaths including performing psychological autopsies, restriction in the availability of lethal means to commit suicide, monitoring of psychic trauma sequelae, improvement of follow-up of suicide attempters, establishment of help-lines for individuals in crises, information activities at schools, participation of the media, etc. (Rojas 2008).

Although some prevention programmes on the regional level have already been examined, the evaluation of those programmes are not yet known, with the exception of a programme conducted in 2005 in the southern province of Chile by a research team of the School of Public Health, University of Chile, in collaboration with the Mental Health Service at the Hospital of Ancud (a programme in which Rubén Alvarado, the second author of this chapter, was involved, and Dr Pamela Eguiguren was a leading participant). This 9-month programme aimed to reduce depression and suicide ideation among youth population in the city of Ancud. The programme established psychologist led 'groups for personal development', drama activities with plays created by the youngsters themselves, and a mental health centre was made available for consultation and treatment. The programme reported a decrease of suicide ideation among young males (66 per cent) and in young women (59 per cent).

Other researchers have put forward, however, that in order to improve the efficacy of prevention programmes in Chile, a substantial design shift would be needed. Prevention programmes should move forward from designs centred mainly on individual/clinical aspects of prevention and treatment, to a more comprehensive multilevel perspective model, which extends from the biological and genetic risk factors to the macro structural factors that have been proven to be associated with an increased risk of committing suicide (Florenzano 2008). This model conceived to include the detection and monitoring of high-risk groups, as well as community interventions in the populations affected. A key factor in this model is the identification of social factors underlying suicidal behaviour.

## Conclusion

The reasons that the suicide rate in Chile has notably increased with regard to other countries in the region deserves further attention. A deeper study of both risk and protective factors, and particularly the impact of ethnicity, demographic changes, and socio-economic factors, would perhaps provide some answers on this complicated phenomenon.

## References

Carvajal C (1994). Variations of the frequency of the diagnosis of depression in Chile. *Acta Psiquiatr Am Lat*, **40**, 301–307.

Castillo B, González J, Schiattino I (1997). Medical certification of deaths by trauma in the Chilean health services. *Rev Med Chil*, **125**, 1389–1398.

Ferrada-Noli M, Åsberg M, Ormstad K (1996). Psychiatric care and transcultural factors in suicide incidence. *Nordic Journal of Psychiatry*, **50**, 21–25.

Ferrada-Noli M (1997). A cross-cultural breakdown of Swedish suicide. *Acta Psychiatrica Scandinavica*, **96**, 108–117.

Florenzano F (2008). Investigación y Prevención del Sucidio en Chile: contribución de los aspectos contextuales y sociales. [Research and Prevention Suicide in Chile: contribution of contextual and social aspects]. Presentation at the the Conference El Suicidio en Chile: perspectivas actuales. Catholic University of Chile, April.

García-Alvarez R (1986). Epidemiology of depression in Latin America. *Psychopathology*, **19**(Suppl), 22–25.

Harlem Brundtland G (2001). *Mental Health in our World: The Challenges Ahead*. World Health Organization Council for Mental Health Seminar, Oslo.

Heerlein A, Valeria C, Medina B (2006). Seasonal variation in suicidal deaths in Chile: its relationship to latitude. *Psychopathology*, **39**, 75–79.

Ministry of Health (2008). *Vital Statistics-Main causes of death*. Department of Statistics and Health Information, Chile

Rojas I (2008). Plan Nacional de Prevención del Suicidio. [National Suicide Prevention Program] Presentation at the the Conference El Suicidio en Chile: perspectivas actuales. Catholic University of Chile, April.

Solimano CG and Mazzei PM (2007). Which are the causes of death among Chileans today? Long-term perspectives. *Rev Med Chil*, **135**, 932–938.

Vicente B, Kohn R, Rioseco P *et al.* (2006a). Lifetime and 12-month prevalence of DSM-III-R disorders in the Chile psychiatric prevalence study. *American Journal of Psychiatry*, **163**, 1362–1370.

Vicente B, Kohn R, Rioseco P *et al.* (2006b). Regional differences in psychiatric disorders in Chile. *Soc Psychiatry Psychiatr Epidemiol*, **41**, 935–942.

WHO (2008). *Number of suicides by age group and gender. CHILE, 2003*. World Health Organization, Geneva. www.who.int/entity/mental_health/media/chil.pdf

# CHAPTER 132

# Suicide prevention in Cuba

Sergio A Perez Barrero

## Introduction

In Cuba, family and forensic doctors determine the diagnosis for the cause of death as suicide, although in uncertain cases, the police and official services of forensic medicine contribute to the diagnosis. This procedure prevents problems of concealment of suicide death that are connected to religious or life insurance issues, and strengthens the reliability of the diagnosis of the cause of death as suicide in Cuba.

Suicide ranks among the top ten leading causes of death in the country (Perez Barrero 1996), and although suicide rates have decreased substantially, they continue to be high in comparison with other countries in South America (World Health Organization 1999, 2000a). The truth is that suicide rates in Cuba are often misinterpreted. Mortality statistics in Cuba are highly reliable, and this may partially explain why Cuba has higher suicide rates than other South American countries. Moreover, the high suicide mortality dates back to the nineteenth century.

## Risk factors for suicide in Cuba

The causes behind suicide in Cuba are similar to those of other countries. Purportedly, suicide is considered as having multivariate causes, including biological, psychological, social, existential and genetic factors (Perez Barrero 2005; Correa and Perez Barrero 2005, 2008).

The trigger factors for Cubans to commit suicide are similar to those in other countries, and among the most frequent reasons are conflicts among couples, thwarted love, the rupture of a valuable relationship and family conflicts (Perez Barrero and Mosquera 2006).

## Suicide methods

The most common method for Cubans to commit suicide is hanging, burning and the ingestion of pesticides. Suicide by firearms is not a frequent suicide method in Cuba, due to the strict control of the holding of firearms, and the prohibition of their sale to the population. Burning is a common method for suicide in Cuba, and historically was often used because of disappointment in love by adolescents whose parents were immigrants to Cuba from the Far East; however, it is now utilized by adults of both sexes, although it is more prevalent in females (Perez Barrero 1994; Bahram *et al.* 2006).

## Suicide prevention

Since 1989, Cuba, like many countries around the world, has had a National Program for Suicide Prevention (MINSAP 1989).

Cuba is represented among the main international organizations for suicide prevention, such as the International Association for Suicide Prevention (IASP), the International Academy of Suicide Research (IASR), and the International Association of Thanatology and Suicidology.

Cuba has also been represented in the Group of Experts of the World Health Organization for suicide prevention, and has participated in the preparation of documents for the World Health Organization, which are related to the prevention of suicide (World Health Organization 1999, 2000a, b, c).

Cuba initiated the process for the establishment of the Section of Suicidology of the World Psychiatric Association. In Cuba, several events of international character have taken place, in which national investigations regarding suicidal behaviour have been presented, and experiences shared with professionals from other countries. Cuba has also been represented in multinational investigations related to topics on 'survivors of loss due to suicide' and addressing the problems of 'assisted suicide' in projects that were directed by the members of the IASP, Professors Norman Farberow and Michael Kelleher, respectively.

## Conclusion

Finally, the Cuban experience in suicide prevention has been presented in several countries, and has provided good examples on how to prepare suicide prevention programmes (Government State of Puebla 2005; Ministry of Health 2005).

## References

Bahram G, Rossignol AM, Perez Barrero SA *et al* (2006). Suicide behaviour by burns among adolescents in Kurdistan, Iran: a social tragedy. *Crisis*, **27**, 16–27.

Correa H and Perez Barrero SA (2005). Las investigaciones biológicas del suicidio.[Biological research on Suicide] *Aspectos históricos Psiquiátr Biol*, **12**, 14–17.

Correa H and Perez Barrero SA (2008). *Suicídio: uma morte evitável* [Suicide: A preventable death]. (In press. Brasil). Editora Atheneu.

Government State of Puebla (2005). *Programa de Atención y Prevencion a la Violencia Intrafamiliar y el Suicidio* [Programme for the prevention of domestic violence and suicide]. Gobierno del Estado de Puebla, Puebla.

Ministry of Health (2005). *Manual de Salud Mental para Periodistas* [Manual of Mental Health for Journalists]. Ministerio de Salud, Perú.

MINSAP (1989). *Programa Nacional de Prevencion del Suicidio* [National Program for Prevention of Suicide]. Ministerio de Salud Pública, La Habana, Cuba.

Perez Barrero SA (1994). *Suicidio por fuego* [Suicide by fire]. Rev Psiquiatria Pública, España.

Perez Barrero SA (1996). *El suicidio. Comportamiento y prevencion* [Suicide. Behaviour and prevention]. Editorial Oriente, Santiago de Cuba.

Perez Barrero SA (2005). Los mitos sobre el suicidio. La importancia de conocerlos. [Suicide Myths. The Importance of their Knowledge]. *Revista Colombiana de Psiquiatría*, **xxxiv**, 386–394.

Perez Barrero SA and Mosquera D (2006). *El suicidio. Prevencion y Manejo*. Ediciones Pléyades. In press. España.

World Health Organization (1999). *Figures and Facts About Suicide*. Department of Mental Health Social Change and Mental Health, World Health Organization, Geneva.

World Health Organization (2000a). *Informe del taller sobre Prevencion de Suicidio para países de la Región de las Américas* [Suicide prevention for countries in the Americas]. 22–24 de Febrero de 2000. Departamento de Salud Mental y Trastornos Mentales y Comportamentales. MNH/MBD/99.3f. Montevideo, Uruguay.

World Health Organization (2000b). *Preventing Suicide. A Resource for General Physicians*. World Health Organization, Geneva.

World Health Organization (2000c). *Preventing Suicide. A Resource for Media Professionals*. World Health Organization, Geneva.

# CHAPTER 133

# Suicide prevention in Peru

Rossana Pettersén and Freddy Vasquez

## Introduction

Peru has a multi-ethnic population and an estimated 28 million inhabitants spread across a national territory, which comprises three principal regions: the coast, the highlands, and the Amazon rainforest.

Peru has started to recover from the effects of two decades of extensive human rights violations due to civil war, which has mentally affected the entire population. There are at least about 22,000 families or 132,000 individuals in need of mental health care as a result of the violence generated by terrorist and military actions. Psychological effects such as prolonged fear, distrust of neighbours, the breakdown of families, loss of property, postponed grief and desperation (Fraser 2004) have contributed to the deterioration of the mental health of the general population, including increased rates of post-traumatic stress disorder, depression, and associated health disorders. The *Harvard University Gazette* reported that the reduction of the social capital created higher rates of hopelessness, demoralization, diminished quality of life, and waves of forced migration, mainly from rural areas to the cities; and this has had its effect on the mental health of the Peruvian population (*Harvard Gazette Archives* 2006).

## Mental health in Peru

Peruvian mental health professionals are confronted with a population made of grandparents who witnessed the sudden decay of a promising country, parents who lived most of their lives under the years of terror and violence created by the civil war, and children and teenagers who do not know why their parents are so sad, aggressive, defensive or anxious.

In rural areas, the high unemployment rates, gender inequalities, low education, lack of availability of mental health services and generalized poverty make these populations very vulnerable to violence and associated mental health problems.

In urban areas, the high crime and unemployment rates, the high demands on academic performance especially from children in primary and high schools, lack of family support, strict parental styles, and drug and alcohol abuse or sexual and psychological abuse of children and teenagers, makes this population very vulnerable to mental ill health.

## Suicide in Peru

The approximate suicide rate in the country in 2006 was 2–3 per 100,000 inhabitants, which is relatively low compared to the suicide rates in developed countries, and other Latin American countries. Regarding suicide attempts, data from 2005 show a total of 630 reported suicide attempts in the country. The distribution follows the international trend of higher suicide attempts among females, N = 466 (74%), than in males, N = 164 (26%). The National Institute of Mental Health, and its Suicide Prevention Program in Peru, are the entities keeping the registers with the data for mortality and morbidity by suicide and suicide attempt, and reporting them to the Peruvian Ministry of Health (2005) every year.

The scientific study of suicidal behaviour, and the activities concerning suicide prevention in Peru, began in 1994. The National Institute of Mental Health, through its suicide prevention programme, runs a project comprising a multidisciplinary team of professionals who are currently studying the sociodemographic components, and the epidemiology of suicidal behaviour in the country.

This is a large-scale and long-term study. Different patterns of suicidal behaviour in the Peruvian population, and the risk and protective factors present in the various ethnic groups, are just beginning to be understood. At the moment, the project has dispatched study teams to gather epidemiological data on suicidal ideation and suicide attempts in metropolitan Lima, the highlands, the jungle and, most recently, to the settlements along the national borders.

## Suicide prevention

To report suicide completion, or to diagnose suicide attempt, the guidelines from the WHO are followed. The official procedure was approved by the Ministry of Health in its *Guide to suicide prevention and treatment* (2006). The intervention strategies are decided according to the SAFE-T model (American Psychiatric Association Practice Guidelines for the Assessment and Treatment of Patients with Suicidal Behaviors), which recommended five points for easy and fast assessment, and interventions for suicide attempters.

After this diagnostic phase, therapeutic psychological intervention for individuals, groups and families, as well as therapeutic coaching and art therapy to suicide attempters and individuals with suicidal ideation, is offered. A suicide-prevention hotline in Lima, which gives psychological support, follow-ups and referrals, and is managed by professionals specifically trained in crisis intervention, is in use.

The media educates the public about suicide, basically, on how to recognize individuals at risk, and to provide referrals to mental health hospitals. The Ministry of Women and the People's Defence Agency (a Peruvian organization that defends the rights of women, children and teenagers) are involved in promoting fast and adequate treatment of individuals who have suffered sexual and/or physical abuse and are at risk for suicide.

At the moment, the primary and secondary school teachers, pedagogues, and tutors are trained to recognize students at risk. Once a year, public and free of charge depression screenings in Lima, and in other large cities, are performed, and people who are considered to be at higher risk for suicide are contacted.

## Conclusion

The main obstacles that suicide prevention activities encounter in Peru are the lack of a permanent budget from the government, undiagnosed and untreated depression in the population, a policy for depression and suicide prevention campaigns, the under-reporting of suicides and suicide attempts (especially in cities far from Lima), the lack of trained personnel for preventive activities, and the stigmatization of suicidal behaviour.

### References

Fraser B (2004). Slow recovery in Peru. World report. *The Lancet*, **364**, 1115–1116.

Harvard Gazette Archives (2006). *Program Combats Peru's Mental and Social Health Problems*. Accessed at: http://www.news.harvard.edu/gazette/2006/02.23/31-peru.html.

Peruvian Ministry of Health (2005). *Protocolo Integral para la atención de la Conducta Suicida* [Comprehensive Protocol for the Treatment of Suicidal Behaviour]. Resolución Ministerial, Lima.

# CHAPTER 134

# Suicide prevention in Uruguay

Silvia Pelaez Remigio

The suicide rate in Uruguay is very high in comparison with other Latin American countries, and ranks only second to Cuba (WHO 2000a, b). There are multiple reasons for this, however, the main ones concerning economic aspects are high unemployment rates, a poor economy (very low incomes and high debts), forced retirement, and the emigration of young people and professionals, etc. Other reasons include domestic violence, sexual abuse, alcoholism, isolation, and the insufficient treatment of psychiatric patients.

In university courses (e.g. psychology, medicine, etc.), suicide is not a theme in the curriculum. Last Resource (Ultimo Recurso), is the only organization that works with suicide prevention in the country. It is a non-governmental organization founded by the Franciscan Order in 1989, represented by Pedro Frontini and the author. This organization assists people in suicidal crises from all social categories, regardless of age, sex, religion and ethnicity, and also helps the 'survivors' of suicide victims in their struggle to come to terms with their loss. The association organizes conferences, courses and workshops for psychiatrists, psychologists, physicians, social workers and educators who work in suicide prevention and counselling groups for survivors. The organization also pursues research in suicide prevention.

Staff of the Last Resource organization is responsible for the only available crisis telephone hotline. In addition, Ultimo Recurso sets up personal meetings in the office for suicidal persons to receive crisis therapy. Ultimo Recurso is the co-organizer of the XXV IASP International Congress, which will take place in Montevideo in 2009.

Until 2004, all the activities conducted during the fourteen years of Ultimo Recurso's service were performed on a voluntarily basis, without any funding. However, in 2004, Ultimo Recurso was chosen by the City Council of Montevideo to implement a suicide prevention programme. This project is described below.

## An Ultimo Recurso programme for the prevention of suicide in western Montevideo

Since 2002, suicide has increased in Montevideo, especially in the western and poorest part of the city, and this is due to the economic crisis.

First, qualified informants from the diverse neighbourhoods of western Montevideo were interviewed, in order to combine historical, sociological and other sources of information. In this way, the different causes of suicide and attempted suicide, as well as the corresponding protective factors, were mapped in this particular part of the city.

The following important factors were disclosed:

♦ Famine (in one of the neighbourhoods);

♦ Domestic violence (in all areas);

♦ Sexual abuse (in all areas);

♦ Discrimination on the labour market (in several neighbourhoods).

The protective factors were:

♦ High self-esteem (Cerro area);

♦ Solidarity (all areas);

♦ High values of friendship (Cerro area).

Additionally, it was found that in the areas where there is a strong tradition of trade unionism (for example, in the cold storage plants of the meat processing industry, which have been shut down), the people possessed higher self-esteem, pride and awareness, and were less likely to resort to suicide, despite being victims of unemployment and poverty.

In this project, the following methodology was used:

♦ Study workshops;

♦ Instructions for telephone operators working with helplines;

♦ Crisis therapy at the clinic;

♦ Psychotherapy;

♦ Group work with survivors of suicide loss in various places of the neighbourhood;

♦ Workshops for children at schools in relevant areas;

♦ Contact with the media and others.

The staff involved the inhabitants in this project, not only as passive bystanders, but by teaching them how to react in crisis situations and how to prevent suicide. The neighbours were trained in workshops to detect signs of suicidal risks, and apply the psychological first aid methods, and they always were told to contact one of the health professionals in the project emergency rooms, which are located all around western Montevideo, for the purpose of consultation and support. The working conditions in the project included listening attentively to patients, as well as to the neighbours from the area who actually became multipliers of knowledge gained through this project.

The number of consultations and persons seeking help for suicide crisis is steadily increasing. This project caught the attention of professionals from many regions, and we were visited by Brazilian Health authorities and received invitations from several parts of Latin America (e.g. Puerto Rico).

## The Latin American and Caribbean Suicidology Association (ASULAC)

The Latin American and Caribbean Suicidology Association (ASULAC) was created in Montevideo, in 2000, during the Mercosur Suicidology Congress. Argentina, Puerto Rico, Cuba, Paraguay and Brazil were the first member countries in ASULAC, later followed by Mexico, Costa Rica and Chile. Dr Peláez from Uruguay was chosen as ASULAC's first President, followed by Dr Parrilla from Puerto Rico.

ASULAC stimulates research in the region, and has organized two regional Congresses: one in Montevideo, Uruguay in 2005, and Belo Horizonte, Brazil in 2007; and the XXV IASP International Congress in Montevideo in 2009.

## References

World Health Organization (2000a). *Health Statistics in the Americas, Year 2000*. Available at: http://www.paho.org. World Health Organization, Geneva.

World Health Organization (2000b). *Informe del taller sobre Prevencion de Suicidio para países de la Región de las Américas. 22-24 de Febrero de 2000. Departamento de Salud Mental y Trastornos Mentales y Comportamentales*. [Report on the workshop on suicide prevention for countries in the Americas. 22-24 February 2000. Department of Mental Health and Mental and Behavioural Disorders.] MNH/MBD/99.3f. Montevideo, Uruguay.

# Index